Lecture Notes in Computer Scie... P9-BUI-999

Commenced Publication in 1973
Founding and Former Series Editors:
Gerhard Goos, Juris Hartmanis, and Jan van Leeuwen

Editorial Board

Christian Barillot David R. Haynor
Pierre Hellier (Eds.)

Medical Image Computing and Computer-Assisted Intervention – MICCAI 2004

7th International Conference
Saint-Malo, France, September 26-29, 2004
Proceedings, Part II

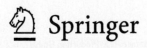 Springer

Volume Editors

Christian Barillot
IRISA-CNRS, VisAGeS Team
Campus de Beaulieu, 35042 Rennes Cedex, France
E-mail: Christian.Barillot@irisa.fr

David R. Haynor
University of Washington
Department of Radiology
Seattle, WA 98195-6004, USA
E-mail: haynor@u.washington.edu

Pierre Hellier
IRISA-INRIA, VisAGeS Team
Campus de Beaulieu, 35042 Rennes Cedex, France
E-mail: Pierre.Hellier@irisa.fr

Library of Congress Control Number: 2004111954

CR Subject Classification (1998): I.5, I.4, I.3.5-8, I.2.9-10, J.3, J.6

ISSN 0302-9743
ISBN 3-540-22977-9 Springer Berlin Heidelberg New York

Springer is a part of Springer Science+Business Media

springeronline.com

© Springer-Verlag Berlin Heidelberg 2004
Printed in Germany

Typesetting: Camera-ready by author, data conversion by PTP-Berlin, Protago-TeX-Production GmbH
Printed on acid-free paper   SPIN: 11317791   06/3142   5 4 3 2 1 0

Preface

The 7th International Conference on Medical Imaging and Computer Assisted Intervention, **MICCAI 2004**, was held in Saint-Malo, Brittany, France at the "Palais du Grand Large" conference center, September 26–29, 2004. The proposal to host **MICCAI 2004** was strongly encouraged and supported by IRISA, Rennes. IRISA is a publicly funded national research laboratory with a staff of 370, including 150 full-time research scientists or teaching research scientists and 115 postgraduate students. INRIA, the CNRS, and the University of Rennes 1 are all partners in this mixed research unit, and all three organizations were helpful in supporting **MICCAI**.

MICCAI has become a premier international conference with in-depth papers on the multidisciplinary fields of medical image computing, computer-assisted intervention and medical robotics. The conference brings together clinicians, biological scientists, computer scientists, engineers, physicists and other researchers and offers them a forum to exchange ideas in these exciting and rapidly growing fields.

The impact of **MICCAI** increases each year and the quality and quantity of submitted papers this year was very impressive. We received a record 516 full submissions (8 pages in length) and 101 short communications (2 pages) from 36 different countries and 5 continents (see figures below). All submissions were reviewed by up to 4 external reviewers from the Scientific Review Committee and a primary reviewer from the Program Committee. All reviews were then considered by the **MICCAI 2004** Program Committee, resulting in the acceptance of 235 full papers and 33 short communications. The normal mode of presentation at **MICCAI 2004** was as a poster; in addition, 46 papers were chosen for oral presentation. All of the full papers accepted are included in these proceedings in 8-page format. All of the accepted 2-page short communications are also included; they appeared at the meeting as posters. The first figure below shows the distribution of accepted contributions by topic, topics being defined from the primary keyword of the submission.

To ensure that these very selective decisions was made as fairly and justly as possible, reviewer names were not disclosed to anyone closely associated with the submissions, including, when necessary, the organizers. In addition, to avoid any unwanted pressure on reviewers, the general chair and program chair did not co-author any submissions from their groups. Each of the 13 members of the Program Committee supervised the review process for almost 50 papers. The members of the Scientific Review Committee were selected based both on a draft and on an open volunteering process and a final list of 182 reviewers was selected based on background and expertise. After recommendations were made by the reviewers and the Program Committee, a final meeting took place during two days in early May in Rennes. Because of the overall quality of the submissions and because of the limited number of slots available for presentation, about one quarter of the contributions were further discussed in order to form the final program. We are especially grateful to Nicholas Ayache, Yves Bizais,

Hervé Delingette, Randy Ellis, Guido Gerig and Wiro Niessen, who attended this meeting and helped us make the final selections. We are grateful to everyone who participated in the review process; they donated a large amount of time and effort to make these volumes possible and insure a high level of quality.

It was our great pleasure to welcome this year's **MICCAI 2004** attendees to Saint-Malo. Saint-Malo is a corsair city (a corsair was a kind of official "pirate," hired by the king) and the home city of Jacques Cartier, the discoverer of Canada and Montreal, the site of last year's **MICCAI**. The city is located on the north coast of Brittany, close to Mont Saint-Michel and to Rennes. Saint-Malo is often compared to a great vessel preparing to set out to sea, always seeking renewal and adventure. We hope that the attendees, in addition to attending the conference, took the opportunity to explore the city, the sea shore, particularly at high tide (which was unusually high at the time of the conference), and other parts of Brittany, one of France's most beautiful regions. For those unable to attend, we trust that these volumes will provide a valuable record of the state of the art in the **MICCAI 2004** disciplines.

We look forward to welcoming you to **MICCAI 2005**, to be held next year in Palm Springs, CA, USA.

September 2004   Christian Barillot, David Haynor and Pierre Hellier

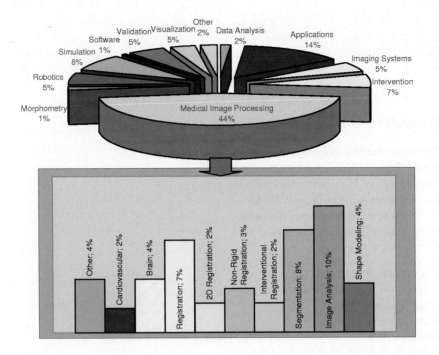

Fig. 1. View at a glance of **MICCAI 2004** contributions based on the declared primary keyword

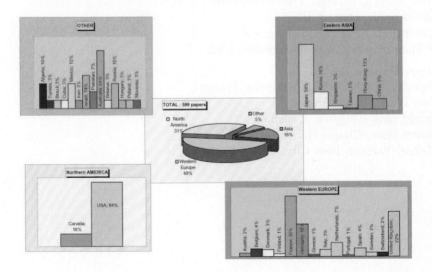

Fig. 2. Distribution of **MICCAI 2004** submissions by region

Organization

Executive Committee

Christian Barillot (General Chair), Rennes, France
David Haynor (Program Chair), Seattle, USA
Pierre Hellier (Program Co-chair), Rennes, France
James Duncan, New Haven, USA
Mads Nielsen, Copenhagen, Denmark
Terry Peters, London, Canada

Program Committee

Long Papers
Brian Davies, London, UK
Hervé Delingette, Sophia-Antipolis, France
Gabor Fichtinger, Baltimore, USA
Guido Gerig, Chapel Hill, USA
Nobuhiko Hata, Tokyo, Japan
David Hawkes, London, UK
Wiro Niessen, Utrecht, The Netherlands
Alison Noble, Oxford, UK
Gabor Szekely, Zurich, Switzerland
William (Sandy) Wells, Cambridge, USA

Short Papers
Nicholas Ayache, Sophia-Antipolis, France
Yves Bizais, Brest, France
Randy Ellis, Kingston, Canada
Steven Pizer, Chapel Hill, USA
Michael Vannier, Iowa City, USA

MICCAI Board

Alan Colchester (General Chair), Canterbury, UK
Nicholas Ayache, Sophia-Antipolis, France
Christian Barillot, Rennes, France
Takeyoshi Dohi, Tokyo, Japan
James Duncan, New Haven, USA
Terry Peters, London, Canada
Stephen Pizer, Chapel Hill, USA
Richard Robb, Rochester, USA
Russell Taylor, Baltimore, USA
Jocelyne Troccaz, Grenoble, France
Max Viergever, Utrecht, The Netherlands

Tutorial Chair

Grégoire Malandain, Sophia-Antipolis, France

Poster Coordination

Sylvain Prima, Rennes, France

Industrial Exhibition Co-chairs

Jean-Loïc Delhaye, Rennes, France
Bernard Gibaud, Rennes, France

Student Awards Coordination

Karl Heinz Höhne, Hamburg, Germany

Conference Secretariat/Management

Edith Blin-Guyot, Rennes, France
Caroline Binard, Rennes, France
Elisabeth Lebret, Rennes, France
Valérie Lecomte, Rennes, France
Nathalie Saux-Nogues, Rennes, France
Marina Surbiguet, Rennes, France

Proceedings Management

Laure Aït-Ali, Rennes, France
Arnaud Ogier, Rennes, France
Cybèle Ciofolo, Rennes, France
Valérie Lecomte, Rennes, France
Anne-Sophie Tranchant, Rennes, France
Sylvain Prima, Rennes, France
Romain Valabrègue, Rennes, France

Local Organization Committee

Christine Alami, Rennes, France
Annie Audic, Rennes, France
Yves Bizais, Brest, France
Patrick Bourguet, Rennes, France
Patrick Bouthemy, Rennes, France
Michel Carsin, Rennes, France
Pierre Darnault, Rennes, France
Gilles Edan, Rennes, France
Jean-Paul Guillois, Rennes, France
Pascal Haigron, Rennes, France
Pierre Jannin, Rennes, France
Claude Labit, Rennes, France
Jean-Jacques Levrel, Rennes, France
Eric Marchand, Rennes, France
Etienne Mémin, Rennes, France
Xavier Morandi, Rennes, France
Gérard Paget, Rennes, France
Jean-Marie Scarabin, Rennes, France

Reviewers

Purang Abolmaesumi
Faiza Admiraal-Behloul
Marco Agus
Carlos Alberola-López
Elsa Angelini
Neculai Archip
Simon R. Arridge
John Ashburner
Fred S. Azar
Christian Barillot
Pierre-Louis Bazin
Fernando Bello

Marie-Odile Berger
Margrit Betke
Isabelle Bloch
Thomas Boettger
Sylvain Bouix
Catherina R. Burghart
Darwin G. Caldwell
Bernard Cena
Francois Chaumette
Kiyoyuki Chinzei
Gary Christensen
Albert C.S. Chung

Philippe Cinquin
Jean Louis Coatrieux
Chris Cocosco
Alan Colchester
D. Louis Collins
Isabelle Corouge
Olivier Coulon
Patrick Courtney
Christos Davatzikos
Brian Davis
Benoit Dawant
Marleen De Bruijne
Michel Desvignes
Simon Dimaio
Etienne Dombre
Simon Duchesne
Ayman El-Baz
Alan Evans
Yong Fan
J. Michael Fitzpatrick
Oliver Fleig
Alejandro Frangi
Ola Friman
Robert Galloway
Andrew Gee
James Gee
Bernard Gibaud
Maryellen Giger
Daniel Glozman
Polina Golland
Miguel Angel Gonzalez Ballester
Eric Grimson
Christophe Grova
Christoph Guetter
Pascal Haigron
Steven Haker
Makoto Hashizume
Stefan Hassfeld
Peter Hastreiter
Pheng Ann Heng
Derek Hill
Karl Heinz Höhne
Robert Howe
Hiroshi Iseki
Pierre Jannin

Branislav Jaramaz
Sarang Joshi
Michael Kaus
Peter Kazanzides
Erwin Keeve
Erwan Kerrien
Charles Kervrann
Ali Khamene
Sun I. Kim
Tadashi Kitamura
Karl Krissian
Gernot Kronreif
Frithjof Kruggel
Luigi Landini
Thomas Lange
Thomas Lango
Rudy Lapeer
Rasmus Larsen
Heinz U. Lemke
Shuo Li
Jean Lienard
Alan Liu
Huafeng Liu
Jundong Liu
Marco Loog
Benoit Macq
Mahnaz Maddah
Frederik Maes
Isabelle Magnin
Sherif Makram-Ebeid
Gregoire Malandain
Armando Manduca
Jean-Francois Mangin
Marcos Martín-Fernández
Calvin Maurer Jr.
Tim McInerney
Etienne Memin
Chuck Meyer
Michael I. Miga
Xavier Morandi
Kensaku Mori
Ralph Mosges
Yoshihiro Muragaki
Toshio Nakagohri
Kyojiro Nambu

Table of Contents, Part II

LNCS 3217: MICCAI 2004 Proceedings, Part II

Robotics

Simulation and Rendering

Interventional Imaging

Brain Imaging Applications

Cardiac and Other Applications

Short Communications

Table of Contents, Part I

LNCS 3216: MICCAI 2004 Proceedings, Part I

Brain Segmentation

Cardiovascular Segmentation

Segmentation I

Segmentation Methods

Segmentation II

Registration I

Registration II

MARGE Project: Design, Modeling, and Control of Assistive Devices for Minimally Invasive Surgery

Etienne Dombre[1], Micaël Michelin[1], François Pierrot[1], Philippe Poignet[1], Philippe Bidaud[2], Guillaume Morel[2], Tobias Ortmaier[2], Damien Sallé[2], Nabil Zemiti[2], Philippe Gravez[3], Mourad Karouia[4], and Nicolas Bonnet[4]

[1] LIRMM, 161 rue Ada, 34392 Montpellier Cedex 5, France
{dombre, michelin, pierrot, poignet}@lirmm.fr
[2] LRP, BP61, 92265 Fontenay-aux-Roses Cedex, France
{bidaud, morel, ortmaier, salle, zemiti}@robot.jussieu.fr
[3] CEA/SRSI, BP6, 92265 Fontenay-aux-Roses Cedex, France
gravez@cea.fr
[4] Groupe Hospitalier Pitié Salpêtrière, 47-83 Bd de l'Hôpital, 75651 Paris Cedex 13, France
{nicolas.bonnet, mourad.karouia}@psl.ap-hop-paris.fr

Abstract. MARGE is a joint project in the framework of the interdisciplinary national program in Robotics, called ROBEA, launched by the French National Research Center (CNRS) in 2001. The focus is on the development of design methodologies and on the control of high mobility and dexterity assistive devices for complex gesture assistance in minimally invasive surgery, especially for coronary artery bypass grafting. This paper presents the main results of this two-year project.

1 Introduction

Minimally invasive surgery (MIS) is now widely used in different specialities. However, it adds several well known difficulties in the surgical procedure. Among them, the penetration point reduces the tool orientation capabilities and the amplitude of motion; the available intracorporal workspace is reduced and cluttered; the friction at the trocar level limits drastically the natural haptic feedback to the surgeon; fine and precise tasks are more difficult to realize, as compared to open surgery, due to the length of instruments, the inversion of motions induced by the trocar, the indirect vision of the scene through a screen monitor, etc. These drawbacks are strengthened in cardiac surgery, in which extremely fine and delicate structures are manipulated. Additionally the motion of the trocar is almost totally constrained by the presence of ribs. Therefore, at least two additional degrees of freedom (dof) must be provided on the distal part of the instruments, which makes the surgical tools difficult to operate manually. This has motivated the development of master-slave surgical robots such as Zeus from Computer Motion or Da Vinci from Intuitive Surgical.

However, the performance of these robots is still rather poor and many advanced functions have to be provided to enhance the surgeon dexterity. Besides, the potenti-

C. Barillot, D.R. Haynor, and P. Hellier (Eds.): MICCAI 2004, LNCS 3217, pp. 1–8, 2004.

alities of robotics have not yet been fully exploited: robots may be used together with new instruments in new surgical procedures aiming at performing less invasive surgery, such as beating heart surgery for instance. These objectives still require research works. The MARGE project contributes to some of them [1]. Its focus was on the development of design methodologies and the control of high mobility and dexterity devices for complex gesture assistance in MIS, especially for coronary artery bypass grafting (CABG). A first step of the project has consisted in the modeling of the CABG gesture. It is presented in section 2 of the paper. The data obtained have then been used for the optimal design of intracorporal dexterous instruments (Sect. 3). Several control algorithms have also been proposed that allows the surgeon to (tele) manipulate the instrument with a conventional robotic arm while respecting the constraint of moving it within the trocar (Sect. 4). Finally, an active trocar has been designed which cancels friction forces at the trocar level and then reflects real interaction force to the surgeon (Sect. 5).

MARGE is a 2-year joint project in the framework of the interdisciplinary program in robotics, called ROBEA (standing for ROBotics and Artificial Entities), launched by the French National Research Center (CNRS) in 2001 [2].

2   Modeling of the CABG Gesture

The CABG surgery derives the blood from a healthy artery to the coronary artery downstream the lesion, so that the cardiac muscle remains irrigated. This is achieved by harvesting the internal mammary artery and by suturing it on the coronary artery. The grafting process, called anastomosis, is the most difficult and important part of the surgical procedure. The anastomosis is described as a continuous elliptic suture around the section of the graft. The length of the incision on the artery varies from *7* to *10 mm*. The anastomosis may end with a knot between the 2 extremities of the thread.

In order to design an intracorporal dexterous instrument, it was necessary to collect data on the 3D motion of the needle during anastomosis as well as on the interaction forces with the coronary. Two surgical instruments have been modified (Fig. 1, left) to record 3D position data and force data, using a magnetic 3D positioning sensor (Minibird from Ascension Technologies Inc.) and a 6-axis force sensor (Nano17 from ATI). The experiments have been carried out by surgeons on sheep and pig hearts.

Fig. 1 (right) shows the interaction force (bottom) between the artery and a curved needle during the insertion in a coronary artery, as well as the corresponding position change of the needle tip (top). Position and force are given in a frame attached to the needle tip and on the axis tangential to the needle curvature. During the insertion phase, the exerted force increases due to the elastic behavior of the artery. When perforation of the artery wall occurs, the force exerted on the needle decreases rapidly due to a relaxation process. Then, viscous friction of the artery wall on the needle is observed. Elastic behaviour and sticking of the tissues on the needle create positive forces on the instrument at the end of the motion. From these experiments, it can be stated that the motion for each suture point is done in a plane, locally normal to the contour of an elliptic incision made on the coronary artery. In this plane, the motion is a rotation of the needle of about *120°*. The perforation force is up to *1.5 N*.

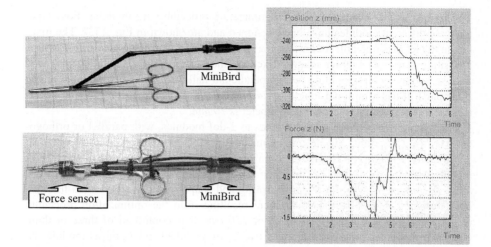

Fig. 1. Modified surgical instruments (*left*). Perforation of a coronary artery (*right*).

3 Optimal Design of Dexterous Modular Instruments

Designing an instrument for MIS requires taking into account several objectives: small size; sufficient number of dof to minimize contacts with organs and circumvent dangerous areas; high resolution in velocity and force; sufficient workspace, making possible to attain all points of a given path with a desired orientation. These environmental, mechanical and control constraints are often conflicting, which make the design difficult, requiring the help of an optimization procedure. We will qualify the resulting instrument as dexterous.

An optimization procedure has been developed. It is based on evolutionary algorithms, which are well suited for optimization over large and non continuous search spaces. A multi-objective genetic algorithm has been implemented that individually evaluates the solutions with respect to every objective and returns a set of best solutions in terms of a given combination of objectives. The evaluation is performed thanks to a realistic simulation including the organs and the models of the surgical gesture (Sect. 2). From the resulting set of solutions, the designer chooses the optimal design according to *a posteriori* criteria [3].

Practically, each instrument candidate is evaluated with respect to four local criteria, calculated at every simulation step, *i.e.* at each of the n points of a given path (for instance to realize anastomosis on the intra ventricular artery). They are:

- Capability to perform the gesture (accuracy of path tracking),
- Manipulability of the instrument (resolution in force and velocity),
- Maximum joint torques,
- Minimal distance to organs.

The instruments evaluated by the optimization procedure are modular. Four kine-maticaly different modules have been designed and are shown in Fig. 2 [3]. The module on the left has one dof. It consists in a micro-motor, a worm and gear transmission, a position sensor (a bipolar magnet fixed on the gear, creating a rotating magnetic field sensed by a chip including two perpendicular hall sensors rigidly mounted on the fixed part). It has a minimal length of *24 mm*, a rotation range of ± *110°*, and gener-ates a *6 mN.m* maximum torque. Its diameter is *10 mm*.

Combining two of these modules leads to 2-dof modules, with parallel or orthogo-nal axes (Fig. 2, right). Their minimum length is *36 mm* with a rotation range of ± *110°*, and a maximum torque of *6 mN.m*. The module on the right shows a 2-dof module with one rotation about the main axis (more than *270°* and *8 mN.m* about this axis). A gripper using a compression spring and shape memory alloy wires has also been designed. The dexterous instrument resulting from the optimization procedure (Fig. 3) has five dof and a total reach of *130 mm*. It is composed of three of these elementary modules (one 1-dof module, two 2-dof modules) and a gripper module. To increase the instrument free-workspace within the chest cavity, it is inserted between the 3rd and 4th ribs, and the left lung is not insufflated. The distal module is parallel to the heart surface during most of the anastomosis procedure while the other modules move to achieve the correct position and orientation of the needle.

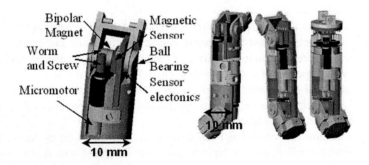

Fig. 2. 1-dof module (*left*). Various 2-dof modules (*right*).

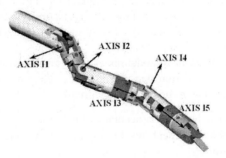

Fig. 3. An optimal dexterous 5-dof instrument for minimally invasive CABG.

4   Control of Assistive Devices for MIS

The dexterous instrument described in section 3 is intended to be held by a robot providing enough dof to align the main axis of the first module of the instrument with the trocar axis and to control its penetration depth. Therefore, at least five extracorporal dof are mandatory (six, if we assume that the rotation about the trocar axis should also be controlled by an extracorporal joint).

Only a small number of such robots are effectively used in the operating room for MIS. They have been mainly involved so far to assessment purpose and training (few CABG operations have been reported in the literature). The main feature of these robots is to mechanically create a fixed point that coincides with the penetration point of the trocar. The Zeus robotic arm makes use of a passive universal joint. The arm holds a tube penetrating the patient through the trocar that creates the kinematic constraint for the passive joint. An additional distal wrist is fixed on the tube. The system provides 6-dof within the patient. The Da Vinci robotic arm and other prototypes such as FZK Artemis [4] and UCB/UCSF RTW [5] systems offer the same service but their kinematics are designed as remote center devices. Another way to create a fixed point is to implement an appropriate force-position control: then, the tool is position-controlled within the patient while respecting a zero force constraint on the trocar [6].

We have explored alternate algorithmic approaches to satisfy the trocar constraint, whose advantage is to not require a dedicated robot [7]. One approach is based on a geometric description of the constraint that is resolved by an optimization procedure. It states that the position of the tool tip must coincide with the desired current position P^d, and that simultaneously the instrument must be aligned with the segment joining P^d and the trocar position P^{tr} (Fig. 4, left).

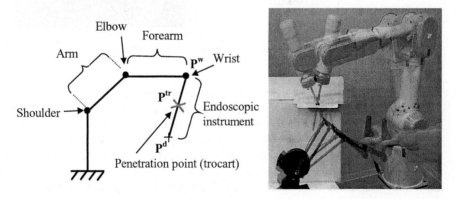

Fig. 4. Principle of the geometrical approach (*left*). Tele-operation under the constraint of penetration point (*right*).

We have validated this approach on a Mitsubishi PA-10 robot. A Phantom 1.5 arm was used as a master device to generate the desired tool tip position of the PA-10 (Fig. 4, right). The experiment is the following: the tool tip of the robot is driven via the Phantom until the contact with the trocar is reached; the instrument is inserted; then, we commute to the aforementioned control algorithm and, again via the Phantom, we realize random motions while satisfying the trocar constraint. We have verified that the distance between the trocar and the instrument shaft is smaller than a few millimeters for translation motion up to 0.3 m.s^{-1}. It is worth noting that this approach might be combined with force control techniques.

Another approach is based on the dynamic decoupling of the control torque into a task behavior control and a posture behavior control [8]. In fact, by minimizing the contact force or, equivalently, by forcing to zero the distance between the instrument passing through the trocar and the current location of the trocar (or the desired location, if the goal is to control it), we compute the posture behavior torque as the gradient of a cost function representing the distance. This approach allows us to dynamically control the penetration point required during MIS.

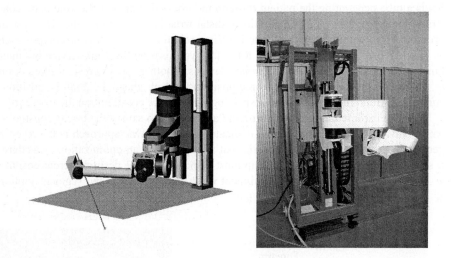

Fig. 5. The D2M2 platform: CAD view of the slave arm holding the instrument (*left*). The prototype of the slave arm (*right*).

We are currently designing a platform for development and assessment of advanced robotic functions for beating heart MIS. A 5-dof slave arm D2M2 (standing for Direct Drive Modular Manipulator) has already been designed (Fig. 5), with a 6-axis force sensor mounted at the tip of the wrist. An intracorporal 3-dof instrument can be attached to the wrist force sensor, providing full mobility to the tool tip. To cope with the high dynamics of the beating heart together with the low friction requirements for haptic interface, direct drive actuators have been preferred. The joint ranges are such that the instrument can be manipulated as the surgeon does it manually. An open control architecture has been developed to allow several autonomous and master-slave operating modes via a Phantom 1.5. The architecture has also been specified to control two or three master-slave devices. We are working on a procedure which will optimize the relative placement of these cooperating robots to reduce the collision risks during surgery while satisfying accessibility and manipulability constraints.

5 High Fidelity Tele-operation

Force control and haptic feedback are two major functions that are still missing in master-slave surgical robots. The main reason is that in MIS the interaction forces between tool and tissues cannot be sensed by the surgeon due to the friction forces in the trocar. One solution would be to measure interaction forces with a sensor mounted very near the tool tip, but such necessarily small and sterilizable device to be inserted into the patient is not yet available. However, force control could be very useful to prevent unintentional damage of tissues or to compensate for organ motion in case of contact between instrument and organ. To compensate for the absence of haptic feedback, the surgeon naturally uses tissue deformation as a visual substitute for sensation of the remote interaction forces. This does not work when he has to perform complex interaction gesture such as knots for instance. The outcome is that MIS requires long training period.

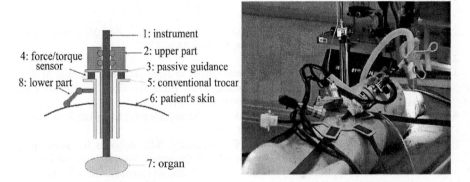

1: instrument
2: upper part
4: force/torque sensor
3: passive guidance
8: lower part
5: conventional trocar
6: patient's skin

7: organ

Fig. 6. Active trocar principle (*left*). *In vivo* tests with the MC^{2}E device (*right*).

An original solution has been proposed in which the sensor is integrated to the trocar, but fixed outside the patient [9]. The instrument is placed inside a passive guidance tube (Fig. 6, left), which increases the rigidity of the system. The passive guidance tube is attached to the upper part of the force/torque sensor. The lower part of the sensor is placed on a conventional trocar. This set up makes it possible to measure the tool-tissue interaction forces by adding mobilities to the trocar. Writing the generalized forces on the different moving parts, it can be shown that the interaction forces may be easily inferred from the force sensor data if the gravitational forces are known and if the forces due to dynamics are known or negligible. A dedicated device, called MC^{2}E (a French acronym for compact manipulation for endoscopic surgery) has been designed. It is lightweight and can be mounted directly on the patient. It is a 4-dof actuated mechanism providing an invariant centre at the fulcrum point, a rotation and a translation respectively about and along the instrument axis. An animal experiment with the active trocar is shown in Fig. 6 (right).

6   Conclusion

This paper has summarized major results of a French national two-year project aiming at the improvement of robotized minimally invasive surgery. The results obtained in modeling of the CABG gesture have clearly shown the need for dexterous motion and high-fidelity tele-operation; we have addressed those need by proposing on one hand a design methodology for intra-corporal devices, and on the other hand the concept of active trocar. Moreover, we have shown a new way for guiding MIS tools inside a trocar without resorting to dedicated robot arms; the proposed method is based on algorithms only, and thus is compatible with multi-purpose (then versatile) arms. Additional work is now required to integrate all the above mentioned technologies into a single system.

References

1. Dombre E. et al.: Projet MARGE: Modélisation, Apprentissage et Reproduction du Geste Chirurgical. Proc. Journées Robea. Toulouse, France (2004) 17-25
2. http://www.laas.fr/robea
3. Sallé, D., Bidaud, P., and Morel, G.: Optimal Design of High Dexterity Modular MIS Instrument for Coronary Artery Bypass Grafting. Proc. IEEE Int. Conf. on Robotics and Automation (ICRA). New Orleans, USA (2004) 1276-1281
4. Rininsland, H.: ARTEMIS: a Telemanipulator for Cardiac Surgery. European J. of Cardio-Thoracic Surgery, Vol. 16 Suppl. 2 (1999) S106-S111
5. Cavusoglu, M.C., Williams, W., Tendick, F., and Sastry, S.S.: Robotics for Telesurgery: Second Generation Berkeley/UCSF Laparoscopic Telesurgical Workstation and Looking Towards the Future Applications. Proc. 39th Allerton Conf. on Communication, Control and Computing. Monticello, USA (2001)
6. Krupa, A., Doignon, C., Gangloff, J., de Mathelin, M., Soler, L., and Morel, G.: Towards Semi-autonomy in Laparoscopic Surgery Through Vision and Force Feedback Control. Proc. Int. Symp. on Experimental Robotics, ISER'00. Waikiki, USA (2000) 189-198
7. Michelin, M., Poignet, P., Dombre, E.: Geometrical Control Approaches for Minimally Invasive Surgery. To appear in Proc. Workshop on Medical Robotics Navigation and Visualization (MRNV), Remagen, Germany (2004)
8. Michelin, M., Poignet, P., Dombre, E.: Dynamic Task / Posture Decoupling for Minimally Invasive Surgery Motions. Submitted 9th Int. Symp. on Experimental Robotics (ISER). Singapore (2004)
9. Zemiti, N., Ortmaier, J., Vitrani, M.-A., Morel, G.: A Force-Controlled Laparoscopic Robot Without Distal Force Sensing. Submitted 9th Int. Symp. on Experimental Robotics (ISER). Singapore (2004)

Crawling on the Heart: A Mobile Robotic Device for Minimally Invasive Cardiac Interventions

Nicholas A. Patronik[1], Marco A. Zenati[2], and Cameron N. Riviere[1]

[1]The Robotics Institute, Carnegie Mellon University, Pittsburgh, PA, USA
[2]Division of Cardiothoracic Surgery, University of Pittsburgh, Pittsburgh, PA, USA

Abstract. This paper describes the development and preliminary testing of a robotic device to facilitate minimally invasive beating-heart intrapericardial interventions. We propose the concept of a subxiphoid-inserted mobile robot (HeartLander) with the ability to adhere to the epicardium, navigate to any location, and administer therapy under physician control. As compared to current laparoscopic cardiac surgical techniques, this approach obviates cardiac stabilization and eliminates access limitations. Additionally, it does not require lung deflation and differential lung ventilation, and thus could open the way to outpatient cardiac therapies. The current HeartLander prototype uses suction to maintain prehension of the epicardium and wire actuation to perform locomotion. A fiber optic videoscope displays visual feedback to the physician, who controls the device through a joystick interface. A working channel provides access for the insertion of various therapeutic tools. This prototype has demonstrated successful prehension and walking during open-chest beating-heart porcine trials.

1 Introduction

Minimally invasive cardiac surgery has become a major objective of the field due to the desire to avoid the morbidity associated with median sternotomy and cardiopulmonary bypass [1]. Sternotomy can be obviated by endoscopy. There are many cardiac surgical procedures that could conceivably be performed endoscopically, but in most cases the necessary instrumentation does not yet exist. The obstacles include not only miniaturization for endoscopic application, but also gaining access to certain hard-to-reach parts of the heart. Current instrumentation generally relies on rigid endoscopes, which can only reach a limited area on the epicardial surface from a given incision [2]. The multi-arm robot systems that are commercially available (at prices around US$1,000,000) provide much of the needed dexterity for the realization of endoscopic heart surgery, but the problem of access remains unresolved for certain areas, such as the posterior wall of the left ventricle [2].

The challenges of minimally invasive access are further complicated by the goal of avoiding cardiopulmonary bypass. This requires surgery on the beating heart, greatly increasing the difficulties involved in worksite access and precise manipulation [3]. Instrumentation is needed that can provide stable manipulation of an arbitrary

C. Barillot, D.R. Haynor, and P. Hellier (Eds.): MICCAI 2004, LNCS 3217, pp. 9–16, 2004.

location on the epicardium while the heart is beating [4]. Thus far, progress in mini-mally invasive beating-heart surgery has been hindered by the need for endoscopic immobilization of the beating heart [2]. In open-heart surgery, immobilization is frequently accomplished using mechanical stabilizers such as the Acrobat (Guidant, Santa Clara, CA), TR^{3}IPOD (Chase Medical, Richardson, TX), and Octopus (Med-tronic, Minneapolis, MN), which grasp a portion of the epicardial surface and hold it steady. Some endoscopic versions of such devices have now been developed. How-ever, the resulting forces exerted on the myocardium can cause changes in the electro-physiological and hemodynamic performance of the heart, and care must be taken to avoid hemodynamic impairment or life-threatening arrhythmia [5]. As an alternative, several researchers in surgical robotics are investigating active compensation of heart-beat motion by visually tracking the epicardium and servoing the tool tips accordingly [6]. Such an approach, however, requires considerable expense for high-bandwidth actuation to manipulate in at least three degrees of freedom over a relatively large workspace [6].

All of these solutions address a problem that exists only because the tools are held by a robot (or surgeon) that is fixed to the table or the floor. We have taken a differ-ent approach: rather than trying to immobilize the heart surface to stabilize it in the (fixed) frame of reference of a table-mounted robotic device, the endoscopic device is mounted in the (moving) reference frame of the beating heart. This is accomplished using HeartLander, an innovative miniature robotic device that enters the pericardium through a minimally invasive port, attaches itself to the epicardial surface, then travels under its own power to the desired location and establishes a stable platform for sur-gery (Fig. 1). The problem of the beating-heart motion is thus avoided by attaching the device directly to the epicardium, and the problem of access is resolved by incor-porating the capability for locomotion.

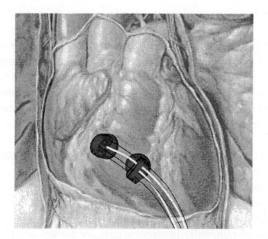

Fig. 1. Illustration of the HeartLander concept. The device is introduced using a subxiphoid approach, adheres to the epicardial surface, travels to the desired operative site, and administers the therapy under the control of the physician with video feedback

Improved access and precise manipulation are not the only benefits of this approach. Port access for minimally invasive cardiac surgery has typically been transthoracic, primarily in order to accommodate the rigid endoscopes generally used for both manual and robot-assisted procedures. Transthoracic access to the heart requires the deflation of the left lung, which necessitates general endotracheal anesthesia and differential lung ventilation. But among both established procedures and innovative ones there is a considerable number that conceivably could be performed entirely within the pericardium; i.e., they do not intrinsically require access to the pleural space or anywhere else outside the pericardium. Examples include, but are not limited to:

- cell transplantation [7];
- gene therapy for angiogenesis [8];
- epicardial electrode placement for resynchronization [9];
- epicardial atrial ablation [10];
- intrapericardial drug delivery [11];
- ventricle-to-coronary artery bypass (VCAB) [12].

Minimally invasive instruments are not currently available for most of these procedures, and those that do exist are typically designed for transthoracic access. However, all of these procedures could be performed without deflating a lung if suitable instrumentation were available.

The ability of HeartLander to move to any desired location on the epicardium from any starting point enables minimally invasive cardiac surgery to be independent of the location of the pericardial incision. HeartLander can therefore be introduced via transpericardial rather than transthoracic access, through an incision below the xiphoid process. This subxiphoid transpericardial approach not only obviates sternotomy and cardiopulmonary bypass, but avoids entering the pleural space altogether. As a result, deflation of the left lung is no longer needed and it becomes feasible to use local or regional rather than general anesthetic techniques. This has the potential to open the way to ambulatory outpatient cardiac surgery.

A HeartLander prototype has been constructed and preliminary tests have been performed, including locomotion on exposed beating porcine hearts. This paper describes the design of the device and the results obtained from testing.

2 Design

Under direct control of the physician, HeartLander will facilitate cardiac interventions by attaching directly to the epicardial surface, crawling to any desired location, and administering the therapy. The current prototype consists of a distal drive mechanism and proximal support system, connected through a 1-m long tether. The drive mechanism is the miniature mobile portion of the robot that enters the patient and performs the aforementioned functions. The support system is the large stationary portion that is externally located and contains all active components that control the drive mechanism. These include the motors for actuation, the pump to supply vacuum pressure, and the PC for visual feedback and control. The tether transmits the functionality of the support system to the drive mechanism. This tethered design allows the therapeutic portion of the robot (drive mechanism and tether) to be passive, lightweight, inexpensive, and largely disposable.

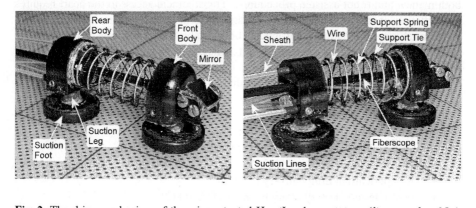

Fig. 2. The drive mechanism of the wire-actuated HeartLander prototype (*lines mark a 25.4-millimeter grid and the dots are spaced 2 millimeters apart*)

At the start of the procedure, HeartLander will be placed directly on the epicardial surface, beneath the pericardium, using a rigid endoscopic tool specifically designed for this purpose. This instrument will be introduced into the thoracic cavity through an incision made just below the xiphoid process of the sternum. The front and back modules of the drive mechanism are each 16 mm tall and have circular footprints 13 mm in diameter, thus allowing the device to pass through a 20-mm cannula. Once the treatment is complete, HeartLander will be retrieved by manually retracting the tether back through the endoscope. This also serves as the recovery method should the device become dislodged during the procedure.

The drive mechanism adheres to the epicardium using suction. Suction has proven to be effective for epicardial prehension in surgical stabilizers such as the Octopus™ and Starfish™ (Medtronic, Minneapolis, MN), as well as general prehension in mobile robotics [13]. The suction forces are applied by two independent suction feet that are attached by compliant legs beneath the front and rear body sections of the drive mechanism. The vacuum pressure is supplied to the feet by the external support system pump through two vacuum lines that pass through the tether (Fig. 2). The pump provides a vacuum pressure of -0.08 N/mm^2, which was found to be effective and safe for use in FDA-approved cardiac stabilizers. The suction forces generated by this pressure have proven effective for our application as well, and did not damage the epicardial tissue (see Sect. 3). The compliant legs allow the suction feet to conform to the curvature of the epicardial surface during locomotion. Fluids and small biological particles drawn through the suction feet and vacuum lines are safely collected, while larger particles are blocked by mesh grates covering the bottoms of the feet to avoid clogging the system. During locomotion, the vacuum pressure is monitored by external pressure sensors and regulated by computer-controlled solenoid valves, both located in the support system.

HeartLander achieves inchworm-like locomotion by coordinating prehension cycles and wire-actuated translations between the two modules of the drive mechanism. The distance and orientation between the two modules are controlled by three superelastic nitinol wires. The wires are linearly actuated by electric motor-driven belts in the support system. They pass freely through the tether and rear body section, and are attached distally to the front body section. The translations of the wires by the motors are transmitted to the modules at the drive mechanism by three plastic sheaths that enclose the wires in the tether. The sheaths are attached proximally to the stationary motor stage, and distally to the rear body section. The super-elasticity of nitinol allows the wires to support tension and compression (i.e. pulling and pushing) without permanently deforming. This eliminates the need for shape-restoring components (like springs) that are required in cable-drive transmissions. Locomotion is a cyclic process, one cycle of which is schematically illustrated in Fig. 3(a). The front module is advanced by pushing on the wires while the rear module has active suction. Retraction of the rear module to the advanced front module is accomplished by pulling back on the wires while the front module has active suction. Although the configuration of the sheaths and enclosed wires is unconstrained during locomotion, some slack must be maintained between the support system and the rear module in order for this locomotion scheme to work (i.e. the tether must not be taut). Turning is achieved by differentially changing the lengths of the side wires, illustrated in Fig. 3(b). The wires pass through triads of eyelets attached to a support spring between the front and rear body sections. This prevents the wires from bowing outward during turning and ensures that the wires maintain equal distances from one another (Fig. 3(c)). The support spring has a very low spring constant (k = 0.012 N/mm), thus the restoring force is negligible as compared to that of the wires. The three independently actuated wires provide three degrees of freedom (DOF) between the modules, two angular and one translational. The two angular DOF allow the device to adapt to the curvature of the heart (i.e. pitch) as well as turn laterally (i.e. yaw).

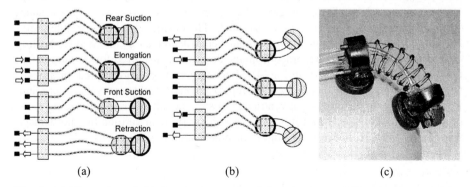

(a) (b) (c)

Fig. 3. (a) Illustration of the locomotion cycle of the wire-actuated HeartLander prototype (*dark ring indicates the module that has active suction at each step of the process*). (b) Illustration of steering. (c) HeartLander prototype with spring to allow sharp turns without bowing of the wires (*90° shown here*). 3 DOF allow the device to conform to surface curvature

The locomotion of the device and operation of the surgical end-effector are controlled by the physician using a PC-based graphical user interface that provides video feedback. A joystick controls the direction of travel and offers two speeds of travel (shown in Fig. 6). The previously described mechanical details of the locomotive process are handled by the computer, and thus are transparent to the user. Visual feedback from the front module is relayed to an external video camera by a 1.6-mm diameter fiber optic endoscope running through the tether, and displayed to the user on the monitor. A mirror is mounted to the front module in order to angle the view of the scope toward the surface of the heart. Along with a channel for the scope, both modules contain a 3-mm working port through which tools can be deployed for a variety of epicardial interventions.

3 Testing

3.1 Prehensile Testing with a Poultry Model

The support system pump provides a vacuum pressure of -0.08 N/mm^2, which was found to be effective and safe for use in FDA-approved cardiac stabilizers. Based on this pressure, the normal and tangential forces calculated to dislodge one of the modules are 1.76 N and 0.87 N, respectively. Bench testing using a force gauge to dislodge the device from a poultry model verified normal and tangential forces of 2.01 N and 0.86 N. The tangential force that can be resisted by the device will be increased significantly by reducing the profile of the next design.

3.2 Locomotion on the Beating Heart Using a Porcine Model

The wire-actuated HeartLander prototype was tested on three open-chest, beating-heart porcine models. The pericardium had been removed entirely and HeartLander was placed directly on the epicardium by hand. The device was able to maintain prehension on the exposed epicardium without being dislodged by the natural beating motion of the heart. Video recorded from the device was displayed for the surgeon on the computer monitor (shown in Fig. 4). Locomotion was also captured on a hand-held video camera as the device traveled approximately 50 mm across the epicardium from the left ventricle to the right ventricle, crossing the left anterior descending coronary artery (LADA), as shown in Fig. 5. A cardiac surgeon verified that no damage was done to the epicardium as a result of the prehension or locomotion.

4 Discussion

The results presented herein demonstrate the feasibility of adhering to and maneuvering on the epicardium of a beating heart using the HeartLander prototype. Future porcine tests will proceed from open-heart testing to minimally invasive testing using a subxiphoid approach.

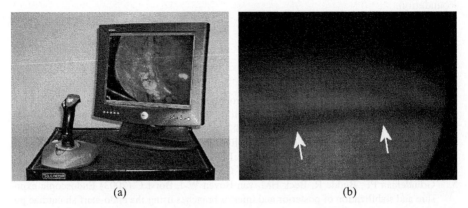

(a)   (b)

Fig. 4. (a) The HeartLander control interface: joystick for control of locomotion, and monitor to display video from the device camera. (b) View of the left anterior descending artery (LADA) through the device camera (*arrows highlight LADA*)

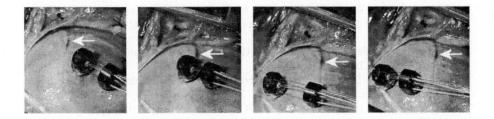

Fig. 5. A time sequence of photographs showing the HeartLander prototype crossing the left anterior descending artery (LADA) on a beating porcine heart (*arrows highlight a reference point along the LADA for comparison between frames*)

By employing a modular design for end-effector attachment, HeartLander will be capable of performing a variety of surgical treatments. The first application planned for evaluation is epicardial lead placement for resynchronization [9]. The actuation for the end-effectors will either be provided directly by an on-board motor or transmitted from an external motor through the tether.

As the research continues, we plan to develop end-effectors for HeartLander for more innovative procedures, such as epicardial delivery of myoblasts or stem cells for regeneration of the failing myocardium. Ultimately, we envision adoption of HeartLander-based intrapericardial therapies not only by minimally invasive cardiac surgeons, but also by interventional cardiologists and electrophysiologists [14,15].

Acknowledgments. Funding provided by the Simeon M. Jones, Jr. and Katharine Reed Jones Fund and the John D. Schaub's Sons Memorial Fund of the The Pittsburgh Foundation.

References

1. Mack MJ (2001) Minimally invasive and robotic surgery. *JAMA* 285:568-572.
2. Falk V, Diegler A, Walther T, Autschbach R, Mohr FW (2000) Developments in robotic cardiac surgery. Curr Opin Cardiol 15:378–387.
3. Borst C, Gründeman PF (1999): Minimally invasive coronary artery bypass grafting: an experimental perspective. *Circulation* 99:1400-1403.
4. Zenati, MA (2001) Robotic heart surgery. Cardiol Rev 9:287-294.
5. Gründeman PF, Budde R, Beck HM, van Boven W-J, Borst C (2003) Endoscopic exposure and stabilization of posterior and inferior branches using the endo-starfish cardiac positioner and the endo-octopus stabilizer for closed-chest beating heart multivessel CABG: hemodynamic changes in the pig. *Circulation* 108:11-34.
6. Çavuşoğlu MC, Williams W, Tendick F, Sastry SS (2003) Robotics for telesurgery: second generation Berkeley/UCSF laparoscopic telesurgical workstation and looking towards the future applications. *Industrial Robot* 30(1):22-29.
7. Li R-K, Jia Z-Q, Weisel RD, Merante F, Mickle DAG (1999) Smooth muscle cell transplantation myocardial scar tissue improves heart function. *J Mol Cell Cardiol* 31:513-522.
8. Losordo DW, Vale PR, Isner JM (1999) Gene therapy for myocardial angiogenesis. Am Heart J 138(2) Pt 2: S132-41.
9. Leclercq C, Kass DA (2002) Retiming the failing heart: principles and current clinical status of cardiac resynchronization. *J Am Coll Cardiol* 39:194-201.
10. Lee R, Nitta T, Schuessler RB, Johnson DC, Boineau JP, Cox JL (1999) The closed heart MAZE: A nonbypass surgical technique. *Ann Thorac Surg* 2:1696-1702.
11. Gleason JD, Nguyen KP, Kissinger KV, Manning WJ, Verrier RL (2002) Myocardial drug distribution pattern following intrapericardial delivery: an MRI analysis. *J Cardiovasc Magn Reson* 4(3): 311-316.
12. Boekstegers P, Raake P, Al Ghobainy R, Horstkotte J, Hinkel R, Sandner T, Wichels R, Meisner F, Thein E, March K, Boehm D, Reichenspurner H (2002) Stent-based approach for ventricle-to-coronary artery bypass. *Circulation* 106:1000-1006.
13. Siegel M, Gunatilake P, Podnar G (1998) Robotic assistants for aircraft inspectors. *Instrumentation Measurement Mag*, 1(1):16-30.
14. Schweikert RA, Saliba WI, Tomassoni G, Marrouche NF, Cole CR, Dresing TJ, Tchou PJ, Bash, D, Beheiry S, Lam C, Kanagaratna L, Natale A (2003) Percutaneous pericardial instrumentation for endo-epicardial mapping of previously failed ablations. *Circulation* 108:1329-1335.
15. Sosa E, Scanavacca M, D'Avila A, Oliveira F, Ramires JAF (2000) Nonsurgical transthoracic epicardial catheter ablation to treat recurrent ventricular tachycardia occurring late after myocardial infarction. J Am Coll Cardiol 35:1442-1449.

High Dexterity Snake-Like Robotic Slaves for Minimally Invasive Telesurgery of the Upper Airway

Nabil Simaan[1], Russell Taylor[1], and Paul Flint[2]

[1] Department of Computer Science
NSF Engineering Research Center for
Computer-Integrated Surgical Systems and Technology
The Johns Hopkins University
3400 North Charles Street – NEB B26 #7, Baltimore, Maryland, 21218
{nsimaan, rht}@cs.jhu.edu
http://www.cisst.org

[2] Department of Otolaryngology - Head & Neck Surgery
Johns Hopkins School of Medicine
601 North Caroline Street, Baltimore, Maryland, 21287
pflint@jhmi.edu
http://www.hopkinsmedicine.org/otolaryngology

Abstract. This paper reports our efforts to develop an integrated system for telesurgery of the throat and upper airway. The system is described while focusing on the novel design of its slave robot. The slave robot is a 3-armed robot that implements novel Distal Dexterity Units (DDU's). These DDU's are dexterous robots for surgical tool manipulation and suturing in confined spaces. Each DDU is composed from a Snake-Like Unit (SLU) and a detachable Parallel Manipulation unit (PMU). The proposed design of the DDU's provides an enhanced downsize scalability and distal dexterity that are crucial for medical applications such as laryngeal surgery where simultaneous manipulation of 2-3 long tools through a narrow laryngeoscope is required. The paper presents the design of these units and the experimentation results with a 4.2 mm diameter SLU to be used for constructing the first DDU for the 3-armed slave robot.

1   Introduction

Previous work on telerobotic systems for MIS (Minimally Invasive Surgery) has focused on endoscopic surgery of the chest and abdomen while using several different mechanical architectures for slave robots. These mechanical architectures included remote-center-of-motion mechanisms (e.g., [1, 2]), serial-link robots with passive joints [3], and mini-parallel robots (e.g., [4, 5]). A recent survey of these works has been presented in [6]. A fundamental challenge for these robots is the kinematic constraint imposed by the passage of the surgical tools through fixed entry ports into the

C. Barillot, D.R. Haynor, and P. Hellier (Eds.): MICCAI 2004, LNCS 3217, pp. 17–24, 2004.

patient's body. If more than four Degrees-of-Freedom (DoF) are required in manipulating a surgical instrument, then some form of distal dexterity mechanism is required.

The purpose of this work is to develop a system for MIS of the upper airway including the throat and larynx - an unusually challenging task due to the shape of the airway and position of the larynx, the need to perform complex procedures on or beyond the vocal folds, and the need to simultaneously manipulate 2-3 long instruments through a predetermined entry port. This aim includes developing down-sizable Distal Dexterity Units (DDU's) for precise surgical tool manipulation in confined spaces where the required diameter of these units is less than 4.5 mm.

2   Clinical Relevance, Setup, and Requirements

The upper airway is a long, narrow, and irregularly shaped organ that includes the pharynx (throat), hypopharynx, and larynx, commonly referred to as the voice box. These areas are subject to a variety of benign and malignant growths, paralysis, and scar tissue formation requiring surgical interventions for excision and/or reconstruction. These procedures (e.g. partial or total laryngectomy, vocal fold repositioning, and laryngotracheal reconstruction) are routinely performed using open surgical techniques on the expense of damaging the integrity of the framework supporting the laryngeal cartilage, muscle, and the connective tissue vital to normal function. Minimally invasive endoscopic procedures are generally preferred over open procedures, thereby, preserving laryngeal framework integrity, promoting faster recovery and frequently overcoming the need for tracheostomy.

Figure 1 shows a typical MIS setup for laryngeal surgery. The internal regions of the airway are accessed by using an array of long instruments (usually ranging between 240 to 350 mm long) through a laryngoscope that is inserted into the patient's mouth and serves as a visualization tool and a guide for surgical instru-

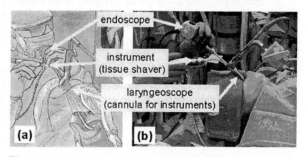

Fig. 1. A typical surgical setup for MIS of the throat (a) artist rendering (b) actual surgical setup

mentation. The laryngeoscope is typically 180 mm long with an oval cross-section usually ranging between 16-20 mm in width at its smallest cross section. This surgical setup requires the surgeon to manipulate several long tools (for example one tool for suction and another for tissue manipulation) that are constrained to 4 DoF motions and lacking tool-tip dexterity. For these limitations, laryngeal MIS is currently limited to simple operations such as microflap elevation, excisional biopsies, and removal of papilloma using laser or powered microdebrider. Functional reconstructive procedures (e.g. tissue flap rotation or suturing), are not performed in throat MIS; although, reconstruction of the vocal fold structures as accurately as possible is crucial for maintaining the voice characteristics. Suture closure of surgical defects has been shown to reduce scar tissue, shorten healing time, and result in improved laryngeal function and sound production [7, 8]. This seemingly simple operation is very difficult, if not impossible, to perform in laryngeal MIS. This work addresses these needs by developing a system to allow surgeons to perform complex functional reconstruction tasks and suturing in MIS of the upper airway.

We use suturing to define the required workspace and force application capability of our system. The goal reachable workspace is a cylindrical work volume about 40 mm in diameter and 50 mm in height and located 180-250 mm axially down the throat. The Distal Dexterity Units (DDU's) should be able to bend 90° sideways in any direction of while maintaining their ability to apply 1 Newton at its tip for tissue manipulation/suturing purposes.

3   Snake-Like Robots for Dexterity Enhancement in MIS

Several approaches to distal tool dexterity enhancement have been reported. Many systems (e.g.,[2]) use wire actuated articulated wrists. Other systems use snake-like active bending devices. For example, [9] used bending SMA (Shape Memory Alloy) forceps for laparoscopic surgery. Dario et al [10] presented an SMA actuated 1 DoF planar bending snake device for knee arthroscopy and Reynaerts [11] designed a hyper-redundant SMA actuated snake for gastro-intestinal intervention. Recently, Piers et al. [12] presented a two DoF 5 mm diameter wire-driven snake-like tool using super-elastic NiTi flexure joints and Ikuta et al. [13] reported a ∅3 mm wire-actuated articulated robot attached at the tip of a flexible stem for microsurgery inside deep and narrow spaces.

Cavusoglu et al. [14] analyzed alternative designs of a 3 DoF wrist for MIS suturing. They proposed a method to determine the workspace and to optimize the position of the entry port in the patient's body to provide optimal dexterity. Faraz and Payendeh [15] recently analyzed three architectures of endoscopic wrists: a simple wire actuated joint, a multi-revolute joint wrist, a tendon snake-like wrist. They compared these joints in terms of dexterity and showed the superiority of the snake-like wrist over the other two wrists in terms of dexterity.

In chest and abdomen MIS, the entry portals for surgical instruments are usually placed some distance apart, and the instruments approach the operative site from somewhat differing directions. This makes it possible (though sometimes inconvenient and limiting) for telesurgical systems such as the DaVinci or Zeus use rather large robotic slave manipulators for extracorporeal instrument positioning. The optimal placement of entry portals based on dexterity requirements for particular procedures is an important subject and has recently been addressed by several authors including Adhami et al. [16] and Cannon et al. [17]. In MIS of the throat, the entry port is predetermined and no such optimization is possible. The slave robot presented in the next section is designed to answer this limitation.

4   The Design of the 3-Armed Slave

Fig. 2 presents the system we are currently developing for throat MIS, [18]. This system has the same master-slave architecture as the DaVinci® [2] or any other telesurgical robot. Although this system is specialized for throat surgery, some components (such as the DDU's) are suitable for minimally invasive microsurgery in confined spaces in general. This paper will focus on presenting the slave robot of Fig. 3.

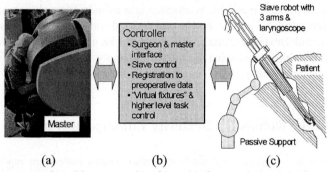

(a)   (b)   (c)

Fig. 2. System overview: (a) a master interface with force and visual feedback (b) a smart controller used for master-slave integration and control of the redundant degrees of freedom offered by the slave robot (c) a 3-armed slave robot for simultaneous manipulation of 2-3 robotic arms equipped with distal dexterity units

The slave robot is a three-armed robot working through a laryngeoscope, Fig. 2-(c). Our design includes a laryngoscope, a base link, two similar DDU's for tool/tissue manipulation, and another DDU for suction. Each DDU is a 5 DoF robot mounted on a corresponding DDU holder, which is manipulated by a corresponding 4 DoF tool manipulation unit (TMU) that controls the angle of approach, the rotation about and the position along

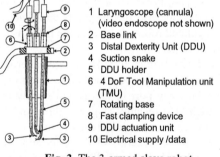

1 Laryngoscope (cannula)
   (video endoscope not shown)
2 Base link
3 Distal Dexterity Unit (DDU)
4 Suction snake
5 DDU holder
6 4 DoF Tool Manipulation unit
   (TMU)
7 Rotating base
8 Fast clamping device
9 DDU actuation unit
10 Electrical supply /data

Fig. 3. The 3-armed slave robot

the axis of the DDU holder. The TMU's are mounted on a rotating base unit (RBU) permitting the system to be oriented within the throat so as to minimize collisions between DDU holders. The DDU holders are thin tubes (about 4 mm in outside diameter) providing an actuation pathway for the DDU and possibly a light-source or a suction channel. Each TMU is equipped with a fast clamping device for adjusting the axial location of the DDU. The actuation unit of each DDU is located at its upper extremity and the actuation is by super-elastic tubes operated in push-pull mode.

This system implements actuation redundancy in the design and control of the DDU's. Each DDU has 7 actuated joints and each TMU has 4 DoF. The total number of actuated joints for the slave is 34.

The DDU (Distal Dexterity Unit). The DDU is composed from a snake-like unit and a detachable parallel manipulation unit attached at its tip, Fig. 4. It is designed to bypass obstacles (such as the vocal folds) and to perform suturing by transforming the rotation of the DDU holder about its axis into rotation about its backbone axis.

The multi-backbone snake-like unit. The SLU of Fig. 4.-(a) is a 2 DoF robot composed from a base disk, an end disk, several spacer disks, and four super-elastic NiTi tubes. These tubes are called the backbones of this SLU. The central tube is the *primary backbone* while the remaining three tubes are the *secondary backbones*. The secondary backbones are equidistant from the central backbone and from one another. The central backbone is attached to both the base and end disks and to all spacer disks while the secondary backbones are attached only to the end disk and are free to slide and bend through properly dimensioned holes in the base and spacer disks. These secondary backbones are used for actuating this snake-like device and they pass through guiding channels in the DDU holder to allow their actuation in both push and pull modes. The spacer disks prevent buckling of the central and secondary backbones and keep an equal distance between them.

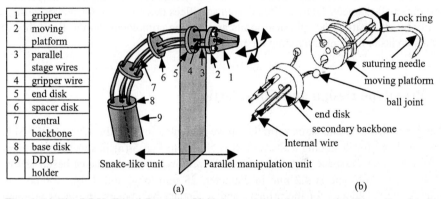

1	gripper
2	moving platform
3	parallel stage wires
4	gripper wire
5	end disk
6	spacer disk
7	central backbone
8	base disk
9	DDU holder

(a)   (b)

Fig. 4. (a) The DDU (Distal Dexterity Unit) is composed from a snake-like unit and a detachable parallel manipulation unit (b) detachable parallel manipulation unit for precise wrist-like and axial motions; and surgical tool interchangeability

This design has several advantages over standard designs using discrete backbones (articulated serial chains). By using flexible backbones, the dependency on small universal joints and wires is removed. This reduces manufacturing costs and enhances downsize scalability. The use of tubes for the backbones provides a secondary application for them as suction channels, actuation channels for the tool mounted on the SLU distal end or as a source of light for imaging. By using three push-pull secondary backbones for actuation, it is possible to satisfy the statics of the structure while preventing buckling of the backbones as was proposed in [18]. This further enhances the downsize scalability while maintaining the force application capability of these SLU's on a level large enough for tool manipulation for delicate tasks (1-2 Newton).

The detachable milli-parallel unit. The SLU is capable bending sideways in any direction, hence, providing 2 DoF for distal dexterity. To enhance it with surgical tool interchangeability and additional precise wrist action and axial motion, we are currently designing and constructing the detachable parallel unit of Fig. 4-(b). The parallel mechanical architecture has been chosen for providing precise and high-accuracy motions in a small workspace while utilizing its inherent rigidity [4, 5].

The detachable milli-parallel unit is constructed from super-elastic actuation wires passing through the secondary backbones, spherical joints, and a moving platform to which a gripper of a tool is affixed, Fig. 4-(b). The moving platform is machined with matching groves such that the balls attached to the end of the actuation wires match its diameter and a flexible locking ring is placed around the circumference of the moving platform to maintain these balls inside their grooves. To detach the gripper/tool one removes the lock ring and removes the moving platform.

There are two possible operation modes using the detachable milli-parallel unit. In the first operation mode, the actuation wires are used only to extend axially in order to attach a new moving platform equipped with another tool. Once the tool is attached, then the actuation wires are retrieved until the moving platform is secured on the end platform of the SLU. In the other mode, for operations requiring small workspace and fine motions, the actuation wires are used to actuate the moving platform as a three DoF parallel platform with flexible extensible links.

We are also considering another alternative design for this parallel manipulation unit for small-diameter DDU's. This design sacrifices detachability for downsize scalability by eliminating the spherical joints and relying completely on the flexibility of the superelastic links manipulating the moving platform.

5   Prototype Design and Construction

Using the kinematic and static formulation we presented in [18], the action of the SLU was simulated for designing a ∅4 mm SLU shown in Fig. 5-(a) in several configurations inside its workspace. Fig. 5-(b) shows the prototype we constructed based on this design. This prototype is 4.2 mm in diameter, 28 mm long, and it uses ∅0.66 mm superelastic backbones for the primary and secondary backbones. In our experiment we manually actuated only two out of three secondary backbones. The unit is able to bend more than 70° sideways in any direction while applying forces at its tip larger than 1 Newton. Once the actuation unit is constructed, we will implement

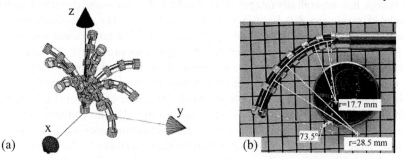

(a)   (b)

Fig. 5. Snake like unit: (a) simulation for design purposes (b) the ∅4.2 mm snake-like prototype based on the parameters of the simulation in (a)

actuation redundancy to actuate all three secondary backbones in push-pull operation. This will help bend the SLU in larger bending angles while keeping the strain in the backbones within a 4% limit for guarding against degradation of the backbones' superelastic properties in repeated operation. The figure shows the total bending angle and the radiuses of curvature of the primary backbone along two different sections. This non-constant radius of curvature is due to the elongation of the secondary backbones due to actuation forces and due to the manufacturing tolerances of the disks. The variable spacing of the disks was used to reduce this effect and to prevent buckling at the base of the SLU that is shown doing spatial motion in Fig. 6.

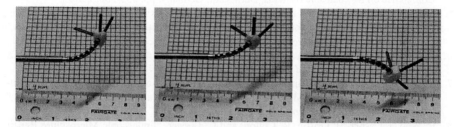

Fig. 6. The snake-like unit of Fig. 5-(b) performing spatial motions. This unit was able to apply more than 1 Newton at its tip and to bend more than 70° sideways in any direction by actuating only two out of its three available secondary backbones

6   Conclusions

This paper presented our work on designing a high dexterity, high accuracy slave for tele-operated MIS of the throat and upper airway. This clinical application was discussed and the benefits of distal dexterity enhancement for functional reconstruction of tissue and suturing inside the larynx were highlighted. These seemingly simple operations are currently extremely difficult to perform in a MIS.

Although this system is not yet finalized and clinically demonstrated, we believe it includes two components that will enhance throat MIS in particular and microsurgery in general. These components are the 34 DoF three-armed slave robot capable of manipulating through a narrow laryngeoscope and the novel Distal Dexterity Units (DDU's) that are useful for precise dexterous operations in small confined spaces. Each DDU is a dexterous robot composed of a SLU and a detachable parallel manipulation unit – all designed to enhance downsize scalability to diameters smaller than 5 mm. The design of this SLU implements several flexible tubular backbones. This allows it to be used for visualization purposes, aspiration, micro drilling and to be easily downsized to diameters smaller than 4 mm. Finally, we presented our first prototype of a Ø4.2 mm SLU. It was shown to have the ability to exert forces larger than 1 Newton at its tip and to bend more than 70° in any direction.

Acknowledgments. This work was partially funded by the National Science Foundation (NSF) under Engineering Research Center grant #EEC9731478, NSF grant #IIS9801684, and by the Johns Hopkins University internal funds.

References

1. R. Taylor, J. Funda, B. Eldridge, S. Gomory, K. Gurben, D. LaRose, M. Talamini, L. Kavoussi, and J. Anderson, "A Telerobotics Assistant for Laparoscopic Surgery," *IEEE Engineering in Medicine and Biology Magazine*, vol. 14, pp. 279-288, 1995.
2. G. Guthart and K. Salisbury, "The Intuitive™ Telesurgery System: Overview and Application," IEEE International Conference on Robotics and Automation, pp. 618-621, 2000.
3. J. M. Sackier and Y. Wang, "Robotically assisted laparoscopic surgery from concept to development," *Surgical Endoscopy*, vol. 8, pp. 63-66, 1994.
4. N. Simaan and M. Shoham, "Robot Construction for Surgical Applications," The 1st IFAC Conference on Mechatronic Systems, Darmstadt, Germany, pp. 553-558, 2000.
5. M. Shoham, M. Burman, E. Zehavi, L. Joskowicz, E. Batkilin, and Y. Kunicher, "Bone-Mounted Miniature Robot for Surgical Procedures: Concept and Clinical Applications," *IEEE Transactions on Robotics and Automation*, vol. 19, pp. 893-901, 2003.
6. R. Taylor and D. Stianovici, "Medical Robotics in Computer-Integrated Surgery," *IEEE Transactions on Robotics and Automation*, vol. 19, pp. 765-781, 2003.
7. D. J. Fleming, S. McGuff, and C. B. Simpson, "Comparison of Microflap Healing Outcomes with Traditional and Microsuturing Techniques: Initial Results in a Canine Model," *Ann Otol Rhinol Laryngol.*, vol. 110, pp. 707-712, 2001.
8. P. Woo, J. Casper, B. Griffin, R. Colton, and C. Brewer, "Endoscopic Microsuture Repair of Vocal Fold Defects," *J. Voice*, vol. 9, pp. 332-339, 1995.
9. Y. Nakamura, A. Matsui, T. Saito, and K. Yoshimoto, "Shape-Memory-Alloy Active Forceps for Laparoscopic Surgery," IEEE International Conference on Robotics and Automation, pp. 2320-2327, 1995.
10. P. Dario, C. Paggetti, N. Troisfontaine, E. Papa, T. Ciucci, M. C. Carrozza, and M. Marcacci, "A Miniature Steerable End-Effector for Application in an Integrated System for Computer-Assisted Arthroscopy," IEEE International Conference on Robotics and Automation, pp. 1573-1579, 1997.
11. D. Reynaerts, J. Peirs, and H. Van Brussel, "Shape memory micro-actuation for a gastrointestinal intervention system," *Sensors and Actuators*, vol. 77, pp. 157-166, 1999.
12. J. Piers, D. Reynaerts, H. Van Brussel, G. De Gersem, and H. T. Tang, "Design of an Advanced Tool Guiding System for Robotic Surgery," IEEE International Conference on Robotics and Automation, pp. 2651-2656, 2003.
13. K. Ikuta, K. Yamamoto, and K. Sasaki, "Development of Remote Microsurgery Robot and New Surgical Procedure for Deep and Narrow Space," IEEE International Conference on Robotics and Automation, pp.1103-1108, 2003.
14. M. Cavusoglu, I. Villanueva, and F. Tendick, "Workspace Analysis of Robotics Manipulators for a Teleoperated Suturing Task," IEEE/RSJ International Conference on Intelligent Robots and Systems, Maui, HI, pp. 2234-2239, 2001.
15. A. Faraz and S. Payandeh, "Synthesis and Workspace Study of Endoscopic Extenders with Flexible Stem," (online report) Simon Fraser University, Canada 2003.
16. L. Adhami and E. C. Maniere, "Optimal Planning for Minimally Invasive Surgical Robots," *IEEE Transactions on Robotics and Automation*, vol. 19, pp. 854-863, 2003.
17. J. W. Cannon, J. A. Stoll, S. D. Sehla, P. E. Dupont, R. D. Howe, and D. F. Torchina, "Port Placement Planning in Robot-Assisted Coronary Artery Bypass," *IEEE transactions on Robotics and Automation*, vol. 19, pp. 912-917, 2003.
18. N. Simaan, R. Taylor, and P. Flint, "A Dexterous System for Laryngeal Surgery - Multi-Backbone Bending Snake-like Slaves for Teleoperated Dexterous Surgical Tool Manipulation," IEEE International Conference on Robotics and Automation, New Orleans, pp.351-357, 2004.

Development of a Robotic Laser Surgical Tool with an Integrated Video Endoscope

Takashi Suzuki[1], Youhei Nishida[1], Etsuko Kobayashi[1], Takayuki Tsuji[1], Tsuneo Fukuyo[2], Michihiro Kaneda[3], Kozo Konishi[4], Makoto Hashizume[4], and Ichiro Sakuma[1]

[1] Institute of Environmental Studies, Graduate School of Frontier Sciences, The University of Tokyo, 7-3-1, Hongo, Bunkyo-ku, Tokyo, 113-8656, Japan
{t-suzuki, nishida, etsuko, tsuji, sakuma}@miki.pe.u-tokyo.ac.jp
http://bme.pe.u-tokyo.ac.jp/index_e.html
[2] Shinko Optical Co.,Ltd., 2-12-2, Hongo, Bunkyo-ku, Tokyo, 113-0033, Japan
shinko-koki@par.odn.ne.jp
[3] Sparkling Photon Inc., 1154-1, Kotta, Tama City, Tokyo, 206-0014, Japan
kaneda@phton.co.jp
[4] Department of Disaster and Emergency Medicine, Graduate School of Medical Sciences, Kyushu University, 3-1-1, Maidashi, Higashi-ku, Fukuoka, 812-8582, Japan
konizou@surg2med.kyushu-u.ac.jp, mhashi@dem.med.kyushu-u.ac.jp

Abstract. Integration of new surgical devices with surgery assisting robots is required by surgeons. We have developed a novel robotic laser coagulator with a charge coupled device (CCD) video endoscope and a bending joint. The endoscope visualizes the detail of the target, and bending joint realizes the irradiation in a selected direction. We adopted two laser diodes for this purpose: an infrared semiconductor laser ($\lambda = 980$ nm) for coagulation, and a visible wavelength laser ($\lambda = 635$ nm) acting as a pointer for the target. The technical originality of this work is the mounting of a laser module on the forceps without using an optical fiber or mirror guide. This reduces the danger of laser leakage at the bending joint, and realizes miniaturization in the multiarticular robot. The clinical significance is the precise positioning and intuitive operation of the laser coagulator through future integration of this tool with a master–slave robotic system. An *in vivo* study achieved necrosis of liver tissue, and demonstrated the feasibility of the robotic laser coagulator using a CCD video endoscope.

1 Introduction

Recently, laparoscopic surgery has been widely performed as a minimally invasive surgery technique. In this method, the surgeon cuts 3 – 4 holes in the abdominal wall, and the entire procedure is carried out inside the abdominal cavity. This has advantages in reducing pain, discomfort, medication, and the time needed for recovery[1]. However, this technique requires the surgeon to have much skill and experience. Various surgical instruments, such as electric cautery, ultrasonic vibration scalpels, laser knives, and laser coagulators have been developed, and

C. Barillot, D.R. Haynor, and P. Hellier (Eds.): MICCAI 2004, LNCS 3217, pp. 25–32, 2004.
© Springer-Verlag Berlin Heidelberg 2004

are widely used in the operating theater. The increasing use of these devices has shown their potential advantages as new surgical tools.

On the other hand, surgery assisting robots (Zeus^{TM}, da Vinci^{TM} [2]) have been applied clinically, and have contributed to an improvement in the quality of surgery. Bending forceps with two degrees of freedom (DOF) can trace the surgeon's operational procedure, and an intuitive operation and enhanced dexterity have been realized that could not be achieved using conventional forceps.

Both new surgical devices and robots have enabled remarkable performance to be achieved. Integration of advanced surgical tools with surgical robots, however, is still not satisfactory. Surgeons have the limited options in choosing advanced surgical tools using current surgical robotic systems. Some robotized systems using lasers have been developed in prostatectomy[3,4]. Their flexibility, however, is not adequate for general abdominal surgery, as irradiation of laser light from an arbitrary direction is required to treat lesions at various locations in the abdominal cavity. Thus, providing advanced surgical instruments with additional motional degrees of freedom will enable further advancement of surgical robot technology.

We have integrated a miniaturized high power surgical laser and a CCD endoscope for target observation using robotic bending forceps. This paper discusses a prototype robotic miniaturized surgical laser and its performance as a laser surgical instrument. We also present preliminary results of animal experiments where a porcine liver was coagulated using the developed system.

2   Materials and Methods

2.1   System Configuration

We aimed to integrate robotic forceps with laser coagulator for carrying out thermal therapy resulting in a necrosis of a tumor or for abdominal surgery hemostasis. An infrared laser with an output wavelength of around $\lambda = 1\mu m$ can penetrate into deep areas of an organ, resulting in coagulation and not ablation. For example, neodymium yttrium aluminum garnet (Nd:YAG) lasers ($\lambda = 1,064$ nm) are widely used in the operating room for photocoagulation. The infrared light is introduced into the abdominal cavity through an optical fiber. A light guiding optical fiber, however, is unsuitable for bending robotic forceps, because cracks in the fiber would occur after repeated bending at a joint. We also have to consider the bending radius that the optical fiber would be subjected to, because the laser light would leak at small radius bends.

We used an infrared semiconductor laser chip for coagulation, and mounted the laser chip on the tip of forceps. The advantages of this laser module are:(1) the need for a light guiding fiber was eliminated, and so any danger of laser light leakage was avoided; (2) any unintended coagulation associated with laser light leakage was avoided; (3) miniaturization was realized. Because infrared light is invisible, we needed a targeting device to operate the laser device. We used a semiconductor laser chip that operated in the visible spectrum, as used in laser pointers. The control box of the laser module was newly developed, based on the idea of remote control for future telesurgery. This had a serial RS232C communication interface, and thus, we could send commands (output power and coagulating time) to the unit from a personal computer.

At the same time, the problem with a conventional rigid laparoscope was highlighted: it provides a limited and narrow view for the surgeon. On laser coagulation using the bending forceps, a rigid scope may not always show the front view of the target. An inadequate view will obstruct any appropriate operation by the surgeon. Therefore, we tried to integrate a video endoscope onto the surgical instrument to provide a detailed view of the nearest point to the target and from the far-side view of the organ, which cannot be seen by a rigid laparoscope[5]. Thus, we mounted a compact charge coupled device (CCD) camera acting as a video endoscope to provide the close-up or far-side view of an organ.

A conventional laparoscope uses an optical fiber to illuminate the abdominal cavity. However, we identified the risk of cracking in the fiber, and so used a white light emitting diode (LED) for illumination, so eliminating the use of an optical fiber for the light source, and in the robotic forceps system, we integrated the above modules: laser, pointer, CCD camera, and LED.

2.2 Semiconductor Laser Module

We used an infrared semiconductor main laser for coagulation (InGaAs/GaAs, $\lambda = 980$ nm , output power = 20 W) (Sparkling Photon, Inc. Japan) that was equivalent to a normal Nd:YAG laser. We assembled a linear array of ten laser diode chips with 2 W output power each to realize a combined output power of 20 W. The alignment of the laser chips is shown in Fig. 1. The main laser bar had an area of 1×5 mm^2. The laser beam output was collimated to ensure the beams were parallel. To point to the target, we mounted a red laser ($\lambda = 635$ nm, output power = 10 mW), as is used in a commercial laser pointing device (see Fig. 2). We circulated physiologic saline inside the base of the laser chips' mount to act as a coolant. We developed our own control unit to control the laser module(Fig. 3). This controlled the current, the coagulating time, the safety lock, the red laser for pointing, a white LED, and a foot switch, and had two input interfaces: a local mode using a nearby controller, and a remote control mode via an RS232C communication interface. This arrangement allows for future adaptation for remote control during telesurgery.

2.3 CCD Camera

We used a compact CCD camera (Shinko Optical Co. Ltd., Japan) as the second scope. The camera dimensions were: diameter = 5 mm; length = 15 mm; and weight = 3 g. The area of the CCD images was 3.30×2.95 mm^2, and this contained 410,000 pixels. In contrast to a fiberscope, the CCD camera produced good quality images. It also had the advantage of being able to be adaptable to the bending forceps, because it did not require optical fibers to function.

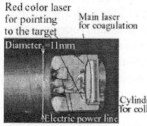

Red color laser
for pointing   Main laser
to the target   for coagulation

Diameter = 11mm

Cylindrical lens
for collimation

Electric power line

Fig. 1. Alignment of the laser chip for co-agulation and pointing.

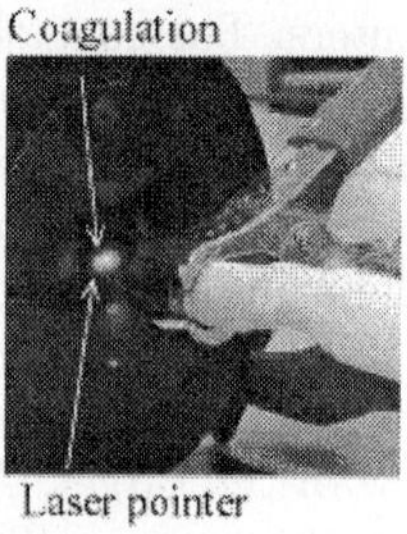

Coagulation

Laser pointer

Fig. 2. The infrared semiconduc-tor laser ($\lambda = 980$ nm) and the red laser ($\lambda = 635$ nm).

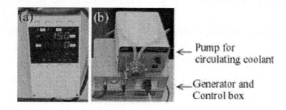

← Pump for
circulating coolant

← Generator and
Control box

Fig. 3. The original control unit for laser module: (a) the controller; (b) the pump for circulating the coolant, and the generator.

Although optical fibers are usually used to transmit light from a light source into the abdominal cavity, we used a white LED (NSPW300BS, Nichia Corporation, Japan) as an additional light source to illuminate the target along with the main light for the laparoscope. This is because a bright light source was necessary to obtain good quality images when using the CCD camera as the second scope. We used a white LED because of its small size and the fact that no optical fiber was required. We did encounter problems with the LED color characteristics, in the red objects, such as arteries, appeared dark because of the LED's wavelength characteristics, which are different from those of conventional light bulbs[6]. In addition, the light intensity of the LED was much lower than a conventional light bulb. However, we found that the LED could be used as a light source in the limited area near the target, and that the problems associated with the spectrum would not be severe, because of the lower intensity of the LED source.

2.4 Bending Forceps and Integration

We developed the robotic forceps as an end effector of the forceps manipulator with four DOF[7,8]. The forceps required two bending joints that were equivalent to the wrist of a surgeon, so that the forceps could trace the operational procedure using six DOF. However, as the laser instrument can be considered to be symmetrical around the longitudinal axis, we eliminated one DOF (the rotational motion around the longitudinal axis). Thus, the forceps had only one DOF (the bending motion of the tip). The prototype device is shown in Fig. 4. The bending joint was driven by a linkage mechanism using a geared stepper motor (Turbo Disk P010, Portescap, USA) and a ball screw. The range of the bending joint was 0 – 90°. The tip of forceps, on which the laser module and CCD camera were mounted, is shown in Fig. 5.

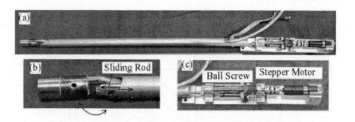

Fig. 4. The prototype: (a) full view; (b) linkage mechanism for the bending motion of the tip; (c) the driving unit using a stepper motor and a ball screw.

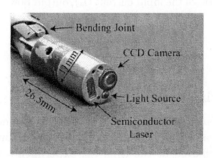

Fig. 5. The tip of the forceps: diameter = 11 mm; length = 26.5 mm; weight = 15 g.

3   Results

3.1   Laser Diode

The area of coagulation was measured to be 0.55×4.75 mm^2 at a distance of 10 mm from the tip of the forceps. This coagulation area was measured using laser alignment paper (Zap-It[R], Zap-It Corp., USA).

We also measured the characteristics of the input current (A), the output power (W), and the temperature of the coolant (°C), shown in Fig. 6. The initial temperature of the coolant was 22°C, and the coolant was circulated a rate of at 60 ml/s during the laser irradiation.

The maximum output power of the laser module was 20.0 W for an input current of 25 A. However, the collimating lens and the glass window in front of the lens reduced the power of the laser to 11.8 W. The temperature of the coolant increased from 22 to 43°C, a temperature of 21°C, showing that the cooling efficiency was high enough for the system to cope.

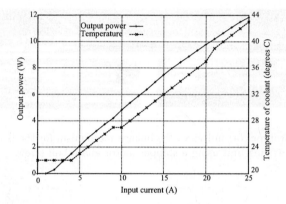

Fig. 6. The characteristicsof the input current (A), output power (W), and temperature of the coolant (°C).

3.2 *In Vivo* Experiments

We carried out *in vivo* experiments on a porcine liver under laparotomy rather than laparoscopy, because the mounting of the laser module on the robotic forceps had not been achieved at the time the experiments were conducted. The laser module was held in place using a clamp that fixed its position near the liver.

The red pointing laser was invisible under the direct high power surgical light, but as it was relatively dark inside the abdominal cavity, this would not be a problem for laparoscopic surgery. The white LED was evaluated as being a suitable point light source, but the effects of the tin white color of the LED could not be ignored, and medical doctors have commented that the color of the white LED needs to be changed.

We evaluated the coagulating performance using an output power of 9.8 W at a current of 20 A, and using an irradiation time of 10, 20, and 30 s. During coagulation, we stopped the respirator in use to eliminate any motion of the organ caused by the action of breathing; the result is shown in Fig. 7. During coagulation, laser bursts occurred in periods lasting around 15 s, and the effect of these showed that the laser had sufficient power for coagulation. On the other hand, bursts inside the abdominal cavity in this manner would cause a rapid increase in air pressure. This may be dangerous for laparoscopic surgery. Even though we will be able to determine the necrosis and carbonization of the tissue from the compact CCD camera images, an adjustment in the laser power is necessary to realize safe and stable coagulation. Thus, it is important to know the relationship between the input energy and volume of necrosis, and to quantify the appropriate input energy before bursts are carried out. As an example of how to achieve this quantification, we measured the volume of denaturation. Using the experimental conditions of power = 7.5W, current = 15 A, and the irradiation period = 20 s, the denaturation volume was 29 mm^3 (see Fig. 8). Collecting this type of data will clarify the characteristics of laser coagulation and enable us to quantify it.

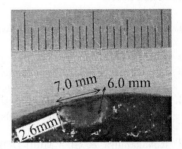

Fig. 8. A cross-sectional view of the liver. The volume was calculated using an approximated elliptical cone. Major axis length = 7 mm; minor axis length = 6 mm; depth = 2.6 mm.

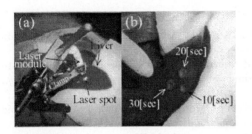

Fig. 7. The *in vivo* experiment on a porcine liver: (a) coagulation; and (b) the result.

4   Discussion and Conclusions

We have realized a robotic laser coagulator with an integrated CCD endoscope. The unit had mounted semiconductor laser chips for coagulation and for pointing to the target. A white LED used for lighting had sufficient light intensity, but its tin white color presented a problem. The advantages of using a semiconductor laser without an optical guide were: (1) miniaturization of the laser module; (2) elimination of laser light leakage causing unintended coagulation at the bending joint; (3) integration of the laser instrument and robotized forceps with a bending joint without any risk of laser light leakage; and (4) realization of a better maintained coherent light source that enables deep penetration into the tissue of an organ compared to a conventional laser instrument using light guiding through an optical fiber.

We have yet to fully evaluate the total sterilization of the system, but we believe that the entire system can be sterilized using ethylene oxide gas (EOG). This is because each individual module of the system, such as the laser, LED, CCD camera, and mechanical part of the forceps is able to be sterilized using EOG.

In future, we will integrate this bending forceps system with a forceps manipulator that has four DOF (rotational motion around the trocar port, and insertion into the cavity) into the slave robotic system, which can realize an intuitive operation based on commands from the surgical console.

This study was supported by the Research for the Future Program JSPS-RFTF99I00904.

References

1. Daijo Hashimoto, editor. *Advanced Technique in Gasless Laparoscopic Surgery.* World Scientific., 1995.
2. http://intuitivesurgical.com/.
3. Mei Q et al. PROBOT - a computer integrated prostatectomy system. *Visualization in biomedical computing. Springer,* pages 581–590, 1996.
4. Gideon Ho et al. Computer-Assisted Transurethral Laser Resection of the Prostate (CALRP): Theoretical and Experimental Motion Plan. *IEEE Biomed. Eng.,* 48(10):1125–1133, 2001.
5. R.Nakamura et al. Multi-DOF Forceps Manipulator System for Laparoscopic Surgery. In *MICCAI2000,* pages 653–660, 2000.
6. Junichi Shimada et al. Medical lighting composed of LED arrays for surgical operation. In *Proc. of SPIE,* pages 165–172, 2001.
7. Takashi Suzuki et al. A new compact robot for manipulation forceps using friction wheel and gimbals mechanism. In *CARS2002,* pages 314–319, 2002.
8. Takashi Suzuki et al. Development of forceps manipulator for assisting laparoscopic surgery. In *CARS2004,* page 1338, 2004.

Micro-Neurosurgical System in the Deep Surgical Field

Daisuke Asai[1], Surman Katopo[1], Jumpei Arata[1],
Shin'ichi Warisawa[1], Mamoru Mitsuishi[1],
Akio Morita[2], Shigeo Sora[2], Takaaki Kirino[2], and Ryo Mochizuki[3]

[1] School of Engineering, The University of Tokyo
7-3-1, Hongo, Bunkyo-ku, Tokyo 113-8656, Japan
{daisuke,surman,jumpei,warisawa,mamoru}@nml.t.u-tokyo.ac.jp
[2] School of Medicine, The University of Tokyo
{amor-tky,sora-tky,tkirino-tky}@umin.ac.jp
[3] NHK Engineering Services, Inc.
1-10-11, Kinuta, Setagaya-ku, Tokyo 157-8540, Japan
r-mochi@cyborg.ne.jp

Abstract. In neurosurgery, surgeons have to perform precise manipulations with poor visibility due to the presence of blood or cerebrospinal fluid and it is particularly difficult to operate in the deep surgical field. The authors have developed a microsurgical system for neurosurgery in the deep surgical field that addresses these difficulties. The authors succeeded in suturing the carotid artery of a rat under a glass tube 120 [mm] in depth and 50 [mm] in diameter. In this paper, the authors propose the concept of robotic-assisted micro-neurosurgery. The design and the system are presented. Furthermore, the performance of the system and *in-vivo* experiments on rats are also reported.

1 Introduction

Neurosurgery has progressed rapidly since surgical microscopes were introduced and widely used in the 1970s. The development of the microscope provided an environment where microsurgery could be routinely executed in an enlarged operation field, enabling surgeons to perform various kinds of operative techniques which had been impossible in conventional surgery safely and precisely. However, it is still a challenge to reduce the invasiveness of microsurgery while protecting normal brain tissue during surgery. Many systems to support operative techniques in neurosurgery [1][2], including master-slave systems to support microsurgery [3][4], have been developed. The master-slave systems designate the operation site as the master and the surgical site as the slave. Micro-manipulation is performed by scaling the master and the slave manipulator motions [5]. The HUMAN system is a master-slave microsurgery system for neurosurgery [6][7]. Its insertion probe is 10 [mm] in diameter and contains a stereoscopic endoscope and three micro-manipulators each of which is 3 [mm] in diameter and has 3 D.O.F. However, the motion range is limited to a 10 [mm] cube, which

C. Barillot, D.R. Haynor, and P. Hellier (Eds.): MICCAI 2004, LNCS 3217, pp. 33–40, 2004.
© Springer-Verlag Berlin Heidelberg 2004

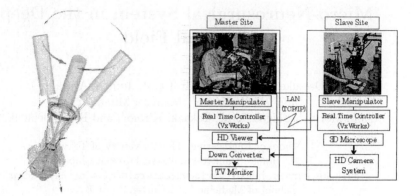

Fig. 2. Overview of the system

Fig. 1. Concept for the forceps

is not enough to complete a surgical operation, such as suturing and removing tumors. Da Vinci [8] and ZEUS [9] are already available commercially and have been used in many clinical applications. However, they are not appropriate for minimally invasive neurosurgery because they were developed to support laparoscopic or heart surgery and their insertion probes are more than 10 [mm] in diameter. To solve the problems, the authors developed a microsurgical system for neurosurgery to assist micro-manipulation in the deep surgical field.

2   Design of a Neurosurgical System

2.1   Concept

To decrease the invasiveness of neurosurgery, it is necessary to provide a sufficiently enlarged image of the target and precise maneuverability to the surgeon. The former requirement is fulfilled with by higher-powered surgical microscope. However, the latter requirement depends mostly on surgeon's personal skill, which is acquired by specialized training and refined through experience and continual application. Therefore, the robotic surgical assistance system is expected to be used in difficult operative procedures. The requirements and necessary conditions for a robotic surgical assistance system for neurosurgery are as follows:

- Precise maneuverability sufficient to suture a micro blood vessel,
- Insertion through a small craniotomy hall to decrease invasiveness,
- Sufficient maneuverability in the deep surgical field,
- To provide the expanded surgical field to a surgeon,
- To assure the mechanical safety of patients, and
- To adapt to the current neurosurgery environment.

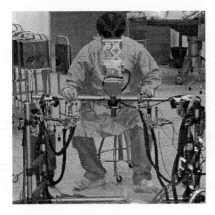

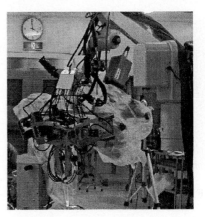

Fig. 3. Master manipulator   **Fig. 4.** Slave manipulator

2.2   System Requirement

Based on requirements and necessary conditions mentioned above, the authors set the following specifications for the microsurgical system:
  – Positioning accuracy of better than 50 [μm],
  – Diameter of the forceps less than 5 [mm],
  – The forceps have 1 bending D.O.F. and a range of motion from -90 [deg] to +90 [deg],
  – There is a fixed point at the insertion part of the forceps,
  – 100 [mm] translational motion range in the inserting direction,
  – The forceps can be changed easily, and
  – The forceps can be sterilized and irrigated easily.

3   Implementation of the System

3.1   Overview of the System

Fig.2 shows a block diagram of the microsurgical system for neurosurgery in the deep surgical field. The system consists of three parts: the master manipulator which the surgeon operates, the slave manipulator which performs actual surgical operations on the patient, and the 3-dimensional surgical microscope system.

3.2   Master Manipulator

The master manipulator is an interface device that a surgeon operates. The surgeon can control the slave manipulator by applying motion to the device. Fig.3 shows an overview of the master manipulator. It consists of left and right arms. Each arm has 3 translational D.O.F., 3 rotational D.O.F., and 1 grasping D.O.F. In addition, it has 3 foot switches to assist operation.

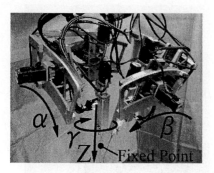

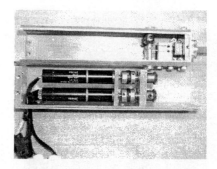

Fig. 5. Mechanism of the slave arm

Fig. 6. Detachable actuators for the forceps

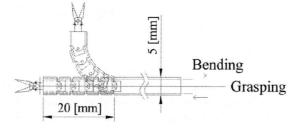

Fig. 7. Mechanism of the forceps

3.3   Slave Manipulator

The slave manipulator performs a surgical pocedure on a patient according to the commands from the master manipulator. Fig.4 shows an overview of the slave manipulator. It consists of three parts: the arm part which holds and moves surgical tools, the forceps part which is inserted in the brain, and the base part which determines the position of the arm.

1. Arm part
   The arm part consists of two arms (left/right) to hold surgical tools (Fig.5). Each arm has 3 rotational D.O.F. (α,β,γ), and 1 translational D.O.F. along the insertion axis (Z). Radius guides were adopted for the rotational motion around α and β-axis. The axes intersect at the mechanical fixed point on the insertion axis. Safe, minimally invasive surgery is achieved by setting the point at the narrowest part of the pathway to the affected area, where the maximum motion limitation is required. The motion ranges of α, β, γ and Z-axis are from −15 to +15 [deg], from −15 to +15 [deg], from −270 to +270[deg], and from 0 to 90 [mm], respectively. Each axis is actuated by a stepping motor.

2. Forceps part
   The micro-active forceps with a diameter of 5[mm] is detachable from the arm part. It has 1 bending D.O.F. and 1 grasping D.O.F. The length of the

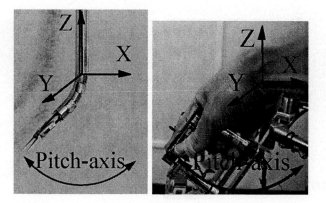

Fig. 8. Correspondence of D.O.F. between the master and the slave manipulator

bending part is 20 [mm], the bending motion range is from −90 [deg] to +90 [deg]. The forceps has enough motion range to suture or to remove a tumor in the deep surgical field. Stainless wires transmit driving forces to bend and to grasp at the head of the forceps (Fig.7). An easily detachable mechanism between the insertion part and the motor of the forceps enables sterilization and irrigation of the insertion part (Fig.6). Each motion is actuated by a small DC motor.

3. Base part
   The base part has 6 passive D.O.F. It determines the position of the arm part and the forceps part before the operation.

3.4   Visual System

To achieve micro-neurosurgery, an enlarged surgical field has to be provided to the surgeon who operates the master manipulator. In addition, good depth peception is crucial to successful operation in the deep surgical field. In the developed system, a high definition surgical view, which is obtained by the surgical microscope and a high definition camera for 3-dimensional display at the slave site, is presented on the 3-dimensional display system at the master site. Using the developed system, the surgeon can operate more safely and precisely.

3.5   Coordination Between Master and Slave Manipulator

In an asymmetrical master-slave manipulator system, hand-eye coordination, which means how the slave manipulator in the display is to be moved according to the motion of the master manipulator by the surgeon, is very important. It is required for the system that the information obtained from the visual display and the operation sensation at the surgeon's hand should correspond. Therefore, a coordinate system transformation is performed between the master and the

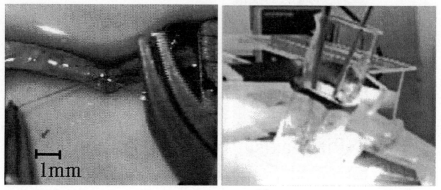

(a) Suturing a carotid artery   (b) A rat under a glass tube

Fig. 9. *In-vivo* experiment on a rat

slave manipulators shown in 8. The bending motion at the head of the slave manipulator corresponds to a rotation around the surgeon's wrist. It enables the surgeon to operate the forceps as if he/she held its tip directly. It also reduces the force sensation felt by the surgeon.

4   *In Vivo* Experiment by a Surgeon

4.1   Method

To verify the effectiveness of the system for the exposure, dissection and suturing of a micro blood vessel in the deep surgical field, experiments were performed using rats (Fig.9). Exposure, dissection, and complete anastomosis of a common carotid artery were conducted on 10-week old male Wister rats by setting a glass tube (Fig.9(b)), whose depth and the diameter are 90 [mm] and 40 [mm], respectively, to simulate an actual minimally invasive neurosurgery on a human brain and to limit the motion range of the forceps. A carotid artery was intentionally cutted off in advance and was sutured 10 to 13 times using a 10-0 needle and suture.

4.2   Result and Discussion

Exposure, dissection and complete anastomosis of the common carotid artery were successfully performed. The blood flow was confirmed without any leaks after suturing. During the suturing, at first the needle was grasped using the right forceps (needle handling) and then was stuck into the arterial wall (needle placement). It was pulled out by the left forceps, and was passed through the other arterial wall (arterial wall passing). Finally, the suture was knotted. The sum of the every operation time is shown in Fig.10. The average time to complete

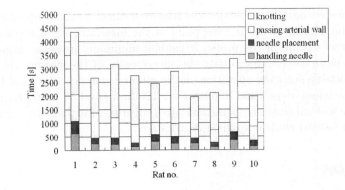

Fig. 10. Operation time

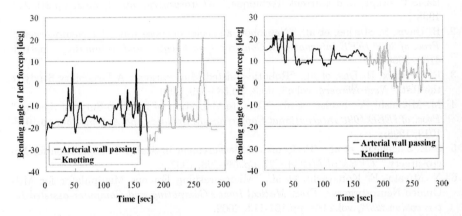

Fig. 11. The bending motions of right and left forceps in the *in vivo* experiment

anastomosis is 42.4 [min.]. Knotting required the longest and the most varied time. The target time is 20 [min.]. Fig.11 shows the bending angle of the left and the right forceps during each task. From the figure, it was determined that the suturing operation was performed by the cooperation of the left and the right forceps. Therefore, the effectiveness of the bending function was proved. Furthermore, blood flow could be confirmed after suturing 10 to 13 times. This demonstrates that the needle was inserted into the intended position around the incision. The experimental results show that the developed system has enough capability for micro-manipulation in deep and narrow spaces.

5   Conclusion

The authors have developed a microsurgical system for neurosurgery in the deep surgical field. The slave manipulator has two forceps, each of which has 1 D.O.F. in bending and 1 D.O.F. in grasping at its head. The length and the diameter of the insertion part are 190 [mm] and 5 [mm], respectively. The developed system provides an environment to suture and remove a tumor in the deep surgical field of the brain. The mechanical fixed point of the insertion probe was located at the narrowest section of the probe. It enables minimally invasive surgery to be performed more safely. To evaluate the effectiveness of the system, the authors have conducted a suturing operation on the common carotid arteries of 10 rats in a glass tube whose depth and diameter are 120 [mm] and 50 [mm], respectively. Blood flow was successfully confirmed after suturing. Further improvements of the system toward clinical application continue.

References

1. A. Perneczky and G. Fries, "Endoscope-assisted Brain Surgery: Part 1-Evolution, Basic Concept, and Current Technique," *Neurosurgery*, vol.42, no.2, pp.219-224, 1998.
2. B. Davis, S. Starkie, et al., "Neurobot: a special-purpose robot for Neurosurgery," *Proc. of 2000 IEEE International Conference on Robotics and Automation*, pp.4103-4108, 2000.
3. P. Le Roux, H. Das, et al., "Robotic-assisted Microsurgery: A Feasibility Study in the Rat," *Neurosurgery*, vol.48, no.3, pp.584-589, 2001.
4. M. Mitsuishi, Y. Iizuka, et al., "Remote Operation of a Micro-Surgical System," *Proc. of IEEE 1998 International Conference on Robotics and Automation*, pp.1013-1019, 1998.
5. S. E. Salcudean, et al., "Performance Measurement in Scaled Teleoperation for Microsurgery," *CVRMed-MRCAS'97*, pp.789-798, 1997.
6. N. Miyata, E. Kobayashi, et al., "Micro-grasping Forceps Manipulator for MR-Guided Neurosurgery," *Proc. Medical Image Computing and Computer-assisted Intervension 2002*, vol.2488, pp.107-113, 2002.
7. K. Hongo, S. Kobayashi, Y. Kakizawa, et al., "Neurobot:Telecontrolled Micromanipulator System for Minimally Invasive Microneurosurgery–Preliminary Results," *Neurosurgery*, vol.51, no.4, pp.985-988, 2002.
8. G. Guthart and JK. Salisbury, "The Intuitive Telesurgery System: Overview and Application," *Proc. of 2000 IEEE International Conference on Robotics and Automation*, pp.618-621, 2000.
9. http://computermotion.com

Dense 3D Depth Recovery for Soft Tissue Deformation During Robotically Assisted Laparoscopic Surgery

Danail Stoyanov[1], Ara Darzi[2], and Guang Zhong Yang[1,2]

[1] Royal Society/Wolfson Foundation Medical Image Computing Laboratory,
[2]Department of Surgical Oncology and Technology
Imperial College of Science, Technology and Medicine, London SW7 2BZ, UK
{d.v.stoyanov,a.darzi,g.z.yang}@imperial.co.uk
http://vip.doc.imperial.ac.uk

Abstract. Recovering tissue deformation during robotic assisted minimally invasive surgery is an important step towards motion compensation and stabilization. This paper presents a practical strategy for dense 3D depth recovery and temporal motion tracking for deformable surfaces. The method combines image rectification with constrained disparity registration for reliable depth estimation. The accuracy and practical value of the technique is validated with a tissue phantom with known 3D geometry and motion characteristics. It has been shown that the performance of the proposed approach compares favorably against existing methods. Example results of the technique applied to *in vivo* robotic assisted minimally invasive surgery data are also provided.

1 Introduction

With recent advances in robotic assisted Minimally Invasive Surgery (MIS), it is now possible to perform closed-chest cardiothoracic surgery on a beating heart to minimize patient trauma and certain side effects of cardiopulmonary bypass. For robotic assisted MIS, dexterity is enhanced by microprocessor controlled mechanical wrists, which allow motion scaling for reducing gross hand movements and the performance of micro-scale tasks that are otherwise not possible. So far, two commercially available master-slave manipulator devices are specifically designed for MIS cardiac surgery [1]. Both systems improve the ergonomics of laparoscopic surgery and provide high dexterity, precision and 3D visualization of the operating field. One of the significant challenges of beating heart surgery is the destabilization introduced by cardiac and respiratory motion, thus severely affecting precise instrument-tissue interactions and the execution of complex grafts. Mechanical stabilizers [2] permit off-pump procedures by locally stabilizing the target area while the rest of the heart supports blood circulation. Despite this, residual motion remains, which complicates delicate tasks such as small vessel anastomosis.

Thus far, a number of techniques have been proposed for resolving intraoperative tissue deformation. Intraoperative 3D tomographic techniques offer precise information about soft tissue morphology and structure, but they introduce significant challenges to instrument design, integration and computational cost. A more practical al-

C. Barillot, D.R. Haynor, and P. Hellier (Eds.): MICCAI 2004, LNCS 3217, pp. 41–48, 2004.
© Springer-Verlag Berlin Heidelberg 2004

ternative is to use optical based techniques to infer surface deformation in real-time. In animal experiments, Nakamura *et al* [3] used a high-speed camera to track a fiducial marker on the epicardial surface. The trajectory changes of the markers were used to identify the frequencies due to cardiac and respiration motion by using an autoregressive model. A region based, reduced affine tracking model was used by Gröger *et al* [4] in robotic assisted MIS heart surgery for computing the local motion of the epicardial surface. Thakral *et al* [2] used a fiber optic displacement sensor to measure the motion of a rat's chest for motion modeling with weighted time series. While these techniques demonstrate the feasibility of providing motion compensation, they generally do not consider detailed 3D deformation. With the use of a stereoscopic laparoscope for robotic assisted MIS, the feasibility of recovering the 3D structure of the operating field based on computer vision techniques has also been investigated [5]. Previously, monocular shading was used to infer surface shape in less interactive endoscope diagnostic procedures [6]. Although the recovery of the depth of a 3D scene based on different visual cues is one of the classic problems of computer vision, dense disparity measurement for deformable structure with high specularity is a difficult task. The purpose of this paper is to present a robust dense 3D depth recovery method with a stereoscopic laparoscope for motion stabilization. The method combines image rectification with constrained disparity registration for reliable depth recovery. The accuracy and practical value of the technique is validated with a tissue phantom with known 3D geometry and motion characteristics. Example results of the technique applied to *in vivo* robotic assisted MIS data are also provided.

2 Methods

2.1 Stereo Camera Model and Calibration

One of the first steps towards depth recovery is to compute both the intrinsic and extrinsic camera parameters of the stereoscopic laparoscope. In this study, the standard pinhole model is assumed and an upper triangular matrix $\mathbf{K}$ is used to describe the internal optics of the camera. Denoting the camera's position and orientation with respect to a world coordinate system by a rotation matrix $\mathbf{R}$ and translation vector $\mathbf{t}$, the camera matrix can thus be defined as:

$$\mathbf{P}^k = \mathbf{K}^k \left[\mathbf{R}^k \mid -\mathbf{R}^k \mathbf{t}^k \right] \tag{1}$$

Without loss of generality, the camera matrices for the stereoscopic laparoscope can be represented by the following equation by taking the left camera as the reference:

$$\mathbf{P}^L = \mathbf{K}^L \left[\mathbf{I} \mid \mathbf{0} \right] \ and \ \mathbf{P}^R = \mathbf{K}^R \left[\mathbf{R} \mid -\mathbf{R}\mathbf{t} \right] \tag{2}$$

In practice, laparoscope cameras deviate from ideal perspective projection and induce a high level of distortion. We consider henceforth the first three terms of the radial distortion, k_1^k, k_2^k, k_3^k and two tangential distortion terms, p_1^k and p_1^k [7].

For MIS, the stereo cameras are usually pre-calibrated before the surgical procedure and then remain unchanged during the operation. Off-line calibration by using objects with known geometry is therefore sufficient [8]. In this study, the intrinsic and extrinsic parameters of the cameras were derived by using a closed form solution as proposed in [9]. Following the initial estimate, the parameters were refined subject to the mean squared error between the measured image points $\mathbf{m}$ and the re-projected world points $\mathbf{M}$. By parameterizing the rotation matrix $\mathbf{R}$ as a vector of three parameters $\mathbf{r}$, the minimization criteria for a set of n images with m grid points can be written as:

$$\sum_{i=1}^{n}\sum_{j=1}^{m}\left\|\mathbf{m}_{ij} - \mathbf{m}\left(\mathbf{K},\mathbf{r}_i,\mathbf{t}_i,k_1,k_2,k_3,k_1,p_2,\mathbf{M}_j\right)\right\|^2 \tag{3}$$

The optimization problem formulated above is non-linear and the Levenberg-Marquardt algorithm was used to derive the above parameters iteratively. After each camera has been calibrated, the relative pose of the two cameras is then introduced such that the following equation is minimized. This allows the use of the solution derived for each individual camera as the initial solution for the Levenberg-Marquardt algorithm.

$$\sum_{i=1}^{n}\sum_{j=1}^{m}\left[\begin{array}{l}\left\|\mathbf{m}_{ij}^L - \mathbf{m}\left(\mathbf{K}^L,\mathbf{r}_i^L,\mathbf{t}_i^L,k_1^L,k_2^L,k_3^L,p_1^L,p_2^L,\mathbf{M}_j\right)\right\|^2 \\ +\left\|\mathbf{m}_{ij}^R - \mathbf{m}\left(\mathbf{K}^R,\mathbf{r}_i^R,\mathbf{t}_i^R,k_1^R,k_2^R,k_3^R,p_1^R,p_2^R,\mathbf{M}_j,\mathbf{r},\mathbf{t}\right)\right\|^2\end{array}\right] \tag{4}$$

2.2 Image Rectification

For reliable dense depth recovery, image rectification based on epipolar geometry is an important step for enhancing the robustness of the algorithm as this effectively restricts the search space for disparity to 1D. For common robotic MIS settings, the cameras are slightly verged to permit both positive and negative disparities so as to enhance the overall 3D depth perception. To ease the fusion of the stereo images for the observer, the stereo cameras are generally in near vertical alignment. However, this arrangement may not be perfect in practice and therefore a planar rectification process is applied to the stereo image pairs before dense correspondence is sought [10]. By definition, the intrinsic matrices of the two rectified images must be the same. Without changing the centers of the cameras, the new projection matrices can be defined through the same rotation matrix such that

$$\mathbf{P}_r^L = \mathbf{K}_r\left[\mathbf{R}_r \mid \mathbf{0}\right] \; and \; \mathbf{P}_r^R = \mathbf{K}_r\left[\mathbf{R}_r \mid -\mathbf{R}_r\mathbf{t}\right] \tag{5}$$

In the above equation, $\mathbf{R}_r$ may be computed by assuming that the new image planes are parallel to the baseline. As the camera centers remain unchanged so does the optical ray through each image point, the original and rectified camera matrices can therefore be written as:

$$\mathbf{P}^k = \left[\mathbf{Q}^k \mid \mathbf{q}^k\right] \ and \ \mathbf{P}_r^k = \left[\mathbf{Q}_r^k \mid \mathbf{q}_r^k\right] \tag{6}$$

Subsequently, the rectifying transformations can be computed from the original and rectified camera matrices through the following pair of equations:

$$\mathbf{T}^L = \lambda^L \mathbf{Q}_r^L (\mathbf{Q}^L)^{-1} \ and \ \mathbf{T}^R = \lambda^R \mathbf{Q}_r^R (\mathbf{Q}^R)^{-1} \tag{7}$$

Although this method does not directly minimize the distortion or resampling effects caused by the transformations [11], in the context of the current work the warping introduced above is inherently small due to the general settings of the stereoscopic laparoscope cameras.

2.3 Stereo Correspondence with Constrained Disparity Registration

Traditional computer vision techniques for dense stereo correspondence are mainly concerned with rigid objects and much emphasis is placed on issues related to occlusion and discontinuity [12]. Occlusion and object boundaries make stereo matching a difficult optimization problem, as disparity is not globally continuous and smooth. Existing techniques include winner-takes-all, graph-cuts, and dynamic programming approaches [13]. For soft tissue as observed in MIS, the surface is generally smooth and continuous and the difficulty of dense depth recovery is usually due to the paucity of identifiable landmarks. Explicit geometrical constraints of the deformation model is therefore required for ensuring the overall reliability of the algorithm. For this study, the free-form registration framework proposed by Veseer $et\ al$ [14] was used as it provides a robust, fully encapsulated multi-resolution approach based on piece wise bilinear maps (PBM). The lattice of PBM permits non-linear transitions, which is suitable for temporally deforming surfaces and it easily lends itself to a hierarchical implementation. With image rectification, the search space for each iteration is constrained on scan lines and the number of PBM forming the image transformation is increased, refining the registration of finer structures. Within this framework, the disparity obtained at low-resolution levels are propagated to higher levels and used as starting points for the optimization process. To cater for surfaces in laparoscope images that have reflectance properties dependent on the viewing position, normalized cross correlation (NCC) was used as a similarity measure. The NCC of two image regions I^L and I^R of dimensions (u,v) is defined as:

$$NCC\left(I^L, I^R\right) = \frac{\sum_{u,v}\left(I^L(u,v) - \overline{I}^L\right)\left(I^R(u,v) - \overline{I}^R\right)}{(uv)^2 \sqrt{\sum_{u,v}\left(I^L(u,v) - \overline{I}^L\right)^2 \left(I^R(u,v) - \overline{I}^R\right)^2}} \tag{8}$$

For deriving disparity values of the soft tissue, the gradient of the given metric can be computed directly which permits the use of fast optimization algorithms. For this study, the Broyden-Fletcher-Goldberg-Shano (BFGS) method can be used. This is a quasi-Newton technique, which uses an estimate of the Hessian to speed up the iterative process [15].

2.4   Experimental Design and Validation

To model the real stereoscopic laparoscope, a stereo camera rig was built by using a pair of miniature NTSC cameras. Each camera has a physical diameter of just over 5mm and therefore it is possible to setup a configuration with a small baseline of just over 5mm. The described calibration procedure was employed by using a 5×7 square grid with a checked black and white pattern. Corners were detected through a semi-automated procedure, where the user indicates guidance positions and sub-pixel re-finement is performed automatically. The pixel re-projection error after calibration was measured at less than half a pixel. We also measured the reconstruction error af-ter triangulation at an average magnitude of 1mm. This can be improved by taking into account errors in the measured coordinates and refining the measurements [16].

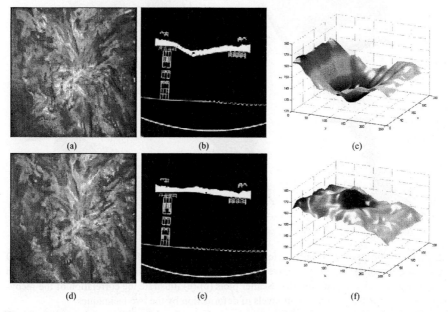

(a)   (b)   (c)

(d)   (e)   (f)

Fig. 1. A stereo image pair of the tissue phantom captured by the stereo rig. (b, e) CT cross sections of the phantom corresponding to two different phases of the deformation and their re-spective 3D surface representation (c, f).

In order to assess the accuracy of the proposed algorithm, a tissue phantom made of silicone rubber and painted with acrylics was constructed. The surface was coated with silicone rubber mixed with acrylic to give it a specular finish that looks similar to wet tissue. The tomographic model of the phantom was scanned with a Siemens So-maton Volume Zoom four-channel multi-detector CT scanner with a slice thickness of 0.5 mm and in-plane resolution of 1mm. To allow the evaluation of temporal surface deformation, the model was scanned at four discrete and reproducible deformation levels. Fig. 1 illustrates a pair of images captured by the stereo cameras and cross sectional images of two different time frames of the tissue phantom captured by CT scanning. The corresponding 3D surface plots are shown in Figs. 1 (c) and (f), re-spectively.

3 Results

Fig. 2 represents the reconstructed surfaces at four different levels of deformation as captured by CT and the proposed algorithm for dense 3D depth recovery. Figs. 2(c)-(e) demonstrate the regression of relative depth change over time as extracted by the two techniques. It is evident that the overall quality of the stereo reconstruction is good, but the scatter plots also show a certain level of deviation. This was largely due to the specular highlights, which were not explicitly modeled in the proposed method.

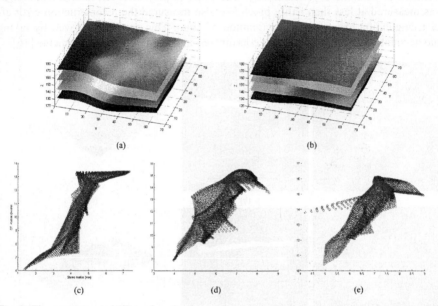

Fig. 2. The reconstructed 3D surface for four different levels of deformation as captured by 3D CT (a) and the proposed depth recovery method based on combined image rectification and constrained disparity registration (b). Scatter plots (c)-(e) illustrate the correlation of the recovered depth change between different levels of deformation by the two techniques.

To demonstrate the potential clinical value of the proposed technique, Fig. 3 illustrates three of the reconstructed depth maps from an *in vivo* stereoscopic laparoscope sequence. Both the depth maps and their associated 3D renditions illustrate the quality of the reconstruction technique. However, it is also evident that specular highlight represent a major problem to the proposed algorithm, as evident from the reconstruction errors indicated by the arrows.

In this study, we also compared the relative performance of the proposed method against existing depth recovery techniques. Fig. 4 shows a comparison of the results obtained from several popular stereo algorithms on an image pair of the phantom model. It is clear that due to the lack of texture these techniques perform poorly in comparison to the proposed technique.

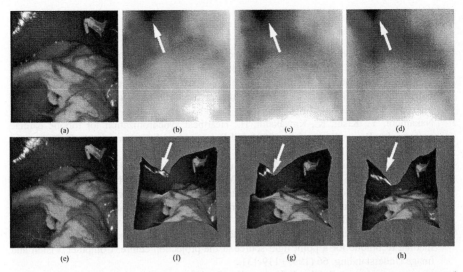

Fig. 3. A pair of stereo images (a, e) from an *in vivo* stereoscopic laparoscope sequence, and three temporal frames of the reconstructed depth map (b-d) and their corresponding 3D rendering results (f-h).

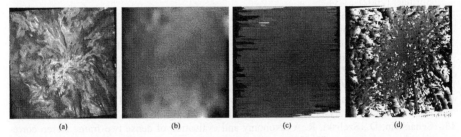

Fig. 4. Comparison of disparity results with popular stereo algorithms (a) rectified left image of a stereo pair of the phantom model (b) the proposed algorithm (c) dynamic programming [17] (d) SSD [13]

4 Discussion and Conclusions

In conclusion, we have developed a practical strategy for dense 3D structure recovery and temporal motion tracking for deformable surfaces. The purpose of the study is to capture real-time surface deformation during robotic assisted MIS procedures such that effective motion stabilization can be deployed. The method uses image rectification to simplify the subsequent free-form disparity registration procedure. Both phantom validation and *in vivo* results demonstrate the potential clinical value of the technique. It has been shown that the performance of the proposed method compares favorably against existing techniques, but the result also indicates the importance of handing specular highlights before depth reconstruction. For robotic assisted MIS procedures, it is possible to exploit the restricted lighting configuration imposed by the laparoscope to filter out these artifacts.

References

1. Ballantyne, G.: Robotic surgery, telerobotic surgery, telepresence, and telementoring. Surgical Endoscopy. 2 Springer (2002) 1389-402.
2. Thakral, A., Wallace, J., Tomlin, D., Seth, N., Thakor, N.: Surgical motion adaptive robotic technology (S.M.A.R.T): taking the motion out of physiological motion. In: Proc. of MICCAI. Volume 2208 of LNCS Springer (2001) 317-325.
3. Nakamura, Y., Kishi, K., Kawakami, H.: Heartbeat synchronization for robotic cardiac surgery. In: Proceedings of the 2001 IEEE International Conference on Robotics and Automation. (2001) 2014-2019.
4. Gröger, M., Ortmaier, T., Sepp, W., Hirzinger, G.: Tracking local motion on the beating heart. In: Proc. of SPIE Medical Imaging Conference. Volume 4681. (2002) 233-241
5. Mourgues, F., Devernay, F., Coste- Manière, E.: 3D reconstruction of the operating field for image overlay in 3D-endoscopic surgery. In: Proceedings of International Symposium on Augmented Reality. (2001).
6. Okatani, T., Deguchi, K.: Shape reconstruction from an endoscope image by shape from shading technique for a point light source at the projection centre. Computer Vision and Image Understanding. 66 (1997) 119-131.
7. http://www.vision.caltech.edu/bouguetj/calib_doc/
8. Morgues, F., Coste-Manière, È.: Flexible calibration of actuated stereoscopic endoscope for overlay in robot assisted surgery. In: Proceedings of MICCAI. Volume 2488 of LNCS. Springer (2002) 24-34.
9. Zhang, Z.: A flexible new technique for camera calibration. IEEE Transactions on Pattern Analysis and Machine Intelligence. 22 (2000) 1330-1334.
10. Fusiello, A., Trucco, E., Verri, A.: A compact algorithm for rectification of stereo pairs. Machine Vision and Applications. 12 (2000) 16-22.
11. Loop, C., Zhang, Z.: Computing rectifying homographies for stereo vision. In: Proceedings of Computer Vision and Pattern Recognition. (1999) 125–131.
12. Brown, M., Burschka, D., Hager, G.: Advances in computational stereo. IEEE Transactions on Pattern Analysis and Machine Intelligence. 25 (2003) 993-1008.
13. Scharstein, D., Szeliski, R.:A taxonomy and evaluation of dense two-frame stereo correspondence algorithms. The International Journal of Computer Vision. 47 (2002) 7-42.
14. Veeser, S., Dunn, M., Yang, G.-Z.: Multiresolution image registration for two-dimensional gel electrophoresis. Proteomics. 1 (2001) 856-870.
15. Nocedal, J., Wright, S.: Numerical optimization. Springer Verlag. (1999).
16. Hartley, R., Zisserman, A.: Multiple view geometry in computer vision. Cambridge University Press. (2000).
17. Birchfield, S., Tomasi, C.: Depth discontinuities by pixel-to-pixel stereo. In: Proceedings of The 6th International Conference on Computer Vision. IEEE Computer Society, IEEE Computer Society Press. (1998) 1073–1080.

Vision-Based Assistance for Ophthalmic Micro-Surgery

Maneesh Dewan[1], Panadda Marayong[2], Allison M. Okamura[2], and
Gregory D. Hager[1]

[1] Department of Computer Science
{maneesh,hager}@cs.jhu.edu
[2] Department of Mechanical Engineering
{panadda,aokamura}@jhu.edu
Johns Hopkins University, Baltimore, MD

Abstract. This paper details the development and preliminary testing
of a system for 6-DOF human-machine cooperative motion using vision-
based virtual fixtures for applications in retinal micro-surgery. The system makes use of a calibrated stereo imaging system to track surfaces
in the environment, and simultaneously tracks a tool held by the JHU
Steady-Hand Robot. As the robot is guided using force inputs from the
user, a relative error between the estimated surface and the tool position
is established. This error is used to generate an anisotropic stiffness matrix that in turn guides the user along the surface in both position and
orientation. Preliminary results show the effectiveness of the system in
guiding a user along the surface and performing different sub-tasks such
as tool alignment and targeting within the resolution of the visual sys-
tem.The accuracy of surface reconstruction and tool tracking obtained
from stereo imaging was validated through comparison with measurements made by an infrared optical position tracking system.

1 Introduction

Age-related macular degeneration (AMD), choroidal neovascularization (CNV),
branch retinal vein occlusion (BRVO), and central retinal vein occlusion (CRVO)
are among the leading causes of blindness in individuals over the age of 50 [2,
15]. Current treatments include laser-based techniques such as photodynamic
therapy (PDT) and panretinal laser photocoagulation (PRP). However, these
treatments often result in high recurrence rate or complications in certain cases,
leading to loss of sight [10]. Recently, alternative approaches employing direct
manipulation of surgical tools for local delivery of a clot-dissolving drug to a
retinal vein (vein cannulation) or chemotherapeutic drugs to destroy a tumor
have been attempted with promising results. However, these procedures involve
manipulation within delicate vitreoretinal structures. The challenges of small
physical scale accentuate the need for dexterity enhancement, but the unstructured nature of the tasks dictates that a human be directly "in the loop." For
example, retinal vein cannulation [17] involves the insertion of a needle of approximately 20-50 microns in diameter into the lumen of a retinal vein (typically

C. Barillot, D.R. Haynor, and P. Hellier (Eds.): MICCAI 2004, LNCS 3217, pp. 49–57, 2004.
© Springer-Verlag Berlin Heidelberg 2004

100 microns in diameter or less–approximately the diameter of a human hair). At these scales, tactile feedback is practically non-existent, and depth perception is limited to what can be seen through a stereo surgical microscope.

In a recent series of papers [1,7,11], our group in the Engineering Research Center for Computer Integrated Surgical Systems (CISST ERC) has been steadily developing systems and related validation methods for cooperative execution of microscale tasks. The primary motivation for these techniques has been to develop assistance methods for microsurgery. The basis of these systems is a specific type of virtual fixture, which we term "guidance" virtual fixtures. Other virtual fixture implementations, often called "forbidden-region virtual fixtures," are described in [8,12,14]. Guidance virtual fixtures create anisotropic stiffness that promotes motion in certain "preferred" directions, while maintaining high stiffness (and thus accuracy) in orthogonal directions.

In this paper, we describe our recent progress at developing vision-based virtual fixtures that provide closed-loop guidance relative to (visually) observed surfaces as well as features on those surfaces. Although, in principle, a direct application of our previously developed guidance fixtures, the implementation of these methods for realistic situations requires attention to significant practical issues. In the remainder of this paper, we describe the structure of our testbed system, detail the vision and control algorithms used, and present data from preliminary demonstrations and validation of the system.

2   System Description

In our previous work, we have described several methods whereby it is possible to create guidance virtual fixtures from image data [4,11]. In this paper, we have chosen to employ algorithms that use relative measures derived from reconstructed 3D geometry. Our goal is to create fixtures that aid in moving tools relative to observed surfaces and surface features in a surgical environment.

2.1   Surgical Field Modeling

Accomplishing the aforementioned goal makes it necessary to detect and track both the underlying surface as well as the operative tool. For both problems, we assume a calibrated stereo camera system. We briefly describe how the vision system recovers both surface and tool geometry.

In our application, the surface is assumed to be smooth to the second order with no self-occlusions. The surface reconstruction is done by first modeling the disparity with third-order tensor B-splines using least squares minimization methods and then reconstructing the disparity surface to obtain the 3D reconstruction. For further details of the method, we refer to [13].

The tool tip position and orientation in 3D characterize the tool geometry, which is computed in a two-step tracking algorithm. The first step involves cue segmentation and maintaining robust cue statistics, similar to the one used in [18]. The second step localizes the tool in the segmented image. The algorithm used for localization is discussed in detail in [5]. The tool is localized in both left and right images and finally reconstructed to obtain its 3D geometry.

2.2   Virtual Fixtures

The virtual fixtures (described in [4]) provide guidance by eliminating the component of the user's applied force in directions orthogonal to the preferred direction. Intuitively, the preferred direction is task-dependent. The preferred direction, $D(t)$, is a $6 \times n$, $0 < n < 6$, time-varying matrix representing the instantaneous preferred directions of motion. Introducing an admittance gain $c_\tau \in [0, 1]$ that attenuates the non-preferred component of the force input, we define a velocity controller which guides the user along the direction parallel to the preferred direction of motion as

$$\mathbf{v} = c(\mathbf{f}_D + c_\tau \mathbf{f}_\tau), \tag{1}$$

where $\mathbf{f}_D$ and $\mathbf{f}_\tau$ are the force components along and orthogonal to the preferred directions, respectively. By choosing c, we control the overall admittance of the system. Choosing $c_\tau < 1$ imposes the additional constraint that the robot is stiffer in the non-preferred directions of motion. Hard virtual fixtures guidance can be achieved by setting c_τ to zero, maintaining the tool motion strictly in the preferred direction.

In our implementation, we consider five different sub-tasks:

- **Free Motion:** The user can freely move the robot to any desired pose. This is equivalent to setting c_τ to 1.
- **Surface Following:** The tool is constrained to move along the surface with a specified offset and, optionally, the tool can maintain an orientation orthogonal to the surface.
- **Tool Alignment:** The user can orient the tool along a preferred direction which is the desired tool orientation.
- **Targeting:** The only motion allowed is toward a fixed target specified on the surface.
- **Insertion/Extraction:** The only motion allowed is along the axis of the tool. In this case, only a separate insertion mechanism of the robot is activated.

The tasks are designed to simulate the sub-steps in performing a more complicated procedure. For example, in a retinal vein cannulation procedure, the surgeon may want to move freely until the tool comes close to the retinal surface, follow with some safe distance along the surface, move to a specified target, align the needle to a desired orientation, then insert and extract the needle for drug delivery into the vein.

We compute the preferred direction by establishing the normal to the surface at the point closest to the tool tip on the reconstructed B-spline surface. The instantaneous preferred direction of motion is then along a plane determined by the span of orthogonal tangents. In order to implement this, the closest point, the normal, and the tangents to the surface at the closest point are determined from the algorithm described in [3]. A relative position error and orientation error can be calculated from the tool tip position and tool orientation estimated from the tool tracker. Position error is a signed vector from tool tip to the intersection point on the surface. Orientation error between the tool orientation and the desired orientation is just their cross product. Hence, the preferred direction, D, and the control, u, can be written for the closed-loop velocity control law for each task (see [4] for detailed derivation).

3   Experimental Setup

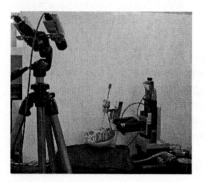

Fig. 1. Experimental setup.

In retinal micro-surgical procedures, the surgeon views the retina and manipulates the tool inside the eye through a microscope. As a preliminary testbed for the application of virtual fixture guidance to real surgery, we developed a scaled experiment, shown in Figure 1. We used the Steady-Hand robot [16] with stereo cameras located approximately 0.6 m away from the robot. A tool is attached to the end-effector of the robot through a 6 DOF force/torque sensors. The user applies force directly at the tool handle. Two types of surfaces were tested, a slanted plane and a concave surface to simulate the back of the human retina. For the latter, we used a concave surface of approximately 15cm in diameter covered with an enlarged gray-scale image of a human retina. The stereo system was comprised of two digital color cameras with 12mm focal length. During manipulation, the user has a direct view of the surface. The user is allowed to change the state of manipulation (Free motion, Tool insertion/extraction, Tool alignment, Targeting, and Surface following) from the GUI. To test the effectiveness of the virtual fixtures, only hard constraints ($c_\tau = 0$) were implemented. The desired offset for the surface tracking task was set at a constant value of 3mm above the surface.

Robot-to-camera and stereo calibration are integral steps in the experimental setup. The resolution and accuracy of the calibration determines the accuracy of the virtual fixture geometry. The 3D coordinates of the surface and the tool pose are computed in the camera coordinate frame by the visual system. The preferred directions and errors are hence first calculated in the camera frame and then converted to the robot frame, where the virtual fixture control law is implemented to obtain the desired Cartesian tip velocity.

The Optotrak, an infrared optical position tracking system, was used for robot calibration and validation of the imaging process. The robot's fixed frame is computed in the Optotrak frame of reference by first rotating the robot about the fixed remote-center-motion point in both the X and Y axes and then translating it along the X, Y, and Z axes with a rigid body placed at the last stage of the joint. In order to obtain the robot-to-camera transformation, the transformation

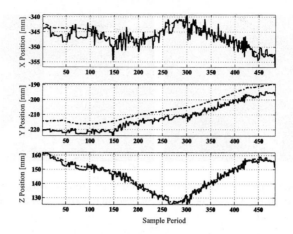

Fig. 2. $X, Y,$ and Z positions of the tool tip estimated by the tool tracker (solid line) and estimated by the Optotrak (dashed line). Calibration error introduced a constant offset of 5 mm in the transformation as shown in the Y position plot.

between the Optotrak and the camera is computed by observing Optotrak LED markers rigidly attached to a planar rigid body in both the camera and the Optotrak frame of reference.

All transformations are computed with reference to an independent fixed rigid body in order to avoid any noise from the motion of the Optotrak. Using a least squares technique to compute rigid body transformations, the average error for the transformation was approximately 2mm with a standard deviation of +/- 1.5mm. We believe that the most significant source of error is due to difficulty of segmenting the centers of the LED markers in the images. However, it is known that slight errors in calibration do not affect the accuracy of the visual servoing system.

3.1 System Validation

First, the accuracy of the tool tracker was validated with the Optotrak. The tool tip positions obtained from the Optotrak were converted to the camera frame using the transformation between the Optotrak and the camera computed earlier. Figure 2 shows the comparison of the $X, Y,$ and Z positions obtained by the Optotrak and the tool tracker. Note here that there is a constant offset of approximately 5mm in the Y coordinates. We believe that this constant offset is due to an error in the Camera-Optotrak calibration. The tool tracking has about 1 pixel error when the offset is accounted for. To validate the accuracy of the reconstructed surfaces (a plane and a concave surface), we compare the reconstructed surfaces with the ground-truth surfaces observed from the Optotrak estimated by tracing the surfaces with a pointed rigid body to obtain points on the surfaces expressed in the Optotrak reference frame. Figure 3 shows the overlay of the data points obtained from the Optotrak (black dots) on the reconstructed surfaces (with texture). The error in the plane reconstruction (left) is

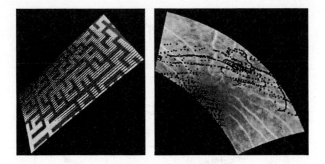

Fig. 3. Textured surface reconstruction overlaid with ground-truth surface data (black dots) obtained from the Optotrak. (Left) Slanted plane and (Right) Portion of the eye phantom.

quite low. For the concave surface (right) however, the reconstruction from the camera shows some errors, especially toward the boundary where the neighborhood information is sparse. The reconstruction covers an area of approximately 6.5cm x 17cm and 6.5cm x 11cm for the plane and the concave surface, respectively.

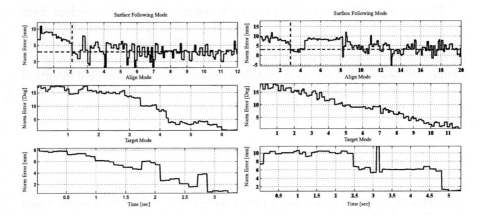

Fig. 4. The signed magnitude of error between the tool tip position and its intersection on a plane (left) and a concave surface (right).

4   Results and Discussion

Figure 4 shows the magnitude of position error over time for manipulation in Surface following, Alignment, and Targeting modes with hard virtual fixtures. Note here that the small steps shown on the plot are the result of the update-rate difference between the cameras and the robot. Sources of noise in the magnitude

Table 1. Resolution estimation of different visual systems.

Systems	Disparity Range [Pixel]	Resolution [mm/pix]
Sony X700 with 12mm lens	275-300	3.07-2.58
Endoscope (Olympus OTV-3D2)	76-86	0.49-0.389
Microscope (Zeiss OPMI1-H)	1992-2036	0.13-0.125

plot may be due to inaccuracy of the surface reconstruction, error in the estimation of tool tip position, and error in calibration. In addition, the width of the tool can introduce some error in the tool tracker's estimation of the tool center as the tool is viewed from different angles. In Surface following mode, we use 3mm as the desired offset above the actual surfaces. The average magnitude of error was approximately 3mm with a standard deviation of +/- 2mm, which is within the 1 pixel error envelope shown in Table 1. The dashed vertical and horizontal lines indicate the time when the tool reached the surface and the average (at 3mm), respectively. We believe that the few negative errors in the surface following error plots are the result of the noise in the system mentioned above. Note that the user started above the desired surface and then the error decreased when the tool moved closer to the surface. The decays of the error as the tool approaches a specified orientation (Alignment mode) and target (Targeting mode) can be clearly seen. In Alignment and Targeting modes, the virtual fixture control law allows movement along the direction of the error vector (forward and backward motion toward the desired orientation/target). However, gain tuning is used to minimize the motion in directions away from the desired pose. Similar results can be seen for the concave surface. We also performed the surface following task in free motion. The performance with virtual fixture guidance in the surface following and targeting tasks do not show significant improvement over free motion, especially with the level of noise and the resolution of the system. However, performance with virtual fixture guidance surpasses free motion in the alignment task.

The accuracy of the calibration and the limitations of the experimental setup are important factors affecting the system performance.Table 1 provides an estimate of the resolution of the current setup (Sony X700) along with an endoscope and a microscope system. Based on our implementation in the current setup and some preliminary experiments, we believe that the method is extendable to the high resolution systems to perform tasks at micro-scale. In order to achieve the required accuracy for vascular procedures in the eye, it appears that it will be necessary to compute tool and surface locations to sub-pixel accuracy. Recent results in this direction appear to promise depth resolution on the order of 1/10 pixel, which is sufficient for the applications described above [9]. Also we would like to incorporate fine motion tracking techniques like SSD and kernel-based methods to obtain subpixel accuracy for tool tracking.

One of the limitations of the system is the slow update rate of the cameras (10-15Hz) with respect to the robot (100Hz). To deal with this, we plan to explore the use of estimation techniques, such as Kalman filtering, in order to obtain smoother tool positions.

5   Conclusion

This work is, to our knowledge, the first example of a human-machine cooperative system guided entirely based on a visual reconstruction of the surrounding
environment. This general approach of creating systems that are able to sense
and react to the surgical environment is central to our goal of creating effective
human-machine systems.

The preliminary demonstration outlined in this paper will be further refined
and ported to work with a stereo endoscope (courtesy of Intuitive Surgical, Inc)
and a stereo microscope available in our laboratory. Our objective is to demonstrate the system working at scales of 10's to 100's of microns on deforming
biological surfaces. Once this is accomplished, the four-step procedure for retinal cannulation will be implemented using our task control architecture [6] and
tested on an eye phantom to determine its efficacy for that procedure.

Acknowledgment. We would like to thank Anand Viswanathan and William
Lau for their help. This material is based upon work supported by the National Science Foundation under Grant Nos. IIS-0099770, IIS-0205318, and EEC-
9731478.

References

1. A. Bettini, P. Marayong, S. Lang, A. M. Okamura, and G. D. Hager. Vision assisted
   control for manipulation using virtual fixtures. *IEEE ITRA*. To appear.
2. N. Bressler, S. Bressler, and S. Fine. Age-related macular degeneration. *Survey of
   Ophthalmology*, 32(6):375–413, 1988.
3. J. Corso J. Chhugani and A. Okamura. Interactive haptic rendering of deformable
   surfaces based on the medial axis transform. *Eurohaptics*, pages 92–98, 2002.
4. G. D. Hager. Vision-based motion constraints. *IEEE/RSJ IROS, Workshop on
   Visual Servoing*, 2002. http://www.cs.jhu.edu/CIRL/new/publications.html.
5. G. D. Hager and K. Toyama. The "XVision" system: A general purpose substrate
   for real-time vision applications. *CVIU*, 69(1):23–27, January 1998.
6. D. Kragic and G. Hager. Task modeling and specification for modular sensory
   based human-machine cooperative systems. *IEEE/RSJ IROS*, 4:3192–3197, 2003.
7. R. Kumar, G. D. Hager, P. Jensen, and R. H. Taylor. An augmentation system
   for fine manipulation. In *MICCAI*, pages 956–965. Springer-Verlag, 2000.
8. F. Lai and R. D. Howe. Evaluating control modes for constrained robotic surgery.
   In *IEEE ICRA*, pages 603–609, 2000.
9. W. Lau, N. A. Ramey, J. J. Corso, N. Thakor, and G. D. Hager. Stereo-based
   endoscopic tracking of cardiac surface deformation. *MICCAI*, 2004. To appear.
10. M.P.S. Group. Argon laser photocoagulation for neovascular maculopathy. 5 yrs
    results from randomized clinical trial. *Arch Ophthalmol*, 109:1109–14, 1991.
11. P. Marayong, M. Li, A. Okamura, and G. Hager. Spatial motion constraints: Theory
    and demonstrations for robot guidance using virtual fixtures. *IEEE ICRA*, pages
    1954–1959, 2003.
12. S. Payandeh and Z. Stanisic. On application of virtual fixtures as an aid for
    telemanipulation and training. *Symposium on Haptic Interfaces For Virtual Envi-
    ronments and Teleoperator Systems*, pages 18–23, 2002.

13. N. Ramey. Stereo-based direct surface tracking with deformable parametric models. Master's thesis, Dept. of Biomedical Engineering, Johns Hopkins University, 2003.
14. L. Rosenberg. Virtual fixtures: perceptual tools for telerobotic manipulation. *IEEE Virtual Reality International Sympsoium*, pages 76–82, 1993.
15. I. Scott. Vitreoretinal surgery for complications of branch retinal vein occlusion. *Curr Opin Ophthalmol*, 13:161–6, 2002.
16. R. Taylor, et al. Steady-hand robotic system for microsurgical augmentation. *IJRR*, 18(12):1201–1210, 1999.
17. J. N. Weiss. Injection of tissue plasminogen activator into a branch retinal vein in eyes with central retinal vein occlusion. *Ophthalmology*, 108(12):2249–2257, 2001.
18. C. R. Wren, A. Azarbayejani, T. Darrell, and A. Pentland. Pfinder: Real-time tracking of human body. *IEEE PAMI*, 19(7):780–785, 1995.

Robot-Assisted Distal Locking of Long Bone Intramedullary Nails: Localization, Registration, and In Vitro Experiments

Ziv Yaniv and Leo Joskowicz

School of Engineering and Computer Science
The Hebrew University of Jerusalem, Jerusalem 91904, Israel.
{zivy,josko}@cs.huji.ac.il

Abstract. We are developing an image-guided robot-based system to assist orthopaedic surgeons in performing distal locking of long bone intramedullary nails. The system consists of a bone-mounted miniature robot fitted with a drill guide that provides rigid mechanical guidance for hand-held drilling of the distal screws' pilot holes. The robot is automatically positioned so that the drill guide and nail distal locking axes coincide using a single fronto-parallel fluoroscopic X-ray. This paper describes new methods for accurate and robust drill guide and nail hole localization and registration and reports the results of our in-vitro system accuracy experiments. Tests of 17 runs show a mean angular error of $1.3°$ (std = $0.4°$) between the computed drill guide axes and the actual locking holes axes, and a mean $3.0mm$ error (std = $1.1mm$) in the entry and exit drill point, which is adequate for successfully locking the nail.

1 Introduction

Closed medullary nailing has become the procedure of choice for reducing fractures of the femur and the tibia [2]. It restores the integrity of fractured bone without surgically exposing the fracture with a nail inserted in the medullary canal. The surgeon reduces the fracture by percutaneously manipulating the proximal and distal bone fragments until they are aligned, inserts a guide wire into the medullary canal and drives the nail in. To prevent fragment rotation and bone shortening, the surgeon inserts lateral locking screws. The procedure is performed with a C-arm under X-ray fluoroscopy, which is used to view the position of bone fragments, surgical tools, and implants.

The insertion of the distal interlocking screws is the most challenging step of the procedure. It requires aligning the drill with the nail hole axis by repeatedly imaging the nail and drill with anterior-posterior and lateral fluoroscopic X-ray images. Once the drill is aligned, drilling proceeds incrementally, with each advance verified with new images. Complications include inadequate fixation, malrotation, bone cracking, cortical wall penetration, and bone weakening due to multiple or enlarged screw holes. The surgeon's direct exposure to radiation is 3–30 minutes per procedure with 31-51% spent on distal locking alone [11].

C. Barillot, D.R. Haynor, and P. Hellier (Eds.): MICCAI 2004, LNCS 3217, pp. 58–65, 2004.

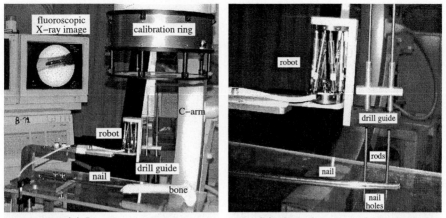

(a) In-vitro setup   (b) aligned axes configuration

Fig. 1. Photographs of (a) the in-vitro setup and (b) the MARS robot in its desired configuration, where the drill guide and nail holes axes are aligned, as shown by the two rods passing through them.

Many devices have been developed for distal locking including proximally mounted targeting devices, mechanical guides, and stereo fluoroscopy [8]. However, all have drawbacks: they are hard to use, are not accurate enough, or cannot always be used. Surgical navigation systems [5] allow the surgeon to position and orient the hand held drill with a few augmented fluoroscopic X-ray images showing in real time the drill position. However, without a mechanical guide, they cannot prevent the drill from slipping or deviating from the desired trajectory. These drawbacks motivate our work.

2   System Concept

We propose to use the miniature robot MARS [10] to provide mechanical guidance for manual drilling of the holes [6]. MARS is directly mounted on the nail head or on the bone and holds a drill guide whose axes are automatically aligned with the distal nail hole axes based on a single lateral fluoroscopic X-ray image (Fig. 1). Since the robot forms a single rigid body with the bone and the nail, there is no need for leg immobilization or real-time tracking during surgery. To achieve accurate results, the fluoroscopic X-ray C-arm must be calibrated and its images corrected for distortion.

MARS is a 5x5x7cm^3, 150–gram 6dof parallel manipulator whose work volume is about 10cm^3 and whose accuracy is better than 0.1mm. When locked, it is rigid and can withstand forces of a few kilograms. The drill guide is a Delrin block with two guiding holes 30mm apart (the spacing between the nail holes). It has a pattern of 28 3mm stainless steel fiducial spheres asymmetrically placed on two planes 20mm apart that are used for its spatial localization (Fig. 2(a)). For a detailed description of MARS and the system setup see [10].

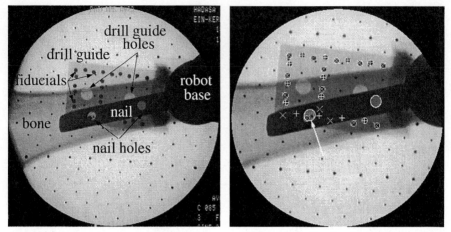

(a) before image processing   (b) after localization

Fig. 2. (a) Fluoroscopic X-ray image in fronto-parallel setting showing the robot base and drill guide, the nail and its locking holes, and the bone; (b) same image after distortion correction with the detected drill guide fiducials and pattern marked in white. The fiducials from each of the two target planes are marked as + and ×. The arrow indicates the correct detection of drill guide target fiducial and nail hole despite the partial occlusions.

The surgical protocol is as follows. Once the fracture has been reduced and the nail has been inserted, the surgeon mounts the robot on the nail head or on the bone. The X-ray technician mounts a calibration ring on the C-arm image intensifier and, with the help of a guidance program, orients the C-arm so that it is in a fronto-parallel setting, where the nail holes appear as circles. The localization and registration software automatically determines from the X-ray image the locations of the drill guide and nail holes and computes the robot transformation that aligns their axes. The robot is positioned according to this transformation and locked in place. The surgeon then manually drills the holes and completes the surgery as usual.

3   Localization and Registration

Accurate and robust computation of the transformation that aligns the drill guide and the nail hole axes is a challenging image processing and pose estimation task. Localization of the nail holes and the drill guide is difficult because partial occlusions are inherent to the setup (the robot is mounted close to the nail holes and the image includes the nail, bone, and soft tissue). The nail holes are small (5mm diameter, about 20 pixels), nearby (30mm), and appear as ellipses in the images, so the accuracy with which their axes can be determined is limited. Furthermore, only one fluoroscopic X-ray image can be used, since there

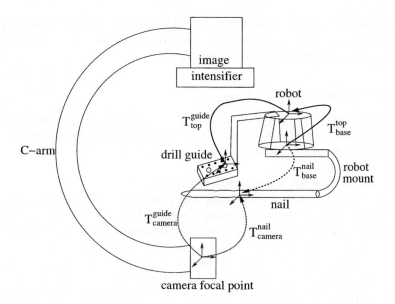

Fig. 3. Robot base to nail holes registration chain.

is no tracking of the C-arm pose. Finally, the C-arm imaging system exhibits orientation-dependent distortions and internal imaging parameters variations.

To cope with these challenges, we have developed a novel model-based approach for robust and accurate localization of the drill guide target and nail holes and for the spatial registration of their axes. To facilitate robust nail pose estimation, we assume a fronto-parallel setup between nail and C-arm. A nearly perfect fronto-parallel pose can be obtained after a few trials by the X-ray technician with guidance from a program that scores the quality of the pose according to hole circularity and the angle between the normal of hole supporting plane and the camera viewing direction [7]. When the pose is fronto-parallel, the ellipse aspect ratio is 1 (a circle) and the angle is 0 (perfect axis alignment).

We model the fluoroscopic camera as a pin-hole camera with distortion [9]. In that work, we developed a robust automatic C-arm calibration algorithm that includes fiducial localization, distortion correction, and camera calibration with an overall submillimetric accuracy even when only 60% of the fiducials are detected. The nail is modeled as a planar object with two circular holes.

To align the robot so that the drill guide axes coincide with the nail hole axes, we compute the spatial transformation between the nail and the robot base, which is given by the following transformation chain (Fig. 3):

$$T_{base}^{nail} = T_{base}^{top} T_{top}^{guide} (T_{camera}^{guide})^{-1} T_{camera}^{nail}$$

where T_{base}^{top} and T_{top}^{guide} are known from design and T_{camera}^{guide} and T_{camera}^{nail} are computed from the C-arm internal camera parameters and the fluoroscopic image.

Our method consists of four steps: 1) C-arm distortion correction and calibration; 2) drill guide identification; 3) nail hole identification; 4) drill guide and nail pose estimation. We describe the later three next.

3.1   Drill Guide Identification

Drill guide identification is performed by first detecting the circular fiducials in the image and then finding the correct correspondence with their 3D model. The key issues are handling partial occlusions and missing fiducials, and minimizing positional inaccuracies.

The target fiducials are detected in two steps: 1) localization and 2) circle fitting. Localization is performed using a modified circle Hough transform and a model-based analysis of the transform accumulator. Since the circular fiducials are darker than the image background, the Hough transform voting scheme is constrained so that edge pixels will only cast their vote if the vector connecting them to the hypothesized circle center is in the opposite direction of the gradient at the edge location. The contents of the transform accumulator are examined to identify the k > #target fiducials which received the most votes. Considering a few more candidate circles is necessary since the accumulator may contain multiple peaks for the same fiducial (these are higher than the peaks for other fiducials). The algorithm then computes the average radius and number of votes of the five circles with the most votes and selects all circles whose radius is within ± 2 pixels of the average radius and which have received more than half of the average votes. These circles, with very high probability, belong to the target.

The selected set of circles may contain overlapping circles, which are due either to multiple responses for the same fiducial or to fiducial overlap. In our imaging setup, there can be at most two overlapping fiducials. Thus, for each set of overlapping circles, we only retain the two circles with the highest number of votes. These pairs of overlapping circles correspond either to two overlapping fiducials or to a single fiducial. When the overlap area between the pair of circles is larger than 60% of the circle's area, it is a single circle, otherwise it is two. Circle fitting is performed using the Random Sample Consensus paradigm [3]. For each circle, the algorithm collects all edge elements contained in its circumscribing square and fits a circle to them. This removes the dependency on the Hough transform discretization accuracy.

The correspondence between the detected fiducials and their 3D model is computed using homographies. Correctly pairing the detected fiducials and the 3D model fiducials is difficult, as there are always missing fiducials which are occluded by the nail. To overcome these problems, we use the geometry of the drill guide target: we use lines instead of points, since lines are less sensitive to partial occlusions.

Since the fiducials are distributed on two planes, the goal is to find the pair of homographies which minimizes the distance between the detected circles and the result of applying the homographies to the target fiducials. The pair of homographies is computed in three steps. First, we identify the line which passes through the maximal number of detected circles. This line is one of the pattern axes. Next, we find all lines which are parallel or perpendicular to this line (within $\pm 5°$) and that pass through two circles only. The target is built such that the two spheres on these lines are on the same plane. Finally, the best match among the small set of possible lines is selected by trying all combinations. The target fiducials are then mapped with the homographies to the image and the detected circles are identified accordingly (Fig. 2(b)).

3.2 Nail Hole Identification

Distal locking nail holes identification is performed by first locating the nail's longitudinal contour and then locating its holes from their expected position with respect to this contour.

To locate the nail longitudinal contours, we use a 3D Hough transform in which the nail is modelled as a band consisting of two parallel lines at a known distance between them. The Hough transform voting scheme is constrained so that pixels which are on parallel lines will only cast their vote if the gray level values between them are lower than the gray level values outside the band. All the pixels outside the contours are discarded.

The search for the nail holes is then performed on the pixels contained between the nail's contours. The algorithm sweeps a parallelepiped window whose sizes are equal to the nail width along the nail's medial axis. The two locations containing the maximal number of edge elements correspond to the locations of the distal locking nail holes. The algorithm then fits an ellipse to the edge data contained inside the parallelepipeds. The edge elements originate from the nail holes, the drill guide target and the C-arm calibration target (Fig. 2(b)). The ellipse parameter estimation is performed by using only the edge elements which belong to the convex hull of the set of elements. This is because ellipses are convex shapes and because the nail is opaque, so outlying edges can only be present in the interior of the ellipse. Next, an ellipse is fitted to the edge elements with a non-linear geometric least squares method initialized with the estimate computed using an algebraic least squares method [4].

3.3 Drill Guide and Nail Pose Estimation

The drill guide pose is computed by non-linear minimization of the projection distances between the known fiducial projection coordinates (x_i, y_i) and the expected ones $(\widehat{x}_i, \widehat{y}_i)$:

$$\mathbf{v}^* = \arg\min_{\mathbf{v}} 0.5 \left(\sum_{i=1}^{n} (x_i - \widehat{x}_i(\mathbf{v}))^2 + (y_i - \widehat{y}_i(\mathbf{v}))^2 \right)$$

where $\mathbf{v}$ is the rigid transformation parameterization. We use the Levenberg-Marquardt method with an initial estimate obtained with a linear method [1].

The nail pose is computed using the fronto-parallel setup assumption, in which the projective transformation applied to the nail holes is a similarity. The pose is computed directly from the nail holes coordinates in the image, $(\mathbf{p}_x, \mathbf{p}_y)$ and $(\mathbf{q}_x, \mathbf{q}_y)$, their average diameter on the image d_{im}, their real diameter d, and the camera focal length f. The nail location is:

$$
\mathbf{t} = \begin{bmatrix} \frac{z}{f}\mathbf{p}_x \\ \frac{z}{f}\mathbf{p}_y \\ z \end{bmatrix}
$$

where $z = fd/d_{im}$ is the nail distance from the camera focal point. The nail orientation relative to the camera is:

$$
R = \begin{bmatrix} \mathbf{p}_x - \mathbf{q}_x & \mathbf{p}_y - \mathbf{q}_y & 0 \\ \mathbf{p}_y - \mathbf{q}_y & \mathbf{q}_x - \mathbf{p}_x & 0 \\ 0 & 0 & -1 \end{bmatrix}
$$

The nail's X axis direction depends on the order in which $(\mathbf{p}, \mathbf{q})$ are chosen. It is set so that its angular deviation from the drill guide's X axis is minimal.

4   Experimental Results

We conducted three sets of experiments to quantify the accuracy and robustness of the proposed method. To test the robustness of the drill guide and nail hole identification, we manually placed the robot and C-arm in random positions. We then acquired 67 fluoroscopic X-ray images. The drill guide and nail holes were correctly identified in 61 images. There were no false positives, i.e., the detection was correct in all images for which our software stated that the drill guide and nail holes were detected. All six failures were automatically detected by the software. They were caused by occlusion of many drill guide target fiducials, which prevented its proper localization.

To quantify the accuracy of the whole system for the task at hand, we define two error measures: the angular deviation of the drill guide axes and the distance between axes entry and exit points, which is the in-plane distance between the intersection points of the axes and two planes located at $100mm$ and $120mm$ from the robot base (the nail is located between these planes).

Next, the robot was manually placed in a pose in which two $4mm$ diameter cylindrical rods with tapered ends pass through the $5mm$ diameter drill guide and nail holes as shown in Fig. 1(b). This pose guarantees successful locking and constitutes the robot's reference pose. To quantify the variability of the reference poses, we placed the robot in 17 different poses in which the two rods passed through the drill guide and nail holes and computed the two error measures. We found an angular variation of $0° - 0.9°$ and a translational variation in the entry and exit points of $0 - 3.9mm$. This means that a registration accuracy of about $1°$ and $\pm 2mm$ will guarantee successful distal locking.

Next, under the guidance of our software, we oriented the C-arm so that it formed a fronto-parallel setup with the nail holes. We placed the robot in 17 random poses, acquired fluoroscopic X-ray images for each pose, and computed the robot alignment transformation for each pose (in all cases, the drill guide target and nail holes were correctly detected). Comparing the 17 computed robot poses to the reference pose our results show a mean angular error of $1.3°$ (std = $0.4°$) between drill guide axes, and a mean $3.0mm$ error (std = $1.1mm$) in the entry and exit points, which is adequate for successfully locking the nail.

5   Conclusions

We have presented a robust, automatic method for aligning the drill guide and the nail holes axes based on a few fluoroscopic X-ray images. The method is part of a new image-guided miniature robot-based system to assist orthopaedic surgeons in performing distal locking of long bone intramedullary nails. Our experimental results show that the automatic localization is feasible within the required accuracy. We are currently working on mechanical and algorithmic improvements to increase the accuracy of the system.

References

1. Ansar A., Daniilidis K., "Linear pose estimation from points or lines", *IEEE Trans. on Pattern Analysis and Machine Intelligence*, **25**(5), 2003.
2. Brumback R.J., "Regular and special features – the rationales of interlocking nailing of the femur, tibia, and humerus", *Clinical Orthopaedics*, **324**, 1996.
3. Fischler M. A., Bolles R. C., "Random sample consensus: a paradigm for model fitting with applications to image analysis and automated cartography", *Communications of the ACM*, **24**(6), 1981.
4. Fitzgibbon A., Pilu M., Fisher R. B., "Direct least square fitting of ellipses", *IEEE Trans. on Pattern Analysis and Machine Intelligence*, **21**(5), 1999.
5. Joskowicz L., Hazan E., "Computer-assisted image-guided intramedullary nailing surgery of femoral fractures" (in French), *Monographie des Conferences d'Enseignement de la SOFTCOT*, Vol. 80, Elsevier, 2003.
6. Joskowicz, L., Milgrom, C., Shoham, M., Yaniv, Z., Simkin, A., "A robot-assisted system for long bone intramedullary distal locking: concept and preliminary results", *Proc. of the 17th Int. Congress on Computer-Assisted Radiology and Surgery*, CARS'2003, H.U. Lemke *et. al.* editors, Elsevier 2003, pp 485–491.
7. Kanatani K., Liu W., "3D interpretation of conics and orthogonality", *Image Understanding*, **58**(3), 1993.
8. Krettek C. et al., "A mechanical distal aiming device for distal locking in femoral nails", *Clinical Orthopaedics*, **384**, 1999.
9. Livyatan H., Yaniv Z., Joskowicz L., "Robust automatic C-arm calibration for fluoroscopy-based navigation: a practical approach", *Proc. of Medical Image Computing and Computer Assisted Intervention*, 2002.
10. Shoham, M., Burman, M., Zehavi, E., Joskowicz, L., Batkikin, E., Kunicher, Y., "Bone-mounted miniature robot for surgical procedures: concept and clinical applications", *IEEE Trans. on Robotics and Automation*, **19**(5), 2003.
11. Skjeldal S., Backe S., "Interlocking medullary nails - radiation doses in distal targeting", *Archives of Orthopaedic Trauma Surgery*, **106**, 1987.

Liver Motion Due to Needle Pressure, Cardiac, and Respiratory Motion During the TIPS Procedure

Vijay Venkatraman[2], Mark H. Van Horn[1], Susan Weeks[1], and Elizabeth Bullitt[1]

[1]CASILAB, University of North Carolina, Chapel Hill, NC
{mvanhorn, sue_weeks, bullitt}@med.unc.edu
http://casilab.med.unc.edu
[2]North Carolina A&T State University, Greensboro, NC
vkvenkat@ieee.org

Abstract. TIPS (Transjugular Intrahepatic Portosystemic Shunt) is an effective treatment for portal hypertension. However, during the procedure, respiration, needle pressure, and possibly other factors cause the liver to move. This complicates the procedure since the portal vein is not visible during needle insertion. We present the results of a study of intraoperative liver motion.

1 Introduction

This paper characterizes intraoperative hepatic motion caused by respiration and needle pressure during Transjugular Intrahepatic Portosystemic Shunt (TIPS) creation. Endovascular procedures are typically guided by fluoroscopic, projection images. These images generally show only the connected portions of the vasculature "downstream" of the catheter tip. The interventionalist thus cannot simultaneously visualize other important anatomical structures or vascular structures that are either "upstream" or disconnected from the vascular anatomy shown in any particular image.

The goal of TIPS is to relieve portal hypertension in patients with liver failure by creating a permanent connection (shunt) between the portal vein and the hepatic vein. During TIPS, the interventionalist obtains access to the internal jugular vein in the neck, and then selectively catheterizes distally into the hepatic vein. The catheter is exchanged for a needle, which is then advanced through the liver parenchyma into the portal vein. This is considered the most difficult part of the procedure [1]. Up to 10 needle passes may be required to achieve portal vein access [2].

There are numerous difficulties associated with TIPS. For example, during needle advancement, other organs bordering the liver such as the kidney, gallbladder, colon, and stomach as well as the hepatic vein or hepatic artery can be inadvertently punctured [3]. To guide the needle and identify the portal vein, a static image is obtained in one or two image planes after hepatic vein catheterization. This is used to estimate portal vein location for the remainder of the procedure. Needle pressure and respiration can displace both the liver and the attached portal vein by an unknown

C. Barillot, D.R. Haynor, and P. Hellier (Eds.): MICCAI 2004, LNCS 3217, pp. 66–72, 2004.

amount. Needle advancement is therefore done "blindly" under conditions in which the portal vein location is unknown and may change during the procedure.

Our group is developing methods of three-dimensional image guidance of the TIPS procedure. The most critical issue is the determination of portal vein position at each moment in time relative to the interventionalist's needle. Two facts ease the problem. First, TIPS patients possess livers that are hard, dense, fibrotic, and generally non-deformable. This means that although both needle pressure and respiration may displace the liver, neither is likely to deform it. A rigid body transformation should therefore be sufficient to indicate change in liver (and thus attached portal vein) position during the procedure. The same transformation can be applied to other portions of the hepatic and portal venous systems relevant to TIPS, which are located within this rigid liver. Second, the liver is bounded on three sides by the bony ribcage and superiorly by the diaphragm. It is additionally tethered by the left and right triangular ligaments and by the falciform ligaments, all of which limit rotation. We therefore assume that liver movement can be described by tracking a single point within the liver, and that the liver can be modeled as a rigid body.

As one of the initial steps in designing a 3D image guidance system, it is desirable to determine the likely range of liver motion during the procedure. Previous analyses of liver motion have examined only the motions likely to occur as a result of respiration. The current report examines displacement of the liver during the TIPS procedure with analysis of the effects of respiration, needle pressure, and possibly heartbeat.

2 Background

A comprehensive assessment was reported in a recent paper [4], which surveyed previous reports on hepatic motion due to respiration during percutaneous minimally invasive procedures. The paper analyzed nine previously published studies of respiratory-associated hepatic motion using different imaging modalities (fluoroscopy, scintigraphy, ultrasound, optical tracking, and MRI). This paper reports that all studies agreed that rostro-caudal motion is the most significant and that measurements of movement in both the anterior-posterior (AP) and lateral directions vary markedly with the assessment technique used.

Korin et al. [5] and Davies et al. [6] suggested that clinically significant liver motion could be approximated effectively by rostro-caudal movement (10-38 mm) alone with minimal motion in the other axes of motion (2.5 mm). Recent studies by Herline et al. [7], Shimizu et al. [8] and Rohlfing et al. [9] suggest that translations along the other axes (anterior-posterior translation: 1-12 mm and lateral translation: 1-9 mm) are significant and cannot be neglected. Based on these considerations, it is clear that lateral and AP translations are significant, particularly when tracking discrete targets within the liver. However, none of these reports examined liver displacement as a result of needle pressure or heartbeat during the TIPS procedure.

3   Methods

Our approach to tracking intraoperative liver motion employs a contrast-filled, ovoid balloon that is inserted into a hepatic vein at the beginning of each procedure. The operation is guided by determining the balloon location in simultaneously acquired AP and lateral fluoroscopic views separated by approximately $90°$. Given prior knowledge of the relationship between the two fluoroscopic views, this pair of 2D points representing the balloon centroid in each projection image can be then reconstructed into 3D. Under the two assumptions that the diseased liver is a predominantly rigid structure and that rotation is limited by the liver's restraining ligaments, this 3D point can then be tracked over time to provide information about liver (and thus portal vein) displacement during the procedure.

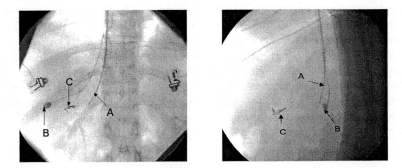

Fig. 1. Typical fluoroscopic images showing the (A) TIPS needle, (B) balloon, and (C) surgical clips. Note that the portal vein is not visible in either image

The current report examines 3D balloon excursion during thirteen image sequences obtained in four subjects undergoing a TIPS procedure. We examined the displacement induced by respiration and needle insertion by using paired image sequences for each study. Image sequences were captured using two synchronized PCs at 15 frames per second with a resolution of 884-by-884 pixels. Each image was time-stamped and stored for post-processing.

Balloon locations within each image were detected automatically on each fluoroscopic image. The algorithm detected the balloon projection by convolving each 2D image with a Laplacian of a Gaussian (LoG) kernel, thresholding the output image, and providing a probability distribution function that includes such features as area, area-to-perimeter ratio, and eccentricity. This probability function was used to identify the correct image feature. The tracking process automatically calculated the pixel (x,y) coordinates representing the centroid of each balloon projection using a connected component algorithm. Subsequent balloon tracking was performed in similar fashion throughout the time sequence with an ROI of 192-by-192 pixels centered on the previously estimated balloon location, thus allowing real-time tracking of the balloon on each image.

In order to make 3D measurements from the biplane views, projection matrices for each view must be computed. For calibration, we used a Plexiglas phantom containing an array of metallic spheres in known locations, and assumed a pinhole camera model. Using the known control point locations and an x-ray image of the phantom, the projection matrices are computed by minimizing the distance between the ideal projections and the observed pixel coordinates of the control points [10, 11].

Given each pair of pixel coordinates for the balloon and the projection matrices for each camera system, the 3D point can be reconstructed by triangulation [10, 11]. A pair of points in correspondence is considered from the biplane images: $m=(u,v)^T$ and $m'=(u',v')^T$ and reconstructed into a 3D point $(X=[x,y,z,t]^T)$. For this paper, we report balloon motion in a coordinate system where the x-axis represents motion from the patient's left-to-right (lateral), the y-axis represents motion from caudal-to-cranial, and the z-axis represents motion from back-to-front (anterior-posterior). For each image pair, balloon motion was tracked over time in x, y, and z; the maximum excursion was also calculated along each axis.

As previously noted, this work has proceeded with the assumptions that the liver (and all structures within it) move rigidly and that rotation is minimal. If these assumptions are correct, point tracking of an intrahepatic balloon may provide a reasonable estimate of the displacement of other structures within the liver, such as the portal vein. We tested these assumptions in one TIPS patient who had surgical clips within the liver, where the relative motion between these clips and the tracking balloon was used to check the validity of the assumptions. Two paired image sequences were used. In the first sequence, only respiration was involved. In the second, images were acquired during needle insertion.

4   Results

The graphs below show typical movement of the liver in the three independent axes due to respiration and needle push in a typical subject studied.

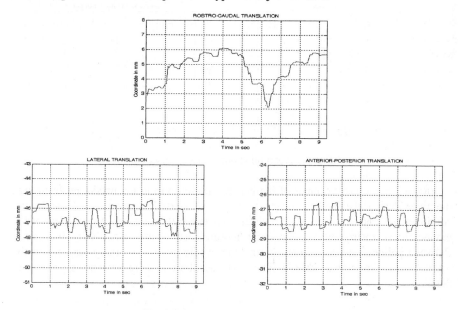

Fig. 2. Liver motion during respiration

Figure 2 shows the hepatic motion due to respiration in the three axes. Note that with respiration the predominant displacement occurs rostro-caudally (Table 1). However, the graph also shows oscillations at 1 Hz, which are consistent with the cardiac cycle. The frequency of the oscillations was verified using power spectral density analysis.

Table 1. Liver Displacement due to respiration

	Displacement (mm)	Mean (mm)	Standard Deviation (mm)
Lateral	1.2 - 2.5	1.9	0.4
Rostro-Caudal	3.9 - 12.3	7.3	3.0
Anterior-Posterior	1.9 - 3.6	2.5	0.7

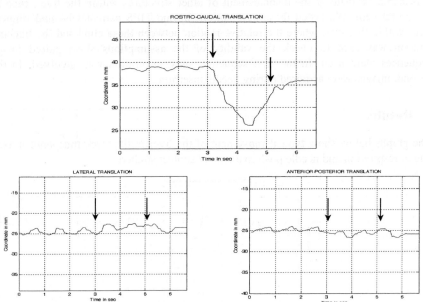

Fig. 3. Liver motion during needle insertion

Figure 3 shows an example of the hepatic motion during the needle push through the liver during the TIPS Procedure. The push started at around 3 seconds and continues for approximately 2 seconds as indicated by the arrows. Again, most of the movement is rostro-caudal, but slight motion also occurs along the other axes. Between patients, the movement during the needle push was highly variable in the rostro-caudal direction (Table.2). The 1 Hz oscillations were present as previously noted.

Table 2. Liver displacement during needle insertion

	Displacement (mm)	Mean (mm)	Standard Deviation (mm)
Lateral	1.4 - 3.1	2.2	0.7
Rostro-Caudal	2.7 - 13.2	7.4	3.9
Anterior-Posterior	1.1 - 2.8	2.2	0.7

From tables 1 and 2, we can deduce that the rostro-caudal translation is the predominant motion but the anterior-posterior and lateral translations may produce several millimeters displacement. The magnitude of the displacement varies from patient to patient.

To validate our assumptions regarding the rigidity of the liver and modeling liver motion with translation only, we analyzed the relative 3D positions of the tracking balloon and a set of surgical clips in one patient. These results are summarized in table 3. While there is a slight variation, the surgical clips and the balloon move in similar directions indicating that our assumptions are generally valid.

Table 3. Mean/standard deviation of balloon-to-clip measurements in mm

	Lateral (mm)	Rostro-Caudal (mm)	Anterior-Posterior (mm)
Respiration	35.7/0.3	1.7/0.4	37.7/0.4
Needle push	35.8/0.4	1.5/0.2	39.2/0.2

These data suggest that the 3D position of a region of interest within the liver such as surgical clips or the portal vein may be estimated to within 2 mm given the 3D position of the tracking balloon and initial offset to the region.

5   Discussion

This paper studies motion of a point within the liver during the TIPS procedure. Our results are consistent with those of other groups who have studied the effect of respiratory motion on liver displacement, concluding that translation along all the axes are significant with the rostro-caudal translation being the predominant translation.

This paper also reports on liver motion during needle pressure. We are unaware of another group reporting a similar study. We conclude that needle pressure displaces the liver primarily rostro-caudally, but can produce displacement of several millimeters along the other two axes.

An unexpected finding is the approximately 1 Hz oscillations along all axes. These oscillations are consistent with the cardiac rhythm. Such motion is less than the predominantly rostro-caudal motion induced by respiration or needle pressure, but the induced motion can be significant when the radiologist's goal is to reach a target that cannot be seen.

A limitation of our approach, in common with the majority of other studies of liver motion, is that we track motion of only a single point within the liver. Rotational movement and deformations therefore cannot be assessed. However, as discussed earlier, it is reasonable to assume that rigid body transformations may be sufficient when analyzing the rigid, diseased liver in patients undergoing TIPS procedures, and that the liver's attached ligaments are likely to preclude major rotational movement. Support for this hypothesis is provided by our analysis of the motion of implanted surgical clips with respect to the tracking balloon wedged within a hepatic vein. Although further studies are required, the current report suggests that tracking a balloon visualized on intraoperative, biplane fluoroscopic views can be an effective means of tracking structures within the liver, such as the portal vein, during respiration, heartbeat, and needle pressure.

Acknowledgments. This work was supported by R01 HL69808 NIH-HLB.

References

1. LaBerge JM. Transjugular Intrahepatic Portosystemic Shunts Technique Using the Wallstent Endoprosthesis in Portal Hypertension: Options for Diagnosis and Treatment. Society of Cardiovascular & Interventional Radiology (1995)
2. Rees Cr, Niblett RL, Lee SP, Diamond NG, Crippin JS. Use of Carbon Dioxide as a Contrast Medium for Transjugular Intrahepatic Portosystemic Procedures. JVIR (1994), 5:383-386
3. LaBerge JM. Hepatic Anatomy Relevant to Transjugular Intrahepatic Portosystemic Shunts in Portal Hypertension: Options for Diagnosis and Treatment. Society of Cardiovascular & Interventional Radiology (1995)
4. Clifford MA, Banovac F, Levy E, Cleary K. Assessment of Hepatic Motion Secondary to Respiration for Computer Assisted Interventions. Computer Aided Surgery, 7:291–299 (2002)
5. Korin HW, Ehman RL, Riederer SJ, Felmlee JP, Grimm RC. Respiratory Kinematics of the Upper Abdominal Organs: A Quantitative Study. Magn Reson Med (1992), 23:172–178
6. Davies SC, Hill AL, Holmes RB, Halliwell M, Jackson PC. Ultrasound Quantitation of Respiratory Organ Motion in the Upper Abdomen. Br J Radiol (1994), 67:1096–1102
7. Herline AJ, Stefansic JD, Debelak JP, Hartmann SL, Pinson CW, Galloway RL, Chapman WC. Image Guided Surgery: Preliminary Feasibility Studies of Frameless Stereotactic Liver Surgery. Arch Surg (1999), 134:644–649; discussion 649–650
8. Shimizu S, Shirato H, Xo B, Kagei K, Nishioka T, Hashimoto S, Tsuchiya K, Aoyama H, Miyasaka K. Three-Dimensional Movement of a Liver Tumor Detected by High-Speed Magnetic Resonance Imaging. Radiother Onco (1999), 50:367–370
9. Rohlfing T, Maurer CR, O'Dell WG, Zhong J. Modeling Liver Motion and Deformation During the Respiratory Cycle Using Intensity-Based Free-Form Registration of Gated MR Images. In: Medical Imaging: Visualization, Display, and Image-Guided Procedures. Proceedings of SPIE, vol 4319. SPIE (2001), 337–348
10. Gang X and Zhengyou Z. Epipolar Geometry in Stereo, Motion and Object Recognition. Kluwer Academic Publishers (1996)
11. Faugeras O. Three-Dimensional Computer Vision: A Geometric Viewpoint. MIT Press (1996)

Visualization, Planning, and Monitoring Software for MRI-Guided Prostate Intervention Robot

Emese Balogh[1,6], Anton Deguet[1], Robert C. Susil[2], Axel Krieger[3],
Anand Viswanathan[1], Cynthia Ménard[4], Jonathan A. Coleman[5], and
Gabor Fichtinger[1,3]

[1] Engineering Research Center, Johns Hopkins University, Baltimore, MD, USA
emese@cs.jhu.edu
[2] Dept. of Biomedical Engineering, Johns Hopkins University, Baltimore, MD, USA
[3] Dept. of Radiology, Johns Hopkins University, Baltimore, MD, USA
[4] Urologic Oncology Branch, NCI, National Institutes of Health, Bethesda, MD
[5] Radiation Oncology Branch, NCI, National Institutes of Health, Bethesda, MD
[6] Dept. of Informatics, University of Szeged, Szeged, Hungary

Abstract. This paper reports an interactive software interface for visualization, planning, and monitoring of intra-prostatic needle placement procedures performed with a robotic assistant device inside standard cylindrical high-field magnetic resonance imaging (MRI) scanner. We use anatomical visualization and image processing techniques to plan the process and apply active tracking coils to localize the robot in real-time to monitor its motion relative to the anatomy. The interventional system is in Phase-I clinical trials for prostate biopsy and marker seed placement. The system concept, mechanical design, and in-vivo canine studies have been presented earlier [6,10,14]. The software architecture and three-dimensional application software interface discussed in this paper are new additions. This software was tested on pre-recorded patient data.

1 Introduction

With an estimated annual incidence of 221,000 cases, prostate cancer is the most common cancer in men in the United States and it is responsible for about 29,000 deaths annually [8]. Numerous studies have demonstrated the potential efficacy of needle-based therapy and biopsy procedures in the management of prostate cancer, but contemporary needle delivery techniques still present major limitations. The "Gold Standard" of guiding biopsy and local therapies has been transrectal ultrasound (TRUS) [9]. It is popular due to its real-time nature, low cost, and ease of use, but its limitations are also substantial. Conventional unassisted freehand biopsy techniques have resulted in a low detection rate of 20%-30% [12]. TRUS has been widely applied in guiding the insertion of metal seeds used for therapeutic irradiation (brachytherapy) and targeting external beam radiation therapy [11], although it fails to visualize the fine details of prostatic tissues. MRI is an attractive choice for image-guidance, because it

C. Barillot, D.R. Haynor, and P. Hellier (Eds.): MICCAI 2004, LNCS 3217, pp. 73–80, 2004.

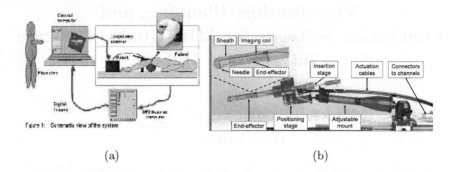

(a)   (b)

Fig. 1. System concept (a) [6], Robot assembled prior to treatment (b) [10]

can clearly visualize the prostate and its substructure [1]. MRI can also show
the distribution and buildup of injected liquid agents, implanted solid capsules,
and can monitor the progress of thermal therapies, all in real-time. All facts
considered, supplanting TRUS in prostate biopsy and therapy with a better-
suited image guidance modality such as MRI is a logical imperative. However,
the strong magnetic field and extremely confined physical space in conventional
high-field MRI scanners present formidable physician/patient access challenges.
D'Amico et al. manually performed targeted biopsy and brachytherapy inside a
0.5T open MRI scanner [3,4] that tends to have suboptimal image quality. With
the use of 1.5T conventional MRI, Beyersdorff et al. applied transrectal needle
guide [2] and Susil *et al.* used transperineal template [13]. They both used passive
fiducial registration and the patient was moved between imaging and the manual
needle insertion. In contrast to prior works, we designed a robot to perform the
procedure in closed MRI scanner. (We note, however, that for increased safety,
in our current protocol we insert the needle outside the magnet.) The robot is
operated with real-time tracking and servo control.

2   System Design

In our concept (Fig. 1a), the device is secured to the table of the scanner with
an adjustable mount. The patient is positioned on the table in prone position
with elevated pelvis, the device is introduced to the rectum, and then the patient is moved into the scanner's magnet. The MRI scanner produces signal with
the patient and device in the field, at the same time. We determine the spatial
relationship between the device and the coordinate system of the MRI scanner
using magnetic coils. The images are transferred to a computer that produces
a 3D representation of the device superimposed on the anatomic images. The
physician selects the target point for the needle and the computer calculates the
kinematic sequence to bring the needle to the selected target position. The computer displays the three motion parameters to the physician who controls the
device from outside the magnet. While the actuation of the device is in progress,

we continue to track the robot's end-effector in real-time. The application computer visualizes the scene with an updated model of the robot, thereby allowing the physician to monitor the motion of the device relative to the anatomy. The robot (Fig. 1b) has three degrees of freedom: (1) a cylindrical end-effector translates in and out the rectum, (2) rotates around the central axis of the translation, and (3) finally the needle is inserted into the prostate. The needle exits on the side of the end-effector and it is inserted into the prostate through the rectum in an oblique angle, along a predefined trajectory, to a predefined depth. There is a rigid stationary sheath around the tubular end-effector. Only the sheath makes contact with the rectum, while the end-effector can freely move inside the sheath, thereby preventing any mechanical distortion to the rectum wall and prostate. The sheath contains an exit window for the needle and imaging coil winding around the window. We employ several guiding channels in the end-effector, providing multiple alternative exit angles. During path planning, the physician can select the optimal angle, depending on the location of the target.

For registration of the robot, we use three active tracking coils attached to the end-effector. The position of each coil in the end-effector is known through calibration. When real-time readings of the coil positions arrive, fast calculation produces the pose of the end-effector in MRI space with an accuracy of 1 mm in less than 60 ms time. MRI is a true real-time imaging modality that makes it possible to manipulate the robot's end-effector in a visual servo loop without encoding the joints. The joints are decoupled and non-backdrivable, their motion is linear, smooth, slow, and their relative pose can be estimated with good accuracy. These conditions make it possible to close the visual servo loop through the physician who handles the actuators, without applying encoders or motors on the joints. The physician moves the joints sequentially. The end-effector is registered in real-time and the updated motion parameters tend to zero as the end-effector is approaching the preplanned position. The joints are independently adjusted to finalize the position. This yielded a safe, simple, inexpensive, and versatile system with which an accuracy of 2.0 mm in-vivo was achieved [10,14].

3   Software Architecture

The architecture of the software system is shown in Fig. 2a. The complete software is distributed between two computers. One is an SGI Octane (Silicon Graphics, Paolo Alto, CA) that serves as a front-end to a GE 1.5T CV/I MRI scanner (GE Medical Systems, Waukesha, Wisconsin) and the other is a Windows XP laptop (Dell Products, L.P., Round Rock, TX.) that serves as an Application Computer. The Tracking Server and DICOM Server both run on the scanner's front-end. When new data becomes available on the scanner's front-end computer, the servers automatically push the data to the client side where they are captured in a dedicated storage area. The physician works at the Application Computer running the top-level Slicer-based Application Program that automatically detects the arrival of tracking and image data. The Tracking Server computes the location of the three tracking coils in MRI image space. It is a C/C++ application that receives MRI signal data from the scanner. To determine the position and orientation of these coils, twelve 1D dodecahedrally spaced

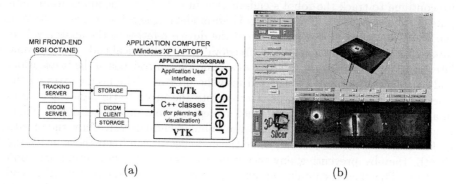

(a)   (b)

Fig. 2. Software archtiecture (a) and Slicer-based application program interface (b)

readouts are collected (TE 2.3 msec, TR 5.0 msec, BW +/-64 KHz, FA 1o, FOV 40cm, 256 readout points), allowing for coil localization, as described previously in [5]. Microcoil location errors due to gradient nonuniformity are removed using gradient dewarping algorithms obtained from the vendor (GE Medical Systems, Waukesha, Wisconsin). At the end of the pipeline, the Tracking Server produces 9 coordinates and 3 error values for its client through a TCP/IP connection with a frequency of about 2 Hz. When new data arrives to the tracking data storage, the robot's current position and inverse kinematics are recalculated and presented to the physician. The vendor's DICOM Server on the MRI front-end is programmed to send all newly created DICOM series through a local network to the Application Computer specified by an IP address. When new data arrives to the DICOM data storage, the physician can decide whether or not to load the new series into the Slicer viewer.

4   The Application Program Interface

The top-level visualization, control, and planning software is implemented within the 3D Slicer package that provides a unified environment for modeling, planning, and monitoring of image guided surgery applications [7]. Slicer integrates into a single environment many aspects of visualization, planning, and monitoring used in image-guided therapies. It provides capabilities for registration, semi-automatic segmentation, generating 3D surface models, and quantitative analysis (measuring distances, angles, surface areas, and volumes) of various medical scans. The 3D Slicer (www.slicer.org) is an open-source software package developed primarily by the Brigham and Women's Hospital. Slicer is extendable due to its modular structure. Each module has its own panel in the Slicer graphical user interface that the developer then flushes out to create his/her own user interface using Tcl/Tk (www.tcl.tk). Modules have access to a wide range of visualization capabilities since Slicer is built on VTK, the Visualization Toolkit (http://www.vtk.org).

After starting the Slicer-based Application Program, the Menu and the Viewer windows appear (Fig. 2b). The Menu window provides menus for accessing the features of Slicer, while the Viewer window displays volumes, image slices, and models. The upper part of the Viewer window is the 3D viewer, while the lower part displays 2D slices. The 2D images can be either original or reformatted images along orthogonal cutting planes across the MRI volume. The 2D images can also be texture-mapped onto a plane and rendered in the 3D view in their correct location; that is, where the reformatted voxels exist in the volume. Each 2D image and the 3D view may be zoomed independently. A graphical representation of the robot's end-effector (Fig. 3a) appears superimposed in the 3D view. At any time during planning and intervention, the physician can visualize the robot relative to the 3D volume of the patient's image. We enhance these visual effects by the built-in visualization tools and routines of VTK and Slicer packages, such as changing transparency of objects and so forth. The robot's position is also projected onto the slices in the 2D windows. The target and intersection of the needle's trajectory with the slice are both presented, thereby giving the physician yet another visual clue whether the needle is being correctly oriented toward the target.

When the target is selected by the physician on a 2D axial slice, the program immediately computes the inverse kinematics of the robot to reach the selected target. The motion parameters are calculated for all alternative needle exit angles and program generates a warning message if the target cannot be reached by one of the needles due to exceeding the allotted range of motion or major anatomical constraints. The physician then selects the appropriate needle channel and the rotation, translation, and insertion are displayed, so that the motion of the robot can commence. The computer can also simulate the sequence of motions by moving a 3D model of the device, to allow the physician to verify that the calculated sequence of motions would indeed take the needle from its current position to the pre-selected target position.

During the robot movements, tracking coil positions are refreshed at a frequency of about 2 Hz. The inverse kinematics is also recalculated and presented to the physician. The robot's position is updated in the 2D and 3D viewers. As the physician moves the device, the end-effector's model appears to be moving toward the target in the 3D view (Fig 3b). When all motion parameters reach zero and the needle points toward the target (Fig 3c), the physician may start inserting the needle to the predetermined depth. In the current embodiment, the needle insertion is not encoded, but the needle can be observed in real-time MRI images. A full volume is also acquired after the needle is inserted, but before the biopsy sample is cut or the marker seed is released. The visualization, motion planning, and monitoring workflow and software were designed to uniformly support a plurality of needle-based interventions. This approach even allows the physician to perform combined interventions. For example, the physician can use the system to place marker seeds into the prostate, and in the same session can also collect biopsy samples if suspicious nodes are detected in the MRI images since the last imaging or biopsy session. (It is never too late to update the staging of the disease, which is the decisive factor in selecting the right course of treatment.)

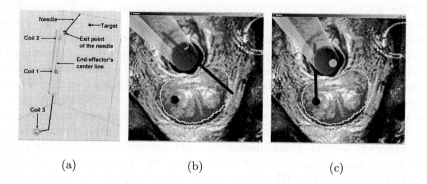

(a)   (b)   (c)

Fig. 3. Model of the end-effector (a). Robot tracking in the 3D viewer. The model of the end-effector and trajectory of needle are superimposed on the pre-segmented target image. When the needle's trajectory intersects with the target (c) the robot can stop.

5   Validation

The accuracy of tracking was verified with the use of a precisely machined mechanical frame that allowed for controlled translations and rotations. This allowed us to move the tracking coils through predefined trajectories and verify whether the Tracking Server correctly rectifies these trajectories. The three tracking coils were fixed to form a triangle that we tracked through a series of poses in the MRI scanner. We calculated the trajectory of the centroid and plane normal vector of the triangle and compared those to the a priori known trajectory. The differences for the centroid and plane normal were 0.41 mm and 1.1 degree, respectively. The fully assembled robot was placed in the MRI scanner and ascertained that incremental motions of the rotation and translation joints correspond to the incremental rotations and translations rectified from the tracking coils. On the client side, we measured an update rate of 2 Hz, which sufficed the polling rate in the top-level application software and was also adequate for the speed of the robotic assistance device. The functionality, speed, robustness, and correctness of the DICOM client/server interface were tested on multiple series of phantom and patient data. Each new DICOM series appeared on the Application Computer with an acceptable delay, considering the amount of data transferred. The contents of the DICOM series were compared between the server and client sides. No loss of information occurred during the transfer and interpretation of the images. The Tracking and DICOM Server-Client units have been integrated under a simplified 2D application interface and deployed first in canine experiments [14] and in Phase-I human trials for prostate biopsy and marker seed placement.

The Slicer-based Application Program Interface has been tested in a simulated environment using the Tracking and DICOM Servers with pre-recorded data from human and phantom cases. The goal was to demonstrate that the Slicer-based Application Program Interface performs as accurately and reliably as the previously clinically commissioned 2D application interface. First we ascertained that the 3D program provides at least the same numerical accuracy, visual realism, and clinical functionality as the simpler 2D version, and then we verified that the new 3D functions produce correct results. In particular, we conducted the following series of tests. (1) We verified that all 2D images and pixels coordinates presented in the Slicer-based interface corresponded to the images and pixel values on the MRI scanners console, which we considered ground truth. (2) By running the inverse kinematics of the robot through the same series of targets as in the pre-recorded cases, we verified that the calculation of robot motion parameters were correct. (3) By cutting through the MRI volume with texture mapped planes in canonical and oblique angles, we verified that all reconstructed surface models of the anatomy (prostate, urethra, nerve bundles, bladder, and rectum) corresponded to the MRI volume. (4) By superimposing the bright spots produced by the Gadolinium fiducials built in the robot and the graphical model of the robot, we verified that the tracking server provided spatially accurate information and that they appeared correctly in the 3D viewer.

6   Conclusions

The 3D visualization, planning, and monitoring system based on the 3D Slicer has been found to be a functionally viable solution. The current embodiment of the application interface software appears to be applicable in clinical use. Currently, we are in the process of migrating the ongoing biopsy and marker seed placement clinical trials from a 1.5T GE scanner to a 3T machine of an other vendor, which necessitates further customization in the software. We have found that the application of active tracking coils for robot guidance is a most accurate and versatile solution, but it also requires significant interaction and exchange of proprietary information with the scanner's vendor. The 3D Slicer system, although it is highly customizable, was not created with the primary intention of clinical use and thus some aspects of its ergonomics still needs further tuning. For the clinicians, handling reconstructed 3D views is a departure from conventional 2D slices, requiring off-line practice. We have determined in the ongoing clinical trials that organ deformation and motion still remains a significant factor. These negative effects could be reduced by a model predicting the deformation and dislocation of the target and thereby allowing for compensation in the planning phase. This, however, is a long-term objective that also involves rapid anatomical segmentation and signal inhomogeneity correction.

Acknowledgments. We are grateful to L.L. Whitcomb and E. Atalar for their contribution. Support was provided by NIH R01 EB002963, HL57483, HL61672, NSF 9731478, US Army PC 10029.

References

1. S. Adusumilli and E.S. Pretorius. Magnetic resonance imaging of prostate cancer. *Semin Urol Oncol*, 20(3):192–210, 2002.

2. D. Beyersdorff, A. Winkel, P. Bretschneider, B.K. Hamm, S.A. Loening, and M. Taupitz. Initial results of MRI-guided prostate biopsy using a biopsy device in a closed MR imager at 1.5T. In *The 88th Scientific Assembly and Annual Meeting of the Radiological Society of North America, Chicago*, page 629, 2002.
3. A.V. D'Amico, C.M. Tempany CM, R. Cormack, N. Hata, M. Jinzaki, K. Tuncali, M. Weinstein, and J.P. Richie. Transperineal magnetic resonance image guided prostate biopsy. *J. Urol*, 164(2):385–387, 2000.
4. A.V. D'Amico, R. Cormack, C.M. Tempany, S. Kumar, G. Topulos, H.M. Kooy, and C.N. Coleman. Realtime magnetic resonance image-guided interstitial brachytherapy in the treatment of select patients with clinically localized prostate cancer. *Int J Radiat Oncol Biol Phys*, 42(3):507–515, 1998.
5. J.A. Derbyshire, G.A. Wright, R.M. Henkelman, and R.S. Hinks. Dynamic scan-plane tracking using MR position monitoring. *J Magn Reson Imaging*, 8(4):924–932, 1998.
6. G. Fichtinger, A. Krieger, R.C. Susil, A. Tanacs, L.L. Whitcomb, and E. Atalar. Transrectal prostate biopsy inside closed MRI scanner with remote actuation, under real-time image guidance. In *Fifth International Conference on Medical Image Computing and Computer-Assisted Intervention*, volume 2488 of *Lecture Notes in Computer Science*, pages 91–98. Springer Verlag, 2002.
7. D.T. Gering, A. Nabavi, R. Kikinis, N. Hata, L.J. O'Donnell, W.E. Grimson, F.A. Jolesz, P.M. Black, and W.M. Wells 3rd. An integrated visualization system for surgical planning and guidance using image fusion and an open MR. *J Magn Reson Imaging*, 13(6):967–975, 2001.
8. A. Jemal, T. Murray, A. Samuels, A. Ghafoor, E. Ward, and M. Thun. Cancer statistics, 2003. *CA Cancer J Clin*, 53:5–26, 2003.
9. J.C. Presti Jr. Prostate cancer: assessment of risk using digital rectal examination, tumor grade, prostate-specific antigen, and system biopsy. *Radiol Clin North Am*, 38(1):49–58, 2000.
10. A. Krieger, R.C. Susil, G. Fichtinger, E. Atalar, and L.L. Whitcomb. Design of a novel MRI compatible manipulator for image guided prostate intervention. *IEEE 2004 International Conference on Robotics and Automation, (accepted)*, 2004.
11. A.J. Nederveen, J.J. Lagendijk, and P. Hofman. Feasibility of automatic marker detection with an a-si flat-panel imager. *Phys Med Biol*, 46(4):1219–1230, 2001.
12. K.A. Roehl, J.A. Antenor, and W.J. Catalona. Serial biopsy results in prostate cancer screening study. *J. Urol*, 167:1156–1161, 2002.
13. R.C. Susil, K. Camphausen, P. Choyke, E. Atalar, C. Coleman, and C. Menard. A system for transperineal prostate biopsy and HDR brachytherapy under 1.5T MRI guidance. techniques and clinical experience. In *The 89th Scientific Assembly and Annual Meeting of the Radiological Society of North America (RSNA), Chicago*, page 644, 2003.
14. R.C. Susil, A. Krieger, J.A. Derbyshire, A. Tanacs, L.L. Whitcomb, E.R. McVeigh, G. Fichtinger, and E. Atalar. A system for MRI guided diagnostic and therapeutic prostate interventions. *Journal of Radiology*, 228:886–894, 2003.

Robotic Strain Imaging for Monitoring Thermal Ablation of Liver

Emad M. Boctor[1], Gabor Fichtinger[1,3], Ambert Yeung[1,2], Michael Awad[2], Russell H. Taylor[1], and Michael A. Choti[2]

[1]Engineering Research Center, Johns Hopkins University, Baltimore, MD, USA
[2]Department of Surgery, Johns Hopkins Hospital, Baltimore, MD, USA
[3]Department of Radiology, Johns Hopkins University, Baltimore, MD, USA
eboctor@ieee.org

Abstract. This report describes our initial *in vitro* results with robotically-assisted strain imaging for intraoperative monitoring of hepatic tumor thermal ablation. First, we demonstrate a strong correlation between thermal ablation of liver tissue and changes in elastic properties. Second, we present an experimental environment to provide controlled robotically-assisted compression of liver tissue with concurrent ultrasonic reading. Third, we present B-mode strain images of thermally treated liver samples, where the strain images corresponded to the boundaries of histologically confirmed necrosis.

1 Introduction

Primary and metastatic liver cancer represents a significant source of morbidity and mortality in the United States and worldwide [1]. An increasing interest has been focused on thermal ablative approaches, particularly radiofrequency ablation (RFA). These approaches utilize image guided placement of a probe within the target area within the liver parenchyma. Heat created around the electrode is conducted into the surrounding tissue, causing coagulative necrosis at a temperature between 50°C and 100°C [2]. Key problems with this approach include localization/targeting of the tumor and monitoring the ablation zone. The first problem has been previously addressed through developing robotic 3DUS system for guidance of liver ablation [3]. The second problem, the subject of this paper, is monitoring the necrosis zone during ablative therapy.

Monitoring the ablation process in order to document adequacy of margins during treatment is a significant problem which often results in either local failure or excessively large zones of liver ablation. Some ablative devices employ temperature monitoring using thermisters built within the ablation probes. However, these temperatures only provide a crude estimate of the zone of ablation. Magnetic resonance imaging (MRI) can monitor temperature changes (MR thermometry), but is expensive, not available in many sites, and difficult to use intraoperatively [4]. Ultrasonography (US) is the most common modality for both target imaging and is also used for ablation monitoring. However, conventional ultrasonographic appearance of ablated tumors only reveal hyperechoic areas from microbubble and outgasing but cannot sufficiently visualize the margin of tissue coagulation. Currently, ablation adequacy is

C. Barillot, D.R. Haynor, and P. Hellier (Eds.): MICCAI 2004, LNCS 3217, pp. 81–88, 2004.
© Springer-Verlag Berlin Heidelberg 2004

only estimated at the time of the procedure and primarily based on the probe position and not the true ablation zone.

The purpose of this study was to assess the ability of US strain imaging to more accurately visualize thermal ablation in the liver. We propose to capitalize on the changes in tissue elastic properties which occur during tissue heating and protein denaturation. It is known that thermal ablation causes significant changes in tissue mechanical properties, including elasticity [5]. Until recently, internal organs such as the liver were not clinically accessible to compression imaging because of the relative resistance of the body wall, and respiratory and cardiac motion artifacts added further difficulties. However, recent trial has been reported performing elasticity imaging of the liver in vivo based on internal cardiovascular motion as a source of compression [6]. Liver tumor ablation is being performed with increasing frequency using operative and laparoscopic approaches. These methods may allow for direct organ compression during therapy, thereby opening the door for more accurate in vivo strain imaging.

2   Elasticity Imaging

The main goal of elasticity imaging is remote and non-invasive representation of mechanical properties of tissues. The elastic properties of tissues cannot be measured directly, so a mechanical disturbance must be applied and the resulting response is then evaluated. We can categorize elasticity imaging approaches into static (strain based), dynamic (wave based), and mechanical (stress based) methods [8]. Strain based approach is imaging internal motion under static deformation; dynamic approach is imaging shear wave propagation; and mechanical approach is measuring surface stress distribution. The main components of these approaches: 1) Data capturing during externally or internally applied tissue motion or deformation, 2) Tissue response (displacements, strain, or stress) evaluation, and if needed 3) reconstruction of the elastic modulus based on the theory of elasticity.

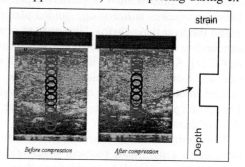

The imaging method adopted in this project is ultrasound strain based approach known as elastography, first introduced in 1991 by Ophir et al. [7]. Elastographic imaging techniques have proved that mechanical properties information can be derived from radiofrequency (RF) US images. The objective is to acquire RF US data from a tissue in both rested and

Fig. 1. 2D representation of strain based imaging model. The overlay represents an A-line with 1D cascaded spring system of unequal spring constants.

stressed states, then to estimate the induced strain distribution by tracking speckle motion (Figure 1). The Young's modulus and Poisson's ratio completely describe the elastic properties of an elastic, linear, homogeneous, and isotropic material. Moreover, most soft tissues are incompressible (Poisson's ratio is nearly 0.5) and the Young's modulus can describe the elastic properties. According to Ophir et al. [7], larger compressors cause more uniform axial stress fields which allows strain to provide a first order estimate of the Young's modulus. This explains why most elastographic investigations rely on the estimation of the strain distribution.

In the following sections we will focus our discussion on elastography and more specifically, on the signal processing methods used to estimate the strain distribution. Estimating the local strain is therefore an essential step, which requires a high level of accuracy, since the amplitude of tissue deformation is relatively small. So far, the most common signal-processing techniques used in elastography have been gradient-based methods that estimate strain as a derivative from of displacement. These techniques uniformly assume that the medium deformation results in delays between the ultrasound footprints. The echo signal acquired after compression is thus assumed to

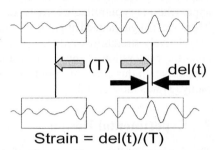

Fig. 2. Illustration of the displacement estimation algorithm applied to an A-line deformation.

be a delayed replica of the pre-compression signal. The local tissue displacement is in this case (Figure 2) a simple shift that can be computed as the location of the maximum of the cross-correlation function of gated pre- and post-compression echo signals [8] or as the zero of the phase of the complex correlation function of the corresponding base-band signals [9]. Irrespective to any given Time Delay Estimation (TDE) technique, these methods remain accurate only for very small deformations [0-2%] and fail rapidly with increasing strains, because they ignore the signal shape variation induced by the physical compression of the medium. One improvement has been to stretch the entire post-compression signal temporally by an appropriate constant factor prior to time delay estimation [10]. This pre-processing has been demonstrated to compensate fairly well for the effect of compression at low strains. However two fundamental limits arise. First, the value of the proper temporal stretching factor requires an a priori knowledge of the strain magnitude. Second, this factor depends on the local deformation and cannot be constant over the signal. Alam et al. [11] took into account these changes in the shape of signals and considered the signal after compression as a locally delayed and scaled replica of the signal before deformation. The local scaling factor is estimated over each segment of study as the factor that maximizes the correlation between the pre-compression and stretched post-compression signal segments. This study showed that using local scaling factors leads to a method that is more robust in terms of de-correlation noise.

Our implementation, as shown in Figure 2, is based on two techniques. One utilizing the maximization of normalized cross-correlation between pre- and post-compression RF signal after applying 1D companding as described in [10]. The second is more robust and is based on information theoretic delay criterion. Elastography techniques have the potential to be extended into real-time 3D elasticity imaging. The application of pressure field is independent from the imaging array, which provides an opportunity for real-time performance. Other techniques like acoustic radiation force imaging (ARFI) rely on the same array to generate the force pulses (60-70 per line) and to image these responses with 50 tracking beams per pulse [12]. In ARFI, the identification of boundary conditions and the extension of the technique to real-time 3D elasticity reconstruction are serious research challenges. It has been known to be of key importance how the compression is actually generated. Freehand elastography is significantly noisier compared to the images from mechanically controlled elastography [14]. Robot-assisted elastography offers several advantages over free-hand approaches: (1) controllable compression to guarantee a strain within the optimal 0.5-2% range, (2) guaranteed alignment of the direction of strain and the image plane, and (3) relatively straightforward extension to 3D, possibly in real-time. All facts considered, the exploration of robotic assistance in strain imaging appeared to be a logical imperative. In this endeavor, prior expertise of our group in robot-assisted ultrasonography [3] was most useful.

3   Experimental Design

The first part of this work was intended to study the variation of liver elastic properties with thermal ablation. A number of researchers have already studied the elastic properties of liver tissues using both healthy and diseased liver tissue excised from experimental animals [13]. However, mechanical elastic testing and modeling of liver tissue undergoing different radio frequency treatment protocols is still lacking. Our study was aimed at measuring the elasticity, i.e. elastic modulus and shear modulus. For these studies, fresh calf liver at room temperature was subjected to focal thermal ablation using RFA (RITA Medical Systems, Inc., Mountainview, CA, XL probe). The liver was cut in 4x4x2 cm cubes following ablation to testing of tissue elasticity. For these studies, a tensile testing (MTS) machine was used at rate of 30 mm/min to produce quasi-static compression up to 20 % strain. Forces were simultaneously recorded both numerically and graphically. In addition, pathological studies were carried out to characterize histologic changes at various stages in the progression of tissue heating. Figure 3 shows the axial compression stress vs. strain curves. These studies demonstrated a trend of increasing slopes and hence increasing Young's modulus values from 20 $^\circ$C up to 100 $^\circ$C. Figure 4 shows the graphical results of the average dynamic shear modulus. The horizontal axis is the frequency of dynamic os-

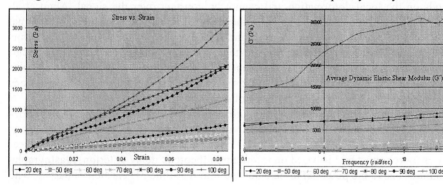

Fig. 3. The axial compression stress vs. strain curves from 20 – 100 degrees C.

Fig. 4. Average dynamic shear modulus

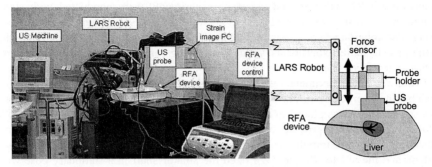

Fig. 5. The overall robotic strain based imaging system (L) and schematic drawing of the robot's end-effector holding the US probe (R). The large probe serves as a compression plate.

cillations in a logarithmic scale. The vertical axis is the dynamic elastic shear modulus (G'). The shear modulus curve also exhibits a positive correlation with temperature. (The details of this elasticity study exceed the limits of this paper.)

The preliminary experiments described above led us to the second phase of this project by designing and implementing a robotic strain imaging acquisition system as shown in Figure 5. We used a Siemens Antares US scanner (Siemens Medical Solutions USA, Inc. Ultrasound Division, Issaquah, WA) with an ultrasound research interface (URI) to access raw RF data. A Siemens VF 10-5 linear array was used to acquire data. The tracking beams were standard B-mode pulses (6.67 MHz center frequency, F/1.5 focal configuration, apodized, pulse repetition frequency (PRF) of 10.6 KHz, with a pulse length of 0.3μs). The US system utilizes dynamic focusing in receive such that a constant F/number of 1.5 is maintained. The robot used was a Laparoscopic Assistance Robotic System (LARS) [15]. The LARS is a kinematically redundant manipulator composed of a proximal translation component with a distal remote center of motion component, which provides three rotations and one controlled insertion motion passing through the RCM point. The LARS end-effector, also shown in Figure 5, contained a six degrees-of-freedom force/torque sensor, a translation stage to induce tissue compression with an accuracy of 0.05 mm, and a rotation stage to sweep an US volume. In earlier research, we demonstrated substantial improvements in the 3DUS volume quality, repeatability, planning and targeting with robotic 3DUS vs. freehand scanning [3]. In this project the LARS plays a dual role by helping generate controlled 3D strain data. The thermal ablation system was an RFA generator (RITA Medical Systems, Inc., Mountainview, CA) with XL probe. A Windows 95 laptop recorded real-time temperature readings via thermisters built in the RFA probe. A dual processor workstation interfaced to all system components and capable of controlling LARS to generate 3DUS data with controlled pressure.

4   Experiments and Results

Experiments were conducted in triplicate. First, a set of phantom studies were conducted on a gel-based object with a hard spherical inclusion (higher gel concentration) in soft gel background. We have collected 3D strain data by sweeping the robot while collecting 2D RF data. Second, a set of experiments were conducted with static monitoring, in which we created 1-2 cm ablated lesion several hours prior to monitoring. The ablation protocol was heating at $100\,^{\circ}$C for 10 minutes. Although both the phantom and static experiments yielded intriguing results, limitation of space excludes their analysis here.

Third, a set of experiments was based on dynamic monitoring of strain in whole fresh bovine liver, ex vivo. The specimen was soaked in degassed water to remove air pockets, and then was placed in a metal tank to facilitate the grounding for the RFA device (Figure 5.) The protocol of the dynamic study was as follows: (1) System Initialization comprised initializing the robot, Antares in URI mode, the dual processor system, and the ablator device. (We fixed the ablator shaft in a stationary pose with respect to the robot and opened up the tips gradually during the study. (2) Alignment comprised setting the robot arm at 0 degree such that a part of the ablator shaft is always present in the US image. The 90 degree orientation then captures the formed lesion at tip of the RFA device. This way we can study the effect of the ablator shaft and its subsequent shadowing it causes in the strain image. (3) Data collection at room temperature, for reference purposes, at 50, 75, and 100 degrees, for 7 minutes. During acquisition phase the robot moves in multiple compression steps and records force and displacements (boundary conditions) measurements. Displacements have been used to optimize the TDE problem while the force data was not utilized in the calculations. (The force reading will be used at a later stage of the project for the inverse reconstruction problem.)

As we mentioned earlier above, the most decisive component in any elastography processing pipeline is handling time delay estimation (TDE). Advanced TDE algorithms have been implemented by others in the frequency domain, but spectral estimation in case of short signal segments has been an apparently strong weakness of those implementations. R. Moddemeijer searched for a time-domain implementation of a TDE algorithm and defined the so called information theoretic delay criterion [16]. Since this work, however, is still incomplete and no further research has been published toward this direction. In contrast, we used two straightforward TDE estimation algorithms implemented in time-domain, using mutual information and standard normalized cross-correlation. Figures 6 and 7 show consistency of the lesion extracted by these two TDE measures

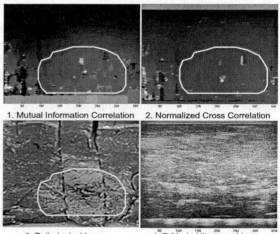

1. Mutual Information Correlation   2. Normalized Cross Correlation

3. Pathological Image   4. B-Mode Ultrasound Image

Fig. 6. Strain images with corresponding pathology and B-mode images at 100°C, with the RFA device in plane. The white contour is created on the pathological picture and matches with the determined strain images.

and a good matching with the actual pathological images. It is worth noting that the B-mode US images appear to be completely useless in the identification of the ablated region. The perpendicular view in Figure 6 shows decorrelation noise due to the shadowing effects of the needle shaft. In Figure 7, the strain images also show the presence of a large blood vessel that in actual patients would act as a heat sink. The vessel, that represents a small zone of soft structure, caused strongly visible artifacts in the strain images. Also strong correlation can be seen

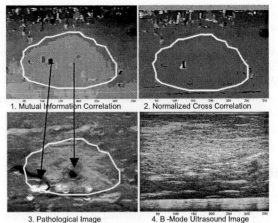

Fig. 7. Strain images with corresponding pathology and B-mode images at 100°C, with the RFA device perpendicular to the plane of imaging. The white contour is created on the pathological picture and matches with the determined strain images.

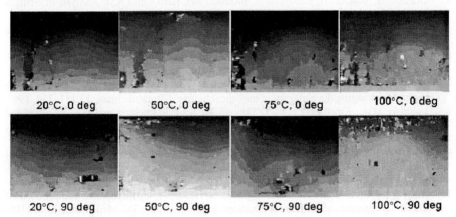
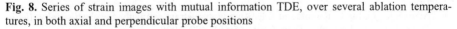

Fig. 8. Series of strain images with mutual information TDE, over several ablation temperatures, in both axial and perpendicular probe positions

between the strain images and the location of the tip of the ablator. Again none of the above discussed fine details could be deduced from the B-mode US images. Figure 8 shows the progression of ablation from room temperature, through 50 °C, 75°C, to 100°C ablation temperature, with the use of mutual information TDE. The 20°C images show reference strain images that reflect defects due to the presence of the ablator shaft or near by vessel. Moving from 50°C, 75°C, to 100°C we can easily recognize the flower pattern for the Rita device (75°C). We can also notice the beginning of ablation near to grounding pads (bottom of the images at 50 °C).

In summary, robotic strain imaging appears to be promising, while still many particulars of it are under investigation. For TDE, our preference is the mutual information (ME) approach. It needs further optimization for which a strain simulator software framework is being developed.

Acknowledgements. We are grateful to Carol Lowery, Levin Nock, and David Gustafson at Siemens Medical Solutions USA, Inc. Ultrasound Division, Issaquah, WA for providing the Ultrasound Antares unit with the research interface. We also extend our thanks to the JHU Biomechanical Research Laboratory for assistance in tissue compression measurements. This work was supported by NSF EEC 9731478 and an intramural grant from the Johns Hopkins University.

References

1. Nakakura EK, Choti MA: Management of hepatocellular carcinoma. Oncology (Huntingt). 2000 Jul;14(7):1085-98; discussion 1098-102. Review.
2. Buscarini L, Rossi S: Technology for radiofrequency thermal ablation of liver tumors.Semin Laparosc Surg 1997;4:96–101.
3. Emad M. Boctor, Gregory Fischer, Michael A. Choti, Gabor Fichtinger, Russell H. Taylor: A Dual-Armed Robotic System for Intraoperative Ultrasound Guided Hepatic Ablative Therapy:A Prospective Study. Accepted ICRA 2004.
4. Graham SJ, Stanisz GJ, Kecojevic A, Bronskill MJ, Henkelman RM: Analysis of changes in MRI properties of tissues after heat treatment. Magn Reson Med 1999;42(6):1061-71.
5. Wu T, Felmlee JP, Greenleaf JF, Riederer SJ, Ehman RL: Assessment of thermal tissue ablation with MR elastography. Magn Reson Med 2001 Jan;45(1):80-7.
6. Alexander F. Kolen, Jeffrey C. Bamber, Eltayeb E. Ahmed: Analysis of cardiovascular-induced liver motion for application to elasticity imaging of the liver in vivo. MIUA 2002.
7. Ophir J., Céspedes E.I., Ponnekanti H., Yazdi Y., Li X: Elastography: a quantitative method for imaging the elasticity of biological tissues. Ultrasonic Imag.,13:111–134, 1991
8. Lubinski M.A., Emelianov S.Y., O'Donnell M: Speckle tracking methods for ultrasonic elasticity imaging using short time correlation. IEEE Trans. Ultrason., Ferroelect., Freq., Contr., 46:82-96, 1999.
9. Pesavento A., Perrey C., Krueger M., Ermert H: A Time Efficient and Accurate Strain Estimation Concept for Ultrasonic Elastography Using Iterative Phase Zero Estimation. IEEE Trans. Ultrason., Ferroelect., Freq., Contr., 46(5):1057-1067, 1999.
10. Alam S.K., Ophir J: Reduction of signal decorrelation from mechanical compression of tissues by temporal stretching: applications to elastography. US Med. Biol., 23:95–105, 1997.
11. Alam S.K., Ophir J., Konofagou E.E: An adaptive strain estimator for elastography. IEEE Trans. Ultrason. Ferroelec. Freq. Cont., 45:461–472, 1998.
12. Fahey BJ, Nightingale KR, Wolf P and Trahey GE: ARFI Imaging of Thermal Lesions in Ex Vivo and In Vivo Soft Tissues. Proceedings of the 2003 IEEE US Symposium. 2003.
13. Wen-Chun Yeh, Pai-Chi Li, Yung-Ming Jeng, Hey-Chi Hsu, Po-Ling Kuo, Meng-Lin Li, Pei-Ming Yang and Po Huang Lee: Elastic modulus measurements of human liver and correlation with pathology. US in Med. Biol. 28(4), 467-474, 2002.
14. M.M. Doyley, J.C. Bamber, P.M. Meany, F.G. Fuechsel, N.L. Bush, and N.R. Miller: Reconstructing Young's modulus distributions within soft tissues from freehand elastograms. Acoustical Imaging, volume 25, pp 469-476 2000.
15. Taylor RH, Funda J, Eldridge B, Gruben K, LaRose D, Gomory S, Talamini M, Kavoussi LA, and Anderson JH: A Telerobotic Assistant for Laparoscopic Surgery. IEEE EMBS Magazine Special Issue on Robotics in Surgery. 1995. pp. 279-291
16. Moddemeijer, R., Delay-Estimation with Application to Electroencephalograms in Epilepsy (Phd-thesis), Universiteit Twente, 1989, Enschede (NL), ISBN: 90-9002668-1

A Tactile Magnification Instrument for Minimally Invasive Surgery

Hsin-Yun Yao[1], Vincent Hayward[1], and Randy E. Ellis[2]

[1] Center for Intelligent Machines, McGill University, Montréal, Canada,
{hyyao,hayward}@cim.mcgill.ca
[2] School of Computing, Queen's University, Kingston, Canada
ellis@cs.queensu.ca

Abstract. The MicroTactus is a family of instruments that we have designed to detect signals arising from the interaction of a tip with soft or hard objects and to magnify them for haptic and auditory reproduction. We constructed an enhanced arthroscopic surgical probe and tested it in detecting surface defects of a cartilage-like material. Elastomeric samples were cut at different depths and mixed with blank samples. Subjects were asked to detect the cuts under four conditions: no amplification, with haptic feedback, with sound feedback, and with passive touch. We found that both haptic and auditory feedback significantly improved detection performance, which demonstrated that an enhanced arthroscopic probe provided useful information for the detection of small cuts in tissue-like materials.

1   Introduction

Minimally invasive surgery benefits patients by the small size of incisions, less pain, less trauma and shorter healing periods; the surgeon, however, must cope with loss of direct tactile information and reduced visual information. It has been demonstrated that even partial restoration of the sense of touch improves performance in teleoperation and virtual environments [2,4,3,5]. "Augmented reality" can be used to improve human performance in surgical applications, however systems often have features in the graphics domain but provide little in terms of haptic feedback [1]. With this in mind, we have designed and tested a new tool to improve the sense of touch during minimally invasive surgical procedures.

During arthroscopic surgery in a joint, a surgeon inserts a small camera in one incision and a surgical instrument in another. It is common for cartilage to be damaged in regions that cannot be seen arthroscopically, in which cases a surgeon must rely completely on haptic feedback obtained from a surgical instrument. One common arthroscopic instrument has a metal tip and a handle. The tips may have many different shapes, but the "arthroscopic hook" with a tip bent to a 90-degree angle is commonly used. With this instrument, a surgeon probes the surface of tissues, including ligaments, menisci and cartilage, to find anomalies.

C. Barillot, D.R. Haynor, and P. Hellier (Eds.): MICCAI 2004, LNCS 3217, pp. 89–96, 2004.
© Springer-Verlag Berlin Heidelberg 2004

We have developed an integrated system designed to improve the sense of touch of a surgeon holding an instrument during tissue examination. Our device is an arthroscopic instrument that actively enhances the tactile experience of interacting with objects by amplifying the mechanical interaction signal. The same signal can also be transformed into sound to heighten sensitivity to small details even further.

We have fabricated an arthroscopy hook shown in Fig. 1, integrated an accelerometer near the tip, and custom-designed an actuator that was embedded in the handle. The complete system was simple and easy to manufacture. We conducted preliminary experiments in which an acceleration signal was amplified and processed with bandpass filtering to test our device in a tear-detection task. The results indicated that with even rudimentary signal processing in the haptic and auditory domains, tear-detection performance was significantly improved.

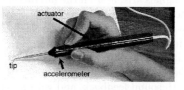

Fig. 1. Application of the MicroTactus concept to an augmented arthroscopic probe.

2   The MicroTactus Touch Magnification Instrument

We determined which signal(s) to detect and amplify by considering the motion of a probe as it interacts with a surface. Motion depends on the forces applied, which for a probe are (1) interaction contact forces and (2) user's grip forces. These combined forces are the forcing term of the probe's dynamics, which in turn are its rigid-body dynamics and structural dynamics. The user's tactile information is derived entirely from the deformation of the tissues of the hand holding the probe, whether the action is to press on, drag over, or tap a surface; this deformation is highly dependent on the dynamics of the probe, and on the size and shape of the probe's tip. Each of these actions, or any combination thereof, informs the user of the probe of properties of the tissues under test.

From this analysis we concluded that the sensory function of the probe is to transfer the movements of its tip to movements of the tissues at the interface with the hand. Since acceleration signals entirely describe the movement of any object (with appropriate integration constants) we concluded that the information to be amplified for tactile enhancement purposes is embodied in the acceleration of the tip of probe, and that sensing force and/or strain is unnecessary.

This analysis also suggested that the appropriate tactile transducer is an actuator that can accelerate the handle. Moreover, because the acceleration signal is highly structured and spectrally rich, if it is converted into an acoustic signal then it might be usefully processed by the auditory system for multi-modality interpretation.

Hardware Design. We applied these principles to the design of an active arthroscopic probe, which we wanted to be similar in structure and use to a conventional probe. As shown in Fig. 2, a biocompatible metal hook was attached to a handle made from carbon fiber tubing that was 15 mm in diameter. An accelerometer was mounted where the probe's metal tip connected to the handle. Preliminary trials indicated that scratching a soft surface produced accelerations of about ±2 g; for harder surfaces, such as wood or plastic, the scratching acceleration was about ±5 g. Knocking on a wooden surface or scratching it at high speed could yield up to ±10 g. A 2 g dual-axis accelerometer (Analog Devices, ADXL311) was selected for a tear-detection task.

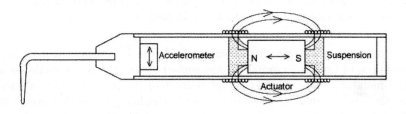

Fig. 2. Main structural components of the probe. The digital signal processing hardware and software is not shown here.

The tactile transducer demanded special attention. After numerous design iterations, we converged on a structure comprising a cylindrical rare earth magnet (NdFeB) elastically suspended inside the handle. To a good approximation the field lines escaping the magnet crossed the loops of two coils at right angles, thereby developing a Lorentz force between the magnet and the handle when current flowed. Although there may be numerous alternative designs (e.g., using variable reluctance actuators) or optimized designs (e.g., using a tubular soft-iron magnetic return), this simple "open magnetic circuit" design was appropriate to our immediate needs.

Maximizing acceleration of the handle's shell required (1) minimizing the mass of the shell, (2) maximizing the mass of the moving part, and (3) maximizing force. We found that our prototype met an appropriate tradeoff: a mere 10 W of electrical power caused vibrations large enough to numb the fingers in wide range of frequencies. This low power consumption, and the modest spectral requirements, enabled us to use an ordinary audio amplifier to drive the device.

We designed the device so that the accelerometer detected the radial components of the acceleration, whereas the actuator would create axial accelerations. This had the effect of dynamically decoupling the input from the output, which was necessary because forces would be transferred through the probe's structure. The device thereby remained stable, even with high feedback gains.

Signal Processing. A digital signal-processor subsystem (Analog Devices Blackfin533) was used to perform filtering and signal shaping. The processor also enabled us to conveniently record and play tactile signals. Accelerations were sampled with 16-bit resolution at 48 kHz.

The signal was first anti-aliased by digital filtering with oversampling. The anti-aliasing filter was a low-pass Finite Impulse Response filter of order 64, with a 3 dB cut-off frequency at approximately 500 Hz and a stopband attenuation of approximately 50 dB. The stopband was needed to filter out high frequency components that contributed little to tactile sensation, while keeping the passband as flat as possible. After anti-aliasing, the signal was down-sampled to 2,400 Hz. Downsampling increased the stability of the feedback system and eased the design of filters, which targeted only the frequency range of tactile sensations. Much remains to be done however to improve system performance and increase robustness in the presence of imperfect decoupling.

Configurations. Because the actuator was driven by a signal to some degree independent of (and orthogonal to) the sensed signal, the probe could be used as a stimulator *independent of actual contact of the probe tip with a surface.* Thus, the probe could be used as a "tactile display" device that could fit in an "augmented reality paradigm": with a second identical probe of the same design, it was also possible to sense surfaces remotely. For example, we could use one hand to manipulate the probe and the other to experience the surface; alternatively, it was possible to have an assistant scratch and tap a surface while a user experienced this physical interaction remotely. The device could also be used as a surface-recording tool so that, for example, we could record what a surgeon experienced during arthroscopy and play back the experience to one or several trainees for instruction. Because of its spectral characteristics, the signal could also be recorded, played back, or monitored with an ordinary audio system.

3   Preliminary Study

To demonstrate the utility of the probe, we tested it during the difficult task of superficial tear detection. In this task, the probe tip was dragged gently on the surface of a cartilage-like material. If there was a crack in the surface the tip would dip slightly in the crack, producing a transient signal that could be detected by touch. If the crack was sufficiently deep relative to the radius of the probe tip, and/or if the normal force was sufficiently high, the tip would catch the lip of the crack and produce a large transient. These, and perhaps other cues, could be used by surgeons to detect and characterize surface anomalies. Typical examples of signals are shown in Fig. 3.

We tested the ability of subjects to detect such cracks under various uses of the MicroTactus arthroscopy probe.

Surface Preparation. In order to approximate the conditions of tear detection during arthroscopy, we prepared 3 mm-thick-pads made of Viton, a high-

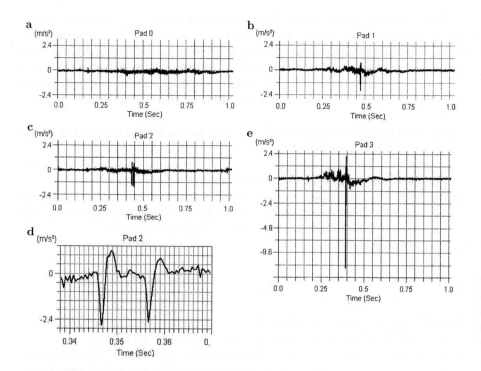

Fig. 3. a) Texture amplitude was modulated by varying the pressure of the probe on the surface. **b)** A small crack produced a single transient. **c)** A double crack produced a double transient. **d)** Enlarged view of **c. e)** A large transient given by a deep cut.

performance fluoroelastomer that resembles cartilage. Four 10×30 mm pads were glue-mounted on small boxes for easy handling. Cuts were made on the surface of the pads with a sharp blade protruding by a set distance out of a block of hard rubber. One pad had no cut, another had a 1.5 mm-deep-crack, another had two 1.5 mm-deep-cracks, and yet another was completely cut 3 mm-deep.

Subjects. We recruited 8 healthy individuals of age 22 to 28. Two of them were physicians and six were students from the Electrical Engineering Department of McGill University. Four subjects were completely unfamiliar with our work, and the other four subjects had used the device before the experiments but did not not know the details of its design.

Procedure. Two identical MicroTactus probes were connected to the signal-processing system. Subjects sat at a table, held one probe with their dominant hand, and used the probe to explore the surface of the samples while using the other hand to hold the sample mounted on the boxes. The subjects were trained in the task under the guidance of the experimenter.

During the trials, the lights of the windowless room were dimmed so that it was no longer possible to see the cuts but the pads could be found on the table. A sequence of 24 pads was given to each subject in a randomized order, each pad being presented 6 times. Subjects were asked to detect if there was a cut in the pad. They had to decide rapidly and answered by pressing keys labeled YES and NO. Trials were done under four conditions in the following order:

1. Haptic: subjects explored the pads with tactile feedback activated on the same probe used for exploration.
2. Audio: subjects explored the surface with the probe, but instead of tactile feedback, audio feedback was relayed through a loudspeaker.
3. Passive: the experimenter explored the pads with a first probe, attempting to keep a constant speed. The tactile feedback from the first probe was sent to the second probe which was passively held by the subject.
4. Off: The subjects use a probe without tactile or audio feedback.

The duration of each testing session was less than one hour.

Results. Fig. 4 summarizes the results (a) by condition and (b) by pad. Fig. 4a shows that the performance of the subjects improved with haptic and sound feedback. A significance test confirmed that the haptic and sound feedback both influenced the performance. Sound feedback improved the performance by approximately 20%, and haptic feedback by 10%. One-way analysis of variance (ANOVA) of the three conditions Off, Haptic and Audio confirmed the significance of the differences ($p = 0.015$, $p < 0.05$). The ANOVA test applied to pairs of conditions yielded $p = 0.015$ between the Audio and Off, and $p = 0.055$ between Haptic and Off conditions. There was no significant difference between Haptic and Passive conditions ($p = 0.15$, $p > 0.05$). The difference in performance between naive and non-naive subjects was not significant as indicated by a 2-way ANOVA test ($p = 0.53$, $p > 0.05$). There was no significant difference between the physicians and the other subjects ($p > 0.05$).

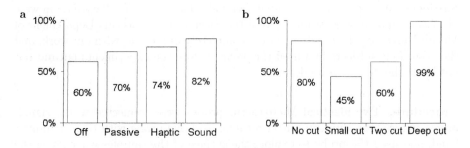

Fig. 4. Results summarized (**a**) by condition, (**b**) by pad.

More detailed data is presented in Table 1. Deep cuts were almost perfectly detected, and most subject also responded correctly for the surface with no cuts. For pads with small cuts, the performance in `Haptic`, `Sound`, and `Passive` was better than in the `Off` condition. When there was no feedback, the subjects failed to detect the presence of small cuts most of the time.

Table 1. Pooled results in percentile in the 4 conditions and for the different cuts.

Condition	No cut	small cut	two cuts	deep cut
Off	92	15	33	100
Haptic	90	44	65	100
Audio	90	63	77	100
Passive	50	60	65	98

Discussion. The results for each pad are presented in Figure 4b and Table 1. For the uncut and the deeply cut pads, the performance was well above chance. The deep cut was almost perfectly detected under all conditions. The haptic and audio feedback did not have a negative influence on detection of a deep cut, and the subjects performed at least as well with feedback as without. Furthermore, in passive detection, the haptic signal was adequate for the correct detection of a deep cut. Without haptic or audio feedback, remote detection would of course be impossible and yet our subjects performed remarkably well: the 2% miss rate for remote detection may well have been due to a single error made when the subject entered the data.

Figure 4b also showed that with one or two small cuts, performance without enhanced feedback was not far from the rate predicted by chance. This suggested that the dimensions of the cuts were close to the threshold of detection. From figures in Table 1, we concluded that without feedback, the existence of cuts were hard to detect. With either auditory or haptic feedback, the detection rate increases. Thus the system was able to improve the performance of subjects in detecting superficial cuts in a cartilage-like material.

Figure 4a summarizes the performance for each condition. The test of significance indicated that haptic and auditory feedback had positive influences on the performance. As for passive cut-detection task, the performance is at least as good as with active exploration without augmentation. In the passive condition, subjects had no control of the probe and could not see how the experimenter explored the surface. When subjects used the probe actively, they could vary the speed and the pressure applied by the probe. However, subjects were still able to detect the cuts well, as shown in Table 1. For pads with small cuts, the performance in the `Remote` condition is similar to `Off` and `Haptic` conditions.

Performance with audio feedback was consistently better than with haptic feedback, and most subjects spontaneously contributed an opinion to this effect. The simplest explanation is that our auditory system is more able to detect small transients out of a noisy background than is our tactile system. It is also possible that, using the two combined modalities of touch and audition, sensitivity may increase. Another possible explanation is that some useful information was lost in the filtering process. The signals to the speakers were not processed, but for haptics the signals were filtered and downsampled in an attempt to attempt to eliminate sensor noise. Even though the 400 Hz threshold was imposed during the filtering, there may be some useful information above this frequency. Signal enhancement techniques beyond plain magnification in a frequency band may be useful.

4   Conclusion

We have introduced the first example of a family of instruments designed to enhance touch while probing a surface. Our preliminary study found that significant task improvement happened when either haptic or auditory feedback were presented. The device also made it possible to experience a surface remotely. The device can be used as a texture-recording/play instrument, with considerable potential for use in surgical simulation and training. The device might also be useful for other judgment and detection tasks.

This project is still at an early stage, and many improvements are possible building on the basic principle described here. The device's structural dynamics might also be modeled and quantified, and a toolbox of signal processing algorithms can be developed to enhance the performance of specific tasks.

Acknowledgments. This research was supported in part by the Institute for Robotics and Intelligent Systems, the Ontario Research and Development Challenge Fund, and the Natural Sciences and Engineering Research Council of Canada.

References

1. Dario, P., Hannaford, B., and Menciassi, A. 2003. Smart Surgical Tools and Augmenting Devices, *IEEE T. on Robotics and Automation*, 19(5):782–792.
2. Kontarinis, D. A., and Howe, R. D. 1995. Tactile Display of Vibratory Information in Teleoperation and Virtual Environments, *Presence*, 4(4):387–402.
3. Rosen, J., Hannaford, B., MacFarlane, M.P., and Sinanan, M.N. 1999. Force controlled and teleoperated endoscopic grasper for minimally invasive surgery-experimental performance evaluation, *IEEE T. on Biomedical Engineering*, 46(10):1212–1221.
4. Okamura, A. M., Cutkosky, M. R., and Dennerlein, J. T. 2001. Reality-Based Models for Vibration Feedback in Virtual Environments. *IEEE/ASME T. on Mechatronics*, 6(3):245–252.
5. Pai, K. and Rizun, P. R. 2003. The WHaT: A Wireless Haptic Texture Sensor. Proc. *Eleventh Symposium on Haptic Interfaces for Virtual Environment and Teleoperator Systems*.

A Study of Saccade Transition for Attention Segregation and Task Strategy in Laparoscopic Surgery

Marios Nicolaou, Adam James, Ara Darzi, and Guang-Zhong Yang

Royal Society/Wolfson Medical Image Computing Laboratory & Department of Surgical Oncology and Technology, Imperial College London, London, United Kingdom.
{m.nicolaou, a.james, a.darzi, g-z.yang}@imperial.ac.uk

Abstract. The advent and accelerated adoption of laparoscopic surgery requires an objective assessment of both operative performance and perceptual events that lead to clinical decisions. In this paper we present a framework to extract the underlying strategy through the analysis of saccadic eye-movements that lead to visual attention, and identification of intrinsic features central to the execution of basic laparoscopic tasks. Markov modeling is applied to the quantification of the saccadic eye movements for elucidating the intrinsic behaviour of the participants and the spatial-temporal evolution of visual search and hand/eye coordination characteristics. It has been found that participants adopted a unified strategy but the underlying disparity in saccadic behaviour reflect temporal and behavioural differences that could be indicative of the mental process by which the task was executed.

1 Introduction

Minimal Invasive Surgery (MIS) has been an important technical development in surgery in recent years. It achieves its clinical goals with reduced patient trauma, shortened hospitalisation and improved diagnostic accuracy and therapeutic outcome. Laparoscopic surgery is a subset of the general field of MIS and relates to most procedures performed in the abdomen in which the surgeon is required to operate by remote manipulation, using specially designed, elongated instruments inserted into port sites that are located through small incisions at specific points in the abdominal wall. The operative field is viewed by means of a laparoscope in which a small camera relays a video signal to a 2D monitor. During laparoscopic surgery, however, the surgeon's direct view is often restricted, thus requiring a higher degree of manual dexterity. The complexity of the instrument controls, restricted vision and mobility, difficult hand-eye co-ordination, and the lack of tactile perception are major obstacles in performing laparoscopic procedures. To date, a number of techniques have been developed for objective assessment of operative skills during laparoscopic surgery [1]. Most existing techniques are concentrated on the assessment of manual dexterity and hand-eye coordination with the combined use of virtual and mixed reality simulators. These environments offer the opportunity for safe, repeated practice and

C. Barillot, D.R. Haynor, and P. Hellier (Eds.): MICCAI 2004, LNCS 3217, pp. 97–104, 2004.

for objective measurement of performance. Limited research, however, has been carried out in assessing how attention and different visual cues are integrated. There are a number of adverse events that go unnoticed in the operating room and many of them are not only associated with dexterity but also attention and visual-spatial perception. Both performance and safety are affected due to constraints placed upon the surgeon in laparoscopic surgery [2]. These events are a growing problem for healthcare organizations around the world [3].

During laparoscopic procedures, the primary constraint is vision as the surgeon is limited by the narrow monoscopic field of view and the representation of the operative scene provided by the laparoscope. To navigate the procedure and execute the appropriate motor commands, the surgeon is reliant upon limited cues through perspective changes in anatomy, occlusion, lighting variations and surface textures [4]. The procedure also involves three entirely distinct, spatial environments or "domains" that include internal (the point of operation), external (the external surgical field and the operating theatre) and the 2-D laparoscopic video [5]. To understand the underlying perceptual and cognitive processes involved, it is necessary to examine in detail the visual search behavior during different surgical steps.

Visual search is the act of searching for a target within a scene that involves both eye and head movement. It is a reactive rather than deliberative process for most normal tasks. The best visual acuity of the human eye falls within a visual angle of one to two degrees. This is called foveal vision, and for areas that we do not direct our eyes towards when observing a scene, we have to rely on a cruder representation of the objects offered by non-foveal vision, of which the visual acuity drops off dramatically from the centre of focus. When we try to understand a scene we fixate our eyes on particular areas and move between them. The intrinsic dynamics of eye movements are complex and saccadic eye movements are the most important to consider when studying visual search. It has a fast acceleration at approximately 40,000 degrees/second^2 and a peak velocity of 600 degrees/second^2. The objective of a saccade is to foveate a particular area of interest in a search scene [6].

The manner in which a surgeon assimilates information from different visual cues has been studied at a basic level mainly through video examination and interview. Experienced surgeons seem to have unparalleled capabilities in mastering visual-spatial capabilities by integrating a number of visual and motor cues. They make extensive use of ancillary and corroborative landmarks to plan for each maneuver and compensate for the loss of depth perception due to video projection. The study of the exact mechanism that underpins these behaviours, however, has proved to be difficult as many actions and perceptual filtering that occurs, are rapid and happen at an unconscious level. The process is further hampered by the fact that visual features are difficult to describe and assimilation of near-subliminal information is cryptic. These drawbacks call for the use of eye tracking for assessing detailed visual search behaviour during surgery. It is well understood that the main function of the oculomotor system is to keep the centre of gaze very close to the point of greatest interest being temporally and spatially coupled to the task at hand [7] and analysis of saccades can reveal much about the underlying cognitive mechanisms that guide them [8]. The use of eye tracking has already enjoyed a certain level of success in decision support in radiology [9], and the purpose of this paper is to present a new paradigm of analyzing surgical competence by extracting underlying task strategies through the analysis of saccadic eye movements that lead to visual attention whilst performing laparoscopic tasks.

2 Materials and Methods

2.1 Surgical Task and Experiment Setup

A homogenous sample group of seven second year medical students (3 male, 4 female, mean age=20) were recruited to participate in this study. Ethics approval was granted by St Mary's local research ethics committee (LREC) with informed consent being obtained from all participants. All participants had no prior laparoscopic experience. The elementary surgical task required participants to grasp a colored section of a simulated blood vessel fixed on a plastic skin pad and transect it at a subsequent colored section using real laparoscopic instruments including grasper and scissors, as shown in Figure 1. The skin pad was placed within a custom-made laparoscopic box trainer with laparoscopic ports for the insertion of the instruments. The operative field was recorded using an analog camera fixed within the box and live video footage was streamed via a computer onto a 2D video screen. The participants were required to perform the task by manipulating the instruments and obtaining visual feedback of their actions on the screen. The displayed video was recorded in digital format on the hard disk of a computer for later analysis. The two targets on the simulated blood vessel and both tool tips were differently colored as to allow the automatic extraction and tracking of these 4 features from the recorded video footage. Gaze positions were also recorded during the procedure using an eye tracker. A diagram and a photo of the overall hardware set-up can be seen in Figure 1(a) and (b).

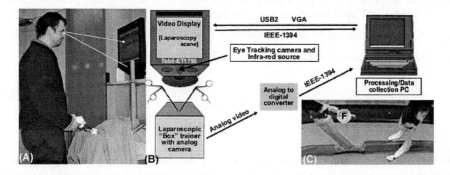

Fig. 1. (a) Experimental setup of the laparoscopic trainer used for this study, and (b) a schematic diagram showing the main data/command flow during real-time eye tracking with a Tobii remote eye tracker. (c) Shows an example of the laparoscopic view of the setup with foveation points super-imposed.

Gaze tracking was performed using a Tobii ET 1750 eye tracker. This is an infra-red video-based binocular eye-tracking system recording the position of gaze in the work plane (screen) at up to 38 samples per second. A fixed infra-red light source is beamed towards the eye whilst a camera records the position of the reflection (known as the Purkinje reflection) on the cornea surface relative to the pupil centre. The infra-red images are real-time digitized and processed. Following a calibration procedure, the point of regard can then be determined with an accuracy of 1 degree across the work plane. This allows accurate tracking of the position of gaze of subjects standing approximately 60cm away from the equipment looking at the video screens as indicated in figure 1a. The system allows a certain amount of head movement, thus providing a realistic setting for the laparoscopic procedure. In this study, we used the screen to feed live video footage of the procedure. Good motion compensation combined with binocular eye tracking allows a seamless integration of eye tracking into the training procedure, and the average calibration time required is twenty seconds approximately [10].

2.2 Analysis of Fixation and Visual Search Strategy

The areas of interest (AOI) for a basic simulated laparoscopic task have been previously assessed [11] and we used this to determine the AOI for the study. The instrument tip (A), the target anatomy (B) and the feature space in-between (C) represented the AOI. For a detailed analysis of visual search and hand/eye strategy, the surgical task was decomposed into two steps: vessel grasping (task 1) and vessel transection (task 2). Each AOI was defined by different colours and automatically tracked by colour segmentation by hue-saturation space filtering previously described [12]. The co-ordinates of each AOI were combined with the gaze data and using developed software we determined which AOI foveal vision (taken as 2° visual angle) was centered. In order to extrapolate intrinsic information of each individual's dynamic eye movements, Markov modeling was used to investigate the sequence of temporal fixations [13] [9]. In this paper we focus on a discrete time, discrete state space model (DTMC) based on a first-order Markov process. The evaluation of a DTMC [14] is achieved by an observation at time i as a random variable X_i, variables $X_0, X_1, X_2, \ldots \ldots X_m$. For all states x_n the following applies:

$$P\left\{ x_{n+1} = x_{n+1} \mid X_0 = x_0, X_1 = x_1, \ldots \ldots x_n = x_n \right\}$$
$$= P\left\{ X_{n+1} = x_{n+1} \mid X_n = x_n \right\}$$

(1)

In this study, areas A,B,C were designated as the states for the Markov model for both the grasping and the transection task. In the first instance, we examined the total number of fixations and transitions between all of the states for i and j for each participant. To further analyse the transition probabilities p_{ij} between the states i and j were calculated by determining the number of fixations per AOI. The total numbers of transitions were normalized for both the task and for each sub task. To observe the transition probabilities between states intrastate transitions were excluded. Only three independent states were considered. The following approach was taken (2):

$$\begin{pmatrix} * & t_{12} & t_{13} \\ t_{21} & * & t_{23} \\ t_{31} & t_{32} & * \end{pmatrix} \longrightarrow \begin{pmatrix} * & p_{12} = \dfrac{t_{12}}{t_{12} + t_{13}} & p_{13} = \dfrac{t_{13}}{t_{12} + t_{13}} \\ p_{21} = \dfrac{t_{21}}{t_{21} + t_{23}} & * & p_{23} = \dfrac{t_{23}}{t_{21} + t_{13}} \\ p_{31} = \dfrac{t_{31}}{t_{31} + t_{32}} & p_{32} = \dfrac{t_{32}}{t_{31} + t_{32}} & * \end{pmatrix} \tag{2}$$

The transition probabilities for the group were further analysed by averaging the sum of the matrices for each task to obtain the arithmetic mean. To demonstrate the spatial-temporal behavior of the individuals in terms of how strategy evolved over the course of the task, we compared the performances of two participants for a single task. The slowest and fastest participants were selected for temporal analysis.

3   Results

For each of the participants we calculated probability transitions matrices for the task as a whole, and the sub-tasks, task 1: grasping and task 2: transection of the vessel. We focused on transitions between states but not self-transitions. All of the other features in the space (C) were classified as a single state.

$$Z_1 = \begin{pmatrix} * & 0.3 & 0.1 \\ 0.2 & * & 0.6 \\ 0.4 & 0.2 & * \end{pmatrix} \qquad Z_2 = \begin{pmatrix} * & 0.7 & 0.3 \\ 0.6 & * & 0.4 \\ 0.6 & 0.4 & * \end{pmatrix} \qquad Z_3 = \begin{pmatrix} * & 0.9 & 0.1 \\ 1 & * & 0 \\ 1 & 0 & * \end{pmatrix}$$

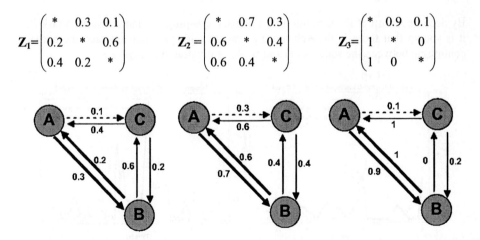

Fig. 2. Example Markov matrices derived for a single participant where Z_1 = Task (1&2) Z_2 = Task 1 (Grasping), Z_3 = Task 2 (transection). Only interstate transitions were considered with the thickness of the line representing the strength of the relationship between states.

The transition data for the participants represents the feature states that formed the underlying strategy. A dominant strategy was observed for the proportion of individuals, with key transitions between A>B and B>A corresponding to both the instrument and the vessel. The eye saccades between the two states, with each feature (A,B) receiving the proportion of fixations. Consequently, each feature receives maximum attention, as the fovea, the area of the eye with highest acuity, is centered on the feature. The mean transitions of the group followed this underlying strategy. Figure 4 illustrates the mean strategy for the task with two states being more dominant more than the rest.

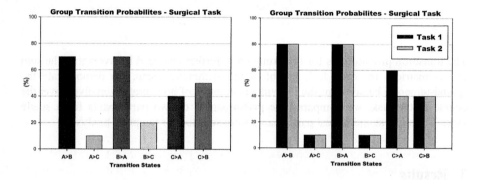

Fig. 3. (a) Mean transition probabilities for the participants performing the surgical task. Transitions between the vessel and instrument were the clear method adopted. There are further saccades between the vessel, instrument and surrounding feature space. (b) Decomposed mean transition probabilities for the group for task 1 and 2. Data clearly illustrates the similarities in strategy for both task one and two.

By decomposition of the task into two subtasks: grasping (1) and transection task (2), it is shown that there is little change in strategy with predominant saccadic activity continuing between the states A>B and B>A, as illustrated in Figure 3.

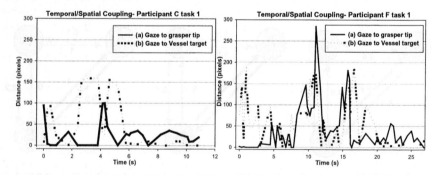

Fig. 4. Data representing the temporal and spatial coupling of eye behaviour for two participants (C) and (F).

The temporal and spatial coupling of saccadic behaviour of the individuals draws out characteristics differences in their underlying strategy and execution of the task. For participant C gaze alternates between instrument (A) and vessel (B) as shown by the waveform of the graph (with a predominant strategy of gazing on the instrument). Six seconds in, fixation concentrates on the vessel whilst the grasper tip is fine tuned into position. A distinct change in behaviour occurs (6s) coupled to the task of executing the grasping of vessel once having attuned the grasper to the correct distance. The behaviour of participant F is distinctly different with most time at the beginning of the task being spent fixating on the instrument. Between 6-16 seconds gaze shifts between the two with some alternate behaviour at 16-20s, guiding the instrument to the vessel. From 20 seconds, like participant C, fixation is concentrated on the vessel, whilst the instrument homes in, void of gaze supervision.

4 Discussions and Conclusions

In conclusion, we have presented a framework for extracting visual search behaviour by the analysis of eye movements and transitions between areas of interest (AOI) within a simple laparoscopic surgical task. The results suggest that there is a definite pattern of transitions within a homogeneous group of laparoscopic novices: a sequence of transitions from the instrument to the vessel and from the vessel to the instrument. This may seem an obvious strategy but it was clear to see that some individuals clearly formed this strategy early on. More importantly temporal analysis revealed intrinsic differences in the process by which the eye of individuals adopts and dictates the strategy. This implies that the underlying mental processes controlling the eye guide the execution of the task. These processes subsequently determine the timely nature by which the task in conducted. Temporal analysis distinguishes the strategic approach and importantly highlights the disparities between individuals that are important to understanding the exact nature of how the task was conducted.

As the surgical profession is in need of a reliable and valid method of assessing operative skill that is distinct from most subjective assessments [7], an understanding of the implicit strategies and features that guide an individual may provide information on the disparities in performance, ultimately quantifying the precise differences between individuals. Understanding the exact nature of these differences may provide a basis by which to attain procedural knowledge critical to optimize task performance. A system that can provide unbiased and objective measurement of surgical precision could help training, complement knowledge based examinations, and provide a benchmark for certification [15] Such a system would have wider implications in guiding the development of safety protocols and the current study is an important step towards the development of such an integrated framework.

Acknowledgements. We would like to thank our collegueas, Rachel King, Michael Rans and Benny Lo from the Royal Society/Wolfson Medical Image Computing Lab. for their support and contribution to the study. We would also like to thank the second year medical students of Imperial Medical School for their support and enthusiastic participation in the study.

References

1. Moorthy K, Munz Y, Sarker SK, Darzi A. Objective assessment of technical skills in surgery. BMJ, 1, 1032-37, 2003.
2. Cao CGL, Mackenzie CL. Task and motion analyses in endoscopic surgery. 1996 ASME IMECE Con Proceed: 5th Ann Sym on Haptic Environment and Teleoperator systems, 583-90.
3. Vincent C, Neale G, Woloshynowych M. Adverse events in British hospitals: preliminary retrospective record review. BMJ, 3, 517-18, 2003.
4. Tendick F, Bhoyrul S, Way L. Comparison of laparoscopic imaging systems and conditions using knot tying task. Computer Aided Surg., 2(1), 24- 33, 1993.
5. Tchalenko J, James A, Darzi A, Yang G-Z. Proceedings ECEM 12, 2003.
6. Yang G-Z, Dempere-Marco L, Hu X-P, Rowe A. Visual Search: psychophysical models and practical applications. Image and Vision Computing, 20, 291-305, 2002.
7. Land M, Mennie N, Rusted J. The roles of vision and eye movements in the control of activities of daily living. Perception, 28, 1311-1328, 1999.
8. Ballard DH, Hayhoe MM, Li F, Whitehead SD. Hand-eye coordination during sequential tasks. Philisophical Trans. of the Royal Society of London , Series B 337, 331-39, 1992.
9. Dempere-Marco L, Hu X-P, MacDonald SLS, Ellis SM, Hansell DM, Yang G-Z. The use of visual search for knowledge gathering in image decision support. IEEE Trans. on Medical Imaging, 21(7), 741-54, 2002.
10. Tobii technology. User Manual, 2003, http://www.tobii.se.
11. Law B, Atkins SM, Lomax AJ, Wilson J. Eye trackers in virtual laparoscopic training environment. Medicine Meets Virtual Reality: J.D Westwood et al (Eds), IOS Press, 184-186, 2003.
12. Lo BP, Darzi A, Yang G-Z. Episode classification for the analysis of tissue/instrument interaction with multiple visual cues. MICCAI, 2878, 230-237, 2003.
13. Hacisalihzade SS, Stark LW, Allen JS. Visual perception and sequences of eye movement fixations: A stochastic modeling approach. IEEE Trans. Syst., Man, Cyber., , 22, 474-81, May/June 1992.
14. Meyn SP, Tweedie RL. Markov chains and stochastic stability. London, UK: Springer-Verlag, 1996.
15. Taffinder N, Smith S, Darzi A. Assessing operative skill. BMJ, 318(3), 887-888, 1999.

Precision Freehand Sculpting of Bone

Gabriel Brisson[1], Takeo Kanade[1], Anthony DiGioia[2], Branislav Jaramaz[2]

[1]The Robotic Institute, Carnegie Mellon University, Pittsburgh PA, USA
{brisson,tk}@cs.cmu.edu
[2]The Institute for Computer Assisted Orthopaedic Surgery, The Western Pennsylvaia
Hospital, Pittsburgh, PA, USA
{tony,branko}@icaos.org

Abstract. The Precision Freehand Sculptor (PFS) is a compact, handheld, intelligent tool to assist the surgeon in accurately cutting bone. A retractable rotary blade on the PFS allows a computer to control what bone is removed. Accuracy is ensured even though the surgeon uses the tool freehand. The computer extends or retracts the blade based on data from an optical tracking camera. Three users used each of three PFS prototype concepts to cut a faceted shape in wax. The results of this experiment were analyzed to identify the largest sources of error.

1 Introduction

Artificial joint replacements must be installed accurately to ensure proper joint biomechanics. Proper installation requires cutting precise shapes out of bone. The Precision Freehand Sculptor (PFS) is a compact, handheld, intelligent tool to assist the surgeon in accurately cutting these shapes (Figure 1). A retractable rotary blade on the PFS allows a computer to control what part of the bone is removed, ensuring accurate results even though the surgeon uses the tool freehand. The surgeon simply glides the tool over the bone surface, where the tool cuts away only the bone that should be removed.

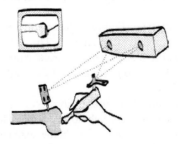

Fig. 1. The PFS system consists of a handheld tool, a tracking system and a display.

To control the tool's retractable blade, the computer compares the tool's current position to a programmed "target shape" for the cut bone. The positions of the tool and the bone are reported to the computer by an optical tracking camera.

C. Barillot, D.R. Haynor, and P. Hellier (Eds.): MICCAI 2004, LNCS 3217, pp. 105–112, 2004.

A computer display shows the tool and current bone surface, as well as the target shape for the bone. It also shows how close the cutter is to the target shape. This allows surgeons to monitor the progress of the cutting task.

Two prototype PFS versions have been completed. To evaluate their performance, each was used by three users to cut a faceted shape in wax. In addition, each user used the more advanced prototype without blade retraction, guided only by the display screen. The resultant surface was digitized with a touch-probe scanner to evaluate the accuracy of the tools. Secondary information such as maximum tool velocity and acceleration was also gathered, and users were observed and surveyed on their use of the display.

The results from this experiment were analyzed to identify major sources of error. This paper focuses on modeling error, which is error in the computer's internal model of where the bone has been cut. Software speed was found to be the largest source of modeling error, while calibration and tracking accuracy also contributed.

We expect the PFS to enable accurate surgery through smaller incisions. A PFS mechanism smaller than the current designs would be ideal for working in small, cramped incisions because the cutter is closely guarded, and because it ensures accuracy even when the surgeon does not have a clear view.

In contrast to robots such as RoboDoc [1] and Acrobot [2], the PFS has a smaller footprint and does not require the bone to be fixed in place. It also features the inherent safety of not being able to move on its own, other than the small motion of blade extension.

The PFS can be seen as an extension of surgical navigation [3]. The PFS extends the capabilities of navigation to allow preparation of more complex shapes. Like navigation, the PFS has the potential to reduce incision size by replacing direct visualization with on-screen visualization [4].

2 System Description

The PFS system consists of a handheld tool, an optical tracking system, a control computer, and a display monitor (Figure 1). Two PFS handheld tool prototypes have been developed.

The earlier "clutch tool" prototype (Figure 2) has a fully exposed spherical blade. The blade starts and stops rotation to control cutting. The clutch tool features a clutch which engages and disengages the blade from the drive shaft. Unfortunately it does not include a brake to stop blade rotation. As a result the blade spins up very fast but takes several seconds to spin down.

The "shaver" prototype (Figure 2) is more advanced. It features a cylindrical rotating blade which extends and retracts behind a guard. The axis of the blade is perpendicular to the long axis of the tool. The blade extends 0.64 mm (0.025 in) beyond the guard to cut, and retracts 0.64 mm (0.025 in) behind the guard to stop cutting, so the transition can be fast and not interfere with the surgeon's motion. Since the blade retracts such a small distance, the opening in the guard must be small to prevent it from cutting. The guard opening is 7.82 mm (0.308 in), which will prevent a sphere with a radius larger than 12.37 mm (0.487 in) from contacting the retracted blade. The blade diameter is 15.2 mm (0.6 in).

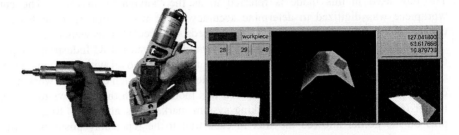

Fig. 2. Clutch tool *(left)* and shaver tool *(right)*   **Fig. 3.** PFS computer display

Both tool prototypes use the same software and tracking system. The position of the tool and bone is tracked by an Optotrak™ camera system (Northern Digital Inc, Waterloo Canada). The nominal accuracy of the Optotrak is 0.1mm RMS at each LED, but small rotational errors can create larger errors away from the marker, e.g. in calculating the position of the blade. With the configuration of markers used in this experiment, we expect the tracking error to be approx +/- 0.3mm, and the tracking latency to be about 4ms.

The shape that the system is instructed to cut, called the target shape, is determined by the implant shape and its planned position. Planning options include preoperative planning on CT scans [5], positioning based on anatomical landmarks the surgeon locates [6], or statistical atlas models of the bone [7]. The PFS is compatible with any of these approaches. It is a tool for executing whatever plan is given it.

The computer display (Figure 3) contains a 3D view, two cross-sectional views, and a bargraph (bottom) that displays the closest distance between the tool's cutter and the target shape. The boxes labeled "tool" and "workpiece" are green when the corresponding Optotrak marker is in view and red when it is not.

The computer maintins a model of the bone surface as it's being cut. In the 3D view, the current bone surface is shown transparently above the target shape. As its distance to the target surface is reduced, the current bone surface changes from red to orange (2mm) to green (0.6mm) and finally disappears in places where the target surface is penetrated. In the 3D view the bone stays fixed and the blade of the tool moves around it. The user may rotate the 3D view by stepping on a footpedal and using the optically tracked tool as an intuitive "3D mouse".

The cross-sectional views show the target shape in white and the waste bone in gray. The cross section planes pass through the center of the blade and are fixed in orientation with respect to the tool. This arrangement dictates that the outline of the tool remains stationary and the bone moves around it, in contrast to the 3D view.

3 Experimental Setup

Three users used each of the two tool prototypes, the "shaver" and "clutch tool", described above to cut a simple faceted target shape in wax. Additionally each user used the shaver tool without blade retraction, where cutting was guided only by the screen display in order to gauge necessity of the blade retraction for accurate cutting. The tool used in this mode is referred to as the "navigated shaver". The cut workpiece was digitized to determine accuracy. The user's motion through each cutting trial was recorded, from which user speeds and accelerations were extracted.

The workpiece used (Figure 4) was CNC validation wax (MSC Industrial Supply Co., Melville, NY, USA), pre-cut to limit bulk material removal without giving away the shape of the underlying target surface. A step milled in each end of the workpiece defined a reference plane. The workpiece was mounted with three screws to a steel holder (Figure 4) to which the tracking system marker was attached. Registration pins on the holder allowed the wax in each trial to be repeatably positioned with respect to the marker.

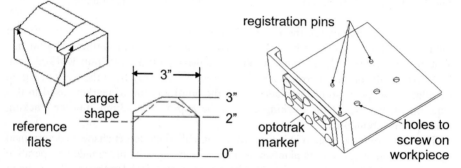

Fig. 4. Wax workpiece *(left)* and workpiece holder *(right).*

The cut workpieces were scanned on a Renishaw Cyclone Series 2 touch-probe scanner (nominal accuracy 0.002 in = 0.051 mm) on a 0.932 mm (0.0367 in) pitch grid, resulting in approximately 1500 samples per wax block. Since the uniform grid produces more samples per surface area on the diagonal facets, points were weighted by the arc-cosine of the facet angle when calculating the accuracy of results.

Subjects were already familiar with the PFS concept. Each subject was given a short orientation based on a written script. Subjects were instructed to try to be as accurate as possible, and were responsible for deciding when to finish the trial. After each trial, subjects completed a survey about their usage of the tool and user interface. Each subject performed the trials in a different order. After initial trials were complete, an error was discovered which required navigated shaver trial to be redone.

While the subject used the tool, the software recorded the blade position, retraction status, and loop time at each software loop. The final 3D model of the cut workpiece surface was also recorded for comparison with the ground truth determined by the touchprobe scanner.

4 Results

The histograms in Table 1 summarize the accuracy results. The left column profiles the error between the actual cut surface and the target surface, with negative numbers indicating that the actual surface was cut too deep. The right column profiles the error between the computer 3D model of the cut surface and the actual cut surface, in effect how much the computer's model of what was cut differs from reality. Negative numbers indicate that the actual surface was cut deeper than the computer model. Note that the clutch tool results are on a larger scale than the others.

Error can be divided into execution error and modeling error. Execution error is that which the computer was aware of but could not prevent: it is reflected in the computer 3D model. Modeling error is that which the computer was unaware of: it is the difference between the final computer model and the actual cut surface, as recorded in the left column of Table 1. As it seems most efficient to worry about execution error only once accurate modeling is achieved, we will discuss execution error briefly and focus on modeling error.

Table 1. Accuracy results.

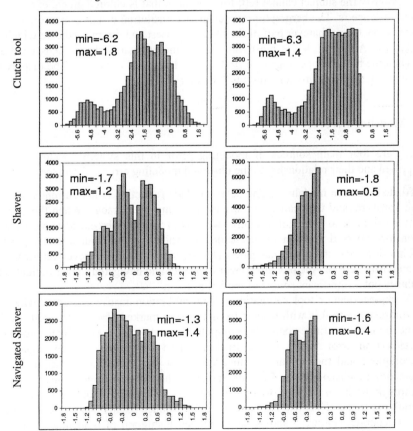

4.1 Execution Error

Execution error in this system has three main causes.

1. Blade retraction speed. (This does not apply to the navigated shaver.) Although the retraction speed of the current prototypes can certainly be improved, almost any PFS mechanism will have a non-negligible retraction time. The solution is for the software to look ahead and retract the blade *before* the tool reaches an area that shouldn't be cut. This is a focus of future work.
2. Lack of partial blade retraction. (This only applies to the shaver.) The software currently extends the blade fully or not at all. For example, if the blade is retracted and passes over an area that needs 0.5mm removed from it, the software will not extend the blade because it extends 0.64mm and would thus violate the target shape. This will be corrected in future software versions.
3. Resolution of target shape coloring. When the current surface of the workpiece is cut to within 0.6mm of the target surface, the display in that area turns green. Where the surface is cut beyond the target shape, the display turns white. Obviously the subject cannot tell, for a point in that is colored green, exactly what the distance is. The bargraph provides higher resolution distance measurement but measures from whatever part of the blade is closest and doesn't indicate which part that is. Although this is most limiting for the navigated shaver, it is used even when the blade is operational to find areas which need to be cut. The display will be changed so that green represents a smaller range.

4.2 Modeling Error

There are four main sources of modeling error in this system. Below they are described and their relationship to the observed modeling error is discussed.

1. Blade retraction modeling. The delay in blade retraction is not currently modeled in software, and thus can contribute to modeling inaccuracy. When the software tells the blade to retract, it instantly switches to updating the cut bone model based on the retracted position of the blade, regardless of the blade's actual position. This does not affect the navigated shaver, since the blade never retracts. The similarity between the modeling error of shaver and navigated shaver indicates that this is not a significant source of modeling error.
2. Workpiece and/or tool calibration. The calibration matrix describes where the workpiece or tool is with respect to its tracking marker. Inaccuracy will result in the tool not cutting where the computer expects. The most likely source of calibration error is the optical-tracking-based procedure used to register the workpiece and tool initially. Since each new workpiece is registered with the positioning pins on the steel holder, and since the tool registration remains constant through trials, errors due to optical tracking calibration should persist through multiple trials. Thus bad calibration would produce results that are repeatable but not accurate. Figure 5 shows the combined histogram of modeling error for all shaver and navigated shaver trials broken down by facet of the target shape. The

modeling error for each facet is more tightly clustered than the aggregate distribution of modeling error, indicating the influence of calibration error.

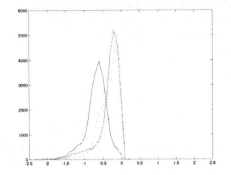

Fig. 5. Combinedshaver/navigated shaver modeling error (mm) broken down by facet.

3. Software cycle time. Each software cycle the computer updates the model of the cut workpiece based on the current position of the tool. Any motion of the tool in between software updates is not reflected in the model of the current workpiece surface. Tables 2 and 3 summarize the software loop times and tool velocities recorded throughout trials. Even for a modest loop time of 80ms and a modest speed of 0.1m/s, the distance of the shaver blade between software iterations is 8mm, which for the 15.2mm diameter blade traveling *across* the surface will result in a modeling error of 1.1mm. This problem is mitigated with the shaver mechanism because the shaver's guard limits the depth of cut so that an area must be passed over multiple times to cut a significant depth. The clutch tool, on the other hand, can make a straight plunging cut and come back up before the software registers its position. This accounts for the difference in modeling error between the shaver/navigated shaver and the clutch tool. Note that modeling error is almost exclusively negative: the computer underestimates how much material has been cut. This is consistent with the modeling errors that can result from slow software.

Table 2. Distribution of software loop times observed in trials.

Software loop time:	40-80ms	80-160ms	160-310ms
# of software cycles:	85912 (73%)	31866 (27%)	10

Table 3. Distribution of tool velocities observed in trials.

Tool velocity:	0-0.1m/s	0.1-0.5m/s	0.5-0.9m/s
# software cycles, (nav)shaver:	131367(85%)	22339 (15%)	150
#software cycles, clutch	35510 (88%)	4869 (12%)	40

4. Tracking system accuracy. We expect tracking accuracy in this experiment to be around +/- 0.3mm. The modeling error seen in the shaver and navigated shaver is small enough to be affected by tracking errors but large enough that tracking error is not the dominant effect. The negative bias of the modeling error supports this conclusion: for a calibrated tracking system, error is usually expected to be centered around zero.

5 Conclusion

The largest sources of modeling error in this experiment were calibration error followed by software speed for the shaver and navigated shaver trials. In the clutch tool trials software speed dominated.

Although the guarded mechanism of the shaver mitigates the problems of slow software, future guarded versions of the PFS will attempt to cut more aggressively than the current shaver and thus will be more affected by software speed. Better synchronization with the tracking system will be necessary to improve software speed and achieve accurate results. Future mechanical prototypes should be designed with calibration specifically in mind.

Improvements to the software to minimize execution error will also be necessary. Some of the execution error problems identified are easy fixes, whereas others, such as predictive retraction of the blade, are difficult and open-ended problems.

References

1. Taylor, et al: An Image-Directed Robotic System for Precise Orthopedic Surgery. IEEE Transactions on Robotics and Automation, 10(3), 1994, 261-274
2. Jakopec, et al: The First Clinical Application of a "Hands-On" Robotic Knee Surgery System. Computer Aided Surgery, 6, 2001, 329-339
3. Simon, D.A., et al: Development and Validation of a Navigational Guidance System for Acetabular Implant Placement. CVRMed-MRCAS'97, 583-592
4. Levinson, T.J., Moody, J.E., Jaramaz, B., Nikou, C., DiGioia, A.M.: Surgical Navigation for THR: A Report on Clinical Trial Utilizing HipNav. MICCAI2000, 1185-1187
5. Jaramaz, B., Nikou, C., Simon, D.A., DiGioia, A.M. III: Range Of Motion After Total Hip Arthroplasty: Experimental Verification Of The Analytical Simulator. CVRMed-MRCAS'97, 573-582
6. Leitner, F., et al: Computer-Assisted Knee Surgical Total Replacement. CVRMed-MRCAS'97, 629-637
7. Fleute, M., Lavallee, S. Julliard, R.: Incorporating a statistically based shape model into a system for computer-assisted anterior cruciate ligament surgery. Medical Image Analysis, 3(3), 1999, 209-222

Needle Force Sensor, Robust and Sensitive Detection of the Instant of Needle Puncture

Toshikatsu Washio and Kiyoyuki Chinzei

Surgical Assist Technology Group, AIST,
1-2-1 Namiki, Tsukuba, Ibaraki, 305-0051, Japan
{washio.t,k.chinzei}@aist.go.jp

Abstract. A force sensor based method to detect the instant of needle puncture to the layers of tissues is proposed. A set of needle and sheath attached to a pair of coaxial force sensors was used to separately measure the cutting force at the needle tip and the sidewall friction. Change of the force profile was observed and marked at the instant of the puncture, and robustly eliminated artifacts caused by body motion such as the respiratory or cardiac motion. The agreement between the subjective feeling of a skilled surgeon and the sensor was good. In several cases the sensor detected the puncture even when the surgeon could not clearly identify it. It was suggested that the sensor is potentially more sensitive than skilled professionals.

1 Introduction

Needle insertion is one of basic medical skills, and also one of the recent technology challenges for robotics. Though image guidance may be applied when inserting a needle to a critical organ, the essential information for good insertion is the subjective feeling from the needle.

Many attempts of robotic needle insertion [1-4] as well as the simulation of puncture [5-8] have been reported in literature. Generally, it is desirable that a robotic needle drive be equipped with at least one monitoring method for safety. The majority of approaches perform the insertion with the aid of an imaging device [1, 2]. Some of them monitor the insertion with a force sensor instead of imaging [3, 4]. Force sensing has no spatial information, though it has advantages over imaging in the view of its ability to sense the dynamic and local properties of tissue [9] and its great cost effectiveness.

The goal of this study is to establish a sensing method of needle insertion that is applicable to robotic needle insertion. In reality, it is not easy to sense the tissue properties using a force sensor, due to the disturbance from body motion, including respiratory and cardiac motion. These can be often dominant in the signal profile of the force sensor.

For this problem, the authors developed coaxial force sensors attached to the coaxial needles. Using this system, we found that the instant of needle puncture was stably detected without being affected by the artifacts. We also examined that the subjective feeling of needle puncture by a skilled medical professional agreed with

C. Barillot, D.R. Haynor, and P. Hellier (Eds.): MICCAI 2004, LNCS 3217, pp. 113–120, 2004.

the sensor's signal pattern. It was also suggested that the sensor could detect the instant of the puncture better than the skillful professional.

This paper is organized as follows: Section 2 outlines the structure and the principle of the sensor system with the underlying assumptions. Section 3 and 4 describe the experiments on the stability against the artifacts, the agreement with the subjective feeling, followed by a discussion and conclusion.

2 Sensor and Needle Structure for Stable Sensing

2.1 What Do Skilled Professionals Feel?

To date, the skill of needle insertion indeed falls in the realm of art. Though it is not trivially clear that skilled professionals sense needle insertion as force, we assume that we can obtain relevant information about needle insertion by force measurement.

The next question is what information they obtain from the force. Skilled professionals can insert a needle from the skin to the epidural space without image guidance. When they do it, they 'monitor' the puncture of layers where they expect to pass through: the skin, the muscle, the ligament, etc. The passage of layers may be detected by two ways: difference of the mechanical properties such as stiffness, or characteristic pattern at the instant of puncture of the membrane between the layers. We consider the latter in this paper and we assume that the break of the membrane is sensed as the force at the needle tip.

Unfortunately, the information through the needle does not carry the force at the needle tip alone. The force is composed of the force at the needle tip and the friction to the needle sidewall. The latter works as noise that occludes the former. As the needle is inserted deeper, it is expected that the friction increases and sensing the needle insertion becomes difficult.

2.2 Structure of the Sensor and the Needle

Based on an early study with our collaborators [10], the authors developed a set of coaxial load cells that can attach a coaxial needle where a sheath covers an internal needle so that only the blade part of the latter interfaces to the tissue (Fig. 1). Both the sheath and the blade are individually attached to the load cells. Since the sheath and the blade are independently attached to the load cells, the sensors basically represent the sidewall friction and the needle tip force respectively.

2.3 Detection of Puncture (Algorithm)

When a needle tip touches a membrane between two different layers of tissues, it reaches the puncture after certain extension. When the membrane breaks, its tension is released and the membrane and the tissues recover the original shape. At the same time, the needle proceeds into the tissue as the consequence of the recovery. Figure 2 illustrates the behavior when a needle breaks the skin, which is a special case of the puncture between two layers.

At the instant of the puncture, both sensors are expected to behave as the following. While the tension of the membrane is released, the needle tip cuts into the tissue. In case of the puncture of soft tissues, the strength of the membrane is usually superior to that of tissue, therefore the total force is expected to decrease. For the sheath, the sidewall friction will steeply increase in accordance to the needle penetrating the tissue.

In summary, at the instant of the puncture, we expect to observe that the tip force decreases and the friction increases. This does not occur due to body motion, since the expected effect of such motion is to either increase or decrease both forces at once.

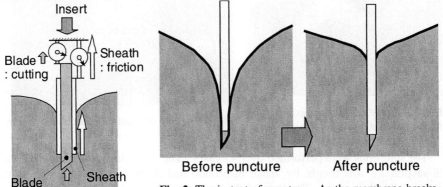

Fig. 1. Structure of the needle force sensor.

Fig. 2. The instant of puncture. As the membrane breaks, the membrane and the tissue recover the original shape. Consequently the needle proceeds into the tissue.

3 Validation

To validate the sensor, two experiments were performed; 1) Specificity of the detection of puncture under the existence of the respiratory and cardiac motion, 2) Sensitivity of the sensor and agreement with the detection to the subjective feeling.

Figure 3 REFshows our prototype of the coaxial load cell. For experimental purposes, the load cell attached to the sheath is a 6-axes force sensor, though in this paper the axial force component alone was used and discussed. Figure 4 shows a coaxial needle attached to the sensor, 130 mm length and 2 mm diameter. It is known that the shape of the needle tip affects the needle insertion. We examined several different needle tips. We examined by preliminary experiments that the shapes of needle tip did not affect the findings in this paper.

3.1 Detection and Its Stability Against Body Motion

The sensor was fixed to a linear motion table. The needle was inserted into a porcine liver under anesthesia. The liver was exposed in advance to the experiment, and was periodically moved by the respiratory motion. The needle was inserted by a constant speed of 5 mm/sec. Since the point where the needle touches was not always visible, a white plastic tube of 2.5 mm inner diameter, 35 mm length and 720 mg weight was placed on the surface of the organ so that the needle went through it. Motion of the tube was observed by video to determine the instant of puncture. It was determined as the puncture when the tube started moving backward according to the recovery of the tissue to its original shape.

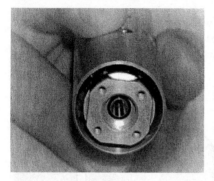

Fig. 3. A prototype of the coaxial sensor, 6-axes (external) + 1-axis (internal).

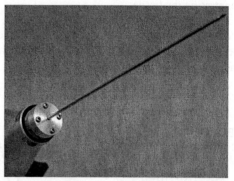

Fig. 4. The coaxial needle attached to the sensor.

The insertions were performed over 45 cases. The characteristic pattern described in section 2.3 was sought by visual inspection and defined as the detection of the puncture by the sensor. The time of the puncture detected by the sensor relative to that of the video observation was examined.

3.2 Agreement with Subjective Feeling

Correlation between the sensor signal and subjective feeling of a skilled surgeon was examined. A skilled neurosurgeon manually inserted the needle by holding the sensor to porcine spleen. We determined the instant of puncture by the video-based detection, i.e., observing the motion of the white tube as stated in section 3.1. When the surgeon felt the puncture occurred, he verbally described it.

The insertions to the spleen were conducted over 59 cases. The instant of the puncture detected by the sensor and declared by the surgeon, both relative to the video-based detection, was examined.

4 Results

4.1 Detection and Its Stability Against Body Motion

A typical profile of the measured forces is shown in Fig..5. The left figure is the measured profile. The profile pattern of the decrease of the tip force and the increase of the side friction appeared at t=8, which corresponds to the video-based detection. There was another similar pattern at t=8.8. We discuss it in a later section.

The right figure is the profile of numerical sum of these forces, which simulates observation using a single sensor. The change at t=8 was minor in contrast to the effect of the artifact by the body motion.

Figure 6 shows an experimental set-up of constant speed insertion. Disparities of the instant of the sensor detection from the video-based detection were in Fig. 7. The sensor detection occurred up to 1 second earlier than the video-based detection.

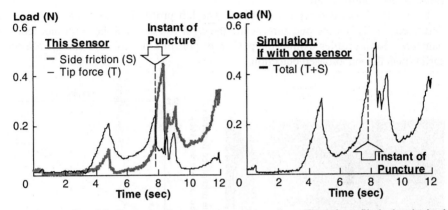

Fig. 5. The profile of the forces by the constant speed insertion. The left profile is the obtained result and the right was the sum of two curves in the left to simulate a single sensor. In the left profile, a periodic change by the respiratory motion mounted in the both curves. At the instant of the puncture (t=8), the tip force reduced and the side friction increased. In contrast, a single sensor would not be able to detect it under the existence of the periodic change.

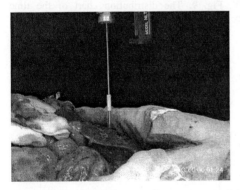

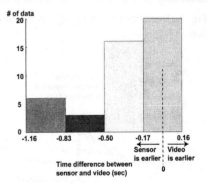

Fig. 6. Experimental set-up of constant speed insertion.

Fig. 7. The histogram of the time difference of the puncture relative to the video detection. The sensor detection started up to 1 second earlier than the surface motion.

4.2 Agreement with Subjective Feeling

Figure 8 shows an experimental set-up of manual insertion. A distribution chart was obtained for 20 of 59 insertions (Fig. 9). The correlation coefficient was 0.88. In the remaining cases, puncture was not clearly felt by the surgeon or the white tube was occluded therefore unable to determine the video detection. These were removed from the distribution chart.

Figure 10 shows two typical profiles. The left profile is a case that the surgeon described clearly felt the puncture, while the right is a case that he could not feel the puncture. Both profiles exhibit the pattern of puncture occurs 0.28 and 0.17 second earlier than the video-based detection.

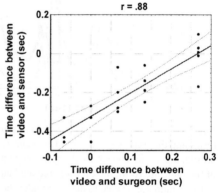

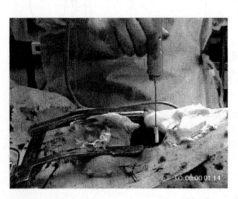

Fig. 8. Experimental set-up of manual insertion.

Fig. 9. The distribution chart of the time difference of puncture detected by the sensor and felt by the surgeon.

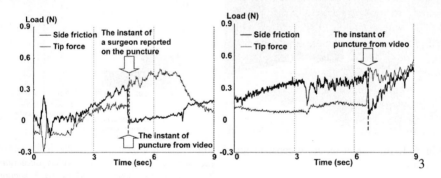

Fig. 10. The profile of the forces by the manual insertion to the spleen. The left profile is a 'clearly felt' case and the right is a 'unclear case he could not find when the puncture occurred'. However, the sensor signal has the pattern similar to the puncture.

5 Discussions

The observed force profile indicated that the artifact from the body motion could easily surpass the change caused by the needle puncture (Fig. 5). The overall performance was excellent in suppressing the effect of the artifacts. There was another similar pattern at t=8.8 in Fig.. 5. Its cause was not identified, though it is estimated that we detected another puncture of the internal structure of the liver.

The agreement between the detection by the sensor and visually determined instant of puncture (Fig. 7) showed that 1) almost all of the sensor detection precedes the video detection, 2) the time difference could reach 1 second. The former fact justified the assumption in Section 2.3. The authors consider that the delay can largely depend on the phase of body motion and the hysteresis of interaction between the needle and tissue. It is suggested that the video detection can be used as the baseline, however it has a window of 1 second in the detection time.

The agreement between the sensor output and the subjective feeling was in general good (Fig. 9). The response of human subject had a constant delay of 0.23 second from the sensor detection. The authors consider it is a typical delay for a human subject responding to a sensory input.

The profile in Fig. 10 shows another interesting event, that the case of the right figure was described as 'unclear when the puncture occurred'. However, there is a pattern of the puncture in the force profile that was 0.28 second preceding to the video based detection of the puncture. It is suggested that the sensor is more sensitive than a skilled surgeon. Regarding the sensitivity, the authors plan different experiments to evaluate the limitations of the sensor.

Since the experiments were performed on the surface of tissues, further study is required to conclude that this method can detect the puncture of layers of different tissues. We also plan to validate the agreement between the sensor and the subjective feeling with more subjects in different situations.

The interpretation of the sensor outputs, one for the cutting force and another for the friction, should be understood as an approximation. Strictly, both the sheath and the needle are in contact with each other; therefore, the separation of these forces is not perfect. When the needle is deflected, the bending force can be applied to both sheath and needle as a counter-force, which can theoretically appear as the pattern of the insertion.

Our detection algorithm needs further improvement. In this study we identified the puncture pattern by observing the force profile. We are currently developing computational method to detect it.

The method described in this paper has potentials in application for safety as well as the logging of manual needle insertion, safety monitoring in combination with robotic tools. For basic science, it will contribute to study the secret of how skilled professionals feel and control the needle insertion.

6 Conclusion

A sensor for detecting the instant of the needle puncture was proposed. A pair of coaxial force sensors attached to a set of needle and sheath was evaluated in terms of its robustness against the artifacts by body motions and the agreement with the subjective feeling of a skilled medical professional.

At the instant of the puncture on the surface of the tissue, the output from the sheath increased while that of the needle decreased. This pattern was observed regardless to the manual or robotic insertion. The sensor detection had a good agreement with the video-based detection. When the surgeon could clearly felt the puncture, the agreement between the sensor and subjective detections were also good. In some cases, while the surgeon could not clearly felt the puncture, the sensor detected the pattern and agreed with the video-based detection. It was suggested that the sensor has the potential to sensitively detect the needle puncture better than skilled professionals.

Remarks

These experiments had been supervised and approved by the internal review board of AIST for animal experiments. Trained veterinarians supported the animal experiments and the animals were treated in the humane manner.

References

1. fichtinger, G., Krieger, A., Susil, R. C., Tanacs, A., Whitcomb, L. L., Atalar, E.: Transrectal Prostate Biopsy Inside Closed MRI Scanner with Remote Actuation, under Real-Time Image Guidance. Proc. MICCAI 2002. (2002) 91-8
2. Hong, J., Dohi, T., Hasizume, M., Konishi, K., Hata, N.: A Motion Adaptable Needle Placement Instrument Based on Tumor Specific Ultrasonic Image Segmentation. Proc. MICCAI 2002. (2002) 122-9
3. Zivanovic, A., Davies, B.L.: A Robotic System for Blood Sampling. IEEE Trans. on Information Technology in Biomedicine. 4(1). (2000) 8-14
4. DiMaio, S.P., Salcudean, S.E.: Needle Steering and Model-Based Trajectory Planning. Proc. MICCAI 2003. (2003) 33-40
5. Brett, P.N., Parker, T.J., Harrison, A.J., Thomas T.A., Carr, A.: Simulation of resistance forces acting on surgical needles. Proc Instn Mech Engrs. 211(H). (1997) 335-47
6. Kwon, D., Kyung, K., Kwon, S.M., Ra, J.B., Park, H.W., Kang, H.S., Zeng, J., Clealy, K.R.: Realistic Force Reflection in a Spine Biopsy Simulator. Proc. IEEE ICRA 2001. (2001) 21-6
7. Popa, D.O., Singh, S.K.: Creating Realistic Force Sensations in a Virtual Environment: Experimental System, Fundamental Issues and Results. Proc. IEEE ICRA 1998. (1998) 59-64
8. Simone, C., Okamura, A.M.: Haptic Modeling of needle Insertion for Robot-Assisted Percutaneous Therapy. Proc. IEEE ICRA 2002. (2002) 2085-91
9. Brett, P.N., Harrison, A.J., Thomas, T.A.: Schemes for the Identification of Tissue Types and Boundaries at the Tool Point for Surgical Needles. IEEE Trans. on Information Technology in Biomedicine, 4(1). (2000) 30-6
10. Kataoka, H., Washio, T., Chinzei, K., Mizuhara, K., Simone, C., Okamura, A.M.: Measurement of the Tip and Friction Force Acting on a Needle during Penetration. Proc. MICCAI 2002. (2002) 216-23

Handheld Laparoscopic Forceps Manipulator Using Multi-slider Linkage Mechanisms

Hiromasa Yamashita[1], Nobuhiko Hata[1], Makoto Hashizume[2], and
Takeyoshi Dohi[1]

[1] Graduate School of Information Science and Technology, The University of Tokyo,
7-3-1 Hongo Bunkyo-ku, Tokyo, 133-8656, Japan
{hiromasa, noby, dohi}@atre.t.u-tokyo.ac.jp
http://www.atre.t.u-tokyo.ac.jp
[2] Graduate School of Medical Sciences, Kyushu University,
3-1-1 Maidashi Higashi-ku, Fukuoka-shi, Fukuoka, 812-8582, Japan
mhashi@dem.med.kyushu-u.ac.jp
http://www.camit.org/hospital

Abstract. This paper proposes a new handheld laparoscopic forceps manipulator using 2-DOFs bending mechanism by multi-slider linkage mechanisms and 1-DOF wire-driven grasping mechanism. Careful design of the linkage channels enables unique and independent bending procedure from −90 to 90 degrees on the horizontal and vertical plane to secure large workspace. The manipulator consists of multi-DOFs end-effector, linear-drive unit, dial-type interface and computer-based control unit. In mechanical performance analyses, 2-DOFs bending mechanism enabled high accuracy of less 1.0 mm manipulation and high bending power of up to 0.85 kgf. In vivo experiments, this manipulator performed laparoscopic surgical tasks, such as raising the liver and the stomach, and suturing the stomach surface tissue in 22.3 ± 5.4 seconds per suture. Furthermore, we operated cholecystectomy with an animal within 45 minutes. In conclusion we were sure of a usefulness of a new handheld laparoscopic forceps manipulator for speedy and dexterous laparoscopic surgery.

1 Introduction

Laparoscopic surgery enables the incision on abdominal wall smaller, thus making invasion to patients minimal. For the sake of this advantage laparoscopic surgery is taken in almost all surgery, such as abdominal surgery, chest surgery, obstetrics and gynecology. After securing space below abdominal wall, surgeons insert special surgical instruments such as forceps and electric cauteries through trocars, and operate instruments under laparoscopic control. However, surgical approaches and manipulations are restricted due to low degree-of-freedom (DOF) instruments . This inflexibility, combined with limited laparoscopic view of the operative field, causes surgeons' mental and physical stress.

To overcome the issues on limited maneuverability in the abdominal cavity, several robotized devices have been proposed to add additional degree-of-motion at the tip of the forceps [1]-[5]. The da Vinci[TM]Surgical System by Intuitive

C. Barillot, D.R. Haynor, and P. Hellier (Eds.): MICCAI 2004, LNCS 3217, pp. 121–128, 2004.
© Springer-Verlag Berlin Heidelberg 2004

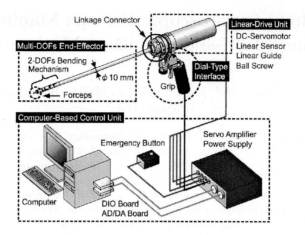

Fig. 1. System configuration of the handheld laparoscopic forceps manipulator.

Surgical Inc. enabled minimal invasive tele-surgery with miniature wire-driven multi-DOFs instruments having near-wrist manipulation [1]. The Mechatronic Arthroscope by Dario et al. enabled unique steering mechanism with two actuating cables, whose external diameter was 4 mm, steering range was 110 degrees and the mean error in the accuracy was 1.1 degrees [2]. These approaches proposed so far utilized wire-driven mechanism to transfer actuation power from actuators outside the abdominal cavity to actuated parts in the tip of the forceps. While this choice wire-driven mechanism is relatively straightforward approach, the issues on wearing and extension of wire has been unsolved.

Our proposal in this paper is to use multi-slider linkage mechanisms instead of wire-driven mechanisms to achieve 2-DOFs motion at the tip of the laparoscopic forceps. The linkage-driven approach is known to have high stiffness, durability and accuracy in manipulation [6][7]. The engineering contribution of this paper is slider-linkage drive to enable robotized motion in the forceps, especially the careful placement design of two slider-linkages while achieving no interference of motion each other. This paper is clinically significant since the highly accurate and stiff 2-DOFs motion of forceps tip possible by newly developed multi-slider linkage mechanisms enable speedy and dexterous laparoscopic tasks such as raising, suturing and ligation. This paper reports 1) newly developed multi-slider linkage mechanism based on our previous preliminary work [8], 2) development of handheld laparoscopic forceps manipulator using this linkage mechanism, 3) in vivo experiments and animal cholecystectomy study for evaluation.

2   Methods

2.1   System Configuration

The system configuration of the handheld laparoscopic forceps manipulator consisted of mainly four parts (Fig. 1). First part was the multi-DOFs end-effector with 2-DOFs bending mechanism and 1-DOF grasping mechanism. Second part was the linear-drive unit consisted of three sets of brushless DC-servomotors (FAULHABER GROUP MINIMOTOR SA, 1628 024 B), linear sensors detecting linkage displacements (ALPS ELECTRIC CO., LTD., RDC1014A09), linear-guides (THK Co., Ltd., RSR3WNUU+36L+) and ball-screws (NSK Ltd., M3 × 0.5). Third part was the dial-type handheld interface with three spindle operated potentiometers (Meggitt Electronic Components Ltd., TYPE 51 SERIES) consisted two dials for the horizontal and vertical bending, a trigger for grasping and a button for straightening the bending mechanisms in getting through a trocar. Fourth part is the computer-based control unit consisted a computer (CPU: Intel Pentium 4 2.00 GHz., RAM: 512 MB, OS: RedHat Linux 7.3) and three servo amplifiers (FAULHABER GROUP MINIMOTOR SA, BLD 3502) calculating displacements of sliding two linkages and one stainless-steel wire by inputted target angles from the dial-type interface.

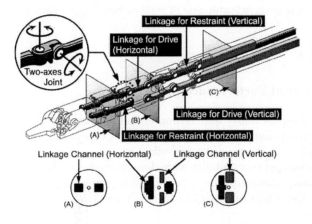

Fig. 2. Perspective view of the 2-DOFs bending mechanism that consists of five frames, two sets of linkages for drive and restraint. Each linkage slides through inner channel shown in sections (A), (B) and (C). Two-axes Joint connects the linkage for drive in horizontal bending mechanism and three links toward the actuator, enabling two-axes rotation responding to the vertical bending angle.

2.2   2-DOFs Bending Mechanism

2-DOFs bending mechanism for the multi-DOFs end-effector was constituted by multi-slider linkage mechanisms. These mechanisms consisted of five outer cylindrical frames, four joints and two sets of linkage mechanisms, one was for the horizontal bending and the other was for the vertical bending (Fig. 2). Each linkage mechanism, furthermore, consisted of two linkages, one was for drive outer frames and the other was for restraint enabling unique driving procedure between ±90 degrees and independent 2-DOFs bending manipulation. Constituent materials of 2-DOFs bending mechanism were all stainless-steel, outer frames and joint-pins were SUS304 and inner linkages were SUS316 (Fig. 3).

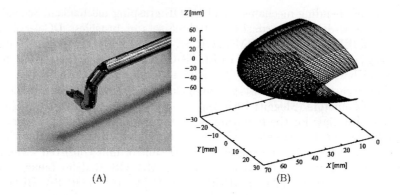

Fig. 3. (A) View of the 2-DOFs bending mechanism bending 90 degrees in horizontal plane and −90 degrees in vertical plane. (B) Workspace of the end-effector with 2-DOFs bending manipulation covering almost half surface of an oval sphere, whose origin of the coordinates is at an actuator-side of vertical bending mechanism.

3   Results

3.1   Mechanical Performance

We examined repeatability and response characteristic of the 2-DOFs bending mechanism using digital video camera (Sony Corporation, DCR-PC110), and generated power at the tip of an end-effector.

Measurements of repeatability were done unloaded with five trials each bending mechanism, examining the actual bending angles against target angles inputted from the computer with five times (Table 1).

Table 1.   Results of repeatability measurement in each bending mechanism.

Measurement item	Horizontal bending	Vertical bending
Repeatability(mean of SD)	$\pm 0.87°$	$\pm 0.91°$
Hysteresis error	less 9.0°	less 5.5°
Error over the theoretical value	less 13.3°	less 10.1°

As response characteristics, we examined actual bending angle against input target angle from dial-type interface to evaluate delay times of 2-DOFs bending mechanisms. Fig. 4 shows results of response characteristics of each bending mechanism between input bending speed and delay time.

3-DOFs generated powers at the tip of an end-effector and calculated torque at the rotational axes are shown in Table 2. Powers of all DOFs and directions fulfilled 0.40 kgf of a requested specification and achieved up to sufficient values of 0.85 kgf for laparoscopic surgery.

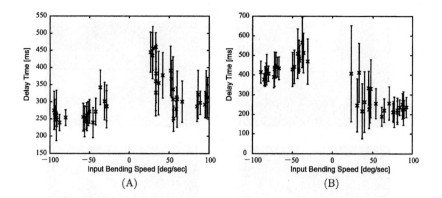

Fig. 4. Response characteristics of (A) the tip-side horizontal bending mechanism and (B) the base-side vertical bending mechanism.

Table 2. Generated power and torque at the end-effector.

DOF	Direction	Power [kgf]	Torque [mNm]
Horizontal	$0° \rightarrow 90°$	0.70	118.6
Horizontal	$0° \rightarrow -90°$	0.85	144.1
Vertical	$0° \rightarrow 90°$	0.40	165.7
Vertical	$0° \rightarrow -90°$	0.50	207.1
Grasp	Closing	0.85	60.8

3.2 In Vivo Experiments

We did usability analyses of the manipulator in near-clinical setting. We had surgeons approach to the liver and the stomach on an animal (swine, 42.5 kg, male) under pneumoperitoneum and do some laparoscopic surgical tasks shown in Fig. 5. Especially in suturing task, we confirmed smooth procedure of one suture in 22.3 ± 5.4 seconds on an average of nine times.

3.3 Cholecystectomy

As an usability analysis of the manipulator for more practical surgical works, we operated cholecystectomy with an animal (swine, 43.0 kg, male) under pneumoperitoneum (Fig. 6). It took 44 minutes and 30 seconds from laparoscope insertion into abdominal cavity to completion of gallbladder ablation.

4 Discussion

4.1 Mechanical Performance

We confirmed that larger workspace of ±90 degrees in 2-DOFs bending mechanism with high repeatability of less ±1.0 degree at the end-effector. Repeata-

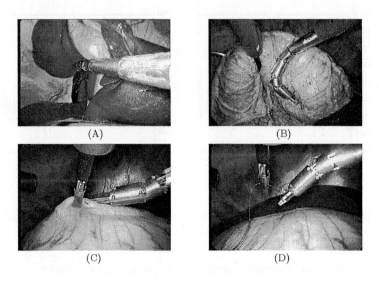

(A)   (B)

(C)   (D)

Fig. 5. (A) Circumventing, holding and raising the liver without flexure and defor-mation of the elements of bending mechanisms. (B) 2-DOF bending angles fit to the stomach curved surface and raising the whole stomach by the safe approach. (C) Stitch-ing the surface tissue before suturing task from appropriate aproach directions with tip side bending motion. (D) Winding a thread around the end-effector, grasping and pulling the thread with tip side DOF manipulation to complete one suture task.

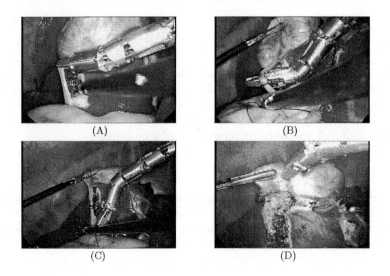

(A)   (B)

(C)   (D)

Fig. 6. (A) Grasping and raising the cystic duct for ablation with the electric cautery. (B) Passing the manipulator's tip part through ablated cystic duct with horizontal swing motion to grasp and pull a thread. (C) Ligation of the cystic duct. One ligation took 26.9 ± 7.11 seconds on an average of seven times. (D) Ablation of the gallbladder with the manipulator, a conventional forceps and an electric cautery.

bility of ±0.87 degrees on the horizontal bending equaled ±0.47 mm and ±0.91 degrees on the vertical bending equaled ±0.89 mm at the end-effector, which demonstrated that plays of multi-slider linkage mechanisms were quite little. Response characteristics varied according to bending DOFs, directions and input bending speed from dial-type interface. Differences affected by the first and second factors were caused by the number of links in 2-DOFs bending mechanism and length of linkage path in cylindrical frames. About third factor, blushless DC-servomotors' operating limit influenced linkage speeds, particularly in case input bending speed was very slow. On the other hand delay time in each DOF often broke 200 ms, which is said to be delay in human perception [9]. Doctors evaluated, however, that they didn't feel noticeable delay in operation of the manipulator. Generated powers of all DOFs and directions fulfilled requested specifications, however, also varied according to bending DOFs and directions. Bending powers from 0 to 90 degrees were 80% of powers from 0 to ±90 degrees, which indicated that the driving efficiency of pushing linkages was 80% of one of pulling linkages. Considering torques at rotational joints, calculated by generated powers, driving efficiency of the tip-side horizontal bending was 70% of one of the base-side vertical bending, which caused the number of links in the linkage for drive.

4.2   In Vivo Experiments

From the results of in vivo experiments we were sure of the usability of a handheld laparoscopic forceps manipulator through some surgical tasks. Bending powers up to 0.85 kgf were sufficient for raising and holding the liver and the stomach from a reverse side. Grasping power up to 0.85 kgf was stronger than conventional forceps to grasp a thin thread in suturing tasks, however, knurled surface, wide and short shape of tooth were not suitable for grasping large tissues and curved needle. As the 2-DOFs bending manipulation, the base-side DOF aided in flexible and safe approaches to target affected area in the abdominal cavity, and tip-side DOF advantaged dexterous work after approaches. However, we confirmed that additional DOFs such as rotation and swing are necessary to the end-effector for more effective, quick and precise operation.

4.3   Cholecystectomy

We operated cholecystectomy in near-clinical setting with an animal within 45 minutes, which was faster than normal operation time of one hour on the average. In the recently reported result of animal study with a surgical robot [5], the average cholecystectomy time for the six animal cases was 47 minutes, we found our handheld laparoscopic forceps manipulator to be useful for more practical clinical application.

5   Conclusion

We were sure of the usefulness of newly developed handheld laparoscopic forceps manipulator with large workspace, high repeatability of less 1.0 mm and sufficient power of up to 0.85 kgf at the end-effector. Especially in vivo experiments we operated a cholecystectomy within 45 minutes, which was speedy compared with conventional surgery, and high mechanical performance of the manipulator enables advanced laparoscopic surgery.

Acknowledgment. We wish to thank Mr. Iimura and Mr. Nakazawa of THK Co., LTD for cooperation in development of the linear-drive unit and the linkage connector. A part of this work is supported by Research for the Future Program "Development of Surgical Robot", administered by Japan Society for the Promotion of Science and Industrial Technology Research Grant Program in '03 from New Energy and Industrial Technology Development Organization (NEDO) of Japan.

References

1. Abbou, C., C., Hoznek, A., Salomon, L., Olsson, L., E., Lobontiu, A., Saint, F., Cicco, A., Antiphon, P., Chopin, D.: Laparoscopic radical prostatectomy with a remote controlled robot. JOURNAL OF UROLOGY. **165** (2001) 1964–1966
2. Dario, P., Carrozza, M., C., Marcacci, M., Attanasio, S., D'., Magnami, B., Tonet, O., Megali, G.: A Novel Mechatronic Tool for Computer-Assisted Arthroscopy. IEEE Trans. Inform. Technol. Biomed. **4(1)** (2000) 15–28
3. Nakamura, R., Oura, T., Kobayashi, E., Sakuma, I., Dohi, T., Yahagi, N., Tsuji, T., Hashimoto, D., Shimada, M., Hashizume, M.: Multi-DOF Forceps Manipulator System for Laparoscopic Surgery - Mechanism miniaturized & Evaluation of New Interface -. Proc. of 4th International Conference on Medical Image Computing and Computer-Assisted Intervention. (2001) 606–613
4. Ikuta, K., Sasaki, K., Yamamoto, K., Shimada, T.: Remote Microsurgery System for Deep and Narrow Space - Development of New Surgical Procedure and Micro-robotic Tool. Proc. of 5th International Conference on Medical Image Computing and Computer-Assisted Intervention. (2002) 163–172
5. Butner, S., E., Ghodoussi, M.: Transforming a Surgical Robot for Human Telesurgery. IEEE Trans. Robot. Automat. **19(5)** (2003) 818–824
6. Peirs, J., Reynaerts, D., Van Brussel, H.: A miniature manipulator for integration in a self-propelling endoscope. Sensors and Actuators A. (2001) 343–349
7. Kobayashi, Y., Chiyoda, S., Watabe, K., Okada, M., Nakamura, Y.: Small Occupancy Robotic Mechanisms for Endoscopic Surgery. Proc. of 5th International Conference on Medical Image Computing and Computer-Assisted Intervention. (2002) 75–82
8. Yamashita, H., Kim, D., Hata, N., Dohi, T.: Multi-Slider Linkage Mechanism for Endoscopic Forceps Manipulator. Proc. of the 2003 IEEE/RSJ International Conference on Intelligent Robots and Systems. **3** (2003) 2577–2582
9. Bate, L., Cook, C.: The Feasibility of Force Control Over the Internet. Proc. of the 2001 Australian Conference on Robotics and Automation. (2001) 146–151

An MR-Compatible Optical Force Sensor for Human Function Modeling

Mitsunori Tada[1,2] and Takeo Kanade[1,2,3]

[1] Digital Human Research Center
National Institute of Advanced Industrial Science and Technology
2-41-6, Aomi, Koto-ku, Tokyo 135-0064, Japan.
m.tada@aist.go.jp
[2] CREST, Japan Science and Technology Agency
[3] The Robotics Institute, Carnegie Mellon University
5000 Forbes Avenue, Pittsburgh, PA 15213, USA.
tk@cs.cmu.edu

Abstract. This paper presents the principle, structure and performance of a newly developed MR-compatible force sensor. It employs a new optical micrometry that enables highly accurate and highly sensitive displacement measurement. The sensor accuracy is better than 1.0 %, and the maximum displacement of the detector is about 10 μm for a range of the applied force from 0 to 6 N.

1 Introduction

Magnetic resonance imaging (MRI) has widely been used in studies of human function because it is non-invasive and has high spatial resolution. However, since MRI requires homogeneous magnetic field and radio frequency (RF) pulse for inducing the nuclear magnetic resonance (NMR), standard mechanical and electrical devices, composed of ferromagnetic materials and electrical circuits, cannot be used in the imaging volume of MRI [1].

The development of mechatronical sensor devices that do not interfere with MRI is one of the key technologies [2,3] in experiments using MRI, especially for studies such as human anatomy [4] and brain functional mapping during motor control and somatosensory perception [5], so that we can quantify the applied load and the voluntary human movement simultaneously while imaging.

Some MR-compatible force sensors have been proposed. Liu *et al.* have developed a hydraulic grip dynamometer [6]. The grip force applied to a hand grip device is transmitted to a pressure transducer outside MRI by a water-filled nylon tube. Due to the friction of a piston built into the hand grip device, the grip dynamometer has a dead zone over a wide range of force, from 0 to 80 N.

We have recently proposed an MR-compatible force sensor [7,8] based on an optical micrometry [9] using an LED and a quadrant photo diode. It achieves MR compatibility by placing both optical elements outside the MRI and extending a light path between them by using fiber optics. It was found, however, that in this design, since the light emitting fiber is fixed on the force detector of the

C. Barillot, D.R. Haynor, and P. Hellier (Eds.): MICCAI 2004, LNCS 3217, pp. 129–136, 2004.
© Springer-Verlag Berlin Heidelberg 2004

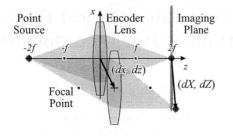

Fig. 1. Principle of the proposed optical micrometry

sensor, mechanical oscillation of the optical fiber easily causes perturbation of the force measurement.

This paper presents a newly designed and developed MR-compatible force sensor that has eliminated the above problem: its principle, structure, and performance. A new optical micrometry is employed that enables highly accurate and highly sensitive displacement measurement. The measurement accuracy is better than 1.0 % and the maximum displacement of the detector is about 10 μm under the applied force ranging from 0 to 6 N. The accuracy and rigidity are comparable to commercially available non-MR-compatible force sensors.

2   Two-Dimensional Optical Micrometry

2.1   Principle

Figure 1 illustrates the principle of the new optical micrometry for measuring minute displacement along one-dimensional direction x perpendicular to the direction of the optical path (along z). The coordinate origin is placed at the position where an optical lens with focal length f, called an encoder lens, is at the rest. A point light source is positioned at $(0, -2f)$, and an imaging plane at $(0, 2f)$. The point source is focused onto the center of the imaging plane $(0, 2f)$ when the lens is at the origin.

When a minute translational displacement (dx, dz) is applied to the encoder lens, it results in a shift of the focused image of the point source by (dX, dZ),

$$(dX, dZ) = \left(2dx - \frac{dxdz}{f + dz}, \frac{dz^2}{f + dz} \right) \tag{1}$$

Neglecting higher order terms,

$$(dX, dZ) = (2dx, 0) \tag{2}$$

Note that the lens has magnified x axial displacement dx two times onto the change in the imaging plane, whereas nullifying the effect of z axial displacement dz. The shift of the focused image location can be measured accurately by using a position detectable photo sensor, such as a segmented photo diode or a position

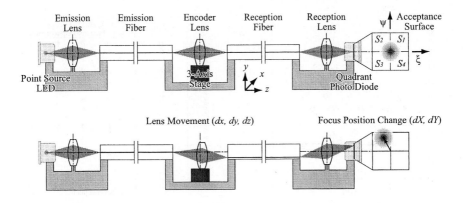

Fig. 2. Experimental set-up for the evaluation of the displacement measurement

sensitive device (PSD). The one-dimensional optical micrometry described above can be generalized to a two-dimensional case; lens displacement within the x-y plane perpendicular to the optical axis (z) can be measured using a quadrant photo diode or a two-dimensional PSD.

It should also be noted that the point source and the imaging plane do not move and can be mechanically connected to the same base, and the encoder lens displaces with respect to the base. In the MRI environment where ferromagnetic materials or electronic circuits are severely restricted, all the electric devices on the base component should be positioned apart from the encoder lens. Such a configuration can be realized by using multi-cored fiber optics to connect a light path from the actual point source to the point source in Fig. 1, and to connect the imaging plane in Fig. 1 to the actual photo detector.

This configuration has distinct advantages over the conventional design [7,8] in which the light source and the sensing device are placed on separate bases and their relative displacement is measured. Firstly, displacement is magnified by a factor of two (higher precision). Secondly, the encoder lens movement along the optical axis has little influence on the displacement measurement (axial independence). Thirdly and equally important for our purpose, there is no need for fiber to be connected to the vibrating component. As a result, oscillation of the fiber optics has no or little effect on the measurement (mechanical independence).

2.2 Experimental Set-Up

We have evaluated the accuracy of the two-dimensional micrometry. Shown in Fig. 2 is the schematic diagram of an experimental set-up constructed for this purpose. Light signal emitted from a point-source red LED (Alpha-One Electronics Co., VS679TM) is condensed by the emission lens (Nihon Sheet Glass Co., W18-S0290-063-ABC) and enters the multi-cored emission fiber (Keyence Co., FU-77) whose end-faces are carefully polished. The light emitted from the other end of the emission fiber, is condensed again by the encoder lens (the same

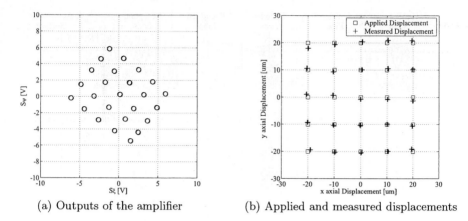

(a) Outputs of the amplifier   (b) Applied and measured displacements

Fig. 3. Evaluation of the two-dimensional optical micrometry

model as the emission lens). The encoder lens is mounted on a three-axis block stage (Sigma Koki Co., TSD-405C), and thus its minute displacement causes the lens to move minutely. As derived in equation (2), translational displacement of the encoder lens results in a shift of the focus location.

The light distribution of imaging plane is transmitted through the reception fiber (the same model as the emission fiber) with multiple cores. Light signal emitted from the other end of the reception fiber is condensed by the reception lens (the same model as the emission lens), and is finally focused onto the quadrant photo diode surface (Moririka Co., MI-1515H-4D). Both emission and reception optical fibers are 10 meters long and have 217 cores.

The output current from each photo diode segment is amplified with the I-V converter composed of an operational amplifier (Analog Devices Inc., OP400). The outputs from these four photo diode segments are fed to instrumentation amplifiers (Texas Instruments Inc., INA105), which compute,

$$\begin{cases} S_\xi = (S_1 + S_4) - (S_2 + S_3) \\ S_\psi = (S_1 + S_2) - (S_3 + S_4) \end{cases} \tag{3}$$

If the shift of the image of the point source is sufficiently minute, (dX, dY) and (S_ξ, S_ψ) are related with a linear transformation, and then (dx, dy) is obtained by the two-dimensional version of equation (2).

2.3   Evaluation

Accuracy of the two-dimensional micrometry was examined by the following procedure.

1. Move the encoder lens within a plane perpendicular to the optical axis, find the position at which both amplifier outputs, S_ξ and S_ψ, become nearly zero, and define that position as the sensor origin.

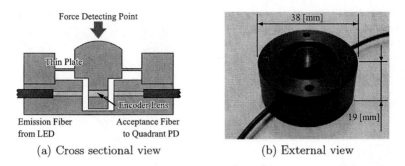

(a) Cross sectional view   (b) External view

Fig. 4. Structure of the developed optical force sensor

2. Move the encoder lens at 5×5 grid positions $(0, \pm10$ and ±20 μm), centered at the sensor origin. At each of 25 positions, outputs of the amplifier are sampled 100 times.

Figure 3-(a) plots the outputs of the differential amplifier at the grid positions. It shows the 100 data samples. Because of the relative rotation between the axes of the three-axis stage and the axes of the quadrant photo diode, there is rotation between the x-y space and the ξ-ψ space.

The lens displacement is modeled by a linear transformation of the outputs of the differential amplifier.

$$\begin{pmatrix} dx \\ dy \\ 1 \end{pmatrix} = \begin{pmatrix} c_{11} & c_{12} & c_{13} \\ c_{21} & c_{22} & c_{23} \\ 0 & 0 & 1 \end{pmatrix} \begin{pmatrix} S_\xi \\ S_\psi \\ 1 \end{pmatrix} = C_m \begin{pmatrix} S_\xi \\ S_\psi \\ 1 \end{pmatrix} \tag{4}$$

The calibration matrix C_m is estimated by least square method using reference data set. Figure 3-(b) shows the result; the relation between the applied displacement and the measured displacement. It also shows the 100 data samples. While there is distortion caused by the large lens displacement in the upper left of the square, the accuracy of the measurement is better than 1.0 % at the other points. We can confirm high linearity, high axial independency and high repeatability of the proposed micrometry from this plot.

3   MR-Compatible Force Sensor

We have designed an MR-compatible force sensor that uses the optical micrometry described in the previous section for displacement sensing. We have evaluated its accuracy and sensitivity in force measurement, and confirmed its MR compatibility.

3.1   Structure

Figure 4-(a) shows the cross sectional view of the force sensor. The force detector at the center is supported by a 0.4 mm-thick annular plate. It converts the

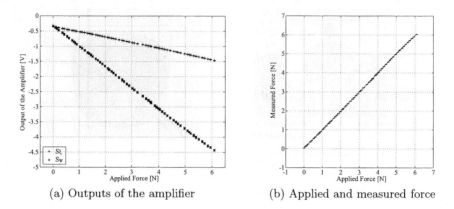

(a) Outputs of the amplifier   (b) Applied and measured force

Fig. 5. Evaluation of the developed optical force sensor

applied force (downward direction in this figure) into minute displacement of the encoder lens that is connected to it at the bottom. For the encoder lens, we use a gradient index (GRIN) lens (Nihon Sheet Glass Co., W18-S0290-063-ABC) because its small dimension and short focal length help reduce the entire size of the force sensor.

Shown in Fig. 4-(b) is the external view of the force sensor. The sensing module is 38 mm in diameter and 19 mm in height. It is made of a polyoxymethylene resin to reduce the affect of the magnetic field and the RF pulse of MRI. Note that this sensor head component corresponds to the middle part in Fig. 2, which is free from any magnetic or electronic elements.

Other optical components (including the fiber optics, LED, photo diode and optical lenses) and the differential amplifier are the same as those of the experimental set-up described in 2.2, except that the light source and the quadrant photo diode are supported by small, two-axis block stages (Sigma Koki Co., TASB-152) for zero-alignment of the optical axis.

3.2   Evaluation

Figure 5-(a) plots the outputs of the differential amplifier with respect to the applied force. It shows the 100 data samples collected in each condition. Figure 5-(b) shows the relation between the applied force and the measured force. It shows the mean and variance of the 100 data samples. The accuracy is better than 1.0 %. The maximum displacement of the encoder lens is less than 10 μm under the applied force ranging from 0 to 6 N.

We have confirmed that the accuracy and the rigidity of the developed force sensor is equivalent to that of commercially available force sensors. However, since the sensor module is made of a polyoxymethylene resin, hysteresis cannot be ignored if the applied force is greater than the rated force. Furthermore, the natural frequency of the force sensor is about ten times lower compared with the force sensors made of metallic materials.

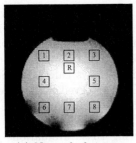   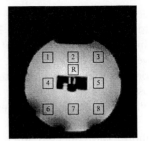

(a) Normal phantom   (b) Sensor-installed phantom

Fig. 6. Cross sectional images of cylindrical phantoms

Table 1. Signal to noise ratio (SNR) of the obtained images and SNR losses induced by the force sensor

Window number	1	2	3	4	5	6	7	8
SNR (Normal phantom)	20.65	15.27	18.26	23.81	35.18	20.99	20.22	26.52
SNR (Sensor-installed phantom)	20.40	14.80	17.93	23.57	34.28	20.42	19.69	26.13
SNR loss (%)	1.21	3.11	1.77	1.03	2.55	2.72	2.63	1.45

3.3   Evaluation of MR Compatibility

We have evaluated the loss of homogeneity of the magnetic field and the losses of signal-to-noise ratio (SNR) of the obtained images caused by the insertion of the force sensor. Two types of phantoms were imaged using 2T experimental MRI with 310 mm bore: one is a normal phantom that is a cylindrical plastic bottle filled with deionized water; and the other is a sensor-installed phantom that is the same as the normal phantom except that the force sensor is installed at the center. The phantoms were placed at the center of the MRI bore. The imaging sequence is gradient echo, TE/TR = 5/500 msec, FOV = 160 × 160 mm, and slice thickness is 2 mm.

The inhomogeneity is defined by the diversity of the observed spectrum. Inhomogeneity of the magnetic field caused by the insertion of the force sensor is 0.61 ppm, which is almost identical to the inhomogeneity 0.54 ppm when the normal phantom is placed.

Figure 6-(a) and (b) show MR images of the normal phantom and the sensor-installed phantom, respectively. In both figures, rectangular image windows for calculation of the SNR are also shown. There is no apparent distortion in the image of the sensor-installed phantom. The SNR is calculated using the following equation,

$$SNR = m_r/\sigma \tag{5}$$

where m_r is the mean value of the 10×10 pixel reference window, and σ is the standard deviation of the 10×10 pixel test window. Though, ideally the reference window should be placed at the center of the phantom, it was selected a little above the center as shown R in Fig. 6 in order to avoid including pixels of the sensor. Test windows are 1 to 8. Table 1 shows calculated SNR values and their losses caused by the force sensor. The observed SNR losses are 1.03 to 3.11 %, which are sufficiently lower than the maximum acceptable SNR loss, 10 % [3].

Furthermore, the collected force data during these evaluations are undisturbed by the magnetic field and the RF pulses. These results indicate that MRI has little influence on the sensor, and also the force sensor has little influence on the imaging sequence of MRI. The developed force sensor is confirmed to be highly MR-compatible.

4   Conclusion

An MR-compatible force sensor based on the new optical micrometry has been developed. Results of the evaluation have indicated that the micrometry is accurate and sensitive enough to be used for force sensing. Correspondingly, the developed force sensor is accurate, rigid and MR-compatible. We expect that the sensor is useful for studying human's force in the area of anatomical and brain functions using MRI.

The authors would gracefully acknowledge Dr. Homma for his assists in conducting experiments for evaluation of MR compatibility.

References

1. Chinzei, K., et al.: MR compatibility of mechatronic devices: Design criteria. In: Proc. of Second Int'l Conf. on MICCAI. (1999) 1020–1031
2. Masamune, K., et al.: Development of an MRI-compatible needle insertion manipulator for stereotactic nuerosurgery. J. of Image Guided Surgery 1 (1995) 242–248
3. Chinzei, K., et al.: MR compatible surgical assist robot: system integration and preliminary feasibility study. In: Proc. of Third Int'l Conf. on MICCAI. (2000) 921–930
4. Chenevert, T.L., et al.: Elasticity reconstructive imaging by means of stimulated echo MRI. J. of Magn. Reson. Med. 39 (1998) 482–490
5. Ehrsson, H.H., et al.: Cortical activity in precision-versus power-grip tasks: An fMRI study. J. of Neurophysiol. 83 (2000) 528–536
6. Liu, J.Z., et al.: Simultaneous measurement of human joint force, surface electromyograms, and functional MRI-measured brain activation. J. of Neurosciece Method 101 (2000) 49–57
7. Tada, M., et al.: Development of an optical 2-axis force sensor usable in MRI environments. In: Proc. of Int'l Conf. on Sensors. (2002)
8. Takahashi, N., et al.: An optical 6-axis force sensor for brain function analysis using fMRI. In: Proc. of Int'l Conf. on Sensors. (2003)
9. Hirose, S., et al.: Development of optical 6-axial force sensor and its signal calibration considering non-linear interference. In: Proc. of Int'l Conf. on Advanced Robotics. (1990) 46–53

Flexible Needle Steering and Optimal Trajectory Planning for Percutaneous Therapies

Daniel Glozman and Moshe Shoham

Medical Robotics Laboratory, Mechanical Engineering Department,
Technion – Israel Institute of Technology, Israel, 32000
{glozmand, shoham}@technion.ac.il
http://robotics.technion.ac.il

Abstract. Flexible needle insertion into viscoelastic tissue is modeled in this paper with a linear beam supported by virtual springs. Using this simplified model, the forward and inverse kinematics of the needle is solved analytically, providing a way for simulation and path planning in real-time. Using the inverse kinematics, the required needle basis trajectory can be computed for any desired needle tip path. It is shown that the needle base trajectory is not unique and can be optimized to minimize lateral pressure of the needle body on the tissue. Experimental results are provided of robotically assisted insertion of flexible needle while avoiding "obstacle".

1 Introduction

The current trend of contemporary medicine is less invasiveness and localized therapy. One of the most common procedures employed in modern clinical practice involves percutaneous insertion of needles and catheters for biopsy and drug delivery. Percutaneous procedures involving needle insertions include vaccinations, blood/fluid sampling, regional anesthesia, tissue biopsy, catheter insertion, cryogenic ablation, electrolytic ablation, brachytherapy, neurosurgery, deep brain stimulation, minimally invasive surgeries and more.

Complications are due, in large part, to poor technique and needle placement [1]. Physicians and surgeons often rely only upon kinesthetic feedback from the tool, correlated with their own mental 3-D visualization of anatomic structures. It was shown in [2], that as the needle penetrates the tissue, the tissue deforms and even straight needles miss the target. Thick and nonflexible needles are easily pointed to the target in the existence of visualization system, but their manipulation causes significant pressure on the tissue. Moreover, straight needles are not suitable for following curved paths, if obstacle avoidance is required.

These problems can be solved by introducing thin and flexible needles. Moreover, it is known that thinner needles cause less pain to the patient. On the other hand, flexible needle navigation deep inside the tissue is very complicated. The system has non-minimum phase behavior and does not lend itself to intuitive control. Path planning for flexible needle insertion and obstacles avoidance inside the body tissue is a challenging problem of mechanics and robotics. Creating an automated system that

C. Barillot, D.R. Haynor, and P. Hellier (Eds.): MICCAI 2004, LNCS 3217, pp. 137–144, 2004.

can plan and perform thin, flexible needle insertion will minimize misplacements, and reduce both risks and patient suffering.

Needle insertion causes the surrounding soft tissues to displace and deform. Di-Maio *et al.* used finite elements simulation for determining such displacements [2]. Using this approach, Alteroviz *et al.* suggest a way to predict needle placement error in prostate brachyterapy procedure and to correct for this error by choosing an appropriate straight needle insertion point [4]. Because of its complexity, the method does not allow online correction of the placement error.

Current methods and techniques all use straight, rigid needles since they are easier to control and their trajectory is well defined. On the other hand, it is known that thinner needles cause less damage and reduce post puncture outcome, as in Post Dural Puncture Headache (PDPH) appearing after spinal anesthesia. As a general rule, the relative risk of PDPH decreases with each successive reduction in needle diameter [5]. Thinner needles are more flexible and thus results in less pressure and damage to the tissue. They allow making curved trajectories and accomplishing easier obstacle avoidance. They are, however, very difficult to control.

An active, flexible steering system using shape memory alloys has been suggested in [6] for a steering catheter. Such a system is not suitable for thin needle navigation because of size limitations. Kataoka *et al.* investigated needle deflection due to the bevel of the tip during linear needle insertion and expressed the deflection as function of driving force [7].

Flexible needle steering was first addressed by DiMaio *et al.* [3]. To solve the inverse kinematics of the needle, iterative numerical computing of the flexible needle's Jacobian is suggested. The computation involves solving for two-dimensional finite element mesh of the tissue and iterative nonlinear flexion of a beam and requires nine independent computations for devising the Jacobian elements. The computation complexity does not allow real-time simulation and control of the system.

The present investigation suggests a simplified model that allows fast path planning and real time tracking for the needle insertion procedure. The future goal of this work is the creation of an image based closed loop system for automatic flexible needle insertion. The concept is described in 2-D space.

2   The Virtual Springs Model

Modeling of a flexible needle is based in this investigation on the assumption of quasistatic motion, so the needle is in equilibrium state at each step. It is known that biologic soft tissue deflection is nonlinear with strain, but for small displacements, locally, we can assume linear lateral force response, based on the work of Simone *et al.* [8] and [9]. The tissue forces on the needle are modeled as lateral virtual springs distributed along the needle curve plus friction forces tangent to the needle. Since the tissue elastic modulus differs as a function of strain, we update the virtual spring's coefficients according to the elastic modulus corresponding to the current strain, and linearize the system at each step. The concept is illustrated in Figure 1.

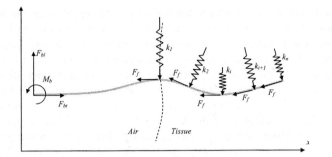

Fig. 1. Virtual springs model: the tissue's reaction is modeled by distributed virtual springs.

As the shape of the needle changes, the location and orientation of the virtual springs change as well. Locally, at each step, the linearized system model yields the shape of the needle at this step. There is no physical meaning for the free length of the virtual springs, and the only important parameter of the spring is the local stiffness coefficient, which expresses the force of the tissue on the needle as a function of local displacement. The stiffness coefficients of the virtual springs are determined either experimentally or by using preoperative images by assuming empiric values for known tissues and organs.

The Linearized System Solution

Initially, assuming small displacements, we approximate the needle by a linear beam subjected to point forces as shown on Figure 2. With appropriate elements spacing, this approximation is close to the flexible beam on elastic foundation model.

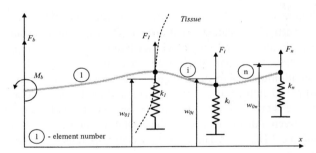

Fig. 2. Linear system model. Flexible beam subjected to a number of virtual springs.

At each joint, the force applied by the virtual spring is proportional to the spring's displacement from its initial position:

$$F_i = k_i \left(w_i - w_{0i} \right) \tag{1}$$

where k_i is the virtual spring coefficient, w_i - displacement at point i, and w_{0i} - is the position of freed spring i.

Since the forces are a function of the deflection, this problem cannot be solved by superposition. It can be solved only globally for all the elements of the beam. We define each element as the part of the beam between two neighboring forces. Thus the first element is the part of the needle outside of the tissue, and the rest of the elements are distributed along the inner part according to the level of discretization. Each element behaves as a linear beam subjected to shearing forces at its borders. Since we assume linear flexible beam, the displacement of each element is given by a third degree polynomial. We adopt the nodal degrees of freedom from finite elements theory, in which the coordinates are specifically identified with a single nodal point and represent a displacement or rotation, having clear physical interpretation. The displacement $y(x)$ will have the form of:

$$y(x) = N_1\phi_1 + N_2\phi_2 + N_3\phi_3 + N_4\phi_4 \tag{2}$$

N_1, N_3 are the coordinates and N_2, N_4 are the slopes at $x=0$ and $x=l$ of an element, respectively. ϕ_i are the shape functions of third degree.

Substituting boundary conditions as displacement and slope at the base and tip of the needle, the result is $4 \times n$ equations - 2 at each side and 4 for each internal node, which yields the global matrix equation:

$$[K]\overline{N} = \overline{Q} \tag{3}$$

where K is the matrix of coefficients of $N_{i,j}$ - elements degrees of freedom. N is the vector of $N_{i,j}$, where i is the number of the element and j is the number of degrees of freedom, Q are the free coefficients.

The 3 DOF Forward Kinematics

The above solution solves for the displacements and rotations of the needle for 2 DOF of needle base - vertical translation y and slope θ. But the main translation of the needle is in x - axial direction. Applying axial translation to the non-compressible needle means that the outside tissue part of the needle becomes shorter by the size of translation x. And an additional element of length x is added to the last element. Assuming that the last $(n+1)$ element is relatively small, and the forces on it create negligible moments, its shape is taken as a straight line, having the slope of the last element.

In summary, given 3 displacements of the 3 DOF of the needle's base, we are now able to calculate the 3 DOF translations of the needle tip, thus completing the forward kinematics solution.

The 3 DOF Inverse Kinematics

In an actual needle insertion problem, the essence is the trajectory following by the needle's tip. First, there is a need to hit the target with the tip; second, the obstacle organs should be avoided. This is the problem of inverse kinematics; namely, for given position and orientation of the tip, calculate the translation and orientation of the needle base.

Let us expand the matrix of equation (3):

$$
\begin{bmatrix}
1 & 0 & \cdots & 0 & 0 \\
0 & -1 & \cdots & 0 & 0 \\
& \tilde{K}_{21} & & \tilde{K}_{22} &
\end{bmatrix}
\begin{pmatrix}
N_{11} \\
N_{12} \\
\vdots \\
N_{n3} \\
N_{n4}
\end{pmatrix}
=
\begin{pmatrix}
Y \\
\theta \\
\vdots \\
\vdots \\
\vdots
\end{pmatrix}
\tag{4}
$$

In the forward kinematics, given the base translation Y and rotation θ, one can solve for $N_{i,j}$. Note that the last two elements of vector N are the translation and rotation of the tip. But in the inverse kinematics problem, the translation and rotation of the tip - N_{n3}, N_{n4} are known and the unknowns are the translation and rotation of the base - Y and θ or N_{11} and N_{12}. Since in the last two equations the two variables are known, we can write (4) as:

$$
\left[\tilde{K}_{21} \right] \tilde{\overline{N}} = \tilde{\overline{Q}} - \tilde{K}_{22} \begin{pmatrix} N_{n3} \\ N_{n4} \end{pmatrix}
\tag{5}
$$

$$
Y = N_{11}
$$

$$
\theta = N_{12}
$$

where $\tilde{\overline{N}}, \tilde{\overline{Q}}$ are the original vectors $\overline{N}, \overline{Q}$ without the last two elements. $\tilde{K}_{21}$ is

(n-2)×(n-2) matrix and equation (5) can be solved for $\tilde{\overline{N}}$ and therefore for Y and θ, which is the solution of the inverse kinematics.

Path Planning

The simple linear path is straightforward. The main challenge is avoiding obstacles, while applying minimal pressure on the tissue, especially vital organs. In the presence of obstacles, the best path should require minimal curvature of the needle. The path planning problem thus reduces to finding the shortest curve, connecting the target and needle insertion point, and avoiding obstacles. It can either be defined by the algorithm or constrained by the doctor.

Trajectory Tracking and Optimization

Trajectory tracking problem means computation of the needle base position and orientation for a given tip trajectory. To solve this problem, full simulation of needle insertion is required, since every step is dependent on the previous history of insertion. Here we will concentrate on one tracking method - moving the tip from one given position and orientation to another position. As explained above, it is possible to reach the desired position with various tip orientations. Since in the needle insertion procedure, orientation of the tip is of less importance, one can reach the desired position with different allowed tip orientations to accomplish the task. For example we require that the needle stay as straight as possible in order to keep minimal pressure on the tissue. The sum of the needle deflections is given by S:

$$S = \min \sum_{i=1}^{n} \left(w_i^2 + \theta_i^2 \right) = \min \sum_{i=1}^{n} \sum_{j=1}^{4} N_{ij}^2 \tag{6}$$

Nodes displacements are a function of desired tip orientation from (5). To get the minimum of S, we differentiate (6) for θ_t and equalize to zero:

$$\frac{dS}{d\theta_t} = \sum_{i=1}^{n} \sum_{j=1}^{4} 2N_{ij} \frac{dN_{ij}}{d\theta_t} = 0 \tag{7}$$

The slope of the last element N_{4n} is not known, hence there is one more unknown than equations. Instead, we add the minimization equation (7), so that the number of unknown variables equals the number of equations.

3 Needle Insertion Simulation

As the needle penetrates deeper into the tissue, additional virtual springs are introduced. The following example simulates needle tip sine wave tracking, thus avoiding an obstacle in the tissue. For simplicity, we draw the virtual springs as a compressible mesh below and above the needle, since the tissue is on both sides. The trajectory, where the tip is forced to be tangent to the trajectory is shown in Figure 3. An optimized for minimal tissue pressure trajectory is shown in Figure 4.

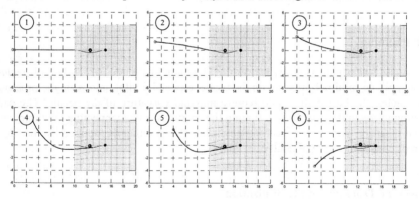

Fig. 3. Simulating needle insertion for tip oriented tangent to the path.

The simulation starts with one element beam of 100 mm length, at step 1. With each advancement of 10 mm into the tissue, the element is subdivided, adding a new element of 10 mm and a virtual spring at the tip of the needle. At the 6th step, there are 6 elements and 6 virtual springs.

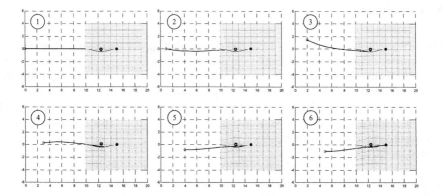

Fig. 4. Simulating needle insertion while minimizing pressure on the tissue.

4 Qualitative Experiment

We performed a qualitative experiment using the RSPR parallel robot [10] as shown in Figure 5. For the tissue we used chicken breast slice of 8mm thickness and the needle is a spinal 22G×90mm – outer diameter 0.711mm, connected through ATI Nano17 6DOF force sensor. With proper lighting it was possible to see through the tissue and to obtain images of reasonable quality. The tissue is placed in a 100mm×100mm frame and constrained in one plane between two glass plates. The stiffness coefficient of the virtual springs was experimentally evaluated by needle force measurement to 60 N/m.

Two metal pieces were inserted into the tissue prior to the experiment – one for the target and one for the obstacle. The robot was required to follow the path, computed with the above algorithm, avoiding the obstacle and hitting the target. The images corresponding to steps 1,3,4,6 of simulation shown in Figure 4 are shown in Figure 5. As can be observed, the path followed by the needle tip is similar to the preplanned.

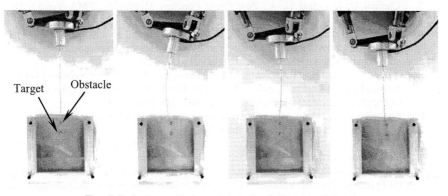

Fig. 5. Robotic needle insertion at simulation steps 1,3,4,6.

5 Conclusion

This investigation develops the planar linearized model approximation for the flexible needle insertion problem with small deflections. Using this model, the inverse and forward kinematics of needle insertion can be solved in one step, solving a low dimensional linear system of equations. Path planning and its optimization for minimal tissue pressure were developed. It was found that this model can be solved in a closed form for a given tip point trajectory. Relaxing the requirement that tip orientation be tangent to path at each point greatly decreases both the base stroke and the pressure exerted on the tissue.

It may also be stressed that the ability to control the needle by its bending decreases deeper in the tissue and other techniques may be suggested.

We performed a qualitative experiment confirming the proposed concept. The needle trajectory was similar to the preplanned, avoiding an obstacle and hitting a target. Future research is focused on nonlinear beam approximation and close loop control utilizing an imaging system.

Acknowledgment. We thank Gábor Kósa and Micha Adler for their assistance with experiments.

References

1. De Andres J., Reina M.A., Lopez-Garcia A., Risks of regional anesthesia: Role of equipment - Needle design, catheters, VII Annual, European Society of Regional Anaesthesia Congress, Geneva Sept. 16 - 19, 1998
2. DiMaio S. P. and Salcudean S. E., Needle Insertion Modeling and Simulation, IEEE Transactions on Robotics and Automation: Special Issue on Medical Robotics, October 2003.
3. DiMaio S. P. and Salcudean S. E., Needle Steering and Model-Based Trajectory Planning, Proceedings of Medical Image Computing and Computer-Assisted Intervention, Montreal, 2003.
4. Alterovitz R., Pouliot J., Taschereau R., Hsu I. J., Goldberg K.. Sensorless Planning for Medical Needle Insertion Procedures. Proceedings of the 2003 IEEE/RSJ International Conference on Intelligent Robots and Systems (IROS 2003), October 2003
5. Chohan U, Hamdani G. A., Post Dural Puncture Headache, JPMA Vol:53, No.8 August 2003.
6. Mineta, T., Mitsui, T., Watanabe, Y., Kobayashi, S., Haga, Y., Esashi, M.: Batch fabricated flat meandering shape memory alloy actuator for active catheter. In: Sensors and Actuators A: Physical. Volume 88. (2001) 112–120
7. Kataoka, H.,Washio, T., Audette, M., Mizuhara, K.: A Model for Relations between Needle Deflection, Force, and Thickness on Needle Penetration. In: Medical Image Computing and Computer Aided Intervention. (2001) 966–974
8. Simone C., Modeling of needle insertion forces for percutaneous therapies, M.Sc. Thesis, Johns Hopkins University, May 2002.
9. Fung Y.C., Biomechanics: Mechanics Properties of Living tissues, 2nd ed., New York: Springer-Verlag, 1993, pp.277.
10. Simaan, N., Glozman, D., Shoham, M., "Design Considerations of New Six Degrees-Of-Freedom Parallel Robots." IEEE International Conference on Robotics and Automation, 1998, Vol. 2, pp. 1327-1333.

CT and MR Compatible Light Puncture Robot: *Architectural Design and First Experiments*

Elise Taillant[1,2], Juan-Carlos Avila-Vilchis[1,3], Christophe Allegrini[1], Ivan Bricault[1,4], and Philippe Cinquin[1]

[1] Laboratoire TIMC-IMAG, Equipe GMCAO, 38706 La Tronche CEDEX, France,
[elise.taillant,philippe.cinquin]@imag.fr
[2] PRAXIM Medivision SA, 38700 La Tronche, France
[3] Universidad Autónoma del Estado de México 50130, Toluca, Mexico
[4] Service Central d'Imagerie Médicale CHU Grenoble. 38700 La Tronche, France [‡]

Abstract. This paper presents a new robotic architecture designed to perform interventional CT/MR procedures, particularly punctures. Such procedures are very popular nowadays for diagnostic or therapeutic purposes. Innovations concerning the robotic architecture, materials and energy sources are exposed. We also introduce the control loop we use to check the movements and the positioning of the robot, including a new method to localize the robot thanks to the images coming from the imaging devices (CT or MRI). Finally, the results of the first experiments are presented.

1 Introduction

CT/MR image-guided interventional procedures are becoming more and more popular, either for diagnostic or therapeutic purposes. Many types of image-guided biopsies are performed routinely, and new percutaneous techniques such as radiofrequency treatment allow efficient tumor ablations with reduced trauma and short recovery time. Nevertheless, even with MR or CT image guidance, the precise insertion of biopsy needles or tumor ablation applicators remains a challenging task. Since it is difficult for physicians to reproduce accurately an oblique 3D path, they often restrict needle trajectories to vertical insertions parallel to the image plane. This can limit the possibility of targeting a lesion while avoiding critical structures. Furthermore, physicians usually do not benefit from a real-time imaging feedback during the procedure, either because they want to avoid CT radiation exposure when they manipulate the needle, or because real-time imaging is not available. As a consequence, the needle insertion procedure requires that physicians switch many times between the patient and the image display room, as they achieve a succession of small needle movements and control imaging acquisitions. This causes an important loss of time. Moreover, without real-time imaging control, it is difficult to adapt the trajectory to soft tissue and

---

[‡] We would like to thank the Radiology Department (Pr. Coulomb) and the Magnetic Resonance Unit (Pr. Le Bas) of Grenoble's University Hospital for their kind assistance in the experiments.

C. Barillot, D.R. Haynor, and P. Hellier (Eds.): MICCAI 2004, LNCS 3217, pp. 145–152, 2004.
© Springer-Verlag Berlin Heidelberg 2004

organ deformations along the needle path. Finally, a precise achievement of the planned trajectory often relies on multiple trials and needle repositioning that may cause more trauma than expected to the patient. Since a few years, systems and methods have been thought up in order to improve needle placement accuracy and to reduce interventions durations as well as radiation exposition. Non-automated methods were invented to help the physicians to perform their task such as the image overlay system with enhanced reality presented in [1] by Masamune et al. or the laser beam guidance for interventional CT by Gangi et al. [2] which allows oblique insertions by aligning the needle with the laser beam. These two methods help physicians to perform a more accurate insertion of the needle but still do not eliminate radiations exposure of the physician.

In the past few years, robots, either guided by physicians with joysticks or autonomous but under physician supervision, have been developped as well as various methods of registration to guide the robot and check its position. In [3], a method for CT guided needle placement is proposed and consists of a localization module (a Brown-Roberts-Well frame) placed on a needle-holding end-effector to localize the effector in the image space using a single CT image. A single cross-section of the frame corresponds to a unique position of the end-effector and allows consequently to know the position of the needle in the body of the patient. This localization method combined with Stoianovici et al. work on a needle driver and a robotic system [4] is used to perform percutaneous interventions [5]. Patriciu et al., in [6], present a robot and needle positioning technique based on laser alignment which does not require any CT image and thus does not expose the patient to radiations but cannot be used to check needle orientation during interventions. Although these methods are proved to work well, most of them were designed for classical robotic arms which are unwieldy in a scanner room, worrisome for the patient and difficult to implement under MR environments.

Several MR compatible devices used to perform biopsies already exist and work well. ROBITOM [7] is a MR compatible robot which works in the isocenter of a closed high-field MR system but it is dedicated only to breast biopsy and therapy and one of its degrees of freedom is manually controlled. Chinzei et al in [8], present a MR compatible surgical assistance robot which is designed to cooperate with a surgeon and position a tool such as a laser pointer or a biopsy catheter. Some drawbacks of this system are that it works only with an opened MR system which implies a bad image quality and that it is quite cumbersome. A MR compatible manipulator for transrectal prostate biopsy with a remote manual actuation is presented in [10] and [9].

The work presented here focuses on a new CT/MRI compatible robotic architecture (LPR for Light Puncture Robot) interdependent of the patient's body, intrinsically compliant, and designed to perform puncture interventions. We also describe the control loop based on images coming from the imaging system and used to check LPR's position and orientation.

Usually punctures are performed for tumoral pathologies. In these cases, lesions smaller than 1cm are hardly characterized and usually followed up rather than treated. Consequently, our goal is to be able to reach targets larger than 1cm.

2   Material and Methods

2.1   Robot Architecture

The LPR possesses 5 DOF (Degree Of Freedom). The platform provides the mechanical support to perform translation thanks to 4 straps bound to the platform on one side and to a support frame on the other side where the actuators for each strap are situated. Translation is performed over the patient's body, which gives a natural orientation to the robot (see fig. 1).

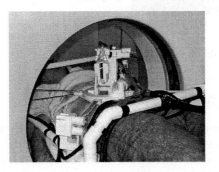

Fig. 1. Robot on Patient Inside CT Gantry

This architecture provides intrinsic compensation of the physiological movements of the patient i.e. the robot follows patient's abdomen movements such as breathing. The robot base can rotate w.r.t. (with respect to) an axis normal to the patient's body thus defining the azimuthal angle $\theta \in [0; 2\pi]$. This rotation is performed in both directions without restrictions. The trocar holder rotates with the base and has a proper rotation (w.r.t the robot's base) defining the polar angle $\phi \in [-\frac{\pi}{18}; \frac{\pi}{3}]$. Each motion is performed by a couple of pneumatic actuators powered by compressed air at the pressure of 3.5 bar. Each actuator is composed of a piston which can drag with an associated sprocket wheel (see fig. 2). This movement is possible only in one direction thus permitting to block the robot in a certain position. Each cylinder possesses two compressed air inlets, one on each of its sides. Air is alternatively injected in each compartment and makes the piston move and push the sprocket wheel by one increment thus the movement is very easily and precisely controlled. A worm is assembled to the sprocket wheel axis and works with its corresponding gear. For each movement the opposite direction is achieved by the complementary actuator. For translation, the actuators have a pulley that allows the straps to be entangled/disentangled. A simple pneumatic actuator is used for the trocar clamping task. In order to perforate the skin, another simple actuator allows a 2cm fast translation of the trocar.

Plastic materials used construct the LPR are MR compatible and completely transparent under MRI, they do not create artifacts under CT scanner. The robot only weighs 1kg. The valving system which controls the actuators is linked to them by 7m long plastic tubes thus allowing it not to be in the CT/MR room.

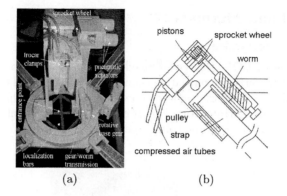

(a)   (b)

Fig. 2. (a)Light puncture robot, main part, (b) Schema of actuators

2.2 Localization Module

Because of LPR's medical applications under CT/MRI environment, it is not possible to use sensors to control its movements and position. Optical or magnetic localizers are not suitable for MRI and furthermore do not give a real feedback as tissues deformations and organ movements are not taken into account. Images coming from the imaging device (CT or MRI) are the best feedback and are consequently used in our application to close the control loop.

Localization is done thanks to the localization module we designed which is totally integrated into the robot architecture and is composed of two parts. The first one is a 7.5cm long and 1.6mm thick square frame (and its diagonals), made of epoxy resin charged with fibreglass. This frame is screwed to the rotating base of the robot so that its center is merged with the entry point. A small drilled ball at the center of the frame allows to let the needle go through the frame's diagonals and to position the needle in the correct direction. That frame is used to determine the position of the entry point of the robot as well as the rotation of LPR's rotating base w.r.t the scanner. The second part is a 1.6cm x 1.6cm x 6.2cm Delrin acetal resin made bar screwed to the needle-holder. It allows to compute the inclination of the needle-holder w.r.t the robot's base and the scanner. For MR applications the same module is used except that all the bars are replaced by small tubes filled with water.

2.3 Image Based Control of the Robot

At the beginning of the procedure, a physician chooses the target he wants to reach and the entry point on a first set of images. Setting these two points implies setting the trajectory the needle will follow and so the orientation/position the robot must take to respect the trajectory. When both the trajectory is defined and a first localization of the robot is done, thus giving the initial position, the shortest trajectory from the initial position to the required position is computed. The robot then moves to the choosen position and orientation. When the movement is done, the position/orientation is checked thanks to the images feedback.

Images are processed and a localization algorithm is applied. If the detected position/orientation is not correct, the robot is moved again and its new position is checked and so on until the desired position is reached.

Image Processing: Depending on the angle between the images and the robot, images will contain either a trace corresponding to the Delrin bar or traces left by the frame (from 2 up to 4 ellipses) or both. As the grey level response of Delrin is different from the grey level response of epoxy, the image processing applied to get the objects depends on the object we want to detect. In both cases, two steps are essential to correctly detect objects. The first step is an estimation of the position of the objects and consists of a hard thresholding followed by morphological operations in order to clear out small objects. We then apply a priori knowledge on the size and on the geometry of the localization device to get the points we are interested in. When the objects' position are approximately found, a second step is performed on the original image to improve the localization in which only small areas around detected points are processed.

Robot Localization: A localization method, using only one slice (as it is done in [3]) which contains both the frame and the Delrin bar, was developed. This method was not used for our application for several reasons. First, using several images improves the precision of the localization. Then, since with MRI, there are no radiations, and since recent multislice CT scanners allow to take several slices at the same time, the acquisition of several images is not a real drawback. Furthermore, it allows the physician to be integrated in the control loop since he is able to see what happens thanks to the multiple slices that were acquired. For these reasons and depending on the position of the robot, we will use a set of images (at least two) to localize it. The only images we can implement are those in which we have detected at least three points for the frame in the image processing step. All the angles and coordinates in this section are to be understood w.r.t the scanner coordinates system, R_S. The angle θ, corresponding to the rotation of the robot's base w.r.t the scanner, is easily calculated from the equations of the diagonals and the sides of the square frame which are computed from the detected points.

The computation of the coordinates of the intersection of the two diagonals gives the coordinates of the entry point. If one of the equations of the diagonals is not possible to compute (only three points on image see fig. 3.a) then the entry point coordinates are computed as follows :

$$(O_X, O_Y, O_Z) = (L \times \frac{\sqrt{2}}{2} - d_2) \times \overrightarrow{V} + (B_{1_X}, B_{1_Y}, B_{1_Z}), \qquad (1)$$

$$\text{with } d_2 = \min(\|\overrightarrow{A_1 B_1}\|, \|\overrightarrow{B_1 D_1}\|) \times (|\cos(\theta)| + |\sin(\theta)|), \text{ (see fig.3.a)} . \qquad (2)$$

with (A_1, B_1, D_1) (respectively (A_2, B_2, D_2)) be the intersections between the first image (respectively the second image) and the frame (see fig. 3).

Finally, the inclination ϕ of the needle-holder w.r.t R_S is calculated. The equation of the line representing the inclination of the needle holder is determined from a set of points belonging both to the localization bar and the needle holder. We then compute the angle between this line and a vertical line. Depending on the

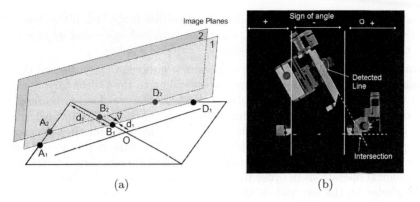

Fig. 3. (a) Image intersecting the frame in 3 points (b) sign of inclination angle

position of the intersection between this line and the base plane of the robot, we are able to determine if this angle is positive or negative (fig. 3.b).

3   Experiments and Results

Open-Loop Performance Experiments: These experiments consist of moving the robot to a particular position/attitude and check its positioning accuracy. They gave the following results assuming that the work surface is a plane. For strap-based translation, accuracy is about 5% of the displacement d (if $d = 20mm$ then the error is about 1mm). Rotation and inclination accuracy are less than 1°. Repeatability is less than 0.5mm for translation and 1° for rotation.

Image-Based Localization Experiments: Experiments on robot localization with CT images were performed to check accuracy. The middle of the frame corresponding to the point where the needle punctures the body is located with an approximate error of 1mm. The base rotation θ is determined with a mean error of 2° while the inclination angle Φ mean error is only 1° .

Phantom Experiments: Our first experiments on phantom took place at the Radiology Department of Grenoble's University Hospital. The CT Scanner used was a Siemens Somatom Volume Zoom. Our phantom is a foam rubber block (see fig. 4) in which we inserted a polyether-cetone disc with a 1cm hole as a target. The experiment consists of trying to reach the target hole from an unknown position and orientation of the robot with the control of images coming from the imaging device, without any intervention of a manipulator and with a limited number of robot movement/localization loop. We tried 6 punctures (2 vertical and 4 with an arbitrary orientation) starting from different initial attitudes/positions. The target point, i.e. the exact pixel that was chosen on the screen, was reached in all the cases with an error smaller than 2mm and the target disc hole was always reached. These results were obtained with a maximum of two image checking/robot movement loop including the initial localization.

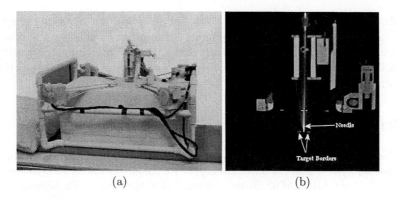

(a)   (b)

Fig. 4. (a) Robot on Phantom on scanner bed , (b) Vertical insertion result

4 Discussion

Open loop translation accuracy of the robot is satisfactory upon small distances (less than 30mm). Over this limit, the displacement is not as much accurate. Since the loop is closed by CT/MR image acquisition, it is possible to remain very accurate, as the the final movement will be less than 30mm.

Some improvements on angle determination with images must be done in order to correctly determine LPR's orientation. A more complex image processing might improve the accuracy.

The experiments on phantom, even if their results are not statistically significant, are very promising. Our goal, which was reaching a 1cm target without human intervention, is achieved in the particular experimental conditions described in sect. 3. It must now be proved that such results could be obtained in more difficult conditions i.e. on a non plane or moving phantom. In such conditions and in addition to problems caused by a non-plane geometry, needle deformations, which are not taken into account for the time being, might occur. In the case of a foam-rubber phantom, these are not significant. In real conditions, the needle curve might alter the precision of punctures.

One of the characteristics of LPR that has not yet been presented in this paper, is the possibility to release the needle from the clamp and grasp it again. This characteristic allows to let the needle follow the movements of patient's target organ while images are acquired, thus avoiding injuries. It also enables the robot to perform a deep insertion (when the target's distance from the entry point is greater than the needle-holder stroke) by releasing the needle and grasping it higher. This possibility has not been tested yet as our phantom is not mobile.

5 Conclusion and Future Work

A new light robot architecture for puncture is proposed in this paper. It is CT and MRI-compatible thanks to materials used to construct the robot and to its remote energy source. This robot uses pneumatic energy to perform translation, orientation and puncture. Experiments gave very promising results.

Future work will concern clinical validation. In a near future, experiments will be done on a non-plane and mobile phantom in order to validate the prototype in almost real conditions. Animals experiments, and later human experiments, will follow as some improvements concerning the easiness of use of the robot will be carried out.

References

1. Masamune, K., Fichtinger, G., Deguct, A., Matsuka, D. and Taylor, R. H.,*An Image Overlay System with Enhanced Reality for Percutaneous Therapy Performed inside CT Scanner*, MICCAI'02, Tokyo, Japan, LNCS 2489, pp. 77-84, September 2002.
2. Gangi, A., Kastler, B., Arhan, J. M., Klinkert, A., Grampp, J.M., Dietemann, J.L., *A compact laser beam guidance system for interventional CT*, J Comput Assist Tomogr. 1994 Mar-Apr;18(2):326-8.
3. Susil, R. C., Anderson, J. H. and Taylor, R. H., *A Single Image Registration Method for CT Guided Interventions*, MICCAI'99,Cambridge, England, LNCS 1679, pp. 798-808, September 1999.
4. Stoianovici, D. Cadeddu, J. A., Demaree, R. D., Basile, H. A., Taylor, R. H., Whitcomb, L. L., Sharpe, W. N. Jr. and Kavoussi, L. R., *An efficient needle injection technique and radiological guidance method for percutaneous procedures*, CVRMed-MRCAS'97, LNCS 1205, pp. 295-298, March 1997.
5. Masamune, K., Fichtinger, G., Patriciu, A., Susil, R., Taylor, R. H., Kavoussi, L. R., Anderson, J., Sakuma, I., Dohi, T. and Stoianovici, D., *System for Robotically Assisted Percutaneous Procedures With Computed Tomography Guidance*, Journal of Computer Assisted Surgery, Vol.6, No.6, pp.370-383, 2001.
6. Patriciu, A., Solomon, S., Kavoussi, L. and Stoianovici, D., *Robotic Kidney and Spine Percutaneous Procedures Using a New Laser-Based CT Registration Method*, MICCAI'01, The Netherlands, LNCS 2208, pp. 249-257, October 2001.
7. Kaiser, WA., Fisher, H., Vagner, J. and Selig, M. *Robotic System for Biopsy and Therapy of Breast Lesions in a High-Field Whole-Body Magnetic Resonance Tomography Unit*, Investigative Radiology, 35(8):513-519, August 2000.
8. Chinzei, K., Hata, N., Jolesz, F. and Kikinis, R., *MR Compatible Surgical Assist Robot: System Integration and Preliminary Feasibility Study*, LNCS 1935, MICCAI 2000, Oct 11-4, Pittsburgh, PA, pp. 921-30, 2000.
9. Fichtinger, G., Krieger, A., Susil , RC., Tanacs, A., Whitcomb, LL. and Atalar, E. *Transrectal Prostate Biopsy Inside Closed MRI Scanner with Remote Actuation, under Real-Time Image Guidance.* MICCAI'02, Tokyo, Japan, LNCS 2488, Part 1, pp 91-98, Springer Verlag, September 2002
10. Susil, RC., Krieger, A., Derbyshire, JA., Tanacs, A., Whitcomb, LL., Fichtinger, G. and Atalar, E., *System for MR Image-Guided Prostate Interventions: Canine Study* Radiology 2003; 228: 886-894.

Development of a Novel Robot-Assisted Orthopaedic System Designed for Total Knee Arthroplasty

Naohiko Sugita[1], Shin'ichi Warisawa[1], Mamoru Mitsuishi[1], Masahiko Suzuki[2],
Hideshige Moriya[2], and Koichi Kuramoto[3]

[1] University of the Tokyo, 7-3-1 Hongo Bunkyo-ku Tokyo, Japan
[2] Chiba University, 1-8-1 Inohana Chuo-ku Chiba, Japan
[3] Nakashima Propeller Co.,Ltd., 688-1 Jotokitakata Okayama, Japan

Abstract. Recently, the number of robot-assisted orthopaedic system which supports surgeon has increased. As one of the background, it is considered the difference between plan and result of the bone cutting is varied because the technique to resect bone is based on the ability of individual surgeon. And authors developed a robot to resect bone which has 9 degree of freedom, and as the result, the accuracy of bone cutting improved. Moreover, we developed a total operation system including pre-operative planning system and intra-operative assist system.

1 Introduction

In the total knee arthroplasty(TKA), the accuracy to set prosthesis affects the inferior limb direction after operation. If the prosthesis is not properly fixed, the post-operative pain, life time reduction of the prosthesis and organization necrosis caused by the abrasion powder may occur. Therefore, it is hoped to improve the accuracy of prosthesis position, and robots to support the bone resection have been introduced rapidly.

In this paper, a developed bone cutting robot which has multiple degrees of freedom is discussed. The movements of this equipment during the bone resection are restricted within the cut plane, and this function is realized by 2 axes for translation and 1 axis for rotation to avoid soft tissue like ligaments. High accuracy and safety are acquired by this technology. And this robot-assisted total knee arthroplasty system has a feature that surgeon can intervene and modify pre-operative plan during operation. It is difficult to judge the state of soft tissue clearly before the operation, and this system allows surgeon to intervene into the system interactively and to modify the pre-operative plan after incising the cutis. Finally, results of the improved bone cutting accuracy with some experiments are presented.

2 Related Work

Computer-assisted orthopaedic system is classified into two categories mainly.[1] One is what guides the portion to resect the bone and the position of prosthesis using navigation system with or without computer tomography .(for

C. Barillot, D.R. Haynor, and P. Hellier (Eds.): MICCAI 2004, LNCS 3217, pp. 153–160, 2004.

example,[2],etc) The other is what supports surgeon with a robot to cut the bone adding into navigation functions.[3]-[5]

This study belongs to the latter. The main robot-assisted orthopaedic systems for lower limb are ROBODOC[3],CASPAR[4],ACROBOT[5]. This system has two main features compared to other systems. First, cartilage and soft tissue can be considered because surgeon can change the pre-operative plan and modify the tool path for the bone resection. And a minimum invasive registration method without any pins is adopted.

On the other hand, some papers report the comparison results in the case of robot-assisted operation and manual operation.[6]-[7] Honl,et al[6] reports that they did THA operation using ROBODOC more than 50 cases, and they compared the accuracy, the condition after operation, time of operation and etc to the manual operation. As the result, it is recognized that the operation with the robot gives the improvement of the accuracy.

3   Pre-operative Assisting System

Overview of the application for total knee arthroplasty we developed is shown in Fig.1. Cross section image, predicted image at any location and projected image are presented on the display, and surgeon decides type and position of prosthesis, and tool path for the bone resection is generated automatically. The determination of prosthesis position is based on the anatomical distinction. Surgeon can decide the position of artificial knee joint considering the total shape of the limb by indicating some points on the display according to the guide of application.

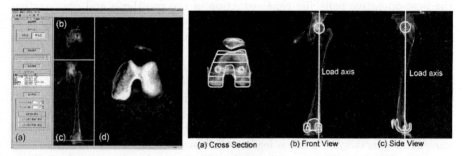

Operation window   Configuration of prosthesis

Fig. 1. Operation Planning Software: Operation window (a)operation window (b)cross section window(c)front view window(d)main window and Configuration of prosthesis

Then, tool path for the bone resection is generated from the information of the planned prosthesis position. First, the area which tool occupies is defined automatically, and surgeon modifies the area to assure safety. And tool path on the cut plane is generated. Coordinates for each cut plane is defined so that plane and area for the bone resection are within the range of U,V,W,A,B and C axes in the bone cutting robot (Fig.2)

4   Bone Cutting Robot

Overview of the bone cutting robot which has 9 degree of freedom(d.o.f) is shown in Fig.2. The size of robot is 810mm x 1500mm x 2050mm,and the weight is approximately 900kg.

4.1   Requirements for Bone Cutting Robot

The requirements for the bone cutting robot are as follows.

- Surface roughness and angle error accuracy between adjacent cut planes
  It is required that the surface roughness and angle error between planes become smaller. And to realize the bone cutting with the high accuracy, a solid structure is desired.
- Assurance of safety during bone resection
  Monitoring of the abnormal state with cutting force, mechanical safety with fail-safe mechanism and emergency button are equipped for this robot. And work space for surgeon should be also considered.

4.2   Characteristics of Mechanism

As mechanical and structural features, the following points are listed.

- Tip position of tool is fixed at the center of 3 rotation d.o.f.
  When the posture of tool is changed, the tip of tool does not move and the safety is kept.
- Movement of tool during resection is restricted within the cut plane
  Axes for bone cutting are defined in advance and the cutting tool is restricted within the cut plane mechanically. And the improvements of safety and cutting accuracy are realized.
- Definition and clarification of role for each axis
  The behavior of robot can be predicted by clarifying the role for each axis, and the motion control like modification of tool path becomes easier.
- Force sensor is equipped
  It is possible to monitor the cutting status by measuring the cutting force.
- Fail-safe mechanism is equipped
  Patient and robot can be protected mechanically.

4.3   Strategy for Layout

The motion of the robot can be predicted by clarifying the role for each axis, and the control like the modification of tool path becomes easier. To resect the bone precisely, axes for approaching to the operation area and axes for resecting the bone are separated respectively. Axes for rough position (X,Y and Z) are located around the base, and axes for fine position (3 rotational and 3 translational axes) are arranged near the tool.

Axes for bone cutting are defined in advance and the cutting tool is restricted within the cut plane mechanically. And the improvements of safety and cutting accuracy are realized.

Axes for the bone cutting is assigned to realize 2 dimensional motion, and the cutting tool is restricted within the plane. More precise cutting is expected by this simple process. Plane inclination is decided by 2 rotational axes (A and B), and 1 translational axis (W) controls the position in radius direction. To cut the plane, 2 translational axes (U and V) and 1 rotational axis (C) to rotate the tool are used.

When the posture of tool is changed, the tip of tool is fixed at the center of 3 rotational axes, and the safety is kept.

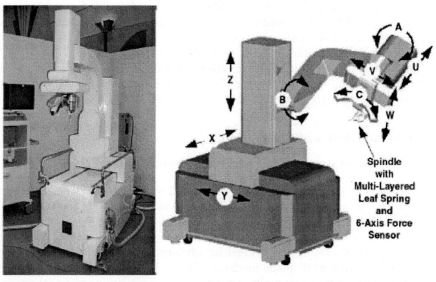

(a) Bone cutting machine   (b) Configuration of axes

Fig. 2. Overview of bone cutting machine: (a)Bone cutting machine (b) Configuration of axes

4.4   Controller

The controller for the bone cutting system consists of a PC for the user interface and a real-time controller. Both computers are connected with LAN. Real time Linux is adopted as a operating system. The controller accepts a command from user interface PC by socket communication on TCP/IP even while it is controlling the cutting machine. The user interface on PC is shown in Fig.3.

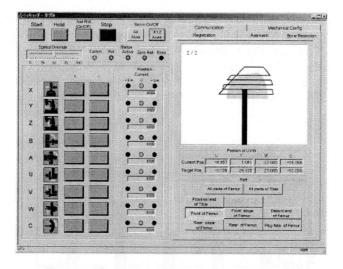

Fig. 3. Operation window for surgeon as user interface

5 Intra-operative Assist System

A registration method which does not need to incise the cutis any more and to use marker pins is introduced. In the registration, the characteristic points which does not depend on individual surgeon are defined as bony landmarks, and the accuracy to probe can be improved. Then, the points indicated on the user interface are identified using the tool part of the robot. The position of the patient on the bed is recognized by the registration, and the approach point for the bone resection and the posture of the robot are decided.

The tool path generated in pre-operative system is based on the image of CT, and it is difficult to consider soft tissue in advance. Therefore, the pre-operative plan can be changed to restrict the area which the tool invades during the operation, and the risk to damage the ligaments, nerves and vessels is lowered. In detail, C axis in Fig.2 is used to rotate the tool posture while cutting and to avoid the hazardous area. Surgeon can configure allowable area which the tool invades, and the tool path is recalculated by the intra-operative system. Finally, the surgeon confirms the represented path.

6 System Evaluation

6.1 Measurement of Surface Roughness and the Angle Accuracy

5 surfaces of model bone for the artificial knee joint were cut using the developed system. The accuracy of the cut surface was compared with that obtained by the conventional method. Each surface was measured by a CMM. The number of sampled points was from 200 to 500, depending on the plane. An approximate

plane was calculated using the sampled point data for each surface. The surface roughness was obtained by calculating the variance of the sampled points from the approximate plane. Fig.4 shows the experimental results. The angle between the desired angle and the experimentally obtained angle is shown in Fig.4. The surface roughness and angle accuracy were improved from 200 to 33.2 μm and 4.49 to 0.125deg., respectively.

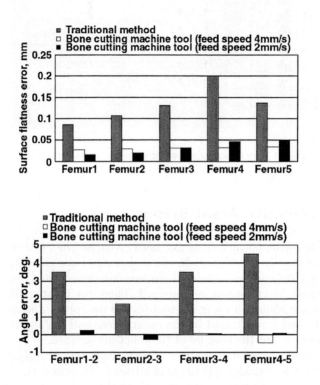

Fig. 4. Comparison of surface roughness(above) and angle accuracy(below)

6.2   Cadaveric Bone Cutting Experiment

Using the developed system, a experiment of the bone cutting was done with cadaver. Regarding the angle of planes to fix the prosthesis, the difference between plan and result was evaluated.

Fig.5 shows the look of this experiment. As the cut plane of femur, two are in front, one in distal end and one in rear. And each plane is connected with curved surface. When the planes are cut, two planes in front are treated as one and each curved surface is approximated as a plane. The evaluation of angle between planes is described in Fig.6

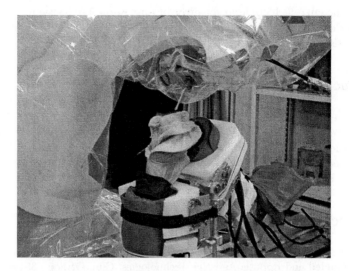

Fig. 5. Cadaveric bone cutting experiment

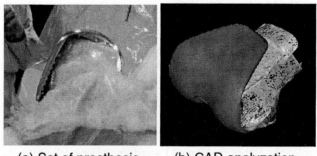

(a) Set of prosthesis   (b) CAD analyzation

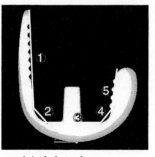

Angle	Plan	Result	Diff.
1 - 3	93.3°	93.8°	0.5°
3 - 5	98.0°	99.0°	1.0°
1 - 3	11.3°	12. 8°	1.5°

(c) Joint planes   (d) Result

Fig. 6. Evaluation of angles between cut planes

With the current technique the error of maximum 4.5 degree may occur, and this experiment showed the error of 1.5 degree at most. From the result, the system is useful for more precise bone cutting.

7   Conclusions

In this paper, a robot-assisted orthopaedic system designed for total knee arthroplasty was described, and the surgeon can modify the pre-operative plan during the operation. And from the result of the experiment with model bone and cadaver, it becomes clear that surface roughness and angle difference between cut planes can be lower than the current operation technique.

References

1. DiGioia AM, Jaramaz B, Colgan BD: Computer Assisted Orthopaedic Surgery: Image Guided and Robotic Assistive Technologies. Clin. Orthop., 354:8-16, 1998
2. Stulberg SD, Loan P, et al: Computer-Assisted Navigation in Total Knee Replacement: Results of an Initial Experience in Thirty-Five Patients. J. Bone Joint Surg.,84-A (2002) S90-98
3. Mittelstadt BD, Kazanzides P, Zuhars J: The Evolution of a Surgical Robot from Prototype to Human Clinical Trial. Proc. Medical Robotics and Computer Assisted Surery (1994)
4. Peterman J, Kober R, Heinze P, Heekt P, Gotzen L: Implementation of the CASPAR System in the reconstruction of the ACL. CAOS/USA. (2000) 86–87
5. Delp SL, Stulbrg DS, David S, Davies B, Picard F, Leitner F: Computer Assisted Knee Replacement. Clin. Orthop. 354 (1998) 49–56
6. Honl M, Dierk O, Gauck C, Carrero V, Lampe F, Dries S, Quante M, Schwieger K, Hille E, Morlock MM: Comparison of Robotic-Assisted and Manual Implantation of a Primary Total Hip Replacement. J. Bone Joint Surg., 85-A (2003) 1470–1478.
7. Krismer M, Nogler M, Kaufmann CH, Ogon M: Revision of Femoral Component: Cement Removal by Robot vs. Manual Procedure. J.Bone Joint Surg. 83-B SI (2001) 80

Needle Guiding Robot with Five-Bar Linkage for MR-Guided Thermotherapy of Liver Tumor

Nobuhiko Hata, Futoshi Ohara, Ryuji Hashimoto, Makoto Hashizume, and
Takeyoshi Dohi

Department of Mechano-Informatics, Graduate School of Information Science and
Technology
The University of Tokyo, Graduate School of Medical Sciences, Kyushu University
{noby, ohara, hashimoto, dohi}@atre.t.u-tokyo.ac.jp,
mhashi@dem.med.kyushu-u.ac.jp

Abstract. This paper reports the robot for horizontal gap open MRI
which controls needle orientation effectively in the vertically limited
gantry space. We locate the robot including actuators wholly in MR
gantry and puncture needle from side of patient's body. The robot has
three Degree-of-Freedom (DOF) and can control needle orientation using five-bar linkage mechanism and gimbal mechanism. Two DOF is to
actuate five-bar linkage and the other DOF to make five-bar linkage up
and down. In experiments, the accuracy of five-bar linkage was 0.89±0.15
[mm] on a whole average and the accuracy of vertical placement of five-
bar linkage was 0.13±0.02 [mm]. MR images had insignificant degradation of 19.4% in attrition rate of S/N ratio at the maximum. We conclude
that the robot can control needle orientation with high repeatability and
high MR compatibility in the limited gantry space.

1 Introduction

Intraoperative Magnetic Resonance Imaging (MRI) is a promising imaging tool
for monitoring and guiding thermal therapy of liver tumor[1]-[3]. In MR-guided
thermal therapies, needle-shaped thermal device is percutaneously inserted to
the target tumor(s) under MRI guidance and coagulates the cancerous tissues
at effector tip under thermal monitoring. Unique imaging capability of MRI is
useful for deliniating tumor tissue, locating thermal probe, and monitoring thermal effect by thermal imaging. MRI guided thermal therapies has been getting
attention since the introductoin of open MRI in clinical practice. The open MRI
allows more unrestricted access to the patient and the operative field than conventional closed-magnet MRI. Up to date, two configurations, i.e. vertical gap
scanner and horizontal gap scanner, of open MRI have been in clinical use to
assess their feasibilities in thermal therapies with laser, microwave, radiowave,
and cryogenic device[1]-[3].

In order to further enhance the capability of MR-guided thermal therapy of
liver tumor, two challenges needs to be addressed. First, the targeting should

C. Barillot, D.R. Haynor, and P. Hellier (Eds.): MICCAI 2004, LNCS 3217, pp. 161–168, 2004.
© Springer-Verlag Berlin Heidelberg 2004

be assisted by intuitive and reliable navigation. Second, actual execution of insertion should be assisted by needle holding device, and possively with active guidance by robot. There are several studies reported to achieve these goals by integrating navigation software, MR compatible robot, and MR scanner [4]-[6]. Most of the studies reported are designed for use in either vertical gap scanner, or conventional close-magnet scanner.

In this paper, we propose a new MR compatible robot specifically designed for use in horizontal gap MR scanner. Specifically, we propose (1) a robot for percutaneous needle puncture from the side opening of the horizontal gap scanner, and (2) five-bar linkage mechanism and gimbal mechanism to achieve both compactness of the robot, maximum degree-of-freedom, and large work-space for needle localization.

The engineering significance of this paper is that the combination of mechanism proposed is, to the authors' best knowledge, the first original contribution for percutaneous robotic needle insertion in horizontal open MR scanner. The paper is also clinically significant since the proposed robot has potential to prevail and impact clinical practice; unlike previously published MR-compatible robot for vertical gap scanner, our robot can be integrated into horizontal gap MR scanner which has been already widespread in clinical sites.

2   Methods

2.1   System Design

Fig.1 illustrates the system configuration of the needle guiding robot proposed in this study. Total system consisted of four components: horizontal gap open MRI, MR compatible robot, console for imaging, control PC for robot. The horizontal gap open MRI and the console are part of commercially available 0.3T MRI (AIRISII, Hitachi, Tokyo, Japan). Upon initial volume scanning for localization of tumor site(s), images are transferred to the control PC for planning of needle placement. A set of software were developed and implemented on the control PC (CPU: Pentium 4, 2.53 GHz, RAM: 1024 MB) using the 3D Slicer. The 3D Slicer is a surgical simulation and navigation software program, which displays multi-modality images three- and two-dimensionally[7],[8]. The 3D Slicer was used in this study to transfer intraoperative images from the scanner and perform tumor segmentation followed by robot control.

Needle guiding robot is placed on the side of the patient to allow horizontal to near-vertical access of the needle to tumor targets in the liver through opening of the Radio Frequency(RF)-coil. The alignment of the robot with respect to the patient (and the targets in the liver) is manual; yet, the needle placement is robotized by three degree-of-freedom (DOF) motion of the needle guiding robot.

2.2   Five-Bar Linkage Mechanism and Gimgal Mechanism

The proposed robot has five-bar linkage mechanism and gimbal mechanism, to achieve three DOF motion of the needle placement. The needle guide is held by

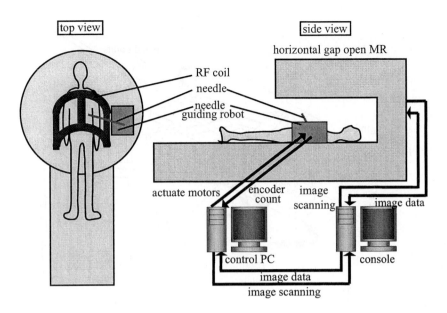

Fig. 1. Schematics illustration of MR compatible needle guiding robot for horizontal gap open MR scanner. Needle guiding robot is placed on the side of the patient enabling horizontal to near-vertical needle placement through opening of the RF-coil.

the top gimbal at the tip of five-bar linkage, and the bottom gimbal at the tip of fixed-bar (Fig.2). Both gimbals enables two rotational motions of the needle guide, though only the bottom gimbal fixes the needle guide to limit the slippage of the needle guide. The five-bar linkage is lifted with respect to the fixed edge unit, to enable vertical rotation of the guide needle.

The five-bar linkage consists of four closed links shown in Fig2. Two links attached to the base stage rotates around the axis on the base and the other two extended links are connected at the tips each other to form closed link. By rotating links at the two 'actuated points' on motor axis, the 'link tip' can be arbitrary placed on horizontal plane formed by the linkages.

The gimbal holds a needle by limiting the freedom-of-motion on two rotation and one slide motion. Specifically, the horizontal rotations of the needle around the gimbal is possible by horizontal motion of five-bar linkage, and the vertical rotation of the needle is possible by lifting the five-bar linkage with respet to the 'fixed edge'. The rotation around the needle axis is prohibited by the fixer on the tail tip.

2.3   Size Specification

Based on the design concept mentioned above, we developed a robot shown in (Fig.3). The height of the robot is 170 [mm] at the lowest state and 240 [mm] at the highest state against the height of MR gantry 420 [mm]. Therefore needle

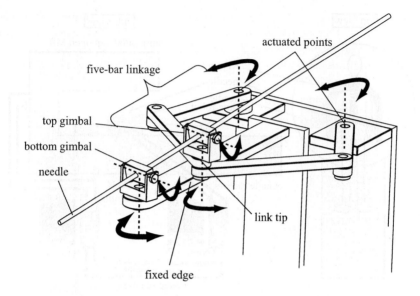

Fig. 2. Five-bar linkage mechanism and gimbal mechanism achieving 3 DOF motion of needle. The needle is held by two gimbals; the top gimbal is attached at the tip of the five-bar linkage manipulator while the bottom one is placed on fixed bar. The needle position and orientation is determined by the in-plane motion of the five-bar linkage.

can tilt up to 36 [degree] against horizontal plane when the robot is in highest state in the gantry, supposing the needle length 300 [mm]. Encoder resolution for motor control was 360/2000 [degree]. Links at the side of 'actuated points' are 75 [mm] long, links at the side of 'link tip' are 95 [mm] long, and diameter between 'actuated points' is 80 [mm]. 'Link tip' can move along superior-to-inferior axis of the patient by stroke of 110[mm], and along left-to-right stroke of 92[mm]. Vertical motion of five-bar linkage is actuated by ultrasonic motor (USR60-E3N, Shinsei kogyo, Tokyo, Japan) and lead screw (stroke; 70 [mm] and resolution; 2 [μm]).

The robot has three passively controlled motion. The first is needle insertion designed to be operated manually by surgeon. The second is vertical motion of the 'fixed edge' with 70 [mm] stroke and the third is whole robot's movement along body axis of the patient. The motion along body axis has stroke of 250 [mm] to cover a whole liver inside needle's target range.

2.4   MR Compatible Materials

Following the detailed report on MR compatibility of robots [?]-[7], we carefully chose stainless-, steel-, aluminium-, resin-, ceramic-based parts for translating unit (lead screw and guide rail), five-bar linkage, gimbals, actuators, and the other constitute.

For lead screw and guide rail in translating unit, we chose stainless steel.Resin was used as a bushing and a nut in translating unit. Ceramic bearing was used as a bushing of lead screw. Five-bar linkage, gimbals and the other constitute consisted of aluminium. Actuators were ultrasonic motors (USR60-E3N and USR30-E3N, Shinsei Kogyo, Tokyo, Japan).

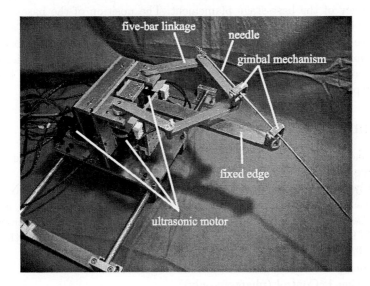

Fig. 3. MR compatible needle holding manipulator

3   Validation Study

Two sets of experiments were conducted to assess the robot in pre-clinical condition. The first study was to assess the reproducibility of needle placement and the second was to investigate the MR compatibility of the robot. The third set of study was performed with phantom in MR scanner to investigate teh usability of the robot in MRI guided therapy. Measurement of accuracy and reproducibility were tested in dry condition in laboratory while MR compatibility test and phantom study were performed clinical MR scanner. No animal or patient were involved.

3.1   Accuracy of Needle Tip Placement

The accuracy and reproducibility of the needle tip placement were assessed in horizontal motion and vertical motion separately. The reproducibility of horizontal motion was tested by setting 2 points as a target and displaced the needle guide tip to the targeted points 10 times in each trial. The motion of the needle guide tip was recorded by a digital microscope (VH-7000C, KEYENCE, Osaka, Japan) placed above the robot. The video images from the digital microscope were later processed to digitize the position of the tips with a resolution of 0.07 [mm]. The result of measured standard deviation indicated from 0.07 [mm] to 0.14 [mm].

The accuracy of vertical needle placement was approximated by measuring the accuracy of the base-stage plamement. The position of the base-stage was measured by a laser gauge(LK-080, KEYENCE, Osaka, Japan) placed above the robot. We set lowest state as a starting position and displaced the base stage from 5 [mm] to 70 [mm] with an interval of 5 [mm]. The result indicated the accuracy of vertical motion was 0.13 ± 0.02 [mm] on a whole average. Errors at each sampling point ranged from 0.11[mm] to 0.14 [mm].

3.2   MR Compatibility Test

The second set of assessment was MR-cmpatibility test to analyze the effect of the needle guiding robot on MR imaging.

A polyethylene cylindrical vessel filled with aqueous solution of NaCl and $MnCl_2$ was used as a phantom. The MR imaging was gradient field echo, a typical imaging sequence for MR-guided thermal therapy, with imaging parameters as follows; TR/TE: 50/20 [ms], FOV: 256 [mm], matrix: 256×128, slice thickness: 10 [mm] flip angle: 90 [degrees].

The images were taken under the following conditions;

Condition 1: Control (phantom only)

Condition 2: The robot installed in the MR scanner and electric power unplugged

Condition 3: The robot installed in the MR scanner actuated (one motor)

Condition 4: The robot installed in the MR sccaner and all axis actuated (linkage actuated).

In order to evaluate the noise, S/N ratio was calculated in eace image using the following equation;

$$S/N ratio = I_{center}/SD_{corner}.$$

I_{center} indicates the average intensity of 120 pixel in diameter at the center of the image and SD_{corner} is the average of standard deviation of the 60 pixel in diameter area at the corner of the image. Imaging and measurement were repeated five time per each of four conditions. Illustrative image for each condition and the measured results are shown in Fig.4. Image degradation in S/N ratio was maximum 19.4 % when all theme actuators were in motion.

3.3   Phantom Study in Clinical MR Scanner

We conducted a set of phantom studies to evaluate the feasibility of the robot in near clinical setting with MR scanner. We also measured the succsess ratio of needle targetting with pseudo tumors (vitamin E capsules 8 [mm] in diameter) placed in an agar phantom(150 [mm] × 250 [mm] × 100 [mm]). Four capsules

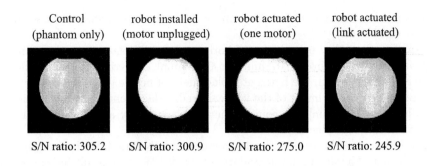

Control (phantom only)	robot installed (motor unplugged)	robot actuated (one motor)	robot actuated (link actuated)
S/N ratio: 305.2	S/N ratio: 300.9	S/N ratio: 275.0	S/N ratio: 245.9

Fig. 4. MR phantom image and S/N ratio from the MR compatibility test. Imaging condition are given on the top of each image.

were placed in the phantom with known geometical correlation, while setting the one capsule as reference point and the other three as pseudo tumors. The needle tip (14-gauge) was first placed at the reference point in the beginning of each trial, and then repositioned to one of the pseudo tumors by the robot. 10 trials were repeated per each target tumor and number of successful hit were counted by observing the MRI. Fig.5 shows an illustrative MR images of a target in the phantom and the same target hit by the needle. We could successfully hit the tumor in all trials.

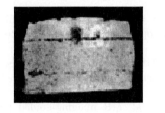
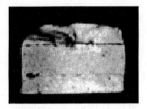

Fig. 5. MR phantom images of needle insertion test. Left image is the image before needle insertion and right image is the image after the needle was inserted.

4   Discussion

We developed a robot specifically designed for use in horizontal gap open MRI and tested the feasibility in near clinical setting. The robot has three DOF and can control needle orientation using five-bar linkage mechanism and gimbal mechanism. The size of the robot is 170 [mm] in the lowest state and 240 [mm] in the highest state to actuate needle in the limited gantry space of MR. And five-bar linkage tip can cover 110 [mm] × 92 [mm] × 70 [mm] volume covering nomal sized liver.

In reproducibility experiment of horizontal needle placement, the standard deviation indicated from 0.07 [mm] to 0.14 [mm]. We conclude the robot has high reproducibility in the horizontal placement of needle guide.In accuracy and reproducibility experiment of the vertical needle placement, the result indicated 0.13 [mm] ± 0.02 [mm]. We could achieve high accuracy and reproducibility in the vertical needle placement.

In MR compatibility test, the degradation of S/N ratio in each condition was insignificant. The maximum degradation was 19.4 %. This result indicates high MR compatibility of the robot and the usability of the robot in MR scanner.

In phantom study in MR scanner, we could successfully hit the pseudo tumors in all trials by observing the MRI. This result indicates that the robot has ability of targetting and hitting the tumor in near clinical setting. Our future work includes development of control theory to hit targets localized in intraoperative MR images, which leads to evalution of the robot in more realistic surgical setting.

Acknowledgement. This study was funded in part by NEDO of Japan. The authors thank Mr. Watanabe of Hitachi Medico for his advice and support on MR imaging.

References

1. Kettenbach J, Silverman SG, Hata N, et al. Monitoring and visualization techniques for MR-guided laser ablations in an open MR system. J Magn Reson Imaging 1998;8:933-943
2. Morikawa S, Inubushi T, Kurumi Y, et al. MR-guided microwave thermocoagulation therapy of liver tumors: initial clinical experiences using a 0.5 T open MR system. J Magn Reson Imaging 2002;16:576-583
3. Silverman SG, Tuncali K, Adams DF, et al. MR imaging-guided percutaneous cryotherapy of liver tumors: initial experience. Radiology 2000;217:657-664
4. Masamune K, Kobayashi E, Masutani Y, et al. Development of an MRI-compatible needle insertion manipulator for stereotactic neurosurgery. J Image Guid Surg 1995;1:242-248
5. Chinzei K, Miller K. Towards MRI guided surgical manipulator. Med Sci Monit 2001;7:153-163
6. Krieger A, Susil R C, Fichtinger G, et al. Design of A Novel MRI Compatible Manipulator for Image Guided Prostagte Intervention. International Conference of Robotics & Automation -ICRA 2004 2004;377-382
7. Gering DT, Nabavi A, Kikinis R, et al. An integrated visualization system for surgical planning and guidace using image fusion and an open MR. J Magn Imaging 2001;13:967-975
8. Hata N, Jinzaki M, Kacher D, et al. MR imaging-guided prostate biopsy with surgical navigation software: device validation and feasibility. Radiology 2001;220:263-268

Computer-Assisted Minimally Invasive Curettage and Reinforcement of Femoral Head Osteonecrosis with a Novel, Expandable Blade Tool

Tsuyoshi Koyama[1], Nobuhiko Sugano[2], Hidenobu Miki[2], Takashi Nishii[2],
Yoshinobu Sato[3], Hideki Yoshikawa[2], Shinichi Tamura[3], and Takahiro Ochi[1]

[1] Division of Robotic Therapy, Osaka University Graduate School of Medicine,
2-2 Yamadaoka, Suita, 565-0871 Osaka, Japan
koyama@cl-comp.med.osaka-u.ac.jp
[2] Department of Orthopaedic Surgery, Osaka University Graduate School of Medicine,
2-2 Yamadaoka, Suita, 565-0871 Osaka, Japan
[3] Division of Interdisciplinary Image Analysis, Osaka University Graduate School of Medicine, 2-2 Yamadaoka, Suita, 565-0871 Osaka, Japan

Abstract. For minimally invasive curettage of femoral head osteonecrosis, we have developed a novel expandable blade tool which can be introduced into the femoral head through the subtrochanteric route under navigation guidance. In this study, we evaluated the effectiveness and feasibility of this tool in comparison with the Cebotome, a conventional bone cutter. A target area in the femoral head of a Sawbone femur model was curetted with each tool through the subtrochanteric route under navigation guidance. The volume of the curetted necrotic lesion was significantly larger and the procedure time was significantly shorter with this tool than with the Cebotome. The compressive strength of the femoral head curetted with this tool and filled with hydroxyapatite blocks was comparable to that of the intact one. This expandable blade tool can be a suggestion for more effective and feasible curettage of necrotic lesions in femoral head osteonecrosis than conventional bone cutters.

1 Introduction

The treatment of femoral head osteonecrosis is still controversial. It has been reported that about 70–80% of hips with femoral head osteonecrosis show progression of collapse of the femoral head if they do not receive any surgical treatment[5] (Fig. 1). In order to halt progression of collapse and to accelerate reparative process of the necrotic lesions, various joint preserving procedures have so far been performed. Core decompression with or without bone grafting[3] is one of the popular procedures in early stages. This procedure is performed through the lateral subtrochanteric route to the proximal femur which is comparatively less invasive than other methods, but this procedure has a limitation in curetting a large lesion through a long narrow hole. It has been reported that 20–40% of hips treated with this procedure in early stages resulted in collapse and needed total hip arthroplasty[1, 3, 4]. On the other hand, the trapdoor

C. Barillot, D.R. Haynor, and P. Hellier (Eds.): MICCAI 2004, LNCS 3217, pp. 169–175, 2004.

procedure[2] enables to curette a large lesion effectively through a trapdoor made in the femoral head. However, this procedure is quite invasive because the hip may need to be dislocated in order to make a trapdoor on the femoral head.

We think that the collapse of the femoral head in femoral head osteonecrosis may be prevented if the necrotic lesions are curetted thoroughly and the deficit is filled with reinforcement materials such as hydroxyapatite ceramics, bone grafts or bone substitutes with sufficient mechanical strength. For minimally invasive curettage of necrotic lesions of femoral head osteonecrosis, we have developed a novel, expandable blade tool which can be introduced into the femoral head through the lateral subtrochanteric route under a surgical navigation system. In this study, we evaluated the effectiveness and feasibility of this tool in comparison with the Cebotome®, a popular conventional bone cutter, with respect to curettage of target necrotic lesions supposed in a Sawbone® femoral head model. Moreover, we evaluated the compressive strength of the Sawbone femoral head after the inside part of the femoral head was curetted with this tool and filled with hydroxyapatite blocks as reinforcement material.

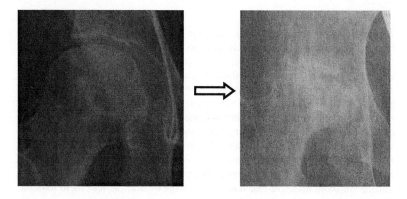

Fig. 1. Course of collapse in femoral head osteonecrosis

2 Materials and Methods

Our novel, expandable blade tool has a mechanism by which a 14–20mm long metal blade housed in the tip of a long 10mm-diameter metal cylinder is made to protrude(Fig. 2 left). The length of the expanding blade is changeable according to the sizes of the femoral head and the necrotic lesions. The blade swings on a hinge and protrudes outwards from the cylinder to an angle of 60 degrees (Fig. 2 right) when a trigger attached to the tool is pulled. This tool is designed to be used after boring a hole into the femoral head from the lateral subtrochanteric portion of the femur with a drill of the same diameter (Fig. 3 B, C). As the cylinder spins at high speed, the blade protrudes gradually, cutting a cone shaped section of bone away.

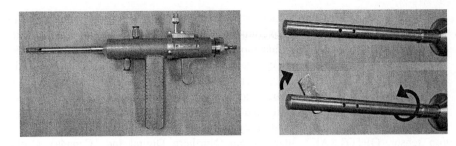

Fig. 2. The expandable blade tool

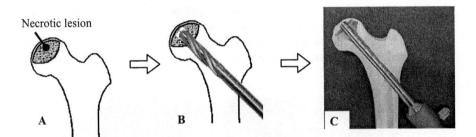

Fig. 3. Usage of the expandable blade tool

A: A typical extensive necrotic lesion of femoral head osteonecrosis
B: Coring a hole into the femoral head with a 10mm-diameter drill using the lateral subtro-
chanteric approach
C: Curettage of the necrotic lesion with the expandable blade tool

Study 1: The effectiveness and feasibility of the expandable blade tool were evalu-
ated in comparison with the Cebotome® (MicroAire Surgical Instruments LLC, USA)
(Fig. 4), a popular conventional bone cutter, using Sawbones® (Pacific Research
Laboratories, USA) femur models.

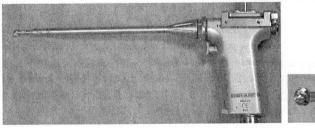
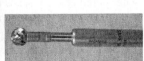

Fig. 4. Cebotome®

A typical extensive necrotic lesion of femoral head osteonecrosis (type C2, by the Classification of the Japanese government investigation group[6]) was created virtually in the three-dimensional surface model of a Sawbone femur on the computer (Fig. 3A). A pre-operative planning to curette the target necrotic lesion with the expandable blade tool or with the Cebotome was carried out on the three-dimensional models on computer so that the target necrotic lesion was curetted maximally with each tool.

The whole procedure of curetting the Sawbone femoral head was performed under a CT-based optical surgical navigation system with an optical three-dimensional position sensor, OPTOTRAK® 3020 system (Northern Digital Inc., Canada). Optical tracking markers were attached to the Sawbone femur and to the surgical tools. First, the surface registration of the Sawbone femur under an optical navigation system was performed. Then, a guide wire was inserted from the lateral subtrochanteric portion of the femur into the femoral head under the navigation guidance according to the pre-operative planning. After drilling with a 10mm-diameter drill over the guide wire to within 4mm of the articular surface of the femoral head, the inside of the femoral head was curetted with the expandable blade tool or with the Cebotome in line with the pre-operative planning (Fig. 5).

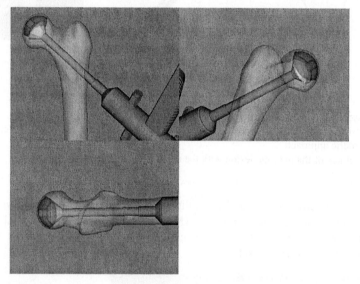

Fig. 5. Curetting the target necrotic lesion with the expandable blade tool under an optical navigation system.

After curettage, CT scans of the curetted Sawbone femur models were carried out. The CT image of the Sawbone femur after curettage was matched to the pre-operative planning image on the computer, and the volume of the actually curetted necrotic lesion and that of the sacrificed normal area of the femoral head were measured from the CT images.

The procedure time taken for the curettage after drilling a hole was also measured. The trials were repeated ten times for each surgical tool. Statistical analyses were performed using the Student's t-test with a significance level of 0.05.

Study 2: After curetting the Sawbone femoral head with the expandable blade tool in Study 1, the cavity in the femoral head was filled maximally with blocks of hydroxyapatite ceramics 3.3 × 3.3 × 5 mm in size (HA Block®, Pentax, Japan) and compressive strength of the femoral head was examined. Compressive strength of the femoral head was measured at the weight-bearing portion of the femoral head with a servohydraulic strength testing system (ServoPulser®, Shimadzu, Japan) (Fig. 6). Five specimens each were tested of: intact Sawbone femur models, models that had been curetted only, and models that had been curetted and filled with the hydroxyapatite blocks. Compression was produced with a 12.7mm-diameter cylindrical indentor attached to the testing machine.

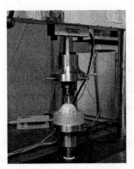

Fig. 6. Compressive strength of the femoral head was measured with a servohydraulic strength testing system.

3 Results

Study 1: The volumes of the curetted necrotic lesion and the volumes of the sacrificed normal area with each surgical tool are shown in Fig. 7.

The procedure time taken for the curettage with each surgical tool after drilling the hole is shown in Fig. 8.

Study 2: The compressive strength of the femoral head of the intact Sawbone femur models, models that had been curetted only, and models that had been curetted and filled with hydroxyapatite blocks are shown in Fig. 9.

4 Discussion

The volume of the curetted necrotic lesion was significantly larger and the procedure time was significantly shorter with the expandable blade tool than with the Cebotome. It can be stated that this expandable blade tool is both feasible and more effective than the Cebotome in curetting the necrotic lesions of femoral head osteonecrosis. The volume of the sacrificed normal area was significantly larger with the expandable blade tool than the Cebotome, however, this sacrificed area is near to the center of the femoral head where the bone mineral density is low, therefore the strength loss of the whole femoral head is supposed to be comparatively small. In fact, the compressive strength test showed that the femoral head that had been curetted with the expandable blade tool and filled with hydroxyapatite blocks had compressive strength comparable to that of the intact femoral head.

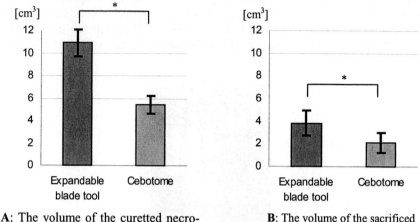

A: The volume of the curetted necrotic lesion

B: The volume of the sacrificed normal area

Fig. 7. The volumes of the curetted necrotic lesion (**A**) and the volumes of the sacrificed normal area in the femoral head (**B**).   (* $P < 0.01$)

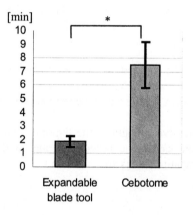

Fig. 8. The procedure time taken for the curettage after drilling the hole. (* $P < 0.01$)

In terms of safety, with the expandable blade tool, only the bone on the side part of the tool can be cut away, therefore the risk of breaking through the surface of the femoral head is low. Moreover, because the diameter of the cylinder of this tool is the same as the drilled long hole, this tool remains stabilized when the cylinder is spinning at high speed.

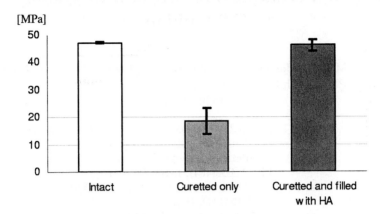

Fig. 9. The compressive strength of the femoral head.

5 Conclusion

Curettage of the necrotic lesion of femoral head osteonecrosis using the novel, expandable blade tool is both feasible and more effective than the Cebotome conventional bone cutter. The femoral head that has been curetted with this tool and filled with hydroxyapatite blocks has compressive strength comparative to that of the intact one. This surgical tool enables minimally invasive and effective curettage of the necrotic lesions in femoral head osteonecrosis.

References

1. Mont MA et al: Core decompression versus nonoperative management for osteonecrosis of the hip. Clin. Orthop. 324:169-178, 1996.
2. Mont MA et al: The trapdoor procedure using autogenous cortical and cancellous bone grafts for osteonecrosis of the femoral head. J. Bone Joint Surg. Br. 80(1):56-62, 1998.
3. Steinberg ME et al: Core decompression with bone grafting for osteonecrosis of the femoral head. Clin. Orthop. 386:71-78, 2001.
4. Stulberg BN et al: Osteonecrosis of the femoral head. A prospective randomized treatment protocol. Clin. Orthop. 268:140-151, 1991.
5. Sugano N et al: Prognostication of nontraumatic avascular necrosis of the femoral head. Significance of location and size of the necrotic lesion. Clin. Orthop. 303:155-164, 1994.
6. Sugano N, Atsumi T, Ohzono K, Kubo T, Hotokebuchi T, Takaoka K.: The 2001 revised criteria for diagnosis, classification, and staging of idiopathic osteonecrosis of the femoral head. J. Orthop. Sci. 7(5):601–605, 2002.

A Parallel Robotic System with Force Sensors for Percutaneous Procedures Under CT-Guidance

Benjamin Maurin[1], Jacques Gangloff[1], Bernard Bayle[1], Michel de Mathelin[1], Olivier Piccin[2], Philippe Zanne[1], Christophe Doignon[1], Luc Soler[3], and Afshin Gangi[4]

[1] LSIIT‡ (UMR CNRS-ULP 7005), Strasbourg I University
Bd. S. Brant, BP 10413, 67412 Illkirch cedex, FRANCE
maurin@eavr.u-strasbg.fr
[2] LICIA(EA3434), INSA-Strasbourg
24, Bd de la Victoire, 67084 Strasbourg, FRANCE
[3] IRCAD, Hôpital Civil,
67000 Strasbourg, FRANCE
[4] Department of Radiology B.,
University Hospital of Strasbourg,
67091 Strasbourg, FRANCE

Abstract. This paper presents a new robotic framework for assisted CT-guided percutaneous procedures with force feedback and automatic patient-to-image registration of needle. The purpose is to help practitioners in performing accurate needle insertion while preserving them from harmful intra-operative X-rays imaging devices. Starting from medical requirements for needle insertions in the liver under CT-scan, a description of a dedicated parallel robot is made. Its geometrical and physical properties are explained. The design is mainly based on the accuracy and safety constraints. A real prototype is presented that is currently tested.

Introduction

Percutaneous medical procedures are among the new minimally invasive techniques that are emerging thanks to the progress of medical imaging and medical devices. Their field of application ranges from the diagnosis of pains to the treatments of tumors inside internal organs. This paper mainly focuses on the biopsies of abdominal organs and the radiofrequency ablations of tumors. These interventions are known to be less painful for the patient than a classical surgical act and thus allows faster recovery.

Given the small size of detectable tumors with current imaging devices, these procedures require high precision targeting during insertion. The success rate of such interventions is highly correlated with the accuracy of the needle positioning. In current manual procedures, the needle is hold by the radiologist and

‡ The authors wish to thank the Alsace Region Council for the financial support of this research project.

C. Barillot, D.R. Haynor, and P. Hellier (Eds.): MICCAI 2004, LNCS 3217, pp. 176–183, 2004.
© Springer-Verlag Berlin Heidelberg 2004

a visual guidance is needed, since freehand guidance with direct tactile feedback is not sufficient. For highly precise interventions (about 1 *mm* of accuracy) computed tomography has proved to be an excellent imaging modality given its resolution and good tissue differentiation. Furthermore, CT guidance is very useful when critical organ areas have to be bypassed, like the portal vein in the liver. While recent CT-scans allow the detection of tumors of 1 *cm* and below, current manual interventions are only made on tumors of 3 to 6 *cm*. The main reason is that destruction of these tumors with freehand insertion is not possible due to accuracy problems. It should be noted also that, during a CT-guided needle insertion, the interventionist may be exposed to X-rays potentially dangerous for his or her health when performing a large number of interventions.

Consequently, given the accuracy needs as well as the necessary X-rays protection, CT-guided robotic systems are gaining more and more attention. CT-guided robotic interventions are not new as discussed by Taylor [1]. Indeed, Kwoh *et al.* [2] have done some early work for neurosurgery, Stoianovici *et al.* [3] on the kidney and they have been followed by other researchers for other organs and procedures. Clinical trials have already been achieved in some cases, but current systems are not well suited for abdominal interventions where the motions and the respiration of the patient create large disturbances.

A general analysis of all existing abdominal procedures is out of the scope of this paper. As an application, we will concentrate on the liver, an organ that is commonly studied because of its importance in numerous pathologies. Furthermore, the internal motions of the liver due to the breathing of the patient makes it a challenging testbed for an image-guided needle insertion robotic system.

1   Percutaneous Procedures of the Abdomen

For a clear description of a typical insertion, we decompose the medical gesture in different steps:

1. Localization of the target using imaging devices;
2. Planning of the trajectory of the needle in the images;
3. Selection of an entry point on the abdomen of the patient with an insertion angle;
4. Small incision at this point and beginning of the procedure;
5. While not on target;
   a) Insertion of a few centimeters, guided by tactile sensing and synchronized with breathing motion;
   b) release of the needle for free motion around the entry point;
   c) New image acquisition for checking;
6. End;
7. Target reached.

Currently, completing all these steps takes about half an hour and accuracy up to 10 *mm* is considered to be good when the depth is about 150 *mm*. The first and second steps are often done with pre-operative scans of the patient. As CT-scans provide good tissue differentiation, the planning for needle trajectories is straightforward for physicians. The third step is then made by the radiologist who holds the needle inside the scanner and valids the entry point by acquiring images with the CT-scan (see Fig. 1).

During the insertion phase (5a), the radiologist uses the tactile feedback to detect transitions between organs. This important source of information helps him to guide the needle through the different layers of tissue while the image checks allows him to follow a specific angle of attack and precisely reach a structure deep inside the organ.

Mainly, for accuracy issues, protection of the radiologist and the medical staff, and faster interventions, is it clear that a robotized system will improve the previous operating scheme.

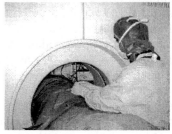

Fig. 1. Check of the needle position during a biopsy under CT guidance

2   Medical Requirements for a Robotic System

The observation of a typical biopsy or radio-frequency ablation gives many constraints that are explained in the following section.

2.1   Patient Safety and Sterilization Issues

Safety and asepsis are critical requirements. For abdominal access, the motion of the patient and the breathing issue are major difficulties. Real-time compensation of motion by hand is obviously what the radiologist is doing during interventions and such analogy should be employed in the design. Furthermore, the robot must remain motionless with respect to the patient in case of a failure, in order to avoid an undesirable motion or twist of the needle. The sterilization has a direct impact on the selection of the structure and its material characteristics, since nearly all radiological instruments are either placed in safe protective bags or sterilized by auto-clave.

2.2   Dimensions and Mobility of the Mechanism

For abdominal interventions, the patient is placed on a translating table that moves in the CT-scan tunnel which is only 700 mm in diameter. The space dimensions are restricted by the patient build and the table. A patient of stout build fills a large volume of the CT gantry and the available space looks like a 200 mm radius half-sphere centered on the entry point.

The insertion gesture made by the radiologist is complex and theoretically requires six degrees of freedom to hold and insert the needle. This can be split in two dissociated mobility: first the positioning and orientation of the supporting axis of the needle, second the insertion along the axis of the needle and the self rotation about its axis. The positioning and orientation is done by the robotic positioning device described in this paper while the descent and self rotation of the needle will be achieved by a special handling device that is not detailed in this document. Consequently, the required mobility of the positioning device corresponds to three degrees of freedom for positioning the entry point and two additional degrees for orientation of the supporting line of the needle about the entry point.

2.3 CT-Scan Compatibility

Metal and electrical devices diffuse X-rays. Thus to avoid a distortion of the reconstructed images, these materials must be avoided in the X-rays plane that slices the body of the patient.

2.4 Exertable Forces and Accuracy

Several recent papers on bovine liver [4] and pigs liver show that a force of about a few Newtons is applied on the needle during real in-vivo insertions. Figure 2 shows typical data measured on the insertion axis during in-vivo acquisitions on a liver of a pig through the skin. The force sensor was attached to a needle and inserted by a robot and a radiologist [5]. To achieve a real improvement over manual insertion, an accuracy of at least 5 mm or better at the tip of the needle is required.

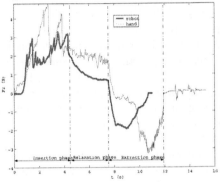

Fig. 2. A typical force measurement on a liver of a pig (by hand and using a robot)

2.5 Tele-operation and Force Feedback

We strongly believe that the mradiologist will remain the principal actor of an intervention and a needle insertion robotic system is necessarily tele-operated on a master-slave basis. Currently, the radiologist feels the different tissue layers while driving the needle. This tactile sense must be given through a sensor-based haptic feedback to the master device. A real-time visual representation of the needle inside the body should be beneficial [6] as CT-image slices are not aquired in real-time.

2.6 Registration of the Needle

CT-scan allows to compute fiducial-to-image registration thanks to stereotaxic fiducials (see [7]). As the configuration of a robotic system can be fully determined by its forward kinematics, the automatic registration of the needle in the operating space may be an advantage over manual intervention. In fact, even if the needle is not completely visible in the image but the fiducial is, the tip position is known.

3 Design and Description of the Robotic System

3.1 Answers to the Previous Medical Constraints

The safety of the patient is undoubtly the most important condition to be favored in the design. Like some recent works done on light robotic systems (see Berkelman *et Al.* or Hong *et Al.* [8,9]) our prototype is also fixed on the abdomen of the patient, so that the motions of the patient and the external motions due to breathing are naturally compensated. Special straps are fastened to the body to avoid involuntary motion of the base support. The robotic device is fixed on the base support. This feature allows to select the best initial configuration according to the intervention objectives. Internal breathing effects can be compensated by synchronisation of the robot and needle driver with the breathing machine.

The size of the robot is small enough to fit in the available space. The weight has been limited to 3 *kg* since the robot has to be on the abdomen which is a typical acceptable value. Sterilization of the actuators and sensors through autoclave is very difficult with usual technology, hence a plastic film will be used to protect all electronic devices that can be directly in contact to a human.

The mobility of the platform of the mechanism, supporting the needle-holder, should be a semi-spherical workspace about the entry point. For each accessible point of this workspace, our device may allow two more degrees of freedom for orientation of the platform. The CT-scan compatibility is ensured by choosing a platform that has no metallic parts crossing the X-rays plane.

To decrease the absolute positioning error, a rigid parallel structure is proposed. As a matter of fact, exerted forces are set to 20 *N* in our design. Rigidity also provides better force measurements from sensors attached to the platform at the interface with the needle driver. This should help the planned tele-operation force control.

Furthermore, patient-to-robot registration is necessary for visual guidance. For this purpose, stereotaxic fiducials (cubes with metals rods) are used to accuratly estimate the position and orientation of the base of the robot.

3.2 Structure Description

The designed structure has three legs, *i.e.*, three serial chains joining the base to the platform. Two opposite legs of the robot are symmetrical chains and form a planar 6-bar linkage. This linkage aims at constraining three degrees of freedom in its plane. Two degrees of freedom remains: the first one is a rotation of the planar 6-bar linkage about the line (Δ_1) passing through the base (see Fig. 3). The second corresponds to the orientation of the platform about the line (Δ_2). According to the classification of Tsai [10], the system we designed is made of a 6-bar linkage joined to a 4-bar linkage by a common platform, which is a parallel structure. The solution of this kinematic problem is done in closed form using a Local Product Of Exponentials Formalism [11,12]. An approximated numerical Jacobian is used to study the workspace and the rigidity of the mechanism since the closed-form solution is not straightforward.

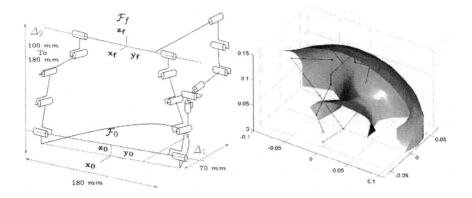

Fig. 3. A kinematic representation of the robot and its reachable workspace

In order to verify the possible motions of the mechanism, a numerical engine in C++ has been build (using Open Dynamic Engine, see Fig. 4). The simulations show that the kinematics models are well solved. The workspace shown on Fig. 3 has been computed using Matlab and shows only the right half space which is compatible with the previous requirements.

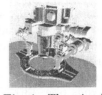

Fig. 4. The simulation environment

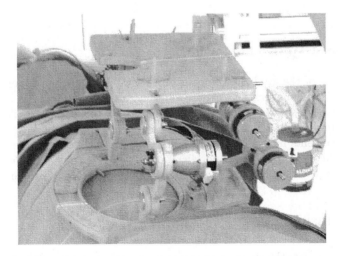

Fig. 5. The robotic system attached to the abdomen, without the needle driver, the cables and the force sensors (1.5 kg)

3.3   Physical Prototype

Starting from the structural description of the robot (mechanism topology, number of bodies type of joints) the robot is modeled in order to define its kinematics skeleton on a CAD system. The material used to build its links is glass-filled polyamide powder to comply with the CT-Scan imaging requirements (see Fig. 5 for the physical prototype). The mechanical design of the links is done using bearings to limit friction and backlash. A special care is taken to increase structural stiffness of the system. This system is designed to maintain a force of 20 N applied to the platform. Each actuation unit comprises a gear housing specifically designed for this application, an Harmonic Drive reduction gearing, an ultrasonic motor and an incremental encoder.

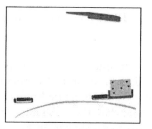

Three force sensors (Sensotec load cells) are symmetrically positioned on the needle driver unit that is attached under the platform. These devices give the force applied along the insertion axis. An haptic interface (Sensable 1.5 PHANToM) is currently used for the feedback needs. The prototype is registered in the CT-scan using stereotaxic fiducials made of $30 \times 30 \times 40$ mm plastic cubes with metal rods (see [13]). The fiducial cubes made for the robot registration are attached to its base (see Fig. 6). For now, an accuracy recontruction of under 1 mm in position is obtained using 512×512 image with 0.5 mm scaling factors.

Fig. 6. CT-scan of a fiducial cube attached to the robot

3.4   Current Work and Limits

The accuracy of the guidance depends on the fastening of the supporting base. This point is under work and a first solution currently explored is based on a deflating bag. It should hold tight the support to the patient while allowing the breathing motion. The current control scheme is position-based and further improvements have to be done for automatic registration of the system. A navigation-like feature (point and click paradigm) is currently implemented in order to help the radiologist to do the initial placement of the needle.

4   Conclusion

This paper presents the strong requirements on a safe robotic assistant for percutaneous procedures on the abdomen under CT-guidance. A novel five degrees of freedom parallel structure is described, intended to help practitioners for guiding and orienting a needle driver. A prototype has been built and is currently tested in a position-based control scheme. Registration of the robot using stereotactic fiducials will allow automatic guidance.

References

1. Taylor, R.H.: Medical robotics and computer aided surgery. In: Proceedings of Medical Image Computing and Computer-Assisted Intervention (MICCAI). (2002) Web PDF Hands-out of presentation.
2. Kwoh, Y.S., Hou, J., Jonckheere, E., Hayati, S.: A robot with improved absolute positioning accuracy for CT guided stereotatic brain surgery. IEEE Transactions on Biomedical Engineering **35** (1988) 153–160
3. Stoianovici, D., Whitcomb, L.L., Anderson, J.H., Taylor, R.H., Kavoussi, L.R.: A modular surgical robotic system for image guided percutaneous procedures. In: Proceedings of Medical Image Computing and Computer-Assisted Intervention (MICCAI), Cambridge, MA (1998) 404–410
4. Simone, C., Okamura, A.M.: Modeling of needle insertion forces for robot-assisted percutaneous therapy. In: Proceedings of the IEEE International Conference on Robotics and Automation (ICRA), Washington, DC, USA (2002) 2085–2091
5. Maurin, B., Barbe, L., Bayle, B., Zanne, P., Gangloff, J., de Mathelin, M., Gangi, A., Forgionne, A.: In vivo study of forces during needle insertions. In: Proceedings of the Medical Robotics, Navigation and Visualisation Scientific Workshop, Remagen, Germany (2004)
6. Gerovichev, O., Marayong, P., Okamura, A.: The effect of visual and haptic feedback on manual and teleoperated needle insertion. In: Proceedings of Medical Image Computing and Computer-Assisted Intervention (MICCAI), Tokyo, Japan (2002) 147–154
7. Susil, R.C., Anderson, J.H., Taylor, R.H.: A single image registration method for ct guided interventions. In: Proceedings of Medical Image Computing and Computer-Assisted Intervention (MICCAI), Cambridge, GB (1999) 798–808
8. Berkelman, P.J., Cinquin, P., Troccaz, J., Ayoubi, J.M., Létoublon, C., Bouchard, F.: A compact, compliant laparoscopic endoscope manipulator. In: Proceedings of the IEEE International Conference on Robotics and Automation (ICRA), Washington DC, USA (2002) 1870–1875
9. Hong, J., Dohi, T., Hashizume, M., Konishi, K., Hata, N.: An ultrasound-driven needle-insertion robot for percutaneous cholecystostomy. Physics in Medicine and Biology **49** (2004) 441–455 IOP Publishing Ltd.
10. Tsai, L.W.: Mechanism Design : enumeration of kinematic structures according to function. Mechanical Engineering series. CRC Press (2001)
11. Murray, R.M., Li, Z., Sastry, S.S.: A Mathematical Introduction to Robotic Manipulation. CRC Press (1994)
12. Yang, G., Chen, I.M., Lim, W.K., Yeo, S.H.: Design and kinematic analysis of modular reconfigurable parallel robots. In: Proceedings of the IEEE International Conference on Robotics and Automation (ICRA), Detroit, MI (1999) 2501–2506
13. Maurin, B., Doignon, C., de Mathelin, M., Gangi, A.: Pose reconstruction from an uncalibrated computerized tomographic device. In: Proceedings of the IEEE International Conference on Computer Vision and Pattern Recognition (CVPR). Volume 1. (2003) 455–460

System Design for Implementing Distributed Modular Architecture to Reliable Surgical Robotic System

Eisuke Aoki[1], Takashi Suzuki[1], Etsuko Kobayashi[1], Nobuhiko Hata[1], Takeyoshi Dohi[2], Makoto Hashizume[3], and Ichiro Sakuma[1]

[1] Institute of Environmental Studies, Graduate School of Frontier Sciences, The University of Tokyo
http://bme.pe.u-tokyo.ac.jp/index_e.html
{aoki, t-suzuki, etsuko, sakuma}@miki.pe.u-tokyo.ac.jp
[2] Graduate School of Information Science and Technology, The University of Tokyo
noby@atre.t.u-tokyo.ac.jp
dohi@miki.pe.u-tokyo.ac.jp
[3] Department of Disaster and Emergency Medicine, Kyushu University
mhashi@dem.med.kyushu-u.ac.jp

Abstract. A method that resolves the two competing requirements for a surgical robotic system (reliability and scalability) is discussed, along with its preliminary implementation in a master-slave system. The proposed method enables an architecture that can be scaled without impairing the performance of the surgical robotic system. Our method uses an optimized architecture consisting of two components: a common object request broker architecture (CORBA) and a master-slave system that typically operates using two-way communication links between a client and a remote server (the dedicated system architecture). In this new architecture, the surgical robotic system can maintain a reliable performance and can integrate with various systems in a transparent manner, regardless of the hardware, operating system, or programming language. Our method was evaluated by recording all the available surgical information, and shows a reliable scalability for a surgical robotic system requiring real-time operation, regardless of the condition of the components of a CORBA-based system.

1 Introduction

Many telerobotic systems using distributed modular architectures have been developed over the last few years. The advantages of using network-based systems built on top of distributed computing systems technology are the reduction in system costs, the arbitrary location of clients, dynamic access to remote expertise as required, and the decreased costs of operator training. Following the current trends in modern distributed system design, open reconfigurable and scalable architectures can be built using standard middleware software for distributed object computing. As one of several standard middleware software packages available, many studies using surgical robotic systems have been reported

C. Barillot, D.R. Haynor, and P. Hellier (Eds.): MICCAI 2004, LNCS 3217, pp. 184–191, 2004.

employing the common object request broker architecture (CORBA) package [1,2]. CORBA uses an Object Request Broker (ORB) as the middleware that establishes a client/server relationship between objects. The client can invoke a method on the server object across a network in a transparent manner without knowing where the application servers are located, or what programming language and operating system are being used. In addition, the components of a CORBA-based system can be implemented and run independently to implement the application, and can be easily integrated into new systems. Schorr et al. reported on the application of a CORBA system to control an image-guided surgical robot, where they controlled an MRI-compatible biopsy robot by sending the control information using CORBA [3,4]. However, there have been several reports that CORBA is not always an effective, flexible, and robust technique for Internet-based robotics systems. One of the technological problems associated with CORBA is how to guarantee stable and reliable control under interference from a CORBA system. Generally, real-time software is required to control mechatronic systems, such as robots, and to develop a stable and reliable control system under limited computational resources, it is important to evaluate the overall system load imposed on the computer system. However, in the distributed modular architecture of a computer aided surgical system, where the system configuration may change depending on the clinical requirements, it is difficult to estimate the system load before the design of the system. In recent years, a master-slave manipulator system has been applied to less-invasive laparoscopic surgery [5]. In contrast to an image-guided control system, the master-slave manipulator system is a relatively slow imaging system, and it requires a higher control frequency. On the other hand, to realize safe and accurate surgical operation, the integration of a surgical navigation system employing a master-slave surgical manipulator is necessary, and for this purpose, a distributed modular architecture is desirable. Thus, it is important to design a control system that meets these two competing requirements, and we set out to resolve these two competing requirements (scalability and reliability) in our surgical robotic system. This paper describes the following system components.

1. The use of an optimized architecture consisting of two components: a dedicated system architecture and CORBA, and
2. The development of an intermediate system to resolve any interference occurring between two architectures.

The above allow a surgical robotic system to maintain a reliable performance and to integrate various systems in a transparent manner, regardless of the hardware, operating system, or programming language used.

2   System Architecture

2.1   System Overview

It is important for a system to have sufficient computational power to handle the necessary information during processing. However, even if a system has sufficient performance, in general, it cannot handle situations that occur at random.

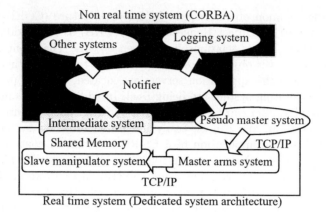

Fig. 1. System architecture

A system needs to function stably under such circumstances, and for the stable transmission of data using a CORBA-based system, the synchronous transmission of data is desirable for reliable communication among distributed objects. It is very difficult to define priorities for multiple objects connected to each other, unless the real time performance of the subsystems is well defined. In the case of a computer-aided surgery system, the configuration of the system may change, depending on the clinical requirements of specific cases. In the design of our prototype system, we prepared an intermediate system that allowed adjustments between the real time master-slave manipulator system and the CORBA-based system to be made. The system we developed consisted of a control system designed for real time control of the surgical master-slave manipulator system, a CORBA-based system that realized a distributed modular architecture, and an intermediate software system that connected these two systems(Fig. 1).

2.2 A Master-Slave Manipulator System with a Dedicated Communication System

The master-slave manipulator system consisted of a pair of master arms (MASTER) and a slave manipulator system (SLAVE). In the MASTER system(Fig. 3), an operator sits in front of a monitor showing a laparoscopic view and controls the master manipulators, using footswitches to command the SLAVE. The SLAVE system uses three slave robotic manipulators with seven degrees of freedom that include a grasping function, and an endoscope with a variable viewing angle [6,7]. The slave robotic manipulators are located on passive positioning arms for easier presetting of the manipulators before surgical operation. The position and orientation of the manipulators and the endoscope were measured using a Polaris optical positioning sensor (Northern Digital Inc., http://www.ndigital.com). The motion of the master arms was recognized as

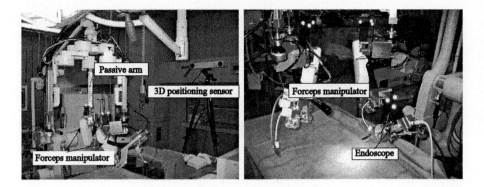

Fig. 2. Surgical slave manipulator system

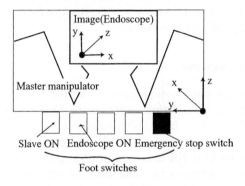

Fig. 3. Master arms system

the motion commands of the endoscope's coordinates, and this motion was transformed to the manipulator's coordinates. The required computation for the SLAVE control was conducted using a real time base. The MASTER and SLAVE were connected using a dedicated communication channel employing TCP/IP protocol. These two systems were tightly connected as a single client device and a server robot. As an alternative to the MASTER, a pseudo-MASTER could be used that could store the time series data from the master arms' motion and related control information, and could relay this data to the SLAVE. The pseudo-MASTER was also connected with the SLAVE using a dedicated communication channel, and in addition, this system was connected to the other distributed objects using CORBA. Using this pseudo-MASTER, the SLAVE could accept motion commands from the other objects using CORBA.

2.3   Common Object Request Broker Architecture (CORBA)

CORBA defines a framework for developing distributed applications. As many implementations support different operating systems, we chose the Adaptic Communication Environment (ACE) and the Object Request Broker (TAO) developed by Washington University, USA [8]. The developed system uses a CORBA-based system to interface with the distributed objects in the system. As an example of a distributed object that could be connected to the master-slave manipulator system, we implemented a logging system that recorded time-series data for the following control information:

- Commands from the master arm system to the slave manipulator system: the position and orientation of the master-manipulators and foot switches (On and Off).
- The status of the slave manipulators: position and orientation of the slave manipulators.
- The viewing direction of the endoscope.
- The set position of the slave manipulators: The set position of each passive arm holding the slave manipulator (the three slave manipulators, endoscope, and Polaris 3-D positioning sensor).

2.4 Intermediate System

We prepared an intermediate system located between the master-slave manipulator system and the communication system using CORBA software. The intermediate system receives data from the master-slave manipulator system in an asynchronous manner by means of a shared memory. It then sends the data to the other objects using CORBA in a synchronous manner to make the communication reliable. Introduction of this intermediate system loosely connected the master-slave manipulator system and the communication system using CORBA software. It prevented any interference with the robot control system due to instantaneous decrease of the system performance caused by communication overload and communication errors. Using this intermediate system, we were able to maintain the performance of the master-slave manipulator system and ensure the reliability of the entire system while keeping connectivity to the communication system based on CORBA. The developed system is shown in Figure 4. To evaluate the system stability under operating conditions, the proposed system design was subjected to the following tests using the experimental conditions shown in Figure 4.

- Logging the system using the proposed system design.
- Carrying out the master-slave experiment using a communication rate of 100 msec.
- Using the total recorded surgical information for evaluation.

3   Results and Discussion

We implemented the system described in Section 2, shown in Figure 4, and we conducted experiments in operating the master-slave surgical manipulator

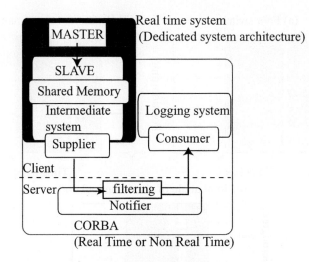

Fig. 4. System architecture in experiment

system. We also recorded the time-series data from the control data of the manipulators using CORBA in the logging system. We could successfully operate the master-slave manipulator and were able to record the control data without any problems. Figure 5 shows examples of the recorded data from the manipulator motion. Figures 5(a) and 5(b) show the position of the slave manipulator. The manipulator was only activated when the foot switch was activated. The data shows the expected behavior of the slave manipulator. Figure 5(c) shows the change in joint angle during operation. We also tested the system without the intermediate system connecting the communication system based on CORBA and the real time control system for the master-slave manipulator in place. Synchronous transmission was used in these experiments to maintain reliable communication. Under these conditions, the real time control system for the manipulator suffered from the influence of coexisting processes of the CORBA communication system, resulting in an unstable system operation. By reinserting the intermediate system, we could successfully interact with the communication processes of CORBA with real time control of the manipulator. The data stored in the logging system was also transferred to the pseudo-master system, and used to repeat the same recorded motions of the manipulator. The slave manipulator repeated the same motions in a stable manner. In the application of the system in a computer aided surgery environment, distributed objects in the system will not always be in a real time system. If we adopt a system with close connections that require a strict real time operation, such as manipulator control, then these non-real time objects can form a bottleneck that will determine the overall system performance. Schorr et al. reported the application of a CORBA-based system to control an image guided surgical robot. They controlled an MRI-compatible biopsy robot by sending its control information

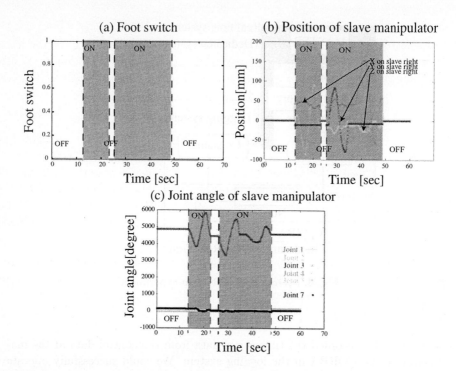

Fig. 5. Log data of logging system;(a)Foot switch, (b)Position of the slave manipulator, (c)Each joint angle of slave manipulator

using CORBA [3,4]. Considering the nature of an MRI scanner, it seems that the required bandwidth for communicating navigation data in that case is not as high as the bandwidth requirements for communicating to our master-arms and slave-manipulators or for the dynamic motion control of our robotic manipulators. Thus, it is effective to utilize CORBA as the communication interface. When we combine the master-slave manipulator system for less invasive surgery, or for a surgical navigation system or surgical simulation system, then in general, the required transmission frequency of the navigation data is not so high. On the other hand, the scalability of a system that allows for the connection of various types of intraoperative imaging devices and instrumentation with positional data is more important. From this consideration, we propose the use of the intermediate system that will compensate for differences in the required real time performance among the distributed objects, while maintaining a reliable and extendable data communication at relatively low frequency using CORBA.

4   Conclusion

We have proposed a method to resolve the two competing requirements of a surgical robotic system: scalability and reliability, and we have shown the following:

- Our system design combined real time objects, such as a master-slave manipulator control system with other non-real time objects used in a computer-aided surgical assistance system. With the proposed system design, the reliability and stability of real time systems and scalability of a CORBA-based system were realized at the same time.
- We developed an intermediate system with real time and asynchronous processing to compensate for the real time and non-real time nature of the distributed objects. This system enabled the coexistence of the dedicated system architectures required for real time processing and CORBA.
- As an example of this function, we developed a logging system for the motion control data from the manipulators and a pseudo master system for the manipulator operation. We confirmed the stable real time control of the surgical master-slave manipulator together with data communication to the other distributed objects.

In future work, we will incorporate a surgical navigation system using the master-slave surgical robotic manipulator to realize safe and accurate surgical operation of this system.

References

1. SONGMIN JIA and KUNIKATSU TAKASE. Internet-based robotic system using corba as communication architecture. *Journal of Intelligent and Robotic Systems*, 34:121–134, 2002.
2. A.Pernozzoli, C.Burghart, J.Brief, S.Habfeld, J.Raczkowsky, J.Muhling, U.Rembold, and H.Worn. A Real-time CORBA Based System Architecture for Robot Assisted Craniofacial Surgery. In *Medicine Meets Virtual Reality 2000 J.D. Westwood et al. (Eds.) IOS Press, 2000*, 2000.
3. A. Bzostek, R.Kumar, N.Hata, O. Schorr, R. Kikinis, and R. H .Taylor. Distributed Modular Computar-Integrated Surgical Robotic Systems:Implementation using modular software and network systems. In *proc, MICCAI '00*, pages 969–978, 2000.
4. Oliver Schorr, Nobuhiko Hata, Andrew Bzostek, Rajesh Kumar, Catherina Burghart, Russel H. Taylor, and Ron Kikinis. Distributed Modular Computar-Integrated Surgical Robotic Systems:Architecture for Intelligent Object Distribution. In *proc, MICCAI '00*, pages 979–987, 2000.
5. G.H.Ballantyne. Robotic surgery,telerobotic surgery,telepresence,and telementoring. In *Springer-Verlag New York Inc.*, pages 1389–1402, 2002.
6. Takashi Suzuki, Eisuke Aoki, Etsuko Kobayashi, Takayuki Tsuji, Kozo Konishi, Makoto Hashizume, and Ichiro Sakuma. Development of forceps manipulator for assisting laparoscopic surgery. In *proc of CARS*, page 1338, 2004.
7. Takemasa Hashimoto, Etsuko Kobayashi, Ichiro Sakuma, Kazuhiko Shinohara, Makoto Hashizume, and Takeyoshi Dohi. Development of wide-angle view laparoscope using wedge prisms. *Journal of Robotics and Mechatronics*, pages 129–137, 2004.
8. David Levine and Sumedh Mungee. The design and performance of real-time object request brokers. *Computer Communications*, 21, 1998.

Precise Evaluation of Positioning Repeatability of MR-Compatible Manipulator Inside MRI

Yoshihiko Koseki[1], Ron Kikinis[2], Ferenc A. Jolesz[2], and Kiyoyuki Chinzei[1]

[1] National Institute of Advanced Industrial Science and Technology,
1-2-1 Namiki, Tsukuba, Ibaraki 305-8564, Japan
http://unit.aist.go.jp/humanbiomed/surgical/
[2] Department of Radiology, Brigham and Women's Hospital,
Francis St. 75, Boston, MA 02115, USA
http://splweb.bwh.harvard.edu:8000/

Abstract. In this paper, we experimentally tested the positioning repeatability of MR-compatible manipulator with a CCD laser micrometer inside MRI. To evaluate the performance of MR-compatible manipulator inside MRI, the measuring system must be confirmed to work correctly inside MRI in advance. Therefore, the measuring system was tested to see if it can measure a specimen similarly regardless to inside or outside MRI. The results inside MRI were different from those outside MRI but the differences were small in comparison with the typical error of our manipulator. With this measuring system, the positioning repeatability of our MR-compatible manipulator was tested inside MRI with image sequence, inside MRI without image sequence, and outside MRI. The results proved that the manipulator performed 0.17[mm] translational and 0.17[deg] rotational positioning repeatability on average, whether inside or outside MRI, whether with or without image sequence.

1 Introduction

1.1 Robotic Assist for MR-Guided Surgery

It has been said for a long time that the combination of intraoperative tomography and robot would promote less invasive surgery, because a manipulator which is numerically controlled referring to the coordinate of tomography can precisely position a surgical tool to a tumor behind normal tissue. In particular among medical tomography, MRI is superior to X-ray CT in terms of its good soft tissue contrast, lack of ionizing radiation, and potential of functional imaging. Therefore, many researchers have been studying MR-compatible robotics, which can work inside and/or nearby MRI.

Masamune has proposed one for stereotactic neurosurgery since 1995[1]. We also have studied MR-compatible mechanics and electronics since 1996 to develop not only robotic manipulators but also other devices, which can work nearby MRI[2]. We have developed 5 d.o.f (degrees of freedom) manipulator for brachytherapy of prostate cancer[3], 6 d.o.f one for general purpose[4], and 4 d.o.f one for trans-nasal neuro-surgery in vertical field open MRI[5]. Kaiser also has proposed one for stereotactic biopsy and therapy of breast cancer since 2000[6].

C. Barillot, D.R. Haynor, and P. Hellier (Eds.): MICCAI 2004, LNCS 3217, pp. 192–199, 2004.
© Springer-Verlag Berlin Heidelberg 2004

1.2 Evalutaions of MR-Compatible Manipulator Inside MRI

Not only the development of MR-compatible manipulator, but the methods to evaluate it are also important. MRI's electromagnetic phenomena are static magnetic field B_0, dynamic magnetic field B_1, and image sequence (RF-pulse sequence). B_1 and image sequence might cause error on sensors and actuators of feedback loop. A movement of a metallic part in B_0 induces resistance force against the movement. Such complications between multi d.o.f manipulator and MRI make it difficult to predict the performance of the manipulator. Therefore, the final performance of MR-compatible manipulator under the influence of MRI's strong magnet must be tested inside MRI.

Measuring the manipulator's performance inside MRI is technically as difficult as developing an MR-compatible manipulator, because the measuring system itself is also under the influence of strong magnet, therefore requires validation of MR compatibility.

1.3 Our Approach

In this paper, we have studied the positioning repeatability of our MR-compatible manipulator inside MRI, because positioning repeatability is one of the most important performances of robot but it has never been precisely measured inside MRI to the extent of the authors' knowledge. This paper is composed from two experiments, the first is validation of the MR-compatibility of our measuring system, and the second is the robot test. A CCD laser micrometer was tested to see if it can measure a specimen similarly regardless to inside or outside MRI. After that, the repeatability of our MR-compatible manipulator was tested in same conditions. The results proved that the manipulator performed 0.17[mm] translational and 0.17[deg] rotational positioning repeatability on average, whether inside or outside MRI, whether with or without image sequence.

2 Materials and Methods

2.1 Measurement System Pretests

A CCD laser micrometer, VG-035/300 (KEYENCE, Osaka, Japan) was used for measurement. It is a pair of laser projector and receiver, and a cylindrical object is placed between them. The projector beams a sheet of laser and the receiver, a line CCD sensor detects the object's shadow. The CCD can detect the edge(s) of the object's shadow. VG-035/300 can measure the position and diameter of the object on the same basics. The summary specifications of VG-035/300 are described in Table 1.

A brass cylinder was prepared and measured by VG-035/300 inside MRI with image sequence, inside MRI without image sequence, and outside MRI. The reference cylinder and sensor heads were set in the gantry of intraoperative MRI, Signa SP^{TM}(GE Medical Systems, Milwaukee, WI, 0.5 Tesla). Signa SP has two magnets with 0.5[m] horizontal opening. Each magnet has an inside

Table 1. Summary specifications of KEYENCE VG-035/300 from its catalog

Sensor head	VG-035
Controller	VG-300
Measuring area	35mm
Repeatability	5 μm
Projector-receiver distance	0 to 300mm
Light source	Semiconductor laser
	(670nm, 38μW, pulse duration: 641μs)
CCD	Resolution: 5000bit
Sensor head's material	Die-cast aluminum

Table 2. Parameters of the MRI and the pulse sequence

Center frequency	21MHz	Bandwidth	62.5Hz
Sequence	Fast spin echo	Repetition time	1200ms
Echo time	96ms	Slice thickness	3.7mm
Matrix	256 × 256	Resolution	1.4mm^2

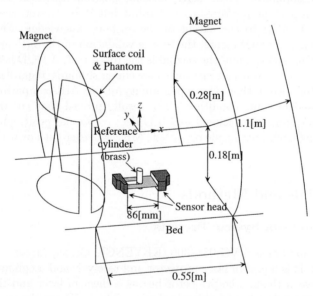

Fig. 1. Setup of measurement system pretest: arrangement of brass cylinder, sensor head, surface coil and phantom inside the gantry of GE's intraoperative MRI

diameter of 0.5[m] and outside diameter of 2.2[m]. The parameters of the MRI and the pulse sequence were shown in Table 2.

Inside the MRI, the reference cylinder was put vertically on the bed. The sensor heads were put horizontally on the bed. A surface coil and phantom were put on the end of imaging area avoiding the conflict with the cylinder and measuring system. In this test, applying image sequence was necessary but MRI imaging was not. However, MRI canceled the image sequence by detecting the absence of the surface coil and phantom. The geometrical setup is shown in Fig. 1. The diameter was measured 30 times for each condition.

2.2 Repeatability Tests of MR-Compatible Manipulator

For the manipulator examination, we used 6 d.o.f manipulator using leverage and parallelogram mechanism introduced in [4]. The leverage and parallelogram mechanism can transmit 3 translational and 3 rotational motions from the outside to the inside of MRI. This remote actuation enables the less MR-compatible and bulky driving units to be set away from MRI.

The driving units form a fixed-linear parallel mechanism, and are set beside the surgical bed, between magnets of Signa SP, above the surgeon. The kinematic parameters are decided to meet the translational workspace of ± 100[mm], and rotational workspace of ± 30[deg].

The linear actuator unit of parallel mechanism consists of ultrasonic motor (USR60-S3N: Shinsei Kogyo Corp., Tokyo, Japan), linear encoder (LM 25CPMM-3S: 0.01[mm] resolution after $\times 4$, Encoder Technology, CA, USA), and limit & home switch (EE-SV3: Omron, Kyoto, Japan). The electrical signals of linear encoder are optically transmitted to the outside of operation room.

The repeatability of our MR-compatible manipulator was tested inside MRI with image sequence, inside MRI without image sequence, and outside MRI. The image sequence parameters were same as before (see Table 2).

VG-035/300 can measure only 1 d.o.f. at a time. Fig. 2 shows how 6 d.o.f were measured with two sets of VG-035/300. The coordinate systems of the manipulator and the manipulator's tool holder were assumed to match that of MRI (See Fig. 1). A long bakelite bar was attached to the tool holder of the manipulator in parallel to $x-$axis of the tool holder. One set of VG-035/300 measured $z-$axis position of one point on the bar (a_x in Fig. 2), and the other set measured $z-$axis position of the different point (b_x in Fig. 2). The sensor heads were fixed on a precisely machined acrylic block, therefore the gap between two sets, $(x_2 - x_1)$, $(y_2 - y_1)$, and $(z_2 - z_1)$ and the gap between sensor heads, d_1 were relatively precise. The bakelite bar and the acrylic block were aligned manually so that the bakelite and the direction of $(x_2 - x_1)$ were parallel to $x-$axis of MRI. x_1, y_1, and z_1 had to be measured by a ruler. Therefore they were relatively imprecise.

The translational positioning error in $z-$axis and rotational positioning error around $y-$axis are calculated as the following equations. Hereafter, E_x, E_y, and E_z are translational positioning errors in $x-$, $y-$, and $z-$axis, respectively. E_p, E_q, and E_r are rotational positioning errors around $x-$, $y-$, and $z-$axis, respectively. $STDEV(a)$ is the standard deviation of group a.

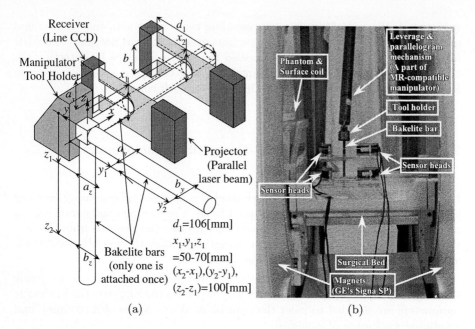

Fig. 2. Setup of the repeatability tests of MR-compatible manipulator: (a) the arrangement of bakelite bars and sensor heads around the manipulator's tool holder, (b) the arrangement of MR-compatible robot arm, sensor heads, bakelite bar, surface coil and phantom inside the gantry of GE's intraoperative MRI

$$E_q = STDEV\left(\tan^{-1}\left(\frac{b_x - a_x}{x_2 - x_1}\right)\right) \tag{1}$$

$$E_z = STDEV\left(\frac{b_x - a_x}{x_2 - x_1}(-x_1) + a_x\right) \tag{2}$$

The manipulator moved the bakelite bar to a specific measurement point from the neighboring random point, and the position of the bar was measured in above-mentioned manner. This procedure was repeated 30 times. After that, the bar's direction was changed to y−axis and z−axis, and x−axis positions and y−axis positions were measured each time. The series of measurement were performed at 5 points, $(x, y, z) = (-60, -60, -60)$, $(60, -60, -60)$, $(0, 0, 0)$ $(-60, 60, 60)$, and $(60, 60, 60)$ and all orientations were $(roll, pitch, yaw) = (0, 0, 0)$. While this experiment, any parts of manipulator including the bar didn't touch with measuring system or surgical bed.

3   Results and Discussion

3.1   Measurement System Pretests

Fig. 3 shows the average and standard deviation of the reference cylinder's diameter, inside MRI with image sequence, inside MRI without image sequence, outside MRI, and the average through all conditions.

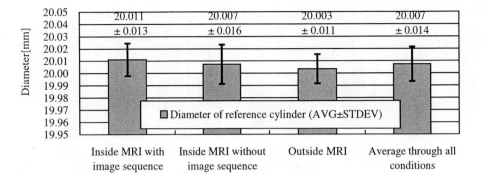

Fig. 3. The average and standard deviation of the reference cylinder's diameter, measured inside MRI with image sequence, inside MRI without image sequence, and outside MRI.

The averages and standard deviations of each condition were slightly different. The results showed that image sequence didn't increase the standard deviation, and that outside MRI, the cylinder measured smaller than inside MRI. However, the standard deviation through all conditions, 0.014[mm] was small in comparison with the positioning error of manipulator.

The possible factors of the difference were the influence of MRI and image sequence, incomplete roundness of the cylinder, and setting of sensor heads and the cylinder. It must be noted that not only electric and/or magnetic influence on measuring systems, but also geometrical imprecision, such as roughness of surgical bed, imprecision of mounting block makes geometrical measurement difficult inside MRI.

This pretest concluded that the MRI's influence on the CCD laser micrometer was negligible, and that the CCD laser micrometer was adequate as the reference of the repeatability test of the MR-compatible manipulator inside MRI.

3.2   Repeatability Tests of MR-Compatible Manipulator

Fig. 4 shows the translational and rotational positioning errors of the MR-compatible leverage and parallelogram manipulator, inside MRI with image sequence, inside MRI without image sequence, outside MRI, and average through all conditions. The errors of each condition were the averages of 5 points. The error ranges were standard deviations of 5 points.

The differences of rotational error between the conditions were minor. The differences of translational error between the conditions were relatively large. The repeatability inside MRI without image sequence was the best and that outside MRI was the worst.

The major possible factors of the error difference between the conditions were the influence of MRI and image sequence on the measuring system and manipulator, setting of the manipulator, bakelite bars, and acrylic block. The results of rotational error indicated that MRI or image sequence didn't influence the

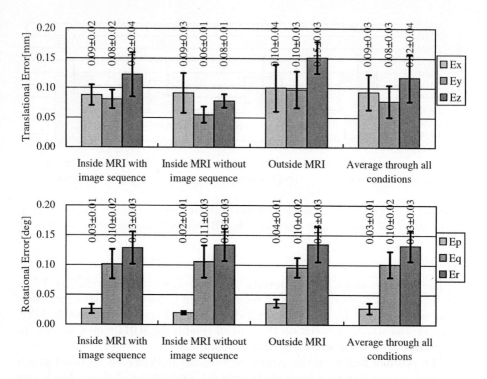

Fig. 4. Translational(upper) and rotational(lower) positioning errors of the MR-compatible leverage and parallelogram manipulator, inside MRI with image sequence, inside MRI without image sequence, outside MRI, and average through all conditions

rotational repeatability. In case of this MR-compatible leverage and parallelogram manipulator, the rotational error and translational error are correlated, because the combination of 6 similar linear driving units determines the position and orientation. Therefore those led that MRI or image sequence didn't influence the translational or rotational repeatability. The rotational error depends on relatively precise parameters (See Eq. (1)). However, the translational error depends on relatively imprecise parameters (See Eq. (2)). So the difference of translational error between the conditions was mainly caused by setting of measuring systems. This experiment indicated that the method to measure the rotational error was precise and adequate to judge if the MRI's influence on the positioning error was minor or not. The method to measure the translational error was relatively imprecise and needs improvement.

In case of rotational repeatability, the order of better repeatability was clear - x-axis was 0.03[deg], y-axis 0.10[deg], and z-axis 0.13[deg] on average through all conditions. The root sum square of average rotational error over all axes was 0.17[deg]. In case of translational repeatability, the order of better repeatability was made unclear by the error of measurement system. The root sum square of average translational error over all axes was 0.17[mm].

4   Conclusion

The engineering significance of this paper is that we have studied how to test the positioning repeatability of MR-compatible manipulator inside MRI. Our method consists of validation of MR-compatibility of measuring system and measurement of the manipulator's repeatability.

Firstly, a CCD laser micrometer was tested to see if it can measured a specimen similarly regardless to inside or outside MRI. The results were different from those outside MRI but the differences were small in comparison with positioning error of manipulator.

Secondly, with this measuring system, the positioning repeatability of our MR-compatible manipulator was tested inside MRI with image sequence, inside MRI without image sequence, and outside MRI. This experiment indicated that the method to measure the rotational error was precise and adequate to judge if the MRI's influence on the positioning error was minor. The method to measure the translational error was relatively imprecise and needs improvement. The results proved that the manipulator performed 0.17[mm] translational and 0.17[deg] rotational positioning repeatability on average, whether inside or outside MRI, whether with or without image sequence.

Acknowledgments. In Japan, this research has been funded by NEDO grant #02A47019b and AIST. In the USA, this research has been funded by NIH grant #P41RR013218, #P01CA067165, and ERC grant #9731748.

We wish to thank Mr. Daniel Kacher for the contribution to this research, as well as the technologists and support staffs of SPL and MRT.

References

1. Masamune K., Kobayashi E., Masutani Y., Suzuki M., Dohi T., Iseki H., Takakura K.: Development of an MRI-compatible needle insertion manipulator for stereotactic neurosurgery. Journal of Image Guided Surgery. **1(4)** (1995) 242–248
2. Chinzei K., Kikinis R., Jolesz F.A.: MR Compatibility of Mechatronic Devices: Design Criteria. Proc. of MICCAI'99, (1999) 1020–1031
3. Chinzei K., Hata N., Jolesz F.A., Kikinis R.: MR Compatible Surgical Assist Robot System Integration and Preliminary Feasibility Study. Proc. of MICCAI 2000 921–930
4. Koseki Y., Koyachi K., Arai T., Chinzei K.: Remote Actuation Mechanism for MR-compatible Manipulator Using Leverage and Parallelogram, Workspace Analysis, Workspace Control, and Stiffness Evaluation. Proc. of ICRA2003 652–657
5. Koseki Y., Washio T., Chinzei K., Iseki H.: Endoscope Manipulator for Trans-nasal Neurosurgery, Optimized for and Compatible to Vertical Field Open MRI. Proc. of MICCAI 2002 114–121
6. Kaiser W.A., Fischer H., Vagner J., Selig M.: Robotic system for Biopsy and Therapy in a high-field whole-body Magnetic-Resonance-Tomograph. Proc. Intl. Soc. Mag. Reson. Med. **8** (2000), 411

Simulation Model of Intravascular Ultrasound Images

Misael Dario Rosales Ramírez[1,2], Petia Radeva Ivanova[2], Josepa Mauri[3], and Oriol Pujol[2]

[1] Laboratorio de Física Aplicada, Universidad de los Andes, Mérida 5133, Venezuela,
[2] Centre de Visió per Computador, 08193 Bellaterra, Barcelona, Spain
[misael,petia,oriol]@cvc.uab.es
[3] Hospital Universitari Germans Trias y Pujol, Badalona, Spain
jmauri@ms.hugtip.scs.es

Abstract. The extraction of quantitative information through Intravascular Ultrasound (IVUS) images is a very important goal for the diagnostic and the therapy in atherosclerotic vessels. The correct interpretation highly depends on what gray level values of the image mean, i.e understanding of IVUS image formation. In this project, we propose a simple physical model for simulating IVUS images, based on a discrete representation of the tissue by individual scatterers elements with given spatial distribution and Backscattering Cross Section. This simulation allows studying the significance and the relation between different tissues and the image. Our model allows to study the physics parameters for the IVUS image generation in order to help to the best interpretation (the study of the visibility and robust discrimination of the different structures) as well as to allow creating image data bases to be used during validation of image processing techniques.

1 Introduction

The introduction of the IntraVascular UltraSound (IVUS) [1,2] as an exploratory technique has made a significant change to the understanding of the arterial diseases and individual patterns of diseases in the coronary arteries. Huge amount of data and difficult interpretation pushed developing of image processing techniques, border segmentation, plaque characterization, multi-modal fusion [3], etc. The question is how to develop robust algorithms that can solve these problems analyzing the artifacts with their multiple appearance in IVUS images. Having a complete set of patient data to present all variance of artifacts appearance in images would mean to dispose of a huge amount of patient cases. A more efficient solution is to develop a simulation model for IVUS data construction so that synthetic data are available in order to "train" image processing techniques. Image study based on modelling the image generation process is a relatively new field, there is a different works [4,5,6] oriented to the simulation of conventional ultrasound images, based on the interaction of sound waves and the biological tissue. Nevertheless, there is no recent investigation about the basic physical principles, as well as the protocols of image processing to obtain intravascular ultrasound images. In this way, different appearance of artifacts can be designed

C. Barillot, D.R. Haynor, and P. Hellier (Eds.): MICCAI 2004, LNCS 3217, pp. 200–207, 2004.

to assure the robust performance of image processing techniques. Differences in IVUS data are caused not only by different morphological structures of vessels but also by different parameters that influence the formation of IVUS images. The images depend on the IVUS apparatus calibration as well as interventional devices, small differences in parameters can lead to different grey-level appearance that can be interpreted in a different way by the physicians. Having a simulation model for IVUS data can help to the training of medical staff as well as can have an important role in designing and testing new interventional devices. At the end, being aware which parameters and in which grade influence to image formation is of unquestionable importance for all persons involved in comprehension of IVUS data and taking final decision for diagnosis and intervention of vessel lesions. The article has been organized as follow: Section 2 we discuss a simple simulation model for formation of 2D IVUS data that explains the complete process of data generation as a result of the interaction between ultrasound signals and vessel morphological structures, section 3 the validation and results are discussed and the conclusions are presented in section 4.

1.1   Formal Definition of the Image Model

IVUS images can be obtained in a simulated form, from a simple physical model based on the transmission and reception of high frequency sound waves, when these radially penetrate a simulated arterial structure (Fig. 1 (a)). Let us consider a ultrasound pulse P_o that is emitted at time t_o with speed c from the point with coordinates (r_o, θ_o, z_o) (Fig. 1 (b)), and that interacts with the scatterer located at the position, (R, Θ, Z) with the spatial distribution of the differential backscattering cross-section, $\sigma(R, \Theta, Z)$. The reflected pulse P_i for the i-th scatterer is an exact replica [7] of the transmitted sound pulse P_o that will return to the point (r_o, θ_o, z_o) at time $(t_i - t_o)$ and will be out of phase temporarily with respect to the pulse P_o by time difference $\delta = t_i - t_o$ between the emitted pulse at t_i and the received pulse at t_o. The time delay δ is given by $\delta = 2|R|/c$. Assuming the Born approximation [8,9], the reflected signal $S(t, \tau)$ for a finite set of N reflecting scatterers with coordinates (R, Θ, Z) and spatial distribution of the differential backscattering cross-section $\sigma(R, \Theta, Z)$ is given by:

$$S(R, \Theta, Z, t, \tau) = \sum_{i=1}^{N} \sigma_i(R, \Theta, Z)\zeta_i(t, \tau) \tag{1}$$

where N is the number of scatterers, $\sigma_i(R, \Theta, Z)$ is the spatial distribution of the Differential Backscattering Cross-section (DBC) of the i-th scatterer located in position (R, Θ, Z), $\zeta_i(t, \tau)$ is the transducer impulse function and τ is the delay time which leads to constructive and destructive contributions to the received signal. We consider a planar transducer that is mounted inside an infinite baffle, so that the ultrasound is only radiated in the forward direction [10,11]. The far field circular transducer pressure $P(r, \theta, t)$ can be written as:

$$P(r, \theta, t) = j\frac{\rho_o c k a^2 v_o}{2r}\left[\frac{2J_1(ka\sin(\theta))}{ka\sin(\theta)}\right]exp(j(wt - kr)) \tag{2}$$

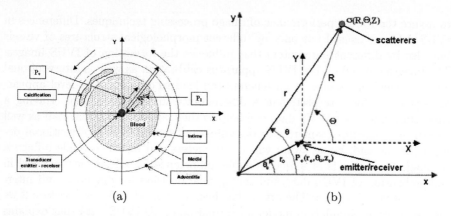

Fig. 1. The disposition (a) of the simulated arterial structures and calcification. The coordinates system (b) used in the model.

where t is the time, ρ_o is the medium propagation density, c is the sound speed for biological tissue, v_o is the radial speed at a point of the transducer surface, a is the transducer radius, $\vec{k}$ is the propagation vector, defined as $k = |\vec{k}| = 2\pi/\lambda$, λ the ultrasound wave length, defined as $\lambda = c/fo$, f_o ultrasound frequency, $\omega = 2\pi f_o$ and $J_1(x)$ is the first class Bessel function. The impulse function $\zeta(t, \delta)$ is generally approximated by a Gaussian which envelopes the intensity distribution and is given by: $\zeta(t, \delta) = I(r, \theta, t) \exp\left(-(t - \delta)^2/2\sigma^2\right)$, where σ is the pulse standard deviation. We consider that the beam is collimated by $\theta = \theta_a$. Hence Eq. (1) in the transducer coordinate system is based on a discrete representation of the tissue of individual scatterer elements with given position and DBC with respect to the transducer coordinates given by:

$$S(R, \Theta, Z, t, \delta) = C_o \sum_{i=1}^{N} \frac{\sigma_i(R, \Theta, Z)}{|R_i|} \zeta(t, \delta) \tag{3}$$

If we consider only the axial intensity contributions, C_o can be written as [10]: $C_o = \rho_o ck^2 v_o^2 A/8\pi$, where A is the transducer area.

The beam ultrasound intensity, as a function of the penetration depth and the ultrasound frequency, is given by [10,11,12]: $I(r) = I_o exp\left(-\alpha(N_\theta)rf\right)$ where I_o is the beam intensity at $r = 0$ and the coefficient, α give the rate of diminution of average power with respect to the distance along a transmission path [16]. It is composed of two parts, one (absorption) proportional to the frequency, the other (scattering) dependent on the ratio of grain, particle size or the scatterer number N_θ located along the ultrasound beam path.

1.2   Determining the Scatterer Number of Arterial Structures

The Red Blood Cells (RBCs) number swept by the ultrasound beam (Fig. 2) can be estimated taking into account the plastic sheathing dimensions of the

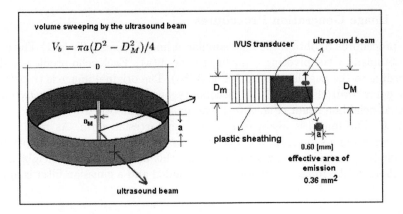

Fig. 2. The scatterers volume for each arterial structure can be calculated taken into account the total volume V_b swept by the ultrasound beam.

transducer and the typical arterial lumen diameter. The scatterer number contained in a sweeping beam volume is given by the difference between the sweeping lumen arterial volume, V_a and the plastic sheathing transducer volume, V_t. $V_b = V_a - V_t = \pi a(D^2 - D_M^2)/4$, where D and D_M are the arterial lumen and the sheathing transducer exterior diameters respectively, and a is the effective emission diameter of the transducer. The numerical values necessary for the evaluation of the DBC scatterer distribution for the intima, media and adventitia were taken from results of L. T. Perelman et. al [13], that give the typical nuclear cells size $l(\mu m)$ distribution for human cells. The "voxel" number for each layer was computed taken into account the typical dimensions of intima, media and adventitia of a normal artery. The voxel number for the sheathing transducer was calculated taking into account the minimal scatterers able to be observed at maximal resolution when the frequency is fixed at $40MHz$, a typical IVUS frequency.

1.3   Generation of the Simulated Arterial Structure

Considering the goal of simulating different arterial structures, we can classify them in 3 groups: Tissue structures, non tissue structures and artifacts. The spatial distribution of the scatterer number with a given DBC, $\sigma(R, \Theta, Z)$ at point (R, Θ, Z) has the following contributions: $\sigma(R, \Theta, Z) = A(R) + B(R, \Theta, Z) + C(R)$, where A(R) are the tissue scatterers, these are determined by the contribution of the normal artery structures, corresponding to: *lumen, intima, media and adventitia*. $B(R, \Theta, Z)$, are non tissue scatterers. These contributions can be originated by structures formed by spatial calcium accumulation, which are characterized because the DBC density is greater than the rest of the arterial structures and C(R) are the artifacts scatterers. In our model we consider only the artefact caused by the sheathing transducer.

1.4   Image Generation Procedures

The procedures to obtain the final simulated image are as follows: 1) The echoes are obtained by the pivoting transducer (Fig. 3 (a)). Each echo profile is ordered according to the angular position (Fig. 3 (b)). The original image is transformed to a polar form (Fig. 3 (c)). 4) Secondary beams are computed between two original neighbor beam (Fig. 3 (c)) The image is smoothed by a 2×2 median filter. 6) The image is again transformed to cartesian form. As result of this transformation a significant number of pixels will be empty. 7) The empty pixels are filled in a recursive way form, using for this an average of the eight nearest neighbors. 8) An image reference reticle is added and a gaussian filter is applied.

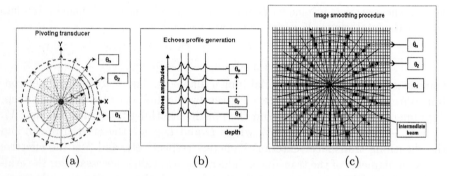

(a)   (b)   (c)

Fig. 3. The transducer emits from the artery center (a), echoes profile (b), the final IVUS image is smoothed (c).

2   Validation of the Image Simulation Model

Once defined the generic basic model of IVUS image formation, we need to compare it to real images contrasting the expert opinion to test its use. In order to compare the real and simulated IVUS images, we have generated 20 synthetic images with morphological structures corresponding to the structures of a set of real images. We have used a real IVUS image with manually delimited lumen, intima, and adventitia to obtain the average radius location, $\overline{R}_k$ for each arterial structure. We applied the optimal frequency of 46 MHz and attenuation coefficient 0.8 [dB/MHZ cm] obtained by cross validation method [14]. Fig. 4 shows an IVUS real image of right coronary artery (a) obtained by a 40 MHz Boston Sci. equipment [15] and simulated (c) cartesian IVUS images and the corresponding real (b) and simulated (d) polar transformations. The global appearance of each image region (lumen, intima, media and adventitia) and their corresponding interface transitions (lumen/intima, intima/media and media/adventitia) are visually well contrasted, compared to the real image. We can see a good gray

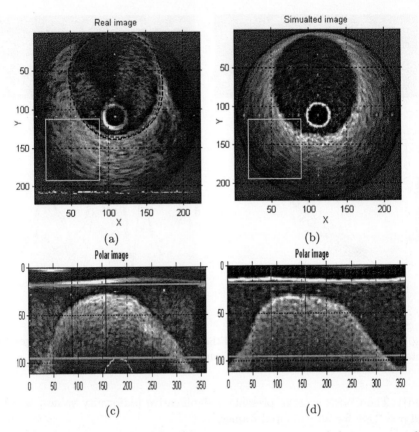

Fig. 4. Real (a) and simulated (b) IVUS images segmentation and their corresponding real (b) and simulated (d) polar transformation. ROIs are given as squares. Manual segmentation of the vessel is given in (a).

level distribution and a soft grey level decay from the center to the peripheries of the IVUS image, produced by the inverse relation between the ultrasound intensity and the penetration depth. Real IVUS images and their corresponding ROIs were selected, the spatial boundaries of the morphological structures of the real data are kept in the synthetic data. Fig. 5 (a) shows 10 real and their corresponding simulated (b) synthetic images. Figure 5 (c) shows the simulated vs real gray level correlation for the polar ROI's images selected as shown in (Fig. 4 (c) and (d)). The linear correlation coefficients show a good gray levels correspondence, being these m=0.90 and b=1.42. The best correspondence is located by low gray levels (20 to 40 gray levels), lumen scatterers, lumen/intima transition, and adventitia. The transition of intima/media and media/adventitia (45 to 60 gray levels) indicate a gradual dispersion. The contrast to noise ratio CNRS as figure of similarity for each arterial validated region is shown in (Fig.

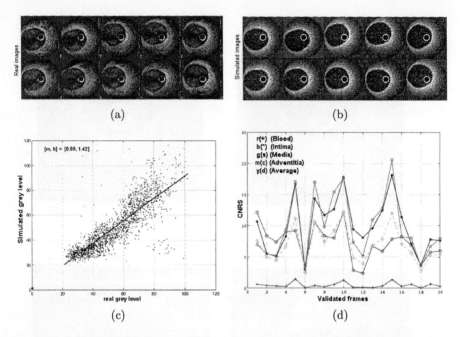

Fig. 5. 10 original IVUS images (a) and the corresponding simulated (b) images. Simulated vs real grey level ROIs values (c) and its CNRS values (c)

5 (d)). The CNRS average presents a significative uniformity values, $\mu = 6.89$ and $\sigma = 2.88$, for all validated frames.

3   Conclusions

Although IVUS is continuously gaining its use in practice due to its multiple clinical advantages, the technical process of IVUS image generation is not known by doctors and researchers developing IVUS image analysis. This fact leads to a simplified use, analysis and interpretation of IVUS images based only on the grey level values of image pixels. In this paper we discuss a basic physical model to generate synthetic 2D IVUS images. The model has different utilities: Firstly, expert medical doctors can generate simulated IVUS images, in order to observe different arterial structures of clinical interest and their grey level distribution in real images. Secondly, medical doctors can use our model to learn and to compare the influence of different physical parameters in the IVUS image formation, for example: the ultrasound frequency, the attenuation coefficient, the beam number influence, and the artifact generations. The obtained results of the validation of our model illustrate a good approximation to the image formation process. The 2D IVUS images show a good correspondence between the arterial structures that generate the image structures and their gray level values. Interested readers are invited to check the generation model in (http://www.cvc.uab.es/∼misael).

References

1. Yock P., Linker D., Saether O., et al., Intravascular two dimensional catheter ultrasound, Initial clinical studies, abstracted, Circulations, No. 78 (suppl II): II-21, 1988.
2. Graham S., Brands D., Sheehan H., et al., Assesment of arterial wall morphology using intravascular ultrasound in vitro and in patient, Circulations, (Suppl II): II-56, 1989.
3. Berry E., and et al, Intravascular ultrasound-guided interventions in coronary artery disease, Tech. Rep., Healt Technology Assesment, NHS R D HTA Programme. A systemac literature review, with decisions-analytic modelling, of outcomes and cot-effectiveness, 2000.
4. Jensen J., A Model for the Propagation and Scattering of Ultrasound in Tissue, J. Acoust. Soc. Am, 1991, 89, 182-191.
5. Jensen J., A Program for Simulating Ultrasound Systems,Paper presented at the 10th Nordic-Baltic Conference on Biomedical Imaging Published in Medical and Biological Engineering and Computing, 1996, Part 1, Supplement 1, 351-353.
6. Trobaugh J., An Image Model for Ultrasound Incorporating Surface Shape and Microstructure and Characteristics of Imaging System, Washington University, Sever Institute of Technology, Departmet of Electrical Ingeniering, 2000, Doctoral thesis.
7. Verhoef, W.A, Cloostermans, M.J, and Thijssen, J.M, The Impulse Response of a Focused Source With an Arbitrary Axisymmetric Surface Velocity Distribution, Journal Acoustic Society American, 1984, 75", 1717-1721.
8. Fontaine I., Bertrand M, Cloutier G., A system-based approach to modelling the ultrasound signal backscattered by red blood cells,Biophysical Journal, Vol. 77, pp. 2387-2399, 1999
9. Fan L., Herrington D., Santiago P., Simulation of b-mode ultrasound to determine features of vessel for image analysis, Computers in Cardiology, Vol. 25, pp. 165-168,1998
10. Cheeke D., Fundamentals and Aplications of Ultrasonic Waves, CRC PRESS, 2002.
11. Kinsler L. , Fundamentos de acústica, LIMUSA, Noriega Editores, 1995.
12. Zagzebski J., Essential of Ultrasound Physics, Mosby A. hardcourt Healt Sciences Company, 1996.
13. Perelman L., and et al, Observation of periodic fine structure in reflectance from biological tissue: A new technique for measuring nuclear size distribution, Physical Review Letters, Vol. 80, No. 3, pp. 627-630, January 1998.
14. Rosales M., Radeva P., A basic model for IVUS image simulation in Handbook of Medical Imaging, Kluwer Academic/Plenium Publishers, 233 Spring Street, New York, NY 10013, USA, (in press), 2004.
15. Boston Scientific Corporation, Scimed division, The ABCs of IVUS, 1998.
16. Arendt Jesen J., Linear Descripcion of Ultrasound Imaging System, Notes for the international Summer School on Advanced Ultrasound Imaging, Tecnical University of Denamark, 2001.

Vessel Driven Correction of Brain Shift

Ingerid Reinertsen[1], Maxime Descoteaux[2], Simon Drouin[1], Kaleem Siddiqi[2], and D. Louis Collins[1]

[1] Montreal Neurological Institute, McGill University, Montréal, Canada
[2] Center for Intelligent Machines, McGill University, Montréal, Canada

Abstract. In this paper, we present a method for correction of brain shift based on segmentation and registration of blood vessels from pre-operative MR images and intraoperative Doppler ultrasound data. We segment the vascular tree from both MR and US images and use chamfer distance maps and a non-linear registration algorithm to estimate the deformation between the two datasets. The method has been tested in a series of simulation experiments, and in a phantom study. Preliminary results show that we are able to account for large portions of the non-linear deformations and that the technique is capable of estimating shifts when only a very limited region of the brain is covered by the ultrasound volume.

1   Introduction

Modern image guided neurosurgery (IGNS) systems enable the surgeon to navigate within the patient's brain using pre-operative anatomical images (MRI, CT) as a guide. The pre-operative images are related to the patient using a rigid body transformation calculated from a number of anatomical landmarks that can be easily identified on both the patient's head and the pre-operative images. By using a computer-tracked probe during the procedure, the surgeon can localize any point in the patient's brain on the pre-operative images. A significant source of error in these systems is brain tissue movement and deformation, so called brain shift, during the procedure. Tissue movement can be caused by gravity, retraction, resection and administration of medication. The amount of movement and its influence on the accuracy of the neuro-navigation system depend on a number of factors including surgical target location, craniotomy size and patient position during surgery. The magnitude of brain shift is estimated to range from 5mm to 50mm [11,6]. Several strategies have been proposed to quantify and correct for anatomical changes during surgery. Model based techniques have shown to recover up to 80% of the error induced by brain deformation[7,12]. One of the main challenges in this approach is to correctly estimate the mechanical properties of brain tissue which may vary significantly between patients and between tissue types.

The more direct solution to the problem is to acquire new images when significant amount of deformation is suspected. The most popular intraoperative imaging modalities for neurosurgery are intraoperative MRI [1,14], intraoperative CT [13] and intraoperative ultrasound (US) imaging. Even though intraoperative MR imaging provides good quality images in reasonable time, this

C. Barillot, D.R. Haynor, and P. Hellier (Eds.): MICCAI 2004, LNCS 3217, pp. 208–216, 2004.
© Springer-Verlag Berlin Heidelberg 2004

solution suffers from a number of limitations. Intra-operative MR imaging is a complex, expensive and sometimes time consuming procedure. The intraoperative images are of lessor quality than pre-operative MR images due to scanner design and short acquisition times. Another major shortcoming of this solution is the substantial investment required for the scanner as well as MR-compatible surgical instruments. In many cases, interventional MRI systems also compromises the surgeon's access to the operating field.

Intraoperative ultrasound imaging does not suffer from many of the limitations associated with interventional MRI. A high-end ultrasound scanner costs less than 10% of a typical MRI system and is already in use by many neurosurgeons. In addition, ultrasound systems are portable and compatible with existing surgical equipment. Despite these advantages, the use of ultrasound in neuronavigation has been limited, probably due to poor image quality and limited skills to interpret such images.

Since the mid-1990's a number of groups have developed systems correlating intraoperative US with pre-operative MR. In a neurosurgical context, intraoperative ultrasound imaging can either be used directly as a surgical guide when brain shift occurs [2] or be used as a registration target for the pre-operative images in order to correct for deformations. Roche et al. [9] estimated the rigid body transform required to linearly align pre-operative MR images and intraoperative US images. They correlated the US intensities with both the MR intensity and the MR gradient magnitude using a variant of the correlation ratio and a robust distance measure. They reported registration errors up to 1.65 mm translation and 1.57 deg. rotation.

In order to correct for non-linear deformation Arbel et al. [3] used a tracking system to reconstruct 3D volumes from a series of US images in the same space as the pre-operative MR-image. From the pre-operative MR images, they created pseudo-US images that closely resembled real US images of the same structures acquired during surgery. They then used an intensity based non-linear registration technique to match tracked intraoperative US images with the pseudo-US images to detect and correct brain deformations. Qualitative results from 12 surgical cases showed that the technique was able to account for a large portions of the deformations.

Registration of intraoperative US with pre-operative MR is a challenging registration problem due to very different underlying physical principles and thus different image characteristics. Image intensities, noise characteristics, contrast, volume coverage and dimensionality are only a few main differences between a typical pre-operative MR image and a corresponding intraoperative ultrasound acquisition.

To try to overcome some of these difficulties, we explore a different approach to this particular registration problem. The idea is to use homologous features in the two datasets. Such features might be any segmented structures present in both images such as edges and other easily identifiable landmarks. In this project we investigate the use of blood vessels segmented from pre-operative angiographic images and Doppler US for registration purposes. Blood vessels are relatively easy to identify and segment from both pre-operative angiographic data such as MR angiograms (MRA) or gadolinium enhanced MR images and from Doppler ultrasound images. The vessels are distributed all over the cortex and inside the brain which means that they will be present in almost any region of interest (ROI). Keeping track of important vessels during surgery also provides the surgeon with important reference points in order to avoid major vessels during the procedure and monitor blood supply to specific areas of the brain.

In this paper we present a method for non-linear registration of pre-operative MR images and intraoperative US data driven by angiographic images. In section 2 we describe the registration technique in detail, and in section 3 and 4 we present a series of simulations and a phantom study in order to test and validate the method. Finally, the results and future work are discussed in the last part of the paper.

2   Methods

The goal of this work is to correct the patient's pre-operative images (anatomical, angiographic, functional,..) for any non-linear brain deformations based on Doppler ultrasound images acquired at different stages during surgery. Before surgery, the patient's angiographic MR images (MRA or gadolinium enhanced MRI) are segmented in order to build a 3D model of the patient's vasculature. Using the 3D model of the vascular tree, we compute a 3D chamfer distance map for use in the registration process. During the surgical procedure, a series of Doppler US images are acquired and reconstructed into a 3D volume using information from the tracking system and the pre-computed probe calibration matrix. The Doppler signal representing the blood vessels is then segmented from the b-mode ultrasound image to obtain a 3D representation of the portion of the vascular tree covered by the US volume. A chamfer distance map is then computed for the US model of the vessels, and used as input to the registration algorithm. Using the two original volumes along with the two chamfer distance maps, we estimate a non-linear deformation field in order to detect any deformation between the pre-operative and intraoperative models of the cerebral vasculature. The resulting deformation field can then be applied to the pre-operative MR images (anatomical and angiographic images) to provide the surgeon with MR images reflecting the surgical reality at any given point during the procedure. These steps will be described in more detail in the following sections.

2.1   Vessel Segmentation

We use a new multi-scale geometric flow for segmenting vasculature in the MR image of the phantom. The method first applies Frangi's vesselness measure [10] to find putative centerlines of tubular structures along with their estimated radii and orientation. This multi-scale measure is then distributed to create a vector field which is orthogonal to vessel boundaries so that the flux maximizing flow algorithm [15] can be applied to recover them. The technique overcomes many limitations of existing approaches in the literature specifically designed for angiographic data due its multi-scale tubular structure model. It has a formal motivation, is topologically adaptive due to its implementation using level set methods, is computationally efficient and requires minimal user interaction. The technique is detailed in [8].

2.2   Chamfer Similarity Function

The chamfer similarity function has been developed and described by Borgefors [4]. The algorithm has since then been applied in a number of different fields as a technique for finding the best fit of edge points from two different images, by minimizing a generalized distance between them. The algorithm takes binary images representing the edges to register as input. It then computes a chamfer distance map corresponding to the source image. This is an image where every non-edge voxel is given a value approximating the Euclidean distance to the closest edge voxel. The target image is then superimposed onto the distance map and translated and rotated in an iterative manner until the root mean square of the voxels in the distance map corresponding to edge points in the target image is minimum.

Another possible approach is to compute chamfer distance maps for both source and target images and then minimize the difference between the two maps. We found this to be more robust than the classic structure-chamfer matching, it is therefore the technique used in the ANIMAL registration procedure described in the following section.

2.3   Non-linear Registration

In this project we use the ANIMAL registration package [5] to compute the non-linear transformation required to map pre-operative MR to intraoperative US images. ANIMAL estimates a dense three dimensional vector field that gives point to point correspondences between the source and target image. The algorithm works in an hierarchical manner, starting with images blurred with a fwhm of 16mm to estimate the largest deformations, and then refining the transformation by using less blurred data. The algorithm builds up a 3D grid covering the target volume, and performs a search within a user-defined local neighborhood around each node. At each resolution level, the optimal displacement vector is stored for each node in the 3D grid. For the most common registration tasks, ANIMAL uses the cross-correlation similarity function to optimize the fit between the source and target image. However, in this project we incorporate the use of chamfer distance maps and minimization of the simple difference between the two distance maps into the algorithm. Both original images and chamfer distance maps were given as input to the registration algorithm, but the optimization was heavily weighted toward the minimization of the difference between the distance maps with a weight of 1 to 100, for the cross-correlation on the original images and difference between chamfer maps, respectively.

3   Simulations

3.1   Method

A patient's gadolinium enhanced MR image used in the simulations was acquired using a Philips 1.5T Gyroscan (The Netherlands) machine and was segmented manually in order to extract the cerebral vasculature. Following the segmentation, we placed anchor points for a thin plate spline transform throughout the volume. Four points on the cortical surface above the tumor were then manually displaced from 3 to 10 mm in the positive and negative x-direction, which represent a smooth expansion or contraction toward the mid-line of the brain. The thin plate spline transform was then computed between the original point set and the pointset containing the displaced points. The resulting transform was applied to the original image and the segmented vessels, and chamfer distance maps were calculated both for the original and transformed volumes. In order to simulate the situation where the Doppler ultrasound data only covers a small portion of the entire brain, we extracted a region of interest (ROI) of $69 \times 75 \times 70 mm^3$ covering the tumor area from the deformed original image and chamfer map. Finally, the original image, the original chamfer map, the ROI of the deformed image and the ROI of the deformed chamfer map were input to the ANIMAL registration algorithm in order to recover the known transformation.

3.2   Results

The results of the simulations for three different displacements are shown in Table 1. Figure 1 shows the initial difference between the original and the transformed image and the corresponding difference image after non-linear registration extimated in the ROI.

Table 1. RMS3D before and after non-linear registration. The RMS3D error is estimated on a regular grid covering the ROI.

Displacement(mm)	RMS3D before registration(mm)	RMS3D after registration(mm)
5.00	2.37	0.60
-5.00	2.49	0.45
-10.00	5.04	1.03

The results of the simulation experiments presented in this section suggest that the registration technique is able to correctly estimate the deformation between an entire brain volume and a ROI covering only a small portion of the brain. This will almost certainly be the situation in most registration tasks between pre-operative MR and intraoperative US, where the US volume only will cover a limited region around the surgical target, and is therefore an important aspect to verify.

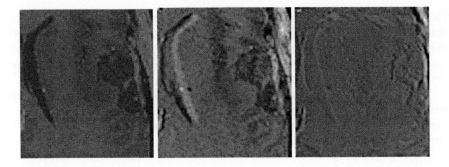

Fig. 1. Left: A transverse slice through the ROI in the original MR image. Middle: Difference image between the original and the transformed image before registration for a displacement of -10 mm. Right: Difference image between the transformed and the deformed original image after registration.

4   Phantom Study

The phantom used in this experiment was made of orange-flavored Jell-o jelly (Kraft Canada Inc., Don Mills, ON). A thin plastic tube was curled and attached to the bottom of a plastic brain mould before filling it with liquid Jell-o. The plastic tube was inserted to simulate the cerebral vasculature. The phantom was then left over night in a fridge to solidify.

4.1   MR Imaging

The phantom was scanned using a Siemens Sonata Vision 1.5T scanner using a standard T1 weighted anatomical scanning sequence with full brain coverage and 1 mm isotropic resolution. The phantom was left in the mould during scanning, and the plastic tube was filled with tap water. Following image acquisition, the vasculature simulated by the plastic tube was segmented from the MR image using the segmentation algorithm described in section 2.1. A surface rendering of the segmented structure is shown in Figure 2. We then computed the chamfer distance map for the segmented MR volume for use in the registration algorithm.

4.2   Ultrasound Imaging and Image Registration

Following MR imaging, the phantom was taken out of the mould and imaged in a container filled with water. Ultrasound images were acquired using an HDI 5000, ATL (Bothwell, WA) ultrasound machine with an ATL P7-4 multi-frequency probe. Tracking was achieved with the use of the Polaris optical tracking system (Northern Digital Inc., Waterloo, ON), a passive reference and an active tracker device (Traxtal Inc., Toronto, ON) attached to the ultrasound probe. We used a physiological pump (Manostat Corp., New York City, NY) to pump water through the plastic tube while we scanned the phantom using color Doppler imaging. Following image acquisition, we masked the images and segmented the Doppler signal from the b-mode images by simple thresholding. We then computed the extent of the scanned volume and resampled and averaged all the 2D images into the resulting 3D volume. A surface rendering of the segmented structure is shown in Figure 2. Finally, we computed the chamfer distance map for the segmented ultrasound volume.

In order to provide a starting point for the non-linear registration algorithm, we linearly registered the two volumes using a series of manually identified homologous landmarks, as done in surgery. We then applied the non-linear registration technique described in section 2.3.

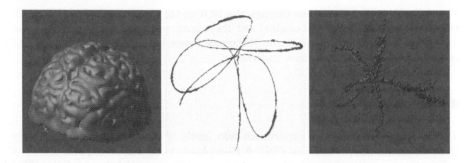

Fig. 2. Surface rendering of the entire phantom to the left, "vessels" segmented from the MR images in the middle and "vessels" from the US volume to the right

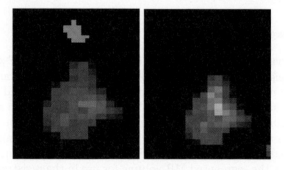

Fig. 3. Cross-section of vessels segmented from MR (white) and Doppler US (color) before (distance=11.36mm) and after (distance=1.41mm) registration.

4.3   Phantom Study Results

Unlike the simulation experiment, the truth is unknown when we register real data. In order to evaluate the performance of the registration in this situation, we measured the distance between vessel centers in MR and US before and after registration. The centers of the vessels were determined manually as the brightest pixel inside the vessel. In the example shown in Figure 3 the distance between the vessel centers is reduced from 11.36mm before registration to 1.41mm after registration. This is comparable with the results shown in the simulation experiments.

5   Discussion and Conclusions

In this paper, we have presented a new method for correction of brain shift based on blood vessel segmentation and registration. The technique has been tested in a series of simulation experiments, and in a phantom study. It has shown to be able to recover large portions of non-linear deformations even when only a very limited region of the MR image is covered by the US acquisition. While more experiments are required to test the method with real patient data, these initial experiments show that blood vessels have the potential of being very useful features for registration of MR and US images. By using segmented blood vessels, we overcome many of the difficulties associated with registration of US data and will hopefully provide the surgeon with a fast and easy way of getting accurate information about the anatomy and vasculature at any given point during surgery. Future experiments will include more realistic simulations in regard to splitting and reconstuction of the ROI and missing vessels, and a more extensive phantom study. The method will also be tested using real patient data in the near future, and this will give us further indication of areas that will need improvement and optimization.

References

1. A. Nabavi et al. Serial intraoperative magnetic resonance imaging of brain shift. *Neurosurgery*, 48(4):787–798, 2001.
2. Å. Grønningsæter et al. Sonowand, an ultrasound-based neuronavigation system. *Neurosurgery*, 47(6):1373–1380, 2000.
3. T. Arbel, X. Morandi, R. M. Comeau, and D. L. Collins. Automatic non-linear MRI-ultrasound registration for the correction of intra-operative brain deformations. *In Proc. MICCAI'2001*, pages 913–922, 2001.
4. G. Borgefors. Hierchical chamfer matching: A parametric edge matching algorithm. *IEEE Trans. on PAMI*, 10(6):849–865, 1988.
5. D. L. Collins and A. C. Evans. ANIMAL: Validation and application of non-linear registration-based segmentation. *IJPRAI*, 11(8):1271–1294, 1997.
6. D. W. Roberts et al. Intraoperative brain shift and deformation: A quantitative analysis of cortical displacement in 28 cases. *Neurosurgery*, 43(5):749–760, 1998.
7. D. W. Roberts et al. Intraoperatively updated neuroimaging using brain modeling and sparse data. *Neurosurgery*, 45(5):1199–1207, 1999.
8. M. Descoteaux, D. L. Collins, and K. Siddiqi. A multi-scale geometric flow for segmenting vasculature in MRI. *In Proc. ECCV*, 2004.
9. A. R. et al.". Rigid registration of 3D ultrasound with MR images: A new approach combining intensity and gradient information. *IEEE TMI*, 20(10):1038–1049, 2001.
10. A. F. Frangi, W. J. Niessen, K. L. Vincken, and M. A. Viergever. Muliscale vessel enhancement filtering. *MICCAI'1998*, pages 130–137, 1998.
11. D. L. Hill, C. R. Maurer, R. J. Maciunas, J. A. Barwise, J. M. Fitzpatrick, and M. Y. Wang. Measurement of intraoperative brain surface deformation under a craniotomy. *Neurosurgery*, 43(3):514–528, 1998.

12. M. I. Miga et al. In vivo quantification of a homogeneous brain deformation model for updating preoperative images during surgery. *IEEE BME*, 47(2):266–273, 2000.
13. N. Haberland et al. Neuronavigation in surgery of intracranial and spinal tumors. *Journ. Canc. Res. Clin. Onc.*, 126:529–541, 2000.
14. C. Nimsky, O. Ganslandt, P. Hastreiter, and R. Fahlbusch. Intraoperative compensation for brain shift. *Surgical Neurology*, 10:357–365, 2001.
15. A. Vasilevskiy and K. Siddiqi. Flux maximizing geometric flows. *IEEE PAMI*, 24(12):1565–1578, 2002.

Predicting Tumour Location by Simulating Large Deformations of the Breast Using a 3D Finite Element Model and Nonlinear Elasticity

Pras Pathmanathan[1], David Gavaghan[1], Jonathan Whiteley[1],
Sir Michael Brady[2], Martyn Nash[3], Poul Nielsen[3], and Vijay Rajagopal[3]

[1] Oxford University Computing Laboratory, Parks Road, Oxford, UK
{pras,gavaghan,jonathan.whiteley}@comlab.ox.ac.uk
[2] Oxford University Department of Engineering Science, Parks Road, Oxford, UK
jmb@robots.ox.ac.uk
[3] Auckland University BioEngineering Institute, Auckland, New Zealand
{martyn.nash,p.nielsen,v.rajagopal}@auckland.ac.nz

Abstract. Two of the major imaging modalities used to detect and monitor breast cancer are (contrast enhanced) magnetic resonance (MR) imaging and mammography. Image fusion, including accurate registration between MR images and mammograms, or between CC and MLO mammograms, is increasingly key to patient management (for example in the multidisciplinary meeting), but registration is extremely difficult because the breast shape varies massively between the modalities, due both to the different postures of the patient for the two modalities and to the fact that the breast is forcibly compressed during mammography. In this paper, we develop a 3D, patient-specific, anatomically accurate, finite element model of the breast using MR images, which can be deformed in a physically realistic manner using nonlinear elasticity theory to simulate the breast during mammography.

1 Introduction

Breast cancer is one of the biggest killers of women in the Western world, killing 400,000 and affecting over a million people each year worldwide. As with all cancers, treatment can be lengthy, extremely unpleasant, and ultimately fruitless. Early diagnosis is the most effective way to improve the prognosis, and so screening programmes have been established in several western countries.

Currently, the imaging modalities used to image the breast are magnetic resonance (MR) imaging, mammography and ultrasound. Due to the highly deformable nature of the breast, and the difference in body position and external forces applied to the breast in the different imaging procedures, the shape of the breast varies massively between images of the different types, hindering attempts at image fusion for more effective diagnosis or predicting tumour location during surgery/biopsy. Various methods have been proposed to model breast deformation. Most are either based on linear elasticity theory, the theory used for

C. Barillot, D.R. Haynor, and P. Hellier (Eds.): MICCAI 2004, LNCS 3217, pp. 217–224, 2004.

small deformations, or to some extent on heuristics. In this paper, we describe the development of a finite element (FE) model of the breast based on the full nonlinear theory of elasticity (also known as finite elasticity). The FE mesh has a geometry determined from MR images of the subject, with an anatomical structure that is determined from segmented MR data. As such, we propose a patient-specific, not generic, model. Such a method models the deformation in a physically realistic manner, hence has a significantly higher likelihood of accurately simulating breast deformation than a linearised or heuristic method. Modelling large deformations with nonlinear elasticity has previously been considered computationally intractable; however, as we shall demonstrate, simulations on a moderately high-resolution mesh can be computed in a reasonable length of time on standard modern PC.

2   Applications of a Physically Realistic Finite Element Model

A robust, accurate deformable model of the breast would have many uses. Firstly, an accurate model could benefit image registration and fusion. For example, during mammography the patient's breast is forcibly compressed (typically 130N), so that fusing mammograms with MR data is extremely difficult. Also, in clinical practice mammograms are taken from different views, the most common being *cranio-caudal* (CC), (head-to-toe), and *medio-lateral oblique* (MLO), (shoulder-to-opposite-hip). Combining the information provided by different mammogram views significantly enhances the detection of tumours, but the large deformation of the breast makes it hard for a radiologist to establish correspondences between these views, hence to reconstruct the tumour (or microcalcification cluster) in 3D. A deformable model of the breast (built from MR data) that can simulate both the CC compressed breast and the MLO compressed breast can be used to match the two types of mammogram. As well as inter-modality matching, the model can be used for temporal matching of images of the same modality.

MR images are generally carried out with the patient in the prone position. During surgery however, the patient will be supine, and a surgeon using MR data to predict the position of a tumour will have to resort to a degree of guesswork. A deformable model of the breast could be used to predict breast shape and tumour location during surgery, enabling minimally invasive surgery. Similarly, the model can be used as a guide during fine-needle or core biopsy, or even eventually to help automate the biopsy procedure.

Finally, the model we develop could be used as a visualisation tool, allowing a doctor to show the patient the position and size of the tumour in 3D, and as a teaching tool for radiologists. An extension of the model could also be used to simulate breast shape after reconstructive surgery.

Current methods used to model breast deformation are often not patient-specific, and/or they embody linear elastic or partially heuristic models of deformation. In [5] the breast edge is assumed to take the shape of quadratic curves, and compression is modelled by assuming that these curves map to new quadratic curves. In [4] the breast shape is obtained from patient data but the fibroglandular region is assumed to be cone shaped, and the tissues are assumed to be linearly elastic. In [1], a deformable MR based model of the breast is developed based on linear elasticity, where the large deformation is considered as a sequence of small linear deformations. However, the deformations the breast undergoes are extremely large and are not in the typical strain range assumed for small-strain linear elasticity (0-10% strains). A physically-motivated nonlinear model is necessary to accurately model such deformations. Nonlinear models have, as far as we are aware, only been considered by *Samani et al* [8]. We aim to develop a fully nonlinear model with the ultimate goal of comparing nonlinear models of varying complexity with linear and simpler models to determine which factors are of greatest importance in breast deformation.

The modelling procedure is as follows: the FE geometry is built using the skin surface and pectoral muscle surface obtained from MR images. The MR images are (easily and accurately) segmented into regions of fat, fibroglandular and tumour tissue, which can be performed to sub-voxel precision. Using the segmented data, each element of the FE mesh is assigned a tissue type. The size of the elements in the mesh determine the potential accuracy of the deformation simulations. With a reasonably refined mesh accuracy to within 2-5mm is possible, assuming the material laws of the tissues are known.

There are three distinct types of deformation which we have to simulate. The first is what we will call the *forward problem*, where body forces (e.g. gravity) are applied to an undeformed (unloaded) state to compute a deformed equilibrium state. This can be used to compute supine breast shape, for example. The second is the inverse problem (the *backward problem*): given a loaded deformed state, compute the unloaded undeformed state. This is necessary because the mesh built from MR data is initially in a gravity-loaded state. The third is modelling the compression of the breast during mammography. Here, the area of the skin in contact with the breast is unknown, and as such the boundary conditions are unknown. Such a problem is known as a *contact problem*.

3   Nonlinear Elasticity

In this section, we briefly formulate the problems which need to be solved. Let Ω_0 be the undeformed state of the elastic body, let $\mathbf{X}$ be the position of a point in the undeformed state, let Ω be the deformed equilibrium state of the body (i.e. when it is loaded under gravity or external tractions), and let the unknown vector field $\mathbf{x} \equiv \mathbf{x}(\mathbf{X})$ be the position of that point in the deformed configuration. The deformation gradient is defined as the tensor $F_{iM} = \frac{\mathrm{d}x_i}{\mathrm{d}X_M}$. The (Lagrangian) strain is defined as $E = \frac{1}{2}\left(F^T F - I\right)$. In nonlinear elasticity theory, a distinction is made between quantities defined in the undeformed coordinate system and those defined in the deformed coordinate system. Force balance equations can only initially be derived in the deformed equilibrium state, whereas the equations to be solved have to be written in terms of the known variables $\mathbf{X}$. It follows that the notion of stress can be defined in a number of ways, the most important being the *Cauchy Stress*, σ_{ij}, defined as the force acting on the deformed body measured per unit deformed area, and the *Second Piola-Kirchoff Stress*, T_{MN}, defined as the force acting on the undeformed body measured per unit undeformed area. σ and T are related by the expression $\det(F)\sigma = FTF^T$. In a gravity-loaded equilibrium deformed state all forces must balance, and it can be shown [6] that this leads to

$$\frac{\partial \sigma_{ij}}{\partial x_j} + \rho g_i = 0 \quad \text{in } \Omega , \tag{1}$$

where ρ is the density in the deformed body and **g** is gravitational acceleration. This equation has to be reformed in terms of the known variables, leading to the following equilibrium equation

$$\frac{\partial}{\partial X_M}\left(T_{MN}\frac{\partial x_i}{\partial X_N}\right) + \rho_0 g_i = 0 \quad \text{in } \Omega_0 , \tag{2}$$

where ρ_0 is the density in the undeformed body.

To relate stress to strain, we need the material dependent constitutive relation between them. Linear stress-strain relationships are often assumed in linear elasticity (small-strain elasticity); however, biological tissues have been shown to exhibit nonlinear stress-strain laws [2] and this is certainly the case for the range of substantial strains involved in breast deformation, so we consider the full nonlinear laws for our model. To do so, we assume there exists a strain energy function $W \equiv W(E_{MN})$ for each tissue which satisfies

$$\frac{\partial W}{\partial E_{MN}} = T_{MN} . \tag{3}$$

Note that in this equation we ignore viscoelastic effects, which we assume to be negligible on the long-timescale problems we are considering. The constitutive law for each tissue can only be determined experimentally. The relative lack of experimentally-determined tissue material laws is perhaps the major factor inhibiting the use of nonlinear elasticity in modelling large biological deformations.

As discussed in Section 2, there are three types of problems which need to be solved:

The Forward Problem: Here the undeformed breast shape is given and the breast shape under gravity (say) is required, a standard elasticity problem. For this, we need to solve (2), together with tissue material laws of the form (3), for **x**, subject to zero displacement boundary conditions on the part of the mesh corresponding to the pectoral muscle and zero surface pressure boundary conditions on the skin surface.

The Backward Problem: A mesh built from MR data will typically be for the breast under the influence of gravity. We initially need to calculate the unloaded state (the shape the breast would take in the absence of gravity) before any other deformation calculations can be computed. This involves solving an inverse finite elasticity problem: we know the deformed position **x** and wish to compute $\mathbf{X}$. This can be accomplished by solving (1), with the material law (3), but writing the strain as $E = \frac{1}{2}((G^{-1})^{T}(G^{-1}) - I)$, where $G = \frac{\partial \mathbf{X}}{\partial \mathbf{x}} = F^{-1}$, so that E is a function of $\mathbf{x}$, and using the relationship between σ and T to obtain σ from the material law.

The Contact Problem: The problem of modelling breast compression has to be considered separately from the other two types of problem. In this case, we do not know which part of the breast will be in contact with the compression plates, and therefore cannot just specify displacement boundary conditions. To derive the contact problem formulation, it is necessary to reformulate (2) as an energy minimisation problem:

$$\min \int_{\Omega_0} W\left(E_{MN}\right) - \rho_0 \mathbf{g} \cdot \mathbf{x} \, dV_0 \quad \text{over } \mathbf{x} \text{ satisfying b.c.s}, \qquad (4)$$

where the boundary conditions (b.c.s) are that the displacement is zero on the pectoral muscle. The (frictionless) contact problem can now be stated as:

$$\min \int_{\Omega_0} W\left(E_{MN}\right) - \rho_0 \mathbf{g} \cdot \mathbf{x} \, dV_0 \quad \text{over } \mathbf{x} \text{ satisfying b.c.s and constraints}, \quad (5)$$

where the constraints are that no point penetrates either compression plate. One method of solving such a problem is to add a *penalty function* to the energy and minimise over unconstrained $\mathbf{x}$:

$$\min \int_{\Omega_0} W - \rho_0 \mathbf{g} \cdot \mathbf{x} \, dV_0 + \int_{\Gamma} \frac{P}{2} \left([-g(\mathbf{x}(\mathbf{X}))]_+\right)^2 dS_0 \quad \text{over } \mathbf{x} \text{ satisfying b.c.s}, \tag{6}$$

where Γ is the skin surface and $g(\mathbf{x})$ is the signed normal distance of a point $\mathbf{x}$ to the nearest plate, and $[z]_+$ is 0 if $z \leq 0$ and z if $z > 0$. $[-g(\mathbf{x})]_+$ is therefore the penetration of a point into the plates, which we wish to be zero. The penalty function penalises violation of the constraint, with greater values of the penalty parameter P leading to greater penalisation.

A well-known drawback of penalty functions is that P needs to be large in order to assure accurate results, but this can lead to badly conditioned matrices when the problem is solved with the finite element method. The *Augmented Lagrangian Method*, which we have used, is an extension of the penalty function method which deals with this problem. For details see [3], but the basic idea is that the penalty function is replaced with

$$\int_{\Gamma} \frac{1}{2P} \left([-\lambda(\mathbf{x}) - Pg(\mathbf{x})]_+\right)^2 dS_0 \ , \tag{7}$$

where λ is an estimate of the Lagrange multipliers associated with the constraint (which are also the compressive forces applied by the plates) that is updated iteratively and converges to the true Lagrange multipliers. With this method P need not be very large to guarantee accurate results.

4   Modelling and Results

A finite element model has been built from MR data of a standing patient. A mesh hexahedral elements was created and adapted to the breast geometry, by fitting the front surface of the mesh to the skin surface and the back surface of the mesh to the pectoral muscle surface. Hexahedral elements are preferred to tetrahedral elements since they have been shown to have better convergence properties [8]. The next stage would be to assign a tissue to each element based on segmented MR data; however with these preliminary results each element has just been considered to be fibroglandular tissue. The final mesh has 5625 nodes and 4608 elements, with trilinear basis functions used to interpolate position, and is shown in Figure 1.

We have assumed the breast tissues are incompressible, since breast tissues are primarily comprised of water. We have currently also made the incorrect assumption that the tissues are isotropic. Breast tissues are likely to be anisotropic, since the connective structures known as Cooper's Ligaments are oriented in the muscle-to-skin direction. In future work, we will investigate the effect of modelling tissues as transverse isotropic or fully anisotropic. If a material is isotropic, the constitutive law for the material simplifies somewhat, in this case the strain energy function W satisfies $W \equiv W(I_1, I_2, I_3)$, where I_1, I_2 and I_3 are the principal invariants[1] of $F^T F$ [9]. We have assumed the exponential constitutive law

$$W(I_1, I_2, I_3) = a \left(e^{b(I_1-3)} - 1 \right) - \frac{p}{2}(I_3 - 1) \ , \tag{8}$$

where a and b are material constants and p is the Lagrange multiplier associated with the incompressibility constraint which can be interpreted as internal pressure. We have estimated a and b using experimental data in [10].

The equations discussed in Section 3 are solved on the mesh using the Galerkin finite element method [7]. For incompressible elastic deformations, the internal pressure p has to be computed together with the displacements. Piecewise constant basis functions are used to interpolate the pressure, as the pressure must be interpolated by lower order basis functions than the position [7]. Since the equations are highly nonlinear, Newton's method has been used.

The results of two simulations on this mesh are shown in Figures 1 and 2. Figure 1 displays the undeformed breast shape which is the result of solving the backward problem on the mesh built from the MR data, together with a supine simulation. Figure 2 is an example of a simulation of CC mammographic compression. The simulations of the supine and compressed breast shape take less than 1.5 hours on a 2 GHz Linux PC. Due to badly-conditioned matrices inherent in the backward problem, computing the undeformed state currently takes significantly longer, up to 24 hours on a 2 GHz Linux PC. Preconditioning the backward problem matrices or finding methods of improving Newton convergence to reduce the time to solve the backward problem is an open problem. In later work will verify these simulations using both phantom models and

---

[1] The principal invariants of a matrix C are $I_1 = \mathrm{tr}(C)$, $I_2 = \frac{1}{2}((\mathrm{tr}(C))^2 - \mathrm{tr}(C^2))$ and $I_3 = \det(C)$.

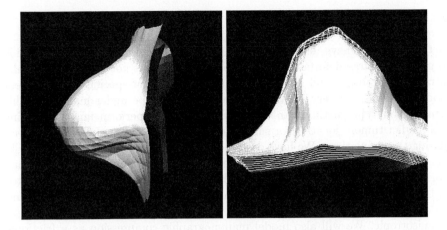

Fig. 1. *Left:* mesh of the breast built from MR images of a standing patient, *right:* the undeformed (gravity-loading removed) breast shape (*wireframe*) and supine patient breast shape (*surface*)

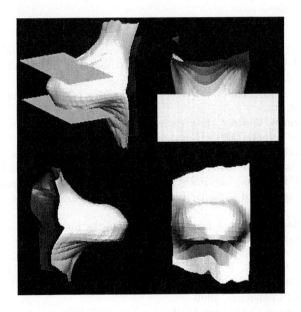

Fig. 2. Various views of the breast under simulated CC mammographic compression

patient data. The latter will involve reproducing supine or compressed breast shape and comparing the surface deformation with photographic results, and simulating the breast shape with a new direction of gravity and comparing with MR images.

5   Conclusions

In this paper we have demonstrated that using the full nonlinear formulation to model the large deformations the breast undergoes is not a computationally intractable problem, and have used a nonlinear patient-specific finite element model to predict surgery breast shape and breast shape under mammographic compression. This method can ultimately be used to perform image matching and predict tumour location for surgery or biopsy. Current work is aimed at validating the simulations. We have described the three types of deformation problem which have to be tackled, and outlined procedures for solving them. In future work we will perform simulations with heterogeneity obtained from segmented MR images, investigate the effect of material parameters on the deformations, and investigate whether the tissues have to be modelled as transversely isotropic or anisotropic. We will also model mammographic compression as a frictional contact problem. Verification using both phantom and patient data studies will be performed.

References

1. F.S. Azar, D.N. Metaxas, M.D. Schnall. A Deformable Finite Element Model of the Breast for Predicting Mechanical Deformations under External Perturbations, Acad. Rad. Oct 2001.
2. Y.C. Fung. Biomechanics: Mechanical Properties of Living Tissues, Springer-Verlag, 1993.
3. G. Kloosterman. Contact Methods in Finite Element Simulations (PhD Thesis), University of Twente, 2001
4. A.M Galea, R.D. Howe. Mammography Registered Tactile Imaging, Surgery Simulation and Soft Tissue Modeling, International Symp. IS4TM 2003 Proc, Springer
5. Y. Kita, R.P Highnam, J.M. Brady. Correspondence between Different View Breast X-Rays Using Curved Epipolar Lines. Computer Vision & Image Understanding 83.
6. M. Nash. Mechanics and Material Properties of the Heart using an Anatomically Accurate Mathematical Model (PhD Thesis), University of Auckland, 1998
7. J.N. Reddy. An Introduction to the Finite Element Method, McGraw-Hill 1993
8. A. Samani, J. Bishop, E. Ramsay, D.B. Plewes. A 3-D Contact Problem Finite Element Model for Breast Shape Deformation Derived From MRI Data. Proc. of ASB, Annual Conference, 1999
9. A. J. M. Spencer. Continuum Mechanics, Longman 1980
10. P. Wellman, R.H. Howe, E. Dalton, and K.A. Kern. Breast Tissue Stiffness in Compression is Correlated to Histological Diagnosis. Technical Report, Harvard Biorobotics Laboratory Technical Report, 1999

Modeling of Brain Tissue Retraction Using Intraoperative Data

Hai Sun[1], Francis E. Kennedy[1], Erik J. Carlson[1], Alex Hartov[1],
David W. Roberts[2], and Keith D. Paulsen[1,2]

[1] Thayer School of Engineering, Dartmouth College, Hanover, NH 03755, USA
{Hai.Sun, Francis.E.Kennedy, Erik.J.Carlson, Alex.Hartov,
Keith.D.Paulsen}@Dartmouth.edu
[2] Dartmouth Hitchcock Medical Center, Lebanon, NH 03766, USA
David.W.Roberts@Hitchcock.org

Abstract. We present a method for modeling tissue retraction during image-guided neurosurgery. A poroelastic brain model is driven by the stereoscopically-measured motion of a retractor to produce a full volume displacement field, which is used to update the preoperative MR images. Using the cortical surface surrounding the retractor as an independent evaluative landmark, we show that our approach is capable of capturing approximately 75% of the cortical deformation during tissue retraction.

1 Introduction

During neurosurgery, the surgeon often employs retractors to intentionally deform the brain tissue in order to gain access to deeper structures. Although the retraction of brain parenchyma during surgery is common, detailed studies of the effects of retraction on tissue are few [1]. Existing simulations are largely limited to qualitative descriptions of the retraction process [2] and are not capable of producing an accurate estimate of the mechanical impact on the parenchyma.

Computational brain models have proven to be powerful in compensating for brain shift [3,4,5], but their success has been largely limited to the initial tissue response to the craniotomy and dural opening. Miga et al. proposed a strategy for digitizing the motion of the retractor and the volume of the resection cavity in order to incorporate these changes into a brain model [6]. In their initial attempt, the intraoperative data were only qualitatively estimated based on preoperative images due to difficulty in tracking surgical tools and the brain surface during surgery. Using porcine subjects, Platenik et al. [7] demonstrated that their brain deformation model is capable of capturing 75% - 80% of the tissue motion generated during interhemispheric retraction.

In order to accurately model the retraction of a human brain, we employ an intraoperative stereo vision (iSV) system constructed by attaching two CCD cameras to the binocular optics of the operating microscope [8]. We have previously shown that this iSV system is accurate to approximately 1mm [9,10].

The project is funded by the National Institute of Neurological Disorders and Stroke (NINDS, R01-NS33900).

Using stereopsis, we have captured the motion of a retractor and continuously monitored the cortical motion during tissue retraction. The measured motion of the retractor is incorporated into the brain model to produce full volume deformation estimates, which are then used to update the preoperative MR (pMR) volume. Using this approach, we have modeled tissue changes both during retraction and after the release of the retractor during a clinical case.

2   Methods

Our technique of modeling tissue retraction involves four basic steps:

1. from preoperative MR scans, generate a finite element mesh of the brain,
2. identify areas of the mesh surface corresponding to both the craniotomy site and the portion of brain tissue under the retractor,
3. track the motion of the retractor using stereopsis,
4. and incorporate the motion of the retractor into the original brain mesh to produce a full volume description of brain deformation.

Each of these steps is described below, and results from one clinical case are presented in the subsequent section.

2.1   Mesh Generation

The modeling process begins with the generation of a computational mesh of the patient's brain using preoperative MR images. The brain is segmented using AnalyzeAVW [1]. The boundary is discretized into triangular patches using the marching cubes algorithm. Custom mesh generation software creates a volumetric mesh consisting of tetrahedral elements [11].

2.2   Sites of Craniotomy and Retraction

This step identifies the portion of the preoperative mesh that corresponds to the sites of both craniotomy and retraction, so that appropriate boundary conditions can be assigned to drive the brain model.

To begin, the coordinate space of the constructed mesh is rigidly registered to the 3-D operating room and the 2-D operating microscope [2] [12]. With these registrations, the coordinates of the surface nodes are first projected into the microscope image. To avoid the inherent ambiguity resulting from this 3-D to 2-D projection, only the surface nodes from the hemisphere of the craniotomy are projected. The boundary of the craniotomy site is manually outlined in the microscope image. The surface nodes that fall within this boundary are identified in the microscope image and hence in the original mesh - this subset of nodes will be referred to as the *craniotomy* nodes.

---

[1] The software ANALYZE was provided by the Mayo Foundation.
[2] The operating microscope, Model M695, Leica USA, Rockleigh, NJ.

The portion of the mesh underneath the retractor can be identified in the same way. A microscope image acquired immediately prior to the retraction is selected for this estimation. The boundary of the retractor in this image is also outlined. The surface nodes that fall within this second boundary are identified - this subset of nodes will be referred to as the *retractor* nodes, which constitute a subset of the craniotomy nodes.

2.3   Tracking the Retractor

When the surgeon retracts the tissue, a stereo pair of the surgical scene is acquired. Using the technique of stereopsis [8,10], we estimate the shape of the retractor, which is represented by a point cloud, which is transformed into the pMR coordinates using registrations established in the previous section.

To track the retractor motion, we regard the retractor nodes (Section 2.2) as the tool location prior to retraction and the iSV-estimated shape as its location after retraction. Given these two point clouds (both in pMR coordinates), we employ the iterative closest point (ICP) algorithm [13] to simultaneously establish the correspondence between the two and estimate the displacement. The resulting displacement is represented as a set of 3-D translation vectors between each retractor node and its corresponding point on the iSV-estimated shape.

2.4   Brain Modeling

We now use the motion of the retractor to guide a computational model for recovering the full volume deformation. To this end, we have adopted a poroelastic brain model, using Biot's consolidation formulation [14] to represent the brain as an elastically deformable porous medium containing cerebrospinal fluid. The partial differential equations and the finite element method (FEM) for solving this mathematical framework can be found in [3]. The solution to the model equations is obtained by applying known boundary and volumetric forcing conditions and solving for the full volume displacement field and the pressure distribution.

These boundary and volumetric forcing conditions include fluid saturation in the bottom half of the brain, the gravitational direction acquired during surgery, stress-free conditions at the craniotomy and at the highest elevation of the brain, zero normal displacement and zero tangential traction beneath the remainder of the cranium, free flow of fluid at the craniotomy site, and no flow of fluid at the walls corresponding to the rest of the cranium.

The estimated retractor motion is incorporated into the brain model as follows. For each retractor node for which a displacement was estimated via stereopsis, the corresponding finite element equations are precisely enforced by this displacement [5,4]. The output of the brain model is a displacement field over the patient brain, which is then used to update the entire pMR volume [10].

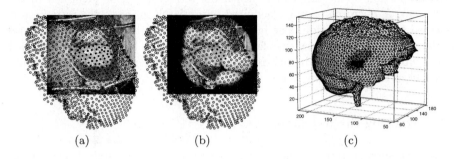

(a)   (b)   (c)

Fig. 1. Shown, from left to right, are (a) the results of projecting the mesh surface nodes onto the surgical scene, where the nodes within the craniotomy boundary are plotted as asterisks and the others as open circles; (b) a second projection of the mesh surface nodes, where those corresponding to brain tissue underneath the retractor are plotted as asterisks and the others as open circles; and (c) the mesh with the craniotomy nodes colored in lighter gray and the retractor nodes colored in darker gray.

3   Results

In this section, a case study is presented to illustrate how we use the motion of the retractor to model the tissue retraction process. The patient was a 52-year-old female with a right sphenoid wing meningioma. Because of the location of the tumor, the surgeon performed a craniotomy at the right temporal region of the skull and retracted the brain tissue at the craniotomy site in order to gain access to the tumor. Two CCD cameras [3] attached to the operating microscope were used to record the surgical field every 10 seconds during the entire procedure.

Prior to surgery, an MRI scan was obtained, and the cranium segmented. A finite element mesh was generated from the resulting segmented brain and registered to the real-time microscope images, Fig. 1(left and middle), acquired at the start of surgery. The surface nodes that correspond to regions of the craniotomy site (lighter gray) and the tissue underneath the retractor (darker gray) are identified, Fig. 1(right).

Shown in Fig. 2(top) is a stereo pair of the retracted brain tissue. From these images, shapes of the retractor and the cortical surface were estimated. These shapes were overlaid with the preoperative mesh to illustrate the tissue deformation, Fig. 2(bottom). As a result of tissue retraction, the anterior portion of the cortical surface collapsed and the posterior portion of the cortical surface distended. From the retractor nodes in Fig. 1 and the shape of this blade in Fig. 2, the motion of the retractor was estimated using the ICP algorithm. Of the 13 retractor nodes, 8 collapsed and 5 distended. The average displacement of collapsing nodes was 9.23mm, with a maximum of 12.34mm and a minimum

---

[3] Sony DFW-x700, Resolution $1024(H) \times 768(V)$, Sony Corp., New York, NY, USA

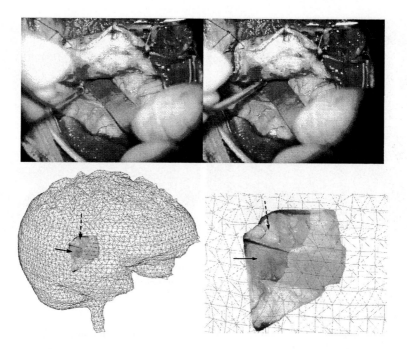

Fig. 2. Shown are: the stereo pair of the retracted brain (top); relative position of the retractor (black arrow) and the deformed cortical surface (dotted arrow) to the preoperative mesh (bottom left) and a close-up view of the same figure (bottom right).

of 4.34mm. The average displacement of distending nodes was 5.42mm, with a maximum of 6.34mm and a minimum of 2.45mm.

The estimated retractor motion was used to guide the brain deformation model, as described in Section 2.4. This model produced a displacement field which was then applied to the pMR volume. Fig. 3 presents the result from this update. The images on the left are the axial slices in the pMR volume with the reconstructed cortical surface (white curves) overlaid. Note the misalignment between the intraoperative and preoperative surfaces. The images on the right display the intraoperative surface overlaid with the updated MR (uMR). Note that these surfaces are now in good alignment.

In order to confirm the viability of our approach in modeling tissue retraction, we compared the model-estimated cortical motion with the same motion captured via stereopsis. Given the accuracy of the iSV system at approximately 1mm [10], we consider the latter estimate as close to the ground truth. The cortical surface surrounding the retractor was used as an evaluative landmark.

To begin, the retractor nodes were subtracted from the craniotomy nodes. The remaining craniotomy nodes, corresponding to the cortical surface surrounding the retractor, were selected for comparison - this set of surface nodes was defined as the *cortical* nodes. As described previously, the brain model had pre-

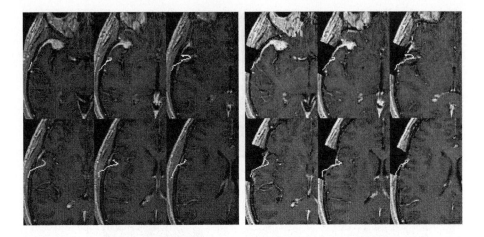

Fig. 3. The retracted cortical surface (white curves) overlaid with axial slices from the pMR volume (left) and the same slices from uMR volume (right).

dicted a displacement for each cortical node. From the stereo pair shown in Fig. 2, the shape of the cortical surface surrounding the retractor was estimated. Using the method described in Section 2.3, the stereo-based estimate of the exposed cortical surface was compared with the corresponding mesh surface, i.e., the cortical nodes, to obtain their displacements. Of 24 cortical nodes, the iSV system estimated that, 15 of those nodes collapsed and 9 distended during retraction. The average displacement of collapsing nodes was 8.76mm, with a maximum of 10.65mm and a minimum of 2.46mm. The average displacement of distending nodes was 4.64mm, with a maximum of 5.64mm and a minimum of 1.83mm.

We next computed, for each cortical node, the absolute difference between the stereo- and model-estimated displacement. The relative difference was determined as the absolute difference divided by the amount of displacement estimated via stereopsis. The final error estimates were cast as the percent capture of tissue motion by subtracting each relative difference from 100 percent. These error estimates were computed in all Cartesian directions (X, Y, Z) and in overall magnitude, Table 1. In this particular case, we have found that our model was capable of capturing approximately 75% of the cortical motion.

In order to further confirm the viability of our approach, we have employed the same strategy to model tissue changes after the release of the retractor. Thirty seconds after the stereo pair in Fig. 2 was acquired, the iSV system recorded another stereo pair shown in Fig. 4 (top). The shape of the cortical surface was estimated using stereopsis and overlaid with the uMR generated during tissue retraction, Fig. 4(bottom left). Note that the cortical surface did not fully recover from the induced tissue deformation. The motion of the retractor nodes was tracked during the recovery phase after blade removal. Of 13 cortical nodes, 4 collapsed and 9 distended after the tissue was released.

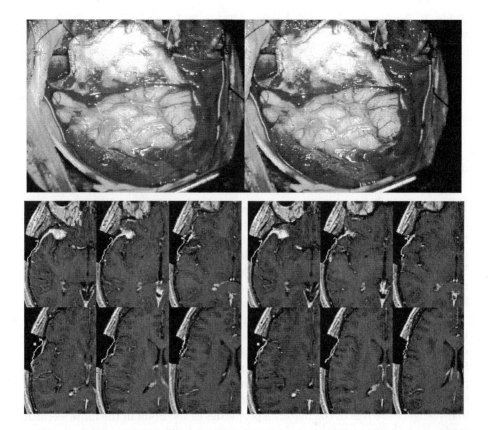

Fig. 4. Stereo pair of the surgical scene taken 30 seconds after the retractor was released (top); The intraoperative cortical surface (white curves) overlaid with axial slices from the uMR volume generated during retraction (bottom left) and the same slices from uMR volume generated after retraction (bottom right).

The average displacement of collapsing nodes was 2.43mm, with a maximum of 4.26mm and a minimum of 1.02mm. The average displacement of distending nodes was 7.32mm, with a maximum of 9.18mm and a minimum of 4.69mm. These retractor nodes displacements were used to guide the brain deformation model for updating the uMR generated during retraction. The images on the right display the current cortical surface overlaid with the uMR generated after 30 seconds during the recovery phase. Note that, compared to the images on the left, the alignment between the intraoperative cortical surface and the surface in the uMR improved as a result of this update. For this modeling step, we also compared the motion of the cortical nodes predicted by the model with the stereo estimation. The model was capable of capturing approximately 72% of the cortical motion during the recovery phase, as shown in Table 2.

Table 1. Percent Capture of Deformation During Retraction

	mean	max	min
X	71.6	97.4	56.7
Y	66.3	89.9	44.3
Z	82.1	98.9	64.4
magnitude	74.8	97.2	53.1

Table 2. Percent Capture of Deformation After Retraction

	mean	max	min
X	69.2	94.3	49.2
Y	78.1	98.4	55.4
Z	65.3	92.1	45.1
magnitude	72.3	96.8	47.9

4   Discussion

We have presented a technique for modeling tissue retraction. By monitoring changes in the surgical field every ten seconds, we have estimated the motion of a retractor and its concomitant cortical surface movement. The retractor motion is then used to drive brain deformation models for updating the preoperative MR volume. Using the cortical surface surrounding the retractor as an independent evaluative landmark, we show that our approach can recover on average approximately 75% of the tissue deformation.

Several extensions and improvements to this work are currently under investigation. First, we plan to further validate our approach through imaging subsurface regions of the brain using co-registered intraoperative ultrasound. Second, in order to improve the modeling results, we plan to test other more sophisticated boundary conditions at the retraction site, in order to produce more realistic tissue motion such as traction along the retractor blade. Finally, we plan to investigate the role of the material properties of the brain in the finite element model. The ability to continuously monitor tissue behavior during the retraction process has the potential of generating more realistic and patient-specific model parameters, which may improve the accuracy of the model estimate.

References

1. Hartkens, T., Hill, D., Castellano-Smith, A., Hawkes, D., Maurer, C., Martin, A., Hall, W., Liu, H., Truwit, C.: Measurement and analysis of brain deformation during neurosurgery. IEEE Transactions on Medical Imaging **22(1)** (2003) 82–92
2. Koyama, T., Okudera, H., Kobayashi, S.: Computer-generated surgical simulation of morpholocial changes in microstructures: Concepts of 'virtual retractor'. Neurosurgery **46(1)** (2000) 118–135
3. Paulsen, K., Miga, M., Kennedy, F., Hoopes, P., Hartov, A., Roberts, D.: A computational model for tracking subsurface tissue deformation during stereotactic neurosurgery. IEEE Transactions on Biomedical Engineering **46** (1999) 213–225
4. Ferrant, M., Nabavi, A., Macq, B., Jolesz, F., Kikinis, R., Warfield, S.: Registration of 3-d intraoperative MR images of the brain using a finite-element biomechanical model. IEEE Transactions on Medical Imaging **20** (2001) 1384–1397
5. Skrinjar, O., Nabavi, A., Duncan, J.: Model-driven brain shift compensation. Medical Image Analysis **6** (2002) 361–373

6. Miga, M., Roberts, D., Kennedy, F., Platenik, L., Hartov, A., , Lunn, K., Paulsen, K.: Modeling of retraction and resection for intraoperative updating of images. Neurosurgery **49** (2001) 75–85

7. Platenik, L., Miga, M., Roberts, D., Lunn, K., Kennedy, F., Hartov, A., Paulsen, K.: In vivo quantification of retraction deformation modeling for updated image-guidance during neurosurgery. IEEE Transactions on Biomedical Engineering **49(8)** (2001) 823–835

8. Sun, H., Farid, H., Rick, K., Hartov, A., Roberts, D., Paulsen, K.: Estimating cortical surface motion using stereopsis for brain deformation models. Medical Image Computing and Computer-Assisted Intervention **2878** (2003) 794–801

9. Sun, H., Roberts, D., Farid, H., Wu, Z., Hartov, A., Paulsen, K.: Cortical surface tracking using a stereoscopic operating microscope. Neurosurgery (in press) (2004)

10. Sun, H., Lunn, K., Farid, H., Wu, Z., Roberts, D., Hartov, A., Paulsen, K.: Stereopsis-driven brain shift compensation. Submitted to:IEEE Transactions on Medical Imaging (2004)

11. Sullivan, J., Charron, G., Paulsen, K.: A three-dimensional mesh generator for arbitrary multiple material domains. Finite Elements in Analysis and Design **25** (1997) 219–241

12. Sun, H., Farid, H., Hartov, A., Lunn, K., Roberts, D., Paulsen, K.: Real-time correction scheme for calibration and implementation of microscope-based image-guided neurosurgery. Proceedings of SPIE Medical Imaging, Visualization, Display, and Image-Guided Procedures **4681** (2002) 47–54

13. Besl, P., McKay, N.: A method for registration of 3-D shapes. IEEE Transactions on Pattern Analysis and Machine Intelligence **14** (1992) 239–256

14. Biot, M.: General theory of three-dimensional consolidation. Journal of Applied Physics **12** (1941) 155–164

Physiopathology of Pulmonary Airways: Automated Facilities for Accurate Assessment

Diane Perchet, Catalin I. Fetita, and Françoise Prêteux

ARTEMIS Project Unit, INT, Groupe des Ecoles des Télécommunications
9 rue Charles Fourier, 91011 Evry Cedex, France

Abstract. In the framework of computer-assisted diagnosis, pulmonary airway investigation based on multi detector computed tomography (MDCT) requires to provide radiologists and clinicians with advanced tools for interactive exploration, quantitative assessment and follow-up. This paper develops a set of automated investigation facilities relying on 3D airway reconstruction, enhanced central axis-based description and accurate meshing. By overcoming the limitations encountered by the current post-processing techniques available in clinical routine, the proposed tools contribute to increase the diagnosis confidence level and provide better insights into the physiopathology of airways.

1 Introduction

Providing radiologist with non-invasive facilities for airway pathology diagnosis and follow-up is still a challenging issue for the medical imaging industry. With the development of multi-detector computed tomography (MDCT), a high resolution imaging of the thorax in a single breath hold is now possible, allowing to assess focal or diffuse, proximal or distal airway diseases [1]. However, an accurate quantitative investigation of the physiopathology of pulmonary airways requires advanced investigation tools which are not available in clinical routine yet. Such tools mainly involve the access to the 3D information on the tracheobronchial tree carried by the MDCT acquisition. In this way, several local analyses become possible: evaluation of the extent of stenosis and bronchiectasis for treatment planning and follow-up, assessment of complex airway abnormalities, study of the airway remodeling in the case of chronic obstructive pulmonary disease (COPD) and asthma, etc.

Starting from an accurate and robust 3D reconstruction of the bronchial tree from MDCT acquisitions, this paper develops additional facilities for local analysis, thus providing new insights into the physiopathology of airways. After an overview of the demanded tools in clinical routine and of the current limitations of the existing techniques (§2), an unified solution relying on a multi-valued central axis-based representation is proposed (§3). The resulting clinical applications are illustrated and discussed in §4.

C. Barillot, D.R. Haynor, and P. Hellier (Eds.): MICCAI 2004, LNCS 3217, pp. 234–242, 2004.

2   Morphofunctional Analysis of Airways: Medical Desiderata and Technical Requirements

The 3D reconstruction of airways from MDCT becomes critical to a full assessment of their physiopathology. In a previous work [2] we have developed a fully-automated 3D segmentation approach which combines a strong morphological filtering (in order to extract a low-order airway subset), and an energy-based aggregation model (able to reconstruct high-order bronchi). The bronchial tree is reconstructed up to the $6^{th} - 7^{th}$ subdivision order, even in the presence of local obstructive pathologies. However, at this stage, such a 3D reconstruction only allows a global analysis of the airways. Additional tools are required for local investigation and quantification: lumen/wall cross-sectional area estimation, surgical planning and analysis via virtual bronchoscopy (VB), computational fluid dynamics (CFD). In this respect, some particular technical aspects have to be considered: (1) local estimation of the bronchus orientation, (2) virtual camera centrality problem in VB automatic navigation, (3) automated and accurate surface mesh generation from the binary 3D reconstruction for VB-based analysis and CFD. While the first two requirements find a solution with the central axis computation, the third one raises several difficulties related to the high branching complexity and to the caliber variability of the airway structure.

The existing algorithms performing the extraction of an object surface mesh from volumetric data can be classified into the following categories: planar contour-based methods [3], deformable models [4,5], and the "Marching Cubes" (MC) algorithm [6,7]. Widely used in medical imaging [8], the MC are better adapted to the bronchial tree structure. However, the MC-based surface meshes engendered directly from the 3D binary segmented data reveals strong irregularities corresponding to the voxel contours as well as some discontinuities in the small caliber branches, Fig. 1.

In order to prevent such effects, the commonly used approach consists in smoothing the binary data by means of a Gaussian filtering prior to applying the MC [8]. The surface mesh smoothness directly depends on the considered filter size. In the case of segmented airways, a large filter size induces geometrical distortions (segment shortening, diameter increasing and branch discontinuities) at the level of small caliber segments, Fig. 2, while a small filter size preserves the surface irregularities for large caliber bronchi. In addition, in the case of pathological configurations, abnormal mesh irregularities may also appear for large caliber segments and large filter sizes. Fig. 3 shows an ectopic bronchus originated from the trachea and generating a tracheal stenosis. The problem results from the subdivision morphology which keeps the segments very close one to another after the bifurcation. When a Gaussian smoothing is applied to such a configuration, local gray level maxima appear near the bifurcation. They may belong to the value range used for MC isosurface generation, which results in "spikes" on the 3D mesh, Fig. 3.

In order to overcome these limitations and to generate a smooth and accurate 3D surface mesh of airways, two requirements are imposed: an adaptive data smoothing according to the bronchus caliber, on the one hand, and an adaptive control of the isosurface values, on the other hand. Such procedure can rely on the information provided by the central axis concerning geometry, topology, segment indexation and local caliber. Hence, central axis computation appears as the key issue in providing local airway investigation and quantification facilities. This issue will be addressed in the following section.

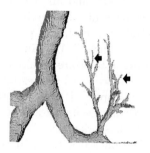

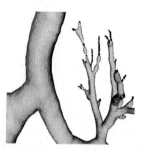

Fig. 1. MC applied to the binary data: irregular surface mesh and local discontinuities at the level of small caliber segments (arrows)

Fig. 2. Smoothed surface mesh by Gaussian filtering prior to MC (light grey) superimposed on the surface mesh from Fig.1 (black)

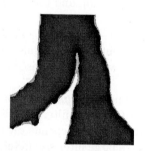

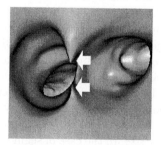

(a) Lateral view. The smoothed surface is displayed in light gray, superimposed on the non-filtered surface

(b) Endoluminal view revealing abnormal spikes

Fig. 3. Mesh generation with Gaussian pre-filtering for a pathological configuration

3   Central Axis Computation

Central axis (CA) algorithms can be classified into three main categories: thinning algorithms, methods based on Voronoi diagram computation and methods using distance maps.

The thinning algorithms iteratively "peel off" the object boundary, layer by layer, until one central layer remains. In 3D, the most challenging issue is the connectivity preservation and such methods fail in preserving both connectivity and geometry, especially in the case of highly branching objects [11].

The second class of methods uses the property that the median axis of a polygon is a subset of its Voronoi diagram [12][13]. Rather adapted to polyhedron-defined objects, these algorithms present limitations in the case of noisy boundary objects: the Voronoi diagram thus obtained is highly complex and therefore imposes a severe skeleton pruning.

The distance map-based algorithms generally use a geodesic distance map or a geodesic front propagation with respect to a source point, and build the central axis by linking the centroids of the successive fronts. To ensure the centrality of the axis, many authors also refer to a distance map with respect to the object boundary in the computation of the centroids. The subdivision of a current front indicates that a branching point has been reached. The algorithm is then recursively applied to each subset of the splited front [14], Fig. 4(a). Since the 3D reconstruction of the bronchial tree reveals a quasi-tubular object with complex branching topology, this latter approach is better adapted to such a structure and was selected for our purpose.

However, the accurate detection of the branch subdivision points remains a key issue. Indeed, the usual criterion based on front splitting is not robust in the case of high caliber bronchi, and may lead to CA geometry distortions and hierarchy errors with respect to the bronchial subdivision order Fig. 4(b), 4(c).

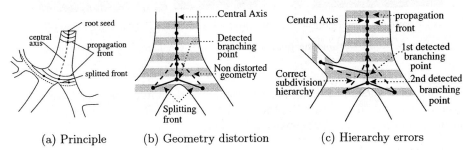

(a) Principle   (b) Geometry distortion   (c) Hierarchy errors

Fig. 4. CA extraction using geodesic front propagation and typical limitations due to branch subdivision detection based on front splitting

3.1 The Developed Approach

In order to overcome these limitations, we propose a robust criterion for subdivision point detection which combines geodesic front propagation and 3D distance map computed with respect to the bronchial wall.

Geometry distortion can be prevented by analyzing the 3D distance map information: the highest value points on the map correspond to the CA location. Thus, the occurence of a branching point can be suspected when several distance map local maxima appear at the level of the current propagation front. Such a technique prevents CA from geometry distortions, Fig. 5(a), but is insufficient to provide the correct configuration of a complex CA subdivision, Fig. 5(b). To achieve the correct hierarchy of the CA subdivision points, we propose a robust criterion based on a space partitioning starting from a possible subdivision point, detected as previously. First, the space partitioning defines the maximum sphere centered at this point and inscribed in the airway set. Then, the points located on the sphere surface propagate toward lower values of the distance map. This will generate a cone-shaped structure associated with each segment of the subdivision, irrespective of the degree of the subdivision (bifurcation, trifurcation, etc.). The geometry of the CA at the subdivision level is then reconstructed by linking the vertex of each cone-shaped structure to the subdivision point, by following the maximum value path on the distance map, Fig. 5(c). The advantage of such a space partitioning is to provide a global information on a subdivision area making it possible to manage any complex geometry.

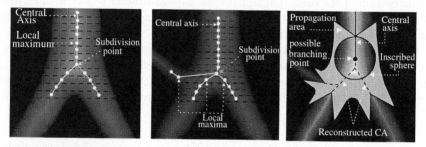

(a) Geometry correction   (b) Hierarchy errors   (c) Space partitioning

Fig. 5. Robust branching point detection with CA hierarchy preservation

The central axis is built up as a hierarchic and multi-valued tree structure: each node carries data related to the geometry, the topology, the caliber and the local orientation of the bronchus at this point.

3.2   Accurate 3D Surface Mesh Construction

Based on the CA information and on the MC algorithm, we propose a simple and efficient approach for accurate surface mesh construction from the binary 3D data. Such an approach consists in implementing an adaptive filtering of the binary reconstructed airways according to the bronchus caliber, and in locally controlling the isosurface values considered by the MC. The adaptive filtering aims at ensuring a constant diameter increasing ratio along the whole bronchial structure. Indeed, as shown in §2, large and small caliber bronchi are differently affected by a same (large size kernel) filter. The idea is to locally adapt the size of the Gaussian kernel to the bronchus caliber, in order to achieve the same diameter increasing ratio of the meshed bronchi with respect to the binary structure. Such an adaptation requires the identification of each bronchial segment, followed by a specific labeling which encodes the segment average radius. In this respect, the bronchial tree volume is divided in disjoint segments by isolating the influence region of each branch of the CA. During the filtering, the smoothed value of each voxel is computed by selecting the kernel size indicated in a look-up table with respect to the bronchus diameter. The look-up table was built up according to simulations carried out on a set of artificial tubular models which diameters vary in the same range as the physiological bronchi. For each model, these simulations determine which kernel size causes a relative radius increasing of 10% (the minimum value able to affect all generations of bronchi), and assign this value to the corresponding bronchus diameter in the table.

In order to avoid mesh irregularities due to pathologies, as shown in Fig. 3(b), the isosurface values resulting from the adaptive filtering should be locally controlled. In this respect, a second look-up table was empirically built up from the set of models previously described. The isosurface value assigned to each diameter is the gray-level value resulting from the adaptive filtering, at the level of the model initial contour. Fig. 6 shows the results provided by the method we proposed. The accuracy of the meshes thus generated has been validated by a radiologist expert who analyzed the mesh contours superimposed on bronchi cross sectional images at different subdivision orders.

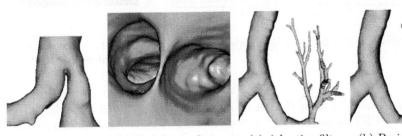

(a) External view   (b) Endoluminal view   (a) Adaptive filter   (b) Basic Gaussian

Fig. 6. Result of the adaptive filtering on the pathological configuration from Fig. 3

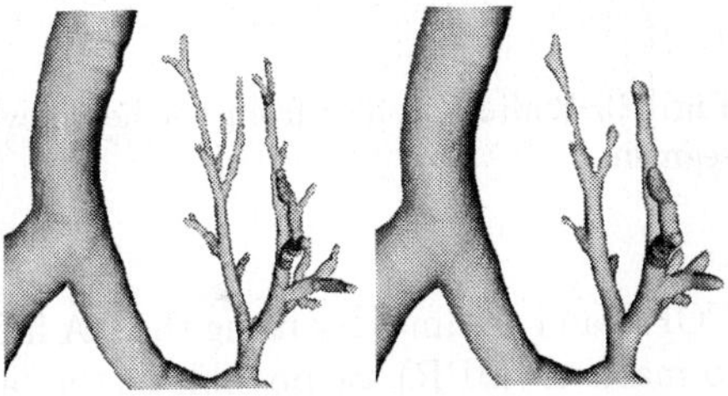

Fig. 7. Result of the adaptive filtering on small caliber bronchi

4   Insights into the Physiopathology of Pulmonary Airways

The combination of the multi-valued information provided by the CA and the accurate reconstruction of the internal airway wall surface enables the development of facilities for local investigation, quantitative assessment, diagnosis and follow-up.

Morphometric information is automatically extracted from the CA structure (branching angles, segment length, Fig. 8). Similarly, the extent of obstructive pathologies, stenosis and bronchiectasis is easily estimated. A particular interest is presented by the accurate evaluation of the bronchial lumen wall surface, orthogonally to the bronchus axis, for the assessment of airway remodeling in

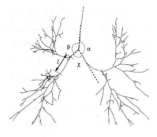

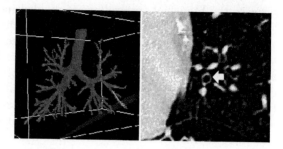

Fig. 8. Morphometric analysis

Fig. 9. Analysis of bronchial wall remodeling

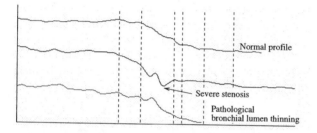

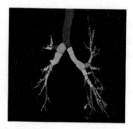

Fig. 10. Radius profiles from trachea down to a terminal segment

Fig. 11.   Bronchial segment indexation

COPD and asthma. By using the CA information, cross-sectional multiplanar reformations (MPR) are possible at the same location, Fig. 9, thus allowing airway comparison pre- and post-intervention (bronchoprovocation, bronchodilatation, therapeutic response).

Investigation paths along the CA are automatically computed starting from the trachea, down to the terminal segment, and bronchus caliber profile displayed with respect to a normal tree profile. Such plots give a first-hand information on the presence of obstructive pathologies, Fig. 10. An automatic procedure for bronchial segment indexation, Fig. 11, makes it possible to perform surgical planning and post-interventional follow-up. With the developments we proposed, airway analysis within virtual bronchoscopy becomes accurate for obstructive pathologies, Fig. 12, and for small caliber distal segments. CA provides automated trajectory computation between two selected points and ensures the centrality of the virtual camera inside the airway structure for an optimal investigation.

The accuracy of the reconstructed surface mesh enables to perform airflow simulations in realistic normal and pathological morphologies, with direct application to inhaled drug delivery [15].

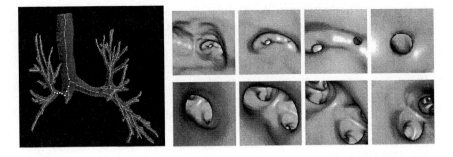

Fig. 12. Virtual bronchoscopy of a severe stenosis in the right upper lobe (RUL) bronchus. The navigation is performed from the right main bronchus down to the RUL bronchus (circles)

5   Conclusion

We have addressed the issue of the MDCT-based investigation of pulmonary airways in a clinical framework. Our objectives were to overcome the limitations encountered by the non-invasive exploration techniques currently available to the medical research and to provide radiologists with complementary tools for an accurate assessment of airway physiopathology.

The developed investigation facilities rely on a fully-automated 3D reconstruction of the bronchial tree from MDCT acquisitions and involve a hierarchic, multi-valued description and an accurate meshing of the complex airway structure derived from robust central axis computation. The resulting exploration tools make it possible to assess a large range of airway pathologies, to increase the diagnostic confidence level and to perform targeted and reproducible quantitative analysis.

Acknowledgement. This study was supported by the French National Project R-MOD.

References

1. Grenier, P., Beigelman, C.: Spiral CT of the bronchial tree. in Medical Radiology: Spiral CT of the Chest, M. Rémy-Jardin, J. Rémy eds., Berlin, Springer Verlag, (1996) 185-199.
2. Fetita, C. I., Prêteux, F., Beigelman-Aubry, C., Grenier, P.: Pulmonary airways: 3D reconstruction from multi-slice CT and clinical investigation. to appear in IEEE Trans on Med Imaging (2004).
3. Kwon, G.H., Chae, S.W., Lee, L.J.: Automatic generation of tetrahedral meshes from medical images. Computers and structures, Vol. 81 (2003) 765-775
4. McInerney, T., Terzopoulos, D.: Deformable models in medical image analysis: a survey. Medical Image Analysis, Vol. 1(2) (1996) 91-108

5. Lachaud, J.-O, Montanvert, A.: Deformable meshes with automated topology changes for coarse-to-fine three-dimensional surface extraction. Medical Image Analysis, 3(2) (1998) 187-207

6. Lorensen, W.E., Cline, H.E.: Marching Cubes: a high resolution 3D surface construction algorithm. Computer Graphics, Vol. 21 (1987) 163-169

7. Wood, Z.J., Schroder, P., Breen, D., Desbrun, M.: Semi-Regular Mesh Extraction From Volumes. in Proc. of IEEE Visualization, (2000) 275-282

8. Summers, R.M., Cebral, J.R.: Tracheal and Central Bronchial Aerodynamics Using Virtual Bronchoscopy. in Medical Imaging 2001: Physiology and Function from Multidimensional Images, Chen, C-T and Clough, AV, Eds., Proceedings of SPIE Vol. 4321,(2001) 22-31

9. Lee, T.-Y., Lin, C.-H.: Growing-cube isosurface extraction algorithm for medical volume data. Computerized Medical Imaging and Graphics, Vol. 25 (2001) 405-415

10. Eck, M., Hoppe, H.: Automatic reconstruction of B-Spline surfaces of arbitrary topological type. ACM SIGGRAPH Proc., (1996) 325-334

11. Ma, C.M., Sonka, M.: A Fully Parallel 3D Thinning Algorithm and its Applications. Computer vision and image understanding, Vol. 64(3) (1996) 420-433

12. Kirkpatrick, D.G.: Efficient computation of continuous skeletons. IEEE 20th annual symphosium on foundations of computer science, (1979) 18-27.

13. Sherbrooke, E.C., Patrikalakis, N.M., Brisson, E.: An algorithm for the medial axis transform of 3D polyedral solids. IEEE transactions on visualization and computer graphics, Vol. 2(1) (1996) 44-61

14. Zhou, Y., Toga, A.: Efficient skeletonization of volumetric objects. IEEE Trans on visualization and computer graphics, Vol. 5(3) (1999) 196-209

15. Vial, L., Perchet, D., Fodil, R., Caillibotte et al: Airflow modeling in a CT-scanned human airway geometry. to appear in European Society of Biomechanics (ESB) Conference, (2004)

A Framework for the Generation of Realistic Brain Tumor Phantoms and Applications

Jan Rexilius[1], Horst K. Hahn[1], Mathias Schlüter[1], Sven Kohle[1], Holger Bourquain[1], Joachim Böttcher[2], and Heinz-Otto Peitgen[1]

[1] MeVis – Center for Medical Diagnostic Systems and Visualization, Bremen, Germany
`rexilius@mevis.de`
[2] Department of Diagnostic and Interventional Radiology, University of Jena, Germany

Abstract. A quantitative analysis of brain tumors is an important factor that can have direct impact on a patient's prognosis and treatment. In order to achieve clinical relevance, reproducibility and especially accuracy of a proposed method have to be tested. We propose a framework for the generation of realistic digital phantoms of brain tumors of known volumes and their incorporation into an MR dataset of a healthy volunteer. Deformations that occur due to tumor growth inside the brain are simulated by means of a biomechanical model. Furthermore, a model for the amount of edema at each voxel is included as well as a simulation of contrast enhancement, which provides us with an additional characterization of the tumor. A "ground truth" is generally not available for brain tumors. Our proposed framework provides a flexible tool to generate representative datasets with known ground truth, which is essential for the validation and comparison of current and new quantitative approaches. Experiments are carried out using a semi-automated volumetry approach for a set of generated tumor datasets.

1 Introduction

Magnetic resonance imaging (MRI) has become an important imaging modality for diagnosis and treatment planning of brain tumors. The main forms of treatment are surgery, radiation therapy, and chemotherapy [1]. A fundamental issue is the accuracy of the calculated quantitative parameters which can have direct impact on therapy. The tumor volume is often used as an objective parameter. However, since brain tumors can largely vary in size, shape, amount of edema, and enhancement characteristics, any quantification of the tumor volume used in clinical routine and in multi-center studies has to be carefully evaluated. Varying acquisition protocols and image quality add to complexity of this task.

Several computer assisted methods have been proposed for the segmentation and quantification of brain tumors [2,3,4,5]. However, due to the absence of a "ground truth" for brain tumors, computation of the exact volume is still a challenging problem. A common approach for the validation of quantitative image analysis methods of brain tumors is based on manual segmentation performed by a medical expert. Since this approach is inherently subjective to interobserver variations and human error, analyses of several experts for the same tumor are usually considered in combination [2].

C. Barillot, D.R. Haynor, and P. Hellier (Eds.): MICCAI 2004, LNCS 3217, pp. 243–250, 2004.
© Springer-Verlag Berlin Heidelberg 2004

Established and representative datasets with known ground truth are essential for the validation and comparison of current and new approaches. A flexible way to generate realistic phantom datasets with exactly known ground truth could be a step towards this goal. Available physical phantoms typically consist of simple objects that are placed in an MR scanner [6]. Digital phantoms can cover a broader range of distributions of shape, size, and contrast behavior. A ditigal phantom for the brain is available from the BrainWeb project [7]. A phantom for Multiple Sclerosis lesions was proposed in [8]. However, there are no suitable phantoms available for brain tumors.

The aim of this paper is to introduce a new approach for the validation of quantitative analyses of brain tumors. We propose a framework for the generation of realistic tumor phantoms of known volumes incorporated in an MRI scan. Brain tumors have a high variabilitly in appearance, size, location, and structure. We focus on glial tumors (gliomas), that constitute the most common group of primary intracranial neoplasms [1]. The biomechanical model used in this paper allows us to simulate deformations that occur due to tumor growth inside the brain. An experimental study is carried out using a semi-automated volumetry approach for a set of generated tumor datasets. In addition, we provide a simulation of contrast agent enhancement characteristics for the tumor phantom.

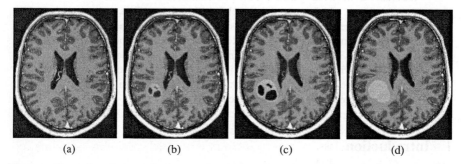

(a)   (b)   (c)   (d)

Fig. 1.   Examples of tumor phantoms without simulation of edema that differ only in size and amount of necrosis in comparison to original MR data. (a) Original T1-weighted image post contrast (T1gd) of healthy volunteer; (b) T1gd image with small tumor; (c) T1gd image with large tumor; (d) T1gd image with large tumor and necrotic tissue scaled to 5%.

2   Modeling Active Tumor Tissue and Necrosis

An issue of specific clinical relevance for a quantitative analysis of brain tumors is the proof of validity of a proposed method. Because of the lack of a "ground truth" for comparison we develop a framework for the generation of datasets with realistic brain tumor phantoms. Essential requirements for the development of our phantoms are (a) a known volume of each tumor to test the accuracy of an investigated method, (b) the possibility to fexibly generate tumors in terms of shapes, sizes, etc., and (c) plausibility with respect to clinical image data. Due to its complex microscopic structure, the tumor phantoms proposed in this work are simulated on a macroscopic level consisting of merely two tissue classes, namely active tumor tissue and necrosis (cf. Figs. 1, 2).

The generation of a phantom dataset consists of two basic steps. In a first step, a high-resolution and arbitrarily shaped tumor phantom with known volume is defined. Then, it is incorporated into an MR scan of the brain of a normal volunteer. A similar concept was used in [8] to generate realistic phantoms of small white matter lesions that occur in patients with Multiple Sclerosis.

2.1 Generation of Brain Tumor Phantoms

Approximation of a continuous volume model. We generate high-resolution binary phantom volumes $i_p : \Theta \to \{0, 1\}$ with signal intensity values $i_p(\mathbf{x}) \in \{0, 1\}$ at voxel positions $\mathbf{x} = (x, y, z)^\top$, $\mathbf{x} \in \Theta$ for the two available tissue classes. A small voxel size is used in order to provide an appropriate approximation of the continuous object volume $V_{i_p} = \int_\Theta i_p(\mathbf{x})d\mathbf{x}$. Different volumes can be easily generated by specifying a different voxel size. To ensure the validity of this assumption, the voxel size for the largest phantom volume is set more than five times smaller than that of the available MR images. In this work we choose tumor volumes between 2 ml and 20 ml.

Both, active tumor tissue and necrosis are drawn non-overlapping on a 256^3 grid with a number of voxels set to gray value 1, so that the underlying ground truth can be extracted for both classes separately. For the figures presented in this work, a shape based on a manual segmentation of a patient dataset with a real brain tumor is used.

Accounting for partial volume effects. In order to incorporate the two previously generated phantom volumes into an MR scan of the brain ($i_b : \Omega \to \mathbb{R}$ with intensity values $i_b(\mathbf{x})$), they are downsampled to the same voxel size as the MR scan, using trilinear interpolation and then reformatted into the coordinate system of the MR scan. This results in a probability map $\tilde{i}_p : \Omega \to \in [0, 1]$ with intensity values $\lambda := \tilde{i}_p(\mathbf{x})$ for each modeled tissue class. Various stages of necrosis can be modeled by scaling each voxel of the original binary image between 0 and 1 (Figure 1 d).

Generation of tumor gray values. We generate volumes i_t for active tumor and necrosis containing reasonable gray values for each available sequence. Furthermore, Gaussian noise is added approximately set equal to the noise of the brain scans. In order to account for a more complex appearance, different noise models could be applied, e.g., based on a Gibbs sampler.

To summarize, this method provides us with a flexible set of rules to generate a realistic tumor phantom with known ground truth that can be incorporated into a dataset of the brain. Tumor phantoms for other organs could be simulated as well using this approach.

2.2 Biomechanical Modeling of Deformations Induced by Tumor Growth

An important aspect in generating a realistic phantom for brain tumors is to simulate the deformation imposed by the tumor growth. A fundamental assumption thereby is that surrounding brain tissue is pushed away from the tumor. In order to gain insight into the process of tumor growth, mathematical modeling has become an increasingly important role and various methods have been proposed. See [9] and references therein. Especially cellular automaton models, that describe the spread and invasion of a tumor on a cell interaction level, have become a popular tool. An approach that simulates the tumor growth on a rather macroscopic level using continuum mechanics was proposed in [10].

In this work, we simulate the three-dimensional tumor growth based on a linear elastic model, which was previously also used to capture shape changes of the brain during neurosurgery [11,12]. Since a rigid model can be assumed for surrounding tissue such as the dura mater, the model is constrained at the boundaries of a brain mask generated by a modified watershed transform [13], so that motion is restricted to areas inside the brain. In order to simulate tumor growth, we place our phantom at an arbitrary position inside the brain with a given radial displacement $u(\mathbf{d}) = \alpha \mathbf{d}, \alpha \in \mathbb{R}^+$ in each direction $\mathbf{d} \in \mathbb{R}^3$. The center of gravity of the tumor phantom is used as point of origin. The computed constraints for both, tumor and brain boundary are then introduced as external forces into the elastic model. Thus, changes in the shape of the brain are modeled to result in an equilibrium state of energy with a displacement u that minimizes the total potential energy given as

$$E(u) = \frac{1}{2} \int_\Omega \sigma^\top \epsilon \, d\Omega \; - \; \int_\Omega F^\top u \, d\Omega \, . \tag{1}$$

The variables are given in terms of the strain vector, σ, the stress vector, ϵ, and the external forces, F [14]. Assuming homogeneous, isotropic material, the mechanical behavior of brain tissue undergoing deformation is described by Young's modulus E ($E = 3kPa$) and Poisson's ratio ν ($\nu = 0.4$). The resulting equation is solved by a finite element approach [14]. A fast parallel implementation was proposed in [12] as part of a nonrigid registration approach.

In order to also simulate the process of tumor growth, we initially start with a deformation restricted to the boundary of a downsampled (factor 5) phantom, with its center of gravity placed at the same position as for the full-scale tumor phantom. Thus, even brain structures very close to or even inside the full-scale phantom's boundaries can be pushed away from the tumor. In a further step, we track the deformation for each voxel by iterating on the deformation field

$$u_n(\mathbf{x}) = u_{n-1}(\mathbf{x}) + u(\mathbf{x} + u_{n-1}(\mathbf{x})) \, . \tag{2}$$

The maximum deformation in the full-scale phantom size is set as stopping criterion for the iteration process. The amount of displacement per iteration varies with the scale factor α as defined above.

It should be noted that although more accurate modeling of tumor growth would be desirable, e.g. [15], it is not essential for the proposed aim of a model for quantitative image analysis.

2.3   Incorporation of a Tumor Phantom into an MR Scan

In a final step, the tumor phantom is incorporated into an MR dataset. Three-dimensional T1-weighted pre and post contrast as well as T2-weighted MR data from a healthy volunteer were used as basis in this work (Siemens Magnetom Vision 1.5T, 256x256 matrix, 1.0mm isotropic voxel size).

In order to simulate the deformation induced by tumor growth as described in the previous section, the generated displacement field is applied to warp the MR data. The resulting phantom dataset is then generated as a linear combination of the deformed MR scan $\tilde{i}_b$ and the tumor volumes $\tilde{i}_t$, containing appropriate gray values for the modeled tumor tissues, i.e. active tumor and necrosis. Thus, new signal intensity values are defined as the convex combination

$$\tilde{i}_b = \sum_{j=1}^{N}(\lambda_j \cdot \tilde{i}_{j,t}) + \left(1 - \sum_{j=1}^{N}\lambda_j\right) \cdot \tilde{i}_b, \qquad \lambda_j \in [0, 1], \tag{3}$$

where N ist the number of modeled tumor tissue classes (here $N = 2$), and the resulting value is assigned to each voxel of the MR dataset. Figures 1 and 2 illustrate some results.

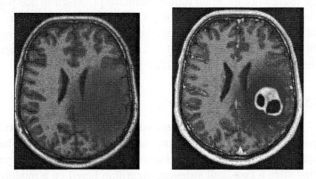

Fig. 2.   Tumor phantom along with a simulation of edema introduced on a T1-weighted image pre and post contrast.

3   Modeling Edema

In addition to the actual tumor, edema is another important structure that should be taken into account for a realistic model of brain tumor phantoms. Brain edema is an inflammatory response to the tumor, which causes, the brain around the tumor to swell and is mostly located in the white matter [1]. Since the brain is located in a confined space and cannot expand, and because the fluid that accumulates cannot easily be carried away, an edema can impair the normal functioning of the brain and causes an increase of intracranial pressure. Therefore, accurate segmentation and quantitative analyses could add valuable information for a physician. Recently, a method for tumor segmentation with an explicit model for edema was proposed in [5].

In order to generate a model for edema we simulate the amount of edema at each voxel, and thus the amount of partial volume, using a geodesic distance transformation [16] starting from the tumor. The basic idea is to constrain the distance computation to remain within a subset of the image volume. As for the edema, we use a white matter mask, since the edema is usually located in the white matter of the brain. To account for tumor growth, we apply the same deformation field as for the MR data before calculating the distance. Depending on the resulting distance map we define a region of pure edema and mixture between pure edema and normal brain tissue, i.e., various degrees of edema dissemination can be simulated this way. The amount of partial volume is scaled accordingly. Further partial volume effects that occur between edema and tumor tissue at the boundary of the tumor are considered as well. A suitable gray value and noise level are defined similar to the method decribed in Section 2.1. In order to finally incorporate edema into the MR scan, Equation 3 is extended by a new tissue class, i.e., $N = 3$.

4   Experimental Results

To evaluate the framework for brain tumor phantoms presented in this paper, we show results for two different applications, namely a semi-automated volumetry method with explicit partial volume modeling and a simulation of contrast enhancement characteristics based on a two-compartment model. All algorithms have been integrated into the research and development platform MeVisLab [17].

4.1   Robust Semi-automated Volumetry

We evaluated 3 phantom MR datasets generated from a brain scan of a normal volunteer. The proposed semi-automated volumetry method combines a 3d marker based segmentation and a multimodal histogram analysis with an explicit model for partial volume effects. In a first step, a fast skull stripping algorithm based on a modified watershed transform is applied to generate an coarse segmentation [13]. Then, the model parameters used for classification are adapted with a maximum likelihood mixture model clustering algorithm on the T1- and T2-weighted images similar to that proposed in [18]. Table 3 compares the semi-automated volumetry method with the known ground truth for each phantom. Our results show an overestimation between 0.15% and 7%.

	Ground Truth	Semi-Automatic
Tumor 1	2.0 ml	2.14 ml
Tumor 2	10.0 ml	10.07 ml
Tumor 3	20.0 ml	20.03 ml

Fig. 3.   Results of semi-automatic partial volume analysis for three different brain tumor phantoms with known ground truth.

4.2   Simulation of Contrast Enhancement Characteristics

Multi-compartment models are commonly used to describe the enhancement of macromolecular contrast agent particles in tumor tissue and thus are an important tool for

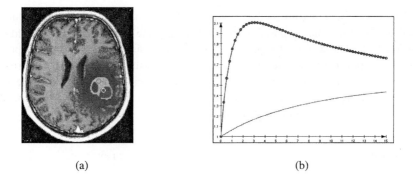

(a)   (b)

Fig. 4.   Results of simulated enhancement characteristics for a T1-weighted gradient echo sequence. The imaging parameters were adapted to the parameters of the real MR scan (TE=5ms, TR=15ms, FlipAngle=30°). (a) Enhancement of tumor tissue. the region drawn in the tumor correspond to the curves in the diagram; (c) enhancement curves for selected regions inside the tumor (horizontal: time in minutes, vertical: relative enhancement). For active tumor tissue the simulation results in a rapidly increasing curve due to high values in the generated permeability parameter map.

computer assisted analysis of dynamic MRI. We have implemented the Tofts&Kermode model [19] in order to generate simulated perfusion datasets. This enables us to combine the prediction of contrast agent enhancement and a known ground truth for a quantitative analyis in simulated brain tumors. In order to apply the Tofts&Kermode model to the tumor phantom, we generate maps for the artificial distribution of physiologic parameters: the permeability of tissue and the extracellular volume fraction which is accessible for the contrast agent. For the permeability we assume an increase from the center to the border of the tumor, where most of the active tumor tissue is usually located. Therefore, an euclidean distance transform is used. A very low permeability is assigned to necrotic tissue using the simulated amount at each voxel as a scaling factor. The extracellular volume fraction is assumed to vary only slightly between $0.7 - 0.8$. Here, we set a higher value for necrosis than for active tumor tissue. Figure 4 exemplary shows the resulting gray values one time-point as well as the enhancement curves for different positions inside the tumor. We generated a simulation of contrast enhancement at a 0.5 minutes scan-interval up to 15 minutes after injection of contrast agent at a dose of 0.1mmol/kg.

5   Discussion and Conclusion

Our main objective in this work has been to develop and test a framework for the generation of realistic phantoms for brain tumors with exactly known volumes for active tumor, necrosis, and edema. Therefore, an arbitrarily shaped high-resolution phantom is incorporated into an MR scan of a normal volunteer. A biomechanical model enables us to simulate deformations that occur due to tumor growth inside the brain. Furthermore, important additional properties such as the amount of edema at each voxel as well as a simulation of contrast enhancement can be provided for the tumor phantom.

Future work will investigate the accuracy and reproducibility of different volumetry methods. Therefore, our proposed framework can provide a realistic basis for validation. New methods that account for preferred tumor dissemination pathways will provide a more accurate basis for the tumor and edema growth, e.g., maps of the principal diffusivity directions derived from diffusion tensor imaging. In order to provide a new tool for comparison in tumor volumetry, our approach could be used to generate a database with a set of brain tumor phantoms.

References

1. A.G. Osborn, K.A. Tong. Handbook of Neuroradiology: Brain and Skull, 2nd edition. Mosby-Year Book, Inc, Missouri, 1991.
2. M. Kaus, S.K. Warfield, A. Nabavi, et al. Automated Segmentation of MR Images of Brain Tumors *Radiology*, 218(2):586-91, 2001.
3. G. Moonis, J. Liu, J.K. Udupa, D.B. Hackney. Estimation of Tumor Volume with Fuzzy-Connectedness Segmentation of MR Images *Am J Neuroradiol*, 23(3):356-63, 2002.
4. J.-P. Guyon, M. Foskey, J. Kim, et al. VETOT, Volume Estimation and Tracking Over Time: Framework and Validation. *MICCAI 2003* vol 2879 of LNCS, pp. 142-149, 2003
5. M. Prastawa, E. Bullitt, N. Moon, et al. Automatic Brain Tumor Segmentation by Subject Specific Modification of Atlas Priors. *Acad Radiol*, 10:1341-1348, 2003.
6. P.S. Tofts, G.J. Barker, M. Filippi, M. Gawne-Cain, M. Lai. An oblique cylinder contrast-adjusted (OCCA) phantom to measure the accuracy of MRI brain lesion volume estimation schemes in multiple sclerosis. *J. Magn Reson Imaging*, 15(2):183-192, 1997.
7. D. Collins, A. Zijdenbos, V. Kollokian, et al. Design and Construction of a Realistic Digital Brain Phantom. *IEEE TMI*, vol. 17, no. 5, pp. 463-468, 1998.
8. J. Rexilius, H.K Hahn, H. Bourquain, H.-O. Peitgen. Ground Truth in MS Lesion Volumetry – A Phantom Study. *MICCAI 2003*, vol 2879 of LNCS, pp. 546-553, 2003.
9. A.R. Kansal, S. Torquato, G.R. Harsh et al. Simulated Brain Tumor Growth Dynamics Using a Three-Dimensional Cellular Automaton, *J Theor Biol*. 203(4): 367-382, 2000.
10. R. Wasserman, R. Acharya, C. Sibata, K.H. Shin. A Patient-Specific In Vivo Tumor Model. *Math Biosci.*, 136(2):111-40, 1996.
11. M. Ferrant, A. Nabavi, B. Macq, et al. Registration of 3D interoperative MR images of the brain using a finite element biomechanical model *IEEE TMI*, vol. 20(12):1384-1397, 2001.
12. J. Rexilius, S.K. Warfield, C.R.G. Guttmann, et al. A Novel Nonrigid Registration Algorithm and Applications. *MICCAI 2001*, pp. 923-931, 2001.
13. H.K. Hahn, H.-O. Peitgen. The Skull Stripping Problem in MRI Solved by a Single 3D Watershed Transform *MICCAI 2000*, pp. 134-143, 2000.
14. O.C. Zienkewickz, R.L. Taylor. The Finite Element Method. McGraw Hill Book Co., 1987.
15. J. Modersitzki. Numerical Methods for Image Registration. Oxford University Press, 2004.
16. P. Soille. Morphological Image Analysis: Principles and Applications, 2nd edition. Springer-Verlag Berlin, 2003.
17. Me*Vis*Lab 1.0, (c) 2004 MeVis gGmbH. Available at: http://www.mevislab.de.
18. A. Noe, J.C. Gee. Partial Volume Segmentation of Cerebral MRI Scans with Mixture Model Clustering. *IPMI 2001*, 423-430, 2001.
19. P.S. Tofts, A.G. Kermode. Measurement of the Blood-Brain Barrier Permeability and Leakage Space Using Dynamic MR Imaging. 1. Fundamental Concepts. *Magn Reson Med*, 17:357-367, 1991.

Measuring Biomechanical Characteristics of Blood Vessels for Early Diagnostics of Vascular Retinal Pathologies

Nataly Yu. Ilyasova[1], Alexander V. Kupriyanov[1], Michael A. Ananin[1], and Nataly A. Gavrilova[2]

[1]Image Processing Systems Institute of Russian Academy of Sciences 151, Molodogvardeiskaya st. 443001, Samara, Russia, ilyasova@smr.ru
[2]Moscow State Medical & Stomatological University

Abstract . A problem of early diagnostics of vascular pathologies is discussed. The method of diagnostic features estimation based on the mathematical model of a retina vessel fragment is presented. The experimental studies of the computa-tion accuracy of the global diagnostic parameters are considered. A technology for localization of the OD region and methods of estimating optic disk parame-ters are proposed. The methods proposed allow a differentiated diagnostics of the retinal diseases.

1 Introduction

Although recent decades have seen obvious advances in diagnostics and treatment of ophthalmologic diseases more people are suffering from retinal impairments of vascular genesis. Since the efficiency of treatment of vascular retinal pathologies essentially decreases with the disease progress the modern research has been focused on ways to enhance informativeness and develop maximally objective methods of early diagnostics, providing prophylactic treatment at the earliest disease stages. Nowadays, diabetes is a major medical & social problem and among the priorities of national health services all over the world. According to the WHO, 150 million people suffer from diabetes throughout the world, with the number increasing by 6-10% every year. Among most frequent and prognostically unfavourable diseases is diabetic retinopathy (DR). Of those suffering from diabetes for over 15 years 80-97 per cent develop DR. Because the early DR stages are marked by retinal vascular changes (changes in absolute and relative diameter ratios of arteries and veins, growth of new vessels, increased vessel tortuosity, etc.) the development of digital and computer technologies for studying the retinal vascular system may show promise in early DR diagnostics. At present, the development of such technologies is associated with im-provement of systems for high-quality retinal image acquisition and development of methods for quantitatively estimating the blood flow status [1, 2]. To get a possibly full insight into the character of vascular changes at early DR stages it is expedient to combine the digital analysis of the retinal vessel routes with examination of the func-tional condition of the vascular wall endothelium. In this paper we introduce and discuss biomechanical characteristics of blood vessels for digital retinal image analysis, which allow the accuracy and informativeness of vascular pathology

C. Barillot, D.R. Haynor, and P. Hellier (Eds.): MICCAI 2004, LNCS 3217, pp. 251–258, 2004.

diagnostics to be enhanced. This paper is a further development of the methods and algorithms for estimating the geometric parameters of vessels proposed in Ref. [3]. Reference [4] deals with estimating one of the parameters (beading) but uses a different approach to extracting vessels from the image.

2   Formation of Retinal Blood Vessels Diagnostic Parameters

To measure the biomechanical vessel characteristics we took a totally new approach to analyzing the retinal image via a tracing vessel segmentation. The method employs a scanning polar frame and allows us to calculate local vessel features (diameter and direction at each point). To determine a set of vascular characteristics and enhance the measurement accuracy we have developed a mathematical model of the vessel (Fig.1) that is defined by the following functions: $x = x(t)$, $y = y(t)$, $r = r(t)$, $0 \le t \le L_v$, where $x(t)$, $y(t)$ $x = x(t)$, $y = y(t)$, $r = r(t)$, $0 \le t \le L_v$, where $x(t)$, $y(t)$ are differentiable functions defining a center line hereafter called the route; $r(t)$ is the branch thickness function (the distance from the route to the vessel boundary reckoned along the perpendicular to the route); t is the distance from the route initial point measured along the route; and L_v is the route length.

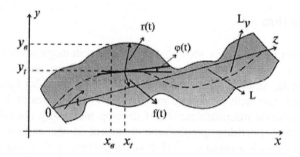

Fig. 1. Mathematical model of a retina vessel fragment

These characteristics uniquely define the route direction function $\varphi(t)$ at each point; the local height function $f(t)$ defined by the distance from the route current point to its projection onto a segment L connecting the initial and final route points (Fig.2); and the configuration of the vessel boundaries hereafter called the walls $x_1^b = x_1^b(t)$, $y_1^b = y_1^b(t)$, $x_2^b = x_2^b(t)$, $y_2^b = y_2^b(t)$, $0 \le t \le L_v$.

The local features involve the route, as well as the distribution of the vessel diameter and the direction along the route. These are calculated immediately from the image using an algorithm for vessel tracing (central line tracing) [3]. The global features include the average diameter, linearity, beading, thickness variation amplitude, thickness variation frequency, thickness tortuosity, route variation frequency, route variation amplitude, and route tortuosity. These serve to characterize the entire vessel on the whole and are later used as diagnostic features.

The vessel *average diameter* $\overline{D}$ is derived from

$$\overline{D} = 2\overline{r} = \frac{2}{N}\sum_{n=1}^{N}r(t_n),$$ (1)

where $t_n = n\Delta$, N is the number of pixels of a local radius measured along the vessel at reliable points, and $\overline{r}$ is the vessel average radius.

The vessel *linearity* P characterizes the vessel deviation from a straight line and is defined as the ratio of length L_v of the vessel medial line to the length L of a straight line connecting the initial and final points of the route:

$$P = L_v/L = \sum_{n-1}^{N-1}\sqrt{(x_n - x_{n+1})^2 + (y_n - y_{n+1})^2}\Bigg/\sqrt{(x_1 - x_N)^2 + (y_1 - y_N)^2}.$$ (2)

The vessel *beading* S characterizes the branch thickness irregularity and is defined as the ratio of the root-mean-square deviation of the vessel radius to its average value:

$$S = \sqrt{\overline{r^2} - \overline{r}^2}/\overline{r},$$ (3)

where $\overline{r}$ is the vessel average radius and $\overline{r^2}$ is the radius mean square.

The vessel *thickness variation amplitude* A_0 characterizes the deviation of the vessel walls from a straight line and is defined as

$$A_0 = \sqrt{2\overline{r^2} - 2\overline{r}^2}.$$ (4)

The vessel *thickness variation frequency* ω_0 characterizes a change in the wall direction per unit length and is defined as

$$\omega_0 = \frac{2\pi}{N}m_0, \quad m_0 = \arg\left(\max_{1<m<N}R(m)\right), \quad R(m) = \left|\sum_{n=0}^{N-1}r(t_n)\exp\left(-i\frac{2\pi nm}{N}\right)\right|,$$ (5)

m_0 is the number of maximal value of Fourier-spectrum of the thickness function.

The *thickness tortuosity* I_0 characterizes the rate of change of the thickness function along the route approximated by a harmonic function of amplitude A_0 and frequency ω_0 and is derived from $I_0 = A_0\omega_0$.

The *route tortuosity* I_1 characterizes the rate of change of the route function at a selected segment, which is approximated by a harmonic function of amplitude A_1 and frequency ω_1, defined as $I_1 = A_1\omega_1$, and derived from

$$P = \frac{2}{\pi}\sqrt{1 + I_1^2}\cdot E(k), \quad k = I_1\Big/\sqrt{1 + I_1^2},$$ (6)

where P is the branch linearity, and $E(k)$ is the total elliptic integral of the 2nd kind.

The *route variation amplitude* A_1 characterizes the degree of deviation of the route trajectory from the straight line and is defined as

$$A_1 = 2\bar{f} \cdot E(k) \bigg/ \left(1 + \ln\left(I_1 + \sqrt{1+I_1^2}\right) \bigg/ \left(I_1\sqrt{1+I_1^2}\right)\right),$$ (7)

where I_1 is the route tortuosity and $\bar{f}$ is the vessel average height.

The vessel fragment *route variation frequency* ω_1 characterizes how often the direction of the branch is changed per unit length and is defined as

$$\omega_1 = I_1/A_1 .$$ (8)

Given below are the experimental studies of the computation accuracy of the following four global parameters: route variation amplitude, route variation frequency, thickness variation amplitude, and thickness variation frequency. In studying the route parameters, images of ideal routes with their trajectories defined as sinusoidal functions of different frequency and amplitude were generated (Table 1). The error in determining the route frequency is caused by the error introduced by the branch tracing algorithm. In studies of the thickness parameters, images of ideal routes with trajectories of their boundaries defined as sinusoidal function of different frequency and amplitude were generated (Table 2). The error in constructing the parameter estimates is caused by the effect of route image discretization.

The studies conducted have shown that the above-discussed features can be used for assessment of the general retinal pathology.

Table 1. The results of the experimental studies of the methods for estimating the route parameters in test images

Route	Amplitude		Frequency	
	Ideal	Estimated	Ideal	Estimated
	10	10.13	1.5	1.500
	10	10.26	2.0	1.789
	20	21.10	2.5	2.049
	20	20.16	4.5	4.127
	20	20.22	5.5	5.176

Table 2. The results of the experimental studies of the methods for estimating the route thickness parameters in test images

Route	Amplitude		Frequency	
	Ideal	Estimated	Ideal	Estimated
	2.5	2.430	3.0	3.002
	8.0	7.918	2.5	2.441
	2.0	2.102	12.5	12.478
	7.0	7.041	9.5	9.482

3 Methods for Estimating Optic Disk Parameters

In the literature there are numerous reports about optic disk impairments caused by the elevated intraocular pressure. The system to autoregulate circulation in the blood vessels feeding the optic disk (OD) is a key mechanism that supports the normal circulation in the optic nerve (ON) head. Disturbance of this function is a risk factor in the progressive development of glaucoma-related ON atrophy [5,6].

Decreased OD vascularization in glaucoma patients and atrophic changes in peripapillar vessels confirm that vascular pathologies have their part in development of optical neuropathy. In this connection, ophthalmologists doing their research with Moscow State Medical & Stomatological University (Ophthalmology Department) commissioned our team to estimate the OD diagnostic parameters. The key characteristics of vascular pathology are the ratio of the total diameter of thin vessels on the OD edge to its perimeter, as well as the total area of the aforementioned vessels in the OD region.

3.1 Localization of the OD

The automated system developed for OD analysis involves the following stages of retinal image processing: localization of the OD region, profiling along the OD edge, vessel detection on the OD edge, estimation of the vessel local features (direction and diameter), and calculation of the diagnostic parameters. The pre-processing stage is aimed at obtaining a binary image of the OD region and determining parameters approximating the OD edge contour.

Based on the data of the original full-color retinal image and the OD contour parameters we can build a profile along the OD edge and perform the subsequent processing using a smoothing filter. The algorithm for obtaining a binary image can be broken down into three stages: profiling the brightness function to get a binary preparation, rank filtration of the binary image, and elimination of large noise fragments (Fig.2).

To obtain the OD edge parameters we used an algorithm that approximates the OD edge by an ellipse of minimal area that covers the whole (or nearly whole) area OD region. The equation of an ellipse with an arbitrary center and tilt is given by

$$\frac{((x-x_0)\cos\varphi-(y-y_0)\sin\varphi)^2}{a^2}+\frac{((y-y_0)\cos\varphi+(x-x_0)\sin\varphi)^2}{b^2}=1. \tag{9}$$

A five-dimensional parallelepiped defining the range of values of the parameters a, b, x_0, y_0 and φ is broken down into cells. In the grid nodes, the area is calculated and the inclusion condition is checked.

The major stages of the algorithm are: (1) exhaustive search of the values x_0, y_0, φ; (2) for a given triplet (x_0, y_0, φ), determination of the semi-axes (a, b) of a minimal-area ellipse covering the OD region. The result of the OD region localization and obtaining the ellipse parameters is shown in Fig.2.

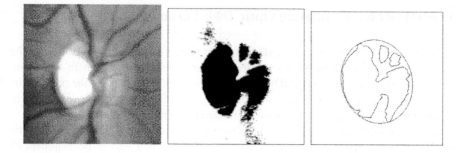

Fig. 2. Operation of the algorithm for the OD region localization: original image; view after brightness profiling; and the OD region contour and the approximating ellipse

3.2 Vessel Detection and Parameter Estimation on the OD Edge

The retinal vessel detection was performed on the basis of analysis of the gray-level profile represented as a brightness function scan along the derived contour of the OD region. In pre-processing, one of the problems consists in bringing the color image profile to the gray-level through transforming the R-, G-, and B-pixels of the original image into the corresponding brightness values. In the course of experimental studies, the red and green components were found to carry a major bulk of information about the background and vessels. Because of this, the arithmetic mean of the red and green components was used as a resulting value of brightness of the current profile point. To suppress noise an averaging filter was used.

The method for vessel detection on the OD edge is based on the analysis of local minima of the derived profile brightness function. The procedure involved a sliding local approximation by a second-order polynomial. The search for minimums corresponding to the vessel centers is carried out analytically, with the subsequent analysis aimed at discarding false minimums. In the algorithm of thickness estimation, the vessel boundaries are given by the profile inflection points nearest to the center. An average relative shift of vessel centers on N neighboring ellipses (similar to the original one, with the coefficient close to 1) allows us to find the vessel direction. The averaging is conducted in the vessel center neighborhood on the major profile. The estimate of vessel thickness is corrected by multiplying by the cosine of the angle between the derived vessel direction and the normal to the OD contour, because the vessels are not perpendicular to the OD region edge.

3.3 Experimental Studies of the Methods

The performance of the algorithm for estimating the vessel local features was checked using test and original OD images. In the course of studies, we examined how the algorithm parameters affected the accuracy of vessel detection and accuracy of diameter estimation on the OD edge. Out of all the experiments conducted, below we discuss only those looking into the impact of noise on the diameter estimation accuracy in test images (Fig.3). The algorithm in question (scheme 1) was compared with the algorithm in which the vessel direction is being sought by using a fan transform [7] (scheme 2). It can be seen from Fig.3 that noise begins to affect the diameter estimation accuracy at the noise-to-signal ratio of 0.216, suggesting that the method shows good robustness.

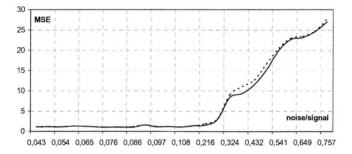

Fig. 3. The error of the vessel thickness estimation vs noise level (solid line – scheme 1, dotted - scheme 2)

Figure 4 shows the result of the algorithm operation for localization of the OD region, contouring and estimating the OD local parameters in an original image. The interface of the OD analysis system allows simultaneously viewing all the necessary data and the results of studies.

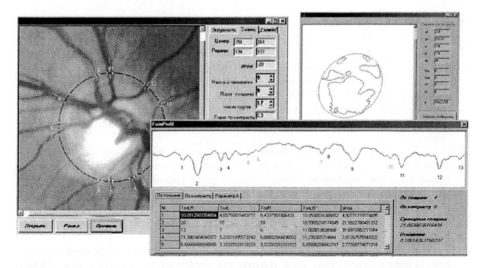

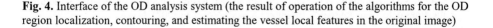

Fig. 4. Interface of the OD analysis system (the result of operation of the algorithms for the OD region localization, contouring, and estimating the vessel local features in the original image)

4 Conclusions

We have developed biomechanical blood vessel characteristics for digital analysis of the retina, which aim to enhance the accuracy and informativeness of vascular pathology diagnostics. The biomechanical characteristics essentially facilitate the expert estimate of the vascular pathology, being capable of detecting slightest pathological changes, its degree, and development probability. The estimation methods discussed have formed the basis for a computerized system for measuring the geometric parameters of biomedical images [3]. The system allows the objective quantitative results to be derived and extends the capabilities of the existing medical methods. The analysis system also includes methods and algorithms for estimating the OD geometric characteristics and a method of searching for vessels on the OD edge and localizing the OD region using peculiarities of the OD color-brightness characteristics and the OD region approximation contouring. Introduction of the developed methods into medical use will enhance its capabilities and allow automatic diagnostics of some diseases and monitoring of pathological retinal changes on the basis of objective quantitative data.

Acknowledgements. This work was financially supported by the U.S. Civilian Research & Development Foundation (CRDF) and the Ministry of Education & Science of the Russian Federation (CRDF project REC-SA-014-02) as part of the Basic Research & Higher Education (BRHE) program; by the Russian Foundation for Basic Research grant under № 03-01-00642; and by the Human Capital Foundation grant.

References

1. Jomier, J., Wallace, D.K., Aylward, S.R.: Quantification of Retinopathy of Prematurity via Vessel Segmentation. Proceedings of MICCAI 2003, LNCS 2879 620-626.
2. Osareh, A., Mirmehdi M., Thomas B., Markham R.: Classification and Localisation of Diabetic-Related Eye Disease. ECCV 2002, LNCS 2353 502-516
3. Ilyasova, N.Yu., Ustinov A.V., Baranov V.G.: An Expert Computer System for Diagnosing Eye Diseases from Retina Images. Optical Memory and Neural Networks, Vol. 9, No. 2 (2000) 133-145
4. Ching-Wen Yang, Dye-Jyun Ma, Shuenn-Ching Chao, Chuin-Mu Wang, Chia-Hsin Wen, Chien-Shun Lo, Pau-Choo Chung, Chein-I Chang: Computer-aided diagnostic detection system of venous beading in retinal images, Optical Engineering, Vol.39, No.5, 2000, pp.1293-1303
5. Mendels, F., Heneghan, C., Thiran, J.P.: Identification of the Optic Disk Boundary in Retinal Images Using Active Contours. Proceedings of the Irish Machine Vision and Image Processing Conference (1999) 103-115
6. Chanwimaluang , T., Fan, G.: An Efficient Algorithm for Extraction of Anatomical Structures in Retinal Images, Proc. IEEE International Conference on Image Processing, Barcelona, Span, September 2003
7. Baranov, V.G., Khramov, A.G.: Discrete fan-shaped Radon transform for net-like structures' centerlines detection. Journal "Computer Optics", Vol. 23 (2002) 44-47

A 4D-Optical Measuring System for the Dynamic Acquisition of Anatomical Structures

Kathleen Denis[1], Tom Huysmans[1], Tom De Wilde[1], Cristian Forausberger[1],
Walter Rapp[1], Bart Haex[1], Jos Vander Sloten[1], Remi Van Audekercke[1],
Georges Van der Perre[1], Kjell Roger Heitmann[2], and Helmut Diers[2]

[1] Division of Biomechanics and Engineering Design, K.U.Leuven,
Celestijnenlaan 200A, B-3001 Leuven, Belgium
[2] Diers International GmbH,
Dillenbergweg 4, 65388 Schlangenbad, Germany

Abstract. This paper presents a novel measuring system for the detection of moving skeletal structures. The system uses white light raster line triangulation in combination with biomechanical modeling techniques. White light raster line triangulation visualizes surfaces (e.g. the back surface) in an accurate and repeatable way, without detrimental effects, and without making contact to the human body. By making use of modeling techniques such as active contour models, active shape models and inverse kinematic models, biomechanically relevant results such as the position of the skeletal segments during motion are obtained.

1 Introduction

1.1 Clinical Relevance

The number of people suffering from musculoskeletal complaints, such as low back pain, is huge. It is by far the most important cause for work absenteeism in Europe, and as the population is increasingly sedentary and ageing, it is a growing problem. Orthopedic physicians and physiotherapists are required to analyze a variety of movements to diagnose pathological or abnormal changes. Therefore, an objective measurement tool to provide the medical examiner or the physiotherapist with clinically relevant data to support the diagnosis and therapy plan is required.

1.2 Innovation of the Measuring System

Standard diagnosis methods for musculoskeletal problems consist of expensive medical procedures (e.g. CT scans), involving potentially harmful ionizing radiation, or require expert operator interaction (e.g. 3D motion analysis based on marker tracing). Most of these methods are aimed at static purposes only and do therefore not involve dynamic measurements. Furthermore they show problems in specific cases (e.g. shift of markers on skin in marker tracing systems). So far, low cost measurement devices for preventive screening, diagnosis or treatment

C. Barillot, D.R. Haynor, and P. Hellier (Eds.): MICCAI 2004, LNCS 3217, pp. 259–266, 2004.

indication and control are not available. The objective was therefore to develop a contact-free measuring system for body surfaces, which is suited for dynamical applications in order to measure the human body in motion. By reconstructing internal anatomical structures, such as the spinal column, the system incorporates functional analysis capacities for medical, ergonomic, and revalidation applications. The reconstruction of internal anatomical structures is based on biomechanical modeling. In this paper, the reconstruction of the spine during stepping and the reconstruction of the shoulder during arm abduction are shown as examples of these techniques.

2   Materials and Methods

2.1   White Light Raster Line Triangulation

White light raster line triangulation (WLRT) enables the scanning of objects in 3D by projecting raster lines on its surface and by capturing these lines under a known and fixed angle with a camera [1] (Figure 1). Based on triangulation algorithms, spatial coordinates of all raster points are calculated, resulting in a dense point cloud of randomly distributed points describing the measured surface. These data points are transformed to a regular grid by using interpolation, which will simplify further calculations. In this way, the system captures and analyzes body motion with a frequency of 15 Hz.

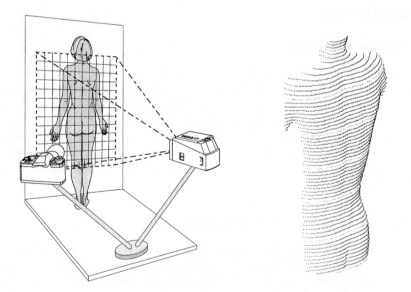

Fig. 1. WLRT acquisition (left) and point cloud describing the back surface (right).

2.2   Active Contour Models (ACM)

The technique of active contours (ACM) or "snakes" was first proposed for outlining purposes [2]: a specific (mathematical) cost is defined in such a way that a minimization of the cost leads to an optimal recognition of a well defined feature. Starting from an initial estimation, the objective is to iteratively move the contour on the image until the cost is minimized and appropriate contour properties are achieved. The cost of an ACM comprises two parts: an external and an internal cost. The external cost guides the contour to a minimal cost position on the surface; the internal costs serve as a smoothness constraint and are defined in such a way that biomechanically incorrect solutions are excluded. The technique of ACM is applied to the extraction of information from the back surface. The external cost that is used for the detection of underlying skeletal structures in movement consists of a surface curvature cost and a symmetry cost. The internal costs include bending and torsion costs, an equidistance cost and a constraint cost. The optimization problem locates an outline with a minimal total cost, starting from an initial ACM.

2.3   Active Shape Models (ASM)

An active shape model (ASM) can be seen as "smart snake" that is only able to deform in ways characteristic of the class of objects it represents [3]. An ASM is built by learning patterns of variability from a training set of correctly labelled points on images. By examining the statistics of the positions of the labelled points a point distribution model can be derived. The model gives the average positions of the points, and has a number of parameters which control the main modes of variation found in the training set. In this way the developed model can only deform in ways found in the training set.

2.4   Inverse Kinematic Models (IKM)

For the shoulder joint, a lot of the skeletal information is hidden underneath the back surface. To reveal this information, a model has been developed to be used together with the surface measurements. The skeletal model contains the sternum, clavicula, scapula and humerus. Between the bones, three joints have been defined: the sternoclavicular joint, the acromioclavicular joint and the glenohumeral joint. These joints are modeled as three-degrees-of-freedom spherical joints. The scapula moves freely with respect to the thoracic wall, to permit scapular winging, which is a condition sometimes caused by nerve injury or another disorder affecting the shoulder. The model has been parameterized; it contains one parameter per bone. The motion of the links is limited in the spherical joints, using limits obtained from biomechanical literature [4]. The bones have been modeled as geometrical primitives. Surface geometry has been added to the model for visualization purposes. Figure 2 shows both.

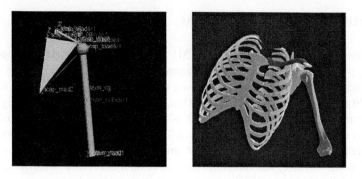

Fig. 2. Shoulder model consisting of geometrical primitives (left) and with surface geometry (right).

3   Results

3.1   Example 1: ASM for the Detection of the Pelvis for a Stepping Motion

ASM's were derived for an objective localization of anatomical landmarks which correspond to the vertebra prominens, the posterior superior iliac spines on the pelvic bone (os ilium) and the sacrum point (the beginning of the rimi ani). At first a point distribution model (PDM) is derived for stepping, based on a few training sets of the movement. The PDM showed clear relations between the anatomical landmarks. Figure 3 shows the first mode shape for a stepping movement. This single mode shape already explains 90% of the total variation in 3D. The PDM is then used to locate the anatomical landmarks on persons who performed a similar movement (ASM). The detection of the four anatomical landmarks for three time steps, using this ASM, is indicated on figure 4.

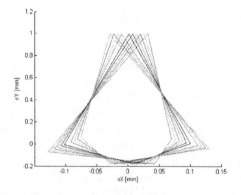

Fig. 3. First mode shape for stepping

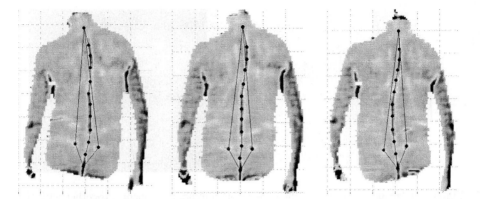

Fig. 4. Detection of the pelvis and the line through the spinous processes based on an ACM and an ASM (stepping, three time steps)

3.2   Example 2: ACM for the Detection of the Line Through the Spinous Processes

The detection of the line through the spinous processes over different measurements can only be made if the cost function is composed of invariant shape properties. Surface curvatures, for example, are an invariant property of the back shape, and can thus be used to analyze the shape of the human back. As a consequence, the positions of the detected anatomical landmarks are independent of the patient's position. An ACM is used for the detection of the line through the spinous processes. The ACM makes use of an asymmetry function, comprising the major part of the external cost for the active contour. The mean curvature is also included - as a minor factor - in order to improve the overall estimation of the line, e.g. to overcome local problems. In order to avoid results that are impossible from a biomechanical point of view, internal costs are added. At first bending and torsion costs are included; these terms are related to the smoothness of the curve, preventing the curve from physically impossible positions. Furthermore, active contour points will mount up during the calculations at places with a high surface curvature and/or symmetry. To avoid this effect, a final internal cost is included to keep all active contour points at an equal distance. A spline describes the ACM. Based on this spline, the internal spine is reconstructed using an anatomical formula, estimating the distance of the skin to the center of a vertebral body [1]. Figure 4 shows the detected line through the spinous processes with the ACM's for different time steps (stepping motion).

3.3   Example 3: IKM for the Detection of the Scapula During Arm Abduction

In case the measurements do not show enough information, an IKM is used. The shoulder IKM is used as follows: in preliminary measurements the person performs standard motions from which the parameters are quantified. After this,

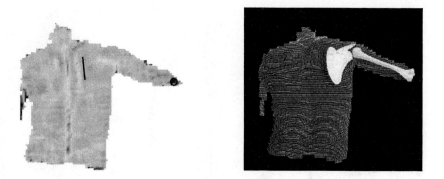

Fig. 5. The mean curvatures of one image from a dynamic sequence, together with the reconstruction of the humerus and scapula.

during the actual measurements, the model is used as extra information. The model calculates the shoulder position using inverse position kinematics. In a dynamic sequence, the model predicts the next position. When an image does not contain the information needed to detect the positions, the information is updated with the model prediction. Figure 5 shows the reconstruction of the scapula and the humerus in one image of a dynamic sequence.

4   Presentation of the Results

Figure 6 shows the user interface to view the results of a dynamic measurement. The left window is the 4D-(three dimensional and time dependent)surface window, the right window gives a graphic representation of selected parameters as a function of time. In the left window, succeeding images of the back surface are shown, with the possibility to show the raster lines, point cloud, mean curvatures, Gaussian curvatures, and 3D-inner skeletal structures in different views. The right window shows clinical parameters such as (for the trunk) trunk imbalance, trunk torsion, trunk inclination, (for the pelvis) pelvic tilt, pelvic torsion, (for the spine) lordotic angle, kyphotic angle, (for the scapula) maximum scapular winging, etc. In this example, the left window shows the Gaussian curvatures of a back surface in frontal view and the lines connecting the left and right dimples with the vertebra prominens and the sacrum point. The right window shows the pelvic tilt and the trunk imbalance as a function of time.

5   Discussion

Systems to detect skeletal structures in movement are mostly marker-based. The described 4D optical measuring system has the following advantages over these systems: there is no preparation time to equip the patient with the markers and there is no expert needed to palpate the patients and find the optimal positions of the markers. No contact is made with the patient, which is more agreeable for

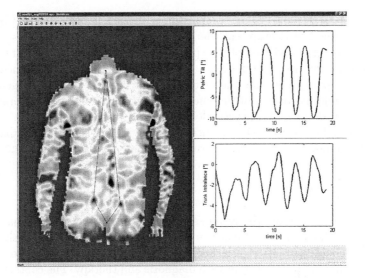

Fig. 6. A screen plot of the presentation of the results.

the patient. This system offers extra information, such as axial rotation of the vertebrae from back shape data. The marker-based systems have the disadvantage that during certain motions the skin with the markers shifts over internal skeletal structures, e.g. the shift of the skin over the scapula during arm elevation, resulting in a non-unique relation between marker and bone position. This source of errors does not exist in the present system. Compared to a marker-based system, the presented system has a limited field of view due to the raster projection, hence limiting the motions that can be investigated. For the moment, a field of view with a width of 1.5 m and a depth of 0.5 m is available. With the current frequency of 15 Hz it is not possible to investigate very fast motions yet; however, slow to medium-fast motions are not a problem. Increasing the frequency would mean an increase of data to be stored and of analyzing time. At present, both measurement time and analyzing time are short since automatic image analysis and processing are applied.

By making use of biomechanical models such as active contour models, active shape models and inverse kinematic models, biomechanically relevant results are obtained. The open structure of the ACM allows the addition of other biomechanical constraint costs, e.g. to examine specific etiological phenomena. In case of scoliosis research, for example, an extra cost is added, describing the observed relation between the lateral deviation and the axial rotation of the vertebrae.

The uniqueness of the presented system makes it difficult to compare the results in 4D. However, the accuracy of the position of the internal skeletal structure has been checked for static purposes using radiographic scans. Drerup and Hierholzer developed an automatic detection of landmarks and spine for static purposes. They obtained an accuracy of 1.3 ± 1 mm for the dimples and the vertebra prominens [5]. The position of the centre of the vertebrae is reconstructed with an accuracy of 3.9 mm [6], in comparison with radiographic scans. Compared with the method of Drerup and Hierholzer, the described system has a similar accuracy: a lateral deviation of the spine of 0.9 mm and an axial rotation of the spine of 0.4° has been obtained [7], and the landmarks are positioned within 2 mm. The main causes for the errors are the noise of the video images and the algorithmic estimation of the line through the spinous processes and of the vertebral rotation (± 3°); nevertheless the error is acceptable for the intended applications. The accuracy is thus better than with marker-based systems, with which the landmarks can be reconstructed with an accuracy of 4.2 ± 1.7 mm [8].

6   Conclusion

The main advantages are the system's ability to reconstruct the internal skeletal structure, without the use of markers or potentially harmful or expensive equipment, as well as its ability to indicate and quantify pathological changes, both at an early stage and in connection with diagnosis and therapy. The contact-free 4D measurement, combined with the automatic detection of anatomical landmarks and the reconstruction of skeletal structures, makes the system unique. The measuring system can be used in public health centers, e.g. for the monitoring of scoliosis when bending sidewards. Ergonomic applications of the measurement device are envisaged as well, e.g. for work task analysis. Revalidation after sports injuries is another application area with a large potential.

Acknowledgement. This research has been supported by the cooperative research project under CRAFT (CRAF-1999-71293).

References

1. B. Drerup and E. Hierholzer. Back shape measurement using video rasterstereography and 3D reconstruction of spinal shape. *Clin Biomech*, 9:28–36, 1994.
2. M. Kass et al. Snakes: Active contour models. *International Journal of Computer Vision*, 1:321–331, 1988.
3. T.F. Cootes et al. Active shape models - their training and application. *Comp Vision Image Underst*, 61(1):38–59, 1995.
4. Engin and Tümer. 3D kinematic modelling of the human shoulder complex - part I. *J Biomech Eng*, 111:107–112, 1989.
5. B. Drerup and E. Hierholzer. Automatic localization of anatomical landmarks on the back surface and construction of a body-fixed coordinate system. *J Biomech*, 20:961–970, 1987.
6. B. Drerup and E. Hierholzer. Assessment of scoliotic deformity from back shape asymmetry using an improved mathematical model. *Clin Biomech*, 7:376–383, 1996.
7. T. Huysmans et al. 3D mathematical reconstruction of the spinal shape, based on active contours. *J Biomech, accepted for publication*, 2004.
8. N. Tardif et al. Evaluation of an integrated laser imaging/x-ray technique for torso asymmetry measurement in scoliosis. *Arch Physiol Biochem*, 108:200, 2000.

An Anisotropic Material Model for Image Guided Neurosurgery

Corey A. Kemper[1], Ion-Florin Talos[2], Alexandra Golby[2], Peter M. Black[2], Ron Kikinis[2], W. Eric L. Grimson[1], and Simon K. Warfield[2]

[1] Massachusetts Institute of Technology, Cambridge, MA 02139
[2] Departments of Neurosurgery and Radiology, Brigham and Women's Hospital, Harvard Medical School, Boston, MA 02115

Abstract. In order to combine preoperative data with intraoperative scans for image-guided neurosurgery visualization, accurate registration is necessary. It has been determined previously that a suitable way to model the non-rigid deformations due to brain shift is via a biomechanical model that treats the brain as a homogeneous, isotropic, linear elastic solid. This work extends that model-based non-rigid registration algorithm to take into account the underlying white matter structure, derived from diffusion tensor MRI, to more accurately model the brain. Experiments performed on retrospective surgical cases were used to evaluate the results of the registration algorithm in comparison to the earlier model.

1 Introduction

Medical imaging has played an increasingly important role in surgical planning and treatment because it provides valuable information about anatomical structure and function. This has been particularly helpful for neurosurgical procedures, where the surgeon is faced with the challenge of removing as much tumor as possible without damaging the healthy brain tissue surrounding it. Regions important to function are often visually indistinguishable and may have been displaced or even infiltrated by the growth of the tumor. However, an abundance of information is available to the neurosurgeon from data derived from a variety of imaging modalities that can address these difficulties.

The development of image-guided neurosurgery (IGNS) methods over the past decade has permitted major advances in minimally invasive therapy delivery. Visualization of the images acquired during IGNS can be enhanced by preoperatively acquired data, whose acquisition and subsequent processing are not limited by any time restriction. For example, conventional MRI provides high resolution anatomical information with increased spatial resolution and contrast, functional MRI provides maps that are correlated with the activation of specific regions of the brain, MR angiography provides the locations of blood vessels, and diffusion tensor MRI (DT-MRI) provides information on the structure of the white matter.

The first issue in utilizing multimodal preoperative data in conjunction with intraoperative images is to correct for patient motion, which is generally limited

C. Barillot, D.R. Haynor, and P. Hellier (Eds.): MICCAI 2004, LNCS 3217, pp. 267–275, 2004.

to rotation and translation of the skull. However, clinical experience has exposed the limitations of these registration and visualization approaches. During neuro-surgical procedures, the brain undergoes non-rigid deformations, and the spatial coordinates of brain structures and adjacent lesions may change significantly.

Most models of deformation either represent the brain as some kind of elastic solid or consolidated material [1,4,6,12]. The most significant limitation at the present time is the computational overhead associated with calculating a Finite Element solution for each update, which limits the complexity of the model that is practical for use in IGNS. Therefore, highly complex models, such as the hyperviscoelastic one described by Miller and Chinzei [7], are not yet appropriate for our application. However, the accuracy of the registration depends on how well the model represents the brain, so we attempt to balance the considerations of accurate modeling and computation time.

The goal of this work was to extend a physics-based biomechanical model for non-rigid registration, designed and developed by Ferrant [2], by incorporating the underlying structure of the brain tissue to better capture changes in the brain shape as it deforms. The deformations estimated by the model were then applied to preoperatively acquired data of different modalities, including fMRI, MRA, and DT-MRI, in order to make the information provided by such data available to the surgeon during the procedure. To meet the real-time constraints of neurosurgery, we utilize a series of scripts [10], which take advantage of high performance computing, to run our registration algorithm.

For validation, the registration algorithm was applied to several surgical cases retrospectively. The registration results were compared to those of the isotropic linear elastic model in order to evaluate the amount, if any, of improvement in registration accuracy was made by extending the model.

2   Method

2.1   Elasticity Model

For the biomechanical model implemented by Ferrant [2] and extended here, the brain is treated as a linear elastic solid. Assuming a linear elastic continuum with no initial stresses or strains, the deformation energy of an elastic body submitted to externally applied forces can be expressed as [13]:

$$E = \frac{1}{2} \int_{\Omega} \sigma^T \epsilon \, d\Omega + \int_{\Omega} F^T u \, d\Omega, \tag{1}$$

where $u = u(x)$ is the displacement vector, $F = F(x)$ the vector representing the forces applied to the elastic body (forces per unit volume, surface forces or forces concentrated at nodes), and Ω the body on which one is working.

In the case of linear elasticity, each stress component (σ) is directly propor-tional to each strain component (ϵ), linked by the elastic stiffnesses, D_{ijkl} which compose a fourth-rank tensor and reduce to a 6x6 symmetric matrix for a general anisotropic material.

In the case of an orthotropic material, the material has three mutually perpendicular planes of elastic symmetry. Hence there are three kinds of material parameters necessary to compute the stiffness matrix: 1) the Young's moduli E_i relate tension and the stretch in the main orthogonal directions, 2) the shear moduli G_{ij} relate tension and stretch in other directions than those of the planes of elastic symmetry, and 3) the Poisson's ratios ν_{ij} represent the ratio of the lateral contraction due to longitudinal stress in a given plane. The determination of these parameters and the assembly of the stiffness matrix are explained in Section 2.3.

2.2   FEM Framework

Within a finite element discretization framework, an elastic body is approximated as an assembly of discrete finite elements interconnected at nodal points on the element boundaries. The continuous displacement field $\mathbf{u}$ within each element is approximated as a function of the displacement at the element's nodal points $\mathbf{u}_i^{el}$ weighted by its shape functions $N_i^{el} = N_i^{el}(\mathbf{x})$. Through such a discretization, and because the integral over the whole domain can be seen as the sum of the integrals over every element, it is possible to evaluate the equilibrium equations separately on every element, and to sum up the contribution of every element to which a vertex is connected to build a global equilibrium matrix system.

For every node i of each element el, we define the matrix $\mathbf{B}_i^{el} = \mathbf{L}_i N_i^{el}$. Using that definition and then minimizing the energy in Equation 1 with respect to the displacement of each element, we have:

$$\int_\Omega \sum_{j=1}^{N_{nodes}} \mathbf{B}_i^{el^T} \mathbf{D} \mathbf{B}_j^{el} \mathbf{u}_j^{el} \, d\Omega = -\int_\Omega \mathbf{F} N_i^{el} \, d\Omega \quad ; \qquad i = 1, \cdots, N_{nodes} \qquad (2)$$

This expression can be written as a matrix system for each finite element, and the assembly of the local matrices then leads to a global system

$$\mathbf{K}\mathbf{u} = -\mathbf{F}, \qquad (3)$$

the solution of which will provide us with the deformation field corresponding to the global minimum of the total deformation energy. Given externally applied forces $\mathbf{F}$ to a discretized body characterized by a rigidity matrix $\mathbf{K}$, solving the previous equation provides us with the resulting displacements.

2.3   Diffusion Tensor MRI

DT-MRI is a technique developed to allow non-invasive quantification of diffusion of water *in vivo*. The directional dependence of water diffusion rates can be closely related to the anisotropy of the structure. Therefore, DT-MRI can be used to infer the organization of tissue components.

In the brain, high anisotropy reflects both the underlying highly directional arrangement of white matter fiber bundles forming white matter tracts and their intrinsic microstructure. This anisotropy can be characterized to distinguish the principal orientation of diffusion, corresponding to the dominant axis of the bundles of axons making up white matter tracts in an given voxel. Because different histologic types of brain white matter demonstrate significant and reproducible anisotropy differences [9], it would be expected that they would deform differently and thus should be modeled differently.

To incorporate the white matter structure into the biomechanical model, the local coordinate system aligned with the fiber direction and its corresponding elasticity parameters must be defined for the stiffness matrix calculation at each tetrahedron. Diagonalization of the corresponding symmetric 3x3 diffusion tensor gives three pairs of eigenvalues and mutually orthogonal eigenvectors. Since molecular diffusion is hindered by encounters with cell membranes and cytoskeletal structures, the water diffusion rate parallel to a fiber is higher than perpendicular to it. The principal eigenvector is therefore parallel to the local tangent of a fiber.

The stiffness matrix for a transversely isotropic material requires 5 independent parameters. Cross-fiber stiffness is approximately 2x to 10x greater than the fiber stiffness for anisotropic brain tissue [8]. We have only limited confidence in using these results for our model because the measurements of fiber stiffnesses are in very specific regions of the brain, such as the corpus callosum and corona radiata, and the stiffness ratios differ throughout. There is currently no measure of how the stiffness ratio relates to anisotropy of diffusion. As an initial attempt to relate the results of DT-MRI and material properties of the brain tissue, we calculate fractional anisotropy (FA) from the eigenvalues of the diffusion tensor and the Young's modulus in the cross-fiber direction p as a linear function of the FA, maximum stiffness ratio (α), and the Young's modulus in the fiber direction f.

$$E_p = (1 + (\alpha - 1)FA)E_f \qquad E_f = E \qquad (4)$$

The Poisson's ratios are assumed to be equal in all three directions because the compressibility of the tissue is not expected to change. The shear moduli are calculated from the Young's moduli and Poisson's ratios as follows:

$$G_f = G_p = \frac{E_p}{2(1+\nu)} \qquad (5)$$

G_f is actually an independent parameter, but it is arbitrarily set equal to the shear modulus in the plane of isotropy because the experiments for the elasticity parameters for anisotropic brain tissue focus do not include the shear moduli.

Once the local stiffness matrix has been determined, it is rotated according to the transformation matrix to the global coordinate system from the local coordinate system, as defined by the eigenvectors.

2.4   Non-rigid Registration Algorithm

The steps of the registration method are summarized as follows: **Preoperative image acquisition, processing and visualization**: Before the surgery, a conventional grey-scale MRI scan, functional MRI, MRA, and DT-MRI datasets are acquired. These images are processed to locate the ventricles, cortical surface, tumor, white matter tracts, and blood vessels, and are manually registered to the grey-scale MRI. 3D Slicer [3], an integrated software tool, is used for visualization and surgical planning. **Intraoperative image acquisition**: The open configuration 0.5 T MR scanner is used to acquire intraoperative scans as necessary. **Intraoperative rigid registration**: The presurgical data is registered to the intraoperative scan using an automated, Mutual Information-based algorithm [11], and is resampled to correspond to the dimensions of the intraoperative data, a 256x256x60 matrix with voxels 0.859375x0.859375x2.5 mm^3. **Intraoperative non-rigid registration**: An active surface matching algorithm deforms the preoperative surface meshes of the brain and ventricles to the corresponding segmentations of the intraoperative target. The resulting surface displacements serve as boundary conditions to the biomechanical model, which solves for the volumetric deformation. Preoperative models and grey-scale image data are deformed according to the resulting displacement field. **Intraoperative visualization**: The combined data is visualized using 3D Slicer, which includes the optical tracking system (Figure 1). Further details on processing and data acquisition parameters are available in [5].

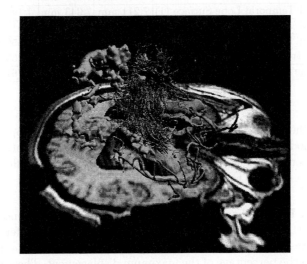

Fig. 1. Preoperative models (white matter tracts are shown in yellow, blood vessels in red, tumor in green, ventricles in blue, and fMRI activation in aqua) deformed according to the FEM calculations and superimposed on an intraoperative axial slice.

3 Registration Results

For the three surgical cases in which DT-MRI data was acquired, the volumetric deformation was applied using both the isotropic and anisotropic linear elastic models given the same initial surface displacement boundary conditions. The default values for the Young's modulus were defined consistently with the previous work ($E = 3000Pa$ for the brain and $E = 1000Pa$ for the ventricles) on the isotropic FEM [2]. Poisson's ratio was set to be 0.35 because that was the closest setting to the previous value of 0.45 that would yield a solution that satified the boundary conditions. The optimal maximum stiffness ratio (α) is 10 using these parameters.

Landmark Displacement Error. Accuracy was evaluated given a set of landmarks indentified by a neurosurgeon in both the preoperative and intraoperative image for one surgical case. These landmarks include the medial tumor margin, 3 points on the lateral temporal lobe surface, and the optic tract. We compared the registration errors of both the isotropic and anisotropic models, as well as the original rigid registration (Table 1). These displacement errors are all very

Table 1. Comparison of error in landmark displacement for rigid registration, the isotropic model, and the isotropic model for one surgical case.

Landmark Location	Rigid Reg.	Isotropic	Anisotropic
Medial Tumor Margin	1.000 mm	0.357 mm	0.357 mm
Lateral Temporal Lobe Surface (1)	7.211 mm	7.343 mm	7.143 mm
Lateral Temporal Lobe Surface (2)	2.236 mm	1.510 mm	1.512 mm
Lateral Temporal Lobe Surface (3)	2.236 mm	2.584 mm	2.559 mm
Optic Tract	2.236 mm	2.236 mm	2.236 mm
Average Error	2.984 mm	2.806 mm	2.761 mm

similar, and there is a limited number of landmarks, but it appears that the anisotropic model does show a minimal amount of improvement. However, to better characterize how the isotropic and anisotropic models differ throughout the volume, we consider the entire deformation fields in the next section.

Deformation Fields. For a quantitative analysis of the differences in the deformation fields, Table 2 shows the maximum displacement difference in each of the three axes, the maximum displacement difference, the mean displacement difference, and the percentage of the maximum displacement. There is a substantial difference in the deformations relative to the displacement when anisotropy is included in the model. The greatest differences in the deformation fields tend to occur in regions of high anisotropy. Though this does not directly show an improvement in accuracy, it does show that including anisotropy does change the registration result.

Table 2. Differences in deformation fields between the anisotropic and isotropic models, over each of the three surgical cases.

	dx_{max}	dy_{max}	dz_{max}	D_{max}	D_{mean}	$D_\%$
Case 1	1.06 mm	1.30 mm	2.60 mm	2.92 mm	0.174 mm	22.6%
Case 2	0.36 mm	0.56 mm	1.14 mm	1.14 mm	0.141 mm	10.7%
Case 3	0.51 mm	0.54 mm	2.08 mm	2.08 mm	0.152 mm	24.5%

3.1 Computation Time Analysis

The time constraints of a neurosurgical procedure require consideration of the additional computation time required to assemble and solve the more complex model. For the purpose of this experiment, we focus only on the assembly and solution time because the additional time required (approximately 9 minutes) for segmentation, rigid registration, applying deformation fields, etc. are unchanged from [10].

Two major factors determine the time required for the Finite Element model. The first is the size and connectivity of the mesh (see [2] for meshing details), which affects both the isotropic and anisotropic computation times. The second is the amount of DT-MRI data available for the mesh. Table 3 shows that in general, the anisotropic model requires about twice as long as the isotropic one to be assembled and solved. However, this only increases the total time required, including pre-processing, assembling and solving the FEM, and revisualizing the data in Slicer, from 12 minutes to 14 minutes, which is still very reasonable, especially considering the rapid increases in computational power.

Table 3. Computation time comparison between anisotropic and isotropic models.

	Isotropic Model	Anisotropic Model	DTI Dataset Size
Case 1	65.6 sec	118.1 sec	256x256x6
Case 2	87.7 sec	175.1 sec	256x256x18
Case 3	97.9 sec	188.3 sec	256x256x19

4 Discussion and Conclusion

We demonstrated that that a biomechanical model of anisotropic white matter elasticity enabled improved localization of white matter tracts during surgical resection. We used a set of landmarks identified by a neurosurgeon to evaluate the relative accuracy of the new model, which showed slight improvement with the anisotropic model. To account for displacement differences that occurred where there were no landmarks identified, we compared the deformation fields directly.

The differences in displacement was between 1 and 3 mm for each surgical case, which is up to nearly 25% of the total maximum displacement due to brain shift. For future surgical cases with greater amounts of brain shift, we expect that the improvement in registration accuracy will be more substantial. Finally, we showed that the computation time required for the anisotropic model was approximately twice that of that of the isotropic model, but still on the order of about three minutes, adequate for near real-time use.

Acknowledgements. This investigation was supported by a research grant from the Whitaker Foundation, by NIH grants R21 MH67054, R01 LM007861, P41 RR13218 and P01 CA67165, and by the NSF ERC grant (JHU Agreement #8810-274).

References

1. C. Davatzikos. Spatial transformation and registration of brain images using elastically deformable models. *Computer Vision and Image Understanding*, 66(2):207–222, 1997.
2. M. Ferrant. *Physics-based deformable modeling of volumes and surfaces for medical image registration, segmentation and visualization*. PhD thesis, Université Catholique de Louvain, April 2001.
3. D. T. Gering, A. Nabavi, R. Kikinis, N.. Hata, L. J. O'Donnell, W. E. Grimson, F. A. Jolesz, P. McL. Black, and W. M. Wells III. An integrated visualization system for surgical planning and guidance using image fusion and an open mr. *Journal of Magnetic Resonance Imaging*, 13:967–975, 2001.
4. A. Hagemann, K. Rohr, H. S. Stiehl, U. Spetzger, and J. M. Gilsbach. Biomechanical modeling of the human head for physically based, nonrigid image registration. *IEEE Transactions on Medical Imaging*, 18(10):875–884, October 1999.
5. C. A. Kemper. Incorporation of diffusion tensor mri in non-rigid registration for image-guided neurosurgery. Master's thesis, Massachusetts Institute of Technology, June 2003.
6. M. I. Miga, K. D. Paulsen, J. M. Lemery, S. D. Eisner, A. Hartov, F. E. Kennedy, and D. W. Roberts. Model-updated image guidance: Initial clinical experiences with gravity-induced brain deformation. *IEEE Transactions on Medical Imaging*, 18(10):866–874, October 1999.
7. K. Miller and K. Chinzei. Mechanical properties of brain tissue in tension. *Journal of Biomechanics*, 35:483–490, 2002.
8. M. T. Prange and S. S. Margulies. Regional, directional, and age-dependent properties of the brain undergoing large deformation. *Transactions of the ASME*, 124:244–252, April 2002.
9. J. S. Shimony, R. C. McKinstry, E. Akbudak, J. A. Aronovitz, A. Z. Snyder, N. F. Lori, T. S. Cull, and T. E. Conturo. Quantitative diffusion tensor anisotropy brain mr imaging: normative human data and anatomic analysis. *Radiology*, 212:770–784, 1999.
10. A. Tei. Multi-modality image fusion by real-time tracking of volumetric brain deformation during image guided neurosurgery. Master's thesis, Massachusetts Institute of Technology, February 2002.

11. W. M. Wells, P. Viola, H. Atsumi, S. Nakajima, and R. Kikinis. Multi-modal volume registration by maximization of mutual information. *Medical Image Analysis*, pages 35–51, March 1996.

12. J. D. West, K. D. Paulsen, S. Inati, F. Kennedy, A. Hartov, and D. W. Roberts. Incorporation of diffusion tensor anisotropy in brain deformation models for updating preoperative images to improve image-guidance. In *International Symposium on Biomedical Imaging*, pages 509–512, 2002.

13. O. C. Zienkewickz and R. L. Taylor. *The Finite Element Method*, volume 1. McGraw-Hill Book Company, 4 edition, 1987.

Estimating Mechanical Brain Tissue Properties with Simulation and Registration

Grzegorz Soza[1], Roberto Grosso[1], Christopher Nimsky[2], Guenther Greiner[1], and Peter Hastreiter[1,2]

[1] Computer Graphics Group, University of Erlangen-Nuremberg,
Am Weichselgarten 9, 91058 Erlangen, Germany
soza@cs.fau.de
[2] Neurocenter, Department of Neurosurgery, University of Erlangen-Nuremberg

Abstract. In this work a new method for the determination of the mechanical properties of brain tissue is introduced. Young's modulus E and Poisson's ratio ν are iteratively estimated based on a finite element model for brain shift and on the information contained in pre- and intraoperative MR data after registration. In each iteration, a 3D dataset is generated according to the displacement vector field resulting from a numerical simulation of the intraoperative brain deformation. This reconstruction is parametrized by elastic moduli of tissue. They are automatically varied in order to achieve the best correspondence between the grey value distribution in the reconstructed image and the intensity entropy in the MR image of the brain undergoing deformation. This work contributes to the difficult problem of defining correct mechanical parameters to perform reliable model calculations of brain deformation. Proper boundary conditions that are crucial in this context are also addressed.

1 Introduction

Computer assisted systems for medical diagnosis, surgery training and therapy require precise computational methods for modeling the deformation of soft tissue. Within the context of neurosurgery, brain shift has been described with various physical and mathematical models. However, even sophisticated algorithms are limited without precise information about the elastic tissue parameters.

Miller *et al.* validated the mechanical properties of swine brain tissue obtained *in vitro* in a series of experiments *in vivo* [9]. Simulated forces were 31% lower than those recorded in experiments, which can be, among others, attributed to the fact that the mechanical properties of deceased tissue are different from those of the tissue *in vivo*.

Biomechanical characterization of living soft tissues has been a subject of intensive investigations in recent years. Different diagnostic imaging modalities have been applied in numerous experiments in order to measure the response of the tissue to various types of loadings. In this context, mainly magnetic resonance imaging (MRI) and ultrasound (US) have been investigated.

Tissue elasticity imaging methods based on US can be divided into two main groups. US waves are considered for detecting internal tissue motion resulting

C. Barillot, D.R. Haynor, and P. Hellier (Eds.): MICCAI 2004, LNCS 3217, pp. 276–283, 2004.

from a static mechanical stimulus [4] (here *in vitro*). Other researchers applied US to observe the behavior of tissue under a low-frequency vibration [12]. MRI has been applied, among others, in investigations of the shear modulus of the brain *in vivo* [5]. A very comprehensive survey of similar works discussing methods for measuring tissue stiffness is given in [10]. Low availability and difficulties with the integration in clinical practice are, however, the main disadvantages of such elasticity imaging techniques.

At the same time, there have been investigations focusing on the implicit estimation of the mechanical properties of the tissue. Various relations between Lamé constants which were reported in the literature for human brain tissue were presented in [1]. The influence of different tissue elasticity values on the accuracy of the simulation was investigated in a comparative study of biomechanical breast models [16]. Also, within the context of mammography, regional measures of image similarity were used by Miga *et al.* in a function minimization framework to reconstruct elasticity images of tissue stiffness [6]. In that work Young's moduli were analyzed for 2D cross sectional MR slice of breast tissue.

However, it is crucial for the simulation to incorporate both, Young's modulus E and Poisson's ratio ν in the reconstructed mechanical properties of tissue since their combination is very important for the behavior of the simulation model. The presented method accounts for this issue and calculates both elastic moduli based on registering the result of a biomechanical simulation and corresponding intraoperative MR data. Furthermore, the approach has been applied for the first time to a 3D brain deformation model.

2   Method

2.1   Model for Parameter Estimation

The model for the automatic determination of the Young's modulus E and the Poisson's ratio ν for the brain tissue is based on an iterative process where a biomechanical model of brain shift interacts with the information extracted from MRI head data acquired before and during craniotomy. In each iteration, a volumetric dataset is reconstructed according to the displacement vector field obtained as a result of the numerical simulation of the intraoperative brain deformation (see Section 2.3). This reconstruction is parametrized by the elastic moduli of tissue E and ν. The main idea of the presented approach for the estimation of the mechanical properties of the brain tissue is to vary these parameters in such a way that the correspondence between the reconstructed volume and the intraoperative dataset is maximized.

The basis for this is the normalized mutual information (NMI) [15] which relates the grey value distributions in both datasets in terms of entropy. We expressed this measure as a function of the elastic moduli E and ν which are free parameters in the optimization procedure. The similarity function denoted by $\mathbf{S_{sim,intra}}$ is formulated as

$$\mathbf{S_{sim,intra}}(E,\nu) = NMI_{sim,intra}(E,\nu) + \alpha_0 < E_{low}, E_{high} > (E) +$$
$$\alpha_1 < \nu_{low}, \nu_{high} > (\nu) , \tag{1}$$

with α_0 representing a penalty term which is defined by

$$\alpha_0 < E_{low}, E_{high} > (E) = \begin{cases} c_0 & : & E \notin < E_{low}, E_{high} > , c_0 \leq 0 \\ 0 & : & E \in < E_{low}, E_{high} > \end{cases} . \tag{2}$$

The search space for E can be constrained by setting the upper and low limits E_{high} and E_{low} and specifying the penalty constant c_0. Thus, expertise about the reasonable interval for this elasticity parameter is incorporated into the optimization process. This reduces the number of iterations required for the determination of the optimal values for E. The same considerations hold for α_1 and ν. Note, that this restriction term can be skipped by setting $c_0 = 0$, thus allowing the optimization in the whole parameter space.

2.2   Numerical Model

During optimization, the similarity between the intraoperative MRI and the volume resulting from the physically-based simulation is computed in each iteration. Generally, the underlying mathematical model of the soft tissue deformation can be chosen arbitrarily. For this purpose, in this work we considered a simplified set of equations describing the behavior of poroelastic materials under load [13]. Thereby, the brain is assumed to be a linearly elastic medium saturated by a viscous fluid. The constitutive equations

$$-\frac{\mu}{1-2\nu}\nabla(\nabla \cdot \mathbf{u}(x,t)) - \mu\Delta\mathbf{u}(x,t) + \alpha\nabla p(x,t) = \mathbf{f}(x,t) \tag{3a}$$

$$\frac{\partial}{\partial t}(d_0 p(x,t) + \alpha\nabla \cdot \mathbf{u}(x,t)) - \nabla \cdot k\nabla p(x,t) = h(x,t) \tag{3b}$$

are coupled. This means that the compression of the solid enhances the fluid flow due to an increased pore pressure. On the other hand, an increasing pore pressure results in stress in the deformable solid matrix. In the equations (3a) and (3b), fluid pressure is referred to by $p(x,t)$ and the displacement vector by $\mathbf{u}(x,t)$. The parameter t expresses the time dependence of the system. Parameters corresponding to the elastic properties of the tissue are Poisson's ratio ν and the shear modulus μ, which is a function of E and ν. The coefficient $\alpha \geq 0$ represents the mechanical coupling of the fluid pressure and the porous solid. The amount of fluid which can be forced into the medium by a pressure increment under conservation of the volume of the medium is expressed by $d_0 \geq 0$. A measure of Darcy flow with respect to the pressure gradient is given by $k \geq 0$.

The presented system of equations is solved by using the finite element method based on the standard Galerkin discretization scheme. As a result, a displacement vector field and a vector of scalar pressure values are obtained, both defined in the nodes of the discretization domain (see Section 2.4).

2.3   Volume Reconstruction

The optimization criterion for the quality of the elasticity parameters is the normalized mutual information function between the image reconstructed from the simulation and the intraoperative dataset. For this purpose, intensities in the deformed volume have to be recalculated in each iteration of the optimization. The direct result of the numerical simulation is a vector field of displacements defined only in vertices of a tetrahedral grid in the computational domain. Therefore, all tetrahedra in the deformed grid are traversed and for each element its inner voxels are considered. The displacement of each voxel is calculated as a scalar product of its barycentric coordinates and of the displacements given in the four nodes of the tetrahedron the voxel belongs to. Finally, a new intensity value is computed by moving back the voxel after the deformation and by trilinear interpolation of the intensities in the preoperative MR volume. This back-projection technique prevents holes in the reconstructed dataset.

2.4   Geometry Generation and Boundary Conditions

Prior to any optimization iteration, the brain surface is extracted from the preoperative MR data. A tetrahedral grid bounded by this triangular surface is then generated. For the numerical stability of further computations, special algorithms are applied to ensure regularity of the grid (for details refer to [14]).

In order to reflect the intraoperative settings in the numerical model, the forces which affect the brain during surgery have to be defined. In [16], non-rigid registration of MR images acquired before and after compressing a volunteer's breast was utilized to derive image-based forces. In our model, the load vector is set according to the location of the skull opening. Since this information is included in the intraoperative dataset only, a rigid registration of the pre- and intraoperative MR scan is performed [2]. In a 3D editor supporting the fusion of the preoperative brain surface and the intraoperative MR data, the respective outer part of the generated volumetric grid is manually marked (see Figure 1). Subsequently, a separate boundary condition is set for the defined surface region.

After the boundary conditions have been set, initial guesses for the parameters E and ν are made and the optimization is started. In each iteration only one parameter is changed and the new volume resulting from the simulation is computed. The process terminates when the similarity function $S_{sim,intra}$ reaches its maximum within a given precision. For the optimization Powell's direction search method was applied [11].

3   Results

In order to assess the quality of the presented method and to determine elasticity parameters for brain tissue, computational experiments were conducted with the biomechanical model described in Section 2.2 and with pairs of T1-weighted pre- and intraoperative MR data. All scans obtained with a Siemens Magnetom

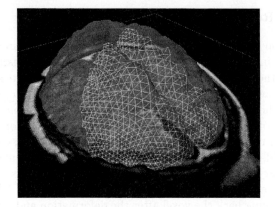

Fig. 1. The region for the boundary condition is manually marked in a 3D editor according to the location of the skull opening. The respective and defined part of the surface is visualized by displaying the underlying grid. The remaining brain surface is shown in a semitransparent representation

Sonata Maestro Class 1.5 Tesla scanner had a resolution of $512 \times 512 \times 160$ voxels and a voxel size of 0.49 mm $\times$ 0.49 mm $\times$ 1.0 mm.

In the first experiment (Experiment 1), the numerical simulation was performed on a very coarse tetrahedral grid consisting of 9952 elements. The corresponding pre- and intraoperative datasets were rigidly registered and appropriate boundary conditions were set. E and ν were initially set to 6500 Pa and 0.40, respectively, while the parameter space was restricted (see Equation (2)) to the interval $< 1300, 12000 >$ for E and to $< 0.3, 0.5 >$ for ν. The corresponding penalty constant c_0 was set to -0.2. The optimization terminated after 89 iterations (979 secs) and the maximal value of NMI was found at $\nu = 0.452$ for the Poisson's ratio and $E = 8863.01$ Pa for the Young's modulus which corresponds to the value of $\mu = 3052$ Pa for the shear modulus (compare Equation (3a)).

For the Experiment 2, a very fine grid was taken. The number of grid elements was 123496. As in the case before, a rigid registration was performed to set proper boundary conditions. The initial values of all parameters were identical to those used in Experiment 1. The optimization returned the value of $\nu = 0.461$ for the Poisson's ratio and $E = 8196.21$ Pa for the Young's modulus ($\mu = 2805$ Pa) in 121 iterations, which took 9780 secs on a 2.66 GHz PIV system. During both optimizations the precision (referring to the value of NMI) was set to 10^{-4}.

Figure 2 shows the similarity function plotted retrospectively as a projection on one of the respective maximal parameters which allows visually assessing the result of both experiments.

4   Discussion

In the experiment performed on the coarse grid one global maximum was observed (see Figure 2a). The resulting Poisson's ratio $\nu = 0.452$ is very close to

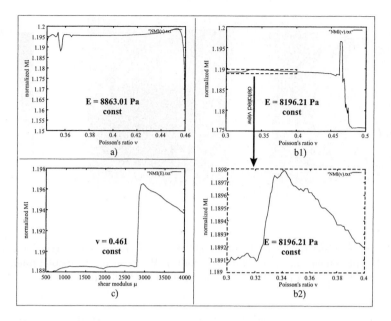

Fig. 2. Plot of the similarity function with one coordinate kept fixed: *a)* Experiment 1 (coarse grid) for $E = 8863.01$ Pa. *b1)* Experiment 2 (fine grid) for $E = 8196.21$ Pa. *b2)* Experiment 2 showing a detailed view of a local maximum in *b1)* with a differently scaled y-axis. *c)* Experiment 2, $\nu = 0.461$ (here NMI as a function of μ)

the value reported in [7] whereas the corresponding Young's modulus is about 4 times bigger. Despite of the coarse grid, the simulation showed good convergence properties, except for ν in the interval $< 0.3, 0.357 >$ (independent of the value of E). Nevertheless, the grid was too coarse to produce reliable results.

In the case of the fine grid, the computations exhibited a numerically more stable behavior. In the vicinity of $\nu = 0.5$ for the Poisson's ratio, however, some problems with the numerical convergence were observed for individual values of ν, which led to local fluctuations in the plot of NMI, see the small peaks in this region in Figure 2b1. The global optimum of $E = 8196.21$ Pa (see Figure 2c) for the Young's modulus is close to the value of $E = 7425$ Pa reported in [8] for the swine brain in an *in vivo* experiment. The corresponding value of $\nu = 0.461$ for the Poisson's ratio is close to the values found in the literature [7] and to the result of Experiment 1.

In the experiment with the fine grid there exists also a local maximum at $\nu = 0.341$ and $E = 1775.48$ Pa (see Figure 2b1 and 2b2). A similar local minimum also appeared as a small peak around the value of $\nu = 0.349$ in the first experiment with the coarser grid (see Figure 2a). Although there are other approaches where $\nu = 0.35$ is used as the elasticity parameter for the brain tissue [3], a reliable confirmation of the existence of such a local maximum requires further analysis since a bad convergence behavior of the numerical computations with our model on the coarse grid could be stated for $\nu \leq 0.357$.

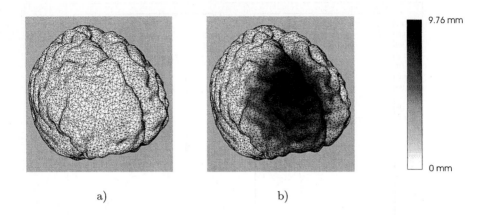

a)   b)

Fig. 3. Surface visualization of the brain *a)* before and *b)* after volumetric deformation. Cortical displacements are coded with grey values. White means no displacement, black corresponds to the maximal displacement, in this case 9.76 mm

In addition to the numerical analysis, a simulation with the use of the calculated optimal values $\nu = 0.461$ and $\mu = 2805$ Pa was performed and the visual results of the deformation are presented in Figure 3.

The mechanical properties of brain tissue obtained with the presented method contribute to a better physically-based simulation by improving the correspondence between the model and the real situation. The results obtained in the different experiments correspond very well to the values given in the literature [3,8,7]. This demonstrates the strength of the proposed strategy and shows that it is a promising alternative to other approaches where the mechanical properties of tissue are directly measured. Moreover, this technique has the advantage that the validation of the results is inherent.

5   Conclusion

A novel approach is presented that uses techniques of numerical simulation and registration for the determination of the mechanical properties of brain tissue. The conducted experiments proved the value of the method and the results correspond very well to the physical parameters in the literature. Thereby, our strategy contributes to solve the difficult problem of estimating the elasticity properties of living tissue. In the future, a statistical analysis will be conducted in order to analyze the obtained parameters.

Acknowledgments. This work was funded by Deutsche Forschungsgemeinschaft in the context of the projects Gr 796/2-1 – 796/2-3. We gratefully acknowledge Stefan Zachow (Zuse Institut Berlin) for his cooperation in the area of grid generation.

References

1. A. Hagemann, K. Rohr, H.S. Stiehl, U. Spetzger, and J.M. Gilsbach. Biomechanical Modeling of the Human Head for Physically Based, Non-Rigid Image Registration. *IEEE Trans Med Imaging*, 18(10):875–884, 1999.
2. P. Hastreiter and T. Ertl. Integrated Registration and Visualization of Medical Image Data. In *Proc. CGI*, pages 78–85, Hannover, Germany, 1998.
3. M. Kaczmarek, R.P. Subramanian, and S. R. Neff. The Hydromechanics of Hydrocephalus: Steady-State Solutions for Cylindrical Geometry. *Bull Math Biol*, 59:295–323, 1997.
4. T.A. Krouskop, T.M.Wheeler, F. Kallel, B. Garra, and T. Hall. The Elastic Moduli of Breast and Prostate Tissues Under Compression. *Ultrason Imaging*, 20:151–159, 1998.
5. A. Manduca, D. S. Lake, S. A. Kruse, and R. L. Ehman. Spatio-temporal Directional Filtering for Improved Inversion of MR Elastography Images. *Med Image Anal*, 7(4):465–473, 2003.
6. M. Miga. A New Approach to Elastography Using Mutual Information and Finite Elements. *Phys Med Biol*, 48:467–480, 2003.
7. M. Miga, K. Paulsen, P. Hoopes, F. Kennedy, and A. Hartov. In Vivo Modeling of Intersitial Pressure in the Brain under Surgical Load Using Finite Elements. *J. Biomech. Eng.*, 122:354–363, 2000.
8. K. Miller and K. Chinzei. Simple Validation of Biomechanical Models of Brain Tissue. In *Proc. European Society of Biomechanics Conference*, volume 31, page 104. Elsevier Science, 1998.
9. K. Miller, K. Chinzei, G. Orssengo, and P. Bednarz. Mechanical Properties of Brain Tissue In-vivo: Experiment and Computer Simulation. *J. Biomechanics*, 33(11):1369–1376, 2000.
10. J. Ophir, F. Kallel, T. Varghese, E. Konofagou, S. K. Alam, T. Krouskop, B. garra, and R. Righetti. Elastography. *Comptes Rendus de l'Acadmie des Sciences - Series IV - Physics*, 2(8):1193–1212, 2002.
11. W. H. Press, S. A. Teukolsky, W. T. Vetterling, and B. P. Flannery. *Numerical Recipes in C++*. Cambridge University, New York, 2002.
12. L. Sandrin, M. Tanter, S. Catheline, and M. Fink. Shear Modulus Imaging with 2-D Transient Elastography. *IEEE Trans Ultrason Ferroelectr Freq Control*, 49(4):426–435, 2002.
13. R. E. Showalter. Diffusion in Poro-Elastic Media. *J Math Anal Appl*, 251:310–340, 2000.
14. G. Soza, R. Grosso, P. Hastreiter, U. Labsik, Ch. Nimsky, R. Fahlbusch, and G. Greiner. Fast and Adaptive Finite Element Approach for Modeling Brain Shift. In *Proc CURAC (Dt. Gesell. Computer and Robotorassistierte Chirurgie)*, 2003.
15. C. Studholme, D. L. G. Hill, and D. J. Hawkes. An Overlap Invariant Entropy Measure of 3D Medical Image Alignment. *Pattern Recogn*, 32(1):71–86, 1999.
16. C. Tanner, A. Degenhard, J. A. Schnabel, C. Hayes, L. I. Sonoda, M. O. Leach, D. R. Hose, D. L. G. Hill, and D. J. Hawkes. A Comparison of Biomechanical Breast Models: a Case Study. In *Proc. SPIE Medical Imaging 2002*, volume 4683, pages 1807–1818, 2002.

Dynamic Measurements of Soft Tissue Viscoelastic Properties with a Torsional Resonator Device

Davide Valtorta and Edoardo Mazza

Institute of Mechanical Systems, ETH Zurich, 8092 Zurich, Switzerland,
`valtorta@imes.mavt.ethz.ch`

Abstract. A new method for measuring the mechanical properties of soft biological tissues is presented. Dynamic testing is performed by using a torsional resonator, whose free extremity is in contact with a material sample. An analytical model of a semi-infinite, homogenous, isotropic medium is used to model the shear wave propagation in the material sample and allows determining the complex shear modulus of the soft tissue. By controlling the vibration amplitude, shear strains of less than 0.2% are induced in the tissue so that the material response can be assumed to be linear viscoelastic. Experiments are performed at different eigenfrequencies of the torsional oscillator and the complex shear modulus is characterized in the range 1-10 kHz. First in vitro experiments on bovine liver confirmed the sensitivity of the proposed technique. The experiment does not damage the soft tissue and allows a fast and local measurement, these being prerequisites for future applications in-vivo during open surgery.

1 Introduction

Measurement of the mechanical properties of biological tissues is required for medical applications, such as diagnostics, surgery simulation and planning [1]. The characterization of the soft tissue mechanical response contributes to a great extent to the reliability of any simulation of organ deformations. Different approaches can be used in testing biosolids, mainly divided in destructive and nondestructive techniques. Destructive testing utilizes material samples extracted from the organ and experiments are performed according to standard methods of material characterization such as tensile tests [2] or compression tests[3]. Non destructive techniques present the great advantage of a possible direct application in-vivo, during open surgery, eliminating the uncertainties due to the alterations of the material in-vitro. Techniques based on tissue indentation are used in in-vivo tests [4,5], the control of the boundary conditions being the major obstacle in data analysis for quantitative evaluations. The aspiration experiment originally developed by Vuskovic [6] provides well defined kinematic and kinetic boundary conditions and allows accurate fitting of material parameters. Application of this quasi static test on soft human organs [7] provided quantitative

C. Barillot, D.R. Haynor, and P. Hellier (Eds.): MICCAI 2004, LNCS 3217, pp. 284–292, 2004.

sets of material parameters for use in large deformation calculations with "slow" deformations.

Testing the materials at high deformation rates provides additional information on the constitutive behavior of the tissue, with applications in diagnostics and trauma research [3]. Dynamic methods for testing soft biological materials range from standard rheometers operating at 0.01 to 10 Hz [8], to devices suitable for modelling the behavior at loading rates up to 350 Hz [9]. Rotary shear tests have been proposed for in-vivo tests by Kalanovic et al. [10] for the low frequency range (up to 20 Hz).

A new non-destructive method for dynamic testing of soft tissues is presented in this paper and is used in our laboratory in order to complement the quasi-static tissue characterization obtained from the aspiration experiments [11]. With the new technique the mechanical properties are derived from the material response to harmonic shear in the linear viscoelasticity range at high frequencies (1-10 kHz). The material is in contact with the free end of a torsional resonator and influences the dynamic behavior of the resonator. The use of a phase locked loop technique provides a high sensitivity to the device. The measurement is fast and, due to the small contact area, a local characterization is achieved. Adherence of soft tissue and torsional oscillator is ensured by vacuum clamping. The soft tissue is modelled analytically as a semi-infinite, homogenous, isotropic medium; a suitable kinematic boundary condition is applied in correspondence of the contact with the resonator. The analytical model consists of a torsional radiating source on a semi infinite space [12,13,14] and is used to extract the material parameters. A mapping procedure and reference tables enable real-time parameter extraction. The results obtained in vitro on bovine liver are reported and discussed, showing the sensitivity and the repeatability of the measurements.

2   Dynamic Torsion Test

2.1   Experimental Details

The Torsional Resonator Device (TRD) is depicted in figure 1. It consists of a rod with circular cross section, excited around the first five torsional eigenfrequencies (in the range of 1-10 kHz) by two electromagnetic transducers, which represent the actuator and the sensor. When the free end of the resonator is in contact with a soft tissues, changes occur in the dynamic properties of the vibrating system. Two parameters, characterizing the dynamic behavior of the system, can be measured: the resonance frequency f_{res}, and the quality factor Q, a measure of damping. Figure 2 shows the typical transfer function of the system, vibrating at resonance during a calibration (without soft tissue contact) and a measurement run (with contact). The damping characteristics and the resonance frequency are inferred from the control variables of a phase stabilization loop, using a technique already employed in viscosimetry [15]. With this method, the measurement can be performed in short time: typically 20 seconds are necessary

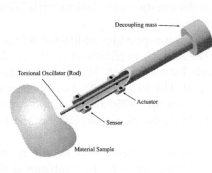

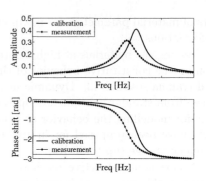

Fig. 1. Torsional Resonator Device (*TRD*)

Fig. 2. Transfer functions of the vibrating system

to analyze each resonance frequency, obtaining the corresponding values of Q and Δf_{res} from the control electronics.

The area of contact with the material sample at the lower extremity of the resonator has a radius $R = 2.55mm$. Despite the small contact area, significant changes occur in the dynamic characteristics of the system, as demonstrated in section 3. It is of course important to prevent sliding between the resonator and the soft tissue sample, since perfect adherence will be assumed in the analytical model for parameter extraction. For this reason, a disc with micro-openings, shown in figure 3, is bonded at the extremity of the resonator. The resonator consists of a tube with controllable internal pressure. By evacuating the internal volume of the tube, adherence between resonator and soft tissues is obtained by vacuum clamping. The small dimensions of the disc openings (width= $30\mu m$, figure 3) and the pressure applied in the tube (0.2*bar* absolute pressure) ensure that no damage occurs in the tissue. The vibration amplitude of the resonator is small so that the material response can be assumed to be linear viscoelastic. To this end the maximum rotation amplitude is kept below 0.001*rad*, therefore limiting the shear strains to $\gamma_{max} = 0.2\%$, for the materials and range of frequencies considered here.

A typical experimental procedure with TRD consists of the following steps: (i) a calibration run is performed; (ii) the resonator is put in contact with the material sample, and the internal pressure of the tube is decreased; (iii) once the contact condition is ensured, the measurement run is performed. The whole procedure takes approximately 20 seconds, and is repeated for the first five torsional eigenfrequencies of the resonator. At the characteristic frequencies of these experiments, the observation time leads to several thousands oscillations periods, so that a steady harmonic response state is reached in the system.

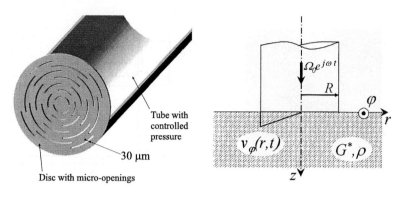

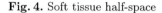

Fig. 3. View of the contact surface   **Fig. 4.** Soft tissue half-space

2.2   Tissue Modelling and Parameter Extraction

An analytical model is applied to determine quantitatively the mechanical parameters of the soft biological tissue. The soft tissue is considered to be homogeneous and isotropic. This assumption is justified for "bulky" soft organs with no or limited reinforcement by muscular fibers, such as liver and kidney.

With reference to figure 4, the tissue is modelled as a semi-infinite viscoelastic space. A cylindrical coordinate system (r, φ, z) is used. The torsional resonator touches the tissue surface, vibrates around the z-axis and excites shear waves with displacement in the r-φ plane (SH-waves) in the tissue. Linear viscoelasticity is employed to describe the tissue behavior in shear deformation:

$$\tau(t) = \left(G(0) + \int_0^\infty e^{-j\omega s} \dot{G}(s) ds \right) \cdot \gamma(t) = G^* \gamma(t) \tag{1}$$

$$\gamma(t) = \gamma_0 e^{j\omega t} \tag{2}$$

$$G^* = G_1 + jG_2 \tag{3}$$

where $\tau(t)$ and $\gamma(t)$ represent the shear stress and strains, respectively, and G^* is the complex shear modulus of the material, with the real and imaginary components G_1 and G_2, called respectively storage and loss shear modulus. Due to the kinematic boundary condition at the tissue surface, the displacement vector in the half space can be described as in equation 4, thus reducing to the azimuthal component u_φ only:

$$\bar{u} = u_r \hat{r} + u_\varphi \hat{\varphi} + u_z \hat{z} = u_\varphi \hat{\varphi} = u_\varphi(r, z, t)\hat{\varphi} \qquad u_r = u_z = 0 \tag{4}$$

$$\frac{\partial^2 u_\varphi}{\partial z^2} + \frac{\partial}{\partial r}\left[\frac{1}{r}\frac{\partial(r u_\varphi)}{\partial r} \right] + \frac{\omega^2}{c_{SH}^2} u_\varphi = 0 \qquad c_{SH}^2 = \frac{G^*}{\rho} \tag{5}$$

The equations of linear momentum and the kinematical relations reduce here to the SH-wave equation in a viscoelastic half-space, equation 5, where c_{SH}

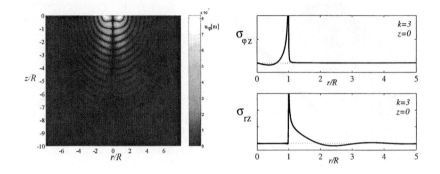

Fig. 5. Example of wave propagation pattern: amplitude of u_φ

Fig. 6. Stresses at $z = 0$

identifies the shear wave speed in the material of density ρ. Considering perfect adherence at the contact location, the boundary conditions are:

$$u_\varphi|_{z=0} = \theta_0 r e^{j\omega t} \qquad \text{for } 0 < r \leq R \qquad (6)$$

$$\tau_{\varphi z}|_{z=0} = 0 \qquad \text{for } r > R \qquad (7)$$

where R is the radius of the contact area. The solution of the boundary value problem with mixed (kinematic and kinetic) boundary conditions of a radiating torsional source, known as Reissner-Sagoci problem [12,13], was derived by Dorn [14], using Hankel Transform methods. The torsional radiation pattern and the torsional mechanical impedance of the medium can be determined for given values of the material parameters G_1 and G_2 for each excitation frequency. In figure 5, an example of the radiation pattern generated by a torsional vibrating source is shown. Colors indicate the amplitude of the azimuthal displacement. The radiation pattern depends on the complex shear modulus $G^*[Pa]$, the exciting angular frequency $\omega[rad/sec]$ and the radius of the contact area $R[m]$, which define a dimensionless wave number k in equation 8.

$$k = \frac{\omega}{\sqrt{G^*/\rho}} R \qquad (8)$$

This number characterizes the wave propagation pattern. For soft tissues and relatively high frequencies, k assumes values higher than 3, leading to waves propagating mainly in z-directions, toward the tissue interior. Typically displacements, for the viscoelastic properties of biological tissues, have negligible amplitude outside a layer of 3 to 4 times the oscillator diameter $2R$, as shown in figure 5. Figure 6 shows the components σ_{rz} and $\sigma_{\varphi z}$ of the stress vector at the tissue surface ($z = 0$). Vacuum clamping, described in section 2.1, ensures that adherence is fulfilled also for $r \rightarrow R$, where large shear stresses $\sigma_{\varphi z}$ occur. By solving the analytical problem described in equations (5), (6) and (7), the torque exerted by the soft tissue on the resonator can be expressed as a function

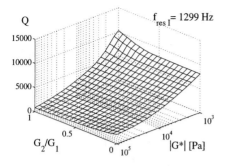
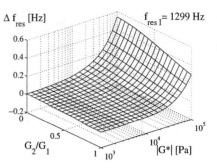

Fig. 7. Quality factor in function of G^*

Fig. 8. Resonance frequency shift in function of G^*

of the material parameters. In this way the changes in the dynamic behavior of the resonator, i.e. the increase in damping and the resonance frequency shift, can be linked to the mechanical properties of the tissue.

The combination of the model of the resonator and the model of a viscoelastic half-space described in section 2.2 leads to the identification of the influence of the material parameters G_1, G_2 and ρ on the system's transfer function. The measured parameters Q and Δf_{res} (Q factor and resonance frequency shift) can be directly correlated to the tissue properties, as shown in figure 7 and 8 for the first resonance frequency. This mapping process allows obtaining an almost real-time measurement of the mechanical properties of soft tissues.

3   Experimental Results and Discussion

The TRD technique was applied for dynamic testing of bovine liver ex-vivo. The main purpose of these experiments was to evaluate the reliability of the TRD measurements. Adult bovine liver samples, obtained from the local abattoir, were tested at ambient temperature. Figure 9 shows the repeatability of the measurements in terms of Q and f_{res}. The first torsional eigenfrequency (1299 Hz) was considered in this analysis. A series of measurements was performed on the same organ at different locations identified by the letters A, B, C, D, E, and F. Three independent measurements have been performed within short time intervals at each location. The repeatability is within 20% and 10% for Q and Δf_{res} respectively, for the measurements at the same location. The variability of the material properties within one single organ is indicated by the comparison of the measurements at different locations and is in line with findings from other studies [3,7]. Figure 10 shows the time evolution of the measurements performed at one single location. The TRD technique is capable of detecting tissue alterations due to dehydration and oxidation, with high sensitivity.

Experiments with bovine liver were performed at different eigenfrequencies of the resonator, in order to show the frequency dependence of the material be-

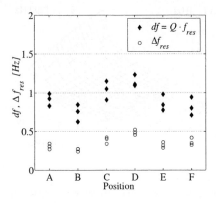

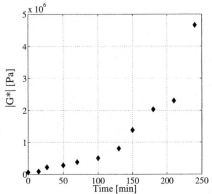

Fig. 9. Repeatability of the measurements on bovine liver capsula

Fig. 10. Time evolution of $|G^*|$ on bovine liver capsula

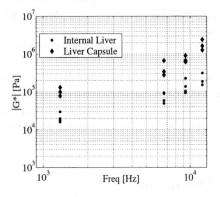

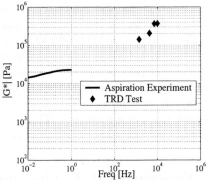

Fig. 11. Frequency dependence of the shear modulus $|G^*|$

Fig. 12. Results from quasi-static experiments [7] and TRD tests

havior. Measurements were taken at one single location. Results are reported for the first, the third, the fourth and the fifth eigenfrequencies. The resulting values of the shear modulus amplitude $|G^*|$ are shown in figure 11, which includes for comparison the results obtained from measurements at the external surface of the liver (contact with the capsule) and at an internal section of liver. Different material responses are obtained from external and internal measurements, acting the capsule as a stiffening membrane. These data show that the shear modulus increases at higher frequencies. The combination of the quasi-static aspiration test [7] and the TRD test yields a characterization of the material response over a wide range of frequencies. Figure 12 shows the results of quasi-static and dynamic experiments on the same bovine liver: in contrast with other studies [2], a significant frequency dependence of $|G^*|$ is demonstrated by these measurements.

4   Conclusions

A new technique has been proposed for dynamic testing of soft biological tissues. The procedure for viscoelastic material properties measurement is fast (results for one frequency are obtained in approximately 20 seconds) and local (a tissue volume of approximately $100mm^3$ is tested). An analytical model allows determining the complex shear modulus of the tissue from the experimental data. Tests on bovine liver have shown the repeatability ($\pm10\%$ and $\pm5\%$ for the target parameters Q and f_{res}) of the experimental technique. The TRD measurements are sensitive enough to detect the influence of the capsule in the mechanical response of the liver as well as the changes in material properties due to dehydration and oxidation. Experiments are ongoing for validation of the reliability of the material properties measurements with TRD: for this purpose, silicone phantoms are used, whose viscoelastic properties are determined with independent wave propagation experiments.

Acknowledgments. This work was supported by the Swiss NSF project Computer Aided and Image Guided Medical Interventions (NCCR CO-ME).

References

1. Szekely, G., Brechbüler, Ch., Hutter, R., Rhomberg, A., Schmidt, P. : Modelling of soft tissue deformation for laparoscopic surgery simulation, medical image computing and computer-assisted intervention. MICCAI '98 Proc. (1998) 550-561
2. Fung, Y. C. : Elasticity of soft tissues in simple elongation. Am. J. Physiol. **213** (1967) 1532
3. Snedeker, J.G., Bar-Bezat, M., Niederer, P.,Schmidlin, F.R., Farshad, M. : Failure behavior of the kidney; quasi-static comparison with human tissue, impact tests on porcine organs, and comparison with a human kidney finite element model, submitted to Journal of Biomechanics (2004)
4. Miller, K., Chinzei, K., Orssengo, G., Bednarz, P. : Mechanical properties of brain tissue in vivo: experiment and computer simulation. J. of Biomech. **33/11** (2000) 1369-1376
5. Ottensmeyer, M.P. and Salisbury, J.K. Jr. : In Vivo Data Acquisition Instrument For Solid Organ Mechanical Property Measurement. MICCAI 2001 Proc. (2001) 975-982
6. Vuskovic, V. : Device for in-vivo measurement of mechanical properties of internal human soft tissues. Diss., ETH No. 14222 (2001)
7. Nava, A. and Mazza, E. : Determination of the mechanical properties of soft human tissues through aspiration experiments. MICCAI 2003 Proc. (2003)
8. Nasseri, S., Bilston, L.E. , Phan-Thien, N.: Viscoelastic properties of pig kidney in shear, experimental results and modeling. Rheol Acta **41** (2002) 180-192

9. Arbogast, K.B., Thibaut, K.L., Scott Pinheiro, B., Winey, K.I.: A high frequency shear device for testing soft biological tissues. J. Biomechanics **30/7** (1997) 757-759

10. Kalanovic D., Ottensmeyer M. P., Gross J., Gerhardt B., Dawson Sl.: Independent testing of Soft tissue viscoelasticity using indention and rotary shear deformation. Medicine Meets Virtual Reality IOS Press (2003) 137-143

11. Nava, A., Valtorta, D., Mazza, E.: Experimental determination of the mechanical properties of soft biological tissues. Proc. 9th Intl. Conf. on the Mechanical Behaviour of Materials, Geneva, Switzerland (2003).

12. Sagoci, H.F.: Forced torsional oscillations of an elastic half-space II. J. of Appl. Phys. **15** (1944) 655-662

13. Robertson, I.A.: On a proposed determination of the shear modulus of an isotropic elastic half-space by forced torsional oscillations of a circular disc. Appl.Sci.Res. **17** (1967) 305-312

14. Dorn, G.A.: Radiation impedance and radiation patterns of torsionally vibrating seismic sources: Ph.D. thesis, Univ. of California, Berkeley (1980)

15. Sayir, M., Goodbread, J., Häusler, K., Dual, J.: Method and device for measuring the characteristics of an oscillating system. Pat. Corp. Treat. PCT/EP95/00761 (1995)

Simultaneous Topology and Stiffness Identification for Mass-Spring Models Based on FEM Reference Deformations

Gérald Bianchi, Barbara Solenthaler, Gábor Székely, and Matthias Harders

Swiss Federal Institute of Technology
Computer Vision Laboratory
ETH Zentrum, CH-8092 Zürich, Switzerland

{bianchi,szekely,mharders}@vision.ee.ethz.ch

Abstract. Mass-spring systems are of special interest for soft tissue modeling in surgical simulation due to their ease of implementation and real-time behavior. However, the parameter identification (masses, spring constants, mesh topology) still remains a challenge. In previous work, we proposed an approach based on the training of mass-spring systems according to known reference models. Our initial focus was the determination of mesh topology in 2D. In this paper, we extend the method to 3D. Furthermore, we introduce a new approach to simultaneously identify mesh topology and spring stiffness values. Linear elastic FEM deformation computations are used as reference. Additionally, our results show that uniform distributions of spring stiffness constants fails to simulate linear elastic deformations.

1 Introduction

Real-time simulation of soft tissue deformation remains a major obstacle when developing surgical simulator systems. One popular approach is based on the mass-spring model (MSM), which consists of a mesh of mass points connected by elastic links. The method requires the setting of system parameters describing deformation behavior. Parameters, such as mass distribution, coefficients of spring transfer functions and overall connectivity have to be determined. In [1], we have suggested an approach based on genetic optimization for the identification of MSM parameters. Our initial focus has been on mesh topology. The main idea is to compare the deformation behavior of a learning model with that of a known reference system and to utilize genetic algorithms to optimize the parameters of the learning model.

In this paper, we first present the extension of our previously described approach to 3D. Then, we introduce a new approach, which merges topology and spring constant parameter estimation. We show the validity of this method by the successful recovery of the topology of a reference MSM. Next, we introduce Finite Element Models (FEM) as the reference model and obtain MSM parameters describing FEM deformation behavior. Several experiments support the

C. Barillot, D.R. Haynor, and P. Hellier (Eds.): MICCAI 2004, LNCS 3217, pp. 293–301, 2004.

validity of the acquired parameters. Finally we show, that linear elastic material cannot be approximated with homogeneous MSM parameters, but requires inhomogeneous parameter distributions.

2   Previous Work

The last ten years have seen a growing interest in research on the stiffness value identification of mass-spring systems. Two main approaches have been proposed so far. The first one focuses on the determination of mathematical relationships in the computation of mesh properties of MSMs based on known values. In [3] stiffness values in triangulated spring meshes were computed proportional to triangle area and Young's modulus. Different generic methods for particle-based systems (referred to as generalized mass-spring systems) have been suggested in [7]. One approach obtains stiffness values in rectangular structures according to angles between diagonal springs. Another method computes the spring constants based on the number of connections attached to a mass-point under consideration. Nevertheless, a general, non-heuristic formulation does not yet exist.

The second approach is based on optimization processes, which try to adapt the behavior of a MSM. A few optimization-based approaches have been proposed in the literature, for instance in [2] the use of simulated annealing for spring constant identification is suggested. Neural networks are used for the simulation of dynamic MSMs by [9]. Furthermore, methods based on genetic algorithms for stiffness value determination were discussed in [4] and [6]. However, all the methods described above only work for predefined topologies such as rectangular or tetrahedral structures. In this paper, we suggest a new solution, which simultaneously focuses on connections and elastic constants to be set in MSM systems. Moreover, our method is based on the comparison of deformation behavior of a MSM with a known, possibly more accurate reference system.

3   Topology Identification in 3D

In [1] we proposed an approach based on genetic optimization to identify the topology of mass-spring systems. A MSM (the *learning model*) was trained by means of a known model (the *reference model*) undergoing stretching and shearing induced by external forces. A cost function measured the difference between the behavior of the learning and the reference model, based on the distance between corresponding point positions in both models. In order to test the method, an MSM was used as reference, since in this case the exact solution was known. Our results for two-dimensional test cases have shown, that the method was able to recover the topology of isotropic and anisotropic reference models

Our first extension is the application of the described approach in 3D. Due to the increasing number of springs in this case, the genetic algorithm has to be optimized in order to converge faster towards the optimal solution. Furthermore, a reasonably limited neighborhood for possible spring connections has to be defined for 3D. Inspired by tightly-packed crystalline structures, we allow at most 26 neighbors (*Moore Neighborhood*) for each node.

3.1 Genetic Algorithm Adaptation

Genetic algorithms (GAs) attempt to mimic natural evolution [8]. They utilize the behaviour of a population of individuals - each one representing a potential solution to a defined problem. The fitness of an individual is determined by a cost function. The optimization principle consists of evolving the population by means of genetic operators such as *mutation* and *crossover*. Mutation applies random changes to the population with a certain probability *pmut*. Crossover creates offsprings by selecting genes from a pair of individuals and combining them into a new one, also with a predefined probability *pcross*. Although GAs do not guarantee a convergence to the global optimum, the reached local optimum may be considered as a good approximation of the exact solution.

Similar to the 2D case, an individual is described by a vector of binary values which represents a potential topology of the mass-spring model. In our experiments we found no significant influence of the population size on the convergence speed of the algorithm as well as on the results. Therefore, a low value was selected for the size to reduce the computation time (*popsize* = 5). While the

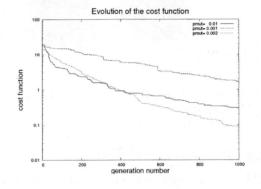

Fig. 1. Comparison of three constant mutation values

crossover operator improves convergence in the early stages of the process, its influence becomes of secondary importance later, when the population is close to the optimum. Therefore, the crossover probability is fixed to a high value (*pcross* = 0.8). In contrast to this, the mutation value has an important effect throughout the whole evolution. Figure 1 depicts the evolution of three trials with different mutation probabilities. While a high value (*pmut* = 0.01) speeds up the convergence at the beginning of the evolution, a lower one (*pmut* = 0.002) gives better results in later stages. Due to this observation, we decided to use an adaptive mutation probability which is inversely proportional to the generation number g: $pmut(g) = \frac{a}{g} + b$. We were able to considerably improve convergence speed with this adaptive mutation strategy. The coefficients a and b are currently determined experimentally - in the case of 3D topology identification, the section $a = 0.2$ and $b = 0.001$ has been found to provide best convergence properties.

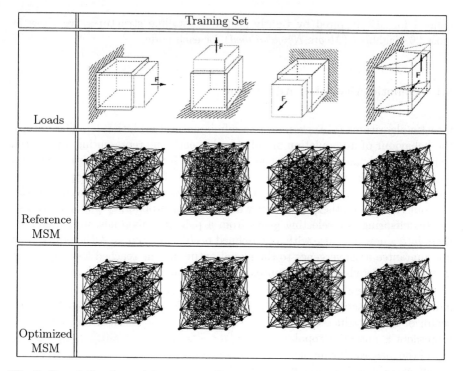

Fig. 2. Row 1: Loads used for training. Row 2: Deformations of reference MSM. Row 3: MSM optimized by genetic algorithm (*generation* = 4000, *popsize* = 5, *pmut* = $\frac{0.2}{g} + 0.001$, *pcross* = 0.8).

3.2   Experimental Results

This section describes the results in the three-dimensional case with a reference mesh consisting of 4x4x4 mass-points and 468 springs. In Figure 2, the first row shows four out of six different load cases used in the training process. The selection of these test cases, including stretching and shearing, was motivated by suggestions made in [2]. The second row depicts the reference MSM deformed by the loads, while row three illustrates the best topology obtained by the genetic algorithm. Here, 5 of 468 springs are missing, however, the normalized difference of point positions between the reference and the learning model is equal to zero. Thus, we were able to very closely approximate the deformation behavior of the reference model and recover almost all connections. Moreover, it proved to be sufficient to use the applied six load cases to obtain the parameters describing the deformation of the reference model.

4   Simultaneous Topology and Spring Constant Identification

In this part we introduce a significant extension of our method. Our focus so far was on the retrieval of mesh topologies. This is now extended by including the identification of individual spring constants into the approach. We achieve this by representing springs in the optimization population as real-valued constants instead of binary connections. Springs are only present, if their stiffness value is greater than a predefined threshold. This approach allows us to determine topology and stiffness values simultaneously. We again start to develop and validate this method with two-dimensional references. Our first step is to use MSM for comparison, however, we also introduce FEM systems as training references.

4.1   Genetic Algorithm

Binary encoding is no longer appropriate for the current method, since the elasticity of springs is a real value. Therefore, a vector of real constants is used to describe the stiffness values, while an interval is defined to limit the range of possible elasticity values. Furthermore, the mutation operator has to be defined differently. Instead of swapping bits, we add a random value x to the current stiffness, where x is limited to an interval I. The value x is normally distributed with zero mean and standard deviation σ. Since a constant σ will cause the random steps to be too high, once the population is close to the optimum, we propose to decrease σ during the optimization process. This can be achieved by defining the deviation according to $\sigma(g) = pmut(g) * sizeof(I)$. The interval size allows $\sigma(g)$ to take on the largest possible value at the beginning of the optimization. Finally, population size and crossover probability are again fixed throughout the evolution.

4.2   MSM as Reference

We performed a comparison between two MSMs with 5x5 points and 72 springs. The goal of this experiment was to test the capability of the method to recover a single stiffness value of a reference MSM. Therefore, we adjusted all the springs of the reference to the same stiffness value of 5. The interval I of the random mutation value x was assigned to $[0.0, 10.0]$. For the same reasons described in Section 3.1, the crossover probability was set to 0.8. Since these tests were done in 2D, we increased the population size to 10 individuals. Our experiments have shown, that greater values did not improve the results, but only increased computation time. Also, we again used an adaptive mutation probability function. The coefficients $a = 2$ and $b = 0$ provided the best results. The experiment was performed with 4000 generations. We were able to recover the complete topology of the reference model. Furthermore, the mean value of the retrieved stiffness was equal to 5.01 with a standard deviation of 0.65. Thus, we were able to simultaneously recover the connections and elasticity values of a reference MSM.

So far we have trained our learning model based on known MSM configurations. However, we would like to use more accurate references which are capable of physically modeling the elastic behavior of real tissue based on continuum

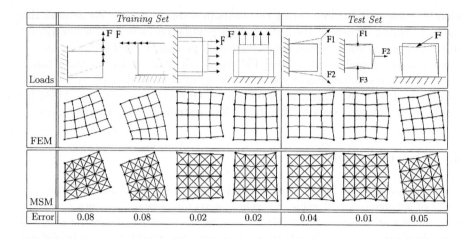

	Training Set				Test Set		
Error	0.08	0.08	0.02	0.02	0.04	0.01	0.05

Fig. 3. Column *Training Set*: Input data and result after training process. Column *Test Set*: Comparison between optimized MSM and additional FEM deformations not used during training for evaluation. Row 1: Test loads used for training MSM and comparison. Row 2: Linear elastic FEM deformations. Row 3: Optimized MSM with both topology and stiffness values obtained. Row 4: Comparison between mean error and smallest rest length of MSM.

mechanics. At the same time it is of primary importance, that the related material parameters can be determined systematically based on actual experiments. This extension will be presented in the next section.

4.3   FEM as Reference

Continuum mechanics based Finite Element Models have been used to accurately simulate soft tissue deformation, however, their high computational demands remain an obstacle for real-time applications. Realistic deformation parameters can be obtained by measurements on real organs. For instance in [5], in-vivo experiments have been introduced to determine appropriate material parameters of complex, non-linear constitutive equations. In order to approximate the behavior of these models, our next step focuses on training a learning MSM based on a reference FEM system. The reference mesh consists of quadrilateral elements, where the vertices correspond to the mass-points in the MSM model. The deformations are computed according to a linear elastic model with Young's modulus $E = 1MPa$ and Poisson coefficient $\nu = 0.3$. For the load cases several training sets were examined including shearing and stretching deformations. Sets of four, eight and twelve different load cases were evaluated. The best results were obtained with the latter set. Similar to the previous experiments, the cost function is based on the distance between the FEM vertices and the MSM mass-points. Population size and crossover probability remain identical to those described in the previous section. The coefficients of the mutation probability function were slightly adapted to $a = 5$ and $b = 0$. The first trial indicated, that all spring con-

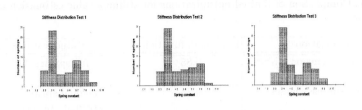

Fig. 4. Comparison of stiffness value distribution obtained by three optimization processes with the same input parameters.

stants were within the interval $[0.0, 10.0]$, therefore, these limits were retained for all experiments. We performed the same optimization steps to obtain the MSM mesh parameters. In order to validate our results, we defined additional load cases and compared the behavior of the previously learned MSM with the corresponding FEM deformations. Figure 3 exemplifies the results of both experiments. The column labelled *Training Set* illustrates the input data as well as the resulting configuration of the training process. The first row depicts four of the twelve test loads applied to the FEM. The second row shows the FEM deformations and the third row contains the learning MSM with the best stiffness values after 3000 generations. In the column *Test Set*, the MSM solution is compared to three elastic linear FEM deformations not included in the training set. The last row shows an error metric for the deformation differences. The mean error distance of the FEM and MSM points is set in relation to the smallest spring rest length of the optimized MSM. As revealed by the error, the stiffness values of the learning MSM seem to be equally well adjusted for both the training and test FEM cases. This experiment shows the capability of our method to finding appropriate stiffness values, allowing us to approximate the deformation behavior of a linear elastic FEM model.

4.4 Stiffness Value Distribution

After obtaining the spring constants from the FEM reference model, we examined the distribution of the stiffness values. Figure 4 shows the results of three trials with the same input data. The plots show that a linear elastic material cannot be approximated with one homogeneous stiffness parameter. Instead, the figures seem to indicate that at least two major classes of stiffness values exist (represented by the two peaks). One possible assumption is that one has to differentiate between diagonal and straight springs. In order to investigate this observation, we performed two additional experiments. The main idea behind these trials is to limit the spring constants to belong to one or two homogeneous classes. In other words, in the first experiment, only one global stiffness value is optimized, while in the second, diagonal and straight springs were optimized as two individual classes. The results of these experiments are summarized in Table 1. It can be observed that the best results are still achieved with our previously performed unlimited optimization experiments with a cost function value

Table 1. Comparison of limited optimizations for stiffness value estimation according to classes.

Limitation	Final cost function	Stiffness values
Single, homogeneous stiffness	0.85	All springs 4.07
Two stiffness classes	0.73	Diagonal springs 3.35, straight springs 4.76
Unrestricted stiffness values	0.58	Spring stiffnesses in interval $[0.0, 10.0]$. Main classes of stiffness values in $[3.0, 4.0]$ and $[6.0, 8.0]$

of 0.58. Assigning only one homogeneous stiffness parameter to all springs gives the worst results. This is also in line with the findings described in [3]. Defining two classes of springs with differing constant values slightly improves the results, however, optimal performance cannot be achieved. Furthermore, both retrieved spring constants of the two-classes belong to the same cluster described by the first peak of the distribution graph. This seems to indicate, that such simple rules based on connection topology might not be sufficient to explain the observed pattern. Besides, due to the small size of the meshes, it is not clear how far boundary effect may explain the observed results. Therefore, larger meshes will be investigated to further analyze the non-homogeneous stiffness distribution.

5   Conclusion and Future Work

We have introduced an extension of our previous work based on genetic algorithms to identify the topology of 3D MSMs. Moreover, a successful simultaneous topology and spring constant identification approach has been described. Our method was able to recover topology and stiffness values of reference MSMs. Moreover, we were able to approximate the behavior of FEM deformations with an optimized MSM mesh. Finally we could show, that homogenous stiffness parameters are not appropriate for simulating linear elastic material.

In future work, we will further evaluate adaptive mutation functions in order to improve the convergence behaviour of the genetic algorithm. We will examine the stiffness value distribution more closely and try to find underlying patterns. Finally, neighborhood selection and the approximation of more complex FEM models will be investigated.

Acknowledgment. The authors would like to thank Stefan Weiss for the FEM deformation calculations. This research has been supported by the NCCR Co-Me of the Swiss National Science Foundation.

References

1. G. Bianchi, M. Harders, and G. Székely. Mesh topology identification for mass-spring models. In *MICCAI 2003*, volume 1, pages 50–58, 2003.
2. Oliver Deussen, Leif Kobbelt, and Peter Tucke. Using simulated annealing to obtain good nodal approximations of deformable objects. In *Computer Animation and Simulation '95*, pages 30–43, 1995.
3. A. Van Gelder. Approximate simulation of elastic membranes by triangulated spring meshes. *Journal of Graphics Tools*, 3(2):21–42, 1998.
4. A. Joukhadar, F. Garat, and Ch. Laugier. Parameter Identification for Dynamic Simulation. In *In Proc. of the IEEE Int. Conf. on Robotics and Automation*, pages 1928–1933, 1997. Albuquerque, US.
5. M. Kauer, V. Vuskovic, J. Dual, G. Szekely, and M. Bajka. Inverse finite element characterization of soft tissues. *Medical Image Analysis*, 6(3):275–287, 2002.
6. J. Louchet, X. Provot, and D. Crochemore. Evolutionary identification of cloth animation models. In *Computer Animation and Simulation '95*, pages 44–54, 1995.
7. A. Maciel, R. Boulic, and D. Thalmann. Deformable tissue parameterized by properties of real biological tissue. In *IS4TM*, pages 74–87.
8. Z. Michlewicz. *Genetic Algorithms + Data Structures = Evolution Programs.* Springer, 1999.
9. A. Nürnberger, A. Radetzky, and R. Kruse. A Problem Specific Recurrent Neural Network for the Description and Simulation of Dynamic Springs Models. In *IEEE IJCNN'98*, pages 468–473, 1998.

Human Spine Posture Estimation Method from Human Images to Calculate Physical Forces Working on Vertebrae

Daisuke Furukawa[1], Takayuki Kitasaka[2] Kensaku Mori[2], Yasuhito Suenaga[2], Kenji Mase[3], and Tomoichi Takahashi[4]

[1] Graduate School of Engineering, Nagoya University
Furo-cho, Chikusa-ku, Nagoya, Aichi, 464–8603 Japan
[2] Graduate School of Information Science, Nagoya University
Furo-cho, Chikusa-ku, Nagoya, Aichi, 464–8603 Japan
[3] Information Technology Center, Nagoya University
Furo-cho, Chikusa-ku, Nagoya, Aichi, 464–8603 Japan
[4] Faculty of Science and Technology, Meijo University
Shiogamaguchi, Tempaku-ku, Nagoya, Aichi, 468–8502 Japan

Abstract. This paper describes a method for estimating a human spine posture from human images using a human spine model to compute the rough approximation of the physical forces working on vertebral bodies. Our method uses the positions of the neck and waist in addition to the positions of the head, torso, and arms estimated from the actual human images. The spine model constructed from 3-D CT images is deformed to place the top and the bottom vertebrae of the spine model to the estimated neck and waist positions. According to the experimental results based on one real MR image dataset of one subject person, our methods estimated the positions of the vertebrae within positional shifts of about 6.3 mm and the rotational variation of about 3.1 degrees. We also confirmed the methods calculated the reasonable estimation of the physical forces working on the vertebral body.

1 Introduction

Recently, there is a growing concern with the physical load analysis of the spine, since diseases such as low back pain due to damage to the spine frequently occur to us in our daily life [1,2,3]. In these studies, local spine models composed of some vertebrae and surrounding muscles are used for numerical computation. Initial conditions and boundary conditions are adjusted to satisfy the situation that we have to analyze such as a subject's posture, external forces, and so on. Under those conditions, internal stress inside the vertebral bodies are calculated using the finite element method. Generally, those conditions are determined manually, hence analyzed posture should be restricted to a simple one.

If we can determine the initial conditions from human images automatically, we can easily compute internal stress for a real posture in which a subject

C. Barillot, D.R. Haynor, and P. Hellier (Eds.): MICCAI 2004, LNCS 3217, pp. 302–310, 2004.

actually holds. To determine the initial conditions, we have to estimate the orientations of the vertebrae and the physical forces working on the vertebrae from human images.

There are few studies on the method that is able to fit a spine model to an actual human image, and to estimate pressure on the vertebrae simultaneously. Some researches on either posture generation or model fitting using a human body model are reported. Badler et al. [4] proposed spine and torso models and a motion generation method using them for computer animation. Otake et al. [5] overlaid a skeletal model of the lower half of the body onto human images using motion capture data. However, it is difficult to apply these methods to physical force computation, since the models are deformed based on kinematics.

We proposed a method for estimating the positions and the orientations of the vertebrae from human images [6]. In this method, the spine model is deformed to place the top and bottom vertebrae on the neck and waist positions obtained from input human images by applying two virtual forces to the top and bottom vertebrae corresponding to the neck and waist. Even though virtual forces were used in our previous method because of the difficulty of obtaining the physically appropriate forces, we were able to estimate the spine postures reasonably.

This paper describes a method for computing the rough approximation of the physical forces working on vertebral bodies as well as for estimating the positions and the orientations of the vertebrae. In Sect. 2, we present the spine posture estimation model. The spine posture estimation process is described in Sect. 3. The physical force computation is also explained briefly. In Sect. 4, we show the experimental results of evaluation of the accuracy of the estimated positions and the orientations of the vertebrae. Then we show the preliminary experimental results of the physical force computation. Section 5 contains conclusions and future works.

2   Spine Posture Estimation Model

The human spine is mainly composed of vertebrae and intervertebral discs. We model the vertebrae and the intervertebral discs as rigid body and elastic body, respectively (Fig. 1). Each vertebra is represented as a surface object since the vertebrae are dealt with as rigid bodies in the model deformation process. An intervertebral disk is modeled as eight springs connecting the adjacent vertebrae. Movement of the vertebrae in the deformation process is constrained by the springs.

A set of X-ray CT images provided by the Visible Human Project [7] is used to construct the model. The surface of the vertebral bodies are determined by applying the marching cubes method to the voxel data obtained by simply thresholding the CT images. The contacting points of the vertebra and the associated springs are manually adjusted considering the center of mass of the vertebra and the symmetry of the arrangement of the springs.

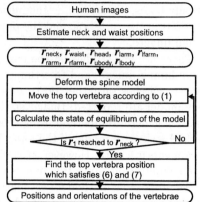

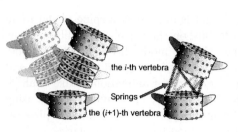

the i-th vertebra

Springs

the $(i+1)$-th vertebra

Fig. 1. Spine posture estimation model.

Fig. 2. Processing flow of the spine posture estimation.

3 Spine Posture Estimation Method

3.1 Neck and Waist Positions Estimation

Figure 2 shows the processing flow of the spine posture estimation method. The input is a sequence of human images of a subject taken by video cameras.

We use the whole body model to estimate the neck and waist positions, and the centers of mass of the head, arms, and upper and lower bodies from the input images. The whole body model consists of eleven parts of ellipsoids that represent the head, upper and lower bodies, upper arms and forearms, and thighs and legs. Although the whole body model was manually registered to the human images in this paper, conventional posture estimation methods such as [10] can be used for registration. After the model fitting, the neck position r_{neck} and the waist position r_{waist} are obtained by the end point of the ellipsoid corresponding to the upper body, and the center of mass of the ellipsoid corresponding to the lower body. The centers of mass of the head, arms, and bodies, r_{head}, r_{larm}, r_{lfarm}, r_{rarm}, r_{rfarm}, r_{ubody}, and r_{lbody} are approximated by the centers of mass of the corresponding ellipsoids.

3.2 Spine Model Deformation

First, the spine model is translated and rotated to make the position and the orientation of the bottom vertebra of the spine model coincide with those of the waist estimated from the inputs. Then the top vertebra is moved toward the neck position by a small distance. This movement is carried out iteratively until the top vertebra reaches r_{neck}. After n iterations, the top vertebra position $r_1(n)$ is expressed by

$$r_1(n) = r_1(n-1) + \delta d, \tag{1}$$

where d satisfies $d = r_{\text{neck}} - r_1(0)$, and δd means the small displacement along the direction of d. $r_1(0)$ is the initial position before the model deformation process.

Each time the top vertebra is moved by δd, the positions and the orientations of the vertebrae except the top and bottom vertebrae are calculated so that the spine model satisfies equilibrium. We consider two types of forces working on the i-th vertebra. The first type is the weight W_i of the body supported by the i-th vertebra. To calculate W_i, we use the information about the positions and the orientations of the ellipsoids that approximate the torso in the whole body model. The weight W_i can be calculated by integrating the volume defined by the surfaces of the ellipsoids and the planes passing through the centers of mass of the $(i-1)$-th and the i-th vertebrae. The second one is the forces of repulsion T_{ij} of the springs connected to the upper and lower side of the i-th vertebra. The spring force is defined by the Hook's law. The parameter k_{ij} denotes the spring constant. Then the force F_i and the torque M_i working on the i-th vertebrae are expressed by

$$F_i = W_i + \sum_j T_{ij}, \qquad (2)$$

$$M_i = r_i \times W_i + \sum x_{ij} \times T_{ij}, \qquad (3)$$

where r_i represents the center of mass of the volume, and x_{ij} the vector that points to the contacting point of the spring from the center of mass of the i-th vertebra. The symbol '$\times$' represents the outer product of two vectors.

As expressed in (2) and (3), F_i and M_i depend on the positions and the orientations of the $(i-1)$-th and the $(i+1)$-th vertebrae as well as the ones of the i-th vertebra. Therefore F_i and M_i can be expressed by the following equations,

$$F_i = F_i(r_{i-1}, \theta_{i-1}, r_i, \theta_i, r_{i+1}, \theta_{i+1}), \qquad (4)$$

$$M_i = M_i(r_{i-1}, \theta_{i-1}, r_i, \theta_i, r_{i+1}, \theta_{i+1}), \qquad (5)$$

where we denote the center of mass of the i-th vertebra as r_i, and the orientation in Euler angle as θ_i. F_i and M_i must satisfy the following equations because of the equilibrium of the model,

$$F_i(r_{i-1}, \theta_{i-1}, r_i, \theta_i, r_{i+1}, \theta_{i+1}) = 0, \qquad (6)$$

$$M_i(r_{i-1}, \theta_{i-1}, r_i, \theta_i, r_{i+1}, \theta_{i+1}) = 0. \qquad (7)$$

Therefore, when we denote the number of the vertebrae as N, the positions and the orientations of the $N-2$ vertebrae except the top and the bottom vertebrae are determined by solving the $2 \times (N-2)$ sets of nonlinear equations. These equations can be solved using the Newton-Raphson method.

We assume that the top vertebra of the model supports the weight of the head and arms as expressed in the following equations,

$$F_1 = W_{\text{head}} + W_{\text{larm}} + W_{\text{lfarm}} + W_{\text{rarm}} + W_{\text{rfarm}} + \sum_j T_{1j}, \qquad (8)$$

$$M_1 = r_{\text{head}} \times W_{\text{head}} + r_{\text{larm}} \times W_{\text{larm}} + r_{\text{lfarm}} \times W_{\text{lfarm}}$$
$$+ r_{\text{rarm}} \times W_{\text{rarm}} + r_{\text{rfarm}} \times W_{\text{rfarm}} + \sum_j x_{1j} \times T_{1j}, \qquad (9)$$

where W_{head}, W_{larm}, W_{lfarm}, W_{rarm}, and W_{rfarm} represent the weight of the head and the arms. F_1 and M_1 do not satisfy the conditions expressed by (6) and (7) because the position of the top vertebra is determined according to (1). Therefore, we find the top vertebra position which satisfies (6) and (7) by translating the top vertebra along the plumb line that passes through its center of mass.

After the spine posture estimation, we can calculate the forces working on the vertebral body by (2) and (3). In these equations, the terms for the forces of repulsion of the spring should be derived by summing only the forces caused by the springs connected to the upper surface of the vertebral body.

4   Experimental Results and Discussion

4.1   Accuracy of the Model Deformation Method Using MR Images

To evaluate the accuracy of the spine model deformation, we compared the positions and the orientations of the vertebrae estimated by our method and the ones measured from actual MR images. We assumed that the neck and waist positions were known so that the whole body model fitting to human images was not carried out.

In this experiment, we used three sets of MR images of healthy subject (Fig.3). The datasets A and B were the coronal and sagittal images in which a subject was lying straightly on the bed of MRI. The dataset C was the coronal images in which the subject was lying with his body bending to the right. To construct and determine the initial posture of the spine model, we measured the sagittal diameters, transverse diameters, and the initial positions of the vertebrae from the datasets A and B. Then the model was deformed to fit it to the neck and waist positions acquired from the dataset C, and we compared the positions and the orientations of the vertebrae resulting from the model fitting with the ones measured from the dataset C. Acquisition parameters of the MR images were: 512×512 pixels, 0.586 mm pixel size, 7 slices. The reconstruction pitch was 15 mm for the image datasets A and C, 8 mm for the image dataset B. We used the T1-weighted images taken by AIRIS-II (Hitachi Medical Corp.). We employed the Young's modulus of 500 MPa and the Poisson's ratio of 0.3 as the material property of the intervertebral discs [8]. The spring constant k_i were determined as the approximations of these values.

We implemented our proposed method on a conventional PC (Pentium 4 2.8 GHz). Total computation time was 77.6 seconds. The model deformation was repeated 65 times until the top vertebra reached the neck position obtained from the MR images. Seventy iterations were performed on average to solve the sets of nonlinear equations (6) and (7).

Table 1 shows the comparison results of the positions and orientations of the vertebrae measured from MR images and the ones estimated by our methods. In this table, Δx and Δy mean the errors along the left-right direction and along the longitudinal direction, respectively. SSD means the sum of squared

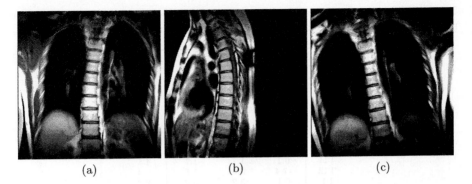

(a)   (b)   (c)

Fig. 3. Typical slices of each of three datasets A, B, and C of MR images to evaluate accuracy of the spine model deformation. The images (a) and (b) are one of the coronal and sagittal images in the datasets A and B. The image (c) is one of the coronal images in the dataset C.

differences. The unit of the values is millimeter. The abbreviation 'T' and 'L' represent thoracic and lumbar vertebrae, respectively.

4.2   Calculation of the Forces Working on the Lumbar Vertebra 'L5'

We calculated the physical force on the upper surface of the lumbar vertebra 'L5' by applying the methods to the real human images, and compared the calculation results with the ones performed by Schultz et al. [9]. In the Schultz's model which did not consider effect of the dorsal muscles, the physical force on the upper surface of the 'L5' was simply calculated by the sum of the weight of the head, torso, arms, and the weight held by a subject. Schultz solved the equation with respect to the force on 'L5' of the subject holding an upright posture and supporting a weight in the right hand. In our experiment, we assumed the conditions similar to Schultz did. The subject was slowly lifting up the weight of about 4.1 kg to his elbow height. The weight of the head, torso, and arm of the subject were about 3.6 kg, 25.7 kg, and 3.3 kg, respectively. The subject was the same person whose MR images were used in the experiment stated in Sect. 4.1. Then the model constructed in the above experiment were used again in this experiment. Fitting the whole human body model to the human images was carried out manually.

Figure 4 shows the examples of the estimated spine postures. The estimated spine postures are overlaid on the figures. The violet ellipsoidal regions represent the whole body model. The computation result of the force working on the lumbar vertebra 'L5' was about 336 N. The experiment was carried out on the same computer resource (Pentium 4 2.8 GHz) used in Sect. 4.1. Total computation time was about 49 seconds.

Table 1. The comparison results of the positions and the orientations of the vertebrae measured from MR images and the ones estimated by our methods.

Vertebra	Δx (mm)	Δy (mm)	SSD (mm)	$\Delta\theta$ (deg)
T2	9.1	1.4	9.3	12.6
T3	11.0	-4.0	11.7	4.3
T4	13.2	-1.7	13.4	2.2
T5	11.7	-1.9	11.8	2.9
T6	10.0	-1.0	10.0	0.2
T7	8.5	-1.4	8.6	0.1
T8	7.0	-0.6	7.0	1.7
T9	4.3	-0.3	4.3	3.1
T10	1.2	0.2	1.2	6.0
T11	0.1	1.7	1.7	4.1
T12	-1.4	0.9	1.6	2.4
L1	0.1	3.2	3.2	3.3
L2	0.4	2.7	2.7	0.9
L3	1.1	3.4	3.5	1.1
L4	1.7	4.3	4.6	1.5
M $\pm\sigma$	5.2 ± 4.9	0.5 ± 2.2	6.3 ± 6.0	3.1 ± 3.0

4.3 Discussion

As shown in Table 1, the average of the positional and rotational variation of the vertebrae were 6.3 mm and 3.1 degrees, respectively. According to our measurement of the position of the vertebra 'T4' based on the MR images, it moved by 68.3 mm from its original position when the subject bent his body. The proposed method estimated its position by 13.4 mm of error. Therefore, the error of the estimation of 'T4' is about 20 %. The computation result of the force working on the lumbar vertebra 'L5' was about 336 N, while the force was about 390 N in the Schultz's simple model which did not have the dorsal muscles [9]. Therefore, it turned out that our model can estimate the physical forces to the vertebrae as accurately as the forces estimated by the Schultz's method.

Compared with the Schultz's and others' methods, the main advantage of the proposed method is that we can understand the state of the spine with respect to real human motions the subject actually takes. The previously proposed methods did not allow such physical force computation based on real postures as our method did. Because the proposed method estimates physical forces from the human images, the proposed method helps us to determine the initial and boundary conditions necessary for precise physical force analyses such as finite element methods.

The dorsal muscles are very important tissues in terms of the forces to the vertebrae. Some experimental results reported by other researchers indicate that more than 1000 N of the forces act on the lumbar vertebrae due to a function of the dorsal muscles. We do not model the dorsal muscles since it is difficult to determine the muscle forces. However, to calculate the forces more precisely, we have to consider the interaction between the dorsal muscles and the vertebrae.

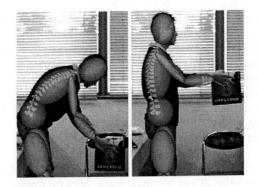

Fig. 4. Examples of the estimated spine postures.

5   Conclusion

In this paper, we have proposed a spine model and a method for estimating the spine posture from human images taken by video cameras. According to the preliminary experiments based on one real MR image data set of only one subject person, the methods estimated the positions of the vertebrae within positional shifts of about 6.3 mm and the rotational variation of about 3.1 degrees. We also confirmed that the methods calculated the reasonable approximation of the physical forces working on the vertebral body. Future work includes: (1) validation of accuracy of the model deformation method using a large set of MR image sets, (2) application to a large set of human images and the discussion about the method for evaluating the estimated spine posture, and (3) precise validation of the calculated physical forces on the vertebra from the viewpoint of anatomy and biomechanics.

Acknowledgements. Authors wish to thank Dr. Hiroshi Iseki and Dr. Kiyoshi Naemura of Tokyo Women's Medical University for cooperating with them to take the MRI images. This study was partly supported by the Grants-in-Aid for Scientific Research and the 21st Century COE Program from Japan Society for the Promotion of Science, Grants-in-Aid for Cancer Research from the Ministry of Health, Labor and Welfare of Japan.

References

1. Chen, C.S. et al.: Stress analysis of the disc adjacent to interbody fusion in lumbar spine. Medical Engineering & Physics. **23** (2001) 483–491
2. Nabhani, F. et al.: Computer modeling and stress analysis of the lumbar spine. J. Materials Processing Technology. **127** (2002) 40–47
3. Pitzen, T. et al.: A finite element model for predicting the biomechanical behaviour of the human lumbar spine. Control Engineering Practice. **10** (2002) 83–90

4. Monheit, G. and Badler, N.I.: A Kinematic Model of the Human Spine and Torso. IEEE Computer Graphics and Applications. (1991) 29–38

5. Otake, Y. et al.: Development of 4-Dimensional Human Model System for the Patient after Total Hip Arthroplasty. Medical Image Computing and Computer-Assisted Intervention. (2002) 241–247

6. Furukawa, D. et al.: Human Spine Posture Estimation from 2D Frontal and Lateral Views Using 3D Physically Accurate Spine Model. IEICE Transactions on Information and Systems. **E87-D** (2004) 146–154

7. National Library of Medicine: The Visible Human Project. http://www.nlm.nih.gov/research/visible/visible_human.html

8. Kumaresan, S. et al.: Finite element modeling of the cervical spine: role of intervertebral disc under axial and eccentric loads. Medical Engineering & Physics. **21** (1999) 689–700

9. Schultz, A.B. and Andersson, B.J.: Analysis of Loads on the Lumbar Spine. Spine. **6** (1981) 76–82

10. Bregler, C. and Malik, J.: Tracking People with Twists and Exponential Maps. Int. Conf. Computer Vision and Pattern Recognition. (1998) 8–15

Modelling Surgical Cuts, Retractions, and Resections via Extended Finite Element Method

Lara M. Vigneron[1], Jacques G. Verly[1], and Simon K. Warfield[2]

[1] Signal Processing Group, Dept. of Electrical Engineering and Computer Science, University of Liège, Belgium
[2] Computational Radiology Laboratory, Surgical Planning Laboratory, Brigham and Women's Hospital, Harvard Medical School, Boston, USA

Abstract. We introduce a new, efficient approach for modelling the deformation of organs following surgical cuts, retractions, and resections. It uses the extended finite element method (XFEM), recently developed in "fracture mechanics" for dealing with cracks in mechanical parts. XFEM eliminates the computationally-expensive remeshing that would be required if the standard finite element method (FEM) was used. We report on the successful application of the method to the simulation of 2D retraction. The method may have significant impact on surgical simulators and navigators.

1 Introduction

Image-guided surgical navigation systems allow the surgeon to follow more precisely his planning by displaying the positions of surgical instruments in preoperative images. However, as surgery progresses, these images become inaccurate due to the deformations of organs. Even though intraoperative images can be acquired, they have limited signal-to-noise ratio and spatial resolution. Additionally, not all imaging modalities (particularly functional ones) are available intraoperatively. Therefore, it is critical to continue using all preoperative images and to update them as organs deform.

Several nonrigid registration techniques could potentially be used for updating preoperative images. One approach is to model mechanical organ behavior based on the finite element method (FEM), as explained in [4][5] for the case of the brain. The idea is to capture the displacement of the surface(s) defining the shape of the organ and to compute the resulting deformation of a volume mesh of this organ by linear elastic finite element (FE) calculations.

Most studies of organ deformation based on biomechanical models have focused on the early stages of surgery, i.e., prior to significant deformations and any cut. The precision achieved for deformation prediction is about 1 voxel [4]. The situation becomes more complex when the surgeon performs cuts, retractions, or resections [4][6]. The last two necessarily involve a cut. Thus, the modelling of cuts and their effects is fundamental. The main difficulty

C. Barillot, D.R. Haynor, and P. Hellier (Eds.): MICCAI 2004, LNCS 3217, pp. 311–318, 2004.

associated with a cut is the discontinuity of matter displacement it involves. Indeed, FEM cannot handle such discontinuities directly.

We model the organs subjected to surgical cuts, retractions, and resections via the extended finite element method (XFEM). This powerful method was introduced in 1999 by Moës *et al* [1] in "fracture mechanics". This field deals with the appearance of cracks, which should be viewed as material discontinuities, and with their progression in mechanical structures such as airplane wings. The hope is that XFEM will reduce computational and memory requirements. Thus, it may hold the key to real-time modelling of deformation in surgical simulation and navigation.

In Sect. 2, we discuss the difficulties encountered with FEM when dealing with cracks. In Sect. 3, we review the main methods used in fracture mechanics. In Sect. 4, we introduce the basic principles of XFEM. In Sect. 5, a preliminary 2D proof-of-concept example, based on real data, is provided for the modelling of brain tissue retraction. Sect. 6 holds the conclusions.

2   Limitations of FEM for Modelling Cracks

Consider a solid, such as an organ, modelled by a volume mesh of elements, typically tetrahedra. The FEM approximation of the displacement $u(x)$ of any point x in this solid is defined by [3]

$$u(x) = \sum_{i=1}^{N} \varphi_i(x)u_i, \tag{1}$$

where i is the node index, N the number of nodes in the mesh, u_i the displacement of node i, and $\varphi_i(x)$ the nodal shape function (NSF) with compact nodal support defined by the space occupied by all elements connected to node i. The u_i's are also referred to as the nodal degrees of freedom (DOF): these are the discrete unknowns solved for in the FEM computation. The NSFs $\varphi_i(x)$ of FEM are defined to be continuous on each element. Thus, FEM has no built-in way of handling a crack going through an element. The only solution is remeshing, which involves the addition of nodes and elements [9] or topology adaptation [7], but these operations are computationally expensive. This makes FEM unsuitable for efficient crack modelling.

3   Methods for Modelling Cracks

Currently, there are three main methods for avoiding the drawbacks of FEM remeshing [10]. The boundary element method (BEM) dates back to the 60's and reached its peak of popularity in the 80's. Originally, it was not designed or used for modelling cracks. BEM is based on the discretization of only the object surface. The size of the corresponding set of equations is thus greatly reduced. However, in contrast to FEM, these equations are non-symmetric and fully populated. BEM takes advantage of the fact that surface meshing is generally easier than volume meshing [13]. When a crack appears and grows, new boundary elements must be added only along the crack. So BEM can avoid much of the remeshing required by FEM. BEM was used to study deformation due to brain shift, thus without any tissue discontinuity [11].

Meshless methods appeared in the 70's but it is only since the 90's that they have received significant attention [15]. Their goal is to address large deformations and cracks [14]. In FEM, the object is represented by a volume mesh. The nodes interact because they are connected via the elements. In meshless methods, the object is represented by a set of non-connected nodes that interact because their NSFs overlap. To model a crack, one cancels the interaction between some nodes by limiting the influence domain of their NSFs. While remeshing is avoided, the computation of the NSFs and the high-order Gauss quadrature required to compute the deformation equations can lead to greater computational requirements than for FEM [3]. Nevertheless, meshless methods are useful when a problem benefits from being solved with a displacement approximation that does not rely on mesh topology [3]. Meshless methods have been used to develop a surgical simulator [16] and to model the often-significant deformations of a biomechanical model of the beating heart [12].

XFEM was developed in 1999 specifically for studying cracks [1]. First, an FEM model, i.e., a mesh and associated NSFs, is built while ignoring the crack. Then, based upon the precise geometry of the crack, simple, auxiliary NSFs are added to some of the existing nodes. The solution of the equations can thus naturally provide a discontinuity in displacement at all points along the crack. The main appeal of XFEM is that it can model, without any remeshing, the deformations due to cracks of arbitrary shapes and also the way they propagate through matter. The equations remain also sparse and symmetric. Since XFEM can be viewed as an extension of FEM, one should be able to add XFEM capabilities to existing FEM frameworks.

4   Introduction to Basic XFEM Principles

XFEM works by allowing the solution of its equations to be discontinuous within mesh elements. Arbitrarily-shaped cracks can then be modelled without any remeshing. To provide a discontinuous solution, the displacement approximation $u(x)$ of Eq. (1) should be expressed, not only in terms of the continuous NSFs $\varphi_i(x)$ of FEM, but also in terms of some auxiliary discontinuous NSFs. The key idea of XFEM is to "enrich" the nodes whose support is fully or partially intersected by the crack: one says that the support contains a "crack interior" and a "crack tip", respectively. Enrichment is performed by adding DOFs and associated auxiliary NSFs, which are the NSFs $\varphi_i(x)$ multiplied by some enrichment function (EF).

If the crack fully intersects the support of a node, this node is enriched with the crack-interior EF given by the Heaviside function, a piecewise-constant function that changes sign at the crack boundary Γ_d, i.e.,

$$H(x) = \begin{cases} 1 & for \quad (x - x^*).e_n > 0 \\ -1 & for \quad (x - x^*).e_n < 0 \end{cases}, \qquad (2)$$

where x is a point of the solid, x^* the point on Γ_d closest to x, and e_n the unit outward normal[1] to Γ_d at x^*. $H(x)$ cannot be used when Γ_d does not fully intersect the support, because one would then effectively extend the discontinuity to the boundary of the support.

Consequently, nodes that have a crack tip within their support are enriched with specific crack-tip EFs that incorporate the radial and angular behavior of the asymptotic crack-tip displacement field, two-dimensional by nature. For an isotropic elastic material, the crack-tip EFs are[2]

$$\{F_l(r, \theta)\}_{l=1}^4 = \{\sqrt{r}sin(\frac{\theta}{2}), \sqrt{r}cos(\frac{\theta}{2}), \sqrt{r}sin(\frac{\theta}{2})sin(\theta), \sqrt{r}cos(\frac{\theta}{2})sin(\theta)\}, \qquad (3)$$

where r and θ are the local polar coordinates. These crack-tip EFs ensure that the crack terminates precisely at the location of the crack tip and that the model possesses a correct near-tip behavior.

The XFEM approximation for a single crack with a single crack tip is thus

$$u(x) = \sum_{i \in I} \varphi_i(x)u_i + \sum_{j \in J} \varphi_j(x)H(x)a_j + \sum_{k \in K} \varphi_k(x)(\sum_{l=1}^4 F_l(x)c_k^l), \qquad (4)$$

where the u_i's are the nodal degrees of freedom (DOFs) associated with the continuous part of the FE solution, the a_j's the nodal enriched DOFs associated with the crack-interior EF, and the c_k^l's the nodal enriched DOFs associated with the crack-tip EFs. I is the set of all nodes in the mesh, J the set of nodes with supports cut by the crack interior, and K the set of nodes with supports cut by the crack tip (Fig. 1). Equation (4) can be generalized to several cracks and crack tips. For details regarding the theory and various implementation issues, refer, e.g., to [1][2][3], and particularly to [2] for equations.

5   Proof-of-Concept Example: Simulation of 2D Retraction

To evaluate the capabilities and potential of XFEM for surgical simulation and navigation, we have performed preliminary tests on 2D objects containing a line-segment crack. The test program was written in MATLAB.

---

[1] "Outward" is defined in an obvious way based upon the relative positions of x and Γ_d.
[2] The first function is discontinuous at the surface of the crack.

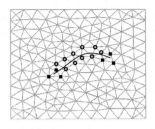

Fig. 1. The mesh and crack geometries are respectively in gray and black. The nodes enriched with the crack-interior EF are represented by circles (set J) while nodes enriched with the crack-tip EFs are represented by squares (set K).

The inputs to the program are the mesh definition and the crack geometry. One begins by identifying the mesh elements that are fully intersected by the crack and the mesh elements that contain a crack tip. One defines the number of DOFs for each node: 2 for a non-enriched node, 4 for a node enriched with a crack-interior EF, or 10 for a node enriched with crack-tip EFs. As with FEM, each elementary stiffness matrix is computed, taking into account the EFs, and the global stiffness matrix is subsequently assembled. Force or displacement constraints are applied in similar ways in both FEM and XFEM.

We conducted a series of experiments. First, we used simple geometric shapes. The triangular mesh was created using the MATLAB PDE toolbox. Our first published example can be found in [18]. Then, we used realistic inputs. In the present case, we start from a segmented 3D image of the cortex and select one of its horizontal slice (Fig. 2(a)). The segmentation is performed as described in [8] (Fig. 2(b)). The mesh is computed using DISTMESH2D[3] (Fig. 2(c)). The linear crack is shown in all images of Fig. 2. It starts at the brain surface and finishes close to the tumor, defining an incision segment (planar facet in 3D). To simulate the effect of a retractor (2D) that spreads out tissue from the incision segment, we compute the points of intersection of the crack with the mesh. Then, we impose an arbitrary displacement of $(-3.5, -1)$ and $(+3.5, +1)$[4] to each intersection, with the mesh, of the left and right crack lips, respectively. The intersection of the crack with the element containing the crack tip was left free to avoid constraints that are too large near the tip. Indeed, we have noticed that element flip causing element overlap can sometimes happen in this situation.

The application of this displacement constraint in XFEM is straightforward. For the intersection (x_{int}) of the crack with an element defined by 3 nodes enriched with $H(x)$, the relations from (4) between the nodal DOFs[5] are

---

[3] Download from http://www-math.mit.edu/~persson/mesh/.

[4] The 1st coordinate is vertical and the 2nd horizontal (with reference to Fig. 2).

[5] We consider the intersection lying on the element boundary between node 1 with DOFs $(u_{x1}, u_{y1}, a_{x1}, a_{y1})$ and node 2 with DOFs $(u_{x2}, u_{y2}, a_{x2}, a_{y2})$.

$$\begin{cases} \varphi_1(\boldsymbol{x}_{int})\, u_{x1} + \varphi_1(\boldsymbol{x}_{int})\, a_{x1} + \varphi_2(\boldsymbol{x}_{int})\, u_{x2} + \varphi_2(\boldsymbol{x}_{int})\, a_{x2} = -3.5 \\ \varphi_1(\boldsymbol{x}_{int})\, u_{y1} + \varphi_1(\boldsymbol{x}_{int})\, a_{y1} + \varphi_2(\boldsymbol{x}_{int})\, u_{y2} + \varphi_2(\boldsymbol{x}_{int})\, a_{y2} = -1 \end{cases} \tag{5}$$

for the left lip, where $H(\boldsymbol{x})$ is equal to $+1$. Similarly, we have

$$\begin{cases} \varphi_1(\boldsymbol{x}_{int})\, u_{x1} - \varphi_1(\boldsymbol{x}_{int})\, a_{x1} + \varphi_2(\boldsymbol{x}_{int})\, u_{x2} - \varphi_2(\boldsymbol{x}_{int})\, a_{x2} = 3.5 \\ \varphi_1(\boldsymbol{x}_{int})\, u_{y1} - \varphi_1(\boldsymbol{x}_{int})\, a_{y1} + \varphi_2(\boldsymbol{x}_{int})\, u_{y2} - \varphi_2(\boldsymbol{x}_{int})\, a_{y2} = 1 \end{cases} \tag{6}$$

for the right lip, where $H(\boldsymbol{x})$ is equal to -1. Finally the discrete displacement solution provided by XFEM calculation was used to warp the brain image according to Eq. (4). The result of warping the image of Fig. 2(a) masked with the region of Fig. 2(b) is shown in Fig. 2(d).

If one attempts to use standard FEM to cope with a material discontinuity, the computation time will increase significantly. Indeed, one must modify the mesh in the vicinity of the discontinuity for the boundaries of the new elements to be aligned with the discontinuity. The nodes on the discontinuity must be identified and duplicated. The matrices representing the system of equations must be updated to take into account the new connectivity. In contrast, XFEM does not require remeshing. However, there are some costs associated with XFEM. While XFEM requires identification of the elements intersected by the crack and the use of $H(\boldsymbol{x})$ requires some geometrical calculations, the primary cost is associated with the calculation of the stiffness matrix of the elements containing the nodes that are enriched. The dimension of elementary stiffness matrices increase from 6×6 for a triangular element with 3 non-enriched nodes to 30×30 for a triangular element with 3 nodes enriched by crack-tip EFs. In contrast, FEM always requires a 6×6 stiffness matrix. The stiffness matrix computation for an element including a node enriched with crack-tip EFs involves analytical computation of their derivatives and Gauss quadrature to numerically integrate over the element.

6   Conclusions

Being able to model the deformations of organs is important both for surgical simulations and for image-guided navigation. This problem becomes complex and computationally intensive if one wishes to model the effects of cuts, retractions, and resections on the deformations of these organs. Current approaches that use a biomechanical model together with FEM to compute deformation require an expensive remeshing as soon as the volume mesh is cut.

This paper introduces a new approach that totally avoids the need for remeshing. In contrast with FEM, the solution provided by XFEM can now contain discontinuities of arbitrary shape inside mesh elements. Since the underlying framework remains that of FEM, the equations remain sparse and symmetric, thereby maintaining the computational efficiency of FEM. Of course, the number of DOFs increases in the case of XFEM because of the node enrichment procedure. Since XFEM can be viewed as an extension of

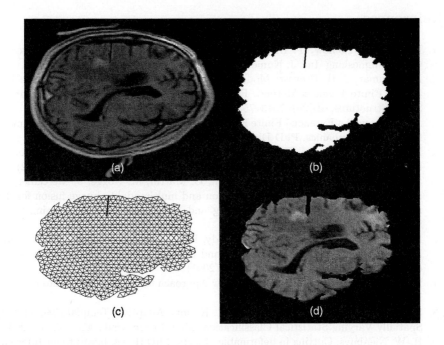

Fig. 2. (a) Original 2D MRI image with cut (discontinuity) leading from top surface to tumor. (b) Binary image of the cortex extracted from (a). (c) Triangular mesh computed from (b). (d) Image showing the result of deforming (a), masked with the region of (b), as specified by the retraction simulation described in the text.

FEM, XFEM techniques should fit well with existing FEM-based codes and applications.

The example of Section 5 confirms that XFEM can elegantly and efficiently take into account displacement discontinuities in the study of the mechanical properties of objects. This and other initial experiments we have performed give us confidence that XFEM may become a key tool for surgical simulation and image-guided navigation. In subsequent work, we will validate the method.

Acknowledgements. This work was sponsored in part by the "Fonds National de la Recherche Scientifique (F.N.R.S.)," Brussels, Belgium, the "Fonds Spéciaux pour la Recherche," University of Liège, Belgium, the "Léon Fredericq Foundation," University of Liège, Belgium, the Whitaker Foundation and by NIH grants R21 MH67054, R01 LM007861, P41 RR13218 and P01 CA67165.

References

1. N. Moës, J. Dolbow, T. Belytschko: A finite element method for crack growth without remeshing. Int. J. Numer. Meth. Engng., **46**: 131–150 (1999)
2. N. Sukumar, J.-H. Prévost: Modeling Quasi-Static Crack Growth with the Extended Finite Element Method. Part I: Computer Implementation. Internat. J. Solids Structures, **40**(26): 7513–7537 (2003)
3. J.E. Dolbow: An Extended Finite Element Method with Discontinuous Enrichment for Applied Mechanics. PhD Dissertation, Northwestern University (1999)
4. M. Ferrant, A. Nabavi, B. Macq, R. Kikinis, S. Warfield: Serial registration of intra-operative MR images of the brain. Med. Image Anal., **6**: 337–359 (2002)
5. J.G. Verly, L.M. Vigneron, N. Petitjean, C. Martin, M. Hogge, J. Mercenier, V. Jamoye, P.A. Robe: Nonrigid registration and multimodality image fusion for 3D image-guided neurochirurgical planning and navigation. Medical Imaging 2004, SPIE Proc. **5367** (Feb 2004)
6. M.I. Miga, D.W. Roberts, F.E. Kennedy, L.A. Platenik, A. Hartov, K.E. Lunn, K.D. Paulsen: Modeling of Retraction and Resection for Intraoperative Updating of Images. Neurosurgery, **49**(1): 75–84 (2001)
7. D. Serby, M. Harders, G. Székely: A New Approach to Cutting into Finite Element Models. MICCAI'01, 425–433 (2001)
8. S.K. Warfield, M. Kaus, F.A. Jolesz, R. Kikinis: Adaptive, Template Moderated, Spatially Varying Statistical Classification. Med. Image Anal., **4**(1): 43–55 (2000)
9. H.-W. Nienhuys: Cutting in deformable objects. PhD thesis, Institute for Information and Computing Sciences, Utrecht University (2003)
10. M. Duflot, H. Nguyen-Dang: A meshless method with enriched weight functions for fatigue crack growth. Int. J. Numer. Meth. Engng., **59**: 1945–1961 (2004)
11. O. Ecabert, T. Butz, A. Nabavi, J.-P. Thiran: Brain Shift Correction Based on a Boundary Element Biomechanical Model with Different Material Properties. MICCAI'03, **2878**: 41–49 (2003)
12. H. Liu and P. Shi: Meshfree Representation and Computation: Applications to Cardiac Motion Analysis. IPMI, 560–572 (July 2003)
13. J.O. Watson: Boundary Elements from 1960 to the Present Day. Electronic Journal of Boundary Elements, **1**(1): 34–46 (2003)
14. T. Belytschko, Y. Krongauz, D. Organ, M. Fleming, and P. Krysl: Meshless methods: An overview and recent developments. Comput. Methods Appl. Mech. Engng., **139**: 3–47 (1996)
15. G.R. Liu: Mesh Free Methods: Moving Beyond the Finite Element Method. CRC Press (2002)
16. S. De, J.W. Hong, K.J. Bathe: On the method of finite spheres in applications: towards the use with ADINA and in a surgical simulator. Comp. Mech., **31**: 27-37 (2003)
17. P.-O. Persson, G. Strang: A Simple Mesh Generator in MATLAB. SIAM Review **46**(2): 329–345 (2004)
18. L. Vigneron, J. Verly, S. Warfield: On Extended Finite Element Method (XFEM) for modelling of organ deformations associated with surgical cuts. Second International Symposium on Medical Simulation (June 2004)

A Collaborative Virtual Environment for the Simulation of Temporal Bone Surgery

Dan Morris[1], Christopher Sewell[1], Nikolas Blevins[2], Federico Barbagli[1], and Kenneth Salisbury[1]

[1] Stanford University, Department of Computer Science
[2] Stanford University, Department of Otolaryngology

{dmorris, csewell, barbagli, jks}@robotics.stanford.edu,
nblevins@stanford.edu

Robotics Laboratory
Gates Building 1A
Stanford CA 94305-9010, USA

Abstract. We describe a framework for training-oriented simulation of temporal bone surgery. Bone dissection is simulated visually and haptically, using a hybrid data representation that allows smooth surfaces to be maintained for graphic rendering while volumetric data is used for haptic feedback. Novel sources of feedback are incorporated into the simulation platform, including synthetic drill sounds based on experimental data and simulated monitoring of virtual nerve bundles. Realistic behavior is modeled for a variety of surgical drill burrs, rendering the environment suitable for training low-level drilling skills. The system allows two users to independently observe and manipulate a common model, and allows one user to experience the forces generated by the other's contact with the bone surface. This permits an instructor to remotely observe a trainee and provide real-time feedback and demonstration.

1 Introduction

1.1 Temporal Bone Surgery

Several common otologic surgical procedures – including mastoidectomy, acoustic neuroma resection, and cochlear implantation – involve drilling within the temporal bone to access critical anatomy within the middle ear, inner ear, and skull base. As computer simulation is becoming a more frequently used technique in surgical training and planning, this class of procedures has emerged as a strong candidate for simulation-based learning.

The time spent on a procedure in this area is typically dominated by bone removal, which is performed with a series of burrs (rotary drill heads) of varying sizes and surface properties. Larger burrs are generally used for gross bone removal in the early part of a procedure, while smaller burrs are used for finer work in the vicinity of target anatomy. Surgeons employ a variety of strokes and contact techniques to precisely control bone removal while minimizing the risk of vibration and uncontrolled drill motion that could jeopardize critical structures. Drills are generally driven by

C. Barillot, D.R. Haynor, and P. Hellier (Eds.): MICCAI 2004, LNCS 3217, pp. 319–327, 2004.
© Springer-Verlag Berlin Heidelberg 2004

pneumatic pressure, which is regulated by a floor-mounted footswitch. A combined irrigation/suction instrument is typically used to keep the contact area moist and to remove accumulated blood and bone dust.

The primary risks to patient safety emerge from drilling in close proximity to the facial and vestibulocochlear nerves, which can be damaged as a result of vibration, heat, and direct contact with instruments. Electrodes are typically placed on the face and neck to monitor nerve activity; these electrodes are critical in allowing surgeons to locate and avoid injury to nerve bundles.

Surgery is typically performed using a binocular microscope. Some soft tissue work is required, including skin incision, muscle retraction, elevation of the tympanic membrane (eardrum), displacement of brain and nerve, and removal of lesions.

1.2 Current Training Techniques

Resident surgical training typically includes dissection of preserved human temporal bones. This allows residents to become acquainted with the mechanical aspects of drilling, but does not incorporate physiological information, continuous feedback for hazard avoidance, or soft tissue work. Temporal bone labs are also costly to maintain, and cadaver specimens can be difficult to obtain in sufficient quantity. This approach also limits the precision with which an instructor can monitor a trainee's drilling performance, as the instructor cannot feel the fine details of the trainee's interaction with the bone surface, and cannot easily share the drill and bone surface for demonstration. A further limitation of cadaver-based training is that instructors have little or no mechanism for controlling anatomic variations or the presence of specific pathology that can lead to challenging training scenarios.

Interactive atlases such as [6] are available for training regional anatomy. Two-dimensional simulations [3] are available for high-level procedure training.

2 Previous Work

Previous work in interactive simulation of temporal bone surgery [2,4,9] has focused primarily on haptic rendering of volumetric data. Agus et al [2] have developed an analytical model of bone erosion as a function of applied drilling force and rotational velocity, which they have verified with experimental data. Petersik et al [9] model their drilling instrument as a point cloud, and use a modified version of the Voxmap-Pointshell algorithm [10] to sample the surface of the drill and generate appropriate forces at each sampled point. Each of these projects has incorporated haptic feedback into volumetric simulation environments that make use of CT and MR data and use volume-rendering techniques for graphical display.

Agus et al [1] describe several enhancements to their simulation environment that incorporate additional skills, including the use of irrigation and suction; and additional sources of intraoperative feedback, including real-time rendering of bone dust.

The system described in this paper draws on the haptic rendering algorithms presented in the above work. In order to extend training efforts beyond physical skills and to focus on clinical decision-making, we extend this work to allow tool-specific haptic rendering, networked interaction among users, realistic auditory feedback based on experimental recordings, and physiological monitoring of simulated nerves. Each of these features represents a key skill or source of feedback required for effective temporal bone surgery training and/or rehearsal. We also incorporate a representation of soft tissues that is not available in purely volumetric simulators.

3 Methods

3.1 Haptic Rendering of Volumetric Data

We use a volumetric representation of bone for haptic rendering, which presents several advantages for drilling simulation. Volumetric data can be derived either from patient-specific CT data or from manually-assembled surface models [7], so this approach generalizes to a variety of data sources. A voxel representation also allows computationally inexpensive collision-detection for points (via direct indexing) and removal or density reduction of solid material. In our system, voxels are stored in a compact hash table; each voxel is associated with color, surface normal, and density information.

Virtual instruments are controlled using a SensAble Phantom [8] haptic feedback device, which provides three-degree-of-freedom force-feedback and six-degree-of-freedom positional input. Users can select from a variety of drills, including diamond and cutting burrs ranging from three to seven millimeters in diameter.

We adopt a haptic feedback approach similar to [9], in which the drill is represented as a cloud of sample points, distributed approximately uniformly around the surface of a spherical burr (we use 82 sample points). At each time step, each sample point is tested for contact with bone tissue. By tracing a ray from each immersed sample point toward the center of the tool, the system can generate a contact force that acts to move that sample point out of the bone volume. The net effect is a realistic sense of mechanical contact between drill and bone [9].

Our system associates a "drilling power" with each sample point; as each traced ray passes through a voxel, it removes an amount of bone density that depends on the drilling power of the sample point and the distance of the voxel from the instrument's main axis. These parameters allow us to simulate key aspects of drill/bone contact, particularly the fact that the equatorial surface of the burr carries a larger linear velocity than the polar surface and thus removes more bone per unit of applied force. The precise distribution of drilling power and the dependence of bone removal on axial distance are varied with the type of drill being used, which allows us to model critical differences among burr types. For example, our model captures the fact that cutting burrs typically show more dependence on drilling angle than diamond burrs do.

Voxels are stored in an in-memory hash table. When a voxel's density reaches zero, it is removed and is no longer accessed for haptic or graphic rendering.

A key aspect of the haptic sensation associated with drilling is the vibration of the instrument, which varies with applied force and with burr type. In order to generate realistic drill vibration frequencies, we outfitted a physical drill with an accelerometer and collected vibration data at a variety of applied drilling forces. These data are summarized in FIGURE 1. The key spectral peaks were identified for each burr type and used to synthesize vibrations during the simulation. Since we are driving our haptic feedback device at only 1 kHz, we are able to preserve only the lower-frequency vibrations identified from these experimental recordings. However, we are able to preserve the variations in vibration associated with changes in burr type and/or changes in applied drilling force.

Our goal in drill modeling is not necessarily to simulate every detail of physical reality, but to allow enough system parameterization for an experienced surgeon to tune the experimentally-based parameters. With this in mind, we have parameterized all of the values discussed in this section – bone removal rate, dependence of bone removal on axial position, and vibration amplitude and fundamental frequency – and made them available via on-screen sliders in a "tuning" version of our system. Initial work with an otologist within our group has allowed us to determine effective values for each of these parameters.

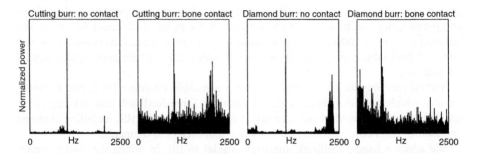

Fig. 1. A spectral representation of drill vibration, collected from cutting and diamond drilling burrs, when in contact with bone and when powered but held away from the bone surface. Only the low spectral peaks have been plotted; those are the vibrations that can be captured with a typical haptic rendering device. The sharp spectral peaks make this data suitable for real-time vibration synthesis.

3.2 A Hybrid Data Structure for Graphic Rendering

Volumetric data is well-suited for haptic simulation of bone removal, as it allows rapid collision detection and efficient removal of material units. However, direct rendering of volumetric data – while appropriate for visualization of transparent volumes – limits the degree to which primarily opaque surfaces (such as bone) can be realistically displayed, due to resolution limitations. Furthermore, a purely volumetric system will be unable to leverage the current trend toward increasingly powerful surface-rendering capabilities in graphics hardware.

With that in mind, our system maintains a hybrid data structure in which voxel data is used for haptic rendering and bone manipulation (as is described above), and triangulated surfaces are used for graphic rendering. Voxel locations are used directly as triangle vertices. When a voxel model is loaded into our system, the following algorithm is performed to isolate a polygonal surface that bounds the underlying voxels:

```
for each voxel v1 that is on the bone surface
  for each of v1's neighbors v2 that is on the bone surface
    for each of v2's neighbors v3 that is on the bone surface
      generate a triangle (v1,v2,v3) oriented away from the bone surface
```

Normals and texture coordinates for each voxel are derived from information embedded in the voxel data file, which is generated by flood-filling a temporal bone surface model [7]. Redundant triangles are eliminated by assigning a unique integer ID to all voxels and rejecting all triangles whose vertex ID's do not appear in sorted order. Further culling of subsurface (and thus invisible) triangles is performed according to [5]. To permit backface culling, each triangle is oriented to face outward by comparing its surface normal with the average of the normals at each vertex.

Each time a voxel is removed, all triangles containing that voxel are removed from the rendering list, and the above algorithm is repeated locally, for each neighbor of the removed voxel that is now part of the bone surface. The local density gradient is also computed at each voxel bordering the removed voxel, to allow normal recalculation, and texture coordinates are propagated to newly-revealed voxels. In this manner, a consistent bounding mesh is maintained, with limited (constant-time) computation performed each time the surface is modified. FIGURE 2 shows a bone surface that has been modified by a drill, along with the underlying volumetric representation.

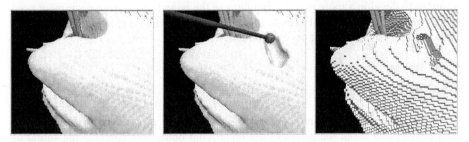

Fig. 2. Interactive bone-drilling simulation. 2a (left): a smooth surface representation of a temporal bone model. 2b (center): virtual drilling of this surface; the surface is re-meshed as voxels are removed. 2c (right): an opaque rendering of the underlying volumetric representation of the surface, which is used for haptic feedback.

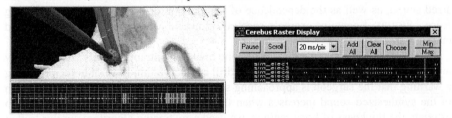

Fig. 3. (a) Left: a virtual drilling procedure that requires drilling in the vicinity of simulated nerves. The bottom of the display represents a virtual neurophysiology monitor; note the bursts of activity resulting from close contact with the drill. (b) Right: A remote system monitors the activity of multiple simulated neurons.

3.3 Neurophysiology Monitoring

Neural electrodes are often used during temporal bone surgery to monitor the facial and/or auditory nerves. The output from these electrodes – typically monitored by a dedicated individual or team – is used to guide navigational decisions. Our system thus incorporates a set of virtual nerves (displayed in FIGURE 3a), whose firing rate increases with proximity of an active drilling tool, but decreases with prolonged drill proximity or direct drill contact. The user can also safely stimulate virtual nerves using an electrical stimulator tool; this is analogous to the direct stimulation performed in the OR in conjunction with electrode monitoring, used to locate critical nerves that are not immediately visible.

An activity monitor can be displayed on the surgeon's display, as is shown in FIGURE 3, and sound can be presented to represent a neural spike train. Since nerve monitoring in certain procedures involves a dedicated neurophysiology team, our system also exports neural activity over a local network for monitoring on another computer. More specifically, our simulator emulates the Cerebus (CyberKinetics, Inc.) neural recording system, a recording amplifier and digitizer used in human and animal neurophysiology research. This allows us to use a variety of visualization tools to present neural activity to users or instructors, who may be monitoring a trainee's performance. Furthermore, the flexible client architecture will eventually allow us to develop a more precise simulator of the neural monitoring equipment used intraoperatively. FIGURE 3b shows a screenshot from the Cerebus client software, demonstrating the activity of several simulated nerves.

3.4 Sound

Sound is a key source of intraoperative feedback, as it provides information about drill contact and about the nature of the underlying bone. We simulate the sound of the virtual burr as a series of noisy harmonics, whose frequency modulates with applied drilling force. Building upon the harmonic-based synthesis approach presented in [4], we have recorded audio data from cutting and diamond drill burrs under a series of drilling forces in order to determine the appropriate frequencies for synthesized sound, as well as the dependence of this data on drill type and applied drilling force. FIGURE 4 contains example spectral information collected from diamond and cutting burrs.

Sound can also be a key indicator of bone thickness intraoperatively; sound quality and frequency change significantly as the drill contacts a thin layer of bone, providing a warning that the surgeon is approaching sensitive tissue. In our simulator, the pitch of the synthesized sound increases when the drilled area becomes thin. In order to estimate the thickness of bone regions, we used a raytracing algorithm similar to that used for haptic rendering. At each voxel that is determined to be on the surface of the bone, the surface gradient is used to approximate the surface normal, and a ray is cast into the bone along this normal. The ray is traced until it emerges from the bone volume, and the thickness is estimated as the distance from the ray's entry point to its exit point. For sound synthesis, this thickness is averaged over all surface voxels with which the drill is in contact. The computed thickness values are also used to visually shade thin bone, which tends to appear red and translucent as the drill approaches soft tissue.

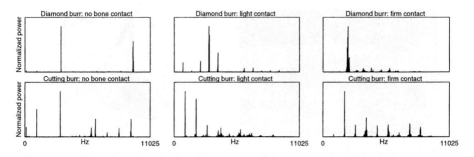

Fig. 4. A spectral representation of audio data collected from diamond (top) and cutting (bottom) drilling burrs. Columns represent no bone contact, bone contact without significant pressure, and bone contact with a typical drilling pressure (applied by an experienced surgeon). The sharp spectral peaks and distinct variation among drill types and contact forces make this data suitable for real-time synthesis.

3.5 Collaborative Networking

A key advantage of simulation-based training is the ability for multiple users to observe and manipulate a common model without interfering with each other's actions. For example, it is useful for an instructor to be able to (possibly remotely) monitor a trainee's performance, and interactively provide feedback and demonstrations.

With this in mind, our system allows a second user to log in via Ethernet and interact with the bone model. We assume that the model is available at both stations, so only model modifications and drill positions/forces need to be sent over the network. We use a private gigabit Ethernet intranet, which allows us to send a continuous stream of position and force data with minimal latency (approximately 5ms).

Additionally, rather than interacting directly with the local model, a user can choose to drive his haptic device using the forces that are generated by the remote user's drill. This allows a surgeon to demonstrate proper drilling technique while a trainee actually experiences the corresponding contact forces, something that is not possible with traditional training techniques. The ability to send forces at haptic update rates allows even high-frequency vibrations to be rendered remotely.

3.6 Soft Tissue Simulation

A training surgeon using a temporal bone simulator will benefit from a logical representation of initial soft tissue incisions and – where appropriate – lesion resection. Our environment uses a system of masses and springs to simulate layers of skin and muscle that can be cut and displaced interactively (see FIGURE 5).

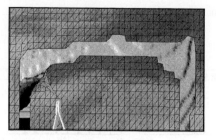
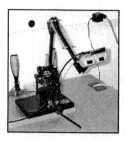

Fig. 5. (left): Skin, modeled as a 3-d mesh of masses and springs, is interactively cut and retracted to reveal the underlying bone volume

Fig. 6. (right): The binocular stereo display and haptic rendering device used for simulation.

3.7 System Architecture

Our simulation environment runs in Windows XP on a 2-CPU 3GHz Xeon with 1GB RAM, using a SensAble Phantom for haptic feedback. OpenGL is used for graphic rendering; each bone surface mesh is rendered as a single vertex array, embedded in a display list. STL hash tables are used to represent voxel information and the mapping from voxels to vertex arrays. A high-priority thread handles all bone interaction, haptic rendering, and networking; reorganizations of the polygon mesh are queued by this thread and performed at graphic update rates by the rendering thread.

The scene is rendered in stereo using either shutter glasses or a binocular display consisting of two small LCD's mounted on an adjustable arm, depicted in FIGURE 6. The latter is analogous to the binocular microscope used intraoperatively.

The virtual drill is enabled and disabled using a floor-mounted switch, which simulates the foot-controlled pneumatic valve that is typically used for regulating drill power. The switch is interfaced via the workstation's parallel port.

4 Conclusion and Future Work

We have collaborated with a Stanford otologist to iteratively refine our simulation. Force and sound data are based on experimental results, but wherever possible, we allow physical parameters to be tuned online. The result is an effective simulation of the haptic and auditory components of drilling.

This paper focuses on novel sources of feedback that are not available in other temporal bone simulation environments; in the next iteration of our simulator, we plan to include additional features that have been previously described in [2], including a particle-based simulation of blood, dust, irrigation, and suction.

Our current source of data is a series of surface models of temporal bone structures, manually created by an otologist in our group. The use of surface models allows us high rendering resolution, provides texture-mapping and normal information for each surface voxel, and will allow us to leverage existing modeling packages as we move toward "scenario training", in which an instructor will be able to modify patient anatomy directly to prepare specific challenges and complications. However, we also plan to incorporate direct use of patient-specific CT data in the next revision of our simulator, a natural extension of our underlying volumetric representation. Also, we are currently applying this work to related procedures and data sets in dental and craniofacial surgery.

Acknowledgements. We thank P. Fong for discussions on rendering, K. Chun for his display mount, and T. Krummel and R. Jackler for consultations. Support was provided by NIH LM07295, BioX 2DMA178, and the NDSEG and Stanford fellowships.

References

1. Agus, M,. Giachetti, A., Gobbetti, E., Zanetti, G., Zorcolo, A.: A multiprocessor decoupled system for the simulation of temporal bone surgery. Comp Vis in Science, 5(1): 35-43, 2002
2. Agus, M,. Giachetti, A., Gobbetti, E., Zanetti, G., John, N.W., Stone, R.J.: Mastoidectomy simulation with combined visual and haptic feedback. Proc of the Medicine Meets Virtual Reality 2002 Conference, Newport Beach, CA, Jan. 23-26, 2002
3. Blevins, N.H., Jackler, R.K., Gralapp, C: Temporal Bone Dissector. Mosby, January 1998.
4. Bryan, J., Stredney, D., Wiet, G., Sessanna, D.: Virtual Temporal Bone Dissection: A Case Study. Proc. of IEEE Visualization 2001, Ertl et. Al., (Eds): 497-500, October 2001.
5. Bouvier, D.J.: Double-Time Cubes: A Fast 3D Surface Construction Algorithm for Volume Visualization. Int'l Conf on Imaging Science, Systems, and Technology, June 1997.
6. Hohne, K.H., Bomans, M., Riemer, M., Schubert, R., Tiede, U., Lierse, W.: A 3D anatomical atlas based on a volume model. IEEE Visualization 1992, 12 (1992) 72-78
7. Kaufman, A., Shimony, E.: 3D Scan-Conversion Algorithms for Voxel-Based Graphics. Proc ACM Workshop on Interactive 3D Graphics. Chapel Hill, NC, Oct 1986, 45-76.
8. Massie, T.H., Salisbury, J.K.: The PHANTOM Haptic Interface: A Device for Probing Virtual Objects. Symp. on Haptic Interfaces for Virtual Environments. Chicago, IL, Nov. 1994.
9. Petersik, A., Pflesser, B., Tiede, U., Hohne K.H., Leuwer, R.: Haptic Volume Interaction with Anatomic Models at Sub-Voxel Resolution. Proc IEEE VR, Orlando, FL, Mar 2002.
10. Renz, M., Preusche, C., Potke, M., Kriegel, H.P., Hirzinger, G.: Stable haptic interaction with virtual environments using an adapted voxmap-pointshell algorithm. Proc Eurohaptics, p149-154, 2001.

3D Computational Mechanical Analysis for Human Atherosclerotic Plaques Using MRI-Based Models with Fluid-Structure Interactions

Dalin Tang,[1] Chun Yang,[2] Jie Zheng,[3] Pamela K. Woodard,[3] Gregorio A. Sicard,[4] Jeffrey E. Saffitz,[5] Shunichi Kobayashi,[6] Thomas K Pilgram,[3] and Chun Yuan[7]

[1]Mathematical Sciences Department, Worcester Polytechnic Institute, Worcester, MA 01609, USA, dtang@wpi.edu
[2]Mathematics Dept, Beijing Normal University, Beijing, China, chyang0@btamail.net.cn
[3]Mallinkcrodt Institute of Radiology, Washington University, St. Louis, MO 63110, USA
Jie Zheng: zhengj@mir.wustl.edu; Pamela Woodard: woodardp@mir.wustl.edu
[4]Department of Surgery, Washington University, St. Louis, MO 63110, USA, sicardg@msnotes.wustl.edu
[5]Dept of Pathology, Washington Universty, St. Louis, MO 63110, USA, saffitz@pathbox.wustl.edu
[6]Dept. of Functional Machinery and Mechanics, Shinshu Univ., Nagano, Japan, shukoba@giptc.shinshu-u.ac.jp
[7]Deparment of Radiology, University of Washington, Seattle, WA 98195, USA, cyuan@u.washington.edu

Abstract. Atherosclerotic plaques may rupture without warning and cause acute cardiovascular syndromes such as heart attack and stroke. It is believed that mechanical forces play an important role in plaque progression and rupture. A three-dimensional (3D) MRI-based finite-element model with multi-component plaque structure and fluid-structure interactions (FSI) is introduced to perform mechanical analysis for human atherosclerotic plaques and identify critical flow and stress/strain conditions which may be related to plaque rupture. The coupled fluid and structure models are solved by ADINA, a well-tested finite-element package. Our results indicate that pressure conditions, plaque structure, component size and location, material properties, and model assumptions all have considerable effects on flow and plaque stress/strain behaviors. Large-scale patient studies are needed to validate the computational findings. This FSI model provides more complete stress/strain analysis and better interpretation of information from MR images and may lead to more accurate plaque vulnerability assessment and rupture predictions.

1 Introduction

Cardiovascular disease (CVD) is the No. 1 killer in the developed countries and is responsible for millions of deaths and disabilities every year. Atherosclerotic plaques may rupture without warning and cause subsequential acute syndromes such as

C. Barillot, D.R. Haynor, and P. Hellier (Eds.): MICCAI 2004, LNCS 3217, pp. 328–336, 2004.

myocardial infarction and cerebral stroke. A large number of victims of the disease who are apparently healthy die suddenly without prior symptoms. Available screening and diagnostic methods are insufficient to identify the victims before the event occurs [4]. Accurate methods are needed to identify vulnerable plaques that are prone to rupture and quantify conditions under which plaque rupture may occur.

MRI technologies have been developed to quantify non-invasively plaque size, shape, and plaque components (fibrous, lipid, and calcification/inflammation) [9]. In addition to plaque morphology and components, mechanical forces clearly play an important role in the rupture process. Mechanical analysis based on MR images has been proposed but is mainly limited to structure-only (2D or 3D) or flow-only (3D) models due to complexity of the problem [3,8]. Accurate flow and stress/strain analysis for plaque rupture predictions using 3D computational modeling with fluid-structure interactions (FSI) based on 3D MRI human plaque morphology and constituents is lacking in the literature.

In this paper, a finite-element 3D FSI model is introduced based on realistic human atherosclerotic plaque morphology and components to perform flow and plaque stress/strain analysis and quantify critical stress/strain conditions under which plaque rupture is likely to occur. 3D plaque geometry will be re-constructed from MR images. Vessel and plaque material properties from our own *in vitro* measurements [6] and existing literature [3,8] are used in the solid models. A typical pressure profile for human internal carotid artery was used to observe stress/strain behavior under pulsating pressure. The coupled fluid and solid models are solved by a finite element package ADINA which is capable of handling multi-physics models with fluid-structure interactions [1,2]. Sensitivity analysis was performed to quantify the effects of controlling factors (pressure condition, material properties, plaque structure, lipid size, plaque cap thickness, calcification, axial stretch) on critical plaque stress/strain conditions (maxima and minima of stress/strain values and their variations corresponding to various changes). Critical stress/strain values were compared with semi-quantitative histopathological plaque vulnerability assessment and some indicative correlation patterns were found.

2   The Computational Model and Method

2.1   3D Re-construction of Plaque Geometry Based on MRI Data

3D *ex vivo* MRI data sets obtained from human atherosclerotic plaques consisting of 32-64 2D slices with high resolution (0.1mm x 0.1mm x 0.5mm) were read by VTK [5] and 3D plaque geometry and mesh were re-constructed following the procedure described in [7]. Intensive interactions and additional programming from the operator/researcher were needed due to the complexity of plaque morphology and components. Boundary lines for various plaque components were generated according to segmentation data ranges validated by histological analysis. Fig. 1 shows 24 MRI slices (selected from a set of 36 slices) of a cadaveric plaque sample, plaque component contour plots based on histological segmentation data, and the re-constructed 3D geometry. The diameter of the vessel is about 5-6 mm. Resolution is

0.25mm × 0.23mm × 0.5mm. Some smoothing was applied. The vessel was extended uniformly at both ends by 3 cm and 6 cm respectively so that it became long enough for our simulations.

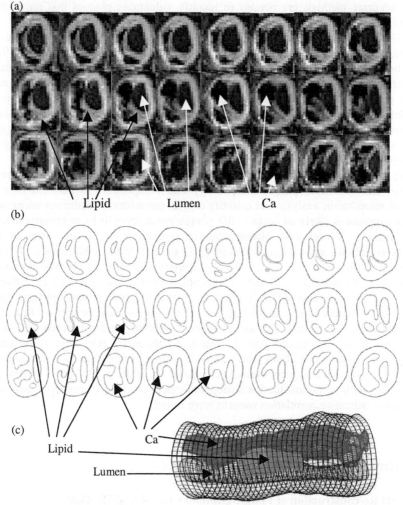

Fig. 1. A cadaveric plaque sample with large calcification block and a lipid pool. a) Selected MR images from a 36-slice set (S9-S33, from left to right); b) Component segmentations of MR images based on histopathological data. Some smoothing was applied; c) Re-constructed 3D plaque geometry. The position of the vessel is rotated for better viewing

2.2 The Solid and Fluid Models

Both artery wall and plaque components in the plaque were assumed to be hyperelastic, isotropic, incompressible and homogeneous. The flow was assumed to be laminar, Newtonian, viscous and incompressible. The incompressible Navier-

Stokes equations with arbitrary Lagrangian-Eulerian (ALE) formulation were used as the governing equations which are suitable for FSI problems with frequent mesh adjustments. No-slip condition was assumed at all interfaces. Putting these together, we have (summation convention is used):

$$\rho(\partial \mathbf{u}/\partial t + ((\mathbf{u} - \mathbf{u_g}) \cdot \nabla) \mathbf{u}) = -\nabla p + \mu \nabla^2 \mathbf{u}, \quad \nabla \cdot \mathbf{u} = 0, \tag{1}$$

$$\mathbf{u}|_\Gamma = \partial \mathbf{x}/\partial t, \quad \partial \mathbf{u}/\partial n|_{inlet, \, outlet} = 0, \tag{2}$$

$$p|_{inlet} = p_{in}(t), \quad p|_{outlet} = p_{out}(t), \tag{3}$$

$$\rho \, v_{i,tt} = \sigma_{ij,j}, \quad i,j=1,2,3; \text{ sum over } j, \qquad \text{(eq. of motion for solids)} \tag{4}$$

$$\varepsilon_{ij} = (v_{i,j} + v_{j,i})/2, \quad i, j=1,2,3, \qquad \text{(strain-displacement)} \tag{5}$$

$$\sigma_{ij} \cdot n_j|_{out\_wall} = 0, \quad \sigma^r_{ij} \cdot n_j|_{interface} = \sigma^s_{ij} \cdot n_j|_{interface}, \tag{6}$$

where $\mathbf{u}$ and p are fluid velocity and pressure, $\mathbf{u_g}$ is mesh velocity, Γ stands for vessel inner boundary, $f_{\bullet,j}$ stands for derivative of f with respect to the jth variable, σ is stress tensor (superscripts indicate different materials), ε is strain tensor, v is solid displacement vector. The 3D nonlinear modified Mooney-Rivlin (M-R) model was used to describe the material properties of the vessel wall and plaque components [1,2]. The strain energy function is given by,

$$W = c_1 (I_1 - 3) + c_2 (I_2 - 3) + D_1 [\exp(D_2 (I_1 - 3)) - 1], \tag{7}$$

$$I_1 = \sum C_{ii}, \quad I_2 = \frac{1}{2} [I_1^2 - C_{ij} C_{ij}], \tag{8}$$

where I_1 and I_2 are the first and second strain invariants [1,2], c_i and D_i are material constants. The stress/strain relations can be found by:

$$\sigma_{ij} = (\partial W/\partial \varepsilon_{ij} + \partial W/\partial \varepsilon_{ji})/2, \tag{9}$$

where σ_{ij} are the second Piola-Kirchhoff stresses, ε_{ji} are the Green-Lagrange strains.

In this paper, the following values were chosen to match experimental data and existing literature [3,6,8]: Artery wall (including fibrous cap): c_1=92,000 dyn•cm^{-2}, c_2=0, D_1=36,000 dyn•cm^{-2}, D_2=2; Lipid: c_1=5,000 dyn•cm^{-2}, c_2=0, D_1=5,000dyn•cm^{-2}, D_2=1.5; Calcification: c_1=920,000 dyn•cm^{-2}, c_2=0, D_1=360,000 dyn•cm^{-2}, D_2=2.

2.3 Solution Method

The fully coupled fluid and structure models were solved by a commercial finite-element package ADINA (ADINA R & D, Inc., Watertown, MA, USA) which has been tested by hundreds of real-life applications [2] and has been used by Tang in the last several years [6,7]. ADINA uses unstructured finite element methods for both fluid and solid models. Nonlinear incremental iterative procedures are used to handle fluid-structure interactions. The governing finite element equations for both the solid and fluid models are solved by Newton-Raphson iteration method. Proper mesh was chosen to fit the shape of each component, the vessel, and the fluid domain. Finer mesh was used for thin plaque cap and components with sharp angles to get better resolution and handle high stress concentration behaviors. The artery was stretched axially and pressurized gradually to specified conditions. Mesh analysis was performed until differences between solutions from two consecutive meshes were negligible (less than 1% in L_2-norm). Details of the computational models and solution methods can be found from Bathe [1,2] and Tang et al [6,7].

3 Results and Conclusion

Simulations were performed using several plaque samples under various conditions to investigate stress/strain behaviors and their correlations with pressure conditions, plaque morphology, plaque structure, and plaque vulnerability as determined by histopathological analysis. Only selected results are presented here.

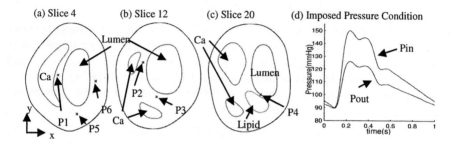

Fig. 2. Normal and critical points are selected to track stress/strain variations. P1: from calcification cap; P2: from a thicker Ca cap; P3: from a thicker Ca cap; P4: from a thin lipid cap (most vulnerable site); P5: normal point to observe stress-xx; P6: normal point to observe stress-yy. (a)-(c) give locations of the 6 points and 3 slices from the plaque sample (Fig. 1); (d) Imposed upstream pressure (Pin) and down-stream pressure (Pout) used for the simulation

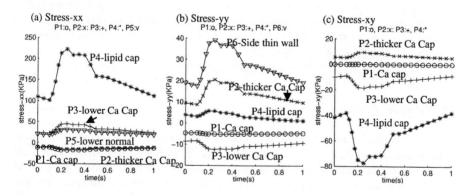

Fig. 3. Tracking of stress components at selected sites under pulsating pressure showing critical point from the thin lipid cap has much greater stress variations. (a) Normal stress in x-direction (Stress-xx); (b) Normal stress in y-direction (Stress-yy); (c) Shear component (stress-xy)

3.1 Unsteady Stress/Strain Behaviors at Critical Sites Under Pulsating Pressure

Blood flow is pulsatile. Blood vessel and atherosclerotic plaque are subjected to strong pulsating pressure conditions and the corresponding stress/strain behaviors are worthy investigating. We hypothesize that relative stress/strain variations in the plaque under pulsating pressure may correlate with plaque rupture risk. Using the plaque sample given by Fig. 1, several critical points were selected from various sites to observe stress/strain variations under pulsating pressure (Fig. 2). A human carotid pressure profile was scaled to 90-150 mmHg range and used in the simulation. Down-stream pressure (Pout) was chosen so that flow rate was physiological (between 2-15 ml/s). Fig. 3 shows that the thin cap point (Point 4) shows much greater (>400%) stress variation than other points. Stress-yy from Point 4 was smaller because of the orientation of the cap. The large stress-yy variation from Point 6 (a normal point) is a false alarm caused by vessel thickness. These initial results indicate that stress/strain variations do carry useful information. However, they must be examined carefully, and plaque structure, cap thickness, component size and shape must be taken into consideration. Relevance of these findings with respect to plaque vulnerability needs to be established using histopathological and clinical data.

3.2 Effect of Material Properties of Arteries and Plaque Components

Using our models, we can change material parameters to perform sensitivity analysis to observe their impact on stress/strain distributions. Since calcification is much stiffer (almost rigid) than normal tissue, lipid is much softer than normal tissue, when their volumes are relatively small compared to the total plaque volume (i.e., they are not the main structure for the whole solid model), their stiffness changes (such as 50% reduction, 100% increase) do not alter stress/strain distributions much (less than 2% from some of our samples [7]); For vessel material test, when vessel stiffness was increased by 100% (by changing c_1 and D_1 values, using the plaque with small lipid pools), maximum stress values were almost unchanged (changes were less than 2%) while maximum strain values were reduced by about 50%. However, for a plaque sample with 30% calcification (shown by Fig. 1), contrary to what was observed from the plaque sample with smaller lipid pools, Fig. 4 and Table 1 show clearly that vessel material properties have considerable effect on maximum values of stress components (50%-100% differences). While calcification did not show much dominance in Stress-P1 and Stress-xx plots, it is dominant in Stress-zz plot due to the 5% axial stretch. Softer vessel case shows greater maximum stress values (about 40-50% increase for most of the components, 65% for Stress-xy, 92% for Stress-yy) because calcification component took more load compared to vessel part. For the same reason, stiffer vessel case shows lower maximum stress values because calcification component was taking less load. It should be noted that these results are still of indicative nature because material properties for the vessel and plaque components were not measured directly for the samples simulated. Direct measurement of plaque component properties will be very desirable and will improve accuracy and reliability of computational findings. However, it is beyond the scope of our current research.

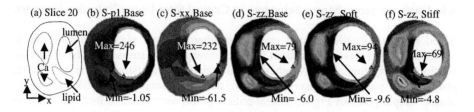

Fig. 4. Plots of selected stress components from the 3D model with different vessel material parameters showing that vessel material properties have considerable effect on stress distributions. Pin=150 mmHg, Pout=126 mmHg, pre-stretch=5%. Material parameters were chosen so that the softer vessel is about 50% softer than baseline vessel and stiffer vessel is about 100% stiffer than baseline vessel. a) Slice 20 showing component shapes and positions; b) Stress-p1 from baseline model showing maximum stress at the thin plaque cap; c) Stress-xx from baseline model; d) Stress-zz from baseline model showing stress concentration in calcified region; e) Stress-zz from soft vessel model; f) Stress-zz from the stiff vessel model

Table 1. Maximum stress values from Slice 20 and Slice 4 of the large calcification plaque sample. Slice 4 is used because it does not contain lipid pool

Cases	S-P1	S-xx	S-xy	S-xz	S-yy	S-yz	S-zz
Case 1: Baseline, 5% stretch	245	231	161	3.3	150	11.2	79.3
Case 2: Softer vessel	373	355	266	4.9	288	16.0	94
Case 3: Stiffer vessel	187	172	85	3.6	75	9.4	69.4
Case 4: Baseline,10% Stretch	247	229	161	4.4	146	13.9	107
Case 5: S4, baseline, no lipid	259	241	82	6.0	51	6.4	51

3.3 Identifying Critical Stress/Strain Indicators for Plaque Vulnerability Assessment

Atherosclerotic plaques have complex structures.   Stress/strain tensors have 12 components (6 each), their distributions in plaque region have complex patterns, and their dynamic behaviors are even more difficult to analyze.   We examine every stress/strain component in the plaque, under steady and pulsating pressures, seeking the right critical indicators.   Some "candidate indicators" are: **i)** Global and local max/min values of each stress/strain component corresponding to maximum pressure condition.   These include local max/min values at thin plaque caps, sharp angle of lipid pools and other possible locations; **ii)** maximum stress/strain variations under pulsating pressure; **iii)** maximum stress/strain space variations (concentration) as represented by the derivatives of stress/strain tensors; **iv)** maximum cyclic stretch and compression as indicated by strain components under pulsating pressure.

The following scheme was used to identify possible critical stress/strain risk indicators.   Histopathological analysis was performed to quantify plaque vulnerability (V) and 5 grades were assigned to each plaque: very stable, V=0; stable, V=1; slightly unstable, V=2; unstable, V=3; and vulnerable, V=4, according to cap thickness, pool size, lumen surface conditions, and various cell counts (Fig. 5). Statistical analysis was performed to find correlation between "critical stress/strain indicators" and plaque vulnerability. Initial results have been obtained from 11 plaques using 2D models [8]. Our results indicate that there are positive correlations between Stress-P1 and plaque vulnerability, lipid pool area ratio, and a negative correlation with plaque cap thickness. More 3D samples are needed to perform the analysis using 3D results.

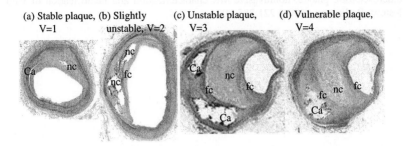

(a) Stable plaque, (b) Slightly   (c) Unstable plaque,   (d) Vulnerable plaque,
V=1   unstable, V=2   V=3   V=4

Fig. 5. Selected histological images of coronary plaques. V value is pathological classification of plaque vulnerability. nc= necrotic lipid core; fc = fibrous cap; m = matrix; Ca = calcification

3.4 Conclusion

Considerably higher stress/strain variations under pulsating pressure are observed at thin plaque cap. Calcification volume and vessel material properties have large impact on stress distributions. With sufficient validations, critical stress/strain indicators may be used for plaque vulnerability assessment.

Acknowledgement. This research was supported in part by NSF grant DMS-0072873 and a grant from the Rockefeller Foundation. J Zheng is supported in part by a Charles E. Culpeper Biomedical Pilot initiative grant 01-273.

References

1. Bathe, K.J.: Finite Element Procedures. Prentice Hall, New Jersey, (1996)
2. Bathe, K.J.: Theory and Modeling Guide, Vol I: ADINA; Vol II: ADINA-F, ADINA R&D, Inc., Watertown, MA, (2002)
3. Huang, H., Virmani, R., Younis, H., Burke, A.P., Kamm, R.D., Lee, R.T.: The impact of calcification on the biomechanical stability of atherosclerotic plaques. Circulation (2001) 103: 1051-1056.
4. Naghavi M, et al. (57 co-authors including C. Yuan): From vulnerable plaque to vulnerable patient: a call for new definitions and risk assessment strategies: Part I. Circulation. (2003) 108(14):1664-72.
5. Schroeder W, Martin K, Lorensen B, The Visualization Toolkit, An Object-Oriented Approach To 3D Graphics, Prentice Hall, 2nd Edition, (1998)
6. Tang, D., Yang, C., Kobayashi, S., Ku, D.N.: Effect of a lipid pool on stress/strain distributions in stenotic arteries: 3D FSI models. J. Biomech. Engng, (2004) In press.

7. Tang, D., Yang, C., Zheng, J., Woodard, P.K., Sicard, G.A., Saffitz, J.E., Yuan, C.: 3D MRI-Based Multi-Component FSI Models for Atherosclerotic Plaques a 3-D FSI model, Annals of Biomedical Engineering. (2004) 32(7):947-960.
8. Williamson SD, Lam Y, Younis HF, Huang H, Patel S, Kaazempur-Mofrad MR, Kamm RD. On the sensitivity of wall stresses in diseased arteries to variable material properties, J. Biomechanical Engineering, (2003) 125, 147-155.
9. Yuan C, Mitsumori LM, Beach KW, Maravilla KR. Special review: Carotid atherosclerotic plaque: noninvasive MR characterization and identification of vulnerable lesions. Radiology. (2001) 221:285-99.

In Silico Tumor Growth: Application to Glioblastomas

Olivier Clatz[1], Pierre-Yves Bondiau[1], Hervé Delingette[1], Grégoire Malandain[1], Maxime Sermesant[1], Simon K. Warfield[2], and Nicholas Ayache[1]

[1] Epidaure - INRIA Sophia Antipolis
[2] CRL - Harvard Medical School

Abstract. We propose a new model to simulate the growth of glioblastomas multiforma (GBM), the most aggressive glial tumors. This model relies upon an anatomical atlas including white fibers diffusion tensor information and the delineation of cerebral structures having a distinct response to the tumor aggression. We simulate both the invasion of the GBM in the brain parenchyma and its mechanical interaction (mass effect) with the invaded structures. The former effect is modeled with a reaction-diffusion equation while the latter is based on a linear elastic brain constitutive equation. In addition, we propose a new equation taking into account the mechanical influence of the tumor cells on the invaded tissues. This tumor growth model is assessed by comparing the virtual GBM growth with the real GBM growth observed between two MRIs of a patient acquired with six months difference.

1 Introduction

1.1 Motivation

The majority of the primitive tumors of the central nervous system are from glial origin, among which the glioblastomas multiforma (GBM) are the most aggressive. Without therapy, patients with GBMs usually die within 10 months. Despite the substantial research effort for improving tumors treatment, patients treated with state-of-the-art therapy have a median survival of approximately 1.5 year.

Relatively little progress has been made toward the construction of a general model describing the growth of these tumors. The interest to carry out a simulation of the tumoral growth for improving the treatment is twofold. First, it could provide additional information about the tumor invasion and help determining the local treatment margins. Second, by quantifying the malignant cell concentration in low contrast areas of MR images, it could also be useful in the selection of the radiotherapy dose.

1.2 Contributions

We propose a patient-specific simulator of glioblastoma growth, including the induced brain deformation (mass effect). The simulation relies upon a Finite

C. Barillot, D.R. Haynor, and P. Hellier (Eds.): MICCAI 2004, LNCS 3217, pp. 337–345, 2004.

Element Model (FEM) initialized from the patient MRIs. Additional information has been included into the patient model to take into account the behavior of different structures with respect to tumor invasion, such as the white matter fiber directions (see [2] for details about the atlas construction). Furthermore, we propose to link the classification of tumors in Gross Tumor Volumes (GTV) proposed in protocols for radiotherapy treatment with different tumor invasion behaviour:

- the GTV1 is associated with the expansion component. By creating new cells, the GTV1 pushes away its surrounding structures. It is therefore responsible for the major mechanical mass effect on the brain. Following cellular expansion models, we propose to use an exponential law to describe the GTV1 volume increase.
- The GTV2 is associated with the diffusion component. It invades adjacent structures by a diffusion process. The GTV2 is thus described in our model with a reaction-diffusion equation. In addition, we propose to link the diffusion process to the mechanical mass effect with a coupling equation.

The model is initialized from an early patient MRI and the simulation is compared to the patient MR images acquired six months later. Compared to

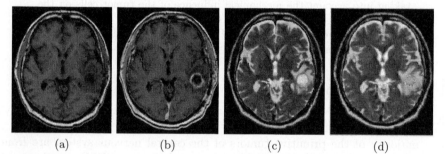

(a)   (b)   (c)   (d)

Fig. 1. MR images of a patient (a) T1; (b) T1 with gadolinium injection; (c) T2; (d) GTV1 (red) and GTV2 (blue) segmentations overlaid on the T2 MRI.

previous works in the tumor growth modeling domain ([7,8,3,4]), our approach includes several improvements:

- the use of diffusion tensor imaging to take into account the anisotropic diffusion process in white fibers.
- The use of the radiotherapy volume classifications to initialize the source of the diffusion component (as opposed to point sources in [7]).
- A new coupling equation between the reaction-diffusion equation and the mechanical constitutive equation.
- Initialization with a patient tumor and comparison with the invasion observed into the later patient MR images.

2   Material and Methods

Our GBM growth simulation consists of two coupled models:

1. a model for the diffusion of the tumor that captures the evolution of the tumor density c over time.
2. A model for the expansion of the tumor that predicts the mass effect induced by the tumor proliferation.

The coupling between these two models is further described in section 3 but it assumes the following behavior : the mass effect is directly related to the tumor density c but the tumor density c is not influenced by the mass effect.

This simple coupling leads to a four steps algorithm:

- **Image segmentation and registration.** The two gross volumes GTV1 and GTV2, are manually delineated by an expert from the patient MR images. The patient MR images are registered with respect to an anatomical atlas. This atlas includes for each voxel the location of the main cerebral structures and a diffusion tensor in the white matter.
- **Meshing and Initialization.** A tetrahedral mesh of the patient's brain is built in the atlas reference frame. Tissue properties are assigned to their associated tetrahedra using the atlas. Furthermore, the value of the tumor density c is initialized based on the GTV1 and GTV2 segmentations by interpolating between the two boundaries.
- **Simulation.** The simulation of the VG (Virtual Glioblastoma) diffusion and expansion is performed on the finite element mesh following the mechanical and diffusion equations.
- **Comparison.** At the end of the growth process, new GTV1, GTV2 and local deformations of the atlas are reported back in the patient images. Therefore, an assessment of the model is performed by comparing the predicted tumor volumes with the ones observed from patient MR image acquired six months later.

3   Glioblastoma Growth Simulation

3.1   Diffusion Model

We rely on the classical reaction-diffusion model ([7]) to account for the growth and the spreading of tumor cells in the GTV2:

$$\underbrace{\frac{\partial c}{\partial t}}_{\text{Tumor density evolution}} = \underbrace{div\left(\underline{D}\,\nabla c\right)}_{\text{Diffusion law}} + \underbrace{S(c,t)}_{\text{Source factor}} - \underbrace{T(c,t)}_{\text{Treatment law}} \qquad (1)$$

In this equation, c represents the normalized cell density ($c \in [0,1]$). The real cell density C is obtained by multiplying c with the carrying capacity of the tissue C_{max} estimated to be equal to $3.5 \times 10^4\,Cells\,mm^{-3}$ [8], $\underline{D}$ represents the local diffusivity of the tissue and depends on the nature of the tissue or, for white matter, of the white fiber directions. Since the goal is only to simulate the tumor growth, we do not consider the treatment term $T(c,t)$ for this model. To minimize the number of tumor-intrinsic parameters, we use a simple linear function to model the source factor, reflecting its aggressiveness: $S(c,t) = \rho c$. The diffusion law 1 can then be written as:

$$\frac{\partial c}{\partial t} = div\left(\underline{\underline{D}}\,\underline{\nabla}c\right) + \rho\,c \tag{2}$$

The local behavior of the tumor therefore only depends on the diffusion tensor $\underline{\underline{D}}$ and the source factor ρ.

Model Parameters and Initialization. We propose the following characteristics for the model:

- since the conductivity of skull and ventricles is null, the flux at the mesh surface is zero: $\underline{J} \cdot \boldsymbol{n} = 0$
- We use the diffusion tensor of the atlas to initialize the diffusion tensor $\underline{\underline{D}}$ in white matter. The intrinsic aggressiveness of the tumor is then controlled by two parameters α and β.
- There are several evidences that glioblastomas diffuse more slowly in the gray matter than in the white matter [7]. Thus diffusivity in gray matter is chosen as a fraction of the maximum diffusivity in white matter $\beta = \frac{D_{white}}{D_{gray}} = \frac{1}{100}$.
- Because tumor cells cannot diffuse through the falx cerebri, we set its diffusivity to zero.
- The GTV1 capacity is fixed to C_{max} as above-defined.
- As discussed in [7], one cannot determine both α and ρ from only two different instants. We thus arbitrarily set $\rho = \frac{\eta}{100}$ (η is defined in section 3.2). The α parameter is then adapted to the GTV2 diffusion speed.

The material diffusivity values are summed up in Table 1. Figure 2 summarizes the diffusion model and the boundary conditions. We use the model of equation 2 to solve the stationary problem, so as to interpolate the c function between the two initial contours delineating the GTV1 and GTV2.

3.2   Mechanical Model

Mechanical Equation. Based on rheological experiments, Miller ([5]) proposed a non-linear constitutive equation for very slow deformations. Since the growing process is extremely slow in our case, and the measured deformation in the parenchyma is in the small deformation range ($\leq 5\%$), we propose to linearize this equation. Choosing the Young modulus $E = 694\,Pa$, the absolute stress error committed on the stress with respect to Miller's model is below $4.2\,Pa$ (see [2] for details). We thus consider linear relationship for both the constitutive equation and the strain computation:

$$\underline{\underline{\sigma}} = \underline{\underline{K}}\,\underline{\underline{\epsilon}} \quad \text{and} \quad \underline{\underline{\epsilon}} = \frac{1}{2}\left(\underline{\nabla}u + \underline{\nabla}u^T\right) \tag{3}$$

- $\underline{\underline{K}}$ is the rigidity matrix (Pa).
- $\underline{\underline{\sigma}}$ the internal stress tensor (Pa)
- $\underline{\underline{\epsilon}}$ is the linearized Lagrange strain tensor expressed as a function of the displacement $\underline{u}$ (no unit).

Table 1. Stiffness and diffusivity properties of the finite element model

Tissue	Young Modulus (Pa)	Poisson Coefficient	Tissue diffusivity $(10^{-3} \, mm^2 \, s^{-1})$
White Matter	694	0.4	$\alpha \cdot$ DTI (anisotropic)
Gray Matter	694	0.4	$\beta \cdot max(\underline{D}(White))$
Falx Cerebri	200.000	0.4	0
Ventricles	0	0	0
Skull	∞	0.5	0

Because the GTV1 is modeled as a pure cell proliferation and since the associated tissue is already considered as saturated, this proliferation directly acts as a volume increase ΔV on the GTV1:

$$\Delta V = V_t - V_0 = V_0 \left(e^{\eta t} - 1 \right)$$

Based on the proposed model, η can be approximated by computing the average volume increase of GTV1 in GBM. We found $\eta = 2.2 \times 10^{-3} day^{-1}$. We use a penalty method to impose this volume variation boundary condition via a homogeneous pressure force into the GTV1.

We propose a new equilibrium equation to model the mechanical impact of the tumor on the invaded structures.

$$div \left(\underline{\underline{\sigma}} - \lambda c \, \underline{\underline{\mathbb{I}_3}} \right) + \underline{f_{ext}} = 0 \qquad (4)$$

This equation is the differential version of the law proposed by Wasserman [9]. It can be locally interpreted as a tissue internal pressure λc proportional to the tumor concentration c. This law is used to describe the mechanical effects of the malignant cells invading the brain parenchyma.

Model Parameters and Initialization. The proposed mechanical model is similar to the one used for predicting intra-operative deformations [1]. It has the following characteristics:

- the skull does not deform and is considered as beeing infinitely rigid. Thus vertices on the surface of the brain mesh are fixed.
- We use the linearized 3D homogeneous version of Miller's constitutive equation (see 3.2 for details), the Young modulus is set to 694 Pa and the Poisson coefficient is thus set to 0.40.

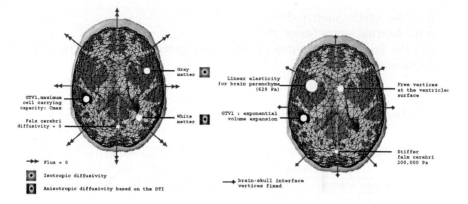

Fig. 2. Summary of the diffusion (left) and the mechanical (right) model.

- We consider that the ventricular pressure is not affected by the tumor growth. Therefore we let ventricular vertices free without additional internal pressure.
- Based on the rheological experiments [6] made on the falx cerebri, we choose its Young modulus equal to $2 \times 10^5 Pa$.
- We choose a coupling factor λ which minimizes the quantitative difference between the model and the real deformations: $\lambda = 1.4 \times 10^{-9} \, N \, mm \, Cells^{-1}$.

The material mechanical properties are summed up in Table 1. Figure 2 summarizes the diffusion model and the boundary conditions.

4   Results

After performing the simulation, we registered both the deformations and the tumor concentration into the first patient MRI (03/2001). Results are presented in two parts, the mass effect and the tumor diffusion.

Mass Effect. Figure 3 shows the displacement of internal tissue due to the mass effect. Even if this major displacements take place close to the GTV1, further away tissues in the same hemisphere are also affected by the tumor growth. The average displacement at the GTV1-GTV2 frontier is 3 mm. The tumor has an influence on the lateral ventricles size (volume variation $\Delta V = 4.6 \, ml$). To quantify the accuracy of the simulation, a medical expert manually selected corresponding feature points on the patient MRIs so as to estimate these landmark displacements between March 2001 and September 2001. These measured displacements can then be compared to the one simulated by the model (complete landmark positions and errors can be found in [2]). The average displacement for selected landmarks is 2.7 mm and the corresponding average error is 1.3 mm. Without recovering the entire deformation, the proposed model captures the largest part of the displacement. The remaining error might be due to different phenomena:

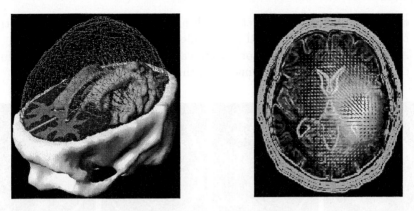

Fig. 3. Displacement of the tissues induced by the tumor mass effect.

- the ratio between the average deformation amplitude (2.7 mm) and the image resolution (1.0 mm) is in the range of manual selection error.
- The deformation phenomenon might be larger in interstitial space than in the brain parenchyma. In such a case, a finer mesh and different constitutive equations would be necessary to model the deformation.

Diffusion. Results on two different axial slices of the diffusion process can be seen on figure 4. The four columns should be read as follow:

- column 1 shows the T2 weighted MRI acquired in March 2001.
- Column 2 shows the same MRI with interpolated contours used to initialize the model.
- Column 3 shows the T2 weighted MRI of the same patient acquired 6 months later.
- Column 4 shows the same MRI with simulated tumor isodensity curves.

5   Perspectives

Model Improvement for Simulation. Previous results have demonstrated the ability of the numerical model to predict the tumor behavior. However, the model could be enhanced with additional characteristics:

- the modification of the fiber structures in the invaded area.
- The model could largely benefit from the use of more patient-specific images. More precisely, patient DTI capturing the white-matter fiber directions could greatly improve the accuracy of the simulation.

Clinical Validation and Applications. We consider the comparison of the simulated VG with the follow-up MR image of the patient as a preliminary step for validating the proposed model. We wish to develop other methods for the identification of parameters and for clinical validation:

- correlation of the VG prediction with histopathological analysis of patient brains, especially in the MRI areas under the threshold of detection.
- Adding functional information into the atlas to allow the prediction of functional loss induced by the tumor growth.

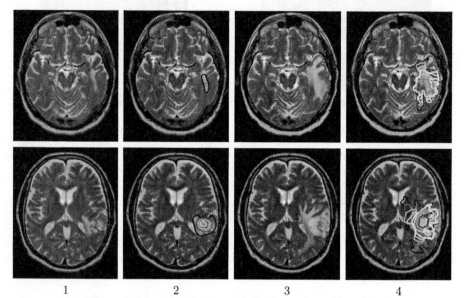

      1   2   3   4

Fig. 4. 1. T2 MRI 03/2001, 2. T2 MRI 03/2001 + GBM initialization, 3. T2 MRI 09/2001, 4. T2 MRI 09/2001 + simulated GBM tumor isodensities

References

1. O. Clatz, H. Delingette, E. Bardinet, D. Dormont, and N. Ayache. Patient specific biomechanical model of the brain: Application to parkinson's disease procedure. In N. Ayache and H. Delingette, editors, *International Symposium on Surgery Simulation and Soft Tissue Modeling (IS4TM'03)*, volume 2673 of *LNCS*, pages 321–331, Juan-les-Pins, France, 2003. INRIA Sophia Antipolis, Springer-Verlag.
2. O. Clatz, P.Y. Bondiau, H. Delingette, M. Sermesant, S.K. Warfield, G. Malandain, and N. Ayache. Brain tumor growth simulation. Research report 5187, INRIA, 2004.
3. B. M. Dawant, S. L. Hartmann, and S. Gadamsetty. Brain atlas deformation in the presence of large space-occupying tumors. *Medical Image Computing and Computer-Assisted Intervention*, volume 1679 of *LNCS*, pages 589–596, 1999.
4. S. K. Kyriacou and C. Davatzikos. A biomechanical model of soft tissue deformation, with applications to non-rigid registration of brain images with tumor pathology. *Proceedings of the First International Conference on Medical Image Computing and Computer-Assisted Intervention*, volume 1496 of *LNCS*, pages 531–538, 1998.
5. K. Miller. *Biomechanics of Brain for Computer Integrated Surgery*. Warsaw University of Technology Publishing House, 2002. ISBN:83-7207-347-3.
6. M. Schill, M. Schinkmann, H.-J. Bender, and R. Männer. Biomechanical simulation of the falx cerebri using the finite element method. In *18. Annual International Conference, IEEE Engeneering in Medicine and Biology*, 1996.

7. K.R. Swanson, E.C. Alvord Jr, and J.D. Murray. Virtual brain tumours (gliomas) enhance the reality of medical imaging and highlight inadequacies of current therapy. *British Journal of Cancer*, 86(1):14–18, Jan 2002.
8. P. Tracqui. From passive diffusion to active cellular migration in mathematical models of tumour invasion. *Acta Biotheoretica*, 43(4):443–464, Dec 1995.
9. R. Wasserman and R. Acharya. A patient-specific in vivo tumor model. *Mathematical Biosciences*, 136(2):111–140, Sep 1996.

An Event-Driven Framework for the Simulation of Complex Surgical Procedures

Christopher Sewell[1], Dan Morris[1], Nikolas Blevins[2], Federico Barbagli[1],
and Kenneth Salisbury[1]

[1] Department of Computer Science, Stanford University
{csewell, dmorris, barbagli, jks}@cs.stanford.edu
[2]Department of Otolaryngology, Stanford University
nblevins@stanford.edu

Gates Building 1A
Stanford, California, USA 94305

Abstract. Existing surgical simulators provide a physical simulation that can help a trainee develop the hand-eye coordination and motor skills necessary for specific tasks, such as cutting or suturing. However, it is equally important for a surgeon to gain experience in the cognitive processes involved in performing an entire procedure. The surgeon must be able to perform the correct tasks in the correct sequence, and must be able to quickly and appropriately respond to any unexpected events or mistakes. It would be beneficial for a surgical procedure simulation to expose the training surgeon to difficult situations only rarely encountered in actual patients. We present here a framework for a full-procedure surgical simulator that incorporates an ability to detect discrete events, and that uses these events to track the logical flow of the procedure as performed by the trainee. In addition, we are developing a scripting language that allows an experienced surgeon to precisely specify the logical flow of a procedure without the need for programming. The utility of the framework is illustrated through its application to a mastoidectomy.

1 Introduction

The traditional method of training surgeons has followed the apprenticeship "see one, do one, teach one" model [1]. However, in recent years simulation-based training has become more commonplace as an adjunct to this method, and its value more widely accepted [2]. It can be a safe, cost-effective, customizable, and easily accessible tool for gaining experience in surgery.

One type of surgical training focuses on developing hand-eye coordination and motor skills necessary for specific tasks, such as grasping and suturing, which are frequently performed in a number of procedures. For minimally invasive laparoscopic operations, such skills have traditionally been developed using box trainers. However,

C. Barillot, D.R. Haynor, and P. Hellier (Eds.): MICCAI 2004, LNCS 3217, pp. 346–354, 2004.

recently computer-based simulations, such as LapSim [3], have been validated and shown to also be effective in developing these skills [4] [5]. Simulators have also been developed to train other specific, isolated tasks, such as catheter insertion [6]. The behavior of such existing surgical simulators tends to be fixed by the program's designers and is not adaptable by the medical schools that purchase them.

In addition to developing specific technical skills, however, a surgeon must also learn the optimal sequence in which to perform these tasks, accounting for differences due to variations in patient anatomy or to consequences of previous actions, and how to respond to unexpected or stressful situations. Recognizing this need, mannequin-based simulations of complex scenarios in specialties such as anesthesiology [7] have been developed. Nevertheless, such simulations are expensive and are limited in use due to the high demands of time and effort needed to prepare and run the simulations. Thus, there is a need for cost-efficient, easily accessible computer-based simulations to provide cognitive training for complex scenarios.

Markov chains have been used to identify specific physical actions in surgical simulations (such as fundoplication), and to objectively rate the skill level with which they were performed [8]. Kumar et. al. used a state machine called a "task graph" to sequence appropriate robotic augmentation computational primitives, such as compliant motion, for surgical fine manipulation tasks based on the history of user control and environmental interactions [9]. In addition, finite state machines have been used to control simulations of digital actors in video games and animated movies, defining actions undertaken by the actors depending upon previous events in the simulation.

We believe that using such models to track the logical flow of events in a surgical simulator will help develop the trainee's cognitive skills in dealing with complex scenarios. Ideally, the program should allow the user to interact with the simulated patient in a free-form manner, while still keeping track of the order in which actions are performed to ensure that safe and effective techniques are taught. In addition, the ability to detect and track discrete events can allow for an increased level of realism without the need for an exceedingly complex real-time physical simulator. For example, by detecting an "incision event" that triggers a "bleed action", the simulation can provide a realistic response to cutting a vein without the physical simulator having to account for the complete dynamics of blood flow through veins. Events could even trigger the loading of an appropriate pre-recorded response from a database, greatly reducing the demands on the real-time simulator.

Furthermore, our system provides the user with control over the design of the simulated procedure. Recognizing the need for customizable surgical simulators, the Teleos authoring tool [10] was designed to make it easier to create new surgical simulation environments. Several frameworks, such as CAML [11] and GiPSi [12], have been proposed to facilitate seamless integration of independently developed physical simulation modules. This idea can be extended to provide scripting tools to allow a professor of surgery using the simulator to easily modify or create scenarios for his/her students, as well as to tailor the performance metrics and logical flow to his/her style and preferences.

2   The Conceptual Framework

Our system can be divided into four domains: the user, the physical simulator, the event engine, and the instructor and performance evaluator. It is a hybrid system with both continuous and discrete components. The framework is illustrated in Figure 1A.

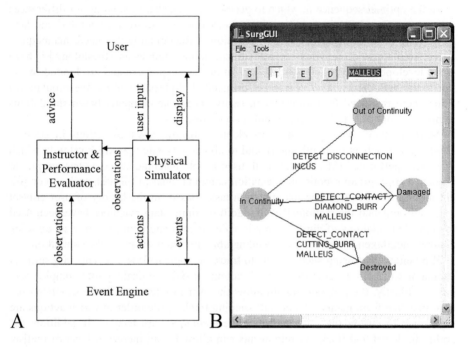

Fig. 1. A) Diagram of the flow of information among the four domains of our simulation conceptual framework, as described in Section 2. B) An example of a simple state machine developed using our graphical scripting environment. Here, the user has specified differing levels of trauma caused by contacting the malleus with two different types of drills. However, if the incus is removed, the hearing chain becomes disconnected, and the malleus enters a state in which there are no such out-transitions, since drill contacts no longer result in hearing loss.

2.1   User and Physical Simulator

The user is the surgeon in training. He/she provides input to the physical simulator, such as movements of a pointing or haptic device. In return, the user may receive graphic, haptic, and auditory feedback from the simulation. The physical simulator is responsible for the rendering of the physical models, which represent the anatomy of the simulated patient, and of the surgical instruments. The rendering should be responsive to continuous interactions between the instruments and the anatomical structures, and among the various structures. Depending on the degree of realism required, a physical simulator of virtually any level of complexity may be used. The only requirement is that it implement the interfaces defined by the other domains.

2.2 Event Engine

In addition to the continuous interactions between the instrument and the anatomical structures, and among the different anatomical structures, there are discrete events that occur during the course of a procedure. These events may trigger specific actions. According to our terminology, "events" are inputs to the engine resulting from interactions with the continuous physical simulation, while "actions" are outputs of the engine that specify a change to the physical simulation. The behavior of the physical simulator can be constrained by the history of past events. For example, if an artery leading into an organ has been cauterized, a subsequent "incision event'" affecting that organ may no longer produce a "bleed action". The relevant aspects of that history, defined by the space of possible current and future events, can be modeled as a state in a finite automaton. Transitions between states (or self-transitions) are triggered by the detection of pre-defined events, and either a transition itself or entry into a state can result in the execution of a specified action.

Once triggered, some action functions may just execute once. For example, positioning an instrument closer than a certain distance from a sensitive structure may result in a warning message being displayed to the trainee. Other action functions place a message in a list that is periodically read by the physical simulator, resulting in a persistent change in the rendering of the physical models. A third type of action function removes messages from the list. For example, detecting an "incision event" at a certain location will result in a message being inserted into the list stating that bleeding should occur at that location. As the physical simulator renders the scene, it reads the list and simulates the bleeding at the given location. Later, detecting a "suture event" at that location will result in the removal of that message, and the physical simulator will no longer render the bleeding.

The event engine receives specifications of events to detect and actions to execute from the input script (described in the following section), and it communicates with the physical simulator through the message list and a standardized API. For action functions that affect the physical simulation, only a few relatively high-level parameters (such as the location and rate of bleeding) are specified in the script and passed on to the physical simulator via the message list by the event engine. The physical simulator is free to implement the requested action in any way. As long as it can read and recognize the messages in the list, any physical simulator, of any degree of sophistication, can be plugged into the system in a modular fashion. Likewise, the event engine passes on only a few high-level parameters (such as the location, length, depth, and force of an "incision event") for events to be detected from the script to the physical simulator. The physical simulator must only implement a specified API, consisting of a number of specific event detection functions that accept these parameters and return true or false.

2.3 Performance Evaluator

A surgical training system should also provide feedback to the user about his/her performance, scoring it and supplying constructive criticisms. Many events may be directly tied to a performance metric, such as contact of a cutting instrument with a nerve resulting in a comment that care needs to be taken around nerves and a reduction in score proportional to the amount of nerve damage. Some such events may only be of evaluation significance and not have a direct effect on the physical simulation, such as using a functional but non-optimal instrument for a certain task. Other metrics may not be tied to events, but rather to an observation of the state of the physical simulation. For example, if the indication for surgery was removal of a tumor, it is obviously relevant how much of the tumor structure remains at the end. Yet other metrics may consider the observed state of the simulation when a specific event occurs, such as the degree of exposure of a structure when it is manipulated or removed.

3 The Scripting Language

A scripting language is being developed to allow surgeons to use the system described in the previous section to design specific procedures and scenarios for training.

The first section of a script in our language simply lists the file names and types (deformable layer, volumetric mesh, or surface mesh) of the models representing the instruments and the anatomical structures, and associates with each a name that can be referenced from elsewhere in the script.

The second section declares variables for metrics to be tracked, which may be given an initial value and ranges for acceptable values. These variables are modified by certain action functions, as described below.

Finite automata are described in the third section. An automaton may be associated with any or all of the structures named in the first section. Associated with each state may be a list of action functions, defined by the event engine's API, that are executed upon entry into the state. These functions may include several parameters, such as a structure name from the first section, a location in Cartesian or spherical coordinates, and/or an expression indicative of something such as rate or severity of the action.

Such expressions may include numerical constants, arithmetic operators, variables declared in the second section of the script, and reserved words (such as FORCE or LOCATION for the haptic force or instrument position at the time of execution of the action function). For example, the BLEED function may be called with three parameters, e.g. "BLEED SKIN LOCATION '5*FORCE'", specifying that the skin will bleed at the current instrument contact position at a rate directly proportional to the force of the contact. More sophisticated parameters of the resulting blood simulation are handled at a lower level, abstracted from the surgeon, by the physical simulator. The "UPDATE_STATUS" function takes as a parameter an expression that modifies a performance metric variable defined in the second section.

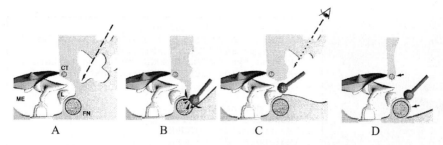

Fig. 2. A) Schematic cross-sectional view of the temporal bone illustrating a lesion (L) within the middle ear (ME) cavity. The goal of this simulation is to access this lesion, in the direction shown by the arrow. The chorda tympani (CT) and the facial nerve (FN) are shown. B) An "injurious" action has occurred, with the burr contacting the facial nerve. C) A "dangerous" action has occurred, when the surgeon has drilled away bone without first establishing clear exposure of the region. D) Correct bone removal has occurred. The nerves have been avoided, and adequate exposure has been established. Failure to adequately thin the bone may be considered a "discouraged" action, since there remains some doubt as to the location of the nerves.

Possible transitions among these states are listed, each associated with and triggered by an event detection function, again defined by the event engine's API. These functions may also take parameters similar to those taken by the action functions. For example, "2 5 DETECT_CONTACT SCALPEL MUSCLE 0.5" indicates a transition from State Two to State Five when the scalpel contacts the muscle layer with a force of at least 0.5 Newtons. Many of these transitions may be self-transitions. For greater specificity, action functions may be associated with a transition rather than with a state. Thus, an action may be taken only when there is a transition into a state from a certain subset of states rather than upon entry into the state from any other state.

A graphical development tool allows the supervising surgeon to "draw" the automata. Variables, reserved words, and action and event detection functions defined by the event engine API can be selected from lists, and templates are provided for parameters. Performance metric variables and models may be defined via dialog boxes. The designed script is then written to a file readable by the simulation program. Figure 1B shows a screen shot of this tool.

4 Application: Mastoidectomy

Our surgical simulation framework and scripting language have been applied to the development of a mastoidectomy training system, similar to [13]. A mastoidectomy is a procedure performed in which a portion of the temporal bone is drilled away in order to provide access to inner regions of the ear. In our simulation, the pathology is a legion located in the middle ear. The logical flow of the operation, and the various potential morbidities, are based on The Temporal Bone Dissector [14]. Our simulator's event engine uses a script of the procedure developed with the aid of an otologist. Examples of "injurious", "dangerous", and "discouraged" user actions relevant to the procedure are illustrated in Figure 2.

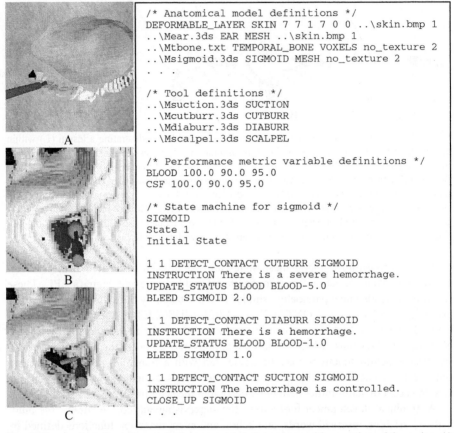

```
/* Anatomical model definitions */
DEFORMABLE_LAYER SKIN 7 7 1 7 0 0 ..\skin.bmp 1
..\Mear.3ds EAR MESH ..\skin.bmp 1
..\Mtbone.txt TEMPORAL_BONE VOXELS no_texture 2
..\Msigmoid.3ds SIGMOID MESH no_texture 2
. . .

/* Tool definitions */
..\Msuction.3ds SUCTION
..\Mcutburr.3ds CUTBURR
..\Mdiaburr.3ds DIABURR
..\Mscalpel.3ds SCALPEL

/* Performance metric variable definitions */
BLOOD 100.0 90.0 95.0
CSF 100.0 90.0 95.0

/* State machine for sigmoid */
SIGMOID
State 1
Initial State

1 1 DETECT_CONTACT CUTBURR SIGMOID
INSTRUCTION There is a severe hemorrhage.
UPDATE_STATUS BLOOD BLOOD-5.0
BLEED SIGMOID 2.0

1 1 DETECT_CONTACT DIABURR SIGMOID
INSTRUCTION There is a hemorrhage.
UPDATE_STATUS BLOOD BLOOD-1.0
BLEED SIGMOID 1.0

1 1 DETECT_CONTACT SUCTION SIGMOID
INSTRUCTION The hemorrhage is controlled.
CLOSE_UP SIGMOID
. . .
```

Fig. 3. Screen shots from the mastoidectomy simulation, along with a portion of the script. A) Detection of an incision event behind the ear triggers an action that changes to the microscope view of the exposed bone. B) Detection of a contact event between the diamond burr and the sigmoid sinus triggers an action that initiates bleeding. C) Detection of a contact event between the suction and the bleeding location triggers an action that controls the hemorrhage.

Many of the events in this simplified procedure relate to contact between a drill and a sensitive structure. Drilling into the sigmoid sinus causes a venous hemorrhage; drilling into the facial nerve results in nerve damage; and drilling into the tegmen mastoidae causes cerebrospinal fluid (CSF) leakage. The severity of such damage is often dependent on whether a cutting burr or diamond burr drill is used. Use of the suction at the location of these problems can result in their removal from the active event list. Some events affect the patient outcome and thus the performance metrics, though there is no perceptible consequence in the physical simulation. For example, drilling into structures of the inner ear can result in vertigo and/or hearing loss. Other events may only be a matter of "style" leading to a message on the final report, such as using the slower diamond burr in "safe" areas that could have been drilled more efficiently with the cutting burr. Examples of several events are shown in Figure 3.

5 Conclusion and Future Work

Both the event-driven conceptual framework and the mastoidectomy simulator remain in development. A progressively more detailed description of the procedure is being generated with the scripting language. A collaborative environment for surgical simulation is also currently under development. After further improvements, clinical validation studies may be performed to determine the utility of the system. Eventually, the simulator may use physical models constructed from patient-specific data, such as CT scans, to provide an opportunity for pre-operative, case-specific rehearsal for even experienced surgeons. We appreciate the help of Tom Krummel, Jean-Claude Latombe, Elena Vileshina, and Phil Fong, as well as NIH Grant R33 LM07295, Stanford BioX Grant 2DMA178, and the NDSEG, NSF and Stanford fellowship programs.

References

1. Gorman PJ, Meier AH, Rawn C, Krummel TM: The future of medical education is no longer blood and guts, it is bits and bytes. *American J Surgery*. 2000 Nov. 180(5):353-356.
2. Haluck RS, Marshall RL, Krummel TM, Melkonian MG: Are surgery training programs ready for virtual reality? *J of the American College of Surgery*. 2001 Dec. 193(6):660-665.
3. Larsson A: An open and flexible framework for computer aided surgical training. *Stud Health Technol Inform*. 2001 81:263-265.
4. Hyltander A, Liljegren E, Rhodin PH, Lonroth H: The transfer of basic skills learned in a laparoscopic simulator to the operating room. *Surg Endosc*. 2002 Sep. 16(9):1324-1328.
5. Seymour NE, Gallagher AG, Roman SA, O'Brien MK, Bansal VK, Andersen DK, Satava RM: Virtual reality training improves operating room performance: Results of a randomized, double-blinded study. *Annals of Surgery*. 2002 Oct. 236(4):458-464.
6. Prystowsky JB, Regehr G, Rogers DA: A virtual reality module for intravenous catheter placement. *American J Surgery*. 1999 177:171–175.
7. Holzman RS, Cooper JB, Gaba DM: Anesthesia crisis resource management: real-life simulation training in operating room crises. *J of Clinical Anesthesiology* 1995 7:675–687.
8. Rosen J, HB, Richards CG, Sinanan MN: Markov modeling of minimally invasive surgery based on tool/tissue interaction and force/torque signatures for evaluating surgical skills. *IEEE Transactions on Biomedical Engineering*. 48 (2001).
9. Kumar R, Hager GD, Barnes A, Jensen P, Taylor RH: An augmentation system for fine manipulation. MICCAI 2000:956-965.
10. Meglan DA, Raju R, Merril GL, Merril JR, Nguyen BH, Swamy SN, Higgins GA: The Teleos virtual environment toolkit for simulation-based surgical educ. MMVR 1996:346-51.
11. Cotin S, Shaffer D, Meglan D, Ottensmeyer M, Berry P, Dawson S: CAML: A general framework for the development of medical simulation systems. *Proc of SPIE* 4037:294-300.
12. Cavusoglu MC, Goktekin TG, Tendick F, Sastry SS: GiPSi: An open source/open architecture software development framework for surgical simulation. MMVR 2004:46-48.

13. Agus M, Giachetti A, Gobbetti E, Zanetti G, Zorcolo A: A multiprocessor decoupled system for the simulation of temporal bone surgery. *Computing and Visualization in Science*. 2002 5(1):35-43.
14. Blevins NH: The promise of multimedia in otology. *American J of Otology*. 1997 May 18(3):283-284.

Photorealistic Rendering of Large Tissue Deformation for Surgical Simulation

Mohamed A. ElHelw, Benny P. Lo, A.J. Chung, Ara Darzi, and
Guang-Zhong Yang

Royal Society/Wolfson Medical Image Computing Laboratory,
Imperial College London, London, United Kingdom
{mohammed.elhelw, benlo, ajchung, a.darzi,
g.z.yang}@imperial.ac.uk

Abstract. With the increasing use of computer based simulation for training and skills assessment, growing effort is being directed towards enhancing the visual realism of the simulation environment. Image-based modelling and rendering is a promising technique in that it attains photorealistic visual feedback while maintaining interactive response. The purpose of this paper is to extend an existing technique for simulating tissues with extensive deformation. We demonstrate that by the incorporation of multiple virtual cameras, geometric proxy and viewing projection manifolds, interactive tissue-instrument interaction can be achieved while providing photorealistic rendering. Detailed steps involved in the algorithm are introduced and quantitative error analysis is provided to assess the accuracy of the technique in terms of projection error through 3D image warping. Results from phantom and real-laparoscope simulation demonstrate the potential clinical value of the technique.

1 Introduction

In minimal invasive surgery, virtual and augmented realities are increasingly being used as new ways of training, preoperative planning, and navigation. Realistic modelling of soft tissue properties in terms of both mechanical and visual characteristics is essential to the perceptual fidelity of the simulation environment. In practice, this is a challenging task due to the diversity of tissue properties and the lack of non-invasive techniques for mapping mechanical indices *in vivo*. For surgical simulation, the nature of the problem strides across both computer graphics for photorealistic rendering and biomechanics for tissue property simulation [1]. Whilst major research has been conducted in the measurement and simulation of soft tissue deformation, increasing effort is being directed towards enhancing the visual realism of the simulation environment.

In our previous work, we have presented an image-based rendering approach for simulating soft tissue deformation due to instrument interaction [2]. The method is based on associating a depth map with each colour texture for modelling surface details. Considering the fact that real-time mechanical simulation of tissue-

C. Barillot, D.R. Haynor, and P. Hellier (Eds.): MICCAI 2004, LNCS 3217, pp. 355–362, 2004.

deformation is normally restricted to a relatively coarse mesh structure, which cannot provide photo-realistic results if it is rendered directly, macro- and micro-surface structures, *i.e.* details, are decomposed during a pre-processing step. During simulation, deformation resulting from tissue-instrument interaction is rapidly calculated by modifying the macrostructure. Microstructures are subsequently added by following the 3D image-warping paradigm [3]. It has been shown that the method significantly reduces the polygonal count required to model the scene whilst offering realistic rendering results. Interactive response can be achieved on a normal PC without dedicated hardware.

The purpose of this paper is to extend the modeling and rendering framework for complex scenes with large tissue deformation. Instead of using one virtual camera to sample the scene for 3D image warping, multiple cameras with overlapping field-of-view are used. This ensures rapid photo-realistic rendering during run time whilst maintaining re-projection accuracy even in the presence of large deformation.

2   Method

The proposed method is divided into preprocessing and interactive phases. During the first phase, tissue geometry and colour information are obtained and made amenable for interactive processing. In the interactive phase, realistic deformation behaviour is achieved by using mass-spring modeling while image-based rendering is used to attain photorealistic visual feedback. In this section we describe in detail the tasks performed at each phase. We also introduce a number of new concepts that make an interactive image-based solution possible for simulating large tissue areas and involve significant deformation. These concepts include the deformable geometric proxy and the viewing projection manifold.

2.1   Pre-processing Phase

The pre-processing step in this study is similar to that of our previous work and involves most of the computationally intensive tasks including the construction of a geometric proxy, *i.e.* a coarse deformable geometric model describing tissue surface and the extraction of surface color and texture details. The output of this stage is the geometric proxy, and a pair of color and microstructure images for each virtual camera.

2.1.1   Geometry and Colour Information Acquisition

Several methods for obtaining tissue or organ geometry and colour can be utilised. We have conducted two experiments to test our technique where different acquisition approaches were used. For the first experiment, an artificial phantom model, mimicking large tissue or organ, was constructed. The phantom was made of silicone rubber and the surface was coated with silicone rubber mixed with acrylic to give it a specular finish that looks similar to soft tissue. The tomographic model of the phantom was scanned with a Siemens So-maton Volume Zoom four-channel multi-detector CT scanner with a slice thickness of 3 mm and in-plane resolution of 1mm. Consequently, model geometry was acquired from the volumetric set by using an isosurface extraction method, namely the marching cubes. The model was also photographed to acquire its colour image.

Subsequently, the colour image of the phantom was aligned with its 3D geometry using 2D/3D registration. An intensity-based pixel-oriented similarity measure employing the normalised cross correlation of the 2D image with the projection of the 3D geometry was optimised until correct alignment was established. The similarity between the colour image (CI) and the projected image (PI) of the volumetric data is given by [4]:

$$R = \frac{\sum_{(i,j)\in T}(I_{CI}(i,j)-\bar{I}_{CI})(I_{PI}(i,j)-\bar{I}_{PI})}{\sqrt{\sum_{(i,j)\in T}(I_{CI}(i,j)-\bar{I}_{CI})^2}\ \sqrt{\sum_{(i,j)\in T}(I_{PI}(i,j)-\bar{I}_{PI})^2}}$$

where $\bar{I}_{CI}$ and $\bar{I}_{PI}$ are the mean values of the two images in the overlap region.

For the second experiment, we have used *in-vivo* data acquired during a laparoscopy procedure. Estimated tissue geometry was attained by using shape-from-shading technique as the surface is assumed to be Lambertian with constant albedo. The depth of the tissue in relation to the camera at each time frame can be estimated with Taylor series expansion, as proposed by Tsai and Shah [5]:

$$Z_t^n(x,y) = Z_t^{n-1}(x,y) + \frac{-f(Z_t^{n-1}(x,y))}{\dfrac{df(Z_t^{n-1}(x,y))}{dZ(x,y)}} \qquad where \qquad Z_0^0(x,y) = 0$$

$$\frac{df}{dZ_t^n} = \left(\frac{(p+q)(pp_s+qq_s+1)}{\sqrt{\left(p^2+q^2+1\right)^3}\sqrt{\left(p_s^2+q_s^2+1\right)}} - \frac{p_s+q_s}{\sqrt{\left(p^2+q^2+1\right)}\sqrt{\left(p_s^2+q_s^2+1\right)}} \right)$$

$$p = \frac{\partial Z}{\partial x} \qquad q = \frac{\partial Z}{\partial y} \qquad p_s = \frac{\cos\tau\sin\sigma}{\cos\sigma} \qquad q_s = \frac{\sin\tau\sin\sigma}{\cos\sigma}$$

where $Z_t^n(x,y)$ represents the depth value of pixel (x, y) at time t after n iteration, and τ is the tilt of the illuminant and σ is the slant of the illuminant.

2.1.2 Geometry Simplification

Because of its complexity, mesh simplification has to be applied to the created geometric model to obtain a coarser representation that allows for real-time processing. To get an idea about shape complexity, the geometric proxy obtained from the scanned phantom model originally consisted of 80,744 polygons. It was reduced to a coarse model of only 80 polygons by naïvely sub-sampling the original mesh, as illustrated in Figure 1. Better approximation results can be obtained by using more advanced mesh simplification approaches. However, when deformation behavior is not of primary objective, high quality visual rendering can still be achieved while using a very coarse proxy. This is one of the main advantages of using the image-based rendering technique to render the deformed tissue.

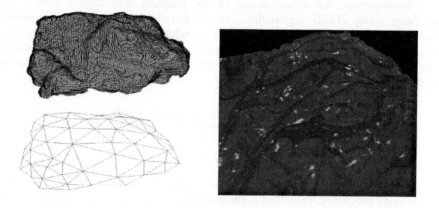

Fig. 1. A mesh reduction technique is applied to the original mesh resulting in a coarser model. Above (left) are the original and coarse meshes. A section of the phantom model rendered by using the image-based technique is shown (right).

After geometry and color information are acquired, the computer-generated model is sampled by a number of virtual cameras with overlapping field-of-view. For each virtual camera, depth and colour information are captured by means of ray casting or by using the graphics hardware depth and color buffers.

2.1.3   Constructing the Deformable Geometric Proxy

The deformable geometric proxy is used to rapidly handle deformations resulting from tissue-instrument interactions. It is constructed by fitting masses to the vertices of the coarse geometric model obtained in the previous step, then connecting them by springs and dampers. Generally, approximate deformation models are well suited for surgical training. However, since the proposed image-based solution completely separates deformation modeling from rendering processes, the mass-spring model can be replaced with a finite element model in case accurate deformations are desired.

2.1.4   Separating Tissue Surface into Macro- and Micro-Structures

3D image warping is used to preserve and enhance the appearance of high-complexity structures on top of tissue surface. As discussed in [2], these details are acquired during the pre-processing phase by using filtering to separate each of the depth or intensity images into macro- and microstructure images then storing the latter. During interactive simulation phase, the macrostructure deformation data is derived from the geometric proxy. Subsequently, microstructures are added to the deformed surface. Thus preserving the microscopic details of the surface undergoing deformation and permitting photorealistic rendering.

2.2 Interactive Simulation Phase

The interactive phase is executed every time step during simulation. It is composed of the five processes described below.

2.2.1 Handling Interactions and Capturing Deformed Surface Information

Surgical simulation involves complex interactions such as tissues-instrument, tissue-tissue and instrument-instrument interactions [6]. Therefore, the majority of simulation loop cycles are spent on computing collision detection and collision responses. The use of the coarse geometric proxy allows for rapid collision detection necessary for realistic visual and haptic responses by reducing the number of collision calculations. In addition, deforming the geometric proxy results in modifying the macrostructure, *i.e.* the depth, captured by the virtual cameras sampling the tissue surface. For each virtual camera, the process of reading modified depth can be efficiently carried out by making use of the available graphics hardware. For instance, OpenGL [7] depth buffer can be used to rapidly acquire depth information.

2.2.2 Adding Microstructure and Rendering Deformed Tissue

The microstructure information is added to the tissue by first distorting the microstructure image to conform to the deformed macrostructure then modulating the latter with the distorted image. This accounts for depth changes resulting from tiny surface details. The procedure is executed for each virtual camera and the view of the deformed tissue is produced as described in [2]. The generated views are then combined together by using a viewing projection manifold (VPM) which is a triangular surface constructed from the intersection of the virtual cameras viewing planes as illustrated in Figure 2.

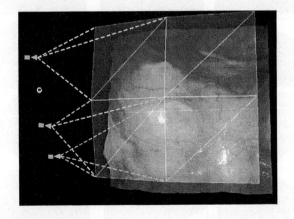

Fig. 2. Viewing projection manifold superimposed over tissue. Also shown several virtual cameras used to capture model depth and colour information

3   Results

3.1   Visual Feedback

The image-based technique has been applied to modelling and rendering an artificial phantom model depicting a deformable bulky tissue or organ. Figure 1 (right) illustrates the results obtained where it can be noticed how photorealistic rendering was achieved with reduced modelling efforts.

Figure 3 shows a number of depth and colour images captured by virtual cameras when the technique was applied to *in-vivo* data. Figure 4 shows a novel view of the tissue. The high fidelity visual feedback using the proposed technique is demonstrated.

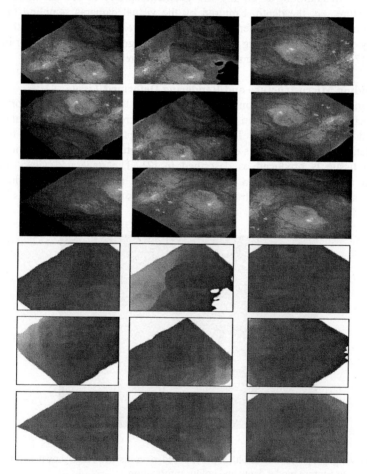

Fig. 3. Colour and depth data captured by virtual cameras. Notice the non-smooth depth resulting from using the shape-from-shading method to extract the geometry of the model [8]

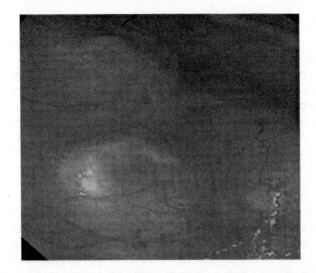

Fig. 4. A novel view of *in-vivo* tissue rendered with the image-based technique.

3.2 Validation

The image-based rendering technique is validated through error analysis by comparing it to the conventional polygonal method. For this study, the "gold-standard" is defined as the screen-space coordinates of the projection of selected original model samples. Thus, error is defined as the deviation, in pixels, of same samples rendered by using the image-based and polygon-based methods. The results of the study are shown in Table 1 where it can be seen that projection errors are minimized when the image-based technique is used. This is expected since the image-based method uses depth images, which provide more faithful representations of the original model, to render the tissue.

Table 1. Error analysis for comparing the accuarcy of image-based and polygon-based methods at different viewing angles

Viewing Angle	Projection Error in Pixels	
(radians)	Image-Based Method	Polygon Method
0.705723	1.41421	9.14112
0.867709	1.52315	3.02655
1.91832	2.34094	16.1307
2.44696	2.20907	10.1193
2.44881	1.20	16.2505

4 Discussion and Conclusions

In this paper we described an image-based rendering method for modelling and rendering bulky tissues and organs. In order to maintain efficient execution, the method is divided into pre-processing and interactive phases. At the pre-processing phase, computationally demanding tasks such as acquiring and constructing the geometric proxy, and separating and storing tissue information are carried out. During simulation, interactivity is sustained by using the coarse geometric proxy to compute tissue instrument interactions, whereas photorealistic rendering is achieved by using image-based rendering to augment 3D surface details and render the final deformed tissue. Although the proposed method provides a photorealistic rendering quality, it assumes fixed tissue topology such that only limited tissue-instrument interaction operations can be simulated. Extending the method to handle other types of interaction such as cutting and piercing is to be investigated. Another area for future research is exploring the use of emerging methods for acquiring *in-vivo* tissue geometry such as the use of projected structured lighting techniques [9] to extract multiple depth images, which can then be combined to obtain model geometry [10].

References

1. Delingette, H. Towards Realistic Soft Tissue Modeling in Medical Simulation. INRIA. Report No 3506 (1998). http://www.inria.fr/Equipes/EPIDAURE-eng.html
2. ElHelw, M.A., Chung, A.J., Darzi, A. and Yang, G.Z. Image-Based Modelling of Soft Tissue Deformation. MICCAI03 (2003) 83-90
3. McMillan, L. An Image-Based Approach to Three-Dimensional Computer Graphics. Ph.D. Dissertation. UNC Computer Science Technical Report TR97-013 (1997)
4. Penney, P.G., Weese J., Little, J., Desmedt, P., Hill, D. and Hawkes, D. A Comparison of Similarity Measures for Use in 2D-3D Medical Image Registration. MICCAI98 (1998) 1153-1161
5. Tsai, P.S. and Shah, M. Shape From Shading Using Linear Approximation. Image and Vision Computing Journal, Vol. 12 No. 8 (1994) 487-498
6. Conference Course Notes on Surgical Simulation. Medicine Meets Virtual Reality (2002)
7. Neider J., Davis, T. and Woo, M. OpenGL Programming Guide. 2nd edn. Addison Wesley (1997)
8. Stoyanov, D., ElHelw, M., Lo, B.P., Chung, A., Bello, F. and Yang, G.Z. Current Issues of Photorealistic Rendering for Virtual and Augmented Reality in Minimally Invasive Surgery. Seventh International Conference on Information Visualization (IV'03), London, England (2003) 350-358
9. Keller, K. and Ackerman, J. Real-time Structured Light Depth Extraction. Three Dimensional Image Capture and Applications III, SPIE proceedings (2000) 11-18
10. Huber, F.D. Automatic 3D Modeling Using Range Images Obtained from Unknown viewpoints. Proceedings of the Third International Conference on 3-D Digital Imaging and Modeling, IEEE Computer Society (2001) 153-160

BurnCase 3D – Realistic Adaptation of 3-Dimensional Human Body Models

Johannes Dirnberger[1], Michael Giretzlehner[1], Thomas Luckeneder[1], Doris Siegl[1], Herbert L. Haller[2], and Christian Rodemund [2]

[1]Upper Austrian Research, Dept. Medical Informatics, AT;
[2]AUVA, Unfallkrankenhaus Linz
info@burncase.at

Abstract. This paper presents the results of the research project BurnCase in the field of realistic and anatomically correct deformations of 3D models of the human body. The project goal is to develop a software system named BurnCase 3D, which supports and enhances the documentation and diagnosis of human burn injuries.

The medical treatment of burn victims strongly depends on size, depth, degree and location of the burnt skin. The size of the affected region is usually expressed as a percentage of the total body surface area (TBSA). Standardized 2D charts (e.g. Lund and Browder, Rule-Of-Nines, etc.) help to determine the percentage of the burnt surface area in relation to the total body surface area. However, body proportions highly influence the distribution of body surface area along the body [Livingston and Lee, 2000]. Thus, standard charts can only give rough approximations of the burnt surface area compared to the real size of an injury on a specific patient.

The software system BurnCase 3D will enhance this commonly applied 2D approximation process by introducing a 3D model of the patient's body. This 3D model provides a higher accordance to the real patient's surface area than any 2D chart does and allows determining the burnt surface areas more exactly. BurnCase 3D is based on an extendable library of currently 7 standard models representing different sex, age and body shape. In order to meet the physical constitution of the real patient, the best fitting model is chosen and has to be adapted according to the patient's height and weight. There exist several possibilities of adapting a 3D model to these parameters. This paper describes the three methods of body adaptations that are realized in the software system BurnCase 3D based on the thesis of Doris Siegl ([Siegl, 2003]).

1   Introduction

Human body shapes show an enormous variability. They are influenced by racial characteristics, alimentation habits and genetic predisposition. We can rely on our sensitivity to the familiar shape of human bodies to recognize correct body forms. Body measurement data, so-called anthropometric data [Flügel et al., 1986], defines the scope of possible proportions more exactly.

C. Barillot, D.R. Haynor, and P. Hellier (Eds.): MICCAI 2004, LNCS 3217, pp. 363–370, 2004.
© Springer-Verlag Berlin Heidelberg 2004

The medical treatment of burn victims strongly depends on size, depth, degree and location of the burnt skin. The size of the affected region is usually expressed as a percentage of the total body surface area (TBSA). Standardized 2D charts (e.g. Lund and Browder, Rule-Of-Nines, etc.) help to determine the percentage of a specific body part in relation to the whole body surface. However, body proportions highly influence the distribution of body surface area along the body [Livingston and Lee, 2000]. Thus, standard charts are not sufficient for reliable surface estimations.

With the aid of a software tool, which uses a three-dimensional model representing the body measurements of the real patient, the burnt surface size can be determined more exactly and leads to enhanced medical treatment and shortened stay in hospital.

2   Research Project BurnCase

The goal of the research project BurnCase is to develop a software system, which supports and enhances the documentation and diagnosis of human burn injuries, thus alleviating the large variations among surgeons regarding approximation of size and depth of burn injuries. The problem of approximations of body surface areas is described in the introduction. Another problem in modern burn care is the large variety in quantity and quality of surveyed data among different burn units as well as the lack of mechanisms to exchange documented data. In order to address this problem, BurnCase 3D offers the possibility of comprehensive documentation of a burn case from admission until discharge.

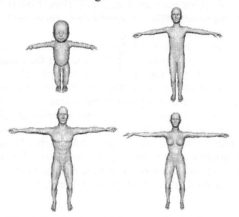

Fig. 1. Standard model library of BurnCase 3D

The strength of BurnCase 3D is the intuitive 3-dimensional graphical user interface that provides direct interaction with a virtual model of the patient's body. Thus, representations of injured regions can be transferred onto this model by using standard input devices like the mouse. Then, the diagnosis is enhanced by modern software technologies involving graphical interaction, complete database support and analysis methods. Accordingly one of the main goals is to provide a user interface which is practicable in a surgeon's daily use.

BurnCase 3D is based on a library of various standard models representing different sexes, ages and body shapes. Figure 1 shows four examples of these standard models. These models have been generated by modern game development software and allow a selection accuracy of one cm^2.

3   Internal Model Representation

The triangle mesh that represents the patient's body in the virtual environment of the BurnCase 3D software system is embedded in an object oriented data structure. The model entity encapsulates the whole model information containing the following types of information:

- Sex and age range
- Axis assignment (which axis defines height, width, breadth)
- Array of 3-dimensional points of the model mesh (vertices)
- Array of triangles that build up the model surface (polygons)

Body surface adaptation algorithms are strongly dependent on the information which axis of the Cartesian coordinate system does represent body height, which one body width and which one body depth. These algorithms use the axis information and transform the 3-dimensional model points. Since the human body does not grow or shrink uniformly on gain or loss of weight these algorithms are non-trivial and have to consider information of location and associated body region's growth behavior.

Thus, triangles do not only know the 3 edge points (addressed by vertex indices) but they contain the following additional information which is necessary for adaptation as well as for visualization and automated medical encoding respectively:

- Anatomical body region (e.g. head, face, thorax, pelvis, etc.)
- Characteristic of injury (e.g. burn degree, necrosectomy, etc.)
- Color for visualization
- Stipple for visualization
- Normal vector for light calculation
- Surface area of the triangle
- Length of longest edge
- Link to neighboring triangles

The normal vector of each triangle gives the direction which side of the triangle lies interior and which one lies exterior regarding the 3-dimensional human model.

4   Realistic Model Adaptation

The different standard models already provide an accurate approach to the real patient's body shape. However, it is necessary to adapt the surface of these standard models to fit the patient's height and weight since all the models are available for one standard height only: 170 cm for adults, 150 cm for children and 60 cm for infants. After choosing an appropriate standard model for the patient the surgeon specifies height and weight of the patient. BurnCase 3D adapts the chosen standard model according to the entered body measurements. This adaptation procedure is described in the following chapters.

4.1   Body Height Adaptation

First of all, the model mesh has to be adapted in terms of body height. This is achieved by simply stretching or shrinking the mesh along the longitudinal body axis (vertical axis along the spine). This is done by simply multiplying every vertex by a factor. Since the model surface area growth is not linearly dependent on this multiplication factor the factor has to be adapted by linear error regression iteration. The factor is thereby calculated as follows:

$$factor_{height} = \begin{cases} \dfrac{h_{dest}}{h_{current}}, & \dfrac{h_{dest}}{h_{current}} \geq 2 \\ 2 - \dfrac{h_{dest}}{h_{current}}, & else \end{cases} \tag{1}$$

This height adaptation is, however, not sufficient for realistic model adaptation. A patient of 180 cm and 70 kg has a completely different body shape than a patient of the same height and 120 kg. Thus, the body surface has to be adapted to the patient's weight too.

4.2   Body Weight Adaptation

In order to correctly adapt the model according to the patient's weight the average body surface area (BSA) is calculated based on several formulas, which approximate the BSA according to age, sex, weight and height based on statistical data. The model adaptation is done by expanding the surface along the normal vectors of the mesh polygons, until the approximated destination surface area is reached. This adaptation must not change the model proportions between corpus and extremities and it takes the varying growing behaviors of different body regions into account.

The following standard formulas for calculating the BSA are integrated into the BurnCase 3D Core system and can be chosen by the surgeon alternatively.

Mosteller [Mosteller, 1987]
A_{BSA} ... Body Surface Area [m²]
H_B ... Body Height [cm]
W_B ... Body Weight [kg]

$$A_{BSA} = \left(\frac{H_B * W_B}{3600} \right)^{\frac{1}{2}} \tag{2}$$

DuBois & DuBois [DuBois&DuBois, 1916] $A_{BSA} = 0.20247 \cdot H_B^{0.725} \cdot W_B^{0.425}$ (3)
   A_{BSA} ... Body Surface Area [m²]
   H_B ... Body Height [m]
   W_B ... Body Weight [kg]

Haycock [Haycock, 1978] $A_{BSA} = 0.024265 \cdot H_B^{0.3964} \cdot W_B^{0.5378}$ (4)
   A_{BSA} ... Body Surface Area [m²]
   H_B ... Body Height [cm]
   W_B ... Body Weight [kg]

Gehan & George [Gehan&George, 1970] $A_{BSA} = 0.0235 \cdot H_B^{0.42246} \cdot W_B^{0.51456}$ (5)
   A_{BSA} ... Body Surface Area [m²]
   H_B ... Body Height [cm]
   W_B ... Body Weight [kg]

Boyd [Boyd, 1930] $A_{BSA} = 0.0003207 \cdot H_B^{0.3} \cdot W_B^{(0.7258-(0.0188 Log(W_B))}$ (6)
   A_{BSA} ... Body Surface Area [m²]
   H_B ... Body Height [cm]
   W_B ... Body Weight [g]

Lam & Leung [Lam&Leung, 1988] $A_{BSA} = 0.007184 * H_L^{0.725} * W_L^{0.425}$ (7)
   A_{BSA} ... Body Surface Area [m²]
   H_L ... Body Height [cm]
   W_L ... Body Weight [kg]

These formulas give good approximations of the BSA for adults in western populations. BurnCase 3D calculates the approximated surface area according to one of these formulas based on the patient's height and weight. After the standard model has been uniformly stretched along the longitudinal axis to fit the body height BurnCase 3D starts the expansion algorithm until the model fits the calculated BSA. Therefore, every triangle's edge vertices are translated along the direction of the exterior normal vector of each vertex.

Let the set of m adjacent triangles T for V_i (triangles that contain V_i) be defined as

$$T(V_i) = \{t_1, t_2, ...t_m | V_i \in t_i\}$$ (8)

Each triangle t_i in T defines a normal vector $\overline{N}$ perpendicular to the triangle's plane. Let the three vertices of t_i be V_1, V_2, and V_3 then the triangle's normal vector is defined as

$$\overline{N}(t_i) = \overrightarrow{V_1 V_2} \times \overrightarrow{V_2 V_3}$$ (9)

Consequently, the normal vector N of vertex V_i is the average vector of all adjacent triangle's normal vectors and can be described as

$$N(V_i) = \left(\sum_{t_i \in T(V_i)} \frac{\overline{N}(t_i)}{|\overline{N}(t_i)|} \right) \frac{1}{m} \tag{10}$$

Where m is the size of $T(V_i)$. The normal vector $\overline{N}$ has to be normalized (division by vector length) in order to receive the correct vertex normal. A linear iteration algorithm computes the factor of translation for every iteration step as

$$factor_{BSA} = \begin{cases} \frac{BSA_{dest}}{BSA_{current}} - 1, & \frac{BSA_{current}}{BSA_{dest}} \geq 2 \\ 1 - \frac{BSA_{current}}{BSA_{dest}}, & else \end{cases} \tag{11}$$

This factor$_{BSA}$ is multiplied by the normal vector of each vertex. The resulting product vector is added to the vertex by vector addition which causes the vertex to move exterior or interior along the direction of its normal vector. The direction is dependent on whether the destination BSA is greater (causing a positive factor$_{BSA}$) or smaller than the current BSA (causing a negative factor$_{BSA}$).

This method converges in most cases, but for extreme values of body height and body weight the iteration may not converge. Thus, BurnCase 3D limits this iterative adaptation to a maximum of 300 iteration steps. The average amount of iterations until the destination height and BSA is reached lies between 4 and 20 steps. For performance reasons the body height adaptation and the body weight adaptation are combined in one iteration procedure. Consequently, less than 20 iterations are needed to adapt both height and BSA of a standard model to a real patient.

4.3   Body Region Growth Behaviors

The adaptation of the model according to body height and weight is described in chapter 4.2. However, the calculation of factor$_{BSA}$ does not take different growth behaviors of different body regions into account. This leads to inappropriate and unrealistic results for patients whose body shapes differ from the body shape of the chosen standard model. In order to avoid these failures each body region additionally defines a growth regression rate. This growth regression rate has a domain of [1, 1000] where 1 means default growth behavior (e.g. chest, stomach, etc.) and 1000 means maximum growth regression (e.g. ear, palpebra).

Thus, a realistic vertex translation along the vertex normal can be applied as follows:

$$\vec{v}_i = \vec{v}_i + \left(\vec{n}_i \frac{factor_{BSA}}{rate_{regression}} \right) \tag{12}$$

Where $\vec{v}$ is the vertex and $\vec{n}$ is the normalized normal vector of this vertex. Without such a growth regulation the model would be deformed unproportionally as depicted in figure 2. Application of equation (12) performs much better and leads to more realistic results as shown in figure 3.

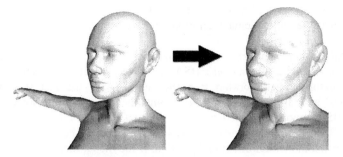

Fig. 2. Unproportional body deformation of the face as consequence of equal growth behaviors of body regions (left: 160cm, 55kg; right: 160cm, 90kg)

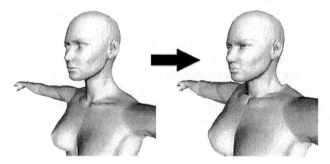

Fig. 3. More realistic body adaptation, taking different growth behaviors of certain body regions into account (left: 160cm, 55kg; right: 160cm, 90kg)

5   Conclusion

The software system BurnCase 3D is already in use in several burn units in Austria and Germany. First results showed up a high reliability of the calculated burnt surface areas on the adapted standard models. In particular, the system is used to determine the surface area of remaining healthy skin that could be used for skin transplantation. The results were verified after the surgery and showed an accordance of only a few square centimeters.

Although the adaptation results are very promising, there are still several drawbacks that have to be overcome. Extreme body shapes cause the adaptation algorithm to build rough edges on the border line between two body regions with different growth behaviors. This can be observed e.g. on the shoulder blade in Figure 3 since shoulders and thorax grow much faster than the neck, resulting in unrealistic edges. [Siegl, 2003] shows that it is possible to refine the deformation results by application of several different smoothing algorithms like iterative smoothing, curve smoothing (sigmoid smoothing) and graded smoothing. These algorithms can smooth the borders between body regions with different growth behaviors. Furthermore, it is suggested to define different types of deformation each defining a specific set of growth parameters. Thus, the typical male type of deformation bulges more stomach and thighs whereas the typical female deformation type applies major growth on buttocks and legs.

The adaptation of the model is performed based on the size of the model's body surface area. As long as the model's BSA does not approximately match a calculated BSA, the deformation algorithm is performed. Due to the fact that these BSA formulas just give approximations which sometimes diverge immensely from a real person's BSA, another approach should be taken into consideration. Not the calculated BSA, but measurements entered by the surgeon should act as termination criterion for the model deformation algorithm. If the model measurements became of greater importance for the deformation process also the measurement methods would have to become more flexible. At present, the measurement methods are only used in order to evaluate the results of the model deformation. However, in clinical practice it is often very difficult to measure parameters like arm perimeter, thigh perimeter, chest perimeter, and many more.

Since July 2003 a first version of the software system is being tested in 3 hospitals in Austria, one hospital in Germany followed February 2004. The results are promising and show that the improved estimation process of injured surface area will have influences in modern burn treatment especially in the application of formulas for fluid donation and planning of skin transplantation. Nevertheless, further investigations on the adequacy and accuracy of the software results are necessary.

References

[Boyd, 1930] Boyd E: Experimental error inherent in measuring growing human body, Am J Physiol 1930; 13:389–432.

[DuBois&DuBois, 1916] DuBois D and DuBois EF: A formula to estimate the approximate surface area if height and weight be known. Arch Intern Med 1916; 17:863–71.

[Flügel et al., 1986] Flügel B, Greil H, Sommer K: Anthropologischer Atlas. Edition Wötzel, 1986.

[Gehan&George, 1970] Gehan EA, George SL: Estimation of human surface area from height and weight. Cancer Chemother Rep part 1 1970; 54:225–35.

[Haycock, 1978] Haycock GB, Schwarta GJ, Wistosky DH: Geometric method for measuring body surface area: A height-weight formula validated in infants, children, and adults. J Pediatr 1978; 93:62–6

[Lam&Leung, 1988] Lam TK, Leung DT: More on simplified calculation of body-surface area, N Engl J Med 1988 Apr 28; 318(17):1130, (letter)

[Livingston and Lee, 2000] Livingston EH, Lee S: Percentage of burned body surface area determination in obese and nonobese patients. J Surg Res. 2000, 91(2):106-10.

[Mosteller, 1987] Mosteller RD: Simplified calculation of body surface area. N Engl J Med 1987; 317:1098

[Siegl, 2003] Siegl D: Virtual Human Body Deformation for Medical Applications. Diploma Thesis, Polytechnic University of Hagenberg, Software Engineering for Medical Purposes, 2003.

Fast Soft Tissue Deformation with Tetrahedral Mass Spring Model for Maxillofacial Surgery Planning Systems

Wouter Mollemans, Filip Schutyser, Johan Van Cleynenbreugel, and
Paul Suetens

Medical Image Computing (Radiology - ESAT/PSI), Faculties of Medicine and
Engineering, University Hospital GasthuisBerg, Herestraat 49, B-3000 Leuven,
Belgium

Abstract. Maxillofacial surgery simulation and planning is an extremely challenging area of research combining medical imagery, computer graphics and mathematical modelling. In maxillofacial surgery abnormalities of the skeleton of the head are treat by skull remodelling. Since the human face plays a key role in interpersonal relationships, people are very sensitive to changes to their outlook. Therefore planning of the operation and reliable prediction of the facial changes are very important. Recently, the use of 3D image-based surgery planning systems is more and more accepted in this field. Although the bone-related planning concepts and methods are maturing, prediction of soft tissue deformation needs further fundamental research. In this paper we present a soft tissue simulator that uses a fast tetrahedral mass spring system to calculate soft tissue deformation due to bone displacement in a short time interval. Results of soft tissue simulation for patients who had a maxillofacial surgery are shown. Finally we truly validated the simulation results and compared our method with others.

1 Introduction

Simulation of the deformation of the facial soft tissues due to bone movement, demands a mathematical model that is able to imitate the behavior of the facial tissues. Various models have been proposed for this simulation.

The Finite Element Method (FEM) [1] [2] is a common and accurate way to compute complex deformations of soft tissue, but conventional FEM has a high computational cost and large memory usage. This makes FEM models inappropriate for realtime simulation. Hybrid models based on global parameterized deformations and local deformations based on FEM, have been introduced to solve this problem[3]. Most of these methods, however, are only applicable to linear deformations and valid for small displacements. Furthermore they rely on pre-computing the complete matrix system and are therefore unable to cope with topological changes when these occur during simulation.

Mass Spring systems (MSS) [4] [5] are widely used to model deformable objects. They are applied to a variety of problems, such as cloth modelling,

C. Barillot, D.R. Haynor, and P. Hellier (Eds.): MICCAI 2004, LNCS 3217, pp. 371–379, 2004.

facial animation or real-time deformation. All approaches use models consisting of mass points and springs. The dynamic behavior of these models is simulated by considering forces at mass points.

A classical mass spring model assumes a discrimination of the object into n points x_i with mass m_i. These points are linked by damped springs. The relation between position, velocity and acceleration for point x_i at time t is defined as

$$m_i \frac{d^2 x_i(t)}{dt^2} + \gamma \frac{dx_i(t)}{dt} + F_i^{int}(t) = -F_i^{ext}(t) \tag{1}$$

with γ denoting a damping factor, $F_i^{int}(t)$ denoting the resulting internal elastic force caused by strains of adjacent springs and $F_i^{ext}(t)$ denoting the sum of external forces, such as gravity or collision reaction forces. Given initial values for $x_i(t)$, $v_i(t)$, $F_i^{int}(t)$ and $F_i^{ext}(t)$ at time t, various methods are commonly applied to numerically integrate through time.

Excellent results can be achieved by applying these numerical integration methods in order to animate deformable models. However, due to numerical problems and slow convergence, these approaches are not very well suited to estimate the rest position of mass spring systems. In maxillofacial surgery this rest position is more important than the exact animation. In previous work [6] we proposed a fast tetrahedral mass spring model to directly estimate the deformation, without calculating the animation.

In the fast tetrahedral mass spring model the object is represented by a number of tetrahedra. A model point p_i is assigned to each vertex and a spring is attached to each edge of the tetrahedra. When a fixed external displacement is applied to some of the points, the new rest position for each point is found by demanding that the total force F_i^{tot} in each point i is minimal. The total force F_i^{tot} in model point i is defined as the sum of forces executed by all springs j that are connected to point i.

$$F_i^{tot} = \sum_{\forall j \in S_i} k_j * (\mid p_j - p_i \mid - L_j) * \frac{p_j - p_i}{\mid p_j - p_i \mid} \tag{2}$$

with S_i denoting the set of all adjacent springs connected to p_i, L_j and k_j denote the initial length and the spring constant of spring j, respectively. As shown in [6] spring constants are determined considering the local mesh geometry and Youngs modulus E of the deformed material.

When comparing this tetrahedral model to a classical mass spring system, one can state some major advantages. Since the model demands that the total force in each soft tissue point is minimal, it is ensured that the outcome of the simulation will be a new rest position for each point. Second as we use a static constraint to find the new rest position, we don't need to know the damping parameter used in a classical mass spring systems. This gives us one parameter less to estimate. Finally our model uses a tetrahedral mesh where classical mass spring systems are layer based [4]. Layer based models consists of several layers with each the same topology: mass points connected by springs to form triangular structures. The consecutive layers are connected by a set of vertical and diagonal inter-layer springs. Obtaining an accurate layer based model starting from volumetric data is certainly not straight froward. Tetrahedral meshes on the other hand, are well studied in classical FEM application and software to automatic generate these meshes, is available.

In this work we present our simulation environment using the fast tetrahedral mass spring system. In the first part the different steps needed for simulation are shown. True validation of the outcome of a simulation is very important and was often lacking in previous work, therefore the validation method is discussed in the second part. Finally we present the results of simulation on real patient data and compare our model to a classical FEM based simulator.

2   The Soft Tissue Simulator

2.1   Acquisition and Bone-Related Planning

When a patient needs to undergo a maxillofacial surgery, pre operatively a CT scan is taken. Out of the CT data we semi-automatic segment the facial soft tissues. First The CT data is treshholded, such that all the soft tissues are segmented. To keep only the outer facial soft tissues, which are important for the soft tissue simulation, a mask is applied to the segmented data. A tetrahedral mesh, that serves as the input for our soft tissue simulator, is created with the Amira software package[1].

Maxilim[2] is a 3D bone-related planning system for maxillofacial surgery, originating from development in our group over the last years [7]. This software allows a maxillofacial surgeon to pre operatively determine the necessary bone movements and see the effect of the procedure.

2.2   Boundary Conditions

If we want to predict the effect of a maxillofacial surgery we have to map the 3D bone-related planning data to the soft tissues. We call this step the determination of the boundary conditions. To do the mapping we presume that the movement of soft tissue points which join at the skull, is equal to the movement of that part of the skull. This way 3 types of points are defined in our soft tissue model:

- Fixed points: All soft tissue points that join at a part of the skull that will not be moved during surgery, are defined as fixed and are not allowed to move during simulation.
- Joint points: All points that join at a part of the skull that will be displaced during surgery due to distraction or repositioning, are called joint points. From the bone-related planning we know the necessary bone displacement and we can define the necessary displacement of the joint points.

---

[1] http://www.amira.com

[2] http://www.medicim.com

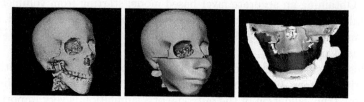

Fig. 1. (a)The planned surgery (created in Maxilim) (b)The planning data is mapped to the soft tissue model (c)Soft tissue model showing the different point types: fixed points (grey), joint points (dark grey) and free points (white).

– Free points: All the other soft tissue points are free. During simulation their movement is completely determined by the resulting force that exists in these points.

The boundary conditions are automatic calculated based on the 3D bone-related planning and the corresponding soft tissue model. Practice has pointed out that the user sometimes wants to define extra boundary conditions, for example by defining extra fixed points. For this purpose we created a coloring module by which the user can interactively select a point or a group of points and define extra conditions for the selected ones.

2.3   Simulation

After preprocessing the patients data, creation of the tetrahedral soft tissue model and determination of the boundary conditions, we can simulate the soft tissue movements due to the bone displacement. The simulator consists of a 3D environment in which the model can be inspected and some interface buttons by which models and boundary conditions can be loaded and simulation can be performed.

It turned out that it is often difficult for a surgeon to immediate see differences between the pre operative and predicted facial skin surface when they are shown together on a workstation. When a dynamic evolution is shown from pre operative to predicted facial surface, the effect of the surgery can much easier be determined. Due to the iterative procedure we use in the fast tetrahedral mass spring system to calculate a new rest position[6], a dynamic transition can easily be generated and shown to the user.

Two main properties for a simulator are its accuracy and the speed of the calculations. Truly validating the accuracy of a simulator is the only way to make a good comparison between two implementations and to see if the approximation goals are reached. Therefore we discuss our validation method in the next section.

3 Validation Procedure

During development of a soft tissue model for surgery planning it is very important to measure how close a prediction is to the real post operative result. The only way to truly measure this accuracy is by comparing post operative data with the predicted data.

To obtain the post operative data, four months after surgery the patient gets a new CT scan. This post operative CT scan is rigidly registered to the pre operative CT data, using maximization of mutual information on a unaltered subvolume[8]. From these co-registered post operative data, a surface representation of the skin is generated. This post operative skin surface will be compared to the predicted skin surface.

We distinguish two different techniques to compare the predicted and post operative skin surface: the first is more qualitative, while the second is a quantitative technique. In the first case we let the user visually compare both surfaces and ask him to give a score value between one and ten, where ten indicates a perfect match. With the second procedure[9] we calculate a distance map between the predicted skin surface and the post operative skin surface. This distance map can be projected on the predicted surface by using a color code or by validating the statistics of the error map. When using the color code, dark grey colors mean that large distances between the predicted and pre operative skin surface were found, while a white color symbolizes areas where both surfaces match perfect. This results in an easily interpretable image of the errors over the entire surface

4 Results

We show results for three patients suffering from unilateral microsomia. All these patients have been treated with unilateral mandibular distraction. The distraction device had two degrees of freedom: unidirectional translation and angular rotation. Figure 2 presents the bone related planning, the pre operative soft tissue model and the predicted new facial outlook. The pre operative facial contour is shown on top of the predicted facial surface to clarify the difference between both surfaces. Simulations were performed on a standard workstation with a 2GHz processor and 1Gbyte of RAM. The soft tissue models contain on average 40000 tetrahedra. All three models were considered as homogenous objects with an elastic modulus $E = 3000Pa$.

In their clinical routine, all patients had a post operative CT scan four months after surgery. These post operative images were also employed to validate our predictions by the above described method. The error images derived from differences between the post operative and pre operative skin surface, are shown in figure 3. As can be seen most errors lie in the range of $-3mm$ and $2mm$. We found that there are two main reasons for the prediction error. In the first place, all patients had a fixation bandage during the pre operative CT, soft tissue deformations due to this bandage result in significant errors in the predicted facial surface. Other large errors occur in regions where the bone has been distracted, we are still searching for a method to compensate this effect.

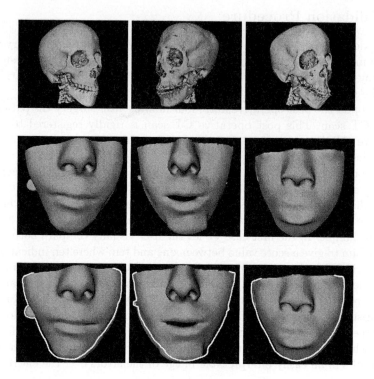

Fig. 2. The pre operative bone-related planning, pre operative facial skin surface and predicted facial surface for the three patients. The pre operative facial contour is shown on top of the predicted facial skin surface.

In the past a FEM based soft tissue simulator has been implemented in our group[2]. To measure accuracy difference between the mass spring system and FEM, we applied the same patient data to the FEM simulator. For the FEM simulations Youngs modulus was chosen at $3000Pa$ and a Poisson coefficient $\nu = 0.45$ was defined. For both methods the histograms of the error map generated by the above described method, are shown in the second row of figure 3. We can notice that our simulator based on the mass spring model and the FEM based simulator, generates a very similar result. The model is clearly capable of giving a good approximation of the soft tissue deformation due to bone distraction.

A second important property of a soft tissue simulator is the time needed to make a prediction. As stated in [6] an iterative procedure is used to find the new rest position of all free points after displacement of the joint points. To validate the speed of this procedure we frequently measured the maximal distance between a temporary result, obtained after a certain number of iterations, and the final stable model. The final stable model is the calculated prediction when no point movement could be noticed anymore between to successive iterations. The maximal distance versus time needed, is shown in figure 4. The graph clearly

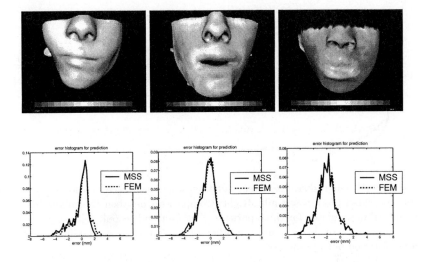

Fig. 3. To validate we measure the distance between predicted and post operative facial skin surface and project these distances on the facial surface with a color code. The scale of the color code ranges from $-8mm$ to $8mm$. A histogram can also be build out of the error data, this is shown in the second row. Histograms of the error data for our simulator that uses the mass spring system and error plots corresponding to deformations calculated with FEM, are shown.

shows that for all three data sets there is an inverse exponential convergence to a stable position. When we take the accuracy of the prediction compared to the real post operative result into consideration, we could state that movements smaller than $1mm$ will have very little influence on the final result. Therefore the iteration procedure can be aborted when maximal movement becomes smaller than $1mm$. The table of figure 4 shows in the first column time needed for each data set to achieve this condition, the second column shows time needed by the FEM based simulator. The maximal and mean distance between the FEM based solution and our solution are shown in column three and four. For our data set, we can conclude that the mass spring system comes much faster to a solution than when the FEM simulator is used. Furthermore the results of both methods are very similar.

5 Conclusion and Discussion

We presented our soft tissue simulator that uses a tetrahedral mass spring system to predict the new facial outlook after maxillofacial surgery. An extensive validation procedure was used to truly measure the accuracy of the model and we compared our simulation results with predictions based on a FEM model. We can conclude that our model is faster and at least as accurate as the FEM simulator and gives a good indication of what the face will look like after surgery.

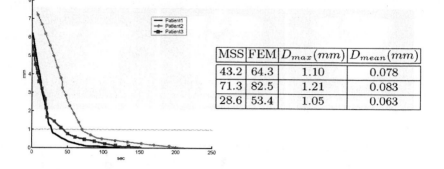

MSS	FEM	$D_{max}(mm)$	$D_{mean}(mm)$
43.2	64.3	1.10	0.078
71.3	82.5	1.21	0.083
28.6	53.4	1.05	0.063

Fig. 4. Left: Maximal distance versus time between the stable prediction and a prediction generated after n seconds. Right: Comparison between the prediction of the MSS and FEM simulator for three patients. The first and second column present time needed for simulation in seconds, the other two columns show maximum and mean distance between both predictions.

However there are still some relative large errors between the predicted and post operative facial outlook. These errors are concentrated around regions where bone was distracted during surgery. Extending our mass spring model so we can compensate for these errors, will be our next challenge. An other field where improvements can be made is determination of the boundary conditions. It would be very useful to know precisely if the soft tissue next to the displaced bone elements stays fixed to it, or what happens exactly. Answers to these questions could influence the prediction result seriously.

Acknowledgements. This work is part of the Flemish government IWT GBOU 020195 project on Realistic image-based facial modelling for forensic reconstruction and surgery simulation and K.U.Leuven/OF/GOA/2004/05.

References

1. Gladilin, E., Zachow, S., Deuflhard, P., Hege, H.: Towards a realistic simulation of individual facial mimincs. In: SPIE Medical Imaging Conference. (2002)
2. Schutyser, F., Cleynenbreugel, J.V., Ferrant, M., Schoenaers, J., Suetens, P.: Image-based 3d planning for maxillofacial distraction procedures including soft tissue implications. Lecture notes in computer science **1935** (200) 999–1007
3. Muller, M.: Stable real-time deformations. In: ACM SIGGRAPH Symposium on Computer Animation (SCA). (2002)
4. Teschner, M.: Direct Computation of Soft-Tissue Deformation in Craniofacial Surgery Simulation. PhD thesis, Friedrich-Alexander-Universitat (2000)
5. Bourguignon, D., Cani, M.P.: Controlling anisotropy in mass-spring systems. In: The 11th Eurographics Workshop on Animation and Simulation. (2000)
6. Mollemans, W., Schutyse, F., Cleynenbreugel, J.V., Suetens, P.: Tetrahedral mass sping model for fast soft tissue deformation. Lecture notes in computer science **2673** (2003) 145–154

7. Poukens, J., Schutyser, F., Cleynenbreugel, J.V., Riediger, D.: 3d planning of distraction osteogenesis with maxilim software. In: Proceedings 4th international congres of maxillofacial and craniofacial distraction. (2003) 251–254
8. Maes, F., Collignon, A., Vandermeulen, D., Marchal, G., Suetens, P.: Multimodality image registration by maximization of mutual information. IEEE transaction on Medical Imaging **16** (1997) 187–198
9. Groeve, P.D., Schutyser, F., Cleynenbreugel, J.V., Suetens, P.: Registration of 3d photographs with spiral ct images for soft tissue simulation in maxillofacial surgery. Lexture notes in computer science **2208** (2001) 991–996

Generic Approach for Biomechanical Simulation of Typical Boundary Value Problems in Cranio-Maxillofacial Surgery Planning

Evgeny Gladilin[1], Alexander Ivanov[2], and Vitaly Roginsky[2]

[1] Zuse Institute Berlin (ZIB), Takustr. 7, D-14195 Berlin, Germany,
[2] Moscow Center of Children's Maxillofacial Surgery,
Timura Frunse 16, 119992 Moscow, Russia

Abstract. In this work, we present a generic approach for biomechanical simulation of two typical boundary value problems arising in cranio-maxillofacial surgery planning, i.e. the prediction of patient's postoperative appearance for a given rearrangement of bones and the reverse optimization of individual facial implants for a desired correction of facial outline. The paper describes the basic methodology for the generation of individual geometrical models from tomographic data, incorporation of the boundary conditions, finite element modeling of tissue biomechanics and experimental results of applied clinical studies.

Keywords: cranio-maxillofacial surgery planning, soft tissue biomechanics, finite element analysis, implant optimization, rapid prototyping

1 Motivation

In cranio-maxillofacial surgery, there is a great demand for efficient computer assisted methods which could enable flexible, accurate and robust simulations of surgical interventions. Modern medical imaging techniques, such as computer tomography (CT) and magnetic resonance imaging (MRI), enable the derivation of useful 3D models of human anatomy. 3D body models provide the information on *geometrical* disposition of different anatomical structures and represent rigid bodies, which only allow rigid and affine transformations. However, the main goal of computer assisted surgery (CAS) is to simulate *physical* interactions with virtual bodies. In particular, the realistic simulation of non-rigid tissue transformations (deformations) under the impact of real or fictitious forces is of crucial importance. Typical boundary value problems arising in the planning of cranio-maxillofacial surgery interventions can formally be subdivided into two major groups:

- "direct problems", e.g. the soft tissue prediction for a given rearrangement of facial bones,
- "inverse problems", e.g. the optimization of individual facial implants for a desired correction of facial outline.

C. Barillot, D.R. Haynor, and P. Hellier (Eds.): MICCAI 2004, LNCS 3217, pp. 380–388, 2004.

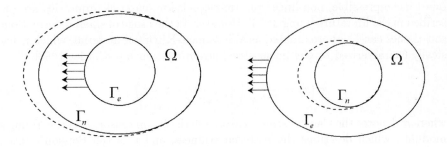

Fig. 1. Typical boundary value problems (BVP) arising in the craniofacial surgical planning: find the deformation of a domain Ω with the natural boundary Γ_n for the boundary conditions given by the prescribed displacements of the essential boundary Γ_e. Left: a direct BVP, e.g. soft tissue prediction for given displacements of bones. Right: an inverse BVP, e.g. find the displacements of bones inducing the desired correction of facial outline.

Both direct and inverse problems are basically of the same nature and can be reduced to a well known boundary value problem (BVP) of structural mechanics: "find the deformation of a domain Ω with the natural boundary Γ_n for the boundary conditions given by the prescribed displacements of the essential boundary Γ_e", see Fig. 1.

In this paper, we present a generic approach for solving typical BVPs of the computer assisted surgery planning (CASP), which is based on the generation of individual geometrical models from tomographic data and the finite element (FE) modeling of deformable biological tissues.

2   Material and Methods

2.1   Geometrical Modeling

Geometrical models of the patient's head are derived from CT data consists of triangulated boundaries between essential soft tissue and bone layers. For the generation of surface models, a standard segmentation technique based on Hounsfield value thresholding as available with Materialise Mimics 6.3 is used [Mimics]. For the subsequent numerical simulation of soft tissue biomechanics, a volumetric grid is required. An unstructured tetrahedral grid for a multi-layer surface model is generated with the help of the multipurpose visualization and modeling system Amira 3.1 [Amira].

2.2   General Soft Tissue Model

Biological tissues exhibit, in general, a very complex biomechanical behaviour. In different experiments with different tissue types, non-homogeneous, anisotropic, quasi-incompressible, non-linear plastic-viscoelastic material properties are described in the literature [Fung 1993]. However, in the range of small deformations soft tissues can be approximated as a St.Venant-Kirchhoff material, which is basically characterized by the linear stress-strain relationship [Ciarlet 1988]:

$$\boldsymbol{\sigma}(\varepsilon) = \frac{E}{1+\nu}\left(\frac{\nu}{1-2\nu}\text{tr}(\varepsilon)\mathbf{I} + \varepsilon\right), \tag{1}$$

where $\boldsymbol{\sigma}$ denotes the Cauchy stress tensor, ε is the strain tensor, E is the Young's modulus, which describes the material stiffness, and ν is the Poisson's ratio, which describes the material compressibility. Typical values for Young's modulus are varying in the range $E \in [2, 200]$kPa. The Poisson's ratio for water-rich soft tissues lies in the range $\nu \in [0.3, 0.5[$. In general, material constants depend on particular tissue type, age, sex and other factors. However, for the quasi-geometrical boundary value problems, i.e. if both boundary conditions and unknowns are the displacements, the simulation results are not sensitive with respect to variation of material constants within "reasonable value ranges" [Gladilin 2003].

The strain tensor in (1) is generally a nonlinear function of the displacement $\mathbf{u}$:

$$\varepsilon(\mathbf{u}) = \frac{1}{2}\left(\boldsymbol{\nabla}\mathbf{u}^{\mathrm{T}} + \boldsymbol{\nabla}\mathbf{u} + \boldsymbol{\nabla}\mathbf{u}^{\mathrm{T}}\boldsymbol{\nabla}\mathbf{u}\right). \tag{2}$$

In the case of small deformations, i.e. $\max|\boldsymbol{\nabla}\mathbf{u}| \ll 1$, the quadratic term in (2) can be neglected, and the strain tensor can be linearized: $\varepsilon(\mathbf{u}) \approx \frac{1}{2}\left(\boldsymbol{\nabla}\mathbf{u}^{\mathrm{T}} + \boldsymbol{\nabla}\mathbf{u}\right)$.

The deformation of a body occupying the domain Ω is obtained as a solution of the boundary value problem (BVP), which is given by (i) the equation of static equilibrium between external loads $\mathbf{f}$ and inner forces (stresses) $\boldsymbol{\sigma}$:

$$\text{div}\boldsymbol{\sigma} + \mathbf{f} = 0 \tag{3}$$

and (ii) the boundary conditions (BC). The boundary conditions in craniofacial surgery simulations are typically given implicitly in the form of node displacements of essential boundaries Γ_e:

$$\mathbf{u}(\mathbf{x}) = \hat{\mathbf{u}}(\mathbf{x}) \quad \mathbf{x} \in \Gamma_e. \tag{4}$$

The essential boundary conditions of structural mechanics correspond to the better known Dirichlet BC of classical potential theory. The Neumann-like BC on "free boundaries" are called the natural BC:

$$\mathbf{t}(\mathbf{x}, \mathbf{n}) = 0 \quad \mathbf{x} \in \Gamma_n, \tag{5}$$

where $\mathbf{t}(\mathbf{x}, \mathbf{n}) = \boldsymbol{\sigma}(\mathbf{x})\mathbf{n}$ is the Couchy stress vector or the traction. In the case of the soft tissue prediction, essential BC are given by the prescribed displacements of rearranged and fixed bones, whereas skin-layer

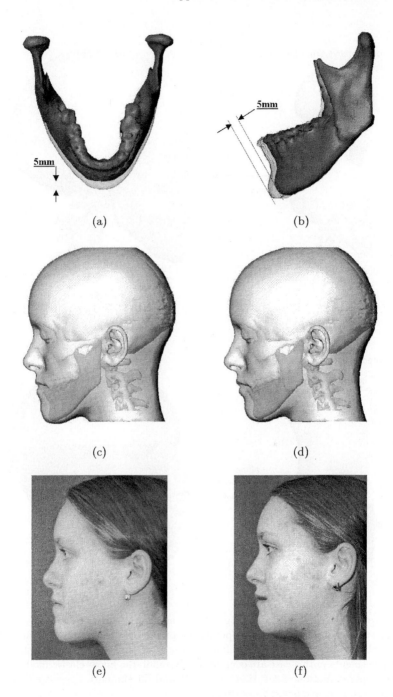

Fig. 2. Setting back mandibula for the correction of lower prognatism (a,b). Geometrical model of preoperative anatomy (c) and the result of the numerical soft tissue prediction (d). Preoperative (e) and postoperative (f) patient profiles, respectively.

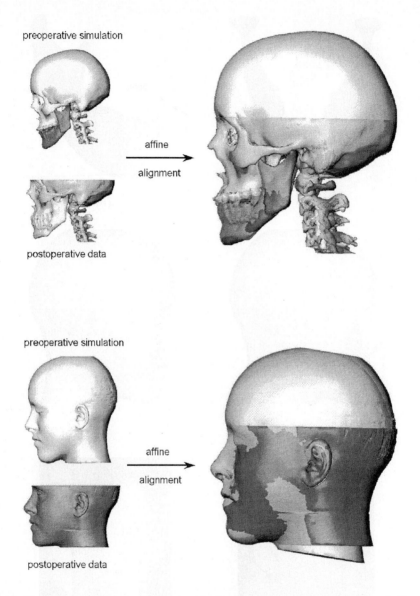

preoperative simulation

affine

alignment

postoperative data

preoperative simulation

affine

alignment

postoperative data

Fig. 3. Top: affine alignment of preoperatively simulated and postoperative skull surfaces. Bottom: superposition of preoperatively predicted and real postoperative facial outlines obtained as a result of the affine alignment of skull surfaces. Since the boundary displacements in this case are comparatively small, the linear elastic model yields a sufficient approximation of soft tissue behavior and the simulation result matches well with the postoperative patient's outline.

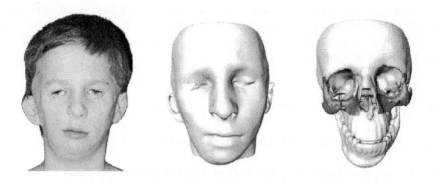

Fig. 4. Left: patient with a Treacher-Collins syndrome. Middle: geometrical model of patient's head with the "virtually corrected" facial outline. Right: initial implant areas.

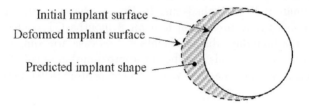

Fig. 5. The volume enclosed by the initial and deformed implant surfaces forms the implant shape, cf. Fig. 1(right).

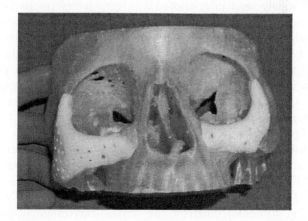

Fig. 6. 3D lithographic model of patient's head including check-bone implants, which were manufactured using the results of the reverse shape optimization.

nodes are set to natural BC. In an inverse BVP, essential boundaries correspond to the warped skin-layer and fixed bones, whereas natural BC are set to the mesh nodes of the initial implant area, cf. Fig. 1(right). To solve the BVP given by (3) and the boundary conditions, the finite element method (FEM) on tetrahedral grids is used [Gladilin et al. 2002].

3   Experimental Results

3.1   Direct Problem. Static Soft Tissue Prediction

In the case of a direct BVP, the patient's postoperative appearance for a given rearrangement of bones has to be predicted. Fig. 2 illustrates the CAS planning for a 15 y.o. female patient with a lower prognatism. The surgical correction consisted in sagittal split osteotomy followed by setting back mandibula by 5mm, see Fig. 2(a,b). The geometrical model derived from CT data consists of a surface mesh corresponding to skin, mandible and skull layers, which has been filled up with approximately 10^6 tetrahedrons. In Fig. 3, the comparison between the result of the soft tissue prediction and an 8 months CT control expertise is shown. Since the boundary displacements in this case are comparatively small, the linear elastic model yields a sufficient approximation of soft tissue behavior and the simulation result matches well with the postoperative patient's outline.

3.2   Inverse Problem. Implant Shape Optimization

In the case of an inverse BVP, the displacements of bones or implants have to be obtained from the prescribed correction of facial outline. Facial implants are nowadays widely used in craniofacial surgery interventions for the correction of facial bones and the improvement of the patient's esthetical appearance [Roginsky et al. 2002]. In Fig. 4, the surgical planning of an inverse craniofacial BVP for a 14 y.o. male patient with a Treacher-Collins syndrome is shown. This patient has already been operated two times within last 5 years with an unsatisfactory outcome. The previous operations consisted of the mandible distraction with the subsequent reinforcement of left and right cheek-bones with the help of implants does not lead to the desired correction of the congenital asymmetry of patient's face. The present surgical impact aims at setting a new, suitably shaped cheek-bone implant over the old one. For the prediction of an optimal implant shape, the methods of reverse biomechanical engineering have been applied. First, the skin-layer of the original 3D mesh near cheek-bones was warped into a desired shape using a 3D sculpture tool as available with Maya 5.0 [Maya], see Fig. 4(middle). Thereby, the "virtual correction" of patient's facial outline has been performed by the maxillofacial surgeon himself. The differences of node coordinates between the warped and original facial meshes yield the displacements, i.e. the boundary conditions for the subsequent FE simulation. Furthermore, the boundary conditions (BC) are given by

- homogenous essential BC on fixed bones,
- non-homogenous essential BC on the displaced skin layer,
- natural BC on initial implant surfaces.

The last condition means that one has to subscribe an initial implant area, where an implant has to be attached to, in order to obtain an unique solution of the inverse BVP, see Fig. 4(right). After assembling the FE system of equations and applying the boundary conditions, the displacement field for the entire mesh has been obtained. The resulting deformation of the initial implant area has been computed by applying the corresponding displacements to the coordinates of the initial implant mesh nodes. The volume enclosed by the initial and deformed implant surfaces forms the implant shape, see Fig. 5. After minor shape improvements, e.g. smoothing some sharp edges, two wax implants (for left and right cheek-bones) have been manufactured with the help of the Stratasys FDM 3000 rapid prototyping system. Subsequently, two biocompatible PMMA/HA[1] implants have been substituted for the wax patterns using the investment casting method, see Fig.6.

4   Conclusion

In this work, a general framework for biomechanical modeling of human head in the craniofacial surgery planning is presented. Our approach is based on the generation of individual 3D models of patient anatomy from tomographic data and the finite element simulation of deformable facial tissues. Two typical boundary value problems arising in the CAS-planning, i.e. the static soft tissue prediction for the surgical planning and the reverse implant optimization, were studied. The results of presented clinical studies are very promising. Further comparative investigations on different patients will help to validate and to fit the underlying biomechanical model of deformable soft tissues. The presented approach can also be applied for the soft tissue prediction and implant optimization in other surgical applications.

References

[Amira] Amira. Indeed - Visual Concepts. URL: http://www.amiravis.com.
[Ciarlet 1988] Ciarlet, P. G. (1988). *Mathematical Elasticity. Volume I: Three-Dimensional Elasticity*, volume 20 of *Studies in Mathematics and its Applications*. North-Holland, Amsterdam.
[Fung 1993] Fung, Y. C. (1993). *Biomechanics - Mechanical Properties of Living Tissues*. Springer, Berlin.
[Gladilin 2003] Gladilin, E. (2003). *Biomechanical Modeling of Soft Tissue and Facial Expressions for Craniofacial Surgery Planning*. PhD thesis, Freie Universität Berlin.

---

[1] PMMA/HA - polymetilmethacrylate and hydroxiapatite.

[Gladilin et al. 2002] Gladilin, E. and Zachow, S. and Deuflhard, P. and Hege, H. C. (2002). Adaptive Nonlinear Elastic FEM for Realistic Prediction of Soft Tissue in Craniofacial Surgery Simulations. In *Proc. of SPIE Medical Imaging Conference*, San Diego, USA.

[Maya] Maya. Alias. URL: http://www.alias.com.

[Mimics] Materialise Mimics. Materialise. URL: http://www.materialise.com.

[Roginsky et al. 2002] Roginsky, V.V. and Popov, V.K. and Ivanov, A.L. and Topolnitzky, O.Z. (2002). Use of stereolithographic and computer biomodeling in children's cranio-maxillofacial surgery. *Journal of Cranio-Maxillofacial Surgery*, 1(1):171–172.

Virtual Unfolding of the Stomach Based on Volumetric Image Deformation

Kensaku Mori[1], Hiroki Oka[1], Takayuki Kitasaka[1],
Yasuhito Suenaga[1], and Jun-ichiro Toriwaki[2]

[1] Graduate School of Information Science, Nagoya University,
Furo-cho, Chikusa-ku, Nagoya 464-8603, Japan
kensaku@is.nagoya-u.ac.jp
[2] School of Computer and Cognitive Sciences, Chukyo University, Toyota, Japan

Abstract. This paper describes a method for generating unfolded views of the stomach based on 3-D gray image deformation. Unfolded views can show the status of the stomach in one image. The previous method approximates the shape of the stomach using a surface model. This approximation is required for the stretching and reconstruction processes. The previous method had the problem that the intensity information inside the stomach wall was not reconstructed appropriately in the unfolded views, because the stretching process was performed by using only the surface information of the stomach. In the proposed method, we generate the approximated shape using a volumetric model. The volumetric model is deformed so as to generate unfolded views of the stomach. We applied the proposed method to five cases of 3-D abdominal CT images. The experimental results showed that the proposed method can unfolded views of the stomach without any undesirable artifacts. Also, it was possible to visualize the progress of unfolding process.

1   Introduction

Virtual endoscopy system (VES) is now widely used for visualizing the insides of anatomical structures[1]. The user of the VES can observe the inside of a target organ from arbitrary viewpoints and view directions. The user also can perform fly-through inside the organ by controlling a mouse. Many medical visualization workstations now have the mode of virtual endoscopy. When we examine the insides of organs having large cavities, such as the colon or the stomach, it is possible to diagnose the status of their internal walls by changing the viewpoint and view direction of the VES. However, we have to frequently change the viewpoint and view direction for observing the entire of a target organ's internal wall. This operation requires much time. Frequent change of the viewpoint and view direction sometimes causes oversight regions that are not observed at all during observation. This also leads oversights of important regions such as lesions. If we could generate unfolded views of a target organ, it would be possible to diagnoses the status of the target organ's wall by only one or a few views. The user does not have to change the viewpoint and direction for observing them.

C. Barillot, D.R. Haynor, and P. Hellier (Eds.): MICCAI 2004, LNCS 3217, pp. 389–396, 2004.
© Springer-Verlag Berlin Heidelberg 2004

We have reported a method for generating unfolded views of the stomach[4]. This method virtually stretches the stomach onto a stretching plane and visualizes the unfolded views. We first extract stomach regions from 3-D abdominal CT images. A set of triangles are generated by applying Marching Cubes method to the extracted regions. The shape model, called the approximated shape, which approximates the shape of the stomach, were constricted from the triangles. It consisted of a set of triangles that represent the outer shape of the stomach. The approximated shape was then stretched onto a stretching plane by elastic deformation of the triangles. The deformed image was reconstructed from the input image by using the geometrical relation between the approximated shape and the deformed approximated shape. This method kept geometrical relation only on the triangles. Since the normals of triangles were crossed around the areas that are close to triangle edges, some artifacts were observed in the unfolded views. Also small fold patterns disappeared in the unfolded views.

For solving these problems, this paper shows an improved method for generating unfolded views of the stomach based on volumetric image deformation. The approximated shape is constructed by a set of hexahedrons. These hexahedrons are deformed by using a node and spring model during a stretching process. The deformed image is reconstructed from the relation between the hexahedrons before and after deformation. Unfolded views are obtained by visualizing the deformed images. Since geometric relation is kept in the deformed image by the proposed method, it is possible to reproduce the fold patterns on the stretched views without causing any artifacts.

There are several researches on generating unfolded views of the colon [2, 3]. Most of these methods basically generate unfolded views by: (a) extracting medial axes and (b) generating unfolded views by casting rays from the medial axes. Because simple ray-casting from the medial axes causes tremendous distortion in the generated views, some researchers reported a method for minimizing distortion in the generated views [3]. However, the target of these methods is the colon. There is no report about unfolded view generation of the stomach. Also, the above stated method cannot be applied to the stomach, because the stomach has large cavity than the colon and its diameter largely changes along its medial axis. Simple unfolding along the medial axis does not give us satisfactory results in the case of the stomach.

In Sect. 2, we present a method for generating unfolded views based on volumetric image deformation. Sect. 3 shows experimental results of virtual unfolding of the stomach. The unfolding process is also visualized in this section. Brief discussion is given in the same section.

2   Method

2.1   Overview

The proposed method consists of four major steps: (1) generation of an approximated shape, (2) deformation of the approximated shape using the node-spring

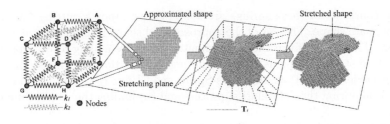

Fig. 1. Elastic modeling and deformation process. (a) Elastic modeling using nodes and springs, (b) unfolding by adding forces that direct to the stretching plane.

model, (3) reconstruction of volumetric image using the relation between the approximated shape and the stretched approximated shape, and (4) visualization of the reconstructed image.

2.2   Generation of Approximated Shape

In this step, we model the shape of a target organ by a set of hexahedrons. First we extract the stomach wall by using the method described in [4]. We shrink the obtained binary image, which stores the extraction result, by simply sampling the image at every d voxels. For each voxel of the shrunk image, a hexahedron is allocated so that its center coincides with the location of the voxel. The length of each edge of the hexahedron is equal to the sample interval d. Two hexahedrons of two adjacent voxels share one surface including four vertices and four edges. The approximated shape is obtained by allocating hexahedrons for all of sample points.

2.3   Deformation of the Approximated Shape

This process stretches the approximated shape by using elastic deformation of the hexahedrons. We allocate nodes at the vertices of the hexahedrons. Here we denote eight vertices of one hexahedron as **A**, **B**, **C**, **D**, **E**, **F**, **G**, **H** (Fig. 1. Springs are allocated on the edges of a hexahedron and on two diagonals on the surface of the hexahedron. Neighboring hexahedrons share nodes and springs. Deformation of the approximated shape is achieved by adding forces, which direct the nodes onto a stretching plane, to the selected nodes. The deformation is computed by iteratively updating the positions of each node based on the force working on each node. The stretching plane is manually allocated by using graphical user interface.

For a hexahedron, we allocate nodes on each vertex and springs on the edges between the vertices **AB**, **BC**, **CD**, **DA**, **AE**, **BF**, **CG**, **DH**, **EF**, **FG**, **GH**, **HE** as illustrated in Fig. 1. The spring constants are set to be k_1 and the natural lengths are the distances between these vertices. Also we allocate springs in the diagonal direction (between the vertices **AC**, **CH**, **AH**, **GE**, **BE**, **BG**. The spring constants of these springs are k_2. Then we input a cutting line on the approximate shape. The cut of the approximated shape is implemented as cut of springs. Then, we deform the approximated shape by adding forces that direct nodes to a stretching plane. For calculating deformation, we choose tne Node-Spring model rather than the Mass-Spring model for: (a) avoiding undesireble oscillation during the deformation process and (b) finding the equilibrium of the forces.

When the stretching force $\mathbf{F}_i(n-1)$ is added to the node i, the position of the node i at the n-th iteration step is described as

$$\mathbf{P}_i(n) = \mathbf{P}_i(n-1) + \rho \mathbf{F}_i(n-1), \tag{1}$$

where ρ is a constant that controls the movement of the node at one iteration step. $\mathbf{F}_i(n)$ is force working on the node i and formulated as

$$\mathbf{F}_i(n) = \mathbf{Fo}_i(n) + \sum_{j \in N_i} \mathbf{Fn}_{ij}(n), \tag{2}$$

where N_i is a set of nodes connecting to the node i. The force $\mathbf{Fn}_{ij}(n)$ is a force caused by the spring between the nodes i and j and represented by

$$\mathbf{Fn}_{ij}(n) = k(\|\mathbf{R}_{ij}(n)\| - l_{ij})\frac{\mathbf{R}_{ij}(n)}{\|\mathbf{R}_{ij}(n)\|}, \tag{3}$$

where l_{ij} is a natural length of the spring between the nodes i and j,k a spring constant, and $\mathbf{R}_{ij}(n)$ a vector that directs from the node i to the node j. $\mathbf{Fo}_i(n)$ is a force for stretching and is working on the nodes that the user specifies. It is formulated as

$$\mathbf{Fo}_i(n) = \alpha \mathbf{T}_i(n), \tag{4}$$

where $\mathbf{T}_i(n)$ is a vector that directs from the node i to the stretching plane. We add the stretching force until the approximated shape becomes a desired shape.

2.4   Volumetric Image Deformation

We deform the input image by using the geometrical relation between the approximated shape and the stretched shape (Fig. 2). All of the hexahedrons of the approximated shape and the stretched shape have one-to-one correspondences. The deformed image is generated by using this relation. We assume that the i-th hexahedron H_i of the approximated shape corresponds to a hexahedron H_i' of the approximated shape. We assume that the vertices $\mathbf{A}$, $\mathbf{B}$, $\mathbf{C}$, $\mathbf{D}$, $\mathbf{E}$, $\mathbf{F}$, $\mathbf{G}$, and $\mathbf{H}$ of H_i correspond to the vertices $\mathbf{A}'$, $\mathbf{B}'$, $\mathbf{C}'$, $\mathbf{D}'$, $\mathbf{E}'$, $\mathbf{F}'$, $\mathbf{G}'$, and $\mathbf{H}'$ of H_i', respectively. When an internal dividing point $\mathbf{P}'$ is in the tetrahedron formed by vertices $\mathbf{A}'\mathbf{C}'\mathbf{D}'\mathbf{H}'$, the point $\mathbf{P}'$ can be represented by

$$\mathbf{P}' = (1-t)\mathbf{A}' + t(s((1-u)\mathbf{C}' + u\mathbf{D}') + (1-s)\mathbf{H}'), \tag{5}$$

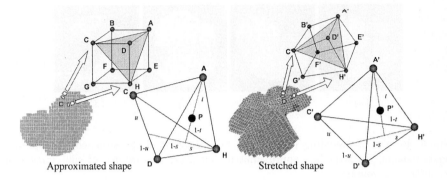

Fig. 2. Geometrical relation between the approximated shape and stretched shape.

where s, u, and t are internal dividing parameters and satisfy $0 \leq s, t, u \leq 1$. The point $\mathbf{P}$ corresponding to $\mathbf{P}'$ can be expressed as

$$\mathbf{P} = (1-t)\mathbf{A} + t(s((1-u)\mathbf{C} + u\mathbf{D}) + (1-s)\mathbf{H}). \qquad (6)$$

If the point $\mathbf{P}'$ is inside a tetrahedron formed by vertices $\mathbf{A}'\mathbf{E}'\mathbf{F}'\mathbf{H}'$, $\mathbf{A}'\mathbf{B}'\mathbf{C}'\mathbf{F}'$, $\mathbf{A}'\mathbf{C}'\mathbf{F}'\mathbf{H}'$, or $\mathbf{C}'\mathbf{F}'\mathbf{G}'\mathbf{H}'$, the corresponding point $\mathbf{P}$ can be calculated in the same way. The gray value at the point $\mathbf{P}'$ in the reconstructed image is computed from the gray values at $\mathbf{P}$ and its neighboring points by linear interpolation. We iterate this process for all points of the reconstruction image.

2.5   Visualization

We visualize the reconstructed image where the target organ is stretched by using a volume rendering method. Virtually stretched image are finally obtained from this visualization process.

3   Experimental Results and Discussion

We have applied the proposed method to five cases of 3-D abdominal CT images. The parameters are set as $\rho = 1$, $k_1 = 0.5$, $k_2 = 0.1$, $\alpha = 0.8$. These values are determined experimentally so that the approximated shapes are stretched on the stretching planes satisfactorily for all cases. Sampling interval in the process of the approximated shape generation is set to be $d = 8$. It took 60 minutes in the approximated shape generation, 15 minutes for stretching, and 30 minutes in volumetric image reconstruction on a conventional PC (CPU: Intel Pentium III 1.0 GHz, Main memory: 1 GB, OS: Windows 2000). Acquisition parameters of CT images are: 512×512 pixels, $150 - 181$ slices, 0.625×0.625 mm of pixel pitch, 1.0 mm in slice intervals, and $1.0 - 5.0$ mm in slice thickness. Figure 3 shows the approximated shape and its unfolded one. The unfolded views obtained by

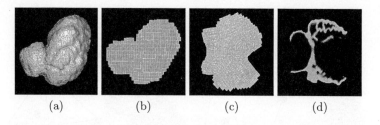

(a)   (b)   (c)   (d)

Fig. 3. Results of unfolding process. (a) Outside view of the stomach, (b) approximated shape, (b) stretched approximated shape, (c) an example of slice images of reconstructed volume.

the previous and the proposed methods are shown in Fig. 4. We visualized the progress of the unfolding process by continuously performing volumetric image reconstruction in Fig. 5.

From the experimental results, it is obvious that the proposed method can generate unfolded views satisfactorily. There are many folds, which have mountain ridge shapes, on the internal wall of the stomach. Because these folds show concentration patterns to lesions in the case of stomach cancer, running directions of folds are very important information for diagnosing the stomach. The unfolded views are quite useful for diagnosing running directions of folds, since it is possible to observe the status of the stomach wall only by one view. Also, the proposed method generates unfolded views basing upon the rule for generating the specimen of a resected stomach defined by Japanese Gastric Cancer Association. Physicians can intuitively understand the status of the stomach by using the generated views.

In the experimental results, the proposed method reproduces small fold patterns very well on the stretched views. Such patterns disappear in the unfolded views obtained by the previous method. Also, some artifacts are observed on the borders of triangles of the approximated shape in the previous method. Such artifacts are not observed on the unfolded views of the proposed method. As illustrated in Fig. 6, although large folds are reproduced well on the unfolded views of the previous method, there are regions that are reproduced with heavy distortion (the part indicated by the arrow in Fig. 6) and some artifacts that do not exist on the original stomach wall. This is because the previous method kept geometric relation only on the triangles. On the other hand, there is no such region in the unfolded views generated by the proposed method. Since the proposed method constructs an elastic model of the stomach wall and then deforms it with keeping its internal geometrical relation by introducing a hexahedron deformation model, few artifacts are observed on the unfolded views.

4   Conclusions

This paper presented an improved method for generating stretched views based on volumetric image deformation. We constructed the approximated shape by

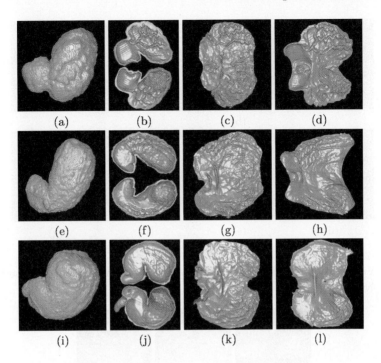

Fig. 4. Unfolded views. (a,e,i) Outside views, (b,f,j) inside views obtained by dividing stomach regions, (c,g,k) unfolded views obtained by the previous method, and (d,h,l) unfolded views by the proposed method.

a set of hexahedrons. We deformed these hexahedrons by using a node-spring model and adding stretching forces to them. The deformed image was reconstructed from the relation between the hexahedrons before and after deformation. Since geometric relation was kept in the deformed image by the proposed method, it was possible to reproduce fold patterns on the stretched views without causing any artifacts. The experimental results showed much improvement in the reproduction of fold patterns on the inner wall of the target organ. Future work includes: (a) quantitative analysis of unfolded views, (b) improvement of computation time, and (c) application to many cases.

Acknowledgments. The authors thank to our colleagues for their useful suggestions and discussions. Parts of this research were supported by the 21st century COE program, the Grant-In-Aid for Scientific Research from Ministry of Education, Sports, Science and Technology and the Japan Society for Promotion of Science, and the Grant-In-Aid for Cancer Research from the Ministry of Health and Welfare of Japanese Government.

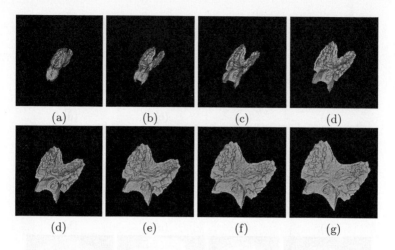

Fig. 5. Visualization results of unfolding process. The unfolding process is performed in time sequence of (a) to (g).

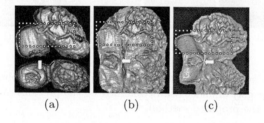

Fig. 6. Comparison of reproduction results of the fold patterns. The regions indicated by the arrows show distorted region reconstructed by the previous method. There exist artifacts of triangles on the view obtained by the previous method inside the area surrounded by dotted line. (a) Inside view, (b) unfolded view by the previous method, and (c) by the proposed method.

References

1. P. Rogalla, J. Terwisscha van Scheltinga, B. Hamm, eds., "Virtual endoscopy and related 3D techniques," Springer, Berlin, pp. 946–950, 2001.
2. G. Wang, E. G. McFarland, B. P . Brown et al., "GI Tract Unraveling with Curved Cross Section," IEEE Trans. on Medical Imaging, 17, 2, pp. 318–322, 1998.
3. S. Haker, S. Angenent, A. Tannenbaum, R. Kikinis, "Nondistorting flattening maps and the 3-D visualization of colon CT images," IEEE Trans. on Medical Imaging, 19, 7, pp. 665–670, 2000.
4. H. Oka, Y. Hayashi, K. Mori, et al. "A method for generating unfolded views of organ and its comparison with virtual endoscopy based on undisplayed region rate," Medical Imaging 2003: Physiology and Function: Methods, Systems, and Application, Proceedings of SPIE, vol.5031, pp. 99-101, 2003.

Cadaver Validation of the Use of Ultrasound for 3D Model Instantiation of Bony Anatomy in Image Guided Orthopaedic Surgery

C.S.K. Chan[1], D.C. Barratt[1], P.J. Edwards[1,2], G.P. Penney[1], M. Slomczykowski[3], T.J. Carter[1], and D.J. Hawkes[1]

[1] Imaging Sciences Division, King's College London, Guy's Hospital, London, UK
carolyn.chan@kcl.ac.uk
[2] Department of Surgical Oncology and Technology, Imperial College London, London, UK
[3] i-Orthopaedics, DePuy a Johnson & Johnson company, Heimstetten, Germany

Abstract. We present cadaver validation of a method that uses tracked ultrasound to instantiate and register 3D statistical shape models (SSMs) of 3 femurs and 2 pelves. The SSMs were generated directly from the deformation fields obtained from non-rigid registration of CT images to a single target CT image. Ultrasound images were obtained from three intact cadavers. These were used to instantiate the model by iteratively minimising the RMS distance between the model surface and the ultrasound-derived bone surface points. The RMS distance between the instantiated model surface and the CT-derived bone surface was less than 3.72mm in the region of the femoral head and acetabulum. We conclude that SSMs of the femur and pelvis may be instantiated and registered to surgical space to within a clinically acceptable accuracy using intra-operative ultrasound. This potentially could reduce the invasiveness of orthopaedic procedures, and remove the requirement for a preoperative CT scan.

1 Introduction

SSMs have recently generated considerable interest for use in orthopaedic surgery, both for image segmentation and for navigation. In particular, it has been shown that a 3D surface model can be instantiated from X-ray images using an SSM [4]. We have recently proposed that instantiation of a 3D model can also be achieved using tracked ultrasound(US)[3]. The present paper describes important modifications to the method described earlier for generating the shape model, and also validation using cadaveric data where an accurate Gold Standard image-to-physical registration transformation (based on bone-implanted fiducial markers) to a high-resolution CT scan was available.

The method uses a statistical shape model (SSM) to generate an anatomically realistic model of bony anatomy given a large number of points on the bone surface extracted from US images[3]. The motivations for this work are to exploit the inherent advantages of accurate image-guided total hip replacement without

C. Barillot, D.R. Haynor, and P. Hellier (Eds.): MICCAI 2004, LNCS 3217, pp. 397–404, 2004.
© Springer-Verlag Berlin Heidelberg 2004

the need for a preoperative computed tomography (CT) scan with its associated radiation dose and expense. The use of US to register the bone also results in a reduction in invasiveness of the procedure compared to conventional methods. In our previous work the SSM was built purely using bone surface points[3]. However, in the present study we have used a 3D vector field, calculated by non-rigid registration of each training CT image onto a template image, in order to establish correspondence between elements of the training set. This approach has the advantage that a complete reconstruction of a synthetic 3D volume can be achieved, including estimates of density changes and the internal structure of bony anatomy that is represented in the training data.

US provides a safe, non-invasive and relatively inexpensive method for locating bone surfaces intraoperatively. Initial phantom studies have demonstrated that US can be used to instantiate and register a femur SSM[2]. This paper describes the validation of the combined instantiation and registration of femur and pelvis SSMs using much more realistic US data collected on 3 cadavers, with corresponding CT volumes providing the ground-truth shape.

At least two other groups have developed shape models for orthopaedic surgery. Yao and Taylor[12] have demonstrated 2D/3D non-rigid registration between a statistical bone density atlas of the hip and a set of X-ray images, and instantiated a deformable hemi-pelvis model with anatomical structures visible in a CT image[11]. Fleute and Lavallee[4], and Fleute et al.[5], instantiated 3D anatomical surfaces of the spine from a point distribution model (PDM) with a few X-rays using a contour-based registration method. To the best of our knowledge, no other groups have attempted to instantiate a 3D model using tracked US apart from [2].

2   Methods and Materials

2.1   Experimental Procedure

Experiments for this study were carried out in the Institute of Anatomy, Ludwig-Maximilians University, Munich using 3 complete female cadavers preserved using the method of W. Thiel[10]. Titanium bone screws were implanted into the femur and pelvis of each cadaver (4 in each femur and 5 in each hemi-pelvis) and fiducial markers, filled with CT contrast agent (Urografin 370, Scherring Health Care Ltd), were attached. A single high-resolution CT scan was then obtained for each cadaver using a spiral CT scanner (Siemans SOMATOM Plus 5). The extent of the CT scan included the whole pelvis and leg down to below the knee, reconstructed with voxel dimensions $0.71 \times 0.71 \times 2 \text{mm}^3$. Following the CT scan, each cadaver was returned to the laboratory and the contrast-filled fiducial markers were replaced with markers which had a 3mm divot, the centre of which is coincident with the centroid of the fluid-filled chamber of the CT-visible markers. This enabled the CT scan to be accurately registered with physical space after using a tracked localiser to measure the 3D positions of the divot centres. All measurements were recorded relative to the 3D coordinate system of a dynamic reference object implanted into the femur or pelvis (see Fig.1).

In this study, a commercial US scanner (Philips-ATL HDI-5000) and high-frequency scan-probe (L12-5, 5-12MHz broadband linear-array transducer) were used to acquire US images. The 3D positions and orientations of US images were measured as the scan-probe was swept slowly across the skin surface. A high-accuracy optical tracking device (Optotrak 3020, Northern Digital Inc., Ontario, Canada) was used to track a custom-built object fixed to the scan-probe, as shown in Fig. 1. This enabled the 3D position and orientation of each 2D ultrasound image to be calculated with respect to the dynamic reference co-ordinate system. The use of a tracked dynamic reference object enabled the position of the cadaver to be changed during US acquisition. This allowed images to be obtained in regions that would otherwise be inaccessible with the cadaver in the supine position.

US images were collected from several approaches so that as many anatomical features as possible were scanned in order to ensure that the model instantiation was well constrained in regions such as the femoral neck and condyles. The number of US image frames acquired was between 248 and 518. The time taken to acquire them was on average 8 minutes and the total number of US points extracted was between 992 and 2107. The US images were segmented manually to extract the bone surface.

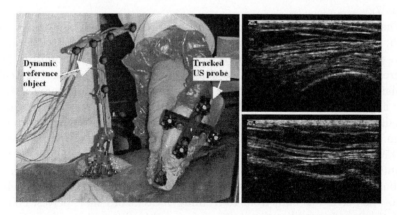

Fig. 1. Tracked US probe scanning the femur (*left*); sample US images in the femur (*top right*) and pelvis (*bottom right*)

2.2   Construction of the Statistical Shape Model

One template image was selected from our database of CT scans and aligned to the other images in the database using a non-rigid registration algorithm[8]. This algorithm uses a combination of global and local transformations: global motion is modelled by both rigid (rotations and translations) and affine (scaling and shearing) transformations. The shapes of the femur and pelvis are challenging for a registration algorithm based on non-rigid registration. Consequently, an initial alignment was defined manually to incorporate rigid movement and scaling (a total of nine degrees of freedom) so that the likelihood of obviously incorrect correspondences was reduced. The local transformation was then modelled by a free-form deformation (FFD) model based on B-splines[8].

The FFD has a potentially large number of degrees of freedom, and is defined by the deformed positions of a regular grid of B-spline node points. The global transformation describes the overall translation and rotation of the bone, while the local transformation is used to describe shape deformation. Normalised mutual information (NMI) was employed as a voxel-based similarity measure [9].

Using the results from the non-rigid registration described above, which registered training CT datasets to one template image, a PDM was built on the node points (also called control points) of the approximating B-splines used to define the FFD. The output of the principal component analysis (PCA) was the mean deformation of the template, with the eigenmodes and eigenvalues representing the deformation fields. The number of node points used for the femur model was about 184, whereas 395 node points were used for the pelvis model. In both cases, a node point spacing of 20mm was used. This method was originally applied to magnetic resonance (MR) images of the brain with encouraging results[7].

The instantiation process generates a high-resolution, 3D grey-level image, which, in this case, has the appearance of a CT scan. In our application this allows propagation of a more densely sampled surface and incorporation of other features, such as variations in bone density, which have important implications for planning prosthesis placement in image-guided orthopaedic surgery. On the other hand, when generating a PDM purely for surface data, there is the problem of finding point correspondence, which can only be achieved by interpolating within the surface, and may give rise to errors in surface shape and texture. The method proposed here provides an estimate of all correspondences within the volume of the bone fully automatically. The femur model used in this study was built from 16 training datasets of mixed male and female femurs, whereas that of the pelvis was built from 10 training datasets of female pelves. Following PCA, the first five modes of variation were used in the model (as a compromise between computational time and population coverage), with individual variation within each mode allowed up to three standard deviations.

2.3   Instantiation of the Statistical Shape Model

US-derived bone surface points were matched to the corresponding SSM surface using the ICP algorithm[1], using the mean shape of each model as the starting estimate. Multiple starting positions for the rigid body registration parameters were used to initialise the instantiation process in order to simulate starting positions which could be obtained in a clinical setting. Three observers were invited to produce 3 starting positions, giving 9 starting positions in total for each instantiation. Given the first 5 modes of variation, the root-mean-square(RMS) point-to-surface distance was then minimised using a multiple layer optimisation strategy. In this scheme, the weight corresponding to each mode of variation was varied and the US points registered to the resulting shape model using the ICP algorithm. A four layer strategy was used, where two modes were considered at layer 1 (modes 1 and 2) and this was increased to five modes by layer 4 (modes 1 to 5). On each iteration, a Golden Section search [6] was used to optimise the shape within one mode alone, with the weight corresponding to all other modes held constant. Visual inspection revealed that one of the pelvic datasets had a number of US points which were obvious outliers. These were removed by aligning the US points with the mean shape and then excluding 5% of the points with the largest RMS point-to-surface distance were excluded from the instantiation.

3   Results

Fig. 2 shows the first mode for the left femur and pelvis models when applying plus or minus three standard deviations to the mean shape. The first mode of the left femur model can be seen to correspond to a change in the femur size and length. Other significant modes of variations include a twisting of the femoral head angle and change of trochanter and condyle sizes.

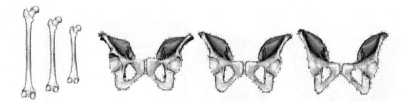

Fig. 2. The left femur PDM (*left*) and the pelvis PDM (*right*) showing the first mode of variation with +/- three standard deviations.

The results of the femur and pelvis instantiations from cadaver 1 are illustrated in Fig. 3 and 4. In each figure, the bone surface segmented from the CT scan was used as the Gold Standard shape model. Results from other cadavers were similar.

Numerical results are given in Table 1 calculated in three different ways. Firstly, the RMS distance was calculated between the instantiated SSM and the US-derived bone surface points registered using the ICP algorithm. Secondly, the RMS distance was calculated between the instantiated SSM and the CT-derived surface, using the Gold Standard (GS) transformation, calculated from point-based registration of the bone-implanted fiducial markers. This measure

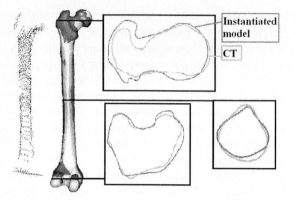

Fig. 3. (*Left to right*) US-derived femur surface points (*left*) and the instantiated SSM overlaid on the CT-derived surface, shown in dark grey. Cross-sectional contours from the instantiated femur model (*black*) with corresponding contours from the CT (*grey*). From top to bottom: the condyles; mid-shaft; and the femoral head.

indicates the combined accuracy of the geometry of the instantiated model and its registration in physical space. Thirdly, the ICP algorithm was used to register the instantiated model and CT surface to provide a measure of the geometric accuracy of the instantiated shape.

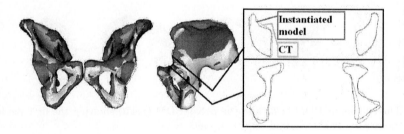

Fig. 4. (*Left to right*) The instantiated SSM (frontal and lateral views) overlaid on the CT-derived surface, shown in dark grey. Cross-sectional contours from the instantiated pelvis model (*black*) with corresponding contours from the CT (*grey*). From top to bottom: near top of acetabulum and middle of acetabulum.

The RMS distance after registering the instantiated model and US points was between 1.52 and 1.96mm for the femur, and between 2.47 and 4.23mm for the pelvis. Since the application area of this study is hip replacement surgery, an RMS distance error was also deter-mined in the region of most clinical relevance: In the femur the RMS distance errors were recomputed in the region of the femoral head and neck, and greater and lesser trochanters, yielding an RMS error in the range 1.83 to 3.69mm for GS and 1.83 to 3.64mm for ICP (See Table 1). In the pelvis, the region around the acetabulum was chosen as having most clinical relevance, with a resulting RMS error in the ranges 3.62 to 3.72mm for GS and 2.61 to 3.71mm for ICP. In each case, all of the 9 starting positions converged to the same RMS distance within 3 significant figures.

Table 1. Average RMS distance for instantiated femur and pelvic surfaces: * Distance between US-derived bone surface points and the instantiated SSM surface; ** distance between the vertices of the surface mesh, which describes the instantiated SSM surface, and the CT-derived bone surface calculated after (i) transforming the CT surface to physical space using the Gold Standard, fiducial-based registration (GS) and (ii) aligning the datasets using the ICP algorithm (ICP); *** as for ** above, but with the measure restricted to regions of clinical interest.

Cadaver & bone	US-Model (mm)*	CT-Model (global)(mm)**		CT-Model (regional)(mm)***	
	ICP	GS	ICP	GS	ICP
1 (femur)	1.96	3.26	2.17	2.90	2.46
2 (femur)	1.54	2.65	1.88	1.83	1.83
3 (femur)	1.52	3.05	2.71	3.69	3.64
1 (pelvis)	4.23	4.95	2.93	3.62	2.61
3 (pelvis)	2.47	5.00	4.88	3.72	3.71

4   Discussion and Conclusion

This work presents the use of US images to instantiate and register a statistical shape model constructed using FFD fields produced using non-rigid registration. In conclusion, preliminary analysis of the data obtained on cadavers suggests that SSMs of the femur and pelvis can be simultaneously instantiated and registered to surgical space with a clinically useful accuracy using intraoperative US data (< 3.72mm RMS for both the femoral head and acetabulum).

One advantage of models produced using FFD fields as opposed to surface points is that they provide much higher resolution. Further work is required to establish this relationship which may then be input as a prior into an automated algorithm. Our plan is to extend this algorithm to one that automatically aligns the US-derived surfaces to the CT surfaces of the model, but to achieve this we need a more accurate model of the precise relationship between the US and CT bone surfaces. Future work includes further automation of the process of US segmentation, and further development of model building and instantiation processes, perhaps including one or two X-rays as additional input data. An algorithm has been suggested by Fleute et al. [4] to reconstruct bones by registering a PDM to X-ray views. One strategy that could be explored is to instantiate the model from one or two X-rays and register using US. Finally, data from the remaining 3 femurs and 1 pelvis is currently being processed and will be reported in due course.

Acknowledgements. This project is funded by the Engineering and Physical Sciences Research Council (EPSRC), United Kingdom (GR/R03525/01 in collaboration with DePuy International and Brainlab AG). The authors wish to thank DePuy International for providing the femur images that were used to build the shape model, Professor Dr. med. R. Putz, Anatomische Anstalt, Ludwig-Maximilian-Universität, München (LMU) for the cadavers and facilities for the cadaver experiments and Philips Medical Systems for advice on US. We also thank the staff of the Radiology Department at LMU for their assistance with CT scanning.

References

1. Besl, P.J., McKay, N.D.: A method for registration of 3D shapes. IEEE Transactions on Pattern Analysis and Medicine Intelligence **14** (1992) 239-256
2. Chan, C.S.K. et al.: Ultrasound-based reconstruction and registration of 3D bone anatomy using statistical shape models. Proceedings of CAOS International, Chicago (2004)
3. Chan, C.S.K., Edwards, P.J., Hawkes, D.J.: Integration of ultrasound based registration with statistical shape models for computer assisted orthopaedic surgery. Proceedings of SPIE Medical Imaging 2003: Image Processing **5032** (2003) 414-424
4. Fleute, M., Lavallee, S.: Nonrigid 3D/2D registration of images using statistical models. Proceedings of MICCAI (1999) 138-147
5. Fleute, M., Lavallee S., Desba, L.: Integrated approach for matching statistical shape models with intra-operative 2D and 3D data. Proceedings of MICCAI (2002) 365-372
6. Press, W.H., Teukolsky, S.A., Vetterling, W.T., Flannery, B.P.: Minimization or Maximization of Functions. In: Numerical Recipes in C, 2nd edn. Cambridge University Press, Cambridge (1992) 394-455
7. Rueckert, D., Frangi, A.F., Schnabel, J.A.: Automatic construction of 3D statistical deformation models using non-rigid registration. Proceedings of MICCAI (2001) 77-84
8. Rueckert, D. et al.: Nonrigid registration using free-form deformations: application to breast MR images. IEEE Transactions on Medical Imaging. **18** (1999) 712-721
9. Studholme, C., Hill, D.L.G., Hawkes, D.J.: An overlap invariant entropy measure of 3D medical image alignment. Pattern Recognition **32** (1999) 71-86
10. Thiel, W.: Ergänzung für die konservierung ganzer leichen nach W. Thiel. Annals of Anatomy **184** (2002) 267-270
11. Yao, J., Taylor, R.: A multiple-layer flexible mesh template matching method for nonrigid registration between a pelvis model and CT images. Proceedings of SPIE Medical Imaging: Image Processing **5032** (2003) 1117-1124
12. Yao, J., Taylor, R.: Deformable registration between a statistical bone density atlas and X-ray Images. Proceedings of CAOS International, Santa Fe (2002) 168-169

Correction of Movement Artifacts from 4-D Cardiac Short- and Long-Axis MR Data

Jyrki Lötjönen[1], Mika Pollari[2], Sari Kivistö[3], and Kirsi Lauerma[3]

[1] VTT Information Technology, P.O.B. 1206, FIN-33101 Tampere, Finland
{Jyrki.Lotjonen@vtt.fi}
[2] Laboratory of Biomedical Engineering, Helsinki University of Technology, P.O.B. 2200, FIN-02015 HUT, Finland
[3] Helsinki Medical Imaging Center, Helsinki University, P.O.B. 281, FIN-00029 HUS, Finland

Abstract. Typically a cardiac MR cine series consists of images over several time points but only from one spatial location. The volumetric information is obtained by combining 2-D slices from different image series. If a patient moves during an MR imaging session, the slices from different image series shift relative to each other, and the 3-D volume reconstructed does not represent the real geometry. In this study, an algorithm was developed to correct movement artifacts simultaneously from short- and long-axis MR cine series. The performance of the algorithm was evaluated by calculating the accuracy of the method against simulated movements imposed on real data, and by visually inspecting the results with real patient images. In both cases, the algorithm reduced significantly movement artifacts.

1 Introduction

Because cardiovascular disease is the most common cause of death in the Western countries, there is a strong need to diagnose and to quantify cardiac diseases. Magnetic resonance (MR) imaging provides detailed anatomical and functional information on the heart. Usually the structures of interest need to be segmented before volumetric measures, such as the ejection fraction, can be computed from the images. As the cardiac function is studied, the segmentation must be performed to images from various phases of the cardiac cycle. Therefore, there have been intense development efforts for automated analysis of the cardiac images during the last years [1]. Several approaches have been proposed for the automated segmentation and volume tracking of the ventricles and myocardium from MR images [2,3,4,5,6].

The use of 3-D data in segmentation is not straightforward because of movement artifacts. Typically, several MR image series are acquired during one imaging session. If a subject moves during an imaging session, the relation between the image series, derived from image headers, is lost and image registration is needed to realign the images. A subject may move because of several reasons, e.g. coughing, breathing or change of inconvenient pose. Breathing is a major source of movement artifacts in cardiac imaging, as the movement due to the heart beating is handled by the ECG gating. McLeish et al. [7] studied the movements of the heart due to respiration. They observed translations up to 23.5 mm in the heart because of breathing. When the cine sequences are used to track the cardiac motion, an image series produced during a breath hold typically contains

C. Barillot, D.R. Haynor, and P. Hellier (Eds.): MICCAI 2004, LNCS 3217, pp. 405–412, 2004.

slices from several time points but only from one spatial location. If the phase of the breathing cycle is not similar during all acquisitions, slices from different image series will be misaligned relative to each other, and a volume built from the image series does not represent the real anatomy of the subject. Although future scanner generations with faster speeds, e.g. fast sampling of k-space using kt-blast, the problem of movement correction is currently relevant in many clinical centers.

The problem has been discussed and reported very little in the literature. Moore et al. [8] recently built a high resolution dynamic heart model from coronal slices acquired from a healthy volunteer. They corrected the breath-hold misalignment by registering a 3-D volume with sagittal and axial scout images. A line-by-line mean squared difference was minimized. In this work, we extended this idea to the registration of two volumes. We optimize the locations of short-axis (SA) slices based on data from long-axis (LA) slices and vice versa. In this work, the movement artifacts are corrected only by translations although the respiration cause also small (typically a couple of degrees) rotations to the heart [7].

2   Methods

2.1   Transformation Between Short- and Long-Axis Images

Since both SA and LA slices are utilized in the movement correction, voxel-by-voxel based correspondence needs to be defined between the image volumes. In the following, the co-ordinates of a voxel in the source volume, denoted by (X, Y, Z), are defined in the co-ordinate system of the destination volume, denoted by (X', Y', Z'). The co-ordinate system of the imaging device is denoted by (X^*, Y^*, Z^*). Next, the parameters for the source volume are defined. Corresponding symbols for the destination volume have a dash. The voxel size of the source volume is (s_x, s_y, s_z). The voxel size in the z-direction is defined to be the distance between neighboring slices, i.e. slice separation. The position of the first voxel of the source volume in the scanner's co-ordinate system is denoted by (o_x, o_y, o_z). In addition, the orientation of x- and y-directions (row and column) are denoted by (r_x, r_y, r_z) and (c_x, c_y, c_z). The normal vector (n_x, n_y, n_z) of the slices can be computed, for example, by subtracting the image positions of the second and the first slices of the volume, and normalizing its length.

The location of a source voxel in the co-ordinate system of a scanner is computed as follows:

$$X^* = s_x X r_x + s_y Y c_x + s_z Z n_x + o_x \tag{1}$$
$$Y^* = s_x X r_y + s_y Y c_y + s_z Z n_y + o_y \tag{2}$$
$$Z^* = s_x X r_z + s_y Y c_z + s_z Z n_z + o_z. \tag{3}$$

The location of the voxel in the co-ordinate system of the destination volume is computed as follows:

$$X' = [(X^* - o'_x)r'_x + (Y^* - o'_y)r'_y + (Z^* - o'_z)r'_z]/s'_x \tag{4}$$

$$Y' = [(X^* - o'_x)c'_x + (Y^* - o'_y)c'_y + (Z^* - o'_z)c'_z]/s'_y \qquad (5)$$
$$Z' = [(X^* - o'_x)n'_x + (Y^* - o'_y)n'_y + (Z^* - o'_z)n'_z]/s'_z. \qquad (6)$$

2.2 Movement Correction

The movement artifacts can be visually observed by forming an image volume from cine series and computing a cross-section of the volume. Fig. 1a shows one original SA and LA slice from a subject having severe movement artifacts. The horizontal lines superimposed on the images indicate the cross-section planes. The cross-sections computed from the SA (six slices) and LA volumes (eight slices) are shown below the original slices. The cross-sections have been interpolated to isotropic voxel size using nearest neighbor interpolation for better visualizing the shifts. The dark, almost vertical stripe in the middle of the images represents the septum, which is normally a smooth and continuous object.

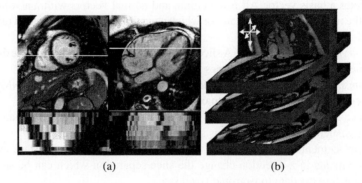

(a)   (b)

Fig. 1. Movement correction. a) The top row shows original SA and LA slices. The horizontal lines represent the location of cross-sections, which are shown on the bottom row. b) The optimization of a LA slice relative to a SA volume. The arrows visualize the degrees of freedom for the movement correction.

The criterium of the smooth and continuous septum could be used to displace the slices in the SA and LA volumes separately. The problem in making the corrections separately is that the comprehensive shape information available in the other volume is not used. In other words, mapping the structures from the SA volume to the LA volume, using Eqs. 1 − 6, could be inaccurate although the shape of the heart may appear to be realistic visually in both volumes separately.

To solve the problem, the normalized mutual information (NMI) [9], denoted by S, is maximized between the 4-D data

$$S(SA, LA) = \frac{H(SA) + H(LA)}{H(SA, LA)}, \qquad (7)$$

where $H(SA)$ and $H(LA)$ are marginal entropies and $H(SA, LA)$ a joint entropy of the data. The voxel-by-voxel correspondence is calculated as described in Section 2.1.

Because all time points related to one spatial location have been acquired during the same breath-hold, data from all time instants can be used to compute the NMI. In other words, the whole image series is displaced simultaneously. The displacement of each image series is assumed to be independent on the displacements of the other image series. The step of displacement at each iteration corresponds to the voxel size in xy-plane (1.4 mm) by default. The basic idea of the registration algorithm is presented in Fig. 1b. Three methods were tested to maximize the NMI:

Gradient maximization. The slices of the two volumes are moved in the direction of an NMI gradient. The gradient of the NMI is computed as follows:

$$\nabla S = \sum_{i}^{N} \left(\frac{\partial S}{\partial \mathbf{r}_i} \mathbf{e}_{\mathbf{r}_i} + \frac{\partial S}{\partial \mathbf{c}_i} \mathbf{e}_{\mathbf{c}_i} + \frac{\partial S}{\partial \mathbf{n}_i} \mathbf{e}_{\mathbf{n}_i} \right) + \sum_{i}^{N'} \left(\frac{\partial S}{\partial \mathbf{r}'_i} \mathbf{e}_{\mathbf{r}'_i} + \frac{\partial S}{\partial \mathbf{c}'_i} \mathbf{e}_{\mathbf{c}'_i} + \frac{\partial S}{\partial \mathbf{n}'_i} \mathbf{e}_{\mathbf{n}'_i} \right), \quad (8)$$

where N and N' denote the number of slices in the SA and LA volumes, respectively, $\mathbf{r}_i$, $\mathbf{c}_i$ and $\mathbf{n}_i$ are the row, column and normal vectors of the SA slice i (see Section 2.1), and $\mathbf{e}$ denotes a basis vector. All row, column and normal vectors within a volume are equal but the index is used to indicate for which slice the gradient is computed (all slices are moved independently).

Random volume maximization. A slice is chosen randomly and moved in the direction of its gradient. The NMI of the volumes is maximized.

Random slice maximization. As *Random volume* maximization, but the NMI of the slice chosen and the other volume is maximized.

The slice locations are iterated until the NMI does not increase more than a user-defined parameter ϵ ($\epsilon = 0.0001$ in this study).

The displacements in x- and y-directions can be easily applied to the stack of slices. The displacements in z-direction change the slice separation which can be seen only after interpolating the data to isotropic voxel size.

2.3   Materials and Evaluation Protocol

The algorithm was developed for correcting the datasets scanned using a 1.5 T Siemens Magnetom Vision and Siemens Sonata imagers (Siemens, Erlangen, Germany) at the Helsinki Medical Imaging Center, University of Helsinki. A standard imaging protocol adopted for cardiac patients in our unit is following: SA images contain ventricles from valve level until the level where the apex is still visible, and LA images contain atria and ventricles. Temporal resolution of 30-40 ms results in 22-30 time points of cardiac cycle, depending on the heart rate of the subject. The pixel size is 1.4×1.4 mm and the slice thickness is 7 mm for the SA and LA images. The corresponding values for the slice separation are 15 mm and 10 mm. The number of SA and LA slices is $4 - 6$ and $4 - 8$ depending on the size of the heart.

The datasets described above can not be used to evaluate the performance of the algorithm because the ground-truth, i.e. movements during the acquisition, is not known. Therefore, we chose a following protocol: 1) We acquired a T1-weighted SA dataset including the atria and ventricles. The pixel size was 1.4×1.4 mm, the slice separation 10 mm and the number of time points 10. No movement artifacts were detected visually. 2) The data were interpolated to isotropic voxel size using shape-based interpolation [10].

3) MR imaging was simulated and a new set of SA and LA slices was generated from the volume using the image parameters (pixel size, gap, slice thickness) of our standard imaging protocol. Although the original SA slices may contain some movement artifacts, the simulated volumes do not include any movement artifacts relative to the original volume. 4) All SA and LA slices were randomly translated in x-, y- and z-directions. The displacements were chosen from an uniform distribution between $[-7.5, 7.5]$ mm in each direction. 5) The correction algorithm was applied and the movements of each slice were compared to the simulated movements. The registration error was defined as follows:

$$e = \frac{\sum_i^N \|\mathbf{s}_i + \mathbf{d}_i\| + \sum_i^{N'} \|\mathbf{s}_i' + \mathbf{d}_i'\|}{N + N'} \tag{9}$$

where $\mathbf{s}_i$ and $\mathbf{d}_i$ are the simulated movement and the correction, respectively, of the SA slice i, and N is the number of the SA slices. The dashed symbols represent corresponding parameters for the LA slices. 6) The steps 4 and 5 were repeated 50 times to evaluate the robustness of the algorithm.

3   Results

Fig. 2a contains the averaged registration errors ($N = 50$) for the simulated SA and LA volumes. The results are shown for the gradient and random maximization techniques, as displacement are allowed either in xy- or xyz-directions of each slice. The root mean square (RMS) and mean errors were computed. In addition, the slice with the maximum error after registration was detected, and a mean ($N = 50$) was defined. Random slice maximization technique computed for all three orientations produced the best results. The difference was statistically significant (paired T-test) as compared with the gradient ($p < 0.00001$) and random volume maximization ($p < 0.01$) techniques.

	RMS	Mean	Mean of max
No correction	6,95	6,6	10,42
Gradient, xy	4,52	3,94	8,37
Gradient, xyz	1,17	0,94	2,76
Random volume, xy	4,64	4,02	8,8
Random volume, xyz	0,85	0,74	1,78
Random slice, xy	4,67	4,04	8,82
Random slice, xyz	0,69	0,64	1,17
Best combination	0,54	0,49	0,89

(a)

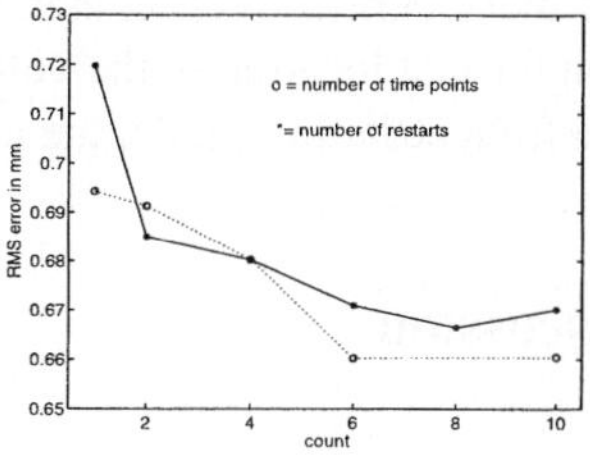

(b)

Fig. 2. a) Registration errors (in [mm]) computed over 50 simulated movements for different parameter combinations. b) The registration error in function of number of time points and restarts as the random slice minimization technique was used.

Several parameter combinations were tested:

The step size of the displacements. The best results were achieved as the registration was iterated first by the step size of one voxel (1.4 mm) and then by the step size of half voxel. Reducing the step size more did not improve the accuracy anymore.

The number of time points. Our hypothesis was that the best results are obtained if all time points are used in registration. However, we noticed that similar accuracy was achieved already with six time points (Fig. 2b).

The number of restarts. If the number of the slices in the SA and LA volumes is altogether 12 and the location of each slice is optimized in all three directions, (x, y, z), the NMI-measure is a function of 36 parameters. Since the function is non-convex containing several local minima, the chosen path from the initial slice configuration to the slice configuration maximizing the NMI has an effect on the result. Because the random maximization technique is a stochastic process, the path is, in practice, different each time the program is run. Therefore, the program can be restarted several times and the path producing the maximum NMI is chosen. We noticed that the RMS error did not decrease considerably after a few restarts (Fig. 2b). The error even increased using ten restarts due to the stochastic variation.

The row *Best combination* presents results for the optimal parameter combination as the random slice minimization technique was used: the step sizes 1.4 and 0.7 mm, six time points and eight restarts were used. Otherwise, the following parameter combinations were used: the step size 1.4 mm, all time points and one restart.

In addition, the algorithm was applied to real patient data. Fig. 3 shows the results from four subjects having severe movement artifacts. The SA and LA volumes are visualized using a chessboard visualization technique before the movement correction (the top row of each subimage) and after the movement correction (the bottom row of each subimage). The first column of each subimage shows the volumes as the LA volume was transformed to the SA co-ordinate system. The second column visualizes the result as the SA volume was transformed to the co-ordinate system of the LA volume. As can be noticed from the images, the edges are more continuous across the chess-boxes with the movement correction than without it. The black boxes indicate that no data is available for that location in the volume, for example, the SA volume does not contain any data from atria. In Fig. 3c, the misalignment corresponds to about 15 mm.

4 Discussion

A novel algorithm was developed for correcting movement artifacts from cardiac short- and long-axis MR images. We applied the algorithm to about 30 data sets. In practice, a subject can normally keep almost an equal breathing phase between the acquisitions and no clear misalignment can be visually detected from the volumes in most cases. However, when movement artifacts existed, the automatic correction performed well. A good indication of successful movement correction was that as we segmented the images after the movement correction, the result (triangulated 3-D surface) fitted well to both SA and LA volumes. The movement correction is a pre-requisite if information from SA and LA images is combined for segmentation and tracking purposes [6].

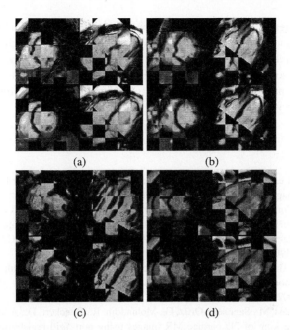

(a)   (b)

(c)   (d)

Fig. 3. Movement correction results for four cases (a,b,c and d) having severe movement artifacts. The chessboard visualization technique was used. The top and bottom rows of each subimage show the SA and LA data before and after, respectively, the movement correction. The left and right columns of each subimage show the data (SA and LA volumes) in the SA and LA co-ordinates systems, respectively.

Image series may contain slices which do not contain any or only small region of the heart, for example, the first or the last slice of the LA volume, or the most apical slice of the SA volume. We found that the algorithm fails often with these slices and produce incorrect results because the slices do not contain enough image features for registration. However, we did not try to develop any automatic method to detect these slices and leave them out from the registration. The movement correction is only a necessary pre-processing step for segmentation of the heart from the volumes. If the slices do not contain data from the heart, they also do not cause problems to segmentation.

The manual correction of the movement artifacts based on visual inspection is relatively time consuming and also very difficult. Although making different cross-sections from the volumes helps considerably the manual correction, often the result is still open to interpretations. The definition of the movements in the z-direction, the direction perpendicular to the slice, was found important in our study but it is almost impossible to obtain it manually in practice. In addition, making manually corrections which produce the similar 3-D geometry in the both volumes, is neither an easy task. For these reasons, an automatic method was needed. The algorithm developed makes the corrections in a few seconds, and it has proved to be robust also to large artifacts.

Acknowledgements. This research was supported by the National Technology Agency, Finland. This study was partly financed by a grant from Helsinki University Central Hospital Research Fund (T181032, TYH 2242), the Radiology Society of Finland, Pehr Oscar Klingendahl Foundation, BIOMEDICUM Helsinki Foundation, the Graduate School "Functional Research in Medicine" (Academy of Finland, Ministry of Education), Waldemar von Frenckell Foundation.

References

1. Frangi, A., Niessen, W., Viergever, M.: Three-dimensional modeling for functional analysis of cardiac images: A review. IEEE Trans. Med. Imag. **20** (2001) 2–25
2. Jolly, M.P.: Combining edge, region, shape information to segment the left ventricle in cardiac MR images. In Niessen, W.J., Viergever, M.A., eds.: Lecture Notes in Computer Science 2208: Medical Image Computing and Computer-Assisted Intervention - MICCAI 2001, Springer (2001) 482–490
3. Mitchell, S., Bosch, J., Lelieveldt, B., van der Geest, R., Reiber, J., Sonka, M.: 3-D active appearance models: Segmentation of cardiac MR and ultrasound images. IEEE Trans. Med. Imag. **21** (2002) 1167–1178
4. Lorenzo-Valdés, M., Sancheez-Ortiz, G., Mohiaddin, R., Rueckert, D.: Atlas-based segmentation and tracking of 3D cardiac MR images using non-rigid registration. In Dohi, D., Kikinis, R., eds.: Lecture Notes in Computer Science 2488: Medical Image Computing and Computer-Assisted Intervention - MICCAI 2002, Springer (2002) 642–650
5. Kaus, M., von Berg, J., Niessen, W., Pekar, V.: Automated segmentation of the left ventricle in cardiac MRI. In Ellis, R., Peters, T., eds.: Lecture Notes in Computer Science 2878: Medical Image Computing and Computer-Assisted Intervention - MICCAI 2003, Springer (2003) 432–439
6. Lötjönen, J., Smutek, D., Kivistö, S., Lauerma, K.: Tracking atria and ventricles simultaneously from cardiac short- and long-axis MR images. In Ellis, R., Peters, T., eds.: Lecture Notes in Computer Science 2878: Medical Image Computing and Computer-Assisted Intervention - MICCAI 2003, Springer (2003) 440–450
7. McLeish, K., Hill, D., Atkinson, D., Blackall, J., Razavi, R.: A study of the motion and deformation of the heart due to respiration. IEEE Trans. Med. Imag. **21** (2002) 1142–1150
8. Moore, J., Drangova, M., Wierzbicki, M., Barron, J., Peters, T.: A high resolution dynamic heart model based on averaged MRI data. In Ellis, R., Peters, T., eds.: Lecture Notes in Computer Science 2878: Medical Image Computing and Computer-Assisted Intervention - MICCAI 2003, Springer (2003) 549–555
9. Studholme, C., Hill, D., Hawkes, D.: Automated three-dimensional registration of magnetic resonance and positron emission tomography brain images by multiresolution optimization of voxel similarity measures. Medical Physics **24** (1997) 71—86
10. Grevera, G.J., Udupa, J.K.: Shape-based interpolation of multidimensional grey-level images. IEEE Trans. Med. Imag. **15** (1996) 881–892
11. Lötjönen, J., Mäkelä, T.: Elastic matching using a deformation sphere. In Niessen, W.J., Viergever, M.A., eds.: Lecture Notes in Computer Science 2208: Medical Image Computing and Computer-Assisted Intervention - MICCAI 2001, Springer (2001) 541–548

Scale-Invariant Registration of Monocular Endoscopic Images to CT-Scans for Sinus Surgery

Darius Burschka[1], Ming Li[2], Russell Taylor[2], and Gregory D. Hager[1]

[1] Computational Interaction and Robotics Laboratory, CIRL
The Johns Hopkins University, Baltimore, USA
{burschka,hager}@cs.jhu.edu
[2] Computer Integrated Surgical Systems and Technology, CISST
The Johns Hopkins University, Baltimore, USA
{liming,rht}@cs.jhu.edu

Abstract. We present a scale-invariant registration method for 3D structures reconstructed from a monocular endoscopic camera to pre-operative CT-scans. The presented approach is based on a previously presented method [2] for reconstruction of a scaled 3D model of the environment from unknown camera motion. We use this scaleless reconstruction as input to a PCA-based algorithm that recovers the scale and pose parameters of the camera in the coordinate frame of the CT scan. The result is used in an ICP registration method to refine the registration estimates.

The presented approach is used for localization during sinus surgeries. It simplifies the navigation of the instrument by localizing it relative to the CT scan that was used for pre-operative procedure planning.

The details of our approach and the experimental results with a phantom of a human skull are presented in this paper.

1 Introduction

Surgery of the frontal sinus can be performed endonasally or through an external approach. In the external approach, with the patient under general anesthesia, the surgeon makes an incision behind the hairline or under the eyebrows. This approach requires large skin incisions and protracted long recovery time. The endonasal approach for surgical treatment of frontal Sinusitis has become increasingly established during the last few years. All information is provided primarily through the endoscope requiring from the surgeon a detailed knowledge of the anatomy. Therefore, Computer Integrated Surgery techniques have been employed in endonasal approach to simplify the procedure. After a registration process, the surgeon can point at a specific structure in 3D and then view the position of the instrument tip in the pre-operative CT-scan [3,4].

Patient motion, imperfections in the surgical instrument or shifts of the reference frame may cause a registration error to a pre-operative registration. Therefore, currently the operating surgeon must update the registration at several

C. Barillot, D.R. Haynor, and P. Hellier (Eds.): MICCAI 2004, LNCS 3217, pp. 413–421, 2004.

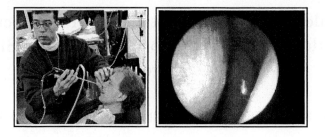

Fig. 1. Endoscopic inspection of the nasal sinus cavities depicting the limited information provided to the surgeon in the current procedures.

points in the operative field throughout the procedure. Typically, registration is verified by localization on known bony landmarks on the skull and in the nasal cavity. In image-guided sinus surgery, registration is performed based on fiducial points or based on the surface parameters [3]. In surface based methods, a probe is used to touch to contours to gather 3D surface data. Typical contours include the medial brow, nasal dorsum, and tragi. In fiducial point based method, radiopaque markers attached to both the patient's face and anatomic landmarks are used.

In this paper, we present a novel method for intra-operative registration directly from the endoscopic images without manual inputs from the surgeon. It is especially useful in revision cases, where the surgical landmarks are usually absent. The paper is structured as follows. In Section 2, we describe the underlying image processing that allows us to recover the 3D-structure and the motion from monocular images of an endoscopic camera and the way we perform the final alignment using a modified ICP approach. In Section 3, we present the experimental results on the phantom skull. We conclude in Section 4 with an evaluation of the presented approach and present our future research goals.

2   Approach

The two major problems that we address in this paper are: 3D reconstruction from monocular camera images and registration of the reconstructed 3D model to a pre-operative CT scan.

Our system reconstructs a scaled 3D model of the environment from a monocular camera. This reconstruction requires knowledge about the motion of the camera, which we assume to be unknown or at least uncertain. That means that, in parallel to model reconstruction, we need to estimate the motion of the camera as well. We discuss the implementation of the vision-based reconstruction in Section 2.1.

The 3D structure estimated from camera images is known up to scale. The correct scale needs to be recovered from the data to align the points roughly with the CT scan. The remaining alignment error between the CT scan data and the reconstructed model is corrected with our modified *Iterative Closest Point* (ICP) estimation with covariance tree optimization (Section 2.2).

2.1   Scaled 3D Reconstruction

Feature Extraction. The algorithm described below assumes that *point features* are extracted from the images. Possible features are: intersections of contours resulting from edge filters [7] or the areas themselves used for template matching in *Sum of Square Differences* (SSD) matching algorithms [5].

The problem in real endonasal images is the sparse density of points that actually can be used for a model reconstruction. Another problem is the moving light source, which is attached to the endoscope (Fig. 2). This violates the brightness constancy assumption used in most common stereo algorithms and thus forces us to switch to a brightness independent image representation.

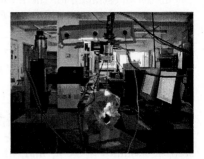

Fig. 2. Our experimental system.

Our current results are based on experiments with a phantom skull. This skull does not have any detectable texture. We added colored points on the surface that we segment in the hue space of the color representation. This way, we are able to identify and track the features in image sequences using a simple color blob tracker despite the changing lighting conditions (Fig. 3).

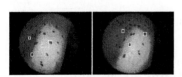

Fig. 3. Example of corresponding points on our phantom.

We obtained preliminary results with real endonasal images using our endoscope camera (Fig. 1). In real images, we compensate the brightness variations by running an edge detector on the original images and doing an SSD search on the resulting gradient images.

Localization and Mapping Step. Since the camera motion needs to be estimated in parallel to the reconstruction, the so called epipolar geometry from the motion between two camera frames needs to be recovered. An approach, commonly used in situations with at least eight point correspondences between images, is the *eight-point-algorithm*. The recovered *Essential Matrix* contains the information about the translation direction T' and rotation R between the images. The translation information can be recovered just up to a scale because of the way, how this matrix is constructed [7].

The number of corresponding (detectable) points between two camera frames varies significantly during the sinus surgery. There are situations, when less than eight points can be matched. The above approach fails in these cases, therefore, we apply here our method for camera localization and mapping requiring merely three point correspondences. We will sketch out the process below. The reader should consult [2] for details of the algorithm.

In this approach, we assume that each 3D point P_i imaged in a unifocal camera frame $p_i = (u_i v_i 1)^T$ can be represented as its direction vector $n_i = p_i/||p_i||$ and the distance to the real point D_i so that $P_i = D_i \cdot n_i$. Since, in typical applications, the scale m of the reconstruction may be unknown, the system works also with a scaled version of the distance $\lambda_i = D_i/m$. This approach calculates an estimate for the rotation $\tilde{\mathbf{R}}$ and the scaled translation $\mathbf{T}'^*$ between the points in the current frame $\{P_i\}$ and the next frame $\{P_i^*\}$ as

$$\bar{P} = \tfrac{1}{n} \sum_{i=1}^n P_i, \quad \bar{P}^* = \tfrac{1}{n} \sum_{i=1}^n P_i^*, \quad P_i' = P_i - \bar{P}, \quad P_i'^* = P_i^* - \bar{P}^*,$$

$$\tilde{\mathbf{M}} = \sum_{i=1}^n P_i'^* P_i'^{\mathbf{T}}, \quad [U\,D\,V^T] = \mathrm{svd}(\tilde{\mathbf{M}}), \tag{1}$$

$$\tilde{\mathbf{R}} = V \cdot U^T, \quad \mathbf{T}'^* = \bar{P}^* - \tilde{\mathbf{R}}^* \bar{P}.$$

The approach requires an initial knowledge of the values for λ_i for the first frame and it estimates a guess for translation $\mathbf{T}'^*$ and rotation $\tilde{\mathbf{R}}$. In the initial step, it assumes $\lambda_i' = \lambda_i$ and, afterwards, it iteratively converges to the true $\tilde{\mathbf{R}}, \mathbf{T}'^*$, and λ_i'. Details and simplifications of the algorithm are discussed in [1]. This algorithm requires only three corresponding points between both images to actually compute the pose difference between two camera frames $(\tilde{\mathbf{R}}, \mathbf{T}'^*)$, which makes it more suitable for the given application.

Eq. (1) updates the distance values for all tracked points P_i' for the new frame. New points can easily be added to the system using the rigid body assumption for the imaged points and solving (2)

$$\left(\tilde{\mathbf{R}}\mathbf{n_x} \quad - \mathbf{n_x^*} \right) \begin{pmatrix} \lambda_x \\ \lambda_x^* \end{pmatrix} = \tilde{\mathbf{R}}\lambda_1 \mathbf{n_1} - \lambda_1^* \mathbf{n_1^*} \tag{2}$$

or in a more robust way from 3 frames to (3)

$$\begin{pmatrix} \tilde{\mathbf{R}}_1 \mathbf{n_x} & -\mathbf{n_x^*} & 0 \\ \tilde{\mathbf{R}}_2 \tilde{\mathbf{R}}_1 \mathbf{n_x} & 0 & \mathbf{n_x^{**}} \end{pmatrix} \begin{pmatrix} \lambda_x \\ \lambda_x^* \\ \lambda_x^{**} \end{pmatrix} = \begin{pmatrix} \tilde{\mathbf{R}}_1 \lambda_1 \mathbf{n_1} - \lambda_1^* \mathbf{n_1^*} \\ \tilde{\mathbf{R}}_2 \tilde{\mathbf{R}}_1 \lambda_1 \mathbf{n_1} - \lambda_1^{**} \mathbf{n_1^{**}} \end{pmatrix}. \tag{3}$$

The pose change from image $1 \to 2$ is annotated here as $(\tilde{\mathbf{R}}_1, \mathbf{T_1})$ and the pose change between images $2 \to 3$ is annotated as $(\tilde{\mathbf{R}}_2, \mathbf{T_2})$. This equation estimates the distance λ_x to a new point P_x in the scale of an already known point P_1 from the currently tracked set of points. This way the newly added points are still measured with the same scaling factor m and the resulting 3D model has a uniform scale.

System Initialization. As mentioned above, our approach requires an initial guess about the structure of at least three landmarks. There are two possibilities for initialization of the surgical system:

- the **eight-point-algorithm** based on the estimation of the *Essential Matrix* of the system from 8 point correspondences that provides the necessary information about $(\tilde{\mathbf{R}}, \mathbf{T}'^*)$;

- **manual feature selection** in the endoscope image, where the surgeon selects three points with known correspondences to the CT-data and the system uses this information to build a map of the entire nose cavity.

The first alternative is completely unsupervised, but it requires a significant initial movement to get a well-conditioned *Essential Matrix*. The second alternative is similar to the current IGS procedure, but it is necessary just for the first frame of the sequence.

2.2 Registration of the Endoscope Data to CT Scan

Scale Recovery for 3D Reconstruction. The scaling factor m in Section 2.1 depends on the scale of the λ_i-values for the initial set of points P_i. In case of the unsupervised bootstrap using the *eight point algorithm* (Sec. 2.1) the resulting reconstruction has an arbitrary scale that depends on the scale of the translation vector $\mathbf{T}'^*$, which is usually assumed as a unit vector in this algorithm. Since the system is continuously updating the position information, it has a rough estimate about the current camera position. We use this estimate to carve out part of the CT data that fall into the expected visibility cone of the camera. This cone is slightly enlarged in all directions to compensate for the unknown camera motion.

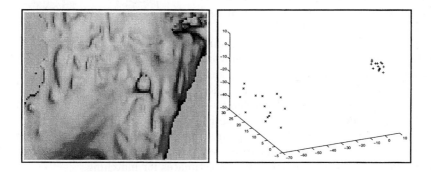

Fig. 4. Scaled reconstruction of surface points: (left) CT scan visualization of the area, (right) matched surface points with ICP {left point cloud}, scaled reconstructed points {right point cloud}.

The visible regions are usually surfaces with two dominant directions of the cavity walls with a third dimension representing the surface structure. We use this for our scale recovery by calculating the covariance matrices of the point clouds in the selected CT scan region and the current reconstruction. In both cases, the smallest eigenvalue (E_{ct}, E_{3d}) represents a metrics for the depth variations in the surface of the CT scan and in the reconstructed point cloud. The normalized eigen-vectors $\{V_{ctx}\}$ and $\{V_{3dx}\}$ and the eigenvalues allow us to calculate the scale m and the rotation $\tilde{R}_{tot}$ between the two data sets to (4). The rotation matrix $\tilde{R}_{tot}$ aligns both dominant surfaces along their normal vectors, which are represented by the eigenvector calculated from the smallest eigenvalue (last column in each of the rotation matrices in (4)). The rotation around the normal vector cannot be restored in this way.

$$m = \frac{\sqrt{E_{ct}}}{\sqrt{E_{3d}}}, \quad V_{p \in \{CT,3D\}} = \begin{pmatrix} V_{px} \\ V_{py} \\ V_{pz} \end{pmatrix}, \quad V_{n-p} = \begin{pmatrix} 0 \\ V_{pz} \\ -V_{py} \end{pmatrix}$$

$$\tilde{R}_{ct} = \left((V_{n-ct} \times V_{ct}) \; V_{n-ct} \; V_{ct} \right), \quad \tilde{R}_{3d} = \left((V_{n-3d} \times V_{3d}) \; V_{n-3d} \; V_{3d} \right),$$

(4)

$$\tilde{R}_{tot} = \tilde{R}_{3d} \cdot \tilde{R}_{ct}^T$$

We apply the scaling and rotation to the zero mean point clouds that were used to calculate the covariance matrices above. This way, we obtain two point clouds with the same alignment, but the CT-scan represents a much larger area because of the expected unpredictable camera movement. Both clouds have a similar scale and alignment of the supporting plane.

We consider now both rotated clouds as sparse "images", where each "pixel" is represented by its distance to the plane calculated from the covariance matrix. We use the reconstructed 3D structure from the current view as template that is matched to the *image* constructed from the CT scan data using standard coarse-to-fine pattern matching techniques. Significant points with large deviation from the supporting plane are identified and matched

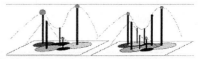

Fig. 5. Three significant points in both images are identified and matched: (left) sparse from the camera, (right) dense from CT scan.

in the *images* with significantly different resolutions (Fig. 5) first. This match is verified and refined based on the remaining points from the reconstruction. The physical position of the sampling points, especially in the 3D reconstruction, does not necessarily correspond to extreme values of the surface hull. We use interpolations between known values as estimates for matching.

The resulting match is used to align the two data sets. The residual error is due to imperfect sampling and the coarse structure of the point sets, especially in the case of the reconstructed data from the phantom skull. The 3D scaling step needs to be performed just in the initial step and in the cases when the system was not able to maintain the minimum number of three features and needs to re-initialize the distance measurements.

ICP. Now, we have reconstructed and localized a 3D dataset with endoscopic images, which has right scale and similar orientation and translation in the coordinate frame of the CT scan.

Rigid registration between CT images and physical data reconstructed by endoscopic images is achieved using the Iterative Closest Point (ICP) algorithm. For some applications in the endoscopic surgery, a deformable registration method can be further applied based on the results of the ICP.

We use a covariance tree data structure to search for the closest point for ICP. A covariance tree is a variant of a k-dimensional binary tree (k-D tree). The traditional k-D tree structure partitions space recursively along principal coordinate axes. In our covariance tree each sub-space is defined in the orthogonal coordinate system of the eigenvectors centered at the center of mass of the point set, and is recursively partitioned along this local coordinate frame. An important advantage of covariance trees is that the bounding boxes tend to be much tighter than those found in conventional k-D trees and tend to align with surfaces, thus producing a more efficient search [6].

3   Experimental Results

The experimental validation of our approach is carried out on the setup depicted in Fig. 2. We track the position of the endoscope with the $OptoTrack^{TM}$ system in the background to verify the motion estimation results from our system.

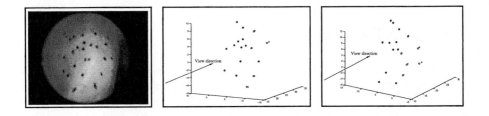

Fig. 6. 3D reconstruction results in camera coordinate frame from 2 consecutive reconstructions: (left) camera view (middle, right) reconstructed points '+', ground-truth from OptoTrack 'o'.

Fig. 6 shows two reconstruction results from a camera motion of $(4.8, 0.2, 5.2)[mm]$ with small and significant rotation between the consecutive frames. The resulting reconstruction errors had a standard deviation of $(0.62, 0.3382)$ for each of the cases. The minimal rotational error expressed as Rodigues vector was r=(0.0017, 0.0032, 0.0004), (-0.0123, -0.0117, -0.0052). The error in the estimate of the translation vector was $\Delta T = (0.05, -0.398, 0.2172)^T, (-0.29, 0.423 - 0.4027)^T [mm]$

We tested our registration with different reconstruction results (patches) that were registered to CT skull images. Because the 3D surface data reconstructed by monocular camera may not cover the whole surface patch, we were interested in the sensitivity to drop-outs. We purposely removed parts of the data from the reconstructed patch. Our experiments with the phantom show that the ICP can accommodate noise levels in the data up to 0.6mm, combined with translational offsets of up to 10mm, and rotational offsets within 10 degrees. The vision-based reconstruction gives us errors an order of magnitude below these limits.

After ICP alignment the average distance error for the sample points is around 0.65mm. By comparison, the fiducial based registration residual error is around 0.40mm for four fiducials that are attached to the surface of the skull.

However, our method directly tells the registration error of the target region for the surgery.

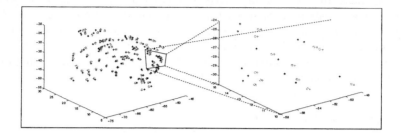

Fig. 7. The relative displacements of the sparse samples (+), their initial position recovered by VGPS(*) and their final position after alignment by ICP (o). Left is the global view of the sample data for a patch. Right is a closer look.

4   Conclusions and Future Work

The presented system performs accurate reconstruction of 3D surface points based on images from an endoscopic camera. The points are successfully aligned with CT scans of our phantom skull in the sinus area. Our major goal is to more extensively test our system in different parts of the skull and on other range images to better evaluate the performance of the system. We are currently investigating the feature type that can be used for a robust estimation and tracking of our *point features* in real endonasal images obtained in a preliminary experiment on a human subject.

Acknowledgments. Partial funding of this research was provided by the National Science Foundation under grants EEC9731748 (CISST ERC), IIS9801684, IIS0099770,and IIS0205318. This work was also partially funded by the DARPA Mars grant. The authors want to thank Dr. Masaru Ishii for his help in obtaining the preliminary data set of real endonasal images.

References

1. Darius Burschka and Gregory D. Hager. V-GPS – Image-Based Control for 3D Guidance Systems. In *Proc. of IROS*, pages 1789–1795, October 2003.
2. Darius Burschka and Gregory D. Hager. V-GPS(SLAM): – Vision-Based Inertial System for Mobile Robots. In *Proc. of ICRA*, April 2004. to appear.
3. Kennedy D.W., Bolger W.E., Zinreich S.J., and Zinreich J. *Diseases of the Sinuses: Diagnosis and Management*. 2001.
4. Olson G. and Citardi M.J. Image-guided Functional Endoscopic Sinus Surgery. *Otolaryngology-Head and Neck Surgery*, 123(3):188–194, 2000.

5. G.D. Hager and P. Belhumeur. Real-Time Tracking of Image Regions with Changes in Geometry and Illumination. *Proceedings of the IEEE Conference on Computer Vision and, Pattern Recognition*, pages 403–410, 1996.
6. Williams J.P., Taylor R.H., and Wolff L.B. Augmented k-D Techniques for Accelerated Registration and Distance Measurement of Surfaces. In *Computer Aided Surgery: Computer-Integrated Surgery of the Head and Spine*, pages 1–21, 1997.
7. E. Trucco and A. Verri. *Introductory Techniques for 3-D Computer Vision*. Prentice Hall, 1998.

Patient-Specific Operative Planning for Aorto-Femoral Reconstruction Procedures

Nathan Wilson[1], Frank R. Arko[2], and Charles Taylor[3]

[1] Stanford University, Clark Center E372, Stanford, CA, 94305-5431
nwilson@stanford.edu
[2] Division of Vascular Surgery, Suite H-3600, Stanford University Medical Center,
Stanford, California 94305-5642
farko@stanford.edu
[3] Stanford University, Clark Center E350B, Stanford, CA 94305-5431
taylorca@stanford.edu

Abstract. Traditionally, a surgeon will select a procedure for a particular patient based on past experience for patients with a similar state of disease. The experience gained from this patient will be selectively used when treating the next patient with similar symptoms. In this work, a surgical planning system was developed enabling a vascular surgeon to create and test alternative operative plans prior to surgery for a given patient. One dimensional and three dimensional hemodynamic (i.e. blood flow) simulations were performed for rest and exercise for operative plans for two aorto-femoral bypass patients and compared with actual postoperative data. The information that can be obtained from one-dimensional (volume flow distribution and pressure losses) and three-dimensional (wall shear stress) hemodynamic simulation may be clinically relevant to vascular surgeons planning interventions.

1 Introduction

Atherosclerosis is a degenerative vascular disease of clinical significance which leads to a narrowing of the flow lumen preventing adequate flow to tissues and organs. In symptomatic patients with occlusive disease of the lower extremities, the infra-renal abdominal aorta and the iliac arteries are the most common sites of obliterative atherosclerosis [1]. Many patients asymptomatic under resting conditions experience ischemic pain under exercise conditions. The primary objective of a surgical intervention for aortoiliac occlusive disease is to restore adequate flow to the lower extremities under a range of physiologic states including rest and exercise. While volumetric flow distribution is of paramount concern initially following a surgical intervention, other quantities such as high particle residence time and low mean wall shear stress are theorized to be flow-related factors in disease progression and impact the long term efficacy of a surgical intervention.

Several major classes of treatment exist for aortoiliac occlusive disease. One technique that may be appropriate for localized occlusive disease is to use catheter-based endoluminal therapies such as angioplasty and stenting. The use of angioplasty

C. Barillot, D.R. Haynor, and P. Hellier (Eds.): MICCAI 2004, LNCS 3217, pp. 422–429, 2004.
© Springer-Verlag Berlin Heidelberg 2004

and stenting has received considerable attention recently due to probable cost savings and decreased morbidity compared to traditional open surgical interventions. The most commonly used procedure for severe cases is direct anatomic surgical reconstruction and is the focus of this work presented here. Direct surgical reconstruction refers to the insertion of grafts replacing or providing alternative pathways to flow through the infra-renal aorta and iliac arteries.

Currently, surgery planning for the treatment of vascular disease involves acquiring diagnostic imaging data to assess the extent of aortoiliac disease in a given patient. The surgeon then relies on his/her past experience, personal bias, and previous surgical training to create a treatment strategy. Initially proposed by Taylor [2], a new paradigm of Simulation-Based Medical Planning (SBMP) for vascular disease has been proposed to utilize computational methods to evaluate alternative surgical options prior to treatment using patient-specific models of the vascular system. Blood flow (hemodynamic) simulations enable a surgeon to see the flow features resulting from a proposed operation and to determine if they pose potential adverse effects such as increased risk of atherosclerosis and thrombus formation.

2 Methods

There are several major steps in the SBMP process for vascular surgical applications [3]. First, patient-specific preoperative geometric models from medical imaging data are created by a technician. Additional imaging processing may occur to obtain physiologic information. This process can take several hours. Next, geometric models representing several surgical alternatives to be evaluated are constructed under the guidance of the attending vascular surgeon. This usually takes on the order of an hour. One and three-dimensional numerical simulations are then performed on the different surgical interventions. Finally, clinically relevant analysis results are then visualized and interpreted. The remaining part of this section summarizes some the important considerations.

2.1 Patient-Specific Geometric Model Construction and Surgical Planning

Magnetic Resonance Imaging (MRI) is a particularly useful technique for SBMP because it can provide both physiologic and volumetric geometric information. In the case studies presented here, the medical imaging data was obtained using a GE Signa 1.5T MRI scanner (General Electric, Milwaukee, WI, USA). Ideally, the scanner creates linearly varying gradients of the magnetic field across the image volume. However, in practice, non-linearity of the magnetic field gradients exists that must be accounted for or significant geometric errors occur in the volumetric image data [4].

It is worthwhile pointing out the advantages and disadvantages of 2-D and 3-D image segmentation since both are available in the system via an integrated multi-dimensional level set kernel [3]. For example, for small regions of interest with high signal to noise acquired with specialized surface coils (e.g. the carotid bifurcation) direct 3-D reconstruction techniques are compelling. In contrast, in the case studies discussed herein, a body coil was used (due to the large extent of the vasculature required to model surgical interventions) reducing the quality of the acquired data. The presence of complex flow and significantly diseased vessels can cause poor signal and vessels only a few pixels in diameter in critical regions of interest (e.g. diseased common iliac arteries). The variability in the level of the contrast agent and noise in the image data can make the constants found in the boundary velocity functions used to do the segmentation a function of position. In addition, the human body contains a vast network of arteries, but it may be desired to simulate only a subset of them. It can be difficult to extract an accurate geometric representation using the level set method in 3-D while preventing the front from advancing into undesired smaller branches (e.g. lumbar arteries). Finally, the 1-D simulation methods described in the next section require medial axis paths and circular cross section segments. Porcine in-vivo studies and other experiment work (see [6]) seem to indicate that that the global impact of approximating three-dimensional junctions with the lofting techniques described above are a second order effect compared to inaccuracies in boundary conditions. See section 4 for further discussion on possible improvements to the image segmentation.

A detailed discussion of the methods used to construct preoperative geometric models in this work from the MRA data can be found elsewhere [3,5]. Briefly, a multi-stage process is used where the first step involves extracting the medial axis paths for vessels of interest utilizing a semi-automatic algorithm. The 3-D data is then sampled in planes perpendicular to the vessel paths at user-selected locations. Several segmentation techniques including thresholding and level set techniques can then be performed on the planar image samples to extract the lumen boundary. A solid modeling operation referred to as lofting is then used to create a 3-D solid from the cross-sections of each vessel. A single 3-D solid representing the flow domain is then constructed by Boolean addition (union) of the individual vessel solid models.

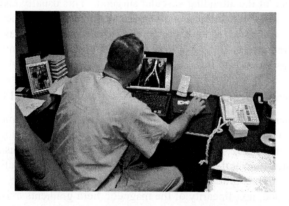

Fig. 1. The software system developed in this work was utilized by a vascular surgeon to create virtual surgical geometric models prior to the patient's actual surgery.

A surgeon can create a patient-specific surgical plan with the system using steps very similar to those used to construct the preoperative model. Specifically, the surgeon defines the path(s) the graft will follow and defines the geometry of the graft flow domain by specifying elliptical and circular cross-sections that are lofted to create a solid model. Fig. 1 shows a vascular surgeon running the software developed as part of this work on his laptop computer to create a surgical plan.

2.2 Boundary Condition Specification from PCMRI Data

When MRA imaging data is acquired for the purpose of SBMP, planar slices of experimental data are also acquired providing temporally and spatially resolved velocity fields (see Fig. 3). The technique used in the present work is known as cine-Phase-Contrast-Magnetic-Resonance-Imaging (PCMRI). With appropriate selection of imaging parameters, the technique can be used to quantify volumetric flow and provide insight into the spatial velocity fields in a given planar slice location. PCMRI was acquired in the case studies presented here to quantify the volumetric flow through several arteries of interest. In addition to the relatively large (with respect to pixel dimension) arteries of interest such as the aorta, aorto-femoral reconstruction planning also requires the quantification of volumetric flow in small (relative to pixel dimension) and diseased vessels such as the common iliac arteries. The software system described in [3] provides multiple segmentation and flow calculating techniques needed for SBMP.

2.3 One-Dimensional Hemodynamic Analysis

Post-operative volumetric flow distribution is of paramount clinical importance in alleviating the symptoms of claudication (i.e. inadequate flow to lower extremity tissue). As discussed in [6], one-dimensional finite element methods can be used to predict volumetric distributions and pressure losses. In addition to simulating resting conditions, volumetric flow distribution during exercise can be estimated by dilation and constriction of the distal vascular beds as described below.

With the assumptions that (1) blood flow velocity along the vessel axis is much greater than the flow perpendicular to the vessel axis, (2) blood can be approximated as a Newtonian fluid, and (3) the velocity profile along the axis is a scaled version of a Poiseuille cross-sectional velocity profile function, a non-linear one-dimensional equation for pulse wave propagation in elastic blood vessels has been derived [6]. The space-time finite element formulation for solving the one-dimensional problem discussed in [6] has been integrated into the present software system (see Fig. 2). The major strength of the one-dimensional method is in its speed (CPU minutes versus CPU days for three-dimensional simulation described below). However, the disadvantage of the method is that it does not account for energy losses associated with secondary flows due to curvature, branching, stenoses, aneurysms, or complex three-dimensional geometric features. As discussed in [6], minor losses due to the pressure losses across a stenosis or due to branching can be incorporated to increase the accuracy of the one-dimensional method.

An impedance boundary condition was utilized to enable simulated exercise. Briefly, a fractal like tree, based on an input root radius, length to radius ratio, and asymmetric branching factor was used to calculate an impedance function of time that produced reasonable physiologic pressures and closely matched the preoperative flow distribution determined experimentally using PCMRI [7]. By adjusting the radii of the resistance vessels in the structured tree of the viscera by constriction and dilating the extremities by an appropriate factor an outlet impedance approximating exercise conditions was obtained [7].

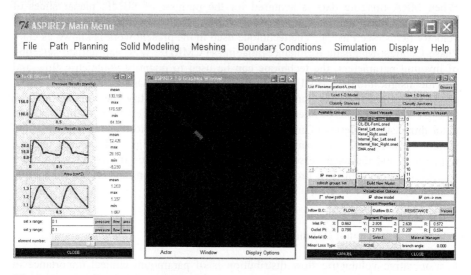

Fig. 2. An example of the graphical user interface (GUI) of the system developed for surgical planning. The "Main Menu" GUI guides a technician through the steps to go from medical imaging data to one and three dimensional hemodynamic simulation. The remaining windows in the figure are examples of controlling and running a one-dimensional analysis.

2.4 Three-Dimensional Hemodynamic Analysis

Mean wall shear stress and particle residence time are theorized to play an important role in disease progression. The patency of the bypass graft and long-term relief of the claudication symptoms are likely determined by flow features which can only be determined from three-dimensional analysis, while the one-dimensional analysis results provide estimates of flow distribution and pressure losses. In the three-dimensional analyses presented here, due to current software limitations it was assumed that the vessel walls were rigid and blood behaves like a Newtonian fluid. The geometric models were discretized using a commercial automatic tetrahedral mesh generator (Simmetrix, Inc., Clifton Park, NY, USA). Inflow velocity boundary conditions were prescribed and volumetric outflow distributions were assigned to the arteries based on the one-dimensional analysis results. A stabilized finite element method was used to solve the Navier-Stokes equations and the results were visualized using custom software built using the Visualization Toolkit (Kitware, Inc., Clifton Park, NY, USA) [3].

3 Results

Two case studies demonstrate the application and limitations of the system for planning an Aorto-Femoral Reconstruction procedure. The first case involves a 67 year-old female patient while the second case involves a 55 year-old male patient.

A preoperative and postoperative MRA for a female patient diagnosed with aortoiliac occlusive disease who underwent a direct surgical revascularization is shown in Fig. 3.   Two different surgical plans were create and hemodynamic simulations were performed. Extremely low (an order of magnitude lower than the preoperative flow rates) volumetric flow was observed in the external iliac arteries during resting conditions in the simulations for the procedures shown in Fig. 3. The simulation results could explain the clinically observed occlusion of these arteries postoperatively.

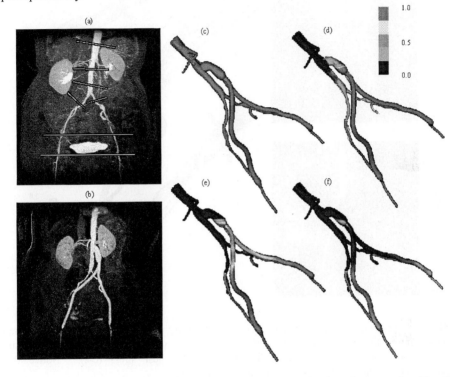

Fig. 3. 67 year-old female AFB patient. Maximum intensity projection of preoperative (a) and postoperative (b) MRA data. Seven PCMRI acquisitions were performed and the slice plane locations as indicated in (a). Notice the postoperative occlusion of the external iliac arteries in (b). A passive scalar transport problem (dye clearance time) was also solved for one of the surgical plans and this indicates area of interesting and stagnant flow (c-f).

A second case study was of a 55-year old male was experiencing severe pain in his legs during mild exercise and was diagnosed with severe aorto-iliac-femoral occlusive disease (see Fig. 4a). An end-to-side aorto-femoral bypass procedure was performed and postoperative MRA data was acquired nine days after the operation (see Fig. 4b). The postoperative MRA clearly indicated a complete occlusion of the distal native aorta. The closure of the native distal aorta was not anticipated and the simulation results for the model shown in Fig. 4 may not be consistent with the occlusion. There are two possibilities to explain the apparent inconsistency of the simulation results with the observed clinical outcome. First, the outflow boundary conditions may not have adequately captured the postoperative flow distribution. Second, it is possible that when the surgeon clamped the native aorta during the operation, thrombus or plaque was dislodged and traveled downstream impeding flow in the distal native aorta. This example illustrates the need for experimental validation studies before SBMP can be used clinically.

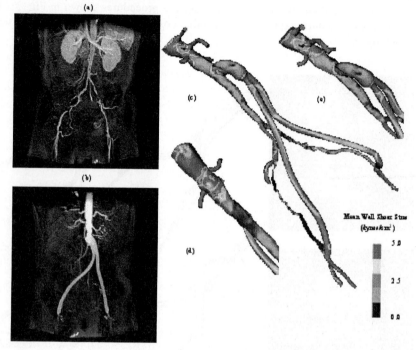

Fig. 4. 55 year-old male AFB patient. Maximum intensity projection of preoperative (a) and postoperative (b) MRA. Evaluating the long-term efficacy of a surgical procedure may require special post-processed quantities such as mean wall shear stress (c-e).   Notice that postoperatively the native distal aorta occluded completely.

4   Conclusions and Future Work

The results presented here demonstrate the first examples of performing the geometric modeling necessary for SBMP in a clinically relevant time frame. Specifically, two case studies were shown where a vascular surgeon was able to preoperatively create geometric models representing alternative surgical procedures for a patient in approximately one hour per plan. In addition, the system enabled the processing of PCMRI data for prescribing velocity boundary conditions needed for hemodynamic simulation. Finally, in certain cases the simulation results appear to be consistent with clinically significant observed postoperative outcomes.

The results of this work indicate several important potential research directions. For SBMP to be clinically applicable, both the geometric modeling and the simulation must be performed prior to the surgery. Integration of one-dimensional and three-dimensional hemodynamic analysis into a common framework was critical given their corresponding tradeoffs for accuracy and computational expense. This motivates improvements in one-dimensional modeling including additional complex downstream boundary conditions and improved minor loss terms for special conditions such as flow in a stenosis or aneurysm. In three-dimensions, relaxing the simplifying assumptions of rigid vessel walls and integration of impedance boundary conditions is underway. Improvements in the area of geometric modeling are focused on integrating 3-D image segmentation and utilizing additional imaging modalities (i.e. CTA) in the SBMP system. Finally, additional experimental validation studies are essential to improve the numerical models and quantify the accuracy of these predictive methods.

References

1. Rutherford, R.B. (ed.): Vascular Surgical Procedures. W.B. Saunders Company, Philadelphia, PA (2000)
2. Taylor, C.A., Draney, M.T., Ku, J.P., Parker, D., Steele, B.N., Wang, K., Zarins, C.K.: Predictive Medicine: Computational Techniques in Therapeutic Decision-Making. Computer Aided Surgery, Vol. 4. (1999) 231-247
3. Wilson, N.M.: Geometric Algorithms and Software Architecture for Computational Prototyping: Applications in Vascular Surgery and MEMS. PhD Dissertation, Department of Mechanical Engineering, Stanford University, Stanford, CA USA (2002)
4. Draney, M.T., Alley, M.T., Tang, B.T., Wilson, N.M., Herfkens, R.J., Taylor, C.A.: Importance of 3D Nonlinear Gradient Corrections for Quantitative Analysis of 3D MR Angiographic Data. ISMRM (2002)
5. Wilson, N.M., Wang, K., Dutton, R.W., Taylor, C.A.: A Software Framework for Creating Patient Specific Geometric Models from Medical Imaging Data for Simulation Based Medical Planning of Vascular Surgery. MICCAI (2001) 449-456
6. Wan, J, Steele B., Spicer, S.A., Strohband, S., Feijoo, G.R., Hughes, T.J.R., Taylor, C.A.: A One-Dimensional Finite Element Method for Simulation-Based Medical Planning for Cardiovascular Disease, Computer Methods in Biomechanics and Biomedical Engineering, Volume 5, Number 3, pages 195-206 (2002)
7. Steele, B.N., Taylor, C.A.: Simulation of Blood Flow in the Abdominal Aorta at Rest and During Exercise Using a 1-D Finite Element Method with Impedance Boundary Conditions Derived from a Fractal Tree. Summer Bioengineering Meeting, Key Biscayne, FL, June 24-29, pages 813-814 (2003)

Intuitive and Efficient Control of Real-Time MRI Scan Plane Using a Six-Degree-of-Freedom Hardware Plane Navigator

Dingrong Yi, Jeff Stainsby, and Graham Wright

Sunnybrook & Women's College Health Sciences Center, Imaging Research,
and University of Toronto, Department of Medical Biophysics, 2075 Bayview Avenue,
Toronto, Ontario, M4N 3M5, Canada
{dingryi,stainsby,gawright}@sten.sunnybrook.utoronto.ca

Abstract. For applications of real-time MRI, it is important but difficult to efficiently prescribe the next scan plane and obtain visual feedback on the prescription. This work addresses these issues with a 6-degree-of-freedom Plane Navigator. The Plane Navigator is a mechanical arm with integrated input and output functionality while being statically balanced. In the input mode, by holding and moving the surface normal of the physical representation of the scan plane, the operator can intuitively place the scan plane at a position with any orientation within a few milliseconds. In the output mode, the Plane Navigator automatically places the physical representation of the scan plane to reflect its position and orientation (pose)[PR1] relative to a patient domain with a maximum delay of half a second. Application examples in MRI cardiac imaging are also described.

1 Introduction

Magnetic resonance imaging (MRI) has long been used to visualize anatomical structures in human patients. The development of new techniques for the rapid acquisition of MR images during the past few years has made it possible to achieve interactive acquisitions at 10-20 frames per second with sub-millimeter resolution [9]. However, one of the major obstacles that prevent real-time MRI from expanding its clinical application is the lack of absolute pointing hardware tools for interactive and intuitive manipulation of the scan plane. The high updating frequency of 10 to 20 frames per second is only feasible at one single location of a scan plane or with automatically prescribed scan planes. Without a suitable hardware device, it is difficult to interactively change the scan plane location quickly enough to fully take advantage of such imaging efficiency.

Most of the current work on interface design focuses on software development to provide graphical tools [1],[3], [6]. Well-designed graphical user interfaces written in software can provide some of the required prescription flexibility by providing a 2D projection of the oblique cut plane corresponding to the current scan plane in the context of a pre-acquired imaging study [6]. However the visual feedback of the location and orientation of the current scan plane provided

C. Barillot, D.R. Haynor, and P. Hellier (Eds.): MICCAI 2004, LNCS 3217, pp. 430–437, 2004.
© Springer-Verlag Berlin Heidelberg 2004

is limited by the flat screen. Meanwhile without a suitable hardware tool it is difficult to precisely control the scan plane in a coordinated manner.

Existing 6-DOF hardware devices such as Spaceball, SpaceMouse and Flock of Birds have been used to improve the efficiency of scan plane prescription [4], [2]. However, none of these device can visually represent a static scan plane position. In this work, we demonstrate how the 6-DOF Plane Navigator can be used to provide intuitive and interactive control of scan plane during real-time MRI.

2   Method

2.1   The Plane Navigator

The Plane Navigator is designed to integrate the following functions in order to provide an intuitive and interactive control of the scan plane: (1) 6-DOF manual inputs, (2) automatic display of a 6-DOF spatial location, and (3) static balance which enables the display of both manual and automatic operations and reduces the required force to be exerted on the stylus for motion during manual operations.

The Plane Navigator is a mechanical arm consisting of a series of mechanical linkages that support a planar surface, referred to as the proxy plane (Figure 1a). A stylus is fixed and perpendicular to the surface to represent its normal. The linkages are connected through 6 rotational joints O_i (i=1, 2,...,6). The Plane Navigator has a spherical workspace of radius $R = 2 * |O_2O_3| = 2 * |O_3O_6|$, centered at O_2. The second joint O_2 is also the origin O_w of world coordinate system. The combined effects of rotating along the A-A, B-B and C-C axes determines the center position O_6 of the proxy plane. The rotation along the D-D, E-E and F-F axes further determines the orientation of the proxy plane. The decoupling of positioning from orientation is realized by setting the cross-point of the axes D-D, E-E and F-F to be the center O_6 of the proxy plane. At each joint an optical encoder is coupled with a motor. Static balance is realized by symmetric design, light weight materials, friction, stabilizing motor torque, and where applicable counter-weight blocks.

The prototyped Plane Navigator is constructed using aluminum alloy, inexpensive components such as 300 count optical encoders E4 (US Digital) and custom modified Hitech servos (Tower Hobby). A single PCI MultiQ I/O board (Quanser) is used to read 6 encoders. The motors are controlled through 6 of the 8 data pins of the parallel port of a personal computer, with real-time linux to precisely control the required timing. Encoder readings are used as feedback for position control. The radius of the spherical work space is 220mm, which allows a 1:1 ratio between the armature and MR scanner dimension for real-time cardiac imaging (Figure 1b). The positioning accuracy for manual mode is 0.8mm and for automatic mode is 1.8mm.[PR2] In automatic mode, the accuracies of rotation along axes D-D, E-E and F-F are 1.5, 0.6, and 0.6 degrees respectively (Figure 1a). There is a cylindrical inaccessible zone along the O_wZ_w axis with radius of 43 mm due to mechanical occlusion (Figure 1a).

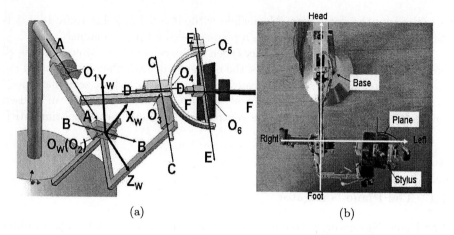

(a)   (b)

Fig. 1. (a) Illustration of the design of the Plane Navigator. A-A through F-F are the rotational axes, O_i (i=1, 2, ..., 6) are the rotational joints, and $O_w X_w Y_w Z_w$ is the fixed world coordinate system used to describe the workspace of the Plane Navigator. (b) Illustrates one way of configuring the workspace of the Plane Navigator to correspond to the coronal view of cardiac MR imaging of a human subject in supine position.

2.2   Registering the Plane Navigator with a MRI Scanner

To demonstrate how the Plane Navigator can be used for real-time MRI, let us consider its application to cardiac imaging, which is one of the major applications of real-time MRI. For imaging the heart, only a portion of the workspace of the Plane Navigator is needed. Therefore the space occupied by the heart in the patient domain is registered with and centered at (0.4, 0.4, 0) of the normalized workspace of the Plane Navigator. Figure 1b illustrates such a configuration of the workspace of the Plane Navigator to match a patient in supine position. The world coordinate system $O_w X_w Y_w Z_w$ of the Plane Navigator matches the scanner's coordinate system in a 1:1 ratio. The axis Z_w is the first linkage. The physical representations of the center O_w and the axis Z_w of the world coordinate system will not change their positions significantly, regardless of the current location and orientation of the proxy plane. Therefore they can serve as the spatial references. For example the physical representation of the Z_w axis can well represent the backbone of a supine patient (Figure 1b).

3   Results

The Plane Navigator is utilized as an input device for MRI scan-plane prescription by having the user hold and maneuver the surface normal (stylus) of the proxy plane, and thus reach an arbitrary position and orientation. Meanwhile, operations involving only rotations at a fixed position are easy to perform. The computer inserts the encoder readings into the forward kinematics to calculate the position and orientation of the proxy plane. This information is constructed into a 4x4 matrix to be sent to the scanner. In such a way the user can simultaneously enter coordinated x, y, z positions as well as pitch, yaw and roll rotations to control the scan plane. The time required to sample the encoders and reconstruct the 4x4 geometric matrix is less than one millisecond.

When the Plane Navigator is activated to take the role of output device the translation vector and 3x3 rotation matrix of a given prescription is converted to the appropriate joint angles using inverse kinematics. These joint angles are then sent to the motors to automatically translate and rotate the proxy plane to physically reflect the position and orientation of the scan plane. The maximum delay in output mode is 500 ms, which corresponds to moving the proxy plane from one edge to the extreme opposite edge of the workspace.

3.1   Interactive Control of Real-Time MRI Scan Plane

The Plane Navigator has been tested to interactively control and automatically represent the scan plane of a 1.5T scanner (GE CV/i). Currently it connects to a personal computer running real-time Linux. A second computer running a real-time MRI interface has direct control of the scanner. The latter sends geometry information such as translation and rotation to the scanner, displays the reconstructed image. etc. The two computers communicate through a socket-based server process to transport the 4x4 geometric matrix containing the position and orientation of the scan plane [8].

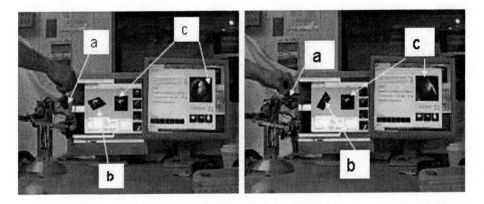

Fig. 2. Two snapshots to indicate how an operator interactively controls the real-time MRI scan plane (b) using the Plane Navigator (a). Image (c) is the resulting real-time MR image of a healthy human subject. The scan plane (b) is graphically displayed in the context of a pre-acquired imaging study of the same human subject [6].

The Plane Navigator provides interactive control of the real-time MRI scan plane in its input mode (Figure 2). The imaging parameters are: GRE sequence with minimum TE, TR=50 milliseconds, Flip angle=30 degree, field of view is

20 cm. Display rate of 15 frames per second was achieved using sliding window reconstruction technique. The update rate of the 4x4 geometric matrix obtained from the Plane Navigator was 200 Hz. However, due to the delay of the socket-based communication between the Plane Navigator and the computer which has direct access to the MRI scanner, currently there is a noticeable delay between the user manipulation of the proxy plane and the appearance of the corresponding image (indicated in Figure 2 as **a** and **c** respectively) . This delay is approximately 200 ms. The delay is anticipated to be reduced to be a few milliseconds longer than the time required for imaging acquisition and reconstruction, which is currently around 70 ms. One way to do this is to let all the processes run within a single computer using shared memory technique or to use simple first-in-first-off buffers for the transportation of the shared geometry matrix. [PR3]

The Plane Navigator's position could be initialized to preset locations, to facilitate subsequent manual fine adjustments to accommodate variability among different subjects. Alternatively the user can use sliders as indicated in [8] to prescribe the next scan plane by translating and rotating the current one. The Plane Navigator can automatically track and follow the prescription. This automatic tracking provides direct visual feedback on the effects of the software-controlled spatial operation. In addition the visibility of the physical representation of the scan plane and its x, y and z axis guides the operator's determination of which direction the current scan plane should move in order to achieve the imaging goal.

3.2   Intuitive Control of the Scan Plane

The Plane Navigator aids the user's intuition in several ways. There is a direct mapping between the workspace of the device and the scanner workspace. Indeed, both spaces can be described by similar coordinate systems. The Plane Navigator provides a physical representation of the current scan plane in a workspace that has a one-to-one correspondence to the subject in the scanner. The capability of holding its pose in a physically visible, fixed reference coordinate system provides the operator with direct visual feedback of the spatial location of the scan plane under manipulation. Such physical correspondence and visual feedback aids comprehension of the location and orientation of the current scan plane relative to patient anatomy.

Holding and manipulating the stylus for 3D inputs is as natural as holding a pen. Delicate[PR4] static balance at each of the joints enables the user to freely manipulate the stylus. The user is not required to expend effort and become fatigued by countering gravity and carrying the device during operation. In addition it is convenient to halt and later resume an unfinished operation.

Cardiologists without training on the Navigator can intuitively manipulate the proxy plane of the device to obtain various standard views of a human heart. Figure 3 illustrates how a cardiologist would place the proxy plane to match standard cardiac views.

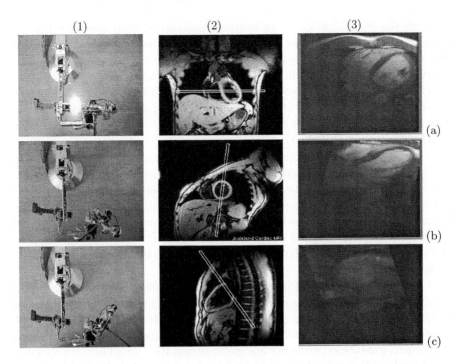

Fig. 3. Illustrating the correspondence between the placements of the proxy plane of the Plane Navigator and the standard cardiac views. Column (1) shows the actual placements of the proxy plane by a cardiologist to match the locations in the patient domain as shown in column (2) to obtain standard cardiac views as shown in column (3). Row (a), (b) and (c) roughly correspond to the axial, long axis and short axis views of a healthy human heart. Column (2) images were borrowed with permission from the anatomy tutorial provided at SCMR official website (http://www.scmr.org/education/atlas/intro).

4   Discussion

There are several advantages of the Plane Navigator over software-based scan plane control tools and other 6-DOF hardware input tools. is that The Navigator can simultaneously provide coordinated scan plane manipulation in the required 6-DOF space in an intuitive and interactive manner within a few milliseconds[PR5]. This capability may eliminate the current bottleneck restricting imaging efficiency in real-time MRI. Meanwhile it presents the user direct visual feedback on the location and orientation of the resulting scan plane in a patient domain. Its capability of automatic tracking of the scan plane enhances visualization when navigating with a software tool. The physical representation of the scan plane and its attached image coordinate system help the user comprehend the anatomy contained in the real-time image in the patient domain.

With the Plane Navigator an operator can interactively navigate the scan plane, guided directly by the individual anatomy and can track the resulting MR images at a display rate of 10 to 20 frames per second. In other words, it is feasible to manually track and visualize moving and deforming anatomical structures regardless of complex dynamic processes. This will certainly improve the diagnostic power of MRI.[PR7] Though designed for the maneuver of real-time MRI scan planes, it can also be used to interactively control the view plane in 3D visualization (Figure 3).

A disadvantage of the Plane Navigator is that the operation space of the proxy plane is constrained within its spherical workspace, hence it is not as flexible as the cable tethered devices nor the wireless handheld components such as the Flock of Birds (Ascension Technology Corporation)[1]. All absolute pointing mechanical armatures such as MicroScribe by Immersion Corp, Freedom6S designed by Hayward [5] and commercialized by MPB[2], Phantom by Sensable[3] and the Plane Navigator suffer this inconvenience due to their fixed-size physical workspaces.

A unique feature of the Plane Navigator is its ability to maintain static balance, whereas other pointing devices will drift in their position and orientation. Preliminary evaluation with cardiologists and real-time MRI researchers indicates that static balance facilitates resuming an unfinished operation. Formal human performance experiments are under preparation to quantitatively evaluate the value of static balance, output functionality and their combination for an absolute-pointing device. Freedom6S to some extent has similar static balance capability. However due to the requirement of high fidelity force output, its stylus may drift away from the position where the user released it. Another difference between the Plane Navigator and haptic devices is that the latter use motors to generate forces instead of precise positions. The most closely related device that the authors are aware of is the slave robot of da Vinci Surgical System designed by Salisbury [7] and commercialized by Intuitive Surgical[4]. The operator can control both manually and automatically the tip position of the surgical tool holder of that robot. Despite this similarity, the Plane Navigator is far more affordable.[PR9]

5   Conclusion

A 6-DOF absolute pointing hardware tool was developed for interactive real-time MRI scanning to enhance the efficiency and intuitiveness of scan plane localization. This system could be applied wherever fast, intuitive localization or tracing in 3D is required.

---

[1] http://www.ascension-tech.com/products/flockofbirds.php
[2] $http://www.mpb-technologies.ca/space/freedom62000/f6s/freedom6s.html$
[3] $http://www.sensable.com/products/phantom_ghost/phantom.asp$
[4] $http://www.computermotion.com/products/index.html$

References

1. Debbins, J.P. and Riederer, S.J. and Rossman, P.J. et al., Cardiac Magnetic Resonance Fluoroscopy, Magnetic Resonance in Medicine, **36** (1996) 588-595
2. Gardstrom, 3D Navigation for real-time MRI using six degrees of freedom interactive devices, Master thesis. Department of Science and Technology, Linkoping University, SE-601M. Sweden, 2003.
3. Kerr, A.B. and Pauly, J.M. and Hu, B.S. et al., Real-Time Interactive MRI on a Conventional Scanner, Magnetic Resonance in Medicine, **38** (1997) 355-367
4. Hardy, C. J.and Darrow, R. D. and Pauly, et al., Interactive Coronary MRI. Magnetic Resonance in Medicine. **40**, (1998) 105-111
5. Hayward, V. and Gregorio, P. and Astley, O. et al., Freedom-7: A High Fidelity Seven Axis Haptic Device With Application To Surgical Training. In Experimental Robotics V, Casals, A., de Almeida, A. T. (eds.), Lecture Notes in Control and Information Science **232**, pp. 445-456, 1998.
6. Radau, P. and Hu, N. and Stainsby, J. and Wright, G.A., Visualization System for Real-time Scan Plane and Catheter Navigation. Accepted to 12th Scientific Meeting and Exhibition of the International Society for Magnetic Resonance in Medicine, 2004.
7. Salisbury, Jr. et al., Master having redundant degrees of freedom, US Patent #6,714,839 (2004).
8. Stainsby, J.A and Hu, N. and Yi, D. and Radau, P and Santos, J.M. and Wright, G.A., Integrated Real-Time MRI User-Interface 12th Scientific Meeting and Exhibition of the International Society for Magnetic Resonance in Medicine, PP. 120. May 5-21, 2004, Japan.
9. Sussman, M.S. and Stainsby, J. A. and Robert, N. and Merchant,N. and Wright, G.A., Variable-Density Adaptive Imaging for High-Resolution Coronary Artery MRI. Magnetic Resonance in Medicine, 2002, 48(5):753-764.
10. Yi, D., Computer Aided Display of 3D Angiograms, Using Graphics and Haptics, Ph.D. dissertation, ECE department, McGill University, Montreal, Canada (2002).

Shape-Enhanced Surgical Visualizations and Medical Illustrations with Multi-flash Imaging

Kar-Han Tan[1], James Kobler[2], Paul Dietz[3], Ramesh Raskar[3], and
Rogerio S. Feris[4]

[1] University of Illinois at Urbana-Champaign, IL, USA
tankh@vision.ai.uiuc.edu,
http://vision.ai.uiuc.edu/~tankh/MultiFlash
[2] Department of Surgery, Massachusetts General Hospital, Boston, MA, USA
james_kobler@meei.harvard.edu
[3] Mitsubishi Electric Research Laboratories, Cambridge, MA, USA
[dietz|raskar]@merl.com
[4] University of California at Santa Barbara, CA, USA
rferis@cs.ucsb.edu

Abstract. We present a novel approach for enhancing images and video used in endoscopic surgery so that they are better able to convey shape. Our method is based on *multi-flash imaging*, in which multiple light sources are strategically positioned to cast shadows along depth discontinuities. We describe designs for achieving multi-flash imaging using multiple endoscopes as well as in single endoscopes. Multi-flash photography can also be used for creating medical illustrations. By highlighting the detected edges, suppressing unnecessary details, or combining features from multiple images, the resulting images convey more clearly the 3D structure of the subject. The method is easy to implement both in software and hardware, and can operate in realtime.

1 Introduction

In many medical applications like minimal-invasive surgery with endoscopes it is often difficult to capture images that convey the 3D shape of the organs and tissues being examined [1]. Perhaps for the same reason, medical textbooks and articles frequently resort to hand drawn illustrations when depicting organs and tissues. In this paper we propose the use of multi-flash imaging to address this problem.

A multi-flash imaging system captures additional shape information compared to traditional cameras and therefore has the potential to enhance visualization and documentation in surgery and pathology. The raw shadowed images can be processed to create finely detailed images that are comparable to medical illustrations or they can be used to enhance edge features for quantitative measurement. Alternatively, the shadowed images can be combined to generate shadowless images, which are often desirable for documentation of specimens in the field of pathology.

C. Barillot, D.R. Haynor, and P. Hellier (Eds.): MICCAI 2004, LNCS 3217, pp. 438–445, 2004.
© Springer-Verlag Berlin Heidelberg 2004

Surgery. Most endoscopic procedures are now performed with the surgeon observing monitor displays rather than the actual tissue. This affords the possibility of interposing image manipulation steps which, if they can run in close to real time, can enhance the surgeon's perception. Depth perception is an obvious deficit when using monocular endoscopes. Three-dimensional imaging using stereoscopic methods has been explored with mixed results. A 1999 study found that stereoendoscopic viewing was actually more taxing on the surgeons than monocular viewing [2]. Structured lighting is also under investigation as a means for calibrating endoscopic images [3,4], but this technique does not provide real-time enhancement of 3-D structures. Application of enhanced shadow information to augment surgical perception has not been exploited previously. Shadows normally provide clues about shape, but with the circumferential ("ringlight") illumination provided by most laparoscopes, this information is diminished. Similarly, the intense multisource lighting used for open procedures tends to reduce strong shadow effects. Loss of shadow information may make it difficult to appreciate the shapes and boundaries of structures and thus more difficult to estimate their extent and size. It may also make it more difficult to spot a small protrusion, such as an intestinal polyp, if there are no clear color differences to set it apart. The ability to enhance the borders of lesions so that they can be measured will become more useful as endoscopes begin to incorporate calibrated sizing features.

Pathology. Documentation of surgical and autopsy specimens is an important service provided by pathology departments. Systems for photography of such specimens involve special methods for eliminating unwanted shadows, usually by placing the specimens on glass plates suspended over black cavities. Using the multiflash system and processing to obtain the MAX composite image produces a view in which almost all shadows are eliminated.

Medical and Biological Illustration. Often it is desirable to generate black and white illustrations of medical and natural history specimens in which salient details are emphasized and unnecessary clutter is omitted [5]. The most important details to emphasize are those that convey the shape of the object. Typically shape is conveyed by emphasizing edges and using stippling for shading. This type of illustration is seen less frequently nowadays because of the expense involved in having artists create these graphics. With multi-flash imaging we found that images very similar to this kind of illustration can be generated quickly and easily. The medical or biological illustrator could use these images as the basis for their graphics.

2   Related Work

The creation of stylized renderings from images without 3D model reconstruction has recently received a great deal of attention. The majority of the available techniques for image stylization involve **processing a single image** as the input applying morphological operations, image segmentation, edge detection and color assignment. Some of them aim for stylized depiction [6] while others enhance legibility. Stereo techniques including passive and active illumination are generally designed to compute depth values or surface orientation rather than to detect depth edges. Depth discontinuities present difficulties for traditional stereo [7]. Active illumination methods have been proposed for depth extraction, shape from shading, shape-time stereo and photometric stereo but are unstable around depth discontinuities [8]. An interesting technique has been presented to perform logical operations on detected intensity edges, captured under widely varying illumination, to preserve shape boundaries [9] but it is limited to uniform albedo scenes. Using photometric stereo, it is possible to analyze the intensity statistics to detect high curvature regions at **occluding contours** or *folds* [10]. But the techniques assume that the surface is locally smooth which fails for a flat foreground object like a leaf or piece of paper, or view-independent edges such as corner of a cube. They detect regions near occluding contours but not the contours themselves.

Techniques for **shape from shadow** (or darkness) build a continuous representation (*shadowgram*) from a moving light source from which continuous depth estimates are possible [11,12]. However, it involves a difficult problem of estimating continuous heights and requires accurate detection of start and end of shadows. Good reviews of shadow-based shape analysis methods are available in [13,14].

3   Multi-flash Imaging

This technique for detecting shape features in images was first described in [15, 16]. For completeness we review the basic idea here. The method is motivated by the observation that when a flashbulb illuminates a scene during image capture, thin slivers of cast shadow are created at depth discontinuities. Moreover, the position of the shadows is determined by the relative position of the camera and the flashbulb: when the flashbulb is on the right, the shadows are create on the left, and so on. Thus if we can shoot a sequence of images in which different light sources illuminate the subject from various positions, we can use the shadows in each image to assemble a depth edge map using the shadow images.

Imaging Geometry. In order to capture the intuitive notion of how the position of the cast shadows are dependent on the relative position of the camera and light source, we examine the imaging geometry, illustrated in figure 1(a). Adopting a pinhole camera model, the projection of the point light source at P_k is at pixel e_k on the imaging sensor. We call this *image* of the light source the *light epipole*. The images of (the infinite set of) light rays originating at P_k are in turn called the *epipolar rays* originating at e_k. We also refer to the images of depth discontinuities as depth edges.

Removing and Detecting Shadows. Our approach for reliably remove and detect shadows in the images is to strategically position lights so that every point in the scene that is shadowed in some image is also imaged without being shadowed in at least one other image. This can be achieved by placing lights strategically so that for every light there is another on the opposite side of the camera so that all depth edges are illuminated from two sides. Also, by placing the lights close to the camera, we minimize changes across images due to effects other than shadows. To detect shadows in each image, we first compute a **shadow-free image**, which can be approximated with the MAX composite image, which is an image assembled by choosing at each pixel the maximum intensity value from among the image set. The shadow-free image is then compared with the individual shadowed images. In particular, for each shadowed image we compute the *ratio image* by performing a pixel-wise division of the intensity by that of the MAX image. The ratio image is close to 1 at pixels that are not shadowed, and close to 0 at pixels that are shadowed. This serves to accentuate the shadows and also remove intensity transitions due to surface material changes.

Algorithm. Codifying the ideas discussed above we arrive at the following algorithm [16]: Given n light sources positioned at $P_1, P_2...P_n$,

- Capture n pictures I_k, $k = 1..n$ with a light source at P_k
- For all pixels x, $I_{max}(x) = \max_k(I_k(x))$, $k = 1..n$
- For each image k,
  - ▷ Create a ratio image, R_k, where $R_k(x) = I_k(x)/I_{max}(x)$
- For each image R_k
  - ▷ Traverse each epipolar ray from epipole e_k
  - ▷ Find pixels y with step edges with negative transition
  - ▷ Mark the pixel y as a depth edge

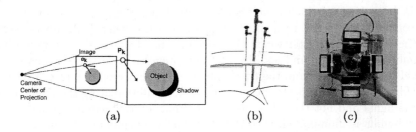

(a)   (b)   (c)

Fig. 1. (a) Imaging geometry. Shadows of the gray object are created along the epipolar ray. We ensure that depth edges of all orientations create shadow in at least one image while the same shadowed points are lit in some other image. Multi-flash imaging setup (b) for minimal-invasive operation (c) for medical illustrations.

4   Multi-flash Imaging with Endoscopes

Unlike many traditional 3D shape recovery methods where the imaging apparatus need to be placed at large distances apart, in multi-flash imaging the light sources can be placed near to the camera. This allows compact designs that can be used in tightly constrained spaces.

Multiple-Instrument Designs. The simplest way to implement multi-flash imaging is to use multiple instruments. One design is shown in figure 1(b), where instead of inserting one endoscope, three are inserted. The middle instrument acts as the camera while the two on the side act as light sources. By synchronizing the light sources with the image capture process for the middle endoscope, the entire setup would act as a multi-flash camera. While it may involve inserting more imaging instruments, it is a way to systematically illuminate the subject, and potentially could reduce the amount of adjustments required during an operation to produce images that convey the required 3D information necessary.

Single-Instrument Designs. In many scenarios, it is more useful to have a single instrument capable of multi-flash imaging. For example in situations where flexible endoscopes are needed, it may be very difficult or impossible to insert and align multiple flexible light sources with the endoscope. Fortunately it is possible to implement multi-flash imaging on a single instrument. Figure 2 shows an R. Wolf *Lumina* laryngeal laparoscope endoscope modified to achieve multi-flash imaging. At the tip of the Lumina, as shown in figure 2(c), there is an imaging lens and two lights on opposite sides of the lens. These lights are made of numerous optic fibers that are bundled together at the base of the laparoscope. By illuminating this fiber bundle, the light is transmitted to the tip, serving as illumination near the imaging lens.

Clearly, if we can turn on each of the two lights independently, the Lumina would be capable of multi-flash imaging. Conventionally, both lights at the tip are turned on and off together, and standard equipment does not make any provisions for turning on only one light. However if one could identify which optic fibers lead to which light, then by only illuminating the fibers leading to one of the lights we can turn one light on without the other. If the fibers leading to the two lights are intertwined at the end of the fiber bundle, one would have to unbundle the fibers and sort them into two bundles manually. Fortunately, we found that the fibers from the two lights are grouped roughly into two parts at the fiber bundle. This is shown in figure 2(b). By illuminating the fibers at one of the lights and not the other, we can see that approximately one half of the fiber bundle is illuminated, with the other half corresponding to fibers leading to the other light. Thus by covering one or the other side of the fiber bundle, we can turn on and off the two lights individually.

5   Multi-flash Imaging for Medical Illustrations

In many traditional medical and biology textbooks and articles, pen-and-ink drawings of organs and tissues are often used in the place of photographs because they are easier to comprehend. However the use of these stylized illustrations is increasingly scarce, primarily because they are more expensive than photographs, and take more time to create. In our experiments with multi-flash imaging, we have observed that the depth edge confidence maps frequently resemble hand drawn sketches. At the same time, since they are created from photographs, they retaining a high degree of realism without overwhelming amounts

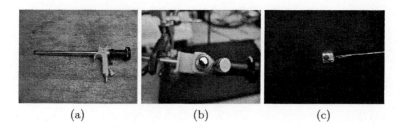

(a)   (b)   (c)

Fig. 2. Single-endoscope Multi-flash Setup. (a) R. Wolf Lumina laparoscope. (b) Fiber bundle with one end illuminated. The tip of the laparoscope shown (c) with left light turned on.

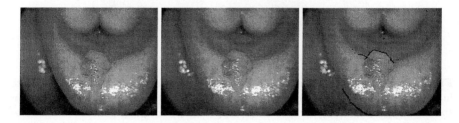

Fig. 3. Calf larynx displayed under (Left) Conventional imaging (Center) MAX composite (Right) enhanced with multi-flash imaging.

of detail. We felt that multi-flash photography may make it faster, easier, and cheaper for artists and researchers to create medical illustrations.

To verify this, we built a multi-flash camera based on a 4 megapixel Canon Powershot G2, as shown in figure 1(c). The 4 flashes mounted around the camera are triggered sequentially by a controller board based on a Microchip PIC16F876 which synchronizes them to the image capture process by sensing the flash signal from the camera hot shoe. Some results generated with this camera are shown in figure 4. The same figure also shows the typical results produced using a conventional intensity edge detector. We showed the results to medical professionals at the Massachusettes General Hospital, and received very positive feedback on the usefulness of these images. In addition, they also found the MAX composite image to be most useful, as it is difficult to take shadow-free images with ordinary cameras. Anatomists and medical illustrators for whom we have demonstrated the system are most interested in the 'depth edge confidence' image, which can be easily converted into a detailed black and white drawing. An example is shown in figure 4(e).

6   Conclusion

We have presented a promising approach to enhancing medical images and video that convey a heightened sense of 3D shape. Using cameras and laparoscopes

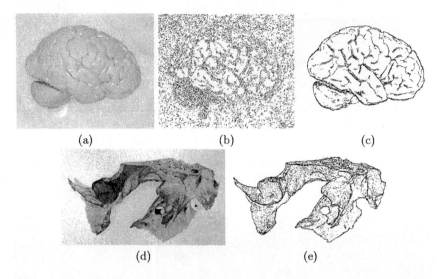

(a)　　　　　　　　　　(b)　　　　　　　　　　(c)

(d)　　　　　　　　　　　(e)

Fig. 4. Creating medical illustrations by multi-flash imaging. (a) MAX Composite image. (b) Canny Edges. (c) Multi-flash Edges. Depicting a fragment of a human sphenoid bone. (d) MAX Composite. (e) Applying a Photoshop pen-and-ink filter to the depth edge confidence image produces an image that resembles a traditional hand drawn illustration.

with multiple sources of illumination, we described methods for computing a MAX composite image that is largely free of shadows and a depth edge confidence map that localize the 3D shape boundaries and provide a qualitative description of the local relative depth. Our contribution to the science of medical imaging are as follows:

▷ A design for implementing multi-flash imaging using multiple endoscopes.
▷ A second design for the same purpose, using a single modified endoscope.
▷ Experimental verification of the two designs.
▷ Experimental verification of the usefulness of both the MAX composite image and the depth edge confidence map for creating medical and biological illustrations and photography.

We believe that we have only scratched the surface of the potential enhancements in medical imaging that are enabled by the use of the multi-flash technique. By using light sources and imaging sensors placed in different spatiotemporal configurations as well as wavelengths, the technique can be adapted to augment many existing methods of medical imaging. We also hope that the technique can serve as a useful tool for medical illustrators and researchers. Additional results can be seen at http://vision.ai.uiuc.edu/~tankh/MultiFlash.

Acknowledgement. Work at Massachusetts Eye and Ear Infirmary supported by the Eugene B. Casey Foundation. We are grateful for support and suggestions from Narendra Ahuja and the Beckman Institute Computer Vision and Robotics Laboratory.

References

1. Vogt, F., Kruger, S., Niemann, H., Schick, C.: A system for real-time endoscopic image enhancement. In: MICCAI. (2003)
2. Mueller, M., Camartin, C., Dreher, E., Hanggi, W.: Three-dimensional laparoscopy. gadget or progress? a randomized trial on the efficacy of three-dimensional laparoscopy. Surg Endosc. **13** (1999)
3. Schade, G., Hess, M., Rassow, B.: Möglichkeit endolaryngealer morphometrischer messungen mit einem neuen laserlichtverfahren. HNO **50** (2002) 753–755
4. Rosen, D., Minhaj, A., Hinds, M., Kobler, J., Hillman, R.: Calibrated sizing system for flexible laryngeal endoscopy. In Schade, G., Müller, F., Wittenbeg, T., Hess, M., eds.: 6th International Workshop: Advances in Quantitative Laryngology (University of Hamburg) Advances in Quantitative Laryngology , Voice and Speech Research (Proceedings), Verlag (2003)
5. Hodges, E.R.S.: The Guild Handbook of Natural History Illustration. John Wiley and Sons (2003)
6. DeCarlo, D., Santella, A.: Stylization and Abstraction of Photographs. In: Proc. Siggraph 02, ACM Press. (2002)
7. Scharstein, D., Szeliski, R.: A taxonomy and evaluation of dense two-frame stereo correspondence algorithms. In: International Journal of Computer Vision. Volume 47(1). (2002) 7–42
8. Sato, I., Sato, Y., Ikeuchi, K.: Stability issues in recovering illumination distribution from brightness in shadows. IEEE Conf. on CVPR (2001) 400–407
9. Shirai, Y., Tsuji, S.: Extraction of the line drawing of 3-dimensional objects by sequential illumination from several directions. Pattern Recognition **4** (1972) 345–351
10. Huggins, P., Chen, H., Belhumeur, P., Zucker, S.: Finding Folds: On the Appearance and Identification of Occlusion . In: IEEE Conf. on Computer Vision and Pattern Recognition. Volume 2., IEEE Computer Society (2001) 718–725
11. Raviv, D., Pao, Y., Loparo, K.A.: Reconstruction of three-dimensional surfaces from two-dimensional binary images. In: IEEE Transactions on Robotics and Automation. Volume 5(5). (1989) 701–710
12. Daum, M., Dudek, G.: On 3-D surface reconstruction using shape from shadows. In: CVPR. (1998) 461–468
13. Yang, D.K.M.: Shape from Darkness Under Error. PhD thesis, Columbia University (1996)
14. Kriegman, D., Belhumeur, P.: What shadows reveal about object structure. Journal of the Optical Society of America (2001) 1804–1813
15. Raskar, R., Yu, J., Ilie, A.: A non-photorealistic camera: Detecting silhouettes with multi-flash. In: SIGGRAPH Technical Sketch. (2003)
16. Raskar, R., Tan, K.H., Feris, R., Yu, J., Turk, M.: Non-photorealistic camera: Depth edge detection and stylized rendering using multi-flash imaging. In: SIGGRAPH. (2004)

Immediate Ultrasound Calibration with Three Poses and Minimal Image Processing

Anand Viswanathan, Emad M. Boctor,
Russell H. Taylor, Gregory Hager, and Gabor Fichtinger

Engineering Research Center, Johns Hopkins University
{anand, rht, hager, gabor}@cs.jhu.edu, eboctor@ieee.org

Abstract. This paper introduces a novel method for ultrasound (US) probe calibration based on closed-form formulation and using minimal US imaging allowing for an immediate result. Prior to calibration, a position sensor is used to track each image in 3D space while the US image is used to determine target location within the image. The calibration procedure uses these two pieces of information to determine the transformation (translation, rotation, and scaling) of the scan plane with respect to the position sensor. We utilize a closed form solution from two motions of the US probe relying on optical digitization with a calibrated pointer to replace with a great extent the traditional segmentation of points/planes in US images. The tracked pointer appeared to introduce significantly less error than the resolution of the US image caused in earlier approaches. Our method also uses significantly fewer US images and requires only minimal image segmentation, or none with a special probe attachment.

1 Introduction

Ultrasound imaging (US) has emerged as a widely popular guidance modality for medical interventions, since it is real-time, safe, convenient to use in the operating room, and inexpensive compared to other modalities such as CT and MRI. Significant research has been dedicated to using US in a quantitative manner. Toward this goal, the main problems are to assemble individual 2D US images into 3D volumes [1] and then to relate the position of surgical tools with respect to the reconstructed US volume. Solution of both problems requires tracking the 2D US probe in 3D space with respect to a stationary frame of reference. Typically, tracking is achieved by rigidly attaching 3D localizers to the US probe. The missing link, however, is the spatial transformation between the US image pixels and the tracking body attached to the US probe, which requires calibration. Hence, calibration is ubiquitously present in all systems where 2D ultrasound is used for quantitative image guidance. Clearly, the accuracy of calibration is the most significant factor in the accuracy of these systems.

In all currently known calibration processes, an object of known geometrical properties (a.k.a. phantom) is scanned by the tracked US probe and then various mathematical procedures are applied to determine the unknown transformation that maximizes the similarity between the US images and the actual phantom. Geometrical phantoms based on points [2, 3, 4, 5, 6] and planes [7, 4, 6] have been developed and

C. Barillot, D.R. Haynor, and P. Hellier (Eds.): MICCAI 2004, LNCS 3217, pp. 446–454, 2004.

compared in terms of accuracy and performance [4, 6].
The cross-wire and three-
wire phantoms require large
numbers of images and are
hard to automate, while the
single-wall phantom as in
Cambridge phantom [4] is a
more automatic, repeatable
method. Typically however,
all of these phantoms are
very complex to create and
to use in calibration. These
complex phantoms also re-
quire segmentation of nu-
merous points per each individual US image. Figure 1
shows a typical formulation
for the coordinate systems
required for the previously
mentioned phantoms.

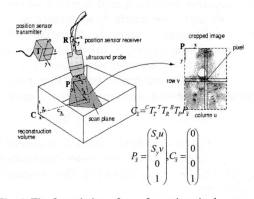

Fig. 1. The formulation of transformations in the cross-wire
phantom. The chain goes from pixel frame P, to receiver
frame R, to transmitter frame T, and to construction frame
C. The (u,v) pixel coordinates are multiplied by (S_x, S_y)
scale factors. The transformed point $C_{\tilde{x}}$ is (0,0,0). (Courtesy
of R. Prager)

There is error associated with each stage of the calibration process (typically
phantom fabrication, image acquisition, spatial co-registration, image processing,
formulation of transformations, and numerical optimization solution) which aggregate
and may induce a prohibitively large final error in the calibration.

2 Mathematical Formulation

In our new framework, we still image a calibration phantom submerged in water bath. We will
demonstrate, however, that in comparison to
standard calibration phantoms, the complexity of
the phantom is minimal and the number of images required for calibration is remarkably low
(3-6 frames). Figure 2 presents the coordinate
systems for mathematical formulation. A_1, A_2
are the transformations of US image coordinate
system (P) with respect to the fixed reconstruction coordinate system (C) at poses 1 and 2, respectively. The actual selection of C is arbitrary
and the only requirement is that it must be rigidly fixed during the calibration process. Using
A_1, A_2, we obtain the transformation between

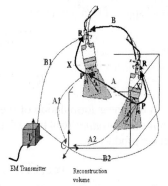

Fig. 2. The coordinate systems formulation for the proposed AX =XB
method.

poses 1 and 2, as $A = A_2 A_1^{-1}$. At the same time, the transformation between the two
poses can be recovered using a calibration phantom or recovered directly by matching

the 2D ultrasound images acquired in these poses to a prior 3D model of the phantom object. To determine the matrix A, we focused on a strategy that minimized the complexity of our imaging phantom. A_1, A_2 are the relative transformations between each of our imaging phantoms. B_1, B_2 are the tracking device readings for the sensor frame (R) with respect to tracker reference frame (T) at poses 1 and 2 respectively. Again, the relative pose between sensor frame (R) at pose 1 and 2 is given by $B = B_2^{-1}B_1$. This yields the following homogeneous matrix equation:

$$AX = XB \tag{1}$$

Where A is estimated from images, B is assumed to be known from the external tracking device, and X is the unknown transformation between the US image coordinate system and the sensor frame (R). The estimated US image frame motion in general is given by:

$$A(\lambda) = \begin{pmatrix} & R_a & & \lambda_x \cdot u_{ax} \\ & & & \lambda_y \cdot u_{ay} \\ & & & \lambda_z \cdot u_{az} \\ 0 & 0 & 0 & 1 \end{pmatrix} \tag{2}$$

Where R_a is the rotation of the US image frame between pose 1 and 2, λ is the unknown scale factor vector that relates the translation vector u_a in voxel space (3DUS, CT, or MRI) to the US image frame translation vector t_a (in mm) such that

$$t_a = \begin{pmatrix} \lambda_x u_{ax} \\ \lambda_y u_{ay} \\ \lambda_z u_{az} \end{pmatrix} = \begin{pmatrix} u_{ax} & 0 & 0 \\ 0 & u_{ay} & 0 \\ 0 & 0 & u_{az} \end{pmatrix} \cdot \begin{pmatrix} \lambda_x \\ \lambda_y \\ \lambda_z \end{pmatrix} = D_{ua}\lambda. \tag{3}$$

It is important to account for the most general case where the scale factor λ, which converts from voxel space to metric coordinates, is not known. Such a scenario could happen if "A" is recovered by registering the US image to a prior acquired model in voxel space. From the homogeneous equation (1) and using (2), one obtains:

$$R_a R_x = R_x R_b \tag{4}$$

$$R_a t_x + D_{ua}\lambda = R_x t_b + t_x \tag{5}$$

In the linear formulation of the problem we will use the linear operator *vec* and the *Kronecker product* ($\otimes$)[10]. Using the following fundamental property of the Kronecker product:

$$vec(CDE) = (C \otimes E^T)vec(D) \tag{6}$$

One can rewrite (4) and (5) into:

$$(R_a \otimes R_b)vec(R_x) = vec(R_x) \text{ , and} \tag{7}$$

$$\left(I_3 \otimes t_b^t\right) vec\left(R_x\right) + \left(I_3 - R_a\right) t_x - D_u \lambda = 0 \tag{8}$$

From (7) and (8), we can transform the whole problem (AX=XB) into a single homogeneous linear system:

$$\begin{bmatrix} I_9 - R_a \otimes R_b & 0_{9*3} & 0_{9*3} \\ I_3 \otimes t_b^t & I_3 - R_a & -D_u \end{bmatrix} \begin{pmatrix} vec\left(R_x\right) \\ t_x \\ \lambda_{3*1} \end{pmatrix} = \begin{pmatrix} 0_{9*1} \\ 0_{3*1} \end{pmatrix} \tag{9}$$

The solution for this homogeneous linear system could be given by finding the null space, which is a subspace in R^{15}. Then the unique solution could be extracted from the null space using the unity constraint to the first 9 coefficients representing the R_x. However, a better solution is described in [9] where the system is solved in two steps: first extract the rotation, and then solve for the translation and scale. The complete algebraic analysis for this problem (where the scale factor is assumed to be constant in three direction) is given in [9], where it is proved that two independent motions with non-parallel axes is sufficient to recover a unique solution for AX=XB. We have extended this solution method to account for inhomogeneous scale in the three coordinate axes.

3   Calibration Setup and Protocol

We have introduced the above closed form formulation before using a modified Z-shape phantom [8], which is tedious to build and process it. In this paper we have replaced the z-phantom with an easier design to build and to process as shown in Figure 3. In our experimental setup, we used the SONOLINE Antares US scanner (Siemens Medical Solutions USA, Inc. Ultrasound Division, Issaquah, WA) with a Siemens VF 10-5 linear array probe held in a rigid attachment mounted on an adjustable arm. The

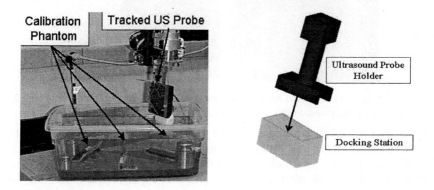

Fig. 3. Calibration setup: Optically tracked probe, which images the calibration phantom (L). A sketch of the planned "docking station" for ultrasound probe calibration.

adjustable arm is used to adjust the spatial position of the tracked US probe to image the calibration phantom. Multiple optical markers were attached to the probe holder, which then were tracked by an OPTOTRAK device (Northern Digital Inc.). The calibration phantom was submerged in a transparent plastic water tank. The calibration phantom consisted of three identical thin (4 mm) plastic plates of irregular shape. The candidate feature from this phantom is simply a single point on a line that can be easily detected by a wide variety of probes and depth settings. The plastic plates were machined together to ensure their congruency. The plates were positioned on a flat surface and fixed in place using Lego blocks and permanent glue for support, as seen in Figure 4. Using an optical pointer, we collected 3D points of each of the plates for offline processing. The pointer was pivoted about each digitized point in order to obtain an accurate estimate of the desired 3D point as shown in Figure 4. These 3D points are registered to provide a local coordinate system for each of the thin plates. From the local coordinate systems, one can calculate the relative transformations between each pair of plates. The poses of the three plates were carefully arranged in order to give the optimal results for the two motions required by the AX =XB formulation, based on previous experiments.

Traditionally in US probe calibration research; arrays of wires have been used to establish the relationship between the coordinate systems of the US and the tracking device. This approach typically involves laborious segmentation to extract the wire points in the US images and then relate these points to the tracking device coordinate system. In this paper, we take a different approach by computing the A_1 and A_2 first by locating prominent feature points of the plates in the US images and then using an optical digitizer (Figure 4) to compute the relative transformation between the plates. We tested two protocols for computing the A_1 and A_2 matrices for our thin plate calibration phantom:

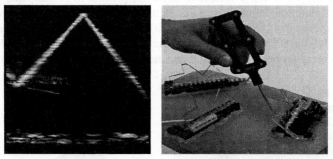

Fig. 4. Optical pointer is used to digitize 3D points prior to calibration on the three clear plastic plates forming the phantom (R), and an ultrasound image of one of the plates (L).

1. Move the US tracked probe such that the probe is parallel to the thin plate and the image plane of the US image shows the middle of the thin plate.
2. Apply the same protocol as above, but collect multiple tracking data from one end of the thin plate to the other end and use an averaging technique to find the "center" of the thin plate.

By using the adjustable arm, we receive consistent and good appearance of the thin plates in the US images. As a practical alternative, we are currently developing a simple probe holder that will dock into the thin plates in a predefined manner, thereby guaranteeing correct alignment between the probe and the plates. This concept can be seen in Figure 3. The same concept (i.e. using a mechanical attachment to the US probe) has been successful in the Cambridge phantom [4]. The consistent placement of the probe on the plates yields predictable and sharp US images that could even be processed automatically. Automatic image processing, however, might not promise a significant advantage, as we only use 3-6 frames and just a single feature point and a line in each.

In Figure 4, An US image of a portion of the calibration phantom is shown. To acquire this image, the probe is placed according to the protocol to make sure that the entire plane of the plate appears in the US image at once. To ensure in-plane alignment of the US probe and a plate being scanned, the contour of the plate is observed as the probe is moved over the plate. The probe and plate being in the same plane forms a constraint from which we assume that the A_1 and A_2 transformation matrices are the relative transformations between the plates of the calibration phantom with a positional offset based on the pixel coordinates of the phantom in the acquired US image. From the US image, we observe the sharp contours of the plates (Figure 4) from which we compute the rotation of the plate within the plane of the US.

Three sets of tracking and US image data are sufficient to solve the mathematical formulation with acceptable accuracy. An additional 3 sets of data can generate 48 calibration datasets, which will ensure a well-conditioned problem and produce comparable results to previous calibration accuracies [4]. Furthermore, when the probe is held in a docking attachment, the US images need to be collected and processed only once during the lifetime of the probe and any future calibration can be performed without relying on any US images.

4 Experiments and Results

To test the numerical stability of the closed form formulation, simulation data was generated. Artificial noise was added to the data points to mimic the error of the tracker and account for the effects of ultrasound image properties. Accordingly, the following protocol aims to simulate these disturbances. First, the missing transformation X is picked by a random choice. Second, a sequence of probe motions is chosen. From the unknown transformation X, the ultrasound image motion can be deduced.

Table 1. Average error and standard deviation of the recovered translation vector for different calibration sequences. The sequences were generated using synthetic data with added noise of .5%, 1%, 5%, 10% respectively.

Noise Level (%)	Average Error (mm)			Standard Dev. (mm)		
0.5	0.0013	-0.00113	-0.0668	0.468	0.125	0.298
1	-0.002	0.00652	0.0356	0.382	0.195	-0.109
5	0.0657	-0.0357	-0.888	8.726	2.132	4.512
10	0.0461	-0.0160	-0.895	13.89	3.459	6.058

Table 2. Average pose and deviation of the recovered calibration matrix using the thin plate calibration phantom with the AX=XB method.

	Average			Standard Dev.(repeatability)		
Position (mm)	93.83	-38.50	38.21	1.31	2.08	2.41
Roll, Pitch, and Yaw Angles (degrees)	177.85	0.29709	2.7751	0.74		

Third, different levels of white noise are added to the ultrasound image motion frame "A's" to simulate a real environment as well as to the simulated tracking readings "B's". The resolution of a tracking device is always in the order of 0.1 % for EM devices and less than 0.001% for an optical based system. The algorithm was executed to recalculate the X transformation under different noise conditions (Table 1.)

In order to check the repeatability of our calibration setup and our phantom's performance, we gathered data using a tracked ultrasound probe. Real US data was acquired in 2 poses for each of the calibration plates. The algorithm was tested on 48 unique combinations of 6 different poses (two poses per plate). Table 2 reports the average recovered pose values of these 48 combinations as well as the standard deviation, which reflect the repeatability of this method. These numbers are comparable to the previously reported repeatability analysis [4]. Right after the data collection (tracking information and the offline processed data), the calibration algorithm executes almost immediately. The major source of expected error stems from the misalignment of the ultrasound probe to the plane of the thin plate. With the addition of the planned docking station, this source of error can be removed from the system.

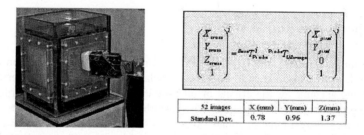

Fig. 5. Reconstruction accuracy setup, acquiring 52 cross wire images from different angles (L), The reconstruction precision framework (R, Top) and the resultant standard deviation in mm (R, Bottom).

Next we performed precision assessment for the calibration, using one of the reported accuracy analysis methods [4, 5]. Reconstruction precision based on 3D reconstruction of the cross wire. The basic idea behind this test is to check how precise the calibration matrix would reconstruct all the cross wire points gathered from different insonification angles into a fixed point in space. The standard deviation of the point cloud reflects the uncertainty in the calibration matrix as well as the manual extraction of the cross wire points, as shown in Figure 5. The resulting calibration precision is highly comparable to [4].

5 Discussion

These preliminary results indicate significant potential in using a simple calibration phantom in conjunction with the AX=XB closed form formulation. The sharp features of thin plastic plates of the calibration phantom appear markedly in US images and it is easy to locate these features based on pixel intensity and gradient. Compared to conventional wire-based calibration phantoms, the simplified design of our phantom and the use of optical digitization of 3D feature points reduced the amount of image processing required and still provided very accurate calibration results. Because conventional calibration methods relied on image information from an US machine, registration accuracy, to a large extent, also depended on the resolution of the US imaging system and the accuracy of feature extraction. Ultrasound noise and beam width problem would normally affect the accuracy of the estimated A matrix. Now, by relying on the OPTOTRAK, which has 0.02 mm resolution and 0.5mm accuracy, we achieved a significantly more reliable calibration. Based on the simulation experiments, the closed formed formulation still produces stable calibration matrix. Therefore if the docking station was used to eliminate the misalignment error between the US probe and the phantom, we should expect sub millimeter reconstruction precision. The simple docking guide mechanism eliminates the need for the currently used adjustable arm and allow for offline image processing leading to immediate calibration.

Acknowledgements. This work is supported by NSF EEC 9731478. We are grateful to Carol Lowery, Levin Nock, and David Gustafson (Siemens Medical Solutions USA, Inc. Ultrasound Division, Issaquah, WA) for providing Ultrasound Antares unit equipped with URI interface.

References

1. A. Fenster, D. B. Downey, and N. H. Cardinal, "Three Dimensional Ultrasound Imaging," *Physics in medicine and biology*, vol 46, pp. 67-99, 2001.
2. P. R. Detmer, G. Bashein, T. Hodges, K. W. Beach, E.P. Filer, D. H. Burns, and D. E. Strandness Jr., "3D Ultrasonic Image Feature Localization based on Magnetic Scanhead Tracking: In Vitro Calibration and Validation." *US in Med. Biol.*, 23(4):597-609, 1996.
3. J. Carr, Surface Reconstruction in 3D Medical Imaging, Ph.D. thesis, University of Canterbury, Christchurch, New Zealand, 1996.
4. R. W. Prager, Rohling R. N., Gee A. H., and Berman L., "Rapid Calibration for 3-D Freehand Ultrasound," *US in Med. Biol.*, 24(6):855-869, 1998.
5. N. Pagoulatos, D. R. Haynor, and Y. Kim, "A Fast Calibration Method for 3-D Tracking of Ultrasound Images Using a Spatial Localizer," *US in Med. Biol.*, 27(9):1219-1229, 2001.
6. Emad M. Boctor, A. Jain, M. Choti, Russell H.Taylor, Gabor Fichtinger, "Rapid calibration method for registration and 3D tracking of ultrasound images using spatial localizer," *Proc. SPIE Medical Imaging*, Vol. 5035,p. 521-532, 2003.
7. F. Rousseau, P. Hellier, C. Barillot, "A fully automatic calibration procedure for freehand 3D ultrasound," *In IEEE Int. Symp. on Biomedical Imaging, Washington D.C, Juillet 2002.*

8. Emad Boctor, Anand Viswanathan, Michael Choti, Russell H. Taylor, Gabor Fichtinger, and Gregory Hager, "A Novel Closed Form Solution for Ultrasound Calibration," *In IEEE Int Symp. On Biomedical Imaging*, 2004.
9. Nicolas Andreff and Radu Horaud and Bernard Espiau, "Robot Hand-Eye Calibration Using Structure from Motion," *International J. of Robotics Research, 20(3), pp 228-248, 2001*.
10. John W. Brewer, "Kronecker Products and Matrix Calculus in System Theory", *IEEE Trans. Circuits and systems, 25(9) Sep.1978*.

Accuracy of Navigation on 3DRX Data Acquired with a Mobile Propeller C-Arm

Theo van Walsum[1], Everine B. van de Kraats[1], Bart Carelsen[2],
Sjirk N. Boon[3], Niels Noordhoek[3], and Wiro J. Niessen[1]

[1] Image Sciences Institute, University Medical Center Utrecht, Heidelberglaan 100,
3508 GA Utrecht, The Netherlands
{theo,everine,wiro}@isi.uu.nl – http://www.isi.uu.nl
[2] Academic Medical Center Amsterdam, Medical Physics Department,
The Netherlands
[3] Philips Medical Systems, Best, The Netherlands

Abstract. Recently, 3DRX imaging has been combined with navigation technology, enabling direct 3D navigation, i.e. navigation on volumetric data without an explicit step to register the image data to the patient coordinate system. In this study, the accuracy of such a navigation setup is evaluated for a mobile C-arm with propeller motion.

1 Introduction

Navigation on preoperative images during therapy requires registration of image data to the patient. In case of navigation on 2D fluoroscopic images, this registration is implicitly obtained by tracking both the patient and the C-arm at the moment of imaging. This approach also requires a geometric calibration and distortion correction of the C-arm images. In practice, tracking is performed by attaching a dynamic reference frame to the patient and to the C-arm. Geometric calibration is generally performed by mounting a calibration phantom, e.g. a plate with radio-opaque spheres, to the image intensifier of the C-arm, and using the pattern of projected spheres to determine the imaging geometry and image distortion.

For 3D image guidance, the solution is less simple, as the imaging is often performed before therapy, and not in the operating room. Registration in this case is conventionally done either using markers which are rigidly attached to the patient and which are visible in the 3D images, or by performing a feature match, e.g. by matching the surface of (exposed) patient anatomy to the corresponding surface in the image. Both methods can be invasive and laborious.

A relatively new approach is to use 3D Rotational X-Ray (3DRX) data for image guidance of therapy. In 3DRX imaging, a 3D volume is reconstructed from a set of fluoroscopic images, obtained with a C-arm that rotates around the subject to image. 3DRX imaging has two distinct advantages, compared to other 3D modalities such as conventional MRI and CT: first, the images can be acquired at the operation theater, and second, the 3DRX image reconstructed

C. Barillot, D.R. Haynor, and P. Hellier (Eds.): MICCAI 2004, LNCS 3217, pp. 455–461, 2004.

is always at the same (or known) location with respect to a fixed position on the C-arm, which implies that, after a calibration step, the 3DRX image can be used for navigation without applying a registration step. This approach has been described earlier, and is called "direct navigation" [1,2,3]. As 3DRX data can also be accurately registered to other 3D imaging modalities such as MRI data [4], intra operative acquisition of 3DRX data can also be used as a replacement of the invasive and laborious conventional registration in image guided surgery on CT and MRI data.

Previously, we have reported on the accuracy of navigation of such a setup when using a fixed, ceiling-mounted C-arm [3]. In this study, we investigate the navigation accuracy of a similar setup when using a mobile C-arm with propeller motion.

In Sect. 2, the concept of direct navigation is described briefly, followed by a description of our experimental setup in Sect. 3. Results and conclusions follow in Sects. 4 and 5.

2 Direct Navigation

The complete process of obtaining 3DRX images for navigation consists of two calibration steps and an imaging step.

The first calibration step is required for 3DRX reconstruction from projection images. In this step, image distortion, imaging geometry and the orientation of the C-arm for each of the fluoroscopic images is determined. First, images are obtained with a bullet-grid attached to the image intensifier of the C-arm. These images are used to determine the imaging geometry (focal distance, etc.) and the image distortion, caused by the pincushion shaped detector and the earth-magnetic field. Subsequently, a special-purpose phantom is scanned to determine the positions from which each of the projection images is taken.

A second calibration step is required to determine the relation between the position of the imaged volume (image space) and some fixed position in the operation room (physical space), e.g. on the C-arm at a known location, see Fig. 1. Hereto, another special-purpose phantom, with a tracker plate attached to it and with fiducials inside, is imaged. The locations of the fiducials w.r.t. the coordinate system defined by the tracker plate are known. After imaging, the image data is imported into the navigation software and the fiducials are pinpointed in the image. Next, the positions of the pinpointed fiducials in the image are registered to the known fiducial locations in the phantom, which yields the relation between image space and the tracker plate. The relation between the C-arm and the phantom tracker plate is determined by attaching a tracker plate to the C-arm, and capturing the relation between the C-arm tracker plate and the phantom tracker plate by means of a camera. This is done with the C-arm in a known (reproducible) position, thus the relation of the image space to C-arm space is known, and can be reused when a patient is imaged.

Both calibration steps need to be performed before imaging of the patient. If the system is calibrated when the patient is imaged, direct navigation without an explicit registration step is possible.

When using direct navigation in practice, a dynamic reference frame must be attached to the patient, and the relation between the reference frame and the C-arm must be stored prior to imaging. As the relation from C-arm to image space is known, because of the calibration step, the relation between the patients dynamic reference frame and the image space is known, which allows direct navigation on the 3DRX image data.

3   Experiments

The accuracy of direct navigation on 3DRX data has been evaluated. For imaging, a prototype mobile C-arm (Pulsera with motorized propeller facility, Philips Medical Systems, Best, The Netherlands) was used to generate the 3DRX images. Navigation was performed using a Treon StealthStation navigation system (Medtronic SNT, Louisville CO, USA) with special software that permits navigation on 3DRX images.

For the accuracy experiments, a special-purpose phantom has been used [5]. The phantom consists of 19 vertical Perspex rods with divots at the top. The locations of the divots on the rods are accurately known from the manufacturing process. The locations of the rods on the phantom have been measured with a precision of $3\,\mu$m. Before imaging, radiodense spheres are put on top of each of the rods, see Fig. 2a. The center of the sphere coincides with the top of the divot, because of the way the sphere and rods are constructed. After imaging, the spheres are removed without moving the phantom, and a navigated pointer is used to touch and store the divot locations in the navigation software (Fig. 2b), in combination with the 3DRX image of the phantom.

Afterwards, special purpose image processing software is used to determine the centers of the spheres with subpixel accuracy. Next, the set of known divot locations is registered rigidly to the sphere centers found (average RMSE for this match is 0.29 mm). This set of divot locations replaces the divot locations found in the image, and is considered to be the gold standard for evaluating the positions touched with a pointer.

Using the gold standard divot locations, the target registration error (TRE), defined as the distance between gold standard divot location and the divot location as stored in the navigation system, for each of the divots can be determined. Both the mean TRE and the standard deviation of the TRE are reported.

Two experiments have been carried out in determining the accuracy: one experiment in which the C-arm did not move in between the calibration steps and the imaging, and one experiment in which the C-arm was moved after calibration and before imaging.

In the first experiment, after imaging of the phantom, all 19 divots were touched ten times, five times using a Passive Planar Blunt probe (Medtronic SNT, Louisville CO, USA) and five times using a Passive Planar Ball probe

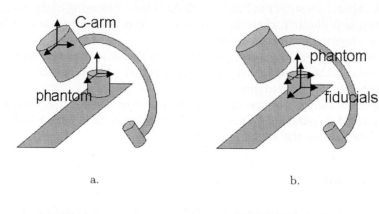

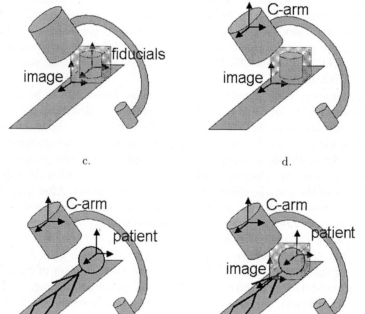

Fig. 1. Transformations involved in direct navigation: a) relation between fixed position on C-arm and phantom tracker plate, captured with camera prior to imaging; b) relation between phantom tracker plate and fiducials in phantom, known by manufacturing; c) relation between fiducials in phantom, and imaged fiducials, known by registering two pointsets; d) combination of a) – c) yields relation between fixed position on C-arm, and the image coordinates; e) relation between patient reference frame and fixed position on C-arm, captured with camera prior to imaging; f) relation between patient reference frame and image, determined from d) and e).

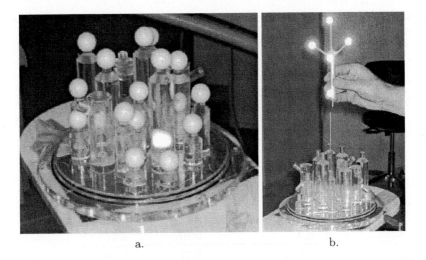

a.   b.

Fig. 2. Phantom for accuracy experiments: a.) phantom to be imaged, with spheres on top of the rods, b.) touching of the divots after the spheres have been removed.

(Medtronic SNT, Louisville CO, USA). For each probe, three observers performed the touching of the divots, one observer three times, and the other two only once. Moving the C-arm around after calibration was expected to affect the accuracy negatively, the results of this first experiment thus should give the optimal accuracy that can be obtained with our setup.

In the second experiment, the C-arm was moved before each imaging step. The phantom was imaged six times, three times after horizontal movement, and three times after vertical movement. Calibration was done twice, once before all horizontal movement imaging, and once (because of an accident with the C-arm tracker plate) before vertical movement imaging. After each imaging step, all divots were touched twice: once by one observer, using the Passive Planar Blunt probe, and once by another observer, using the Passive Planar Ball probe.

4   Results and Discussion

The experiment without moving the C-arm results in a mean TRE of 0.78 mm. This error is determined using 189 points (nineteen divots, five times with one probe, and five times with the other probe; one point was left out, because is was more than 100 mm off). A listing of the errors and standard deviation is shown in Table 1. There is no significant difference between the three observers in this experiment, and there is no significant difference between the two probes used.

The second experiment shows the effect of moving the C-arm around after calibration. Here, the mean TRE is 1.04 mm (220 points: nineteen divots, six images, two probes; eight outliers where removed from the data), which was not significantly different from the mean TRE of the C-arm that has not moved.

Table 1. Mean TRE and standard deviation of the first experiment: no movement of the C-arm.

Probe, Observer	mean TRE (mm)	std. dev. (mm)
Blunt, A	0.79	0.19
Blunt, A	0.68	0.15
Blunt, A	0.85	0.24
Blunt, B	0.73	0.16
Blunt, C	0.81	0.16
Ball, A	0.79	0.25
Ball, A	0.81	0.20
Ball, A	0.89	0.33
Ball, B	0.66	0.23
Ball, C	0.80	0.25
Blunt, All	0.77	0.19
Ball, All	0.79	0.26
Both, All	0.78	0.22

Table 2. Mean TRE and standard deviation of the second experiment: horizontal and vertical movement of the C-arm; A stands for observer A with Passive Planar Blunt probe, B stands for observer B with Passive Planar Ball probe.

Motion	mean TRE (mm)	std. dev. (mm)
Horizontal 1, A	0.99	0.18
Horizontal 1, B	0.73	0.24
Horizontal 2, A	1.59	0.18
Horizontal 2, B	1.19	0.13
Horizontal 3, A	1.61	0.50
Horizontal 3, B	1.39	0.39
Vertical 1, A	1.26	0.31
Vertical 1, B	0.88	0.35
Vertical 2, A	0.52	0.23
Vertical 2, B	0.67	0.19
Vertical 3, A	0.82	0.22
Vertical 3, B	0.84	0.62
All A	1.13	0.49
All B	0.95	0.43
Horizontal, A & B	1.25	0.43
Vertical, A & B	0.83	0.42
All, A & B	1.04	0.47

The mean TRE for navigation after horizontal motion of the C-arm is 1.25 mm (110 points), and the mean TRE for vertical motion is 0.83 mm (110 points). A listing of the errors and standard deviation is shown in Table 2.

From these results it follows that moving the C-arm around does not severely affect the navigation accuracy negatively. As approximate orientation and position of the C-arm are still the same, the 3DRX calibration probably still holds. Furthermore, the C-arm appears to be rigid enough to be moved around after calibration for navigation.

The overall accuracy of 1.0 mm is sufficient for many navigated surgical interventions. When these numbers are compared to the results for a ceiling-mounted C-arm (RMSE 0.7 mm [3]), these numbers show that the mobility of the C-arm system only slightly compromises the accuracy. Furthermore, similar numbers have been reported for the SIREMOBIL Iso-C^{3D} [2]; the average errors for that C-arm range from 1.0 to 1.6 mm, depending on the experimental setup.

Given the propeller motion of the C-arm, imaging and thus navigation is limited to extremities and pediatric, head and neck applications.

5 Conclusion

Direct navigation using a mobile C-arm with propeller motion is accurate. In our experiments, the mean TRE is 1.0 mm, which is sufficient for many applications.

Acknowledgments. Herke-Jan Noordmans is acknowledged for his assistance in extracting the sphere centers from the 3DRX images of the phantom.

References

1. Mitschke, M., Ritter, D.: Direct navigation with an isocentric mobile C-arm. In: Computer Assisted Orthopedic Surgery. (2002) 209–211
2. Ritter, D., Mitschke, M., Graumann, R.: Markerless navigation with the intraoperative imaging modality SIREMOBIL ISO-C3D. Electromedica **70** (2002) 31–36
3. Van de Kraats, E.B., Van Walsum, T., Kendrick, L., Noordhoek, N., Niessen, W.J.: Direct navigation on 3D rotational X-ray images. In: Computer Assisted Orthopedic Surgery. (2003) 382–383
4. Van de Kraats, E.B., Van Walsum, T., Verlaan, J.J., Öner, F.C., Viergever, M.A., Niessen, W.J.: Noninvasive magnetic resonance to three-dimensional rotational X-ray registration of vertebral bodies for image-guided spine surgery. Spine **29** (2004) 293–297
5. Willems, P.W.A., Noordmans, H.J., Berkelbach van der Sprenkel, J.W., Viergever, M.A., Tulleken, C.A.F.: An MKM-mounted instrument holder for frameless point-stereotactic procedures: a phantom-based accuracy evaluation. Journal of Neurosurgery **95** (2001) 1067–1074

High Quality Autostereoscopic Surgical Display Using Anti-aliased Integral Videography Imaging

Hongen Liao, Daisuke Tamura, Makoto Iwahara, Nobuhiko Hata, and
Takeyoshi Dohi

Graduate School of Information Science and Technology, the University of Tokyo
7-3-1 Hongo, Bunkyo-ku, Tokyo 113-8656, Japan
liao@atre.t.u-tokyo.ac.jp

Abstract. This paper presents an autostereoscopic three-dimensional (3-D) surgical display with high quality integral videography (IV) rendering algorithm. IV is an animated extension of integral photography, which provides 3-D images without using any supplementary glasses or tracking devices. Despite IV's many advantages, the quality of its spatial image has thus far been poor. We developed a high quality image rendering method with oversampling technique for enhancing the resolution of elemental IV image and low-pass-filter for smoothing the image. Furthermore, we manufactured a high-resolution IV display for evaluating the feasibility of proposed method. The experimental results show the quality of anti-aliased IV image is improved. We also integrated the developed IV image into image-guided surgery display system. This approach will allow us to acquire the optimum process to produce high quality 3-D image for planning and guidance of minimally invasive surgery.

1 Introduction

The objective of the image-guided surgery is to enhance the surgeon's capability to utilize medical imagery to decrease the invasiveness of surgical procedures and increase their accuracy and safety. The display used for the surgical navigation system is often placed in a nonsterile field from surgeon. These force the surgeon to take extra steps to match guidance information on the display with the actual anatomy of the patient. This hand-eye coordination problem has been discussed as possible cause of the interruption of surgical flow [1]. Furthermore, most of medical information in pre- or intra-operative image to surgeons, as a set of 2-D sectional images displayed away from the surgical area. This reconstructed 3-D information sometimes differs between individual surgeons.

Stereoscopic technique has been taking an important roll in surgery and diagnosis with various modes of visualization on offer [2-3]. Among previous reported stereoscopic techniques use polarized or shuttering glasses to create 3-D image for surgical simulation and diagnosis. This binocular stereoscopic display reproduces the depth of projected objects by using fixed binoculars; because the images for the left and right eyes are formed separately, there is a disparity in the reproduced image. Therefore, different viewers can have inconsistent depth perception [4]. Not much has

C. Barillot, D.R. Haynor, and P. Hellier (Eds.): MICCAI 2004, LNCS 3217, pp. 462–469, 2004.

been done to investigate the negative impact of this inconsistency on the accuracy of surgical navigation.

We have developed an autostereoscopic imaging technique, in contrast to a binocular stereoscopic display, that can be integrated into a surgical navigation system by superimposing an actual 3-D image onto the patient. The autostereoscopic images are created by using a modified version of integral videography (IV), which is an animated extension of the integral photography (IP) proposed by Lippmann [5]. IP and IV record and reproduce 3-D images using a micro convex lens array and photographic film (or a flat display). A high-resolution multi-projection IV display system [6] and a surgical navigation system by IV image overlay [7] are introduced for image-guided surgery. With additional improvements in the display, these systems will increase the surgical accuracy and reduce invasiveness.

Despite IV's many advantages that have been proven in both feasibility studies and clinical applications [6-8], the quality of its spatial image has thus far been poor. Furthermore, a high quality 3-D visualization system must be developed to integrate capabilities for pre-surgical/intra-operative image guidance. In this study, we describe an anti-aliased image rendering algorithm for high quality IV image generation. The high-quality rendering method is developed for each elemental image of IV by using oversampling technique to enhance the resolution of element images and low-pass-filter to smooth the resultant images. We further manufactured a high-resolution IV display for evaluating the feasibility of the proposed method.

2   Materials and Methods

2.1   Original IV Image Rendering Method

IV uses a fast image rendering algorithm to project a computer-generated graphical object through a micro-convex lens array. Each point shown in a 3-D space is reconstructed at the same position as the actual object by the convergence of rays from the pixels of the elemental images on the computer display after they pass through the lenslets in the lens array. The surgeon can see the object on the display from various directions, as though it were fixed in 3-D space.

Because resolution of flat display is much lower than that of photographic film (used in the original method of IP), there is a decrease in the amount of information displayed. Thus, all points on a 3-D object cannot be displayed on flat display, and only the 3-D information of the points most suitable to each pixel of the computer display must be processed.

The coordinates of the points in the 3-D object that correspond to each pixel on the screen must be computed for each pixel on the display (Fig. 1). The procedure is similar to the ray-tracing algorithm, although the tracings in this instance are directly opposite those observed on the screen. Our algorithm creates 3-D objects in the space between the screen and the observer, while the ray-tracing algorithm would place the object behind the screen. Unlike natural objects, information about any point in the original object can be directly acquired in the case of medical 3-D images, making our method free from the pseudoscopic image problems peculiar to IP.

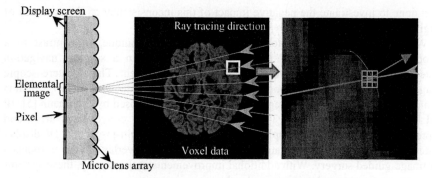

Fig. 1. Fundamental IV rendering algorithm.

2.2 Quality Improvement of IV Elemental Image by Anti-aliased Algorithm

The limited resolution of flat display cause several problems. Because the depth information is encoded into the 2-D image, the projected image of this into 3-D space has a much lower resolution. The aliasing appear when we use a low-density ray tracing (low sampling frequency) algorithm and display resultant IV elemental image in a low-resolution display. There were a large number of different techniques in anti-aliasing in the computer graphics community and medical field [9-11].

The relationship between the pixels in the elemental image is considered for generating the pixel. The entire image information surrounding to the voxel data tracked by ray tracing is used for pixel calculation when the single pixel of the elemental image is rendered (Fig. 2). We introduce a modified oversampling image processing method for anti-aliased IV rendering.

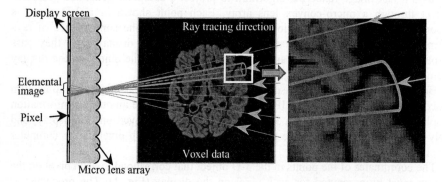

Fig. 2. Oversampling ray tracing method for rendering IV elemental image.

Assuming the lens pitch and the pixel pitch of display to be p and P_p, respectively, and each lens covers N_p pixels, the width of each elemental image is $W_p = N_p \times P_p$. The voxel data is putted in the space with a mm and b mm in front of and behind the lens array, respectively (Fig. 3). The maximum rendering area of the voxel data in position

a for each elemental image is W_v mm, which covers N_v voxel number with each voxel pitch of V_p, then $W_v = N_v \times V_p$.

The focal length of lenslet is h, the relationship between the W_p and W_v is $W_v = W_p \times a/h$. The covered voxel numbers in position a is given by

$$N_v = \frac{W_v}{V_p} = \frac{a \times W_p}{h \times V_p} \tag{1}$$

A signal sampled at a frequency higher than the pixel number of elemental image (Nyquist frequency in the ray tracing) is said to be oversampled β times, where the oversampling ratio of the voxel number to pixel number is defined as

$$\beta = \frac{N_v}{N_p} = \frac{a \times P_p}{h \times V_p}. \tag{2}$$

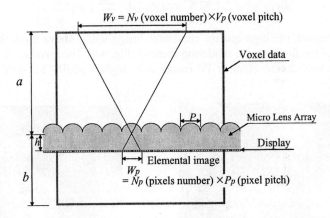

Fig. 3. Relationship between the pixel of elemental image and voxel data.

Considering the maximum position of voxel data corresponding to the lens array and the spatial relationship between the voxel data and the lens array, the oversampling ratio is modified as

$$\beta = \frac{\max(a,b) \times P_p}{h \times V_p \times \cos \theta} \tag{3}$$

where θ is an intersected angle between the voxel and lens array.

Although the resolution of elemental image is increased, the display only provides limited pixels for each elemental image. It is necessary to keep the high quality of image and drop the image resolution as it can be displayed in IV display. A low-pass-filter imaging method with Fourier transform is proposed to solve this problem.

Assuming the resolution of display is $m \times n$ pixels and the oversampling ratio is β, the number of ray tracing for IV image rendering will be $(m \times \beta) \times (n \times \beta)$. A Discrete Fourier Transformation is used for image transform. The spectrum function of $F(u,v)$ is expressed as

$$F(u,v) = \sum_{x=0}^{m*\beta-1} \sum_{y=0}^{n*\beta-1} f(x,y) \exp\left(-j\frac{2\pi x}{m*\beta}u - j\frac{2\pi y}{n*\beta}v\right), \tag{4}$$

where $f(x,y)$ is brightness value function of the pixel in position (x,y), u and v are the frequencies of image in x and y direction, respectively . The output of oversampled elemental image is low-pass filtered and decimated to achieve a necessary frequency component of image with the target pixel count by using

$$F'(u,v) = F(u,v) * \delta_{u,v}, \tag{5}$$

where $\delta_{u,v}$ is a delta function. We extract the central oversampled image to $(m \times n)$ pixels.

$$F(s,t) = F'\left(\frac{m * \beta}{2} - m + 1 + s, \frac{n * \beta}{2} - n + 1 + t\right); \quad (s \in [0, m-1], \ t \in [0, n-1]). \tag{6}$$

Last, transform the resultant spectrum to normal image corresponding to each elemental image by using a Reverse Discrete Fourier Transformation.

$$f(x,y) = \frac{1}{m}\frac{1}{n}\sum_{s=0}^{m-1}\sum_{t=0}^{n-1} F(s,t)\exp\left(j\frac{2\pi s}{m}x + j\frac{2\pi t}{nt}y\right). \tag{7}$$

We compare the high quality elemental image using above algorithm (Fig. 4b) with that of the fundamental rendering method (Fig. 4a). The novel rendering method creates an anti-aliased element IV image with higher quality for spatial IV image formation.

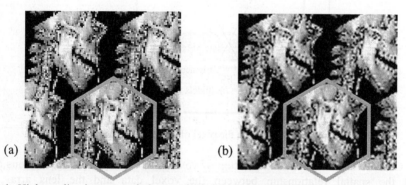

(a)   (b)

Fig. 4. High quality image rendering method for elemental IV image (hexagon lens); a) Fundamental IV rendering method. b) Modified oversampling algorithm for anti-aliased image.

2.3 High-Resolution IV Autostereoscopic Display

The IV display we developed consists of a high-resolution LCD with a micro convex lens array. The quality of the IV image depends primarily on the pixel density of the display (the number of pixels per unit display area) and the lens pitch of the lens array. The LCD display (IBM, T221) is with 3840×2400 pixels on a size of 460.8×288.0 mm (200ppi). The pitch of each pixel on the screen is 0.085 mm. Each lenslet element is hexagonal with a base area of 1.486 mm in width and 1.238 mm in height, which covers 12×10 pixels of the projected image. The focal length of the lenslet is 2.4 mm. Photographs of IV display device and motion parallax of displayed IV image.

3   Experiments and Results

3.1   IV Image Quality Evaluation

We evaluated the feasibility of proposed method by using a zoneplate (Fig. 5a) displayed in front of the lens array. The image brightness of zoneplate is defined as:

$$A \times \sin\left\{\frac{\pi}{2}\left(\frac{(x-a)^2}{\alpha} + \frac{(y-b)^2}{\beta}\right) + \Theta\right\} + B \tag{8}$$

where (x, y) is the position of image, (a, b) is center of concentric circle. (α, β) is the radius of the concentric circle in maximum resolution. A is an amplitude of a sine wave. B is an overlaid gray level of the sine wave. Θ is a phase of sine wave in the concentric circle.

Figure 5c show an IV images of zoneplate by using anti-aliased technique. The aliasing images disappear in area A and B compared with the image using original rendering method as shown in Fig. 5b.

Figure 6 give the measured results between the frequency of observed alias and the oversampling ratio. By analyzing the frequency of IV image processing, we found the IV rendering algorithm can be improved for a high-quality IV image generating.

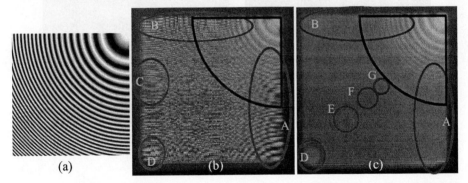

Fig. 5. IV autostereoscopic image: (a) zone plate used for evaluating the image quality. (b) Original IV rendering result, $\beta=1$; the aliasing images appear in area A, B, C, and D. (c) IV image using oversampling and low-pass-filter, $\beta=20$.

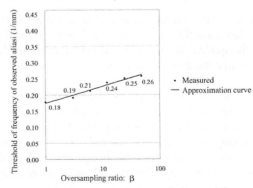

Fig. 6.   Relationship between the frequency of observed alias and the oversampling ratio.

3.2 Feasibility Evaluation for Image-Guided Surgery

We evaluated the usefulness of the developed method. In clinical feasibility study, we performed CT scanning to take photo of in-vivo skull. The volumetric CT images of skull (256×256 pixels × 94 slices, thickness of 2.0mm) were rendered and displayed in high-resolution IV display. Figure 7a show an image with original rendering method. The condylar process of mandible and the mandibular notch shown in the circle can not be distinguished, while the image using anti-aliased method with oversampling and low-pass-liter is improved (Fig. 7b).

Intra-operatively, IV image overlay technique with corresponding image registration can help with the navigation by providing a broader view of the operation field [7]. In combination with robotic and surgical instrument, it even can supply guidance by pre-defining the path of a biopsy needle or by preventing the surgical instruments from moving into critical regions.

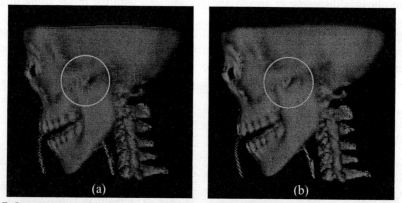

(a)   (b)

Fig. 7. Improvement of IV image quality. (a) with fundamental rendering methods; (b) with anti-aliased rendering algorithm.

4 Discussions and Conclusion

We describe a high quality image rendering for anti-aliased IV imaging by use of oversampling and low-pass-filtering techniques. The merits of developed methods are improvement of the quality of IV elemental image from single pixel to the whole elemental image. These methods directly contribute the remarkable services to the IV image formation.

The methods using for high quality IV image generation have a common weak point of computational cost. Image quality requirement of density or the resolution will increase the rendering time. Especially the IV image based on CG rendering method is time costing compared with normal CG in the same resolution of total pixels, since it is necessary to render the image for each lenslet. There are fewer connections between the rendered images of the adjacent lenses, especial when a complex structure of object is performed. Consequently, the corresponding high speed rendering method must be brought to support the high quality IV imaging.

The display system combined with high quality IV rendering method offer a geometrical accuracy image over the projected objects (esp. depth perspective), without using the extra devices such as the wearing of special glasses. Using the proposed method, IV display enables a safe, easy, and accurate navigation.

In conclusion, we developed a high quality IV imaging algorithm and corresponding display for IV surgical display system. The feasibility study indicated that the oversampling and low-pass-filter technique for anti-aliased imaging can improve the autostereoscopic image quality. The developed display with proposed method is satisfactory and suitable in surgical diagnosis and planning setting.

Acknowledgements. The work of H. Liao was supported in part by the Japan Society for the Promotion of Science (15-11056). N. Hata was supported in part by New Energy and Industrial Technology Development Organization (NEDO) of Japan.

References

1. P. Breedveld, H. G. Stassen, D. W. Meijer, and L. P. S. Stassen, "Theoretical background and conceptual solution for depth perception and eye-hand coordination problems in laparoscopic surgery," *Minim. Invasiv. Ther.*, vol.8, pp.227-234, Aug. 1999.
2. P. Mitchell, I. D. Wilkinson, P. D. Griffiths, K. Linsley, J. Jakubowski: "A stereoscope for image- guided surgery," *British Journal of Neurosurgery*, Vol.16, No.3, pp. 261-266, 2002.
3. H. Seno, M. Mizunuma, M. Nishida, M. Inoue, A. Yanai, M. Irimoto: "3-D-CT stereoscopic imaging in maxillofacial surgery," *Journal of Computer Assisted Tomography*, Vol.23, No.2, pp.76-279, 1999.
4. B. T. Backus, M. S. Banks, R. van Ee, and J. A. Crowell: "Horizontal and vertical disparity, eye position, and stereoscopic slant perception," *Vision Research*, vol.39, pp.1143-1170, 1999.
5. M.G.Lippmann, "Epreuves reversibles donnant la sensation du relief," *J. de Phys* Vol.7, 4th series, pp821-825, 1908.
6. S.Nakajima, K.Nakamura, K.Masamune, I.Sakuma, T.Dohi, "Three-dimensional medical display with computer-generated integral photography," *Computerized Medical Imaging and Graphics*, 25, pp235-241, 2001.
7. H. Liao, N. Hata, S. Nakajima, M. Iwahara, I. Sakuma, T. Dohi, "Surgical Navigation by Autostereoscopic Image Overlay of Integral Videography," *IEEE Trans. Inform. Technol. Biomed.*, Vol.8 No.2, pp.114-121, June 2004.
8. H. Liao, N. Hata, M. Iwahara, I. Sakuma, T. Dohi, "An autostereoscopic display system for image-guided surgery using high-quality integral videography with high performance Computing," *MICCAI 2003*, LNCS 2879, pp247-255, 2003.
9. P. J. La Riviere, X.C. Pan, "Anti-aliasing weighting functions for single-slice helical CT," *IEEE Trans. Med. Imag.*, Vol.21 No.8, pp.978-990 AUG 2002.
10. J. G. Yang, S. T. Park, "An anti-aliasing algorithm for discrete wavelet transform," *MECH SYST SIGNAL PR*, Vol.17, pp.945-954, 2003.
11. K. Mueller, R. Yagel, J. J. Wheller, "Anti-aliased three-dimensional cone-beam reconstruction of low-contrast objects with algebraic methods," *IEEE Trans. Med. Imag.*, Vol.18 No.6, pp.519-537, JUN 1999.

Enhancing Fourier Volume Rendering Using Contour Extraction

Zoltán Nagy, Marcin Novotni, and Reinhard Klein

Department for Computer Science II, Bonn University, 53117 Bonn, Germany
{zoltan,marcin,rk}@cs.uni-bonn.de
http://cg.cs.uni-bonn.de

Abstract. Fourier Volume Rendering (FVR) has received considerable attention in volume visualization during the last decade due its $O(N^2 log N)$ rendering time complexity, where $O(N^3)$ is the volume size. Nevertheless, FVR currently suffers from some quality limiting its usefulness in particular medical applications. The main reason for this is the lack of weighting sample points in dependence of the samples along the integration path. In this work we propose a solution for a special class of problems, namely the extraction and emphasis of contours in volumetric datasets. The accuracy of the illumination of the extracted contours can be derived in an exact manner. Main applications of our method include contour extraction and enhancement of features, noise removal and revealing of important spatial relationships between interior and exterior structures, making it an attractive tool for improved X-ray-like investigations of the given dataset.

1 Introduction

Volume rendering is a technique for visualizing sampled scalar or vectorial volumes of three dimensions by propagation of light in a participating medium. Two main approaches have established in this area: (i) object space and (ii) Fourier space algorithms. The first class of algorithms was originally introduced by Kajiya [6] in 1984. Since then, this model was steadily improved in both speed and quality using global illumination, graphics hardware, pre-integration strategies and Wavelet compression (see e.g. [12], [4] and [7]). Since working in object space, these algorithms allow for modelling light transport in a variety of ways, involving transfer functions and physical parameters like albedo, interreflection, material density, gradients, etc. This class of volume rendering models has in general a rendering time complexity of $O(N^3)$, where N^3 is the volume size, since the whole dataset has to be sampled entirely per frame.

The second class of algorithms work in Fourier space. Introduced by Levoy [8] and Malzbender [9], this method sacrifices some features –which object space algorithms offer– against rendering speed. In FVR, the original dataset is 3D Fourier transformed in $O(N^3 log N)$ time in the preprocessing phase. During rendering, a plane through the center of the Fourier transformed data representation is sampled perpendicularly to the viewing direction and 2D inverse Fourier transformed in $O(N^2 log N)$ time. The Fourier Projection-Slice Theorem tells us, that

C. Barillot, D.R. Haynor, and P. Hellier (Eds.): MICCAI 2004, LNCS 3217, pp. 470–477, 2004.
© Springer-Verlag Berlin Heidelberg 2004

the so obtained image contains an unweighted projection of the sample points of the input dataset from the given view. This leads to occlusion free X-ray like images, since ray attenuation can not be modelled in dependence of the actively cumulated opacity of the voxels. It was soon recognized, that occlusion-free projections are difficult to interpret and a X-ray like linear depth cueing illumination model with directional shading was introduced [8]. The latter method can support the observer in estimating positions of anatomical entities, but projections remain occlusion free.

In this work we eliminate some disadvantages of standard FVR methods. In particular, we extract material boundaries on surfaces in Fourier space. This problem was already considered for medical questions in object space [1,2], rather than Fourier space. In this work, we show, how this technique can be derived and implemented in Fourier space. We show three important applications which makes our technique attractive: (i) extraction of object, rather than screen-space contours, (ii) noise reduction and (iii) removal of non-contributing samples to obtain better visibility of the contours. To accomplish these we adopt the reflection equation for shading in context of FVR [3] formulated in terms of Spherical Harmonics. The main difference is the novel interpretation of the terms appearing in the equation: (i) instead of the incoming light used originally to shade the surface the gradient magnitude is plugged in to emphasize areas of high contrast and (ii) instead of the cosine projection term we use a sine transfer function to highlight surfaces with normals perpendicular to the viewing direction (cf. Section 3 for details). Our technique is of special interest for radiologists who work with X-ray like projections of the given dataset and who want to obtain a better insight to spacial relationships of the investigated medical material.

2   Shading Using Spherical Harmonics

Spherical harmonic (SH) approximation of an illumination model allows for shading of the dataset without recalculating the entire 3D transform per frame. The method derived here is a generalized view on the methods of Entezari et al. [3] and Ramamoorthi and Hanrahan [11]. Their derivation is tailored to lighting voxels/surfaces; we, however, deduce a method for contour extraction.

Normalized SHs are a rotational invariant group of functions that form an orthonormal basis on the unit sphere. While mostly described in complex form, a real representation is available saving memory representing the imaginary part [3]. Any function of finite energy on the sphere may be approximated to any degree of accuracy in terms of SHs $Y_{lm}(\theta, \phi)$ using the expansion

$$f(\theta, \phi) = \sum_l \sum_m f_{lm} Y_{lm}(\theta, \phi) \tag{1}$$

where $f_{lm} = \int_0^{2\pi} \int_0^\pi f(\theta, \phi) Y_{lm}^*(\theta, \phi) \sin\theta d\theta d\phi$. The radiance on a surface (or more specifically, on a voxel position) in its original setting is given by

$$E = \int_{\Omega_i'} L(\omega_i) \rho(\omega_i', \omega_o) max(cos\theta_i', 0) d\omega_i' \tag{2}$$

where subscript i (o) denotes the incoming (outgoing) light direction, the global (local) coordinate system is unprimed (primed), $L(\omega_i)$ is the incoming light, $\rho(\omega_i', \omega_o')$ is the BRDF (bidirectional reflection distribution function) over the upper hemisphere Ω_i' and $max(cos\theta_i', 0)$ is a transfer function preventing the surface from being lit from behind. For the case that diffuse shading is assumed ($\rho = 1/\pi$=const.), and an arbitrary transfer function $f(\theta, \phi)$ is chosen, we obtain omitting ρ

$$E = \int_{\Omega_i'} L(\omega_i) f(\omega_i') d\omega_i' \tag{3}$$

By expanding $L(\omega_i) = \sum_l \sum_m L_{lm} Y_{lm}(\omega_i)$ and $f(\omega_i') = \sum_l \sum_m f_{lm} Y_{lm}(\omega_i')$, substitution into equation (3) leads to the general formulation

$$E = \sum_l \sum_m \sum_p \sum_q L_{lm} f_{pq} \int_{\Omega_i'} Y_{lm}(\omega_i) Y_{pq}(\omega_i') d\omega_i' \tag{4}$$

Note, that two different coordinate systems are assumed here (primed and unprimed). To rotate the primed system into the unprimed one, the canonical rotation formula using the coefficients related to the matrix of the rotation group $SO(3)$ [11]

$$Y_{lm}(\omega_i) = Y_{lm}(R_{\alpha\beta}(\omega_i')) = \sum_{m'=-l}^{l} D_{mm'}^l(\alpha) e^{im\beta} Y_{lm'}(\omega_i') \tag{5}$$

is used, where $R_{\alpha\beta}(\omega_i')$ represents the rotation into the unprimed coordinate system. Applying this rotation in equation (4) leads to

$$E = \sum_l \sum_m \sum_p \sum_q L_{lm} f_{pq} \sum_{m'} D_{mm'}^l(\alpha) e^{im\beta} \int_{\Omega_i'} Y_{lm'}(\omega_i') Y_{pq}(\omega_i') d\omega_i' \tag{6}$$

Due to the orthogonality relationship of SH the integral portion is nonzero iff $l = p$ and $m' = q$. Using the relations $D_{m0}^l(\alpha) e^{im\beta} = \sqrt{\frac{4\pi}{2l+1}} Y_{lm}(\alpha, \beta)$ and $L_{lm} = Y_{lm}(\theta_L, \phi_L)$ [3] we obtain a specialized formulation for functions f with no asimuthal dependence (f_{pq} is zero for $q \neq 0$):

$$E = \sum_{l,m,p} L_{lm} f_{p0} \sum_{m'} D_{mm'}^l(\alpha) e^{im\beta} \delta_{l,p} \delta_{m',0} = \sum_{l,m} \sqrt{\frac{4\pi}{2l+1}} Y_{lm}(\omega_L) f_{l0} Y_{lm}(\alpha, \beta)$$

$$\tag{7}$$

To use latter equation for contour extraction, three requirements have to be met. First, appropriate SH coefficients f_{l0} have to be found which model the brightness of a contour in dependence of the viewing vector and the local gradient. An explicit formula is derived for this in the appendix. Second, note that equation (7) is derived for diffuse shading, i.e. the illumination is independent of the viewer. Fortunately, for contour extraction, we can set the light direction ω_L collinear to the viewing direction ω_V: $\omega_V = \omega_L$, therefore this is implicitly solved. Thirdly, we want to weight a voxel individually, depending on the gradient magnitude, to remove homogeneous regions and to obtain a high degree of visibility of the contours. This is done in the following section.

3   Contour Extraction

Equation (7) is the key equation for general diffuse lighting of a surface, when the lighting distribution and the transfer function can be represented in terms of SH coefficients L_{lm} and f_{lm}, respectively. From this general setting, we can derive a special case, which allows for the enhancement of contours in Fourier space. We regard a sample in the volume as a contour sample, iff $< \omega_V, \omega_N > = 0$, i.e. the viewing vector ω_V is perpendicular to the normal ω_N of the given sample. In the following, a metric of the degree of how much the active sample is likely to be a contour sample is given by the function f:

$$f(\theta_i', \phi_i') = f(\theta_i') = sin(\theta_i')^{2k}, k \in \mathbf{N}_0, \theta_i' = cos^{-1}(< \omega_V, \omega_N >) \qquad (8)$$

In our experiments, we used $k = 8$. The motivation for using this function is to emphasize samples with gradients near-to-orthogonal, in order to induce enough illumination energy for the final projection.

The last thing missing in our considerations is the weighting of the scalar voxel values in dependence of the gradient length. We use a squared version of the gradient length to overemphasize positions with high gradient length:

$$E_{weighted} = E \cdot ||\overrightarrow{\omega_N}||_2^2 = \sum_l \sum_m \sqrt{\frac{4\pi}{2l+1}} ||\overrightarrow{\omega_N}||_2^2 Y_{lm}(\omega_V) f_{l0} Y_{lm}(\omega_N) \qquad (9)$$

where $||\overrightarrow{\omega_N}||_2$ denotes the length of the respective vector N at the surface (or voxel) position.

4   Algorithm

Equation (9) describes the shading at a voxel position in dependence of the local normal N and the global viewing vector V. Applying the Fourier transform operator $\mathcal{F}\{ \}$ results in

$$\mathcal{F}\{E_{weighted}\} = \sum_l \sum_m \sqrt{\frac{4\pi}{2l+1}} Y_{lm}(\omega_V) f_{l0} \mathcal{F}\{||\overrightarrow{\omega_N}||_2^2 Y_{lm}(\omega_N)\} \qquad (10)$$

The usage of this equation is as follows. During preprocessing, volumes V_{lm} are initialized with their respective voxel values $V_{lm}(x, y, z) = ||\overrightarrow{\omega_N}||_2^2 Y_{lm}(\theta_{xyz}, \phi_{xyz})$, $0 \leq l \leq M, -l \leq m \leq l$. The 3D Fourier transform is then applied on every volume V_{lm}. During rendering, we sample slices $S_{lm}(x', y')$ through the origins of every transformed dataset $\mathcal{F}\{V_{lm}\}$ perpendicularly to the viewing direction ω_V. Slice $S_{lm}(x', y')$ is weighted by $\sqrt{\frac{4\pi}{2l+1}} Y_{lm}(\omega_V)$ at every sample point. Finally, the weighted slices are summed up componentwise and the inverse 2D Fourier transform is executed on the result, leading to the desired projection for the current viewing direction.

5   Results and Discussion

In figure 1 we compare rendering results of the conventional FVR algorithm (1st and 3rd row) with our method (2nd and 4th row), using the head, skull (both obtainable from www.volren.org) and the Visible Female dataset. The examples show applications in three main areas.

Hidden feature emphasis. The head dataset (left column) exemplifies how our algorithm is capable of recovering features when the material density of the input dataset is high. We are able to emphasize transitions between air and skull, skull and cerebrospinal fluid, and boundaries around the corpus callosum.

Noise reduction. The skull (middle column) is an example for an extremely noisy dataset. The projection quality is worsened by the fact, that this property is amplified by "ghosting" artifacts of ordinary FVR. Since noise in more likely contained with low gradient portion, our algorithm removes it significantly. Furthermore, the contours of the teeth appear sharper here than with the traditional method.

Boundary and contrast enhancement. Finally, we were able to recognize some important spatial relationships on the Visible Female dataset (right column) using our method. While ordinary FVR leads to strongly diffuse projections of the dataset, we were able to relate exterior structures, like the run of the skin, the ears, the lips, with interior structures like the (upper and lower) jaw and the spinal court using our algorithm.

All three datasets used have a size of 128^3 voxels, where the second and third one were downsampled to this size in order to reduce memory requirements. Rendering times are identical for every view and dataset, with about 3 fps on an 3.06 GHz Intel P IV with 1 GByte RAM.

A little caveat of our method is the somewhat high memory consumption. When using three non-negative SH coefficients, 15 datasets have to be used with 4Bytes at each voxel for the real and the imaginary part, respectively. Since we work with real SHs, the input volumes are real, and according to Fourier theory $F(u, v) = F^*(-u, -v)$, i.e. the Fourier transformed dataset is symmetric with respect to the origin up to conjugation. Thus, memory can be saved by a factor of two. Lossy methods for further memory reduction like vector compression can be incorporated- this is part of future work.

6   Conclusion and Future Work

The intention of this work was to make FVR a more viable alternative in volume visualization, when it comes to explore medical datasets via X-ray like volume rendering techniques. Due to its reduced runtime complexity, the importance of our method in a quantitative sense will grow, when datasets will become larger.

head   skull   Visible Female

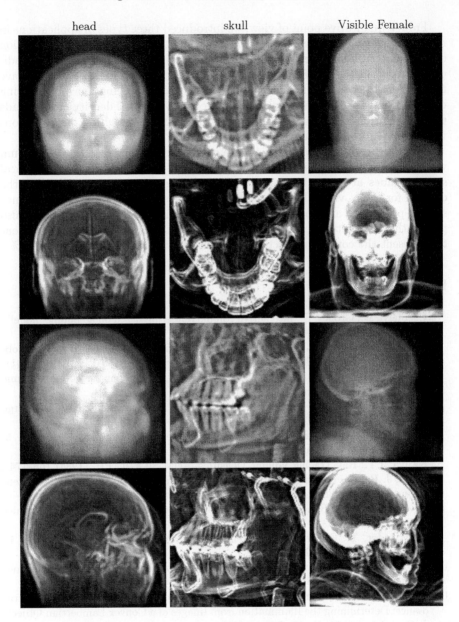

Fig. 1. *Rendering results.* We exemplify our method on three datasets, namely the head (1st col.), skull (2nd col.) and Visible Female dataset (3rd col.). 1st and 3rd row: conventional FVR. 2nd and 4th row: respective counterparts of our method using contour extraction.

From a qualitative point of view, we introduced three types of applications in medical visualization: recovery of hidden features, noise removal, and detection of boundaries. This type of exploration is especially valuable, when the radiologist works with X-ray like projections of the input material. We also have to mention, that the results can not be obtained by applying image processing operators on the respective projections, since high material density mostly leads to a cumulation and hiding of underlying 3D features, resulting in projections with more feature-less, homogeneous areas.

From a theoretical point of view, we created a Fourier projection algorithm, which is capable of lighting features in the dataset in dependence of the local sample values at interactive rates without the requirement to recalculate the dataset for every view. This is a remarkable property of our algorithm, since spatial properties are normally difficult to localize in Fourier space. We also proved that the first three *non-zero* coefficients of the SH expansion are sufficient to represent the contour extraction function with an accuracy of about 94.7%.

References

1. Csébfalvi, B., Gröller, E.: Interactive volume rendering based on a "bubble model". Graphics Interface. (2001)
2. Csébfalvi, B., Mroz, L., Hauser, H., König, A., Gröller, E.: Fast visualization of object contours by non-photorealistic volume rendering. EUROGRAPHICS. (2001).
3. Entezari, A., Scoggins, R., Möller, T., Machiraju, R.: Shading for Fourier Volume Rendering. IEEE Volume Visualization. (2002)
4. Guthe, S., Wand, M., Gonser, J., Strasser, W.: Interactive Rendering of Large Volume Data Sets. IEEE Vsiualization. (2002)
5. Gröbner, W., Hofreiter, N.: Integraltafel, Zweiter Teil, Bestimmte Integrale. 5. Auflage. Springer Verlag. (1973)
6. Kajiya, J.T.: Ray Tracing Volume Densities. ACM SIGGRAPH. (1984) 165–174
7. Kniss, J. Premože, S. Hansen, C., Ebert, D. Interactive Translucent Volume Rendering and Procedural Modeling. IEEE Visualization. (2002)
8. Levoy, M.: Volume Rendering using the Fourier projection-slice theorem. Graphics Interface. (1992) 61–69
9. Malzbender, T.: Fourier Volume Rendering. ACM Transactions on Graphics 12 (3), July 1993. (1993) 233–250
10. Ramamoorthi, R., Hanrahan, P.: An Efficient Representation for Irradiance Environment Maps. ACM SIGGRAPH. (2001) 497–500
11. Ramamoorthi, R., Hanrahan, P.: On the Relationship Between Radiance and Irradiance: Determining the Illumination from Images of a Convex Lambertian Object. J. Opt. Soc, Vol.18, No.10, October 2001.
12. Roettger, S., Guthe, S., Weiskopf, D., Ertl, T., Strasser, W.: Smart Hardware-Accelerated Volume Rendering. Joint EUROGRAPHICS-IEEE TVCG Symposium on Visualization. (2003)
13. Totsuka, T., Levoy, M.: Frequency domain volume rendering. Computer Graphics, 27:(4), August 1993. 271–278
14. Varshalovich, D.A., Moskalev, A.N., Khersonskii, V.K.: Quantum Theory of Angualar Momentum. Irreducible Tensors, Spherical Harmonics, Vector Coupling Coefficients, $3nj$ Symbols. World Scientific. (1988) 130–163

A   Appendix

A.1   Explicit Formula for f_{l0}

f_{l0} can be obtained using equation (5) on p. 143 of [14] by specialization setting $f(\theta,\phi) = f(\theta) = (sin\theta)^{2k}$, and by observing that $Y_{l0}^*(\theta) = Y_{l0}(\theta) = P_l(cos\theta)$:

$$f_{l0} = \sqrt{\frac{2l+1}{4\pi}} \int_0^{2\pi} \int_0^\pi (sin\theta)f(\theta)Y_{l0}(\theta)d\phi d\theta = \sqrt{\pi(2l+1)} \int_0^\pi (sin\theta)^{2k+1} P_l(cos\theta)d\theta, \quad (11)$$

where $P_l(x)$ is the Legendre polynomial of the first kind. By plugging $x = cos\theta$ into Equation (7) on p. 24 of [5] we obtain

$$\int_{-1}^1 x^{2k} P_l(x)dx = \int_0^\pi sin\theta(cos\theta)^{2k} P_l(cos\theta)d\theta = \begin{cases} 0 & 2k < l \text{ or } l \text{ odd} \\ \frac{2(2k-l+2;1;l)}{(2k-l+3;2;l)} & otherwise \end{cases} \quad (12)$$

where $(m;d;\nu) := m(m+d)(m+2d)...(m+(\nu-1)d)$. Thus, using the relationship $sin\theta = \sqrt{1-cos^2\theta}$ and the binomial theorem, we obtain for $2k \geq l$ and l even

$$f_{l0} = \sqrt{\pi(2l+1)} \int_0^\pi (sin\theta)^{2k+1} P_l(cos\theta)d\theta = \sqrt{\pi(2l+1)} \int_0^\pi sin\theta(1-cos^2\theta)^k P_l(cos\theta)d\theta$$

$$= \sqrt{\pi(2l+1)} \sum_{n=0}^k (-1)^n \binom{k}{n} \int_0^\pi sin\theta(cos^{2n}\theta) P_l(cos\theta)d\theta$$

$$= \sqrt{\pi(2l+1)} \sum_{n=0}^k (-1)^n \binom{k}{n} \frac{2(2n-l+2;1;l)}{(2n-l+3;2;l)}$$

and zero, otherwise.

A.2   Quality of the Approximation of $f(\theta)$

The Parseval condition (see p. 144 in [14]) states, that

$$F := \sum_{l=0}^\infty \sum_{m=-l}^l |f_{lm}|^2 = \int_0^{2\pi} \int_0^\pi |f(\theta,\phi)|^2 sin\theta d\phi d\theta \quad (13)$$

If F is finite, the residual error can be determined from this formula when $f(\theta,\phi)$ is approximated with the first t terms only. Plugging the analytical expression for f into equation (13) leads to the residual error

$$R := \int_0^{2\pi} \int_0^\pi (sin\theta)^{4k+1} d\phi d\theta - \sum_{l=0}^t |f_{l0}|^2 \quad (14)$$

In particular, for k=8 and t=4, we obtain F=2.720966695 and R=2.576686223, thus 94.7% of the energy is contained in the expansion using the first three *non-zero* coefficients.

A Novel Approach to Anatomical Structure Morphing for Intraoperative Visualization

Kumar Rajamani, Lutz Nolte, and Martin Styner

M.E. Müller Institute for Surgical Technology and Biomechanics, University of Bern, Switzerland,
kumar.rajamani@MEMcenter.unibe.ch,

Abstract. In computer assisted surgery 3D models are now routinely used to plan and navigate a surgery. These models enhance the surgeon's capability to decrease the invasiveness of surgical procedures and increase their accuracy and safety. Models obtained from specifically acquired CT scans have the disadvantage that they induce high radiation dose to the patient. In this paper we propose a novel method to construct a patient-specific model that provides an appropriate intra-operative 3D visualization without the need for a pre or intra-operative imaging. The 3D model is reconstructed by fitting a statistical deformable model to minimal sparse 3D data consisting of digitized landmarks and surface points that are obtained intra-operatively. The statistical model is constructed using Principal Component Analysis from training objects. Our morphing method then computes a Mahalanobis distance weighted least square fit of the model by solving a linear equation system. The refined morphing scheme has better convergence behaviour because of the additional parameter that relaxes the Mahalanobis distance term as additional points are incorporated. We present leave-one-out experiments with model generated from proximal femors and hippocampi.

1 Introduction

Three dimensional (3D) models of the patient are routinely used to provide image guidance and enhanced visualization to a surgeon to assist in navigation and planning. These models are usually extracted from 3D imagery like CT or MRI. To avoid the high radiation dose and costs associated with such scans, image free approaches have been researched extensively and are becoming popular especially in orthopedic surgery. In an image free approach, building a 3D model that is specific to the patient anatomy is quite challenging as only very sparse patient data is available.

For this purpose, statistical models of shape have been extensively researched. The basic idea in model building is to establish from a training set the pattern of legal variations of shape. The model is adapted to the patient anatomy using digitized landmarks and bone surface points obtained during surgery. The main problem here is to extrapolate this extremely sparse three-dimensional set of points to obtain a complete surface representation. The extrapolation or morphing procedure is done via a statistical principal component analysis (PCA) based

C. Barillot, D.R. Haynor, and P. Hellier (Eds.): MICCAI 2004, LNCS 3217, pp. 478–485, 2004.
© Springer-Verlag Berlin Heidelberg 2004

shape model. Fleute et al fit the morphed model surface to sparse intra-operative data via jointly optimizing morphing and pose [1]. Chan et al [5] optimize morphing and pose separately using an iterative closest point (ICP) method. In our prior work [6] we proposed to iteratively remove shape information coded by digitized points from the PCA model. The extrapolated surface is then computed as the most probable surface in the shape space given the data. Unlike earlier approaches, this approach was also able to include non-spatial data, such as patient height and weight. It is only applicable though for a small set of known points. In our earlier work [7] we presented a novel morphing scheme that computes a Mahalanobis distance weighted least square fit of the model by solving a linear equation system.

We propose a enhanced morphing scheme that has better convergence behaviour. This is achieved by having an additional parameter in the objective function that relaxes the Mahalanobis distance term as additional points are digitized. As more information in terms of additional digitized points is received we relax the constraint on the surface to remain close to the mean and allow it to deform so that the error between the predicted surface and the set of digitized points is minimized as far as possible. In this paper we demonstrate proof of principle of our method using a proximal femur model as well as hippocampus model and evaluate these models using leave-one-out experiments.

2   Method

2.1   Model Construction

The first step is to build a deformable model from a training database. The basic idea of building a statistical model based on PCA is to establish, from the training set, the pattern of legal variations in the shapes for a given class of images. Statistical PCA models were introduced by Cootes et al[2] based on point distribution model (PDM).

A key step in this model building involves establishing a dense correspondence between shape boundaries over a reasonably large set of training images. Our previous comparison study [4] of some of the popular correspondence establishing methods revealed that for modeling purposes the best of the correspondence method was Minimum Description Length (MDL) [3]. Correspondence was initialized with a semi-automatic landmark driven method and then optimized based on the MDL criterion.

We construct a deformable statistical shape model based on the corresponding point positions. Each member of the training population is described by individual vectors $\bar{x}_i$ containing all 3D point coordinates. The aim of building this model is to use several training datasets to compute the principal components of shape variation. PCA is used to describe the different modes of variations with a small number of parameters. For the computation of PCA, the mean vector $\bar{x}$ and the covariance matrix D are computed from the set of object vectors(1). The sorted eigenvalues λ_i and corresponding eigenvectors p_i of the covariance

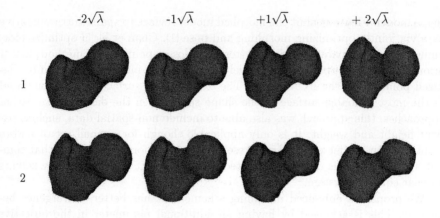

Fig. 1. The first two eigen modes of variation of our proximal femur model. The shape instances were generated by evaluating $\bar{x} + \omega\sqrt{\lambda_k}u_k$ with $\omega \in \{-2, .., 2\}$

matrix are the principal directions spanning a shape space with $\bar{x}$ representing its origin(2). Objects $\mathbf{x_i}$ in that shape space can be described as linear combination with weights $\mathbf{b_i}$ calculated by projecting the difference vectors $\mathbf{x_i} - \bar{\mathbf{x}}$ into the eigenspace(3).

$$D = \frac{1}{n-1}\sum_1^n (\mathbf{x_i} - \bar{\mathbf{x}}) \cdot (\mathbf{x_i} - \bar{\mathbf{x}})^T \qquad (1)$$

$$P = \{\mathbf{p_i}\}; \ D \cdot \mathbf{p_i} = \lambda_i \cdot \mathbf{p_i}; \qquad (2)$$

$$\mathbf{b_i} = D^T(\mathbf{x_i} - \bar{\mathbf{x}}); \ \mathbf{x_i} = \bar{\mathbf{x}} + P \cdot \mathbf{b_i} \qquad (3)$$

Figure 1 shows the variability captured by the first two modes of variation of our proximal femur model varied by ± 2 standard deviation.

2.2 Morphing

Anatomical structure Morphing is the process of recovering the patient specific 3D shape of the anatomy from the few available digitized landmarks and surface points. Our approach uses the statistical based shape model built earlier to infer the anatomical information in a robust way. This is achieved by minimizing the residual errors between the reconstructed model and the cloud of random points, and provides the best statistical shape that corresponds to the patient.

Earlier morphing methods were based on fitting procedures in Euclidean space and have the disadvantage that these are often computationally expensive and only a small set of shape variations can be considered. The morphed model also does not represent the most probable shape given the input data but rather a constrained fit. Our novel morphing method operates directly in the PCA shape space incorporating the full set of possible variations. The method consists of two steps

- Initially a small point-set of anatomical landmarks with known correspondence to the model is digitized. This is used to register the patient anatomy to the model. This also provides an initial estimation of the 3D shape with only a few digitized points.
- To improve the prediction additional points can be interactively incorporated via closest distance correspondence. A color coded feedback is given to the surgeon which shows regions where the prediction is accurate and regions where the prediction could be improved. This assists the surgeon in deciding the location where to digitize extra points.

The morphing computation is based on formulating the problem as a linear equation system and then solving for the shape parameters that best describe the unknown shape. An additional term in the objective function minimizes the Mahalanobis shape distance. The objective function that we minimize is defined as follows

$$
f = \rho * \left\{ \gamma * \sum_{\substack{k=1 \\ j=index_k}}^{N} \|Y_k - (X_j + \sum_{i=1}^{m} \alpha_i p_i(j))\|^2 \right\} + (1-\rho) \left\{ \sum_{i=1}^{m} \frac{\alpha_i^2}{\lambda_i} \right\} \quad (4)
$$

with N the number of points that are digitized, Y_k is the kth digitized point, X_j is the point in the mean model that is closest to Y_k, $p_i(j)$ is the j_{th} tuple of the i_{th} shape basis vector, λ_i the i_{th} eigen value and $\alpha_i's$ are the m shape parameters that describe the shape. The first term of the function minimizes the distance between the predicted shape and the set of digitized points. This is similar to the Euclidean distance term used by Fleute [1] . The second term controls the probability of the predicted shape. This term ensures that the predicted shape has minimal Mahalanobis shape distance. The factor γ is a parameter that weights the two terms of the function and ensures that a valid shape is predicted in the scenario when there are relatively few digitized points. A series of tests with varying values of gamma was carried out to determine the optimal value of gamma. The granularity of gamma was chosen using binary selection scheme where the region containing the current best value of gamma was further divided to find gamma to an acceptable level of accuracy. Our series of tests revealed that for our current application the best results with the least prediction mean and median errors were obtained when the value of gamma was fixed at one. Hence based on our tests the optimal value of γ was empirically fixed at one.

We modified the morphing scheme to one that is enhanced and has better convergence behaviour. This is achieved by having an additional parameter ρ in the objective function that relaxes the Mahalanobis distance term as additional points are digitized. As more information in terms of additional digitized points is received we relax the constraint on the surface to remain close to the mean and allow it to deform so that the error between the predicted surface and the set

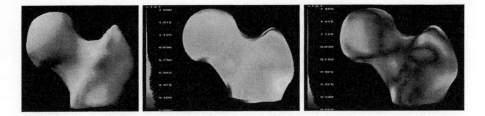

Fig. 2. Left: A typical proximal femur of the population that was used in the leave-one-out test. Middle: The average shape of the population with color coded distance map to the actual shape. The mean error is 3.37 mm and the median is 2.65 mm. Right:The shape based on only 6 digitized points with color coded distance map to the actual shape. The mean error is 1.50 mm and the median error is 1.25 mm

of digitized points is minimized as far as possible. As the error ideally decreases exponentially with the increase in the number of digitized points, we chose ρ to increase logarithmically, and was defined according to the following equation

$$\rho = \begin{cases} 0.5 & N \leq 6 \\ \frac{log\{\frac{N}{MaxN}(g*e-1)+1\}}{2*log(g*e)} + 0.5 & N > 6 \end{cases} \quad (5)$$

where N is the number of digitized points, MaxN is the total number of points g is a factor which determines the rate of growth of ρ. To achieve faster growth rate for ρ, g was empirically set to be the number of members in the population.

To determine the shape parameters α_i that best describe the unknown shape, the function f is differentiated with respect to the shape parameters and equated to zero. This results in a linear system of m unknowns, which is solved with standard linear equations system solvers using QR decomposition.

3   Results

In this paper we demonstrate proof of principle of our method using the proximal femur structure. 14 CT scans of the proximal femur were segmented and a sequence of correspondence establishing methods was employed to compute the optimal PCA model [4]. A series of leave-one-out experiments was carried out to evaluate the new method. Three anatomical landmarks, the femoral notch and the upper and the lower trochanter are used as the first set of digitized points. This is used to initially register the model to the patient anatomy. The remaining points are added uniformly across the spherical parameterization so that they occupy different locations on the bone surface.

Our studies with the two different correspondence methods, MDL and closest correspondence for incorporating additional points along with different error plots are discussed in [7]. Figure 2 shows a example of a very good estimate with mean error of 1.5mm obtained with as few as 6 digitized points using MDL

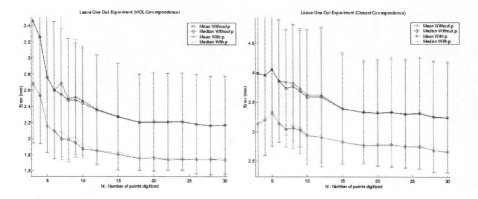

Fig. 3. Statistics cumulated from the different leave-one-out experiments of the proximal femur with and without the ρ factor. The average of the mean error and the average of the median is plotted against the number of digitized points Left: Shows the error plot obtained using MDL correspondence. Right: Shows the error plot using Closest Point Correspondence

correspondence. The color-coded 3D rendering is calculated using Hausdorff's Distance to measure the distance between discrete 3D surfaces[8].

Here we present results using our refined morphing scheme and also compare it to our initial version. Figure 3 shows the cumulative statistics of all leave-one-out experiments with and without ρ factor using the MDL and Closest point correspondence. In both the cases there seemed to be no significant improvement using the ρ factor, mainly due to low number of subjects in our proximal femur study population.

To evaluate the influence of the ρ factor we studied the enhanced morphing scheme in Hippocampus model generated from 172 hippocampus instances[9]. Here the larger population helps us to efficiently capture the shape variability and also helps us to evaluate better the influence of the ρ factor. Figure 4 shows the cumulative statistics from ten randomly chosen leave-one-out experiments with and without ρ factor using the MDL and Closest point correspondence for the Hippocampus population. Here we can clearly see the excellent influence of the ρ factor. The better convergence and the error factor We gain is about 10% in the MDL scenario and about 5% in the closest correspondence case.

4 Discussion

In this paper we have presented a refined novel anatomical structure morphing technique to predict the three dimensional model of a given anatomy using statistical shape models. Our scheme is novel in that it operates directly in the PCA shape space and incorporates the full set of possible variations. It is also fully interactive, as additional bone surface points can be incorporated in real-time. The computation time is mainly independent of the number of points

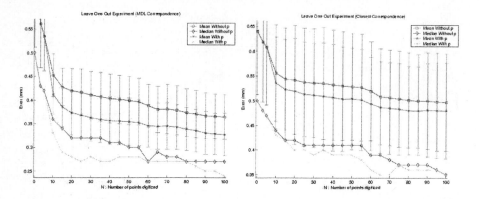

Fig. 4. Statistics cumulated from ten randomly chosen hippocampus leave-one-out experiments with and without the ρ factor. The average of the mean error and the average of the median is plotted against the number of digitized point. Left: Shows the error plot obtained using MDL correspondence. Right: Shows the error plot using Closest Point Correspondence

intra-operatively digitized, and largely depends on the number of members in the population. The enhancement of this scheme compared to our earlier approach is that we achieve smaller errors and better convergence as additional points are digitized.

The gamma parameter plays a vital role in balancing the predictive error term and the probability term. We empirically fixed its value to adapt to the case when small number of points are digitized. The ρ parameter helps us to relax the probability term to get a much better estimate as more points are digitized. The effect of the ρ parameter is not significantly noticed in the case when the population size is small. This is because the error gets stabilized and uniform after the first few points are digitized and there is not much information that could be extracted by adding additional points in this case. Hence the ρ factor seem not to contribute much as was observed in the proximal femur model with a population size of only 14 members. On the contrary in the hippocampus population the effect of the ρ parameter was significantly visible and it contributes in a significant way to decrease the error and achieve better convergence.

Another interesting observation that we can make is that the average mean error in the hippocampus population is far less compared to the proximal femur population. With 20 digitized points the average mean error in the proximal femoral population is about 2.25mm whereas in the hippocampus population it is only 0.37mm. The reason for this is because the hippocampus is a simple shape and we had a large population for the hippocampus model. Interestingly the error reduction that we achieve with 20 digitized points is about 35% for both the models.

There are a number of extensions that we plan to incorporate to this idea. We have a fully developed and validated technology at M.E. Müller Institute to extract bone contours from Ultrasound (US) images. First we plan to this use this large set of bone surface points from US images into the morphing scheme. Using this technique we can non-invasively get a large set of bone surface points intra-operatively. We also plan to incorporate fluoroscopic images into the process to extract surface points.

The concept of anatomical structure morphing has many interesting medical applications. The primary application that we focus is on hip surgery such as total hip replacement (THR) and knee surgery such as total knee arthroplasty (TKA) and anterior cruciate ligament surgery (ACL). Several current navigation systems for TKA/THR do not require preoperative CT or planning. By moving the joint, the center of motion is obtained. The hip, knee, and ankle motion centers give the functional axes of the femur and tibia. The surgeon is usually provided with a digital readout and a single display of the relative bone positions or angles. It is sometimes difficult for surgeons to intuitively understand such displays. The technique of anatomical structure morphing introduces novel navigation concepts wherein reconstructed 3D bony images are overlaid on top of 2D views of the axes. The proposed technology brings a variety of advantages to orthopaedic procedures, such as improved accuracy and safety, often reduced radiation exposure, and improved surgical reality through 3D visualization and image overlay techniques. In particular navigation based on anatomical structure morphing opens the door to larger minimally invasive approaches.

References

1. Fleute, M., Lavallee, S.: Building a Complete Surface Model from Sparse Data Using Statistical Shape Models, MICCAI (1998) 879-887
2. Cootes, T., Hill, A., Taylor, C.J., Haslam, J.: The Use of Active Shape Models for Locating Structures in Medical Images. Img. Vis. Comp. (1994) 355-366
3. Davies, Rh.H, Twining, C.J., Cootes, T.F., Waterton, J. C., Taylor, C.J.: A Minimum Description Length Approach to Statistical Shape Model. IEEE TMI (2002)
4. Styner, M.A., Kumar .T.R., Nolte L.P., Zsemlye G., Szekely, G., Taylor, C.J., Davies Rh.H.,: Evaluation of 3D Correspondence Methods for Model Building, IPMI (2003) 63-75
5. Chan, C.S., Edwards, P.J., Hawkes, D.J., : Integration of ultrasound-based registration with statistical shape models for computer-assisted orthopaedic surgery, SPIE, Medical Imaging (2003) 414-424
6. Kumar T.R., Nolte L.P., Styner M.A.,: Bone morphing with statistical shape models for enhanced visualization, SPIE Medical Imaging (2004)
7. Kumar T.R., Joshi, S.C., Styner M.A., : Bone model morphing for enhanced surgical visualization, IEEE International Symposium on Biomedical Imaging: From Nano to Macro ISBI (2004)
8. Aspert,N., Santa-Cruz, D., Ebrahimi, T.,: MESH:-Measuring Errors between Surfaces using Hausdorff Distance, IEEE ICME (2002) 705-708
9. Styner, M.A., Lieberman, J., Gerig, G. Boundary and Medial Shape Analysis of the Hippocampus in Schizophrenia, MICCAI (2003)

Enhancement of Visual Realism with BRDF for Patient Specific Bronchoscopy Simulation

Adrian J. Chung[1], Fani Deligianni[1], Pallav Shah[2], Athol Wells[2], and Guang-Zhong Yang[1]

[1] Department of Comupting, Imperial College, London
[2] Royal Brompton Hospital, London

Abstract. This paper presents a novel method for photorealistic rendering of the bronchial lumen by directly deriving matched shading and texture parameters from video bronchoscope images. 2D/3D registration is used to match video bronchoscope images with 3D CT scan of the same patient, such that patient specific modelling and simulation with improved visual realism can be achieved. With the proposed method, shading parameters are recovered by modelling the bidirectional reflectance distribution function (BRDF) of the visible surfaces by exploiting the restricted lighting configurations imposed by the bronchoscope. The derived BRDF is then used to predict the expected shading intensity such that a texture map independent of lighting conditions can be extracted. This allows the generation of new views not captured in the original bronchoscopy video, thus allowing free navigation of the acquired 3D model with enhanced photo-realism.

1 Background

With the maturity of minimal access surgery in recent years, there has been an increasing demand of patient specific simulation devices for both training and skills assessment. This is due to the fact that the complexity of the instrument controls, restricted vision and mobility, difficult hand-eye co-ordination, and the lack of tactile perception are major obstacles in performing minimal access surgeries. They require a high degree of manual dexterity from the operator. Computer simulation provides an attractive means of performing certain aspects of this training, particularly the hand eye co-ordination and instrument control. One significant challenge to computer based simulation is the creation of patient specific models combined with photo-realistic rendering so that basic as well as advanced surgical skills can be assessed with these simulation platforms.

For patient specific bronchoscope simulation, a number of techniques have been proposed for co-registering bronchoscope videos with 3D tomographic data such that camera pose in relation to the bronchial tree during video bronchoscope examination can be derived [1,2] With the use of image based modelling and rendering techniques, it is possible to extend conventional texture mapping to support the representation of 3D surface details and view motion parallax in addition to photorealism [3,4,5]. One of the major challenges of combining 2D

C. Barillot, D.R. Haynor, and P. Hellier (Eds.): MICCAI 2004, LNCS 3217, pp. 486–493, 2004.

video with 3D morphological data for patient specific simulation is the extraction of intrinsic surface texture and reflectance properties that is not dependent on specific viewing conditions. This allows the generation of new views with different camera and lighting configurations. For surgical simulation, this permits the incorporation of tissue instrument interaction, and thus greatly enhances the overall realism of the simulation environment. The purpose of this paper is to introduce a novel technique based on BRDF modelling for the recovery of intrinsic visual properties of the surface. An essential part of this process is the factoring of each video image into a surface shading function and texture map, as this enables new viewpoints to be visualised. With the effective use of 2D/3D registration, we demonstrate how the proposed method can be used to generate new renditions that are morphologically accurate and visually photo-realistic during free navigation of the 3D model.

2   Methods

2.1   Image Based Modelling of BRDF

One method for rendering a realistic visualisation of a surface is to solve the complete Rendering Equation[6]:

$$
\begin{aligned}
L_p(\theta_r, \phi_r) = &\ E_p(\theta_r, \phi_r) \\
&+ \int_{\theta_i \in [0, \frac{\pi}{2}]} \int_{\phi_i \in [0, 2\pi]} \rho_p(\theta_i, \phi_i, \theta_r, \phi_r) I_p(\theta_i, \phi_i) \cos(\theta_i) d\phi_i d\theta_i
\end{aligned} \quad (1)
$$

which states that the light exiting, L, from a point, p, in a direction given by spherical polar coordinates (θ_r, ϕ_r), depends on light emitted by that point, E_p, and light reflected, I_p, from all incoming directions (θ_i, ϕ_i) over the hemisphere. Light is not reflected equally from every direction however. It is weighted by a bidirectional reflectance distribution function, $\rho(\theta_i, \phi_i, \theta_r, \phi_r)$, whose properties are determined solely by the material being rendered. A variety of functions have been proposed for ρ that cater for specific classes of materials [7]. These models usually have several parameters to adjust in order to match the characteristics of the target material, and there is often no robust way to ensure accuracy of the values chosen. For some models [8] optimisation techniques can be used for parameter estimation provided the reflectance of the target material can be measured over a range of illumination directions and intensities. This approach requires a great degree of control over lighting conditions to ensure adequate coverage of the high-dimensional domain over which ρ is defined [9]. For this purpose, a special reflectance measurement apparatus can be specifically designed for the task [10]. By extending this strategy to entire images rather than point measurements of reflectance, one can measure not only a single BRDF but an entire set of BRDFs and map them as a texture map over the surface of an object of known geometry [11].

In situations where one has little control over the lighting environment, an approach based on global illumination modelling may be pursued. Given images

captured from a finite number of viewing positions, the outgoing light intensities
for several points in the environment are extracted and then by inverting the
Rendering Equation, the BRDFs are determined [12,13]. Normally a large number of images must be captured from a wide range of directions and viewpoints,
however there are techniques which rely on the uniformity of the materials so
that the number of input images can be significantly reduced [14]. In the case of
bronchoscopy, one has limited control over the lighting conditions and the choice
of viewpoints and viewing angle is restricted by the tubular structure of the airways. For this reason, a certain degree of uniformity of the reflectance in the
bronchial lumen is assumed in subsequent sections. The overall steps involved
in the proposed technique are illustrated in Figure 1 where 2D/3D registration
[2] was applied to the 2D video and 3D CT data sets after radial distortion correction of the video camera[15]. Illumination parameters are extracted through
BRDF and attenuation estimation, which is then used to recover the global texture map. The extracted surface texture and surface illumination characteristics
allow the generation of new views of the 3D model by using the 3D mesh derived
from the 3D CT images.

For this study, patients to undergo bronchoscope examination were scanned
with a Siemens Somaton Volume Zoom 4-Channel Multidetector CT with a
slice thickness of 3 mm and in-plane resolution of 1 mm. The bronchial tree was
segmented from the other anatomy using region growing [16] and morphological
operators. Subsequently, the airway surface was reconstructed as a polygonal
mesh by using the marching cubes algorithm. This mesh was then registered
with the image frames captured from the video output of the bronchoscope
and the end result was a pairing of video frames with camera poses within the
bronchial airway from which each video image had been taken.

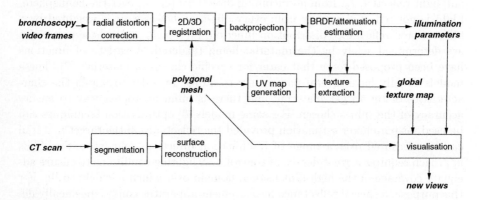

Fig. 1. The CT data and bronchoscopy video must pass through several stages of
processing to create realistic patient specific visualisations from novel view points.

2.2   Simplified Bidirectional Reflectance Distribution Function

In general, modelling the BRDF of any real world material requires the representation of a function over a parameter space of at least four dimensions, $(\theta_i, \phi_i, \theta_r, \phi_r)$. Fortunately the specific lighting configuration imposed by the bronchoscopy examination allows a number of simplifications to be made to the BRDF and the global illumination model.

- There is only one light source and it always coincides with the viewpoint. That is, $\theta_i = \theta_o$ and $\phi_i = \phi_o$.
- The inner airway surface is assumed to be isotropic. Thus, the BRDF is independent of ϕ_i and hence can be modelled as a function of θ_i only.
- The intensity of light incident on a surface depends mainly on distance from light source and the width of the airway.

By taking the above into consideration, the illumination conditions within the airway were modelled by using a cubic curve parameterised on the normalised scalar product of viewing vector $\boldsymbol{V}$ and surface normal $\boldsymbol{N}$.

$$\rho_p(\boldsymbol{V}, \boldsymbol{N}) = \sum_0^3 c_i B_i^3(\gamma) \text{ where } \gamma = \frac{\boldsymbol{V} \cdot \boldsymbol{N}}{|\boldsymbol{V}||\boldsymbol{N}|} \,, \ B_i^n(t) = \frac{n!}{i!(n-i)!}(1-t)^{n-i}t^i \quad (2)$$

Variations in shade cannot all be accounted for by BRDF effects alone, as intensity also depends on distance from light source. This depth dependent variation observed from viewpoint, **p**, was also modelled using a cubic curve:

$$\varrho_p(z) = B_0^3(r) + \sum_1^3 d_i B_i^3(r) \quad (3)$$

where $r = (z - z_{min})/(z_{max} - z_{min})$ and z is the distance of the surface point from the viewpoint. The linear shift of the parameter, z, was needed to avoid errors due to extrapolation. The shade of a surface point observed from viewpoint, **p**, is thus:

$$\Psi_p(\boldsymbol{V}, \boldsymbol{N}, z) = \rho_p(\boldsymbol{V}, \boldsymbol{N})\varrho_p(z) \quad (4)$$

2.3   Back Projection and Parameter Estimation

For each **p** there is a unique set of parameters, $(c_0, c_1, c_2, c_3, d_1, d_2, d_3)$, that determine the intensity of every visible point in the 3D model. These parameters were estimated by backprojecting each registered video image onto the 3D geometry and then fitting Ψ to the pixel intensities. Using the position of the bronchoscope that was determined through 2D/3D registration[1], each pixel in the video image was backprojected onto the 3D geometry to estimate the surface normal and distance from viewpoint. The following cost function is then minimised over all pixels:

$$C_p = \sum_i w_i(\Psi_p(\boldsymbol{V}_i, \boldsymbol{N}_i, z_i) - P_i)^2 \quad (5)$$

where P_i is the pixel intensity. To ensure that Ψ fits the sample points adequately in areas of low sample point density a weighting factor, w_i, was included to compensate for the non-uniform distribution of samples. A histogram was applied to the (γ, z) domain and w_i was set to the inverse of the estimated sample density.

2.4   Texture Mapping and Generating New Views

The polygonal mesh reconstructed from the CT data was used to generate a texture atlas[17] on which a global texture map was constructed. The texture was extracted from each video frame by dividing the pixel intensities by $\Psi(\gamma_i, z_i)$. Multiple textures were combined into a single map using weighted averaging. Weights were initially chosen based on the intensities predicted by the Ψ function since low intensities often yielded unreliable texture values, however this yielded blurry textures. Instead, for each texture pixel the non-maximal weights were suppressed and the resulting weight map was smoothed in the texture domain. This yielded sharper textures while reducing discontinuities. To generate a new view from a view point, $\mathbf{p}_{new}$, the nearest point, $\mathbf{p}$, was found for which Ψ_p had previously been estimated. The 3D geometry was raycast from $\mathbf{p}_{new}$, and the surface normal and depth information were converted to intensities using Ψ_p. This was then multiplied by texture values at corresponding points in the global texture map.

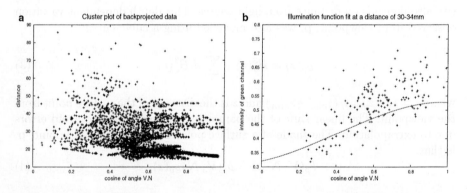

Fig. 2. (a) Cluster plot showing uneven distribution of backprojected samples. To ensure that Equation 4 fits the data over the entire domain and not just in regions of high density, each sample point was weighted inversely to point density. (b) The Ψ function is shown fitting to the data at depth 30-34 mm. The function must fit sample points at all depths.

3   Results and Discussion

To illustrate how Ψ fits the sample points in areas of low sample density through the use of w_i, Figure 2 shows the cluster plot of the backprojected samples and

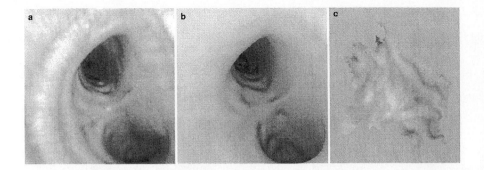

Fig. 3. (a) An original video frame has been corrected for radial distortion in preparation for 2D/3D registration and backprojection. (b) The backprojected intensity values were used to estimate parameters for the Ψ. This illumination model was then used to predict the expected intensities of each pixel in the red, green, and blue channels. A part of the final extracted texture map is shown in (c) after remapping to the domain of the 2D texture map.

an example 2D plot showing the Ψ function is fitted to the data at depth 30-34 mm.

Figure 3(a) shows a video frame to which Ψ has been fitted. The intensities predicted by Ψ were mapped to the geometry when viewed from the same viewpoint as the bronchoscope (b). This was subsequently factored out of the original video frame, resulting in a texture independent of shading variations due to BRDF and global illumination.

To demonstrate how the extracted texture, which is independent of shading variations due to BRDF and global illumination, can be used to generate new views of the 3D structure, Figure 3(c) shows rendering results by using the proposed technique. It is evident that the rendered results retain the photorealism required despite the significant change in viewing angles.

In summary, we have presented a new technique based on BRDF modelling for recovering intrinsic surface properties of the bronchial tree. The method factorises each 2D video bronchoscope image into a surface shading function and texture map so that new views can be rendered with photo-realistic appearance. The method presented here exploits the restricted lighting configurations imposed by the bronchoscope, which significantly simplifies the use of BRDF to predict expected shading intensity so that a texture map independent of lighting conditions can be extracted. The current method assumes the initial 2D/3D registration is accurate, but in reality this is difficult to guarantee particularly in the presence of airway deformation between pre-operative CT and bronchoscope examination. With the advent of miniaturised catheter electro-magnetic trackers, however, it is now possible to achieve relatively accurate camera-pose estimation with 5 degrees-of-freedom, thus significantly enhancing the accuracy of the registration process.

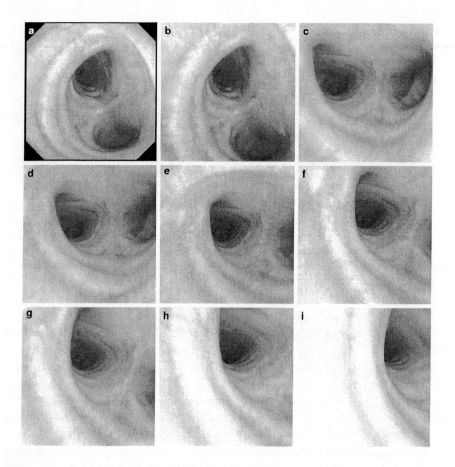

Fig. 4. (a)A typical frame captured from the video stream output of the bronchoscopy video processor is shown here. Radial distortion which must be corrected **b** prior to BRDF estimation. (**c-i**) New views of the bronchial lumen were generated using texture maps merged from the training video frames.

References

1. Mori, K., Deguchi, D., Sugiyama, J., Suenaga, Y., an d C. R. Maurer Jr., J.T., Takabatake, H., Natori, H.: Tracking of a bronchoscope using epipolar geometry analysis and intensity -based image registration of real and virtual endoscopic images. Medical Image Analysis **6** (2002) 321–336
2. Deligianni, F., Chung, A., Yang, G.Z.: pq-space 2d/3d registration for endoscope tracking. In: Conference on Medical Image Computing & Computer Assisted Intervention (MICCAI03). Volume 1. (2003) 311–318
3. McMillan, L.: An image-based approach to three-dimensional computer graphics. Technical Report TR97-013 (1997)
4. Chen, S.E., Williams, L.: View interpolation for image synthesis. In: SIGGraph 1993. (1993) 279–288

5. Debevec, P.E.: Pursuing reality with image-based modeling, rendering, and lighting. In: Second Workshop on 3D Structure from Multiple Images of Large-scale Environments and applications to Virtual and Augmented Reality (SMILE2), Dublin, Ireland. (2000)

6. Kajiya, J.T.: The rendering equation. In Evans, D.C., Athay, R.J., eds.: Computer Graphics (SIGGRAPH '86 Proceedings). Volume 20. (1986) 143–150

7. He, X.D., Torrance, K.E., Sillion, F.X., Greenberg, D.P.: A comprehensive physical model for light reflection. Computer Graphics **25** (1991) 175–186

8. Lafortune, E.P., Willems, Y.D.: Using the Modified Phong BRDF for Physically Based Rendering. Technical Report CW197, Department of Computer Science, Katholieke Universiteit Leuven, Leuven, Belgium (1994)

9. Ward, G.J.: Measuring and modeling anisotropic reflection. In Catmull, E.E., ed.: Computer Graphics (SIGGRAPH '92 Proceedings). Volume 26. (1992) 265–272

10. Dana, K.J., van Ginneken, B., Nayar, S.K., Koenderink, J.J.: Reflectance and texture of real-world surfaces. In: ACM Transactions on Graphics. Volume 18 (1). (1999) 1–34

11. Lensch, H.P.A., Kautz, J., Goesele, M., Heidrich, W., Seidel, H.P.: Image-based reconstruction of spatial appearance and geometric detail. ACM Transactions on Graphics **22** (2003) 234–257

12. Yu, Y., Debevec, P., Malik, J., Hawkins, T.: Inverse global illumination: Recovering reflectance models of real scenes from photographs. In Rockwood, A., ed.: Proceedings of the Conference on Computer Graphics (Siggraph99), N.Y., ACM Press (1999) 215–224

13. Loscos, C., Frasson, M.C., Drettakis, G., Walter, B., Grainer, X., Poulin, P.: Interactive virtual relighting and remodeling of real scenes. Available from www.imagis.imag.fr/Publications RT-0230, Institut National de Recherche en Informatique en Automatique (INRIA), Grenoble, France (1999)

14. Boivin, S., Gagalowicz, A.: Image-based rendering of diffuse, specular and glossy surfaces from a single image. In Fiume, E., ed.: SIGGRAPH 2001, Computer Graphics Proceedings. Annual Conference Series, ACM Press / ACM SIGGRAPH (2001) 107–116

15. Zhang, Z.: A flexible new technique for camera calibration. IEEE Transactions on Pattern Analysis and Machine Intelligence **22** (2000) 1330–1334

16. Schlathölter, T., Lorenz, C., Carlsen, I.C., Renisch, S., Deschamps, T.: Simultaneous segmentation and tree reconstruction of the airways for virtual bronchoscopy. In: Proceedings of SPIE, Medical Imaging 2002: Image Processing. Volume 4684. (2002) 103–113

17. Lévy, B., Petitjean, S., Ray, N., Maillot, J.: Least squares conformal maps for automatic texture atlas generation. In Spencer, S., ed.: Proceedings of the 29th Conference on Computer Graphics and Interactive Techniques (SIGGRAPH-02). Volume 21, 3 of ACM Transactions on Graphics., New York, ACM Press (2002) 362–371

Stereo-Based Endoscopic Tracking of Cardiac Surface Deformation

William W. Lau[1], Nicholas A. Ramey[1], Jason J. Corso[2], Nitish V. Thakor[1], and Gregory D. Hager[2]

[1] Department of Biomedical Engineering, Johns Hopkins School of Medicine, Baltimore, Maryland, USA
{wlau, nramey, nthakor}@bme.jhu.edu
[2] Computational Interaction and Robotics Laboratory, Johns Hopkins University, Baltimore, Maryland, USA
{jcorso, hager}@cs.jhu.edu

Abstract. We propose an image-based motion tracking algorithm that can be used with stereo endoscopic and microscope systems. The tracking problem is considered to be a time-varying optimization of a parametric function describing the disparity map. This algorithm could be used as part of a virtual stabilization system that can be employed to compensate residual motion of the heart during robot-assisted off-pump coronary artery bypass surgery (CABG). To test the appropriateness of our methods for this application, we processed an image sequence of a beating pig heart obtained by the stereo endoscope used in the da Vinci robotic surgery system. The tracking algorithm was able to detect the beating of the heart itself as well as the respiration of the lungs.

1   Introduction

Stereo imaging systems are commonly employed in today's operating rooms. However, these systems usually only provide basic stereoscopic images to the surgeon. Our goal is to process these images to produce a time-varying model of the surgical field. By computing such models, it will be possible to develop control methods that improve safety and provide guidance or enhanced dexterity to the surgeon. For example, one of the major revolutions in medicine is the introduction of cardiopulmonary bypass (CPB), which provides a motionless and bloodless surgical field optimal for anastomosis construction. Arrested heart on-pump surgery has been the gold standard for the last 50 years. However, a number of studies show that CPB is associated with high incidences of morbidity, including systemic inflammatory response and cerebral thromboembolism [1-3]. Driven by the idea of decreasing the trauma related to CPB, recent advancements in stabilization techniques have made coronary artery bypass grafting (CABG) on beating heart technically feasible. In essence, the stabilizer attaches to the beating heart by means of suction to locally immobilize the coronary artery to be bypassed while the rest of the heart beats and supplies blood to the body. Currently approximately one fourth of all CABG

C. Barillot, D.R. Haynor, and P. Hellier (Eds.): MICCAI 2004, LNCS 3217, pp. 494–501, 2004.

performed in the United States are done by beating-heart approaches [4]. With the aid of computer-assisted telemanipulation, totally endoscopic off-pump bypass surgery has also been successfully carried out by several groups [5-6].

Although sufficient stabilization can be achieved, improvement is desired to reduce prolonged operating time due to incomplete immobilization [7]. In robot-assisted surgery, this problem can potentially be addressed by a virtual stabilization system. A virtually arrested heart can be created by dynamic adjustments of the robotic arm to compensate the residual motion so that the orientation between the heart surface and the robot's end-effector remains constant. This leads to the problem of tracking the non-rigid motion of the heart surface in real time.

Traditional brute-force stereo matching techniques using local match measures are time consuming and often have limited accuracy. To provide accurate, real-time visualization of the surgical scene in 3D, we have developed a surface tracking algorithm that can recover a dense set of depth estimates of the objects in the field of view. The algorithm directly infers the 3D structure of the surface by locally adjusting an algebraic surface description. This makes the algorithm both numerically stable and computationally efficient. The ability to process the images online allows our algorithm to be used in a number of surgical applications, including establishing safety regions, developing virtual fixtures, and measuring mechanical properties of various tissues and organs. Our previous work has demonstrated the utility of the algorithm to track respiration with sub-pixel accuracy. In this paper, we focus on investigating its application to tracking the deformation of a beating heart.

2   Materials and Methods

2.1   Experimental Procedures

A cross-bred domestic pig (weight, 19.5 kg) was anesthetized with telazol-ketamine-xylazine (TKX, 4.4 mg T/kg, 2.2 mg K/kg, and 2.2 mg X/kg) and mechanically ventilated with a mixture of isoflurane (2%) and oxygen. Heart rate was continuously monitored by a pulse oximeter (SurgiVet, Waukesha, WI). The da Vinci tele-manipulation system (Intuitive Surgical, Sunnyville, CA) was used for endoscopic visualization. Three small incisions were made on the chest to facilitate the insertion of a zero-degree endoscope and other surgical tools. The pericardium was opened and video sequences of the beating heart from the left and right cameras were recorded at 30 frames/sec. The recording lasted approximately two minutes.

2.2   Surface Representation

B-spline representation is efficient in that the surface can be evaluated continuously at each pixel coordinate using a substantially smaller set of parameters than the size of the surface. Moreover, its spatial uniqueness, continuity, local shape controllability, and parameter linearity make it the best model to represent the surface for our problem.

Consider a collection of scanline locations α and row locations β, with m parameters per scanline and n parameters for row locations, a pth by qth degree tensor B-spline is a disparity function of the form

$$D(p; \alpha, \beta) = \sum_{i=0}^{m} \sum_{j=0}^{n} N_{i,p}(\alpha) N_{j,q}(\beta) p_{i,j} ,$$

(1)

where $\mathbf{p}$ is the set of control points for the B-spline surface. Furthermore, we can formulate B as a matrix of basic functions so that the disparity can be represented by the matrix product of B and $\mathbf{p}$:

$$D(p) = Bp .$$

(2)

Let k donate an indexing linear enumeration of the mn evaluated basis functions, and define $B_{i,k} = N_{k,p}(\alpha_i) * N_{k,q}(\beta_i)$. It follows that B can be defined as

$$B \equiv \begin{bmatrix} B_{1,1} & B_{1,2} & \cdots & B_{1,mn} \\ B_{2,1} & B_{2,2} & \cdots & B_{2,mn} \\ & & \vdots & \\ B_{N,1} & B_{N,2} & \cdots & B_{N,mn} \end{bmatrix} .$$

(3)

If we have the intrinsic and extrinsic parameters of the cameras, we can obtain the depth information in metric coordinates using

$$Z(p, u, v) = f \frac{T}{D(p, u, v)} ,$$

(4)

where u and v are image coordinates, f the common focal length, and T the baseline of the stereo system.

2.3   Stereo Matching

The algorithm has been discussed in detail in [8]. Briefly, stereo matching is computed through minimization of zero-mean sum of squared differences (ZSSD). Correct matching is dependent on the availability of texture on the surface. In addition to the global dc offset that results from differences between the optical characteristics of the two cameras, local dc offsets at parts of the images arise from the fact that the object is viewed from two slightly different angles. Regional illumination difference of the surface is therefore treated by subtracting the image by its convolution with a small Gaussian filter. As the algorithm iteratively updates disparity estimates, it requires some initial disparity estimates to start with. The initial estimates can be the disparity of a sampled point on the surface or they can be obtained by traditional stereo fitting with a complete correspondence search. The cameras are calibrated so that image pairs can be rectified to reduce the dimensionality of the problem.

Let $L(u,v,t)$ and $R(u,v,t)$ denote the left and right rectified image pair at time t, respectively. The disparity map can be considered as a lookup table consisting of a scalar offset for each pixel in the left image so that $L(u,v,t)$ and $R(u+D(u,v),v,t)$ are the projection of the same physical point in 3D space. Our objective is to estimate a set of parameters $\mathbf{p}$ that minimizes the ZSSD of the left and right warped images. Let $\overline{L}$ and $\overline{R}$ be the left and right zero-mean images, respectively, the optimization criterion can be written as

$$O(\mathbf{p}) = \sum_{(u_i,v_i)} (\overline{L}(u_i,v_i,t) - \overline{R}(u_i + D(\mathbf{p};u_i,v_i),v_i,t))^2 .$$
(5)

After some mathematical manipulations, the optimal $\Delta\mathbf{p}$ is the solution to the overdetermined linear system

$$\Delta\mathbf{p} = J(\mathbf{p},t)^t E(\mathbf{p},t) ,$$
(6)

where

$$E(\mathbf{p},t) \equiv \overline{L}(t) - \overline{R}(\mathbf{p},t) ,$$
(7)

and the Jacobian

$$J(\mathbf{p},t) = diag(\overline{L}_\chi(t)) \delta D / \delta \mathbf{p} .$$
(8)

It is obvious that $\delta D/\delta\mathbf{p}$ is equivalent to the N x mn matrix B in the previous section. Since B is a constant matrix and J does not change within an image frame, by using B-spline surface presentation, we avoid the problem of recomputing the Jacobian of the disparity function at runtime, thus speed up the processing significantly.

3   Results

The algorithm was implemented in matlab/mex. We processed the images on a desktop with a 3-Ghz P4 processor and one gigabyte of memory running Linux. A bi-quadratic B-spline surface with three control points in each direction was used. To initiate processing, we employed a standard stereo algorithm with a complete correspondence search.

The subject was ventilated at 15 breaths/min and the mean heart rate was found to be 104 beats/min. Examples of the 3D reconstruction of the heart surface are shown in figure 1. The coronary artery tree provided some natural landmarks for more accurate tracking. Figure 2a shows the motion of the heart surface measured at one pixel point for 12 seconds. The figure consists of two principal components. One component has a frequency of 60 x 3 / 12 = 15 cycles/min, and an amplitude of approximately 15 units of disparity. In figure 2b we subtract off the lower frequency component from the signal. The remaining component has a frequency of 21 x 60 / 12 = 105 cycles/min. The amplitude ranges from 6 to 8 units of disparity.

4   Discussion

Motion of the heart was contributed by the beating of the heart itself as well as the respiration of the lungs. The low-frequency, high-magnitude component represented the subject's respiration, and was consistent with the ventilator setting. The other component resembled the heart beats, and corresponded well to the oximeter measurement. Each heart beat consisted of three peaks. The dominant peak in the middle was caused by the contraction of the left ventricle. When the left ventricle started to relax, the left atrium contracted, which led to the smaller peak at the end of the cycle. We are not certain what the cause of the first peak was. In the future, we will include electrocardiography in our experiments. This will help us verify our data with higher confidence and identify the source of the first peak.

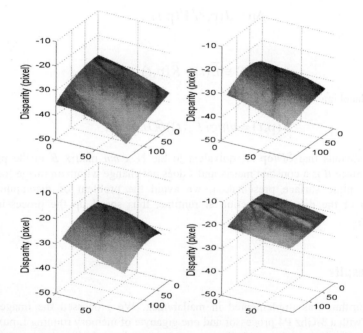

Fig. 1. 3D reconstructions of the heart surface at different phases of the heart beat cycle. The texture is mapped on a bi-quadratic B-spline surface with nine control points. The coronary artery tree serves as natural landmarks for the tracking system.

We measure the performance of the algorithm by its ability to correctly register the left and the right images. A relatively low-order B-spline surface was chosen to construct the disparity map because it sufficiently represented the smooth surface of the selected heart region. Since the region we were tracking was small (158x282 pixels), only nine control points were needed for optimal tracking. For each frame, the initial disparity was adopted from the disparity calculated in the previous frame. The system adjusted this disparity map to fit the current frame until the error or the change of error went below a certain predefined threshold, or the maximum number of iterations had been reached. We plot in figure 3a the percentage improvement of image ZSSD difference between the left and the warped right image for each frame on a representative sequence. The error improvement ranges from about 0% to as high as 70%. Small improvements, e.g. the frame at line 1 in figure 3, do not equate to low performance. The derivative of disparity in figure 3c is indicative of how fast the heart moves. If the movement of the heart is small between two consecutive frames, the initial disparity would be very close to the optimal disparity, thus minimal change is needed. Likewise, substantial improvements (line 2) are often due to the large movement of the heart. Figure 3b shows that the final error in each frame is comparable, falling within a narrow range.

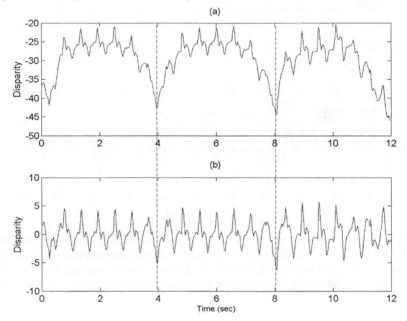

Fig. 2. (a) Shows the tracking of a pixel point on the heart surface. (b) shows the same tracking with the lower-frequency component filtered out.

Because the system essentially tracks the motion of the coronary artery tree, when the tree move away from the region of interest, the ability of the system to accurately track the surface reduces. This situation explains the larger errors in some image pairs. Nevertheless, since we do not explicitly track the motion of points on the surface, the system can be improved by projecting structured light onto the surface. Another practical issue is that during an actual bypass operation various tools will come into the scene and the heart will be occluded from the endoscope's view. Although the effect of occlusion on the stability of heart motion tracking is not assessed here, we have previously showed that the system can handle C^0 discontinuities well [8]. In addition, specular reflections can potentially cause instability to the system because of their inconsistency between the left and right images. Currently we do not account for the specularity in the images as it does not seem to significantly affect the results. In the future, we will incorporate a scheme to detect and mask out specular reflections from the tracking.

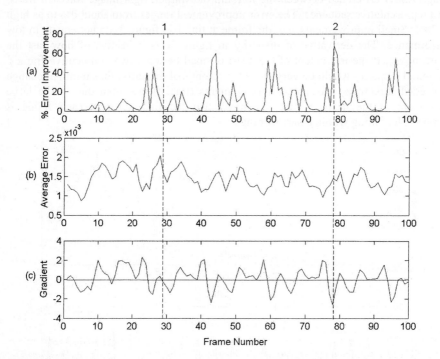

Fig. 3. (a) % Error improvement from the initial disparity to the final disparity in each image pair for 100 frames. (b) The mean image difference between the left and right warped images in the corresponding sequence. (c) Derivative of the heart motion indicates that large error improvements are partly due to considerable difference between the current and the previous frames.

5 Conclusion

The algorithm has demonstrated its ability to track the coherent motion of the heart. We pose the tracking problem as a time-varying optimization of a parametric disparity map describing the depth. The algorithm computes the surface geometry directly from image intensity data. It is robust, accurate, and the image processing can be done in real-time. When couple with the region tracking algorithms described in [9], the package can be used as a virtual stabilization system so that CABG can potentially be performed safely without the need of a heart-lung machine or a mechanical stabilizer. The main issue lies on the robot's ability to react accurately to relatively small motions at high frequencies. In the future, we will also explore the utility of this technique in other clinical areas, with one of them being the assessment of regional myocardial functions.

Acknowledgements. This work is based on work supported by the National Science Foundation under grant EEC-9731478. The authors are grateful to Dr. Randy Brown and his staff in the U.S. Minimally Invasive Surgical Training Center for their surgical assistance and to Dr. David Yuh of Cardiac Surgery for clinical advice.

References

1. Kirklin, J.K., Westaby, S., Blackstone, E.H., et al. Complement and the damaging effects of cardiopulmonary bypass. *J Thorac Cardiovasc Surg* 86:845–57, 1983.
2. Roach, G.W., Kanchuger, M., Mangano, C.M., et al. Adverse cerebral outcomes after coronary bypass surgery. *N Engl J Med* 335:1857-63, 1996.
3. Mack, M.J., Pfister, A., Bachand, D., et al. Comparison of coronary bypass surgery with and without cardiopulmonary bypass in patients with multivessel disease. *J Thorac Cardiovasc Surg* 127(1):167-73, 2004.
4. Mack, M.J. Advances in the treatment of coronary artery disease. *Ann Thorac Surg* 76(6):S2240-5, 2003.
5. Boyd, W.D., Rayman, R., Desai, N.D., et al. Closed-chest coronary artery bypass grafting on the beating heart with the use of a computer-enhanced surgical robotic system. *J Thorac Cardiovasc Surg* 120:807–9, 2000.
6. Mohr, F.W., Falk, V., Diegeler, A., et al. Computer-enhanced robotic cardiac surgery—experience in 148 patients. *J Thorac Cardiovasc Surg* 121:842-53, 2001.
7. Detter C., Deuse T., Christ F., et al. Comparison of two stabilizer concepts for off-pump coronary artery bypass grafting. *Ann Thorac Surg* 74:497-501, 2002.
8. Ramey, N.A., Corso, J.J., Lau, W.W., et al. Real time 3D surface tracking and its applications. Accepted to *Proceedings of Workshop on Real-time 3D Sensors and Their Use (at CVPR 2004)*, 2004.
9. Hager, G.D., and Belhumeur P.N. Efficient region tracking with parametric models of geometry and illumination. *IEEE Trans Pattern Analysis and Machine Intelligence* 20(10):1025-39, 1998.

Online Noninvasive Localization of Accessory Pathways in the EP Lab

Michael Seger[1]*, Gerald Fischer[1], Robert Modre[1], Bernhard Pfeifer[1],
Friedrich Hanser[1], Christoph Hintermüller[1], Florian Hintringer[2],
Franz Xaver Roithinger[2], Thomas Trieb[3], Michael Schocke[3], and
Bernhard Tilg[1]

[1] Institute for Biomedical Signal Processing and Imaging, University for Health
Sciences, Medical Informatics and Technology, Innsbruck, Austria,
[2] Department of Cardiology, Medical University Innsbruck, Austria
[3] Department of Radiology I, Medical University Innsbruck, Austria
michael.seger@umit.at,
http://imsb.umit.at

Abstract. Inverse electrocardiography has been developing during the
last years and is about to become a valuable clinical tool for analyzing
arrhythmias and electrical dysfunction in general. By combining measurements obtained by electrocardiographic body surface mapping with
three-dimensional anatomical data, the electrical activation sequence of
the individual human heart can be imaged noninvasively. This technique
was applied on-line in the electrophysiology lab. The results of four patients, who underwent an interventional electrophysiology study, are presented in this paper. The sites of early activation were compared to the
locations of successful radio-frequency ablation. The location error was
found to be between 13 and 20 mm. This promising finding may bring
this noninvasive method closer to clinical application.

1   Introduction

Atrial and ventricular arrhythmias are of great concern in clinical electrocardi-
ology [1,2]. In clinical practice, the localization of the origins of arrhythmias is
currently achieved by traditional catheter techniques and by catheter mapping
techniques [1,3]. These techniques show significant limitations when it comes
to acquiring single-beat activation maps. In addition, the invasive procedures
cannot be used for screening patients in order to decide the optimal individual
therapeutic procedure (e. g., drug, ablative or hybrid therapy). The simultaneous acquisition of three-dimensional (3D) anatomical and electrocardiographic
(ECG) data of individual patients enables noninvasive imaging of the electrical function in the human heart. Three-dimensional anatomical data from the
human thorax can be obtained, e. g., from magnetic resonance imaging (MRI).
ECG mapping data can be acquired from the patient's chest surface with multi-
channel (32 up to 256 channels) biopotential recording systems. The coupling of

---

* Corresponding author

C. Barillot, D.R. Haynor, and P. Hellier (Eds.): MICCAI 2004, LNCS 3217, pp. 502–509, 2004.

these two modalities in time and space permits the imaging of electrical function when applying bioelectromagnetical field theory and solving an *ill-posed inverse problem* [4,5,6,7]. The primary electrical source in the cardiac muscle is the spatio-temporal distribution of the *transmembrane potential* (TMP) φ_m [4,5,8, 9]. The potential on the chest surface and the potential on all other conductivity interfaces are related to φ_m by a *Fredholm integral equation* of second kind. The relationship between the impressed electrical sources and the potentials at the electrode sites on the torso surface is described by the *leadfield-matrix*, the solution of the *forward problem of electrocardiography* [4,10]. The boundary element method (BEM) – a surface integral equation approach – is, in general, applied to solve this forward problem [4,5,11]. In the *electrocardiographic inverse problem*, the impressed electrical source distribution is estimated from the chest surface ECG mapping data. This imaging technique requires an electrical source model. Because of the generally unknown individual fiber orientation, *electrical isotropy* is assumed in the surface heart model approach based on the *bidomain theory* [5, 6,7]. The most established inverse formulations are the imaging of the *activation time* (AT) map on the entire surface of the atria or ventricles and the imaging of the *epicardial potential pattern* [6,12]. With the AT imaging approach, the time of onset of depolarization at each source node is estimated, whereas the epicardial potential problem aims at estimating the (extracellular) potential on the pericardium. When used in a straightforward manner, the epicardial potential formulation does not allow the imaging of the potentials on the endocardia. The heart model approach employing the bidomain theory, however, is capable of imaging the electrical excitation on the entire atrial or ventricular surface, i. e., on the epicardia as well as on the endocardia. This is of particular interest from a clinical point of view, as most of the catheter interventions in the electrophysiology (EP) lab are performed on the endocardia. The difference of this work to previous studies is, that the noninvasive imaging of cardiac electrical function was performed *on-line* in the EP lab. In former publications, e. g., in [6,7,13], the computation of the AT was performed *off-line* and after the intervention. In order to demonstrate that noninvasive imaging of cardiac electrical function is feasible under clinical conditions, we applied the AT imaging approach *on-line* in the catheter laboratory: During the diagnostic part of the EP study using the electroanatomical mapping system CARTO^{TM} (Biosense Webster Inc.), the AT sequences were computed. The CARTO^{TM} maps were used as 'gold standard' for the resulting AT maps. In this study, the on-line imaging of ventricular preexcitation was investigated as an important example for clinical application.

2   Methods

Four patients[1] (patient A – D; age: 19 – 35 years, 2 female) suffering from Wolff-Parkinson-White (WPW) syndrome were included in the on-line study.

---

[1] Written informed consent was obtained from the patients before any diagnostic and therapeutic treatment. The study protocol was approved by the local ethics committee.

The time schedule for the on-line procedure was organized as follows: Previous to the intervention, the patients were moved to the MRI scanner. Afterwards, the volume conductor model consisting of the lungs, chest, blood masses and the ventricles was generated. In the EP lab, the electrodes were attached on the patients' chest, the locations of the electrodes were digitized and the body surface potentials (BSP) were recorded. Before intervention, the on-line AT map was computed for a couple of single beats. After the diagnostic part with the CARTO^{TM}system and after successful therapy, the computed AT was validated with the CARTO^{TM}solution.

2.1 Preprocessing

MRI scanning. An MRI scan of the patients was made previous to the intervention. Individual anatomical data were obtained from MRI using a Magnetom-Vision-Plus 1.5 T (Siemens Medical Solutions) scanner. The ventricular geometry was recorded in CINE-mode during breath-hold (expiration, short-axis scans, 6 mm spacing). The shape of the lungs and the torso were recorded in T1-FLASH-mode during breath-hold (expiration, long-axis scans, 10 mm spacing). Seven markers (vitamin E-capsules, anatomical landmarks on the anterior and lateral chest wall) were used to couple the locations of the electrodes to the MRI frame. Eleven capsules were attached on the back, in order to tag the positions of the posterior electrodes, which were not accessible during the EP study.

Generation of the Volume Conductor Model. The volume conductor model containing the relevant compartments (i. e., atria or ventricles, chest, lungs, blood masses) of the individual patient was generated using the software package amiraDev^{TM} 3.0 (TGS Europe Inc.) in combination with a semi-automatic myocardial extraction tool [14]. The lungs and chest could be segmented in a straightforward manner. A marching cubes algorithm was applied to the segmented compartments, which resulted in a triangulated surface mesh of the whole volume conductor model. The volume conductor model of patient D is depicted in Fig. 1.

2.2 Online Procedure

When the patient arrived in the EP lab, the posterior, lateral and anterior electrodes were attached on the patient's chest. The positions of the anterior and lateral electrodes were digitized using the Fastrak system (Polhemus Inc.). Additionally, the locations of the 7 anatomical landmarks were digitized in order to allow transformation into the MRI frame. The computation of the leadfield-matrix and of the ATs, respectively, was performed on an INTEL^R Xeon^{TM}dual processor (2.8 *GHz* with 2 *GB* memory for each processor).

Computation of the leadfield-matrix. After transformation of the electrode coordinates into the MRI frame, the leadfield-matrix was computed. The leadfield-matrix **L** with dimension e × s describes the relationship between the impressed electrical sources and the (extracellular) potentials **Φ** in e electrodes for all time steps T [4,10]:

$$\mathbf{\Phi} = \mathbf{L}\mathbf{\Phi}_m, \tag{1}$$

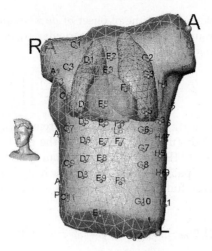

Fig. 1. Volume conductor model of patient D. The ventricles are shown in a transparent style, the blood masses and lungs are outlined. The electrodes are shown with their notation. The WCT defining the reference potential comprises the left arm (LA), right arm (RA) and left leg (LL). Note the head icon for spatial orientation.

with the $s \times T$ matrix $\mathbf{\Phi}_m$ containing the TMPs (electrical sources) in all s nodes of the cardiac surface. Note that $\mathbf{\Phi}_m$ is the time-discretized expression of φ_m. The computation of $\mathbf{L}$ was performed applying the BEM. The chosen conductivity values for the different compartments were chosen according to [4]: ventricles: effective intracellular conductivity: $0.1\ \mathrm{Sm}^{-1}$, bulk conductivity: $0.2\ \mathrm{Sm}^{-1}$; lungs: $0.08\ \mathrm{Sm}^{-1}$, blood masses: $0.6\ \mathrm{Sm}^{-1}$ and chest: $0.2\ \mathrm{Sm}^{-1}$.

Acquisition of the BSP Map. The ECG mapping data was recorded before, during and after the EP study. The BSP map was acquired in 62 channels by the Mark-8 system (Biosemi V.O.F.). The Wilson-Central-Terminal (WCT) defined the reference potential [15]. The sampling rate was 2048 Hz. Signals were bandpass filtered with a lower and upper edge frequency of 0.3 and 400 Hz, respectively. The AC-resolution of the system was 500 nVbit^{-1} (16 bits per channel).

Signal preprocessing. For estimating the AT pattern, the ECG signals representing the depolarization sequences (target ECG waves) were used as input for further computation. In case of imaging ventricular pre-excitation, the QRS complex represents the target wave. The QRS complex was detected manually. The extracted signals were baseline corrected and no additional filtering was applied. Time discretization was set 1 ms.

Estimation of the AT on the Heart Surface. The estimation of the ATs by considering (1) and (2) leads to an ill-posed, nonlinear (the TMP $\varphi_m(t)$ depends nonlinearly on the AT τ [6]), inverse problem. Because of the ill-posedness, *regularization techniques* have to be employed in order to guarantee a stable solution in the presence of modeling errors and measurement noise. As the AT imaging focuses on the estimation of the time of onset of *depolarization*, the time course of the TMP at each source point of the ventricular (or atrial) surface can be approximated employing the analytical formula [6]

$$\varphi_m(\tau, t) = \frac{u}{2}\left\{1 + \frac{2}{\pi}\arctan\left[\pi\frac{t - \tau}{w}\right]\right\} + a, \tag{2}$$

where a represents the resting transmembrane potential (a = − 90 mV), u the action potential amplitude (u = 100 mV) and w the rise time w = 2 ms. Equation (2) determines the TMP time course and can therefore be considered as *temporal regularization*. Spatial regularization is achieved by adding the surface Laplacian [16] in the cost function [6,7], which is to be optimized with respect to τ

$$\|\mathbf{L\Phi}_m - \mathbf{D}\|_F^2 + \lambda^2\|\Delta\tau\|^2 \longrightarrow \min. \tag{3}$$

The surface Laplacian Δ is introduced in (3) in order to avoid an unphysiological AT pattern by smoothing the solution of the AT map. The parameter λ determines the amount of regularization and is calculated employing the *L-curve method* [17], weighting the residual norm on the left hand side of (3) against the spatial regularization term. The e × T matrix **D** contains the measured ECG data in the electrodes and $\|\cdot\|_F$ represents the Frobenius norm. The interval [0, T] reflects the duration of depolarization of the underlying target ECG wave. A Quasi-Newton solver was used for minimizing the functional in (3).

Validation of the computed AT map. The computed AT map was compared with the standard ECG diagnosis approach and with the CARTO[TM] map, respectively. After the intervention had been finished, the position of the 7 anatomical markers were digitized with the ablation catheter, in order to transform the CARTO[TM] map and the catheter ablation points into the MRI frame.

3   Results

The following is given for patient C. Similar computation and handling times were observed for all other patients. The MRI scanning took 1 h 5 min, the segmentation of the volume conductor model was in the order of 1 h 15 min. Another 23 min were used for attaching the electrodes and for digitizing their locations. Within 11 min the leadfield-matrix was calculated and two ECG sequences were recorded. After 4 min of signal preprocessing (determination of the target waves, baseline correction), the AT map was available after additional 11 min. In case of patient C, the location of the accessory pathway due to inspection of the conventional ECG recordings was supposed to be posteroseptal. The achieved inverse solution, however, could clearly reveal the accessory pathway to be located in the left posterior wall. This was also confirmed by the CARTO[TM] map. For the other patients the AT map corresponded to the findings from the conventional ECG and the CARTO[TM] map. The accessory pathway in patient A was located in a postero-septal position, in patient B and D the site was found to be in a left-lateral position. Figure 2 shows the on-line computed

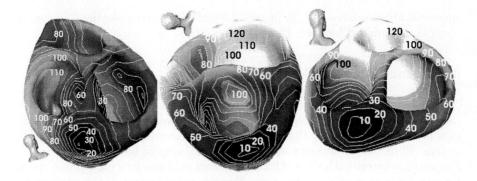

Fig. 2. Estimated electrical activation time sequences in patient A, B and C (left to right). Dark areas indicate early, white late activation. Isochrones are shown in steps of 10 ms.

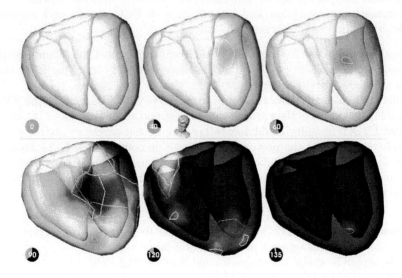

Fig. 3. Time series showing the spread of electrical activation in patient D. Dark areas indicate activated tissue, white areas tissue at resting potential. The isochrones show the site of the wavefronts. The accessory pathway was localized in a left-lateral position. The numbers in the small circles indicate the elapsed time in ms.

AT map of patients A, B and C. Figure 3 shows the time series of the calculated spread of electrical excitation in patient D.

After successful ablation of the accessory pathways, the 7 anatomical markers were digitized using the ablation catheter in the CARTO™ reference coordinate system. The transformation of the CARTO™ ablation points and anatomical markers into the MRI frame was done off-line. The location error between the successful ablation sites and the inversely found locations employing AT imaging could be determined between 13 and 20 mm.

4   Discussion and Conclusion

Noninvasive imaging of the electrical activation was performed with four patients. The overall calculation time for these maps was in the same order as the time necessary for mapping the basal area of the ventricles using the CARTO^{TM}-system. With the AT imaging approach, the AT map of both chambers can be computed, whereas with the CARTO^{TM} system only one or a part of one chamber can be imaged in the same time. Further enhancement of the noninvasive AT imaging approach can be achieved by:

- having anatomical imaging modalities (e. g., MRI) available in the EP lab,
- improving the techniques of semi-automatic segmentation of the electrical relevant compartments for generating the volume conductor model,
- automatic segmentation and classification of ECG signals and automatic determination of the target ECG waves.

Currently, the pipeline for segmenting the compartments of the volume conductor model and classification algorithms for detecting and classifying ECG target waves are under development.

This study clearly shows that on-line noninvasive AT imaging in the EP lab is feasible and supports the cardiologist with important information. In one case (patient C) AT imaging could locate the site of the accessory pathway more precisely compared to the presumed site based on conventional ECG data.

Further research will be about AT imaging for assessment of ablations in the right and left atrium of patients suffering from atrial flutter or fibrillation, as well as the imaging of atrial flutter circuits.

Acknowledgements. The authors would like to thank Sigrid Egger for her experienced technical support in the catheter laboratory.

This research study has been funded by the START Y144-N04 program granted by the Austrian Federal Ministry of Education, Science and Culture (bm:bwk) in collaboration with the Austrian Science Fund (FWF).

References

1. Lesh, M. D., Kalman, J. M., Olgin, J. E., Ellis, W. S.: The role of atrial anatomy in clinical atrial arrhythmias. J. Electrocardiol. **29** (1996) 101–113
2. Sippens-Groenewegen, A., Lesh, M. D., Roithinger, F. X., Ellis, W. S., Steiner, P. R., Saxon, L. A., Lee, R. J., Scheinman, M. M.: Body surface mapping of counterclockwise and clockwise typical atrial flutter: A comparative analysis with endocardial activation sequence mapping. J. Am Coll. Cardiol. **35** (2000) 1276–1287
3. Ben Haim, S. A., Osadchy, D., Schuster, I., Gepstein, L., Haya, G., Josephson, M. E.: Nonfluoroscopic, in vivo navigation and mapping technology. Nat. Med. **2** (1996) 1393–1395

4. Fischer, G., Tilg, B., Modre, R., Huiskamp, G. J., Fetzer, J., Rucker, W., Wach, P.: A bidomain model based BEM–FEM coupling formulation for anisotropic cardiac tissue. Ann. Biomed. Eng. **28** (2000) 1229–1243

5. Greensite, F.: The mathematical basis for imaging cardiac electrical function. Crit. Rev. Biomed. Eng. **22** (1994) 347–399

6. Modre, R., Tilg, B., Fischer, G., Wach, P.: Noninvasive Myocardial Activation Time Imaging: A Novel Inverse Algorithm Applied to Clinical ECG Mapping Data. IEEE Trans. Biomed. Eng. **49** (2002) 1153–1161

7. Tilg, B., Fischer, G., Modre, R., Hanser, F., Messnarz, B., Schocke, M., Kremser, C., Berger, T., Hintringer, F., Roithinger, F. X.: Model-Based Imaging of Cardiac Electrical Excitation in Humans. IEEE Trans. Med. Imaging **21** (2002) 1031–1039

8. Geselowitz, D. B., Miller, III W. T.: A bidomain model for anisotropic cardiac muscle. Ann. Biomed. Eng. **11** (1983) 191–206

9. Henriquez, C. S.: Simulating the electrical behavior of cardiac tissue using the bidomain model. Crit. Rev. Biomed. Eng. **21** (1993) 1–77

10. Mosher, J. C., Leahy, R. M., Lewis, P. S.: EEG and MEG: Forward solutions for inverse methods. IEEE Trans. Biomed. Eng. **46** (1999) 245–259

11. Huiskamp, G. J., van Oosterom, A.: The depolarization sequence of the human heart surface computed from measured body surface potentials. IEEE Trans. Biomed. Eng. **35** (1988) 1047–1058

12. Oster, H. S., Taccardi, B., Lux, R. L., Ershler, P. R., Rudy, Y.: Noninvasive electrocardiographic imaging: Reconstruction of epicardia potentials, electrograms and isochrones and localization of single and multiple electrocardiac events. Circ. **96** (1997) 1012–1024

13. Modre, R., Tilg, B., Fischer, G., Hanser, F., Messnarz, B., Seger, M., Schocke, M. F. H., Berger, T., Hintringer, F., Roithinger, F. X.: Atrial Noninvasive Activation Mapping of Paced Rhythm Data. J. Cardiovasc. Electrophysiol. **14** (2003) 712–719

14. Pfeifer, B., Hanser, F., Hintermüller, C., Modre, R., Fischer, G., Seger, M., Kremser, C., Tilg, B.: Atrial myocardium model extraction. Med. Imaging, Proceedings SPIE 2004 (2004) (in press)

15. Fischer, G., Tilg, B., Modre, R., Hanser, F., Messnarz, B., Wach, P.: On Modeling the Wilson terminal in the boundary and finite element method. IEEE Trans. Biomed. Eng. **49** (2002) 217–224

16. Huiskamp, G. J.: Difference formulas for the surface Laplacian on a triangulated surface. J. Comp. Phys. **95** (1991) 477–496

17. Hansen, P. C.: The L-curve and its use in the numerical treatment of inverse problems. In: Johnston, P. (Ed), Computational Inverse Problems in Electrocardiography, WIT Press, Southampton (2001) 119–142

Performance Evaluation of a Stereoscopic Based 3D Surface Localiser for Image-Guided Neurosurgery

Perrine Paul, Oliver Fleig, Sabine Tranchant, and Pierre Jannin

Laboratoire IDM, Faculté de Médecine, Université de Rennes, 35043 Rennes, France
{Perrine.Paul,Pierre.Jannin}@univ-rennes1.fr

Abstract. This paper reports the performance evaluation of a method for visualisation and quantification of intraoperative cortical surface deformations. This method consists in the acquisition of 3D surface meshes of the operative field directly in the neuronavigator's coordinate system by means of stereoscopic reconstructions, using two cameras attached to the microscope oculars. The locations of about 300 surfaces are compared to the locations of two reference surfaces from a physical phantom: a segmented CT scan with image-to-physical fiducial-based registration, used to compute the overall system performance, and a cloud of points acquired with the neuronavigator's optical localiser, used to compute the intrinsic error of our method. The intrinsic accuracy of our method was shown to be within 1mm.

1 Introduction

Limitations of image-guided neurosurgery systems mainly concern (1) intraoperative visualisation of preoperative data and (2) intraoperative anatomical deformations. Concerning visualisation, most neuronavigation systems offer display of preoperative images in microscope oculars as 2D monochromatic contours whereas preoperative images are 3D and multimodal. Augmented reality with 3D graphics has been proposed by [1] but only for displaying the 3D surface of the lesion. Extending this approach to multimodal images raises the issue of how to display images without obstructing the normal vision of the field of view (FOV). Intraoperative deformations, due to both brain shift and resection, need to be detected in order to update preoperative images. The proposals found in the literature tend to favour the use of surface or volume intraoperative imagery. To account for these limitations, we previously proposed to map preoperative images to direct light images of the intraoperative FOV [2] in the virtual world.We called this approach augmented virtuality. We then applied stereoscopic reconstruction techniques to this approach, in order to acquire intraoperative 3D surface data sets [3]. We call this system a 3D surface localiser. Our approach was initially limited to visualisation features. Our medium term objective is to use this method to quantify the cortical surface shift. Similar proposals, using images acquired by cameras fixed to the surgical microscope,

C. Barillot, D.R. Haynor, and P. Hellier (Eds.): MICCAI 2004, LNCS 3217, pp. 510–517, 2004.
© Springer-Verlag Berlin Heidelberg 2004

have been developed by [4] and [5]. In [6], a laser grid was projected onto the brain surface for surface deformation tracking purposes.

In this paper, we focus on evaluating the performance of our 3D surface localiser using a bone skull phantom. We first briefly summarise the principle of the 3D surface localiser. Two procedures of accuracy testing on a phantom are then described using a standardised framework [7]. The influence of certain input parameters is also evaluated. Lastly, the results obtained from 156 and 292 reconstructed surface meshes are provided and discussed.

2 Material and Methods

2.1 3D Surface Localiser

The method used has already been described in [3]. Briefly, we used a standard neuronavigation system with a pair of stereo cameras attached to the surgical microscope. Colour images were taken alternately from the left and right oculars. A strong calibration process, which was initialised with the results of Tsai's camera calibration, allowed rectification of image pairs and the use of epipolar geometry. Point mapping based on zero-mean normalised sum of squared differences (ZNSSD) of luminance and epipolar geometry provided a disparity map which was used to reconstruct a surface mesh [8]. Owing to microscope position tracking by the neuronavigator, the reconstructed surface mesh was directly expressed into the neuronavigator's coordinate system.

2.2 Performance Evaluation

The performance evaluation procedures were based on a comparison with two different reference surfaces. The first (see Figure 1), used by the FIDSCAN procedure, was the 3D surface segmented from a CT scan of a skull phantom registered to the neuronavigator's coordinate system by means of attached markers. The second reference surface (see Figure 1), used by the LOCCLOUD procedure, was a cloud of points acquired by the pointer of the optical localiser of the neuronavigation system, referred to as the pointer. Reconstructed surface meshes and reference surfaces are in the same coordinate system, that of the neuronavigator. The FIDSCAN procedure was used to study the overall performance of the 3D surface localiser including image-to-physical registration error. The LOCCLOUD procedure was used to measure the error due to the calibration and reconstruction method alone. A standardised framework, as proposed in [7], was applied to describe both procedures (see Table 1).

Validation data sets: For the two validation procedures, the same bone skull phantom (referred to as D_I in Table 1) was used.

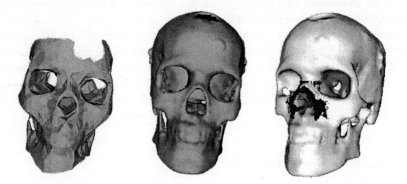

Fig. 1. Left, Reference 2, i.e., surface from the points cloud. Centre, Reference 1, i.e., surface of the CT scan. Right, a reconstructed surface mesh was superposed on Reference 1 (on the nose).

Table 1. Description of the two validation procedures

	FIDSCAN	LOCCLOUD
D_I: Validation data sets	Synthetic skull	Synthetic skull
P_I: Input parameters	FOV type, Light, Focus	FOV type, Light, Focus
F_M: Method to be evaluated	Surface localiser	Surface localiser
$\hat{S}_M$: Surfaces computed by F_M	292 meshes	156 meshes
F_R: Function which computes reference from D_I & P_I	CT scan with fiducial registration	Points cloud acquired with pointer
$\hat{S}_R$: Output data from F_R (i.e., reference)	CT scan volume in neuronavigator's coordinates system	2000 points in neuronavigator's coordinates system
$\hat{E}_R$: Estimated error relative to the computation of $\hat{S}_R$ by F_R	TRE	Pointer precision
F_{NSR}: Function which transforms $\hat{S}_R$ for comparison	Marching Cubes + inner surface removal	Delaunay triangulation
$\hat{S}_{NR}$: Normalised results for comparison	Outer surface of F_R	Front surface of D_I
F_C: Validation metric to compare $\hat{S}_M$ and $\hat{S}_{NR}$	ICP point-to-surface distance	ICP point-to-surface distance
O_C: Discrepancy between $\hat{S}_M$ and $\hat{S}_{NR}$ computed by F_C	i.median[a][b], i.max[a][b] i.stddev[a][b], S_R	i.median[a][b], i.max[a][b] i.stddev[a][b], S_R
O_{QI}:Quality index from O_C	Mean[a], stddev[a], max[a],min[a]	Mean[a], stddev[a], max[a],min[a]
F_H: Statistical tests	Wilcoxon test, ANOVA	Wilcoxon test, ANOVA

[a] in millimetres.
[b] i.* stands for results of ICP.

Input parameters: Influence of the following input parameters (referred to as P_I in Table 1) on method performance was studied:

- FOV type: mat, bright. The bright FOV is obtained by covering the skull phantom with gel.
- Light: weak, average, strong. The amount of light was measured using luminance histogram computed from the images.
- Focus of the microscope: minimal focus (f_{min}), maximal focus (f_{max}). These two focus values corresponded to the two extrema values of possible microscope focus settings.

Reference 1: For the first procedure, FIDSCAN, the skull phantom had a high resolution CT scan, with 8 fiducial markers attached. The positions of these markers were identified in the CT scan images and localised with the tracking system pointer in the neuronavigator's coordinate system. The rigid transformation computed between image and physical space was subsequently applied to the CT scan volume. To obtain an estimate of the registration quality, the *Target Registration Error* TRE [9] was computed over the surface of the skull phantom. The surface of the registered CT scan volume was then extracted using a *Marching Cubes* algorithm. Since the skull had thickness, the extracted surface was made up of an inner and an outer surface. To be comparable with reconstructed surface meshes, Reference 1 (referred to as $\hat{S}_{SNR}$ in Table 1) was defined as the outer surface of the skull phantom.

Reference 2: For the second procedure, LOCCLOUD, a cloud of $2,000$ points was acquired on the skull phantom surface with the pointer. This points cloud was directly expressed into the neuronavigator's coordinate system. Reference 2 was the cloud which was triangulated by the Delaunay method in order to be compared to the reconstructed surface meshes.

Reconstructed surface meshes used for validation: For each of the 12 combinations of P_I (2 FOV type levels $\times$ 3 Light levels $\times$ 2 Focus values), 25 image pairs were acquired, i.e., 25 surface meshes were intended to be reconstructed, with a size of 5×3 cm (obtained for f_{min}) and 8×6 cm (obtained for f_{max}). These 300 image pairs were acquired from different viewpoints, moving the microscope to cover all the facial part of the skull. In fact 8 surfaces (for f_{max}) were not reconstructed. For the FIDSCAN procedure, the 292 reconstructed surface meshes were studied while in LOCCLOUD only 156 meshes which had a covering rate of 100% with $\hat{S}_{NR}$ (see Table 1) were manually selected.

Validation metric: For the two FIDSCAN and LOCCLOUD procedures the validation metric was the distance in millimetres from each vertex of a mesh (more than 30,000 vertices per mesh) to the nearest $\hat{S}_{NR}$ surface point (see Table 1). This was achieved using the *Iterative Closest Point* (ICP) algorithm.

Discrepancy: For each reconstructed surface mesh, ICP was performed with Reference 1 or 2 as the target. As ICP results for one mesh, we kept the median (referred to as i.median), standard deviation (referred to as i.stddev) and maximal value (noted as i.max). We also defined the success ratio S_R as the percentage of points reconstructed at a correct location compared to the total number of points, expressed by $S_R = \frac{R_R * Q_R}{100}$ where: S_R stands for success ratio (as a percentage); R_R stands for the reconstruction ratio (as a percentage), i.e., the number of points which have been reconstructed compared to the total number of points (pixels) studied; Q_R stands for the quality ratio, i.e., the number of points of the reconstructed surface mesh being reconstructed under a threshold compared to the total number of points of the reconstruction. The threshold was determined as the worst i.median.

Quality indices: Quality indices were defined as follow for the three procedures: Precision of our 3D surface localiser is given by standard deviation and the maximal value of i.median, i.max and i.stddev. Accuracy is represented by the mean of the different values of i.median. Robustness is shown by the results obtained for the worst parameter combination and the success ratio S_R. Parameter influence is checked by a variance analysis of i.mean and R_R.

3   Results

Parameter influence. Only 292 surface meshes were reconstructed from 300 image pairs. This failure rate of 3% was only observed for the acquisitions with f_{max}. To study parameter influence, reconstructed surface meshes were grouped by combining parameters into 12 samples. The distribution of median values i.median is shown in Figure 2 for both FIDSCAN and LOCCLOUD procedures. Parameter influence was not related to the procedure. Analysis of variance (ANOVA) of the mean distance i.mean was performed on the samples grouped by focus. Residuals were Gaussian, and the p-value was within 10^{-16}. Consequently, the high impact of focus on accuracy was assumed. The same ANOVA was performed on the f_{min} samples to test the impact of FOV type and luminance level. These two parameters have no significant impact on accuracy (p-value> 0.5). The reconstruction ratio R_R was also studied: only the luminance level and FOV type have an impact on R_R.

Results of the FIDSCAN procedure. The values of i.median, computed for over 30,000 vertices for each of the 150 reconstructed surface meshes with f_{min}, have a mean of 1.88±0.65mm with a Q75 of 2.30mm and a maximal value of 5.4mm. The mean of i.RMS is 3.32 ± 1.20mm. The mean TRE was 4mm on the front part of the skull, where the image pairs were acquired. A Wilcoxon non-parametric test showed that the Q95 of i.RMS for all focus values can be considered as below the TRE. The success ratio S_R for all the focus had a mean of 62.15% with a threshold of 5mm. The minimum of S_R was 24.38%, however 219 out of 292 reconstructed surface meshes had a S_R higher than 55%. The best result of 84.15% was obtained for a bright FOV type and strong luminance.

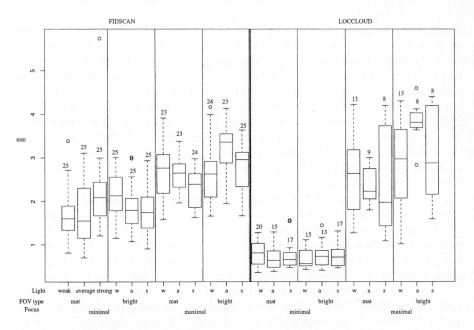

Fig. 2. Distribution of the median of the distance between reconstructed surface mesh and the reference surface for each sample corresponding to a parameters combination, for both procedures. The number of data in each sample is indicated by the number above its box-plot.

Results of the LOCCLOUD procedure. The mean of i.median for all 156 reconstructed surface meshes was 1.53 ± 1.20mm. The results from LOCCLOUD with f_{max} are not significant since there were too few 3D surface meshes per sample (see Figure 2). However, the results seem to show no difference between FIDSCAN and LOCCLOUD procedures with f_{max}, which might be explained by the limitations of the ICP validation metric. Considering the results for f_{min} alone, the mean of i.median was 0.74 ± 0.27mm with a maximal value of 1.56mm. A Wilcoxon test showed that the median can be expected to be within 1mm (p-value 10^{-11}).

4 Discussion

Performance shown by the FIDSCAN procedure included the registration error of the reference surface, estimated by TRE. Therefore, this performance corresponded to a global error, which has been shown to be quite similar to the system error without the 3D surface localiser. In order to check the influence of the image-to-physical registration error on overall 3D surface localiser performance, the FIDSCAN procedure was repeated on the 292 reconstructed surface meshes, by just changing the image-to-physical registration method. The CT scan volume was registered using both fiducials and a surface described by a 2,000 points cloud acquired with the localisation pointer. In [10], this type of registration using a combination of fiducials and surface has been shown to have an error lower than the fiducial-based registration. Our results were consistent since the global error was reduced: the mean value of the i.median for the 150 reconstructed surface meshes with f_{min} was 1.41 ± 0.65mm, in comparison with 1.88 ± 0.65mm, i.e., a performance improvement of 25%. The inherent error of our 3D surface localiser, which was estimated by the accuracy obtained using the LOCCLOUD procedure, was within 1mm. The success ratio S_R was more than 55% for all the reconstructed surface meshes, which demonstrates the robustness of our method. Besides, the similar distribution of samples grouped by focus has shown good repeatability. Precision was given by the standard deviation of results and was within 1mm.

Because of the method point mapping step, based on ZNSSD, the luminance was expected not to have impact. The impact of focus values on performance can be explained by computation of the disparity interval in our method. For the minimal focus value, the computed interval was $[-40, 40]$ whereas for a maximal focus value it was $[-45, 12]$. This aspect of our method leaves room for improvement. However, stereoscopic systems are known to be sensitive to distance.

The fact that local deformations are respected by our 3D surface localiser needs highlighting, given that in [5] the reconstructed 3D surface is fitted to a spherical model. Moreover, local zones which are too dark or have too high specularity do not interfere with the rest of the surface reconstruction, unlike [4]. Studying two performance evaluation procedures allowed to emphasise the different sources of error. Moreover, while in [5] accuracy has been studied with 5 points of one reconstructed surface mesh, our performance evaluation relates to more than 30,000 points for each of the 156 to 292 reconstructed surface meshes.

Some limitations in the performance evaluation require underlining. Firstly, a clinical evaluation would probably be worse than evaluation on a phantom. The 3D surface localiser was tested for 3 clinical cases, but only the reconstruction ratio R_R was computable, since there was no available reference surface. Results with skin, bone, or cortex images were similar to those computed on a phantom. In one clinical case, the reconstructed surface mesh of the skin was compared to the skin surface segmented from a preoperative MRI, and was rigidly registered to the physical space. The results obtained were a promising start: 3.25 ± 1.58mm with a Q75 of 6mm. The second limitation of the 3D surface localiser performance evaluation is that the ICP validation metric might over-evaluate performance, due to the fact that ICP does not give a symmetrical distance, and the homologous point in the reference surface of a reconstructed surface mesh point is supposed to be the nearest point from an Euclidean viewpoint.

5   Conclusion

To conclude, 3D surface localiser performance has been described and demonstrated using a rigorous procedure, which allowed differentiation between overall system error and the inherent error of the 3D surface localiser. This study is a first step towards validation. Indeed, we distinguish between validation and performance evaluation as follows: performance evaluation consists of computing quality indices whereas validation includes analysis of the evaluation results according to specific clinical contexts and objectives [7]. Since our aim is the visualisation and the quantification of the cortical surface deformations, some thresholds would require defining. Visualisation should consist of enhanced virtuality by merging data from the real world (i.e., textured reconstructed surface meshes) and the virtual world. Surface deformation quantification could be used to update the preoperative structures near the surface, or as a constraint for volume approaches (e.g., 3D Ultrasounds). Indeed, further deep structures are subject to deformations which are difficult to predict from surface deformations alone [11].

Acknowledgements. The authors would like to thank Dr. Xavier Morandi for the fruitful discussions about the clinical relevance of the system and for the preliminary clinical results.

References

1. Edwards PJ *et al*. Design and evaluation of a system for microscope-assisted guided interventions (MAGI). *IEEE Trans Med Imaging*, 19(11):1082–93, 2000.
2. Jannin P, Bouliou A, Journet E, and Scarabin JM. A ray-traced texture mapping for enhanced virtuality in image-guided neurosurgery. *Stud Health Technol Inform*, 29:553–63, 1996.
3. Fleig OJ, Devernay F, Scarabin JM, and Jannin P. Surface reconstruction of the surgical field from stereoscopic microscope views in neurosurgery. In *Proc. CARS'2001*, pages 259–64, 2001.
4. Skrinjar O, Tagare H, and Duncan J. Surface growing from stereo images. In *IEEE CVPR'00*, volume II, pages 571–76, 2000.
5. Sun H *et al*. Estimating cortical surface motion using stereopsis for brain deformation models. In *Proc. MICCAI'03*, pages 794–801. LNCS 2878.
6. Audette M, Siddiqi K, and Peters T. Level-set surface segmentation and fast cortical range image tracking for computing intrasurgical deformations. In *Proc. MICCAI'99*, pages 788–97. LNCS 1679.
7. Jannin P *et al*. Validation of medical image processing in image-guided therapy. *IEEE Trans Med Imaging*, 21(11):1445–49, 2002.
8. Devernay F and Faugeras O. From projective to euclidean reconstruction. In *IEEE CVPR'96*, pages 264–69, 1996.
9. Fitzpatrick JM, West JB, and Maurer CR. Predicting error in rigid-body, point-based registration. *IEEE Trans Med Imaging*, 17(5):694–702, 1998.
10. Maurer CR, Maciunas RJ, and Fitzpatrick JM. Registration of head CT images to physical space using a weighted combination of points and surfaces. *IEEE Trans Med Imaging*, 17(5):753–61, 1998.
11. Hartkens T *et al*. Measurement and analysis of brain deformation during neurosurgery. *IEEE Trans Med Imaging*, 22(1):88–92, 2003.

Bite-Block Relocation Error
in Image-Guided Otologic Surgery

J. Michael Fitzpatrick[1], Ramya Balachandran[1],
and Robert F. Labadie[2]

[1] Department of Electrical Engineering and Computer Science
Vanderbilt University, Nashville TN 37212
{j.michael.fitzpatrick, ramya.balachandran}@vanderbilt.edu

[2] Department of Otolaryngology-Head and Neck Surgery
Vanderbilt University Medical Center, Nashville TN 37232
robert.labadie@vanderbilt.edu

Abstract. Otologic surgery is undertaken to treat ailments of the ear including persistent infections, hearing loss, vertigo, and cancer. Typically performed on healthy patients in outpatient facilities, the application of image-guided surgery has been limited because accurate (<1mm), non-invasive fiducial systems for otologic surgery are not available. We have developed such a system, which repeatably attaches to a subject via a dental bite block [1]. In a previous report, ex-vivo validation indicated that mean target registration error ± standard deviation for 234 targets within the surgical field was 0.73±0.23mm with a root mean square of 0.77mm [2,3]. In an effort to further understand the limitations of our system, we undertook, and report herein, a detailed error analysis to determine what portion of the error is attributable to the inaccuracies in relocation fit of the fiducial frame to a subject's dentition. Our analysis shows that the root-mean-square error due to relocation alone is approximately 0.66 mm, while that due to fiducial registration is approximately 0.30 mm.

1 Introduction

Image-Guided Surgery (IGS) has found widespread use in neurosurgery where bone-implanted fiducial markers are used. Such invasive fiducial systems are tolerated by patients with life-threatening diseases such as malignant brain tumors. Ear surgery shares many of the characteristics of neurosurgery, *i.e.,* microscopic surgery performed in the region of the cranium, but differs in that the majority of cases are for non-malignant processes. As such, invasive fiducial marker systems are unacceptable. Non-invasive fiducial systems, such as those based on skin-affixed fiducial markers and laser contouring, have not met the requirement of submillimetric accuracy.

These seemingly paradoxical design criteria, high accuracy and non-invasiveness, can be overcome by means of fiducial frame systems that attach to the teeth [1]. In this paper we report on a fiducial system based on a dental bite-block with an attached rigid frame containing 14 fiducial markers whose configuration surrounds the surgical

C. Barillot, D.R. Haynor, and P. Hellier (Eds.): MICCAI 2004, LNCS 3217, pp. 518–525, 2004.
© Springer-Verlag Berlin Heidelberg 2004

field of interest, the ear. Previous studies have confirmed submillimetric accuracy [2,3]. Figure 1 shows the system attached to a human skull. Because the least reproducible component of our system is the coupling of the fiducial frame to the subject's dentition (Figure 1b), we set out to analyze its contribution to target registration error. The analysis is based on tests with three human skulls.

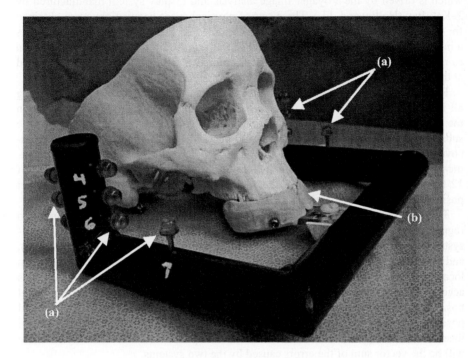

Fig. 1. Fiducial frame system. (a) Fiducials attached to frame. (b) Dental bite block by means of which the frame is attached to the upper dentition of a cadaveric skull.

2   Methods

The three skulls had their temporal bones removed and were retrofitted with an independent registration system, which we call the "target system", attached directly to bone within the region of the temporal bone, the bone encasing the left ear. The target system consisted of a disk with 12 markers placed in a centered cross-hair pattern in the vicinity of the surgical field. This system is named the "target system" because it is located in the vicinity of the surgical targets. Each skull was also affixed with the fiducial system coupled to the skull via a dental bite block [4]. Clinically applicable CT scans (slice thickness=0.5mm) were obtained, and the centroids of all markers (*i.e.*, both the fiducial-system markers and target-system markers) were identified using previously described algorithms [5]. Next, each skull was transported to the laboratory where the bite block was removed from the skull and reattached. The physical location of all markers were then determined using a 3-D localization systems based on a commercially available infrared tracking system, the active Polaris system, manufactured by Northern Digital, Inc. (Waterloo, Ontario, Canada) including a coordinate reference frame (not shown) attached to the fiducial frame and a tracked probe that is brought into contact with the markers (also not shown), all of which is driven by the Voyager image analysis and display system manufactured by Z-Kat, Inc. (Hollywood, FL). Three sets of physical space acquisitions were obtained for each skull. In each case the probe was oriented so as to keep its infrared emitters aimed at the Polaris. The skull with attached frame was re-oriented during localization as needed but with the attached coordinate reference frame kept continuously aimed at the Polaris.

Rigid registration between physical and radiographic space was performed using all 14 fiducial markers and also using nine subsets containing six of the 14 markers on the fiducial system such that the centroid of the six markers varied for each of the subsets. Registration was performed using singular-value decomposition of the cross-covariance matrix to minimize fiducial registration error (FRE), which is the root-mean-square distance between corresponding fiducials after registration [6]. A set of 12 target positions was chosen in the surgical field of the left ear. For each target position, target registration error (TRE) was measured experimentally.

The experimental measurement of TRE was accomplished by comparing two registrations: Registration 1, which is accomplished by aligning either all fiducial-system localizations or a subset of 6 localizations in the two spaces (CT and physical), and Registration 2, which is accomplished by matching the set of 12 target-system localizations in the two spaces. The comparison of the two registrations is accomplished by applying the two transformations in turn to each of the target positions in image space and measuring the disparity between their transformed positions in physical space. Each transformation will suffer error due to fiducial localization error (FLE). Since these errors are independent, the error that we measure will be the vector sum of the errors caused by the two systems.

In addition to the error caused by FLE, repositioning of the bite block relative to the teeth, and hence to the skull, will cause additional error. It is that error that we wish to assess. While it is not possible experimentally to separate the components of error, due to FLE and due to movement of the frame, it is possible to estimate the former error by means of theoretical considerations. The error due to frame movement also adds vectorially, and because it is unrelated to the error due to FLE, its error can be expected to be uncorrelated. As a result, we can expect that for each target position, the errors will add in quadrature, as stated in Eq. (1).

$$\left\langle \text{TRE}^2_{\text{total}} \right\rangle = \left\langle \text{TRE}^2_{\text{FLE}} \right\rangle + \left\langle \text{TRE}^2_{\text{frame}} \right\rangle, \tag{1}$$

where $\langle \cdot \rangle$ means expected value. We assess the frame repositioning error by estimating $\left\langle \text{TRE}^2_{\text{frame}} \right\rangle$. To do that, we employ the formulation given in [6] to calculate the theoretical value of $\langle TRE^2_{FLE} \rangle$. We then repeatedly measure $|TRE_{total}|$ experimentally and average to get an estimate of the left side of Eq. (1). Finally, we estimate $\langle TRE^2_{frame} \rangle$ by subtracting:

$$\langle TRE^2_{frame} \rangle = \overline{|TRE^2_{total}|} - \langle TRE^2_{FLE} \rangle, \tag{2}$$

where the horizontal bar means "average of experimentally measured values".

The calculation of $\langle TRE^2_{FLE} \rangle$ must take into account the errors arising from both Registration 1 and Registration 2. The difference between these two calculations arises from the difference between the configurations of the markers in the fiducial system and in the target system. Since there are no markers in common between these two systems, their target errors are independent. Thus,

$$\langle TRE^2_{FLE} \rangle = \langle TRE^2_1 \rangle + \langle TRE^2_2 \rangle, \tag{3}$$

where the subscripts 1 and 2 refer to Registrations 1 and 2, respectively. The calculation of each of the terms on the right is based on the equation [6,7],

$$\langle TRE^2(\mathbf{r}) \rangle = \frac{\langle FLE^2 \rangle}{N} \left(1 + \frac{1}{3} \sum_{k=1}^{3} \frac{d_k^2}{f_k^2} \right), \tag{4}$$

where $\mathbf{r}$ is the target position, $\langle FLE^2 \rangle$ is the expected value of fiducial localization error, N is the number of fiducials used in the registration (six for Registration 1 and twelve for Registration 2), d_k is the distance of $\mathbf{r}$ from the kth principal axis of the fiducial set, and f_k is the root-mean square distance of the fiducials themselves from their kth principal axis. The value of $\langle FLE^2 \rangle$ is estimated by using the relationship [6,7],

$$\langle FRE^2 \rangle = (1 - 2/N) \langle FLE^2 \rangle, \tag{5}$$

where N is the number of fiducials. For these experiments, Eq. (5) was applied to the fiducial system for each subset of markers (Registration 1) with N equal to 6 and to the target system with N equal 12 (Registration 2).

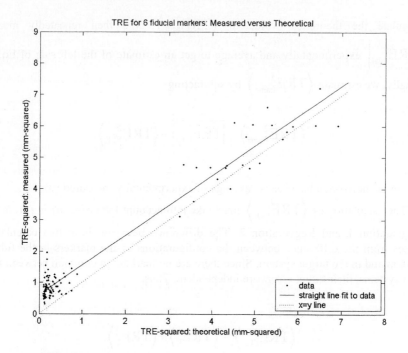

Fig. 2. TRE: Measured versus theoretical for combinations of 6 fiducials

3 Results

Figure 2 shows a plot of $\overline{\left|\text{TRE}^2_{\text{total}}\right|}$ versus $\left\langle\text{TRE}^2_{\text{FLE}}\right\rangle$. There are 108 plotted points, each point representing one of the 12 target positions and one of the nine subsets of markers from the fiducial system (in each case all 12 markers were used for the target system). The value of $\overline{\left|\text{TRE}^2_{\text{total}}\right|}$ was gotten in each case by averaging the squared values of TRE over three measurements on three skulls (9 independent measurements). The value of $\left\langle\text{TRE}^2_{\text{FLE}}\right\rangle$ was gotten in each case by averaging the values calculated from Eqs. (3) and (4) for the three skulls. The value of $\left\langle\text{FLE}^2\right\rangle$ used in Eq. (4) is calculated from Eq. (5).

The solid line is a least-squares regression line. Its slope is 0.95 and its intercept is 0.60 mm^2; $R^2 = 0.96$. The dotted line (slope = 1, intercept = 0) is the ideal, which would be expected if the only contribution to error were that arising from FLE (with no error arising from the relocation error of the bite block). The subsets of the markers of the fiducial system include two that were purposefully chosen to be substandard arrangements for the target positions.   These arrangements are substandard because in each case all 6 markers are located on the right side of the head, while the target positions are on the left side. As a result, the centroid of the marker configuration is far from the target positions. The 24 points at the upper right of the plot were produced by these two combinations. The remaining points, which are clustered at the lower left, were produced by arrangements that included at least one marker on each side of the skull.

The smaller errors of the points at the lower left of Figure 2, as compared with the others show that it is important to position markers used as fiducials for registration such that the centroid of their configuration is near the target region. This point has been emphasized before as has the importance of including a large number of markers [8]. For these reasons, the frame includes 14 markers with 7 positioned on each side of the head. Using all 14 fiducial markers, we observed for $\overline{\left|\mathrm{TRE}_{total}^2\right|}$ a value of 0.53 mm^2 over all three skulls, all three trials for each skull, and all 12 targets for each trial. Using Eqs. (3) and (4), we calculated for $\left\langle \mathrm{TRE}_{FLE}^2 \right\rangle$ a value of 0.09 mm^2 for all three skulls and all 12 targets. Using these two values in Eq. (2), we calculated $\left\langle \mathrm{TRE}_{frame}^2 \right\rangle$ to be 0.44 mm^2. Taking square roots, we find the root-mean-square values given in Table 1.

Table 1. Root-Mean-Square TRE Values

TRE_{total}	0.73 mm
TRE_{FLE}	0.30 mm
TRE_{frame}	0.66 mm

The root-mean-square FRE for all skulls and all trials was also calculated and found to be 0.69 mm; the root-mean-square FLE = 0.74 mm. Contributions to FLE error come from the localization of the markers in the CT images and from the error in physical localization. The latter error comprises two components that combine in quadrature, as described in [9]: the error in tracking the probe and the error in tracking the coordinate reference frame, which is situated at an average distance of 190mm from the targets.

4 Discussion

Other groups have also reported registration errors based on bite-blocks that mount to the patient's maxillary dentition [4,10,11], but none of them has employed theoretical calculations to determine the contribution to error caused by the error in the application of the bite block.

In order to employ the theoretical estimation of TRE_{FLE} in our analysis, it is important to justify its validity for this experiment by demonstrating agreement between measured TRE and theoretical TRE. Figure 2, which is a plot similar to that shown recently by West and Maurer [9], provides this demonstration by including both excellent and poor fiducial combinations so as to provide a wide range of TREs. The obvious correlation of the measured TRE with the theoretical TRE is a strong indication that the theoretical calculation is correct for this application. That correlation provides our justification for using the theoretical value in Eq. (2) to estimate the relocation error. The roughly constant vertical disparity between the least-squares fit line (solid) and the ideal line (dotted) is to be expected because of the relocation error of the dental bite-block. (It is in fact this error that is the major subject of the paper.) The square-root of the intercept of the solid line in Figure 2, which should be approximately equal to TRE_{frame}, is 0.77 mm, which indicates that the frame error may be slightly higher than the value given in Table 1.

5   Conclusion

These results demonstrate that for this system most of the target registration error is caused by error in the repositioning of the dental bite-block. However, the results also demonstrate that, thanks to the small size of this error and the considerably smaller size of the error due to fiducial localization, submillimetric target registration error is achievable with this system, when all fiducial markers are used. The clinical application of this system is currently being validated intraoperatively.

References

1.   Labadie RF, Fenlon M, Devikalp H, et al. Image-guided otologic surgery. Computer Assisted Radiology and Congress and Exhibition (eds: Lemke HU, Vannier MW, Inamura K, Farman AG, Doi K, Reiber JHC) pp. 627-32. Elsevier Science, Amsterdam, The Netherlands, 2003.
2.   Labadie RF, Shah RJ, Harris SS, et al. Image – Guided Otologic Surgery: Submillimeter Accuracy within the Temporal Bone, Oto-HNS (in submission).
3.   Labadie RF, Shah RJ, Harris SS, et al. Submillimetric Target-Registration Error using a Novel, Non-Invasive Fiducial System (the EarMark™) for Image Guided Otologic-Surgery, JCAS (in submission).
4.   Fenlon MR, Jusczyzck AS, Edwards PJ, and King AP. Locking acrylic resin dental stent for image guided surgery. J of Prosthet Dent;**83**:482-5, 2000.
5.   Wang MY, Maurer Jr. CR, Fitzpatrick JM, and Maciunas RJ. An automatic technique for finding and localizing externally attached markers in CT and MR volume images of the head. IEEE Trans Biomed Eng;**43**:627-37, 1996.
6.   Fitzpatrick JM, Hill DLG, and Maurer CR. Registration. *Medical Image Processing, Volume II of the Handbook of Medical Imaging*, M. Sonka and J. M. Fitzpatrick, ed., SPIE Press. 447-513, 2000.

7. Fitzpatrick JM, West JM, Maurer Jr. CR. Predicting error in rigid-body, point-based registration. IEEE Trans Med Imaging **17**, 694-702, 1998.
8. J. B. West*, J. M. Fitzpatrick, S. Toms, C. R. Maurer, Jr.*, R. J. Maciunas, ``Fiducial point placement and the accuracy of point-based, rigid-body registration'', *Neurosurgery* **48**, 810-817, 2001.
9. West JB and Maurer CR. Designing optically tracked instruments for image-guided surgery. IEEE Trans. Med. Imaging **23**: 533-545, 2004.
10. Bale RJ, Burtscher J, Eisner W, et al. Computer-assisted neurosurgery by using a noninvasive vacuum-affixed dental cast that acts as a reference base: another step toward a unified approach in the treatment of brain tumors. J Neurosurg, **93**: 208-13, 2000.
11. Meeks SL, Bova FJ, Wagner TH, et cl. Image localization for frameless stereotactic radiotherapy. Int J Radiat Oncol Biol Phys;**4**,6:1291-9, 2000.

Characterization of Internal Organ Motion Using Skin Marker Positions

Ali Khamene[1], Jan K. Warzelhan[1], Sebastian Vogt[1], Daniel Elgort[2],
Christophe Chefd'Hotel[1], Jeffrey L. Duerk[2], Jonathan Lewin[2],
Frank K. Wacker[2], and Frank Sauer[1]

[1] Imaging and Visualization Dept., Siemens Corporate Research,
755 College Road East, Princeton NJ 08540, USA
<first name>.<last name>@scr.siemens.com
[2] Radiology Department, Case Western Reserve University
11100 Euclid Ave., Cleveland OH 44106, USA
<first name>.<last name>@uhrad.edu

Abstract. Internal organ motion due to breathing is a phenomenon that nullifies the rigidity assumptions in many interventional applications, ranging from image guided needle biopsies to external beam radiation therapy. In this paper, we propose a method to correlate and characterize internal organ motion with the location of skin markers. The method utilizes a MR time sequence along with tracked magnetic marker positions to establish the correlation. We perform a validation study to quantify the degree of the accuracy and the reproducibility of this correlation. The results demonstrate that patient specific correlation of internal motion and skin markers can be established and the target positioning accuracy of better than 15% of the maximum range of the target movement can be achieved.

1 Introduction and Background

Interventional procedures have been performed to localize, biopsy, and treat cancers for several decades. These procedures are gaining increased popularity mainly due to reduced trauma and improved recovery time. In minimally invasive procedures, in contrast to open procedures, there is a dramatic reduction in the surgeon's visual ability. Radiological, ultrasonic, and magnetic resonance imaging (MRI) techniques are employed to map anatomical geometry in intraoperative procedures. Image guidance systems have been devised to provide visualization of both surgical tools and preoperative images with in the same coordinate system [4]. The problem arises in the scenarios, where the guidance system relies on preoperative images, assuming that the anatomical site has not deformed. The assumption is valid for certain anatomical sites (e.g., brain), where the procedures can be performed with high level of accuracy. However, many other organs, specially in thoracic and abdominal areas, are affected by respiratory and heart motion. Periodicity of the heart beat together with a reliable gating signal (i.e., ECG) provide means to address heart motion problem

C. Barillot, D.R. Haynor, and P. Hellier (Eds.): MICCAI 2004, LNCS 3217, pp. 526–533, 2004.
© Springer-Verlag Berlin Heidelberg 2004

[9]. On the other hand, respiratory motion is known to be rather subjective, posing a difficult targeting problem [12]. One approach is to utilize a real-time imaging modality during procedure updating the image guidance system with the most recent state of the anatomy (see e.g. [2], [4]). Real-time imaging modalities, such as ultrasound and x-ray, do not provide high quality images with soft tissue contrast. Therefore, the utilization of such imaging systems is limited to certain procedures. In [1], the authors address this problem by registering a real-time low quality intraoperative set of images with preoperative high quality MR images. The proposed registration problem is then solved using a priori knowledge of organ movement within the preoperative data sets taken at various stages of breathing using the breath-hold technique. There have been also studies where researcher try to model and/or characterize the respiratory motion using realtime imaging [3,7,9,10,11]. The target movement characterization has also been addressed in radiotherapy applications [8,13]. In this application, either the target motion is incorporated in 3D dose calculation and planning [8], or the radiation beam is gated using a sensor indicating the stage of breathing [8]. The effectiveness of the latter method depends on the degree of the dependency and reproducibility of breathing sensor signal to tumor location. Unfortunately, there is little information in the literature with regard to the correlation between internal anatomical and external skin marker movement.

In this paper, we propose a method to infer the internal organ motion (position) by observing the movement of a skin marker set. At first, we employ a realtime modality such as MRI in cine mode. In the pre-procedure phase, we acquire a set of images along with the position of a marker set attached on to the patient's skin surface. We analyze the markers and the target positions within the images for several breathing cycles. Once the sought after relationship is established, in the interventional stage, the skin markers are tracked and according to the position and the motion pattern the image guidance system is updated with the preoperative data, which best represent the current stage of breathing. Our goal is to 1) devise an appropriate technology for both marker and image based target tracking, 2) to design and implement an algorithm to correlate the external (artificial) and internal (natural) landmarks, 3) to evaluate the correlation of target movement and marker position, and 4) to perform patient/volunteer studies and validate the overall approach.

2   Material and Method

The goal is to predict the location of an anatomical target at the time of intervention without performing real-time imaging. It is assumed that the movement of the target lesion is only caused by the diaphragm motion due to breathing. A set of external markers, which are placed on the subject's thorax and can be tracked optically, provides information regarding the patient's respiratory stage during intervention. This requires a patient specific knowledge of the correlation between the skin markers and internal target movements, which has to be established prior to the intervention. The relationship depends on many individual parameters including skin marker position, internal target location, subject weight, height, and most importantly, specific breathing pattern. In the proposed approach, we characterize the relationship shortly before the procedure. During the interventional procedure, the patient specific correlation pattern is used to infer the location of the internal targets from the movement of the skin markers.

2.1   Pre-procedure Stage

In the pre-procedure mode, the goal is to characterize the relationship between the movement of skin markers and internal target. This process requires acquiring a set of images through multiple breathing cycles, in which the target point can be identified and its location be tracked. Furthermore, the locations of the skin markers associated with each image have also to be acquired. We employ a MRI system to acquire both the images and to track the location of magnetic markers. The magnetic markers are tuned coils attached to a plate, which is also instrumented with a set of optical markers. The marker plate is attached to the patient's skin. The optical markers are used to track the position of the magnetic markers once the patient is outside of the MR bore. In order to establish a common coordinate frame between the magnetic and optical markers on the plate, a calibration procedure has to be performed.

Concurrent Imaging and Marker Tracking. Time series are acquired using a MRI TRUE-FISP pulse sequence, which enables the reconstruction of a 25 cm^2 field of view in less than 200 ms. The magnetic markers are LC tuned coils, where their natural frequency is matched to that of the proton resonance of the scanner. One-dimensional projection signals of a fast radial MRI pulse sequence suppress virtually all signals in the imaging volume except that from the magnetic markers. The one-dimensional projections contain peaks, which correspond to each magnetic marker. The projections are acquired in between two consecutive image acquisitions. In [5], the authors describe a method to reconstruct the three-dimensional coordinates of the markers within the imaging volume using a set of one-dimensional peaks. In our application, three magnetic markers are attached to a plate with a fixed geometry. Therefore, there is a strong geometrical constraint regarding the relative positions of the markers. We have incorporated that into the reconstruction algorithm outlined in [5]. The new approach has a non-linear optimization step. The a priori knowledge regarding the geometry of three markers, enables us to formulate an energy functional based on position and orientation (i.e., six parameters) of the coordinate frame assumed to be representing the three magnetic markers.

Let us assume the positions of the three markers are $n_i \in \Re^3$ for $i \in [0, 2]$ within an arbitrary coordinate frame on the marker plate. The positions of the markers in the MR coordinate system can be acquired using the following equation: $m_i = R * n_i + t$, where $R \in \Re^{3\times3}$, $t \in \Re^3$ are the rotation matrix and the translation vector. This translation and rotation maps the local coordinate frame of markers to that of the MR scanner. Given the location of the magnetic markers $\mathbf{m}_i$ within the MR coordinate system, the operators $\mathcal{P}_\theta^{XZ}$, and $\mathcal{P}_\theta^{YZ}$ produce peak locations in a one dimensional projection at the angle θ. The position of these peaks $p_\theta^{XY}(i)$ and $p_\theta^{YZ}(i)$ are functions of six parameters of pose (i.e., rotation matrix $\mathbf{R}$ and translation vector $\mathbf{t}$), and have to coincide with the projection peaks (i.e., $\widetilde{p}_\theta^{XY}(i)$ and $\widetilde{p}_\theta^{YZ}(i)$) acquired through the radial pulse sequence applications. The optimization cost function, which has to be minimized, can be written as follows:

$$[\widetilde{\mathbf{R}}, \widetilde{\mathbf{t}}] = \arg \min_{[\mathbf{R}, \mathbf{t}]} \sum_i \sum_\theta \left\| [\widetilde{p}_\theta^{XY}(i) | \widetilde{p}_\theta^{YZ}(i)] - [p_\theta^{XY}(i) | p_\theta^{YZ}(i)] \right\|^2. \quad (1)$$

The optimization problem in equation (1) can be solved using the Levenberg-Marquart technique. The closed-form solution outlined in [5] is considered as the initial value for the optimization process. The advantage of re-formulation of the problem to form of equation (1) is: first, the geometrical constraints of the markers are inherently included, and second, the projections in two orthogonal scan planes XY and YZ are concurrently used in the reconstruction procedure. By addition of the non-linear optimization step, the accuracy and robustness of the marker tracking and labelling is increased.

Target Tracking in MR image sequence. The next step is to track the region of interest, containing the anatomical target, in a series of MR images. The goal is to build up the trajectory of the target for multiple breathing cycles. In our approach, the user specifies a bounding box around the target area in one of the images. We apply the Laplacian of Gaussian (LoG) operator on the image, first to smooth and decrease the artifacts due to the fast acquisition, and second to enhance the edges in the images and decreases the brightness and contrast variations. A normalized cross correlation technique is then used to extract the pixel movement of the desired region in each of the two consecutive images within a series.

Correlating Internal and External Motion Through PCA analysis. Principal Component Analysis (PCA) has proven to be very useful tool for dimensionality reduction of multivariate data with many application areas in image analysis and time series prediction [6]. The typical definition of PCA calls for a given set of vectors $\mathbf{a}_1, \cdots, \mathbf{a}_k$ in an n-dimensional space with zero mean, arranged as the columns of an $n \times k$ matrix A. The output set of principal vectors are an orthonormal set of vectors representing the eigenvectors of the sample covariance matrix $\mathbf{A}\mathbf{A}^\top$ associated with the $q \leq n$ largest eigenvalues. The matrix $\mathbf{U}\mathbf{U}^\top$ is a projection onto the principal components space with the property that: 1) the projection of the original sample is faithful in a least-square sense. i.e., $min \sum_{i=1}^k \left\| \mathbf{a}_i - \mathbf{U}\mathbf{U}^\top \mathbf{a}_i \right\|^2$, 2) the projection of the sample set onto the lower dimensional space maximally retains the variance, i.e., the first principal vector $\mathbf{u}_j$ maximizes $\sum_i |\mathbf{A}^\top \mathbf{u}_j|$ for $j \in [1, k]$. The representation of a sample point $\mathbf{a}_i$ in the lower dimensional feature space is defined by $\mathbf{x}_i = \mathbf{U}^\top \mathbf{a}_i$, 3) the covariance matrix $Q = \sum_i \mathbf{x}_i \mathbf{x}_i^\top$ of the reduced dimension representation is diagonal, i.e., PCA de-correlates the sample data, and 4) Euclidian distance in the feature space $\mathbf{x}_i$ provides an opportunity to quantify the proximity among the higher dimensional samples $\mathbf{a}_i$.

In our application, we analyze the correlation between skin marker positions and internal target motion using the PCA method. Let us assume that we are given the location of the three skin markers through time $\mathbf{p}_i^1$, $\mathbf{p}_i^2$, and $\mathbf{p}_i^3$ ($\mathbf{p}_i \in \Re^3$), and the corresponding internal marker position $\mathbf{q}_i \in \Re^3$) , where i represents discreet time ($i \leq n$). It is widely known that, because of the hysteresis phenomenon, the target paths through the inhalation and exhalation stages do not coincide[3,11]. Therefore, we incorporate the motion to the sample vector at each time instance i. For the skin markers, we construct the sample vector as follows:

$$\mathbf{a}_i = [\, \mathbf{p}_i^1 \; \mathbf{p}_i^2 \; \mathbf{p}_i^3 \; \Delta\mathbf{p}_i^1 \; \Delta\mathbf{p}_i^2 \; \Delta\mathbf{p}_i^3 \,] \tag{2}$$

where Δ is the consecutive position difference of the point. Based on the same principal , we build up the sample array for the target lesion as $\mathbf{b}_i = [\, \mathbf{q}_i \; \Delta\mathbf{q}_i \,]$. Principal component analysis is performed on the sample vectors with zero mean. Mean of the sample vector of the skin marker set $\bar{\mathbf{a}}$ can be used to recover the rigid patient movement and correct for the patient position.

Let us denote with $\mathbf{U}$ the matrix of principal components of the sample $\mathbf{a}_i - \bar{\mathbf{a}}$, and call the corresponding weights and/or features $\mathbf{w}_i$. The components of the target position and direction samples $\mathbf{b}_i - \bar{\mathbf{b}}$ are denoted by $\mathbf{Y}$, and the corresponding weights by $\mathbf{v}_i$. $\bar{\mathbf{b}}$ is the mean of the target sample vectors. Major modes of variations in both sample marker and target sample vectors can be identified by singling out high magnitude elements of the feature space. Furthermore, a meaningful metric distance can be used in the feature space because of the orthonormality of the feature space basis vectors. Let us consider $\widetilde{\mathbf{w}}_i$ and $\widetilde{\mathbf{v}}_i$ be the features, in which only the elements with larger magnitude is kept (s and r respectively). Our goal here is then to define a relationship between primary modes of the variation represented by $\widetilde{\mathbf{w}}_i$ and $\widetilde{\mathbf{v}}_i$. The function array $\mathcal{F}$ consists of functions $[f_1, f_2, \cdots, f_r]$, where its elements maps $\widetilde{\mathbf{w}}_i$ to an element in $\widetilde{\mathbf{v}}_i$. Domain of the functions are skin marker feature vectors, and the range is the target feature vectors. In order to specify these functions, we first parameterize them by a set of basis functions (e.g., b-splines), and second we recover the parameters, which result in functions minimizing the least-squares error for a set of corresponding features.

2.2   Intra-procedure Stage

At the intra-procedure stage, the patient is moved out of the scanner bore, where is accessible for the intervention. The issue at this time is to be able to update the image guidance system with the correct location of the target lesion, corresponding to the real-time respiratory state of the patient. As mentioned in section 2.1, the skin marker plate includes a set of optical markers, which can be tracked with an optical tracking system. The skin marker plate's magnetic and optical marker locations are known within a single coordinate frame.

Inferring Internal Organ Position. Through optical tracking of the skin markers, we first measure the position and the velocity of the magnetic markers $\widehat{\mathbf{a}}$. The measurement is then mapped into the feature space specified by orthonormal vectors in $\mathbf{U}$. Let us denote $\widehat{\mathbf{w}}$ as the feature vector of the mapped sample. The result of the function array $\mathcal{F}$ operation on $\widehat{\mathbf{w}}$ is the estimate of the target position in feature space $\widehat{\mathbf{v}}$. The final stage is to recover the actual value for the target position using the principal components and the feature vectors.

$$\widehat{\mathbf{b}} = \mathbf{Y}\mathcal{F}(\mathbf{U}^\top\widehat{\mathbf{a}}) + \bar{\mathbf{b}} \tag{3}$$

It is important to mention that in the outlined procedure, we are not assuming any periodicity for the breathing.

3   Experimental Results

We present results of the algorithm for multiple time series acquired from abdominal/thoracic area of two volunteers. The orientation of the MRI scan planes are selected in a way that the anatomical targets, in these cases the portal vein in the liver, moves within the plane. The resolution of the images is 128×128 with square pixels of size $1.9mm$. The slice thickness is chosen to be $10mm$. The scanning time is about $24sec$, providing about 100 images for each study. These studies contain about 12 to 20 breathing cycles. Along with the images, we acquired 1D projections required to track the positions of the three skin markers. Both the images and markers positions are time stamped, which provides a means to relate each marker set (interpolated) position to an image. We use the algorithm specified in section 2.1 to obtain the pose of the magnetic skin markers. The re-projection errors for the optimization are always below 0.6 pixels, which corresponds to $0.59mm$ of mean error. The procedure for the error evaluation of the algorithm is as follows. We first establish the principal feature vectors and the mapping function using all but one time samples. We then find the estimated target location using the established correlation for the sample that was left out. To establish error statistics, we permutate this operation for all the time samples in the data set. We quantify the target registration error (TRE) in terms of millimeters for all data sets. In all the data sets, we only recognize two modes of principal variation for the marker position. These two modes cover more than 98% of the total variation. Also for the target position more than 98% of the variation falls within the first two components of the feature vectors. Therefore, the function array $\mathcal{F}$ has two functions, to be determined based on the sample points.

In Figures 1(b) , a sample image with the overlaid bounding boxes around the structure is shown. Figure 1(a) shows the corresponding trajectory of the

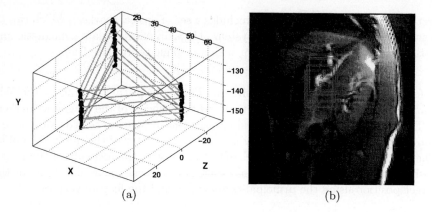

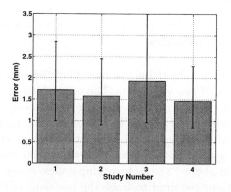

(a)   (b)

Fig. 1. (a) Trajectory of the skin marker set, and (b) MR images overlaid with the tracked target position.

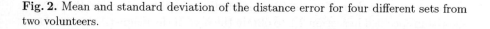

Fig. 2. Mean and standard deviation of the distance error for four different sets from two volunteers.

skin markers. Finally Figure 2, depicts the target registration error analysis for four studies performed on two volunteers, each tested twice. The mean distance error in all the studies is below $1.8mm$. The maximum total target movement in all these data sets was about $24mm$. Hence, for the given data set, the error in recovering the target motion with our proposed method is about 15%.

4   Summary and Conclusion

Understanding the correlation between the movement of skin marker set and internal targets is important for many interventional applications. Based on this correlation, an image guidance system can be used in procedures on anatomical targets affected by diaphragmatic motion. In this paper, we propose a technique to characterize this correlation. The method takes advantage of a preoperative

MRI image sequence, along with the location of tracked markers to establish this correlation. A PCA based method is used, first to identify the primary modes of variation and decrease the effects of outliers in the correlation, and second to establish a mapping function in feature domain, where a distance metric can be used. We present the results of the proposed algorithm using MR image series from two volunteers.

References

1. Blackall, J. M., King, A. P., Penney, G. P., Adam, A. and Hawkes, D. J., A Statistical Model of Respiratory Motion and Deformation of the Liver. In MICCAI 2001, Lecture Notes In Computer Science, vol. 2208, pp. 1338-1340, 2001.
2. Bzostek, A., Inoescu, G., Carrat, L., Barbe, C., Chavanon, O., Troccaz, J. Isolating Moving Anatomy in Ultrasound without Anatomical Knowledge: Application to Computer-Assisted Pericardical Punctures. In MICCAI 1998, Lecture Notes in Computer Science, vol. 1496, pp. 1041-1048, 1998.
3. Davies, S.C., Hill, A.L., Holmes, R.B., Halliwell, M., and Jackson, P.C., Ultrasound Quantitation of Respiratory Organ Motion in the Upper Abdomen. Br. J. Radiol., 67:1096-1102, 1994.
4. Desbat, L., Champleboux, G., et. al., 3D Interventional Imaging with 2D X-Ray Detectors, In MICCAI 1999, Lecture Notes in Computer Science, vol. 1679, pp. 973-980, 1999.
5. Flask, C., Elgort, D., Wong, E., Shankaranarayanan, A., Lewin, J., Wendt, M., and Duerk, J. L., A Method for Fast 3D Tracking Using Tuned Fiducial Markers and a Limited Projection Reconstruction FISP (LPR-FISP) Sequence, Journal of Magnetic Resonance Imaging, 14:617-627, 2001.
6. Jolliffe, I., T., *Principal Component Analysis*, Springer Verlag, New York, 1986.
7. Korin, H.W., Ehman, R.L., Riederer, S.J., Felmlee, J.P. and Grimm, R.C., Respiratory Kinematics of the Upper Abdominal Organs: A Quantitative Study. Magn. Reson. Med., 23:172-178, 1992.
8. Lujan, A.E., Larsen, E.W., Balter, J.M., and Ten Haken, R.K., A Method for Incorporating Organ Motion due to Breathing into 3D Dose Calculations. Med. Phys., 26(5):715-720, 1999.
9. McLeish, K., Hill, D.L.G., Atkinson, D., Blackall, J.M., and R. Razavi, A Study of the Motion and Deformation of the Heart due to Respiration. IEEE Trans. Med. Imaging, 21(9):1142-1150, 2002.
10. Rohling, T., Maurer, C.R., O'Dell, W.G., and Zhong, J., Modeling liver motion and deformation during the repiratory cycle using intensity-based free-form registration of gated MR images. In Medical Imaging 2001: Image Processing, 2001.
11. Suramo, I., Paivansalo, M. and Myllyla, V., Cranio-caudal Movements of the Liver, Pancreas and Kidneys in Respiration. Acta Radiologica Diagnosis, 25(2):129-131, 1984.
12. Sheafor, D.H., Paulson, E.K., Simmons, C.M., DeLong, D.M. and Nelson, R.C. Abdominal Percutaneous Interventional Procedures: Comparison of CT and US Guidance. Radiology, 207:705-710, 1998.
13. Tada, T., Minakuchi, K., et. al., Lung Cancer: Intermittent Irradiation Synchronized with Respiratory Motion - Results of a Pilot Study. Radiology , 207(3), 779-783, 1998.

Augmenting Intraoperative 3D Ultrasound with Preoperative Models for Navigation in Liver Surgery

Thomas Lange[1], Sebastian Eulenstein[1], Michael Hünerbein[1], Hans Lamecker[2], and Peter-Michael Schlag[1]

[1] Department of Surgery and Surgical Oncology
Charité - Universitary Medicine Berlin, Germany
lange_t@rrk.charite-buch.de
[2] Zuse Institute Berlin, Germany

Abstract. Organ deformation between preoperative image data and the patient in the OR is the main obstacle for using surgical navigation systems in liver surgery. Our approach is to provide accurate navigation via intraoperative 3D ultrasound. These ultrasound data are augmented with preoperative anatomical models and planning data as an important additional orientation aid for the surgeon. We present an overview of the whole ultrasound navigation system as well as an approach for fast intraoperative non-rigid registration of the preoperative models to the ultrasound volume. The registration method is based on the vessel center lines and consists of a combination of the Iterative Closest Point algorithm and multilevel B-Splines. Quantitative results for three different patients are presented.

1 Introduction

The resection of tumors from the liver is a demanding and risky surgical intervention. The exact intraoperative location of the tumor, its relative position to important liver vessels and the boundaries of vascular territories would be a benificial support for precise and safe liver surgery. This support can be provided by a 3D ultrasound-based navigation system, like the SonoWand-System [1] or our system [2]. Such systems show the position of surgical instruments in relation to an intraoperative ultrasound volume. The advantage of an ultrasound based system is that it is inexpensive and can be integrated easily into the OR. One of the limitations of intraoperative 3D ultrasound is image quality such that tumor and vessels are sometimes difficulty to delineate. Transmission of models of portal veins, hepatic veins, tumor and liver surface from preoperative CT/MR scans onto the ultrasound images can significantly improve differentiation of these structures. The relation of ultrasound planes to preoperative data or models would increase the orientation ability of the surgeon. In addition the transmission of a preoperative resection plan to the patient in the OR is possible. Several systems have been developed for liver surgery planning in the last couple of years [3,4,5]. But the precise implementation of the plan in the OR is still an

C. Barillot, D.R. Haynor, and P. Hellier (Eds.): MICCAI 2004, LNCS 3217, pp. 534–541, 2004.

open problem. In oncological liver surgery the aim is to completely resect one or several lesions with a security margin and to resect as little healthy parenchyma as possible. In most cases however also healthy parenchyma has to be resected if its blood supply and drainage would be disrupted by the surgery. The purpose of the planning systems is to compute anatomical resection proposals based on the vascular territories as shown in Fig. 1 a) and b).

For transmission of models and resection plans to the patient in the OR it is necessary to register preoperative and intraoperative image data. In contrast to neurosurgery or orthopedic surgery rigid registration via landmarks or surface-matching of bony structures is not possible due to significant organ deformations. Since fast and precise automatic algorithms for non-rigid intraoperative registration of 3D ultrasound data are still under development, for neurosurgery Lindseth et al. [6] suggested only to rigidly register preoperative data, trust on ultrasound navigation and use the preoperative data as an orientation aid. Applications in abdominal interventions which make use of preoperative image data to augment navigated intraoperative ultrasound scans include: laparoscopy [7, 8] for better orientation and thermal ablation of liver lesions [9,10] for precise placement of preplanned applicator positions.

Fast and robust intraoperative registration is the crucial task for augmenting the ultrasound data. Hence automated rigid and non-rigid registration methods, that have been applied or adapted to 3D ultrasound data, are reviewed in the following. Some image-based methods [11,12,10] have been reported to rigidly register 3D ultrasound and MR data. Non-rigid image-based algorithms for registration of two ultrasound volumes are described in [13,14]. These approaches are usually too time-consuming for intraoperative use. Liver vessels are features which can be easily identified in CT/MR and ultrasound data, in particular in Powerdoppler ultrasound. A feature-based rigid approach using correlation between segmented vessel voxels is reported in [15]. In [16] manually identified vessel center lines are rigidly registered via the Iterative Closest Point (ICP) algorithm. Hybrid approaches, which fit preoperatively extracted features directly to intraoperative image data, are promising. The lack of a time constraint in the preoperative phase allows for precise feature extraction yielding fast intraoperative registration. Aylward et al. [17] use vessel models and a special metric for rigid hybrid registration.

We follow the approach to use intraoperative 3D ultrasound for precise navigation and augment it with preoperative data and models. For fast intraoperative non-rigid registration we combine the ICP algorithm and multilevel B-Splines, as in [18]. In contrast to Xie et al. the correspondence determination is not based on surface similarity but on vessel center line points in both modalities.

2   Methods

Preoperatively liver parenchyma, portal veins, hepatic veins and the tumor are segmented from MR/CT data. Portal veins and hepatic veins are imaged in two different acquisitions, because their contrast maximum is reached at different times after contrast agent application. Parts of the portal veins are also imaged in the hepatic vein phase so that they can be registered with our vessel-based

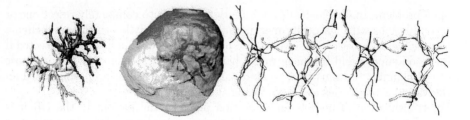

Fig. 1. (a) Portal veins devided into to be resected (light gray) and remaining vessels (dark gray) resulting from tumor location (white). (b) Resulting vascular territories of liver parenchyma. (c) Rigidly and (d) non-rigidly registered portal vein center lines from MR/CT (thin and dark) and 3D US (thick and bright).

non-rigid registration algorithm to get a joint representation of all vessels. Afterwards a resection proposal is automatically computed by our planning software based on the segmented structures. These preoperative models and the resection proposal are transfered to the ultrasound navigation system. In the following we give a short overview of our navigation system, a description of the non-rigid registration procedure and suitable intraoperative visualization methods.

2.1   US Navigation System

In contrast to freehand 3D ultrasound systems, where the volume is compounded from manually moved and tracked 2D ultrasound data, we use the 3D ultrasound device Voluson 730D from Kretztechnik/GE. This system is based on a 3D probe containing a 2D ultrasound transducer, which is mechanically swept by a motor. The advantage of this system is that it is fast and can easily be applied in the OR. Intraoperatively a 3D ultrasound scan consisting of simultaneous B-Mode and Powerdoppler (PD) acquisition is performed in a few seconds. The position of a passive tracker attached to the ultrasound probe is measured during the acquisition by a Polaris tracking system. The data are digitally transferred in high quality to the navigation system via a DICOM interface and not via the video output. Afterwards tracked surgical instruments can be navigated in relation to the 3D ultrasound data. For a more detailed description of the ultrasound navigation system see [2].

2.2   Registration Based on Vessel Center Lines

Before surgery the vessels are segmented from preoperative CT or MR by a region growing algorithm and manual post-processing to assure the segmentation of as many vessels as possible. Next the center lines of the vessels are automatically extracted by the TEASAR algorithm [19]. The intraoperative pre-processing starts with a reformatting of the 3D US data to Cartesian coordinates, because of the specific original imaging geometry. After this reformatting the center lines of the vessels are extracted from the PD US volume like they were extracted from the preoperative data. The first step of the registration procedure is a coarse rigid

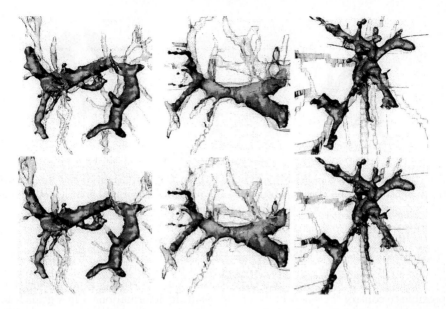

Fig. 2. Rigidly (upper row) and non-rigidly (lower row) registered vessel surfaces from MR/CT data (transparent) to 3D US (opaque) of three different patients (from left too right).

registration of the center lines via 3-4 manually selected paired landmarks near the main branching of the portal vein. The second step consists of an automatic ICP-like rigid registration. In the third step non-rigid transformations modeled by multilevel B-Splines are incorporated into the ICP-like registration.

In contrast to the standard ICP algorithm in each iteration corresponding vessel center line points of reference and model data are determined instead of corresponding points between surfaces. Because of the branching topology of vessels the nearest point of a model point to the reference center lines often does not correspond anatomically. Thus we search for the closest vessel segment with a similar direction. A vessel segment is to be defined as a part of the center line between two branching points. For each point M on the model those vessel segments S_i in the reference are sought for, which have a closest point C_i to M that is inside a given search radius R. All the potential corresponding segments S_i are sorted by increasing distance of M to C_i. Starting with S_1 the closest segment S_c is determined for which the angular difference of the vessel direction at M and C_i is below a given threshold. The direction at a vessel point is computed by the difference vector of the two neighbored points on the vessel. To increase robustness we averaged the directions of 5 neighboring points. If no corresponding segments can be found that fulfill maximal distance ($R = 10mm$) and maximal angle difference ($30°$) constraints no correspondence is introduced for this model point M.

If further improvements can be achieved by applying a rigid transformation in an ICP iteration step it is replaced by a B-Spline transformation. A B-Spline

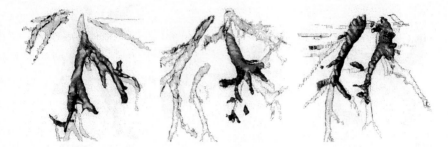

Fig. 3. Non-rigidly registered hepatic veins from CT/MR (transparent) to 3D US (opaque) of three different patients (from left to right). Deformation of hepatic veins is based on B-spline deformation determined by portal vein registration.

approximation of the displacement vectors between corresponding points can be determined directly and fast without need of an optimization algorithm. B-Splines are defined by a uniform control grid. Via the control grid spacing it is possible to control the smoothness of the resulting deformations. Finer grids lead to less smoother deformations. Computations of multilevel B-Splines starts with a coarse grid that is successively refined until a given minimal grid spacing is reached. We start the non-rigid ICP iterations with coarse multilevel B-Splines and refine them if no further improvements can be achieved. The minimal control grid spacing has been set to 15 mm.

2.3   Intraoperative Visualization

We implemented different intraoperative visualization techniques. For direct US navigation two ultrasound image planes, a top view and a perpendicular slice are shown. The planes can be dynamically chosen according to the position of the tip of the surgical instrument or can be frozen and the instrument is shown in relation to the planes. The registered preoperative models of vessels, tumor, liver surface and resection plan can be rendered as different colored intersection lines into the ultrasound planes. In addition the current position of the surgical instrument and one or both ultrasound planes in relation to the preoperative models are visualized in an extra viewer. It is also possible to show corresponding CT/MR slices to the ultrasound planes.

3   Results

We performed the registration algorithm retrospectively on data sets of three different patients. The preoperative CT or MR data were acquired during breath-hold using contrast agents. Patient 1 and 3 got preoperative T1-weighted Flash 3D VIBE MR-sequences with 2.5 mm slice thickness. For Patient 2 a single slice spiral CT with 2 mm reconstructed slice thickness (5mm collimation, pitch 1.5) was acquired. 3D B-mode and Powerdoppler ultrasound was simultaneously acquired transcutaneously for patient 1 and intraoperatively for patient 2 and

3 using a 3.5 MHz abdominal 3D probe. The original resolution of the power-doppler scans was 0.2 mm in scan line direction, 0.5-0.7 degrees in the scan plane and 0.9 degrees between consecutive scan planes. A scanning volume of approximately 2 liters was reached and usually more than half of the liver is imaged. The original data were resampled isotropically to 1 mm Cartesian coordinates. Manual selection of 3-4 landmarks near the portal vein trunk for pre-registration lasts 1-2 minutes. The automatic procedures without interactive segmentation of PD-US data and manual pre-registration is possible in 1-2 minutes. The whole registration process lasts less than 15 minutes and can be significantly accelerated by an improved segmentation step, which seems possible.

Correctness and accuracy determination of non-rigid registration algorithms is a non-trivial task. On the one hand we evaluated the correct assignment of pre- and intraoperative portal vein center lines and on the other hand we measured the deviations of structures which have not been involved in the correspondence determination, like hepatic veins, tumor boundary and liver surface. Vessel center line segments were manually assigned and these assignments were compared with the assignments of the algorithm. We observed only two wrong assignments. In Fig. 1 c) and d) rigidly and non-rigidly registered portal vein center lines of patient 1 are shown. A RMS difference of 5.6, 5.7 and 3.4 mm has been computed between rigidly and non-rigidly registered center line points of the three patients. The resulting portal vein surfaces match well for all three patients as can be seen in Fig. 2. Similarly in Fig. 3 the surfaces of the hepatic veins are shown which have not been used for correspondence determination. Intersections of the preoperative models with the ultrasound data of patient 2 and 3 are shown in Fig. 4. By inspection of these intersections for all three patients we observed 6 to 9 mm maximal deviation for the vessels, 12 bis 15 mm for the tumor and 16 to 20 mm for the liver surface.

To assess the reproducibility of the results the algorithm was run for 50 different starting positions for each patient simulating different manual pre-registrations. The starting positions were uniformly distributed in the range of +/- 5 mm for each of the three translational parameters and in the range of +/- 5 degrees for each of the three Euler angles. The RMS error of all points on the model center lines between disturbed and undisturbed starting position was in almost all cases below 0.3 mm RMS error. We had only 4% failures with RMS errors between 1.7 and 8.3 mm.

4   Discussion and Conclusion

First promising results on augmenting intraoperative 3D ultrasound data of three different patients with preoperative models were shown. The use of portal vein center lines as features for a non-rigid registration approach worked well on all three data sets. While the accuracy in the surrounding of vessels which were involved in the correspondence determination is high the accuracy decreases with increasing distance to those vessels. This indicates that the inaccuracies at the liver surface are caused by the deformations and not by the segmentation or skeletonization process. So far we have used only portal veins for registration, because hepatic veins occur in another time period of contrast agent application.

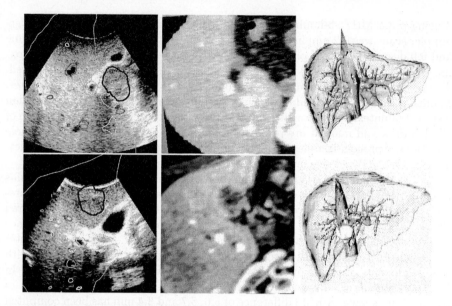

Fig. 4. Intraoperative visualization possibilities for two different patients (upper and lower row). From left to right: US slice with different colored intersection lines of pre-operatively modeled tumor (dark and thick), portal veins (bright), hepatic veins (dark) and liver surface (bright and thin). Corresponding CT (upper row) resp. MR (lower row) slice. Overview image showing portal veins, tumor, liver surface and location of US slice.

But we plan to integrate hepatic veins in the future. A possibility to improve the accuracy for structures lying further away from vessels is to incorporate the liver surface into the registration process. Some parts of the liver surface can be identified in the ultrasound images yet other parts can be determined better by a range scanner like in [20]. We will explore both possibilities. We think that for accurate and robust intraoperative liver registration we need both deep lying structures (vessels) and surface information. By streamlining the registration procedure and reducing interaction time for intraoperative vessel segmentation intraoperative non-rigid registration of the liver seems to be possible in less than five minutes.

References

1. Gronningsaeter A, Kleven A, Ommedal S et al.: SonoWand, an ultrasound-based neuronavigation system. Neurosurgery 47(6):1373–1379, 2000.
2. Eulenstein S, Lange T, Hünerbein M, Schlag PM: Ultrasound based navigation system incorporating preoperative planning for liver surgery. CARS 2004, accepted.
3. Soler L, Delingette H, Malandain G, et al.: Fully automatic anatomical, pathological and functional segmentation from CT scans for hepatic surgery. Computer Aided Surgery 21(11):1344–1357, 2001.

4. Selle D, Preim B, Schenk A, Peitgen HO: Analysis of vasculature for liver surgical planning. IEEE Trans Med Imaging 21(11):1344–1357, 2002.
5. Meinzer HP, Thorn M, Cardenas C: Computerized planning of liver surgery - an overview. Computers & Graphics 26(4):569–576, 2002.
6. Lindseth F, Ommedal S, Bang J, et al.: Image Fusion of Ultrasound and MRI as an Aid for assessing Anatomical Shifts and improving overview and interpretation in Ultrasound Guided Neurosurgery. CARS 2001, 1230:247–252, 2001.
7. Kaspersen JH, Sjølie E, Wesche J, et al.: 3D ultrasound based navigation combined with preoperative CT during abdominal interventions: A feasability study. Cardiovasc Intervent Radiol 26:347–356, 2003.
8. Ellsmere J, Stoll J, Rattner D, et al.: A Navigation System for Augmenting Laparoscopic Ultrasound. MICCAI 2003, LNCS 2879:184–191, 2003.
9. Aylward SR, Jomier J, Guyon JP, Weeks S: Intra-Operative 3D Ultrasound Augmentation. IEEE International Symposium on Biomedical Imaging, 2002.
10. Penney GP, Blackall JM, Hamady MS, et al.: Registration of freehand 3D ultrasound and magnetic resonance liver images. Med Image Anal 8(1):81–91, 2004.
11. Roche A, Pennec X, Malandain G, Ayache N: Rigid Registration of 3-D Ultrasound With MR Images: A New Approach Combining Intensity and Gradient Information. IEEE Trans Med Imag 20(10):1038–1049, 2001.
12. Slomka PJ, Mandel J, Downey D, Fenster A: Evaluation of voxel-based registration of 3-D power Doppler ultrasound and 3-D magnetic resonance angiographic images of carotid arteries. Ultrasound Med Biol 27(7):945–955, 2001.
13. Pennec X, Cachier P, Ayache N: Tracking brain deformations in time sequences of 3D US images. Pattern Recognition Letters 24(4-5):801–813, 2003.
14. Letteboer M, Willems P, Viergever MA, Niessen W: Non-rigid Registration of 3D Ultrasound Images of Brain Tumours Acquired during Neurosurgery. MICCAI 2003, LNCS 2879:408–415, 2003.
15. Porter BC, Rubens DJ, Strang JG, et al.: Three-Dimensional Registration and Fusion of Ultrasound and MRI Using Major Vessels as Fiducial Markers. IEEE Trans Med Imag 20(4):354–359, 2001.
16. Penney GP, Blackall JM, Hayashi D, et al.: Overview of an ultrasound to CT or MR registration system for use in thermal ablation of liver metastases. Proc. Medical Image Understanding and Analysis, 2001.
17. Aylward SR, Jomier J, Weeks S, Bullitt E: Registration and Analysis of Vascular Images. Int J Computer Vision 55(2-3):123–138, 2003.
18. Xie Z, Farin GE: Deformation With Hierachical B-Splines. Mathematical Methods in Computer Aided Geometric Design, 545–554, 2001.
19. Sato M, Bitter I, Bende M, et al.: TEASAR: Tree-structure extraction algorithm for accurate and robust skeletons. Procs. PACIFIC GRAPHICS-00, 281–289, 2000.
20. Cash DM, Sinha TK, Chapman WC, et al.: Incorporation of a laser range scanner into image-guided liver surgery: surface acquisition, registration, and tracking. Medical Physics 30(7):1671–1682, 2003.

Control System for MR-Guided Cryotherapy
– Short-Term Prediction of Therapy Boundary Using Automatic Segmentation and 3D Optical Flow –

Ryoichi Nakamura[1, 2], Kemal Tuncali[2], Paul R. Morrison[2], Nobuhiko Hata[3], Stuart G. Silverman[2], Ron Kikinis[2], Ferenc A. Jolesz[2], and Gary P. Zientara[2]

[1] Institute of Advanced Biomedical Engineering and Science, Tokyo Women's Medical University, 8-1 Kawada-cho, Shinjuku, Tokyo 162-8666 Tokyo
ryoichin@abmes.twmu.ac.jp,
[2] Dept. of Radiology, Brigham & Women's Hospital and Harvard Medical School, 75 Francis Street, Boston MA 02115 USA
{paul, zentai, worku, kikinis, jolesz, zientara}@bwh.harvard.edu,
[3] Dept. of Mechano-informatics, Graduate school of Information Science & Technology, the Univ. of Tokyo, 7-3-1, Hongo, Bunkyo-ku, Tokyo 113-8656 Japan
{ryoichi, noby}@atre.t.u-tokyo.ac.jp

Abstract. During cryotherapy, it is extremely useful for the interventionalists to have available intra-operatively a 3D iceball visualization, to ensure the effectiveness and safety of the procedure. Additionally, it highly beneficial to provide the interventionalists with a best estimate of how the iceball will grow in the future, and an estimate of the extent to which the target region and the tissues around it will be ablated. In this study, we introduce a newly developed control system for cryotherapy using a novel approach for the real-time/future-predicted assessments of the treatment. The system has been validated using results from cryotherapy experiments.

1   Introduction

Cryotherapy (cryocautery, cryosurgery, cryoconization) is the treatment destroying tissue cell by freezing its water component. Cryoprobes containing low temperature circulating liquid are placed in contact with or inside the lesion to be frozen percutaneously. Iceball is created around the tip of the probes and do damage to the tissues. It is percutaneous or interstitials treatment and relatively safe to heat ablation such as laser, RF, so Cryotherapy is very valuable procedure in Minimally Invasive Surgery field. [1,2]

But Cryotherapy often suffers from visualization problems in treating internal tumors unless performed under intra-operative image guidance and monitoring due to its less invasiveness [3]. Non-invasive radiological imaging is useful to evaluate soft tissue properties pre-operatively and to monitor changes during surgery. Notably, cryotherapy is interstitial / percutaneous and iceballs are not visible, these imaging technologies are helpful.

C. Barillot, D.R. Haynor, and P. Hellier (Eds.): MICCAI 2004, LNCS 3217, pp. 542–550, 2004.
© Springer-Verlag Berlin Heidelberg 2004

In our institutes, we perform Cryo procedure under interventional MR monitoring system. High quality MR images produce rich information of iceball and its surroundings. But there still be some limitation to use only 2D MR images for monitoring and controlling. At first, it is difficult to detect the accurate iceball shape and visualize in 3D. Secondly, the problem is the inability to estimate the size and geometry of iceball. It is very important to know what will occur for controlling treatments carefully. However it is difficult to predict the future iceballs because radiation absorption and heating is not uniform spatially due to tissue heterogeneity, blood flow, tissue perfusion, etc.

In this paper, we introduce a novel control system for MR-guided cryotherapy. Previously we developed and evaluated a predictive method for estimating the extent and effectiveness of thermal therapies using 2D optical flow [4]. In this study, we expand the method an implement various newly developed modules for 3D visualization, iceball detection and prediction. We also developed several modules for intra-operative assessments for cryotherapy. These modules provide surgeons rich and important information to assess the treatment in real time or predictively. System evaluation and validation was performed using animal cryotherapy experiments data.

2   Method

2.1   Automatic Iceball Segmentation

The most important module for the control system for cryotherapy is iceball segmentation. It is the base of the software to monitor and validate the thermal effect.

Therapy region on thermal treatment shows tissue intensity changes from light gray (high intensity) to dark gray (low intensity) and finally to black (MR signal void) in MR imaging. Experimental work has shown that within the range of temperatures 37°C to 50°C / 37°C to 0°C T1 varies approximately linearly with temperature at a rate of 1%/°C [5,6]. I use the percentage of the difference of signal intensities (DiffSI) for the segmentation of thermal changed region. In cryotherapy, Signal intensity increases according to the temperature decreasing in 37~0°C. But after starting freezing, intensity changes on another mode.

The DiffSI mapping for thermal region segmentation from T1-w FSE images consist of these steps as described;

1) Image acquisition; access to buffer; data transfer to research workstation
2) FOV definition to enhance the region of interest
3) Image subtraction and division by baseline image
4) Gaussian filtering for noise reduction
5) Adding segmented probe data
6) Segment using region growing method and Image Opening/Closing

The DiffSI-based method is very fast and sensitive, but suffered from SNR. To segment smooth thermal region, we use low-pass Gaussian filtering and image dilation/erosion for noise reduction.

Most of cases in image guided surgery, the lesion is limited and localized region in the whole image field of view (FOV). I use physician-defined FOV for DiffSI mapping to reduce computation load.

Through those procedure iceball can be segmented, but there are often scattered voxels outside the region due to image noises caused by RF noises, motion of tissues and vessels, and blood flow etc. To cut off the scattered voxels outside of iceball, we use region-growing method for the segmentation. Seed Points for the iceball segmentation must be defined before starting segmentation. But all the therapy regions grow from the tip of the thermal probes (Laser fiber, RF probe, and cryoprobe), hence the

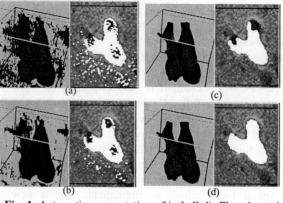

Fig. 1. Automatic segmentation of iceball. l): Flowchart of segmentation procedures. r): results of automatic segmentation using Diff-SI image (in-vivo pig experimental result). (a): original DiffSI map. (b): map(a) w/ Gaussian filtering. (c): map(b) + region growing method & OpenClose Filter. (d): map(c) + segmented probes.

definition of the seed points are not difficult task for the interventionalists.

Finally, adding the segmented crytoprobe volumes, thermal region is created (Fig.1).

2.2   Predictive Iceball Detection – 3D Optical Flow Estimation –

Preliminary study, we use 2D optical flow method using second order derivatives [7] and multi-point based solution with least squares (MPLS) [8] for estimating the growing velocities of therapy region [4]. For the fast prediction of therapy effect during treatment, calculation task must be limited enough to update the prediction information near to realtime. Through the advance of computer architecture, we can use powerful CPU and much memory for image processing and visualization.

Optical Flow
Optical Flow is a mathematical method for estimating the velocity field of voxel motion in the set of images. The gradient-based optical flow constraint equation is described as,

$$I(x,t) = I(x + v \cdot dt, t + dt) \qquad (1)$$

where $\nabla I(x,t) = (I_s, I_y, I_z)$ and I_t are the 1st order partial derivatives of I.

However, as in two or higher dimensional cases, we cannot solve v. The unknown components of v are more than two, constrained by only one liner equation. Further constraints or assumptions are necessary to solve for components of v. There are various technique for solve the optical flow constant equation (OFC, Eq(1)). Detailed comparison of those methods appears in [9] .In thermal therapies, the motion of thermal region is diverging (expansion). In the validation on the report [9], Lucas and Kanade's method [10] produced good result. I use this technique for estimating the velocity of thermal region growing, expanding three-dimensional field.

Prediction Using 3D Optical Flow Information

When the image dataset at timepoint n (t=t(n)) is taken, 3D optical flow information at timepoint n-1 can be calculated using the image datasets at timepoint n, n-1, n-2. Using the DiffSI image and velocity information (DI(x, t(n-1)), v(x, t(n-1))) at

$$DI(x + v(x, t(n-1)) \cdot \Delta t, \quad t(n+k)) = DI(x, \quad t(n-1)) \quad (5)$$

timepoint n-1, future image at timepoint n+k (t=t(n+k))is estimated using this constant equation;

where $\Delta t = t(n+k) - t(n-1)$.

On cryotherapy, the intra-operative MR images are taken every 2~3 minutes but of course the timing of image acquisition is varied. In this study, I use 3minutes (180sec) future prediction as the standard length between the timepoint of last image acquisition and the timepoint for prediction. Surgeon can see the iceball on current image dataset and the region on 3minutes future timepoint on every timepoint.

Using these method and thresholding procedure such as auto-segmentation for actual iceball, future iceball is created.

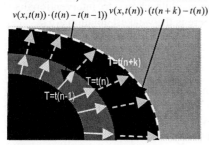

$$v(x, t(n)) \cdot (t(n) - t(n-1)) \quad v(x, t(n)) \cdot (t(n+k) - t(n))$$

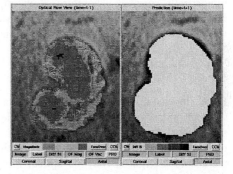

Fig. 2. Prediction method for future iceball. At timepoint n, the velocity of growing of iceball at timepoint n-1 is given by 3D optical flow computing. On assumption of velocity constancy, the voxel on x at timepoint n-1 will move to $x + v(x, t(n-1)) \cdot \Delta t$.

Fig. 3. Optical Flow Estimation and Prediction. Left) Optical Flow vector information is overlaid on the iceball at timepoint t-1. Right) Predicted Iceball Region using the vector information is overlaid the glayscale at t+1. The estimation of iceball region looks pretty good.

2.3   Module for Assessing Therapy

By the development of these key features above, we can take accurate and quantitative iceball information. It is very beneficial to assess the treatment in real time. To validate cryotherapy intra-operatively, we first developed and implemented these modules to the software.

– % Target Coverage (%TC) and Dice Similarity Coefficient (DSC)

%TC is the most general and simple assessment for measuring the effect of ablation therapies. On this module for thermal therapies, it shows how much target volume is ablated using target volume as volume A, therapy volume as B. In thermal therapies, %C must be 100% at the end of procedure. If not, it leaves residual survival tumor cells.

DSC shows the similarity between 2 volumes by voxel-by-voxel classification on MRI segmentation dataset. It is generally accepted that a value of DSC>0.7 represents excellent agreement [11]

The combination of %C DSC shows not only the coverage of target volume by ablation, but also under/over-treatment situation. It is helpful for the treatment validation, including effectiveness and safety [12].

– Alarming module for boundary violation

Violation of protected region by iceball, like ablating vessels, functional region in brain, means critical damage for patient. To avoid such life-threaten or residual damages, boundary violation must be checked throughout the treatment thoughtfully.

One of the main objectives of development of prediction module for iceball is estimate the situation of boundary violation priory.

– Minimum Ablation Margin

In ablation therapy, target must be ablated with some marginal zone to avoid residual tumor cells survival. Therefore, it is important message how much the ablation margin is at least. Minimum Ablation Margin module shows to interventionalists where is the minimum marginal area, that is, where is the weakest ablation area.

2.4   System Overviews

Fig.4 shows the overviews of the software including the modules described. The viewer window (right on Fig.4) has 4 rendering windows, an alarming window, and a spreadsheet for the assessment of the therapy and 3D optical flow prediction. 4 rendering window show 1) 3D view of therapy area (left-up), 2) 2D slice view of therapy area (right-up), 3) 3D optical flow information on iceball (iceball) (bottom left), and 4) 2D slice view of predicted iceball (bottom right). In 3D window, there are 3 volumes, probes, current iceball, and predicted iceball. Almost of all cases where

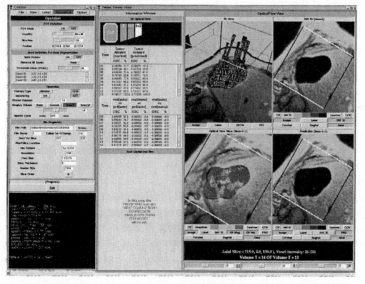

Fig. 4. Overview of the control system for cryotherapy. (Clinical demonstration)

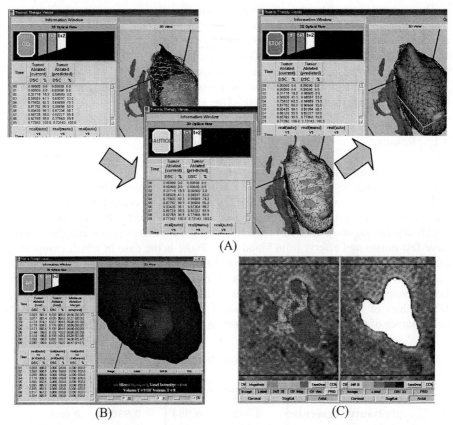

Fig. 5. Functions of the systems. A) Alarming (Protected boundary violation by auto/predicted), B) Margin (Points & lines shows the nearest between tumor surface and iceball surface), C) One prediction example in heterogeneous and noisy case.

this software is used, predicted region is larger than current thermal region, hence I use the mesh surface for the predicted region to see the iceball through the mesh.

Figure 5 shows some demonstration of the Functions of this system.

3   Results

3.1   Experimental Design

The performance of this system mainly depends on the accuracy of auto/predicted iceball detections and the execution speed. We evaluated the accuracy of the segmentation/prediction with the comparison of the generated volumes to manually segmented iceball data which medical experts created. We use 3 in-vivo pig cryo experimental data to validate the accuracy of iceball detection.

The experimental data are performed under the monitoring using 1.5T closed magnet system to have high-resolution datasets for the validation. MR image datasets are taken every 80 second and image acquisition time is 40 second. To evaluate the accuracy of iceball model, we use DSC value with the auto/predicted iceball and manually segmented iceball data by medical experts.

For the assessment of the execution speed, we use several clinical data of cryotherapy and measured the meantime of the execution time.

3.2   Results

− Accuracy of auto/predicted iceball detection

Table 1 shows the results of the comparison between generated auto/predicted iceball and manually segmented iceball data. This evaluation is carried out using all the iceball image data taken during freezing on each experiment. Pig#1 is the case in which cryoprobes are placed in relatively homogeneous liver tissue and the images have few noises and effects from blood flow. Pig#2 is the case in which cryoprobes are located to vessel-rich part of the liver and the iceball images are strongly affected vessel movement and blood flow. Pig#3 is the case at which cryoprobes are located in heterogeneous tissues, such as liver, muscle, and skin. But, these cases have good DSC values of the comparison with manual segmentation data. It shows the high performance of auto/predicted iceball detection module of this control system.

Table 1. DSC comparison results from in-vivo experiments

	lowest	highest	average	sd
pig1:auto segmented	0.758	0.957	**0.937**	**0.051**
pig2:auto segmented	0.748	0.994	**0.930**	**0.063**
pig3:auto segmented	0.850	0.996	**0.907**	**0.039**
pig1:predicted	0.736	0.954	**0.907**	**0.072**
pig2:predicted	0.661	0.938	**0.870**	**0.106**
pig3:predicted	0.735	0.930	**0.871**	**0.062**

We also checked if the performance of iceball prediction is grater than other methods including 2D optical flow, Uras' method. The system we newly developed has significant improvements in accuracy of the prediction.

− Execution time in clinical environment

We evaluate the performance of the guidance information updating.

This evaluation is done using some of the actual therapy data because the pig data used in accuracy evaluation have higher resolution than ordinal clinical cases. Using 256x256x8~20 voxel slab (256x256resolution, 8~20slices for each timepoint) and 64x64x20FOV for computation region around cryoprobes, all the update is carried out in approx *2.5 sec*. Most of clinical cases, it takes about 1 minute for this kind of images on T1-w FSE protocol using 0.5T Interventional MRI. Therefore, this result shows the novel performance of this control system for cryotherapy.

4   Discussion and Conclusions

We developed a novel MRI-based monitoring and control system for cryotherapy. The system shows the interventionalists rich visual and quantitative information of the treatment in real-time and provides highly beneficial predicted information regarding the course of the treatment. Two key components of the system provide accurate quantitative iceball information and the 3D visible model.

Results of animal experiments were used to demonstrate the good accuracy of the system. Noisy, or heterogeneous cases are The results from using our system during animal cryotherapy experiments indicate the system's value in increasing the therapeutic effectiveness of the ablation and the safety of the procedure. We now improve and evaluate the system performance using 1) several different methods for iceball segmentation, and 2) estimation of more accurate "true" iceball shape from the sets of hand segmentation results for more reliable assessment. We are also attempting to assess its clinical ability in real operation field in direct system connection to MR system.

Acknowledgements. This research is supported by NIH R01-CA86879, Harvard University Milton Fund, and Grant-Aid for Research Fellow of the Japanese Society for the Promotion of Science.

References

1.   Balmer A, Gaillound C, De Potter P, Munier F, Chamero J, Treatment of retinoblastoma and results, Lausanne1963-1989 Klin Monatsbl Augenheilkd 1990 May, 196(5), pp.374-376, 1990
2.   Tsuji T, Otake N, Nishimura M, Cryosurgery and topical fluorouracil: a treatment method for widespread basal cell epithelioma in basal cell nevus syndrome, Journal of Dermatology, 20(8), pp507-513, 1993
3.   Muller Lisse UG, Heuck AF, Control and monitoring of focal thermotherapy with magnetic resonance tomography. An overview, Radiology, 38(3), pp.200-209, 1998
4.   Zientara GP, Saiviroonporn P, Morrison PR, Fried MP, Hushek SG, Kikinis R, Jolesz FA. MRI Monitoring of Laser Ablation Using Optical Flow, Journal of Magnetic Resonance Imaging, No.8, pp1306-1318, 1998
5.   Matsumoto R, Oshio K, Jolesz FA. T1-weighted MR monitoring for interstitial laser- and freezing-induced ablation in the liver, Journal of Magnetic Resonance Imaging, No2, pp555-562, 1992
6.   Kuroda K, Chung AH, Hynynen K, Jolesz FA. Calibration of water proton chemical shift with temperature for non-invasive temperature imaging during focused ultrasound surgery, Journal of Magnetic Resonance, No.8, pp175-181, 1998
7.   Uras S, Girosi F, Torre V, A Computational Approach to Motion Perception, Biological Cybernetics, vol. 60, pp. 79-87, 1988.
8.   Nesi P, BimboD, Ben-Tzvi D. Algorithms for Optical Flow Estimation in Real-time on Connection Machine-2, Department of Systems and Informatics Technical Report, Faculty of Engineering University of Florence Italy, DSI-RT 24/92, 1992
9.   Barron JL, Fleet DJ, Beauchemin SS. Performance of Optical Flow Techniques, International Journal of Computer Vision, No.12(1), pp43-77, 1994

10. Lucas B, Kanade T. An Iterative Image Registration Technique with an Application to Stereo Vision, Proc of DARPA Image Understanding Workshop, pp121-130, 1981
11. Bharatha A, Hirose M, Hata N, Warfield SK, Ferrant M, Zou KH, Suarez-Santana E, Ruiz-Alzola J, D'Amico A, Cormack RA, Kikinis R, Jolesz FA, Tempany CMC. Evaluation of three-dimensional finite element-based deformable registration of pre- and intra-operative prostate imaging., Medical Physics, No28, pp2551-2560, 2001.
12. Tuncali K, Morris M, Warfield SK, Morrison PR, Dahm F, Shankar S, Sonnenberg E, Silverman SG. 3D Assessment of Percutaneous MRI-guided Cryotherapy of Liver Tumors, IVth Interventional MRI Symposium of ISMRM, Leipzig Germany, September 2002

Fast and Accurate Bronchoscope Tracking Using Image Registration and Motion Prediction

Jiro Nagao[1], Kensaku Mori[1], Tsutomu Enjouji[1], Daisuke Deguchi[1],
Takayuki Kitasaka[1], Yasuhito Suenaga[1], Jun-ichi Hasegawa[2],
Jun-ichiro Toriwaki[2], Hirotsugu Takabatake[3], and Hiroshi Natori[4]

[1] Graduate School of Information Science, Nagoya University, Japan
{jnagao,ddeguchi,kitasaka,mori,suenaga}@suenaga.m.is.nagoya-u.ac.jp
[2] School of Computer and Cognitive Sciences, Chukyo University, Japan
[3] Sapporo Minami-sanjyo Hospital, Sapporo, Japan
[4] Department of Diagnostic Ultrasound and Medical Electronics,
Sapporo Medical University, Japan

Abstract. This paper describes a method for faster and more accurate bronchoscope camera tracking by image registration and camera motion prediction using the Kalman filter. The position and orientation of the bronchoscope camera at a frame of a bronchoscopic video are predicted by the Kalman filter. Because the Kalman filter gives good prediction for image registration, estimation of the position and orientation of the bronchoscope tip converges fast and accurately. In spite of the usefulness of Kalman filters, there have been no reports on tracking bronchoscope camera motion using the Kalman filter. Experiments on eight pairs of real bronchoscopic video and chest CT images showed that the proposed method could track camera motion 2.5 times as fast as our previous method. Experimental results showed that the motion prediction increased the number of frames correctly and continuously tracked by about 4.5%, and the processing time was reduced by about 60% with the search space restriction also proposed in this paper.

1   Introduction

A bronchoscope is a tool to observe inside the bronchi. A physician inserts a bronchoscope into a patient's airway with watching a TV monitor. During an examination or treatment with a bronchoscope, it sometimes happens that the physician gets disoriented because the lung has complex bifurcation structures. As the body of a bronchoscope can be bent, a positional sensor has to be attached to the tip of it if the position of the tip should be directly measured. However, because bronchi are very narrow, it is hard to attach a positional sensor to the tip. Even if you use one of electro-magnetic types, the measurement does not have sufficient accuracy for the navigation use. To support the physician during a bronchoscopic examination by providing information such as the position and orientation of the bronchoscope tip, we have reported a bronchoscope tracking method [1,2]. This method tracks bronchoscopic camera motion by image registration (IR) between real bronchoscopic (RB) images and virtual bronchoscopic

C. Barillot, D.R. Haynor, and P. Hellier (Eds.): MICCAI 2004, LNCS 3217, pp. 551–558, 2004.

(VB) images generated from 3-D CT images [3,4]. This method tracks broncho-scopic camera motion by sequentially registering RB and VB images frame by frame. Although this method is robust to patient motion caused by breathing, it requires large amount of computation time. Since bronchoscope navigation should work in real time, efficient tracking algorithm is desired.

This paper proposes a fast and accurate bronchoscope tracking algorithm. Since the tracking is based on IR that finds the best camera parameter of VB that maximizes image similarity between RB and VB images, good initial guess of the camera parameter can reduce computation time. For obtaining good initial guess, we predict bronchoscopic camera motion by the Kalman filter [5]. Several research groups are working on developing bronchoscope navigation or bron-choscope tracking [6,7]. However, there exists no report on motion prediction in bronchoscope tracking. In Sect. 2, the proposed method for camera motion tracking is described. The experimental results and a brief discussion are shown in Sect. 3.

2   Camera Motion Tracking

2.1   Camera Parameters of Virtual Bronchoscope

The extrinsic camera parameters of the VB camera at the k-th frame are denoted by:

$$\mathbf{Q}^{(k)} = \begin{pmatrix} \mathbf{R}(\boldsymbol{r}^{(k)}) & \boldsymbol{t}^{(k)} \\ {}^{t}\mathbf{0} & 1 \end{pmatrix} , \tag{1}$$

where $\boldsymbol{r}^{(k)} = {}^{t}(r_x \ r_y \ r_z)$ is the camera orientation represented in Euler angle around the x-, y-, and z-axes in the world coordinate system and $\mathbf{R}(\boldsymbol{r}^{(k)})$ is a rotation matrix constructed from $\boldsymbol{r}^{(k)}$. $\boldsymbol{t}^{(k)} = {}^{t}(t_x \ t_y \ t_z)$ means the camera position. $\mathbf{Q}^{(k)}$ is obtained from $\boldsymbol{q}^{(k)} = {}^{t}({}^{t}\boldsymbol{r}^{(k)} \ {}^{t}\boldsymbol{t}^{(k)})$. It is this parameter vector $\boldsymbol{q}$ that the method we will describe later directly seeks for. When the camera moves from the k-th frame to the $(k+1)$-th frame, the movement is formulated as:

$$\mathbf{Q}^{(k+1)} = \mathbf{Q}^{(k)}\Delta\mathbf{Q}^{(k)}, \quad \mathbf{Q}^{(k)} = \begin{pmatrix} \mathbf{R}^{(k)} & \boldsymbol{t}^{(k)} \\ {}^{t}\mathbf{0} & 1 \end{pmatrix}, \quad \Delta\mathbf{Q}^{(k)} = \begin{pmatrix} \mathbf{R}(\Delta\boldsymbol{r}^{(k)}) & \Delta\boldsymbol{t}^{(k)} \\ {}^{t}\mathbf{0} & 1 \end{pmatrix} , \tag{2}$$

where $\Delta\mathbf{Q}^{(k)}$ is the movement between the k-th and $(k+1)$-th frames. Hence, bronchoscope camera tracking is achieved by continuously finding $\Delta\mathbf{Q}^{(k)}$ con-structed from $\Delta\boldsymbol{q}^{(k)} = {}^{t}({}^{t}\Delta\boldsymbol{r}^{(k)} \ {}^{t}\Delta\boldsymbol{t}^{(k)})$.

2.2   Overview of Tracking Algorithm

The parameters of an RB camera are estimated by means of IR between the RB images and virtual bronchoscopic images. The input of the system is a 3-D chest CT image and a sequence of real bronchoscopic images $\{\mathbf{B}^{(k)}\}$, both of which are obtained from the same patient. The CT image is used for generating VB images. The output is the sequence of tracking results $\{q^{(k)}\}$.

The tracking method consists of two major components: (a) camera motion prediction by a Kalman filter (Motion Prediction Step) and (b) camera parameter estimation by IR (Registration Step). In order to reduce computation time, a restricted search space is configured before each Registration Step. When the camera motion at the 0-th through the k-th frames are tracked, the camera motion tracking process for the $(k + 1)$-th frame is performed as follows:

1. **(Motion Prediction Step)** The camera parameter prediction $\hat{q}^{(k+1)}$ for the $(k + 1)$-th frame, which is used in the succeeding Registration Step, is predicted by the Kalman filter. The Kalman filter outputs $\hat{q}^{(k+1)}$ using $q^{(0)}, \ldots, q^{(k)}$ acquired in the preceding Registration Steps.
2. Configure a restricted search space using $\hat{q}^{(k+1)}$.
3. **(Registration Step)** $q_0^{(k+1)} = \hat{q}^{(k+1)}$ is used as the initial search parameter for IR. Here, $q_0^{(k+1)}$ denotes the initial search parameter for IR at the $(k+1)$-th frame. A series of VB images $\{V(Q^{(k)} \Delta Q^{(k)})\}$ is generated with changing $\Delta q^{(k)}$ that constructs $\Delta Q^{(k)}$. The parameter generating the VB image that is the most similar to $B^{(k+1)}$ is selected as the camera parameter estimation result $Q^{(k+1)}$.

The above process is iterated for each of the subsequent RB frames. We assume that the camera parameters $q_0^{(0)}$ at the starting frame $B^{(0)}$ are known.

2.3   Camera Motion Prediction by Kalman Filter

Kalman Filtering. The Kalman filter is formulated as follows:

$$x_{k+1} = Fx_k + Gw_k \qquad \text{(state equation)} , \tag{3}$$

$$y_k = Hx_k + n_k \qquad \text{(observation equation)} , \tag{4}$$

where x_k is a system state vector at time step k and y_k is an observation vector. Although F, G, H, the state transition, driving and observation matrices, respectively, can change in time, they are assumed to be invariant in our model. The covariance matrices of Gaussian noises n_k and w_k, Σ_{n_k} and Σ_{w_k}, respectively, are assumed to be known.

The Kalman Filter Algorithm. Hereafter, $\hat{x}_{t|t'}$ and $\hat{\Sigma}_{t|t'}$; $((t, t') = (k, k - 1)$, (k, k), $(k+1, k)$ or $(0, -1))$ denote the estimated values of x_t and covariance matrix of x_t, respectively, given the observation signals $y_0, \ldots, y_{t'}$. When y_k is received, $\hat{x}_{k+1|k}$ is predicted by the two steps described below. The iteration starts with $k = 0$, and the starting initial values are $\hat{x}_{0|-1}$ and $\hat{\Sigma}_{0|-1}$.

[**STEP 1**] Estimate $\hat{x}_{k|k}$ and $\hat{\Sigma}_{k|k}$ from y_k, $\hat{x}_{k|k-1}$ and $\hat{\Sigma}_{k|k-1}$.

$$\hat{x}_{k|k} = \hat{x}_{k|k-1} + \hat{\Sigma}_{k|k-1}{}^t H \left(H\hat{\Sigma}_{k|k-1}{}^t H + \Sigma_{n_k} \right)^{-1} (y_k - H\hat{x}_{k|k-1}) , \tag{5}$$

$$\hat{\Sigma}_{k|k} = \hat{\Sigma}_{k|k-1} - \hat{\Sigma}_{k|k-1}{}^t H \left(H\hat{\Sigma}_{k|k-1}{}^t H + \Sigma_{n_k} \right)^{-1} H\hat{\Sigma}_{k|k-1} . \tag{6}$$

[STEP 2] Predict $\hat{x}_{k+1|k}$ and $\hat{\Sigma}_{k+1|k}$ using $\hat{x}_{k|k}$ and $\hat{\Sigma}_{k|k}$.

$$\hat{x}_{k+1|k} = \mathbf{F}\hat{x}_{k|k} \ , \tag{7}$$

$$\hat{\Sigma}_{k+1|k} = \mathbf{F}\hat{\Sigma}_{k|k}{}^t\mathbf{F} + \mathbf{G}\Sigma_{w_k}{}^t\mathbf{G} \ . \tag{8}$$

Camera Motion Prediction by Kalman Filter. We assume that the camera motion is in a constant state of acceleration. The motion is written as:

$$\boldsymbol{v}^{(k)} = \frac{d\boldsymbol{q}^{(k)}}{dt} = \frac{\boldsymbol{q}^{(k)} - \boldsymbol{q}^{(k-1)}}{\Delta t} \ , \tag{9}$$

$$\boldsymbol{a}^{(k)} = \frac{d\boldsymbol{v}^{(k)}}{dt} = \frac{\boldsymbol{v}^{(k)} - \boldsymbol{v}^{(k-1)}}{\Delta t} = \frac{\boldsymbol{q}^{(k)} - 2\boldsymbol{q}^{(k-1)} + \boldsymbol{q}^{(k-2)}}{\Delta t} \ , \tag{10}$$

where $\boldsymbol{v}^{(k)}$ and $\boldsymbol{a}^{(k)}$ represent the velocity and acceleration, respectively, and Δt the interval between time steps. Using (9) and (10), $\boldsymbol{q}^{(k+1)}$ and $\boldsymbol{v}^{(k+1)}$ can be rewritten in terms of $\boldsymbol{a}^{(k)}$ and $\boldsymbol{v}^{(k)}$ as:

$$\boldsymbol{q}^{(k+1)} = \boldsymbol{q}^{(k)} + \boldsymbol{v}^{(k)}\Delta t + \frac{1}{2}\boldsymbol{a}^{(k)}(\Delta t)^2 \ , \tag{11}$$

$$\boldsymbol{v}^{(k+1)} = \boldsymbol{v}^{(k)} + \boldsymbol{a}^{(k)}\Delta t \ . \tag{12}$$

Letting $\boldsymbol{x}_k = {}^t\left({}^t\boldsymbol{q}^{(k)} \ {}^t\boldsymbol{v}^{(k)} \ {}^t\boldsymbol{a}^{(k)}\right)$ and constructing $\mathbf{F}$ from (11) and (12), we obtain:

$$\mathbf{F} = \begin{pmatrix} \mathbf{Id}_6 & (\Delta t)\mathbf{Id}_6 & \frac{1}{2}(\Delta t)^2\mathbf{Id}_6 \\ \mathbf{0}_6 & \mathbf{Id}_6 & (\Delta t)\mathbf{Id}_6 \\ \mathbf{0}_6 & \mathbf{0}_6 & \mathbf{Id}_6 \end{pmatrix} \ , \quad w_k = \begin{pmatrix} w_q \\ w_v \\ w_a \end{pmatrix} \ , \tag{13}$$

$$\mathbf{G} = (\mathbf{Id}_6 \ \mathbf{Id}_6 \ \mathbf{Id}_6) \ , \quad \mathbf{H} = (\mathbf{Id}_6 \ \mathbf{0}_6 \ \mathbf{0}_6) \ ,$$

where $\mathbf{Id}_6$ and $\mathbf{0}_6$ are 6×6 identity and zero matrices, respectively. The predicted camera parameter is given by $\hat{\boldsymbol{q}}^{(k+1)} = \mathbf{H}\hat{x}_{k+1}$ and provided to the Registration Step as the initial search parameter $\boldsymbol{q}_0^{(k+1)}$.

2.4   Camera Parameter Estimation by Image Registration

Image Registration. The parameters of the bronchoscope camera is estimated by using $\boldsymbol{q}_0^{(k+1)} = \hat{\boldsymbol{q}}^{(k+1)}$ as the initial search parameter. IR for finding camera parameter at the $(k+1)$-th frame is formulated as the maximization problem:

$$\Delta\mathbf{Q}^{(k)*} = \arg\max_{\Delta\mathbf{Q}^{(k)}} S\left(\mathbf{B}^{(k+1)}, \ \mathbf{V}\left(\mathbf{Q}^{(k)}\Delta\mathbf{Q}^{(k)}\right)\right) \ , \tag{14}$$

where $S(\mathbf{B}, \mathbf{V})$ is the image similarity between $\mathbf{B}$ and $\mathbf{V}$. The camera parameter at the $(k+1)$-th frame is obtained by

$$\mathbf{Q}^{(k+1)} = \mathbf{Q}^{(k)}\Delta\mathbf{Q}^{(k)*} \ . \tag{15}$$

This maximization problem is numerically solved by Powell method [8]. The search starts from $\Delta\mathbf{Q}_0^{(k)}$ obtained from the predicted camera parameter $\hat{\boldsymbol{q}}^{(k+1)}$ and $\mathbf{Q}^{(k)}$.

Search Space Restriction. Also, we restrict the search space by using the prediction results. The restricted search space is calculated by:

$$\left(\left| t^{(k+1)} - \hat{t}^{(k+1)} \right| \leq \left| t^{(k)} - \hat{t}^{(k+1)} \right| \right)$$
$$\wedge \left(\left| r^{(k+1)} - \hat{r}^{(k+1)} \right| \leq \left| r^{(k)} - \hat{r}^{(k+1)} \right| \right) \quad , \tag{16}$$

where $t^{(k)}$ and $r^{(k)}$ are the position and orientation of the bronchoscopic camera defined by (1).

3   Experimental Results and Discussion

3.1   Experiments

We applied the proposed method to eight pairs of RB video sequences and 3-D CT images. The RB video and the CT image in each pair were obtained from the same patient. The acquisition parameters of the CT images are: 512×512 pixels of slice size, 72-209 slices, 2.0-5.0 mm of slice thickness, 1.0-2.0 mm of reconstruction pitch. A conventional PC hosting two Intel XEON 3.06GHz processors and 2GBytes of main memory was used for this experiment. Table 1 and Fig. 1 show the tracking results of: (1) Our previous method [2] without motion prediction or search space restriction (abbreviated to "Previous" in the table), (2) the proposed method with motion prediction, without the search space restriction ("MP"), and (3) the proposed method with motion prediction and search space restriction ("MP+SSR"). The tracking results were evaluated in terms of the number of frames correctly and continuously tracked by visual inspection. Continuity of the tracking was judged to end when the VB images generated from the estimated camera parameters looked greatly different from the corresponding RB images for several frames, or when the tracking no longer followed the motion of the RB camera. Figure 1 shows examples of RB images and the corresponding VB images generated from the camera parameters calculated by each method.

3.2   Discussion

The number of frames tracked by the "MP" method increased in the six of the fifteen paths used for the experiment, and the total number of tracked frames increased by about 4.5%, reducing the processing time by about 20%. Furthermore, with the search space restriction (i.e. "MP+SSR" method), the computation time was reduced by about 60%, maintaining the larger number of tracked frames compared to those of the "Previous" method. We assumed that the real bronchoscope camera was in a state of constant acceleration. In reality, however, the motion of the camera is not in such a state. Therefore, it is expected that there might be some reduction in the number of frames tracked by the "MP" method; this was the case in the two of the fifteen paths. In this sense, it can be said that there is a tradeoff between speed and accuracy and robustness.

Table 1. The tracking results. The results are shown in [frames]. Figures in the parentheses show the average processing time per frame [sec]

Case	Path	Frames	Number of tracked frames (avg. time [sec])		
			Previous	MP	MP+SSR
	A	500	500 (3.42)	500 (3.21)	500 (2.25)
1	B	257	116 (6.82)	106 (2.63)	106 (1.97)
	C	200	180 (7.08)	180 (5.98)	180 (1.85)
2	A	430	407 (3.68)	407 (4.04)	407 (2.66)
	A	300	255 (6.90)	261 (5.32)	261 (2.54)
3	B	1100	973 (4.74)	973 (4.89)	973 (2.97)
	C	1000	873 (9.05)	873 (4.62)	873 (2.97)
4	A	205	205 (2.21)	205 (2.27)	205 (1.57)
5	A	300	69 (6.93)	70 (2.69)	70 (1.93)
	A	400	300 (7.94)	353 (7.69)	353 (2.05)
6	B	800	715 (7.64)	715 (6.72)	478 (2.29)
	C	524	200 (4.50)	351 (4.97)	351 (1.43)
7	A	225	140 (6.94)	161 (5.62)	161 (1.92)
	B	300	140 (2.96)	141 (3.14)	141 (2.09)
8	A	300	282 (4.59)	263 (1.92)	263 (1.54)
Total (avg. time)			5355 (5.94)	5559 (4.77)	5322 (2.38)

It is considered that the improvement of the tracking performance was owing to the Kalman filter. Because it gives good initial guess for the search by IR, the Powell method can reach the solution more quickly, avoiding undesirable local minima. In Path C of Case 6, the number of tracked frames significantly increased. Since the "Previous" method used the estimation result of the previous frame as the initial search parameters, the search by the Powell method fell into a local minimum. On the other hand, since the Kalman filter gives better initial parameters closer to the correct minimum, the Powell method could find the correct solution.

The number of tracked frames did not increase in some paths. In these paths, the IR might not have been performed properly due to distortion of the bronchus or bubbles appeared in the bronchi. To avoid such tracking failure because of improper IR, skipping IR and merely using the motion prediction result is one solution. Rapid changes of entropy of the RB images might be used to detect appearance of large bubbles.

In Path B of Case 6 with "MP+SSR," the number of tracked frames was fewer than that of the "Previous" method. In this path, the estimation result by IR was affected by the bubbles. Then the Kalman filter used the improper result for motion prediction, and consequently improper restricted search space was configured. On the other hand, the tracking result of the path without search space restriction ("MP" method) was acceptable. Therefore this problem can be solved by detecting bubbles as we mentioned before. In Path B of Case 1, the motion prediction could not give proper prediction when the camera moved

| Frame No. | RB image | "Prev" | "MP" | "MP+SSR" |

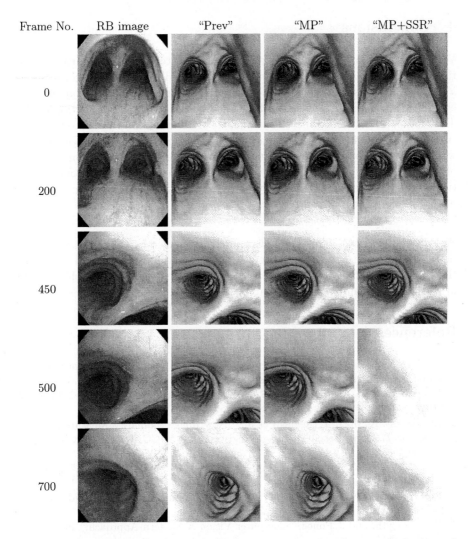

Fig. 1. Examples of tracking results. VB images are rendered using the estimated camera parameters. The columns labeled "Prev," "MP," and "MP+SSR" show the results obtained by the previous method [2], the method using the Kalman filter's output as initial guesses, and the method using restricted search space, respectively.

quickly. Because our Kalman filter assumes the camera to be in a constant state of acceleration, it can not predict the camera parameter properly when the motion violates the assumption too badly. In such cases, we might need another method to estimate the amount of camera motion.

4 Conclusions

We proposed a method for faster and more accurate bronchoscope camera motion tracking by camera motion prediction. To predict camera motion, we used a Kalman filter, assuming that the camera motion is in a constant state of acceleration. Also, the search space for IR was restricted using the prediction results. The motion prediction increased the number of frames correctly and continuously tracked by about 4.5%, and with the search space restriction the processing time was reduced by about 60%. Our future work includes: (1) accuracy improvement of the camera motion prediction by the Kalman filter, (2) reduction of computation time, (3) experiments on many more cases, and (4) quantitative evaluation of the tracking accuracy.

Acknowledgments. This study was partly supported by the Grants-in-Aid for Scientific Research and the 21st Century COE Program from Japan Society for the Promotion of Science, Grants-in-Aid for Cancer Research from the Ministry of Health, Labor and Welfare of Japan.

References

1. K. Mori, Y. Suenaga, J. Toriwaki et al., "Tracking of camera motion of real endoscope by using the Virtual Endoscope System," In H. U. Lemke, M. W. Vannier, K. Inamura et al. (Editors), CARS2000, International Congress Series 1214, pp.85-90
2. D. Deguchi, K. Mori, Y. Suenaga et al., "New Image Similarity Measure for Bronchoscope Tracking Based on Image Registration," MICCAI 2003, LNCS vol.2878, pp.399-406
3. D. J. Vining, R. Y. Shitrin, E. F. Haponik et al., "Virtual Bronchoscopy," Radiology, 193 (P), Supplement to Radiology (RSNA Scientific Program), p.261, 1994
4. P. Rogalla, J. Terwisscha van Scheltinga, and B. Hamm, eds., "Virtual endoscopy and related 3D techniques," Springer, Berlin, 2001
5. D. A. Forsyth, and J. Ponce, "Computer Vision A Modern Approach," Pearson Education, 2003
6. I. Bricault, G. Ferretti, P. Cinquin, "Registration Real and CT-Derived Virtual Bronchoscopic Images to Assist Transbronchial Biopsy," IEEE Trans. on Medical Imaging, 17, 5, pp.703-714, 1998
7. J. P. Helferty, W. E. Higgins, "Technique for Registering 3D Virtual CT Images to Endoscopic Video," Proceedings of ICIP, pp.893-896, 2001
8. W. H. Press, S. A. Teukolsky, W. T. Vetterling et al., "Numerical Recipes in C, The Art of Scientific Computing Second Edition," CAMBRIDGE UNIVERSITY PRESS, pp.321-336, 1999

Virtual Pneumoperitoneum for Generating Virtual Laparoscopic Views Based on Volumetric Deformation

Takayuki Kitasaka[1], Kensaku Mori[1], Yuichiro Hayashi[1], Yasuhito Suenaga[1],
Makoto Hashizume[2], and Jun-ichiro Toriwaki[3]

[1] Graduate School of Information Science, Nagoya University,
Furo-cho, Chikusa-ku, Nagoya, Aichi, 464-8603, Japan
{kitasaka, kensaku, suenaga}@is.nagoya-u.ac.jp
[2] Center for the Integration of Advanced Medicine and Innovative Technology,
Kyushu University Hospital, Fukuoka, 812-8582 Japan
[3] School of Computer and Cognitive Sciences, Chukyo University
101 Tokodachi, Kaizu-cho, Toyota, Aichi, 470-0393, Japan
jtoriwak@sccs.chukyo-u.ac.jp

Abstract. This paper describes a method for generating virtual pneumoperitoneum based on volumetric deformation and its application to virtual laparoscopy. Laparoscopic surgery is now widely performed as a minimum-invasive surgery. Because a laparoscope has a very narrow viewing area, this limits the surgeon's viewable area. Making views that the abdominal wall is virtually elevated (virtual pneumoperitoneum) will be very helpful for intra-operative surgical navigation or pre-operative surgical planning. We deform original 3-D abdominal CT images so that the abdominal wall is virtually elevated. The entire process consists of five major steps: (a) extracting the abdominal wall, (b) elastic modeling, (c) elastic deformation of the model, (d) deformation of the original image, and (e) rendering virtual laparoscopic images. Virtual laparoscopic images are then generated from the deformed image. We have applied the method to three cases of 3-D abdominal CT images. From the experimental results, we confirmed that the abdominal wall was appropriately elevated by the proposed method. Laparoscopic views were very helpful for intra-operative surgical navigation as additional views of a surgeon or pre-operative surgical planning.

1 Introduction

Laparoscopic surgery has been widely performed as one of minimum-invasive surgery methods. Laparoscopic surgery is performed by making a working space (pneumoperitoneum) by infusing CO_2 gas through a needle inserted to the peritoneum and inserting a laparoscope and forceps inside the abdominal cavity. Holes of 1cm diameter are created on the abdominal wall for inserting such equipments. A surgeon performs surgery by watching a TV monitor that displays video images taken by the laparoscope camera. Although laparoscopic

C. Barillot, D.R. Haynor, and P. Hellier (Eds.): MICCAI 2004, LNCS 3217, pp. 559–567, 2004.

surgery does not require to widely open the abdomen and is less invasive, a laparoscope has very narrow viewing area. This limits the surgeon's viewable area. Sometimes it is very difficult for a surgeon to understand the positional relations between abdominal organs and lesions. This significantly increases the surgeon's load of laparoscopic surgery. Surgical planning and intraoperative surgical aid using three-dimensional (3-D) CT or MR images are very important.

Since surgical simulation or surgical planning using preoperative 3-D images are quite useful, there are many researches on these topics[1,2,3,4]. We have also developed a virtual endoscopy system that can be used for preoperative surgical planning and intraoperative surgical guidance[6]. Virtual endoscopy system is now widely used in the clinical field[5]. If we could use a virtual endoscopy system and provide a surgeon virtual laparoscopic images rendered at arbitrary viewpoints and view directions during surgery, it would be very helpful for intraoperative surgical navigation or pre-operative surgical planning. A surgeon can make a surgical plan by checking the insertion points of a laparoscope and forceps by observing virtual laparoscopic views. Also it is possible to observe the positional relations between organs and lesions on virtual laparoscopic views. There are, however, very few reports for creating virtual laparoscopic views that simulates laparoscopy.

The virtual pneumoperitoneum requires to lift the abdominal wall for generating virtual laparoscopic images, since CT images are taken before pneumoperitoneum process in most cases. This paper proposes a method for elevating an abdominal wall based on volumetric deformation. We deform original 3-D abdominal CT images so that the abdominal wall is virtually elevated. Then, virtual laparoscopic images are generated from the deformed image. As far as we know, there is no report on simulating pneumoperitoneum for creating virtual laparoscopic images.

In Section 2, we describes the detail procedures for creating virtual laparoscopic views. Section 3 shows experimental result of virtual pneumoperitoneum. We add brief discussion in Section 4.

2   Method

2.1   Overview

The entire process consists of five major steps: (a) extraction of abdominal wall, (b) elastic modeling, (c) elastic deformation of the model, (d) deformation of the original image, and (e) rendering of virtual laparoscopic images. We explain each steps below.

2.2   Abdominal Wall Extraction

We extract abdominal wall regions from input 3-D images. Abdominal wall regions comprise fat, muscle, and skin regions. Since these regions show very similar CT values, it is very difficult to segment abdominal wall regions based on simple thresholding. Therefore, we manually trace abdominal wall regions on slice

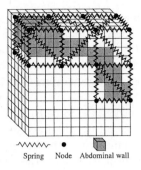

Spring   Node   Abdominal wall

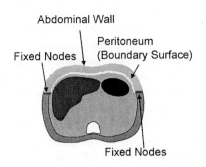

Fig. 1. Illustration of elastic cube allocation. Gray voxels are voxels forming the abdominal wall regions traced manually, while white voxels are non-abdominal wall regions that will not be deformed in the virtual pneumoperitoneum procedure. In this figure, we allocated one elastic cube for $4 \times 4 \times 4$ voxels regions for avoiding the figure becomes complex for understanding.

Fig. 2. An explanation of boundary surface and fixed nodes. thick yellow line shows peritoneum and red lines show the boundaries where nodes are fixed. The nodes on the dark gray boundaries are not forced to be moved during the deformation process.

images. The traced regions are used as the target areas of virtual pneumoperitoneum.

2.3 Elastic Modeling

Tetrahedron Division. In the proposed method we deform only abdominal wall regions for simplification, although underlying organs such as the liver, the colon, or the kidney is also deformed during pneumoperitoneum. In the elastic modeling process, we model the abdominal regions extracted in the above step by using a node and spring model. The node and spring model can compute deformation of the target regions by calculating forces working on each node and then moving the nodes to the directions of the resultant force.

We divide the extracted abdominal region into a set of cubes for reducing the computational time of deformation. Each cube consists of $8 \times 8 \times 8$ voxels. Figure 1 shows an example of elastic cube allocation. We consider vertices of a cube as nodes and assign springs on the edges and the diagonals on the surfaces of a cube (Fig. 1). One cube is divided into five tetrahedrons by this tessellation. Each tetrahedron consists of four nodes and six springs. The natural length of a spring is the distance between two connected nodes. We fix the nodes on the boundary surfaces that exist between the extracted abdominal walls and other regions as shown in Fig. 2.

Forces for deformation. We deform the abdominal wall by adding virtual air pressure to the boundary surfaces. The abdominal lifting is achieved by calculating elastic deformation of tetrahedrons. In this paper, we consider three types of forces working on nodes in the deformation steps: (a) force caused by springs $\mathbf{F}_s$, (b) force that maintains the volumes of tetrahedrons $\mathbf{F}_v$, and (c) forces caused by air pressure $\mathbf{F}_b$. The type (c) force is considered only for the nodes on the boundary surfaces. Here, we denote a set of nodes that are connected to the i-th node by springs as N_i. A set of tetrahedrons that has the i-th node as their vertices is denoted as T_i.

In the n-th iteration step of deformation calculation, the force $\mathbf{F}_i(n)$ working on the i-th node is calculated as the resultant force of: (a) the force caused by the springs between the i-th node and the nodes connected to the i-th node and (force by springs) (b) the force caused by tetrahedrons that have the i-th node (force for preserving volume and force by air pressure). Hence the resultant force $\mathbf{F}(n)_i$ is described as

$$\mathbf{F}_i(n) = \sum_{j \in N_i} \mathbf{F}_{s_{i,j}}(n) + \sum_{t \in T_i} \mathbf{F}_{v_{i,t}}(n) + \mathbf{F}_{b_i}, \tag{1}$$

where $\mathbf{F}_{s_{ij}}$ means the force caused by the spring between the i-th node and the j-th node connected to it, $\mathbf{F}_{v_{it}}$ the force caused by the t-th tetrahedron that has the i-th node as its vertex.

2.4   Iterative Deformation

Each node is moved to the direction of the force working on it at very small distance. Moving distance is in proportion to the magnitude of the calculated force. We iteratively calculate the movement of each node. At the n-th iteration step, the position of the i-th node for the $(n + 1)$-th iteration step $\mathbf{R}_i(n + 1)$ is computed by

$$\mathbf{R}_i(n + 1) = \mathbf{R}_i(n) + \varDelta s \mathbf{F}_i(n), \tag{2}$$

where $\varDelta s$ is a constant that controls the distance of movement at each iteration step. The movements of nodes are sequentially performed along the ordered list that holds the nodes. We iterate this movement step until

$$\sum_{i \in S} \| \mathbf{R}_i(n + 1) - \mathbf{R}_i(n) \| < \beta, \tag{3}$$

where β is a constant for determining convergence of the movement.

2.5   Reconstruction of Volumetric Image

After the deformation process, we reconstruct a volumetric image from the original image by using the relation between tetrahedrons of before- and after-deformation. This process generates a deformed volumetric image where the abdominal wall is elevated.

There is one-to-one relation between vertices of a tetrahedron of after- and before-deformation. We deform the original 3-D image by using this relations.

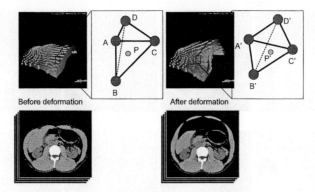

Fig. 3. Geometric correspondence for volumetric image reconstruction. Points **A**, **B**, **C**, and **D** of before-deformation tetrahedron correspond to points **A′**, **B′**, **C′**, and **D′** of deformed tetrahedron. Point **P**, which is inside after-deformation tetrahedron, corresponds to point **P** inside before-deformation tetrahedron.

Let us consider the tetrahedron t and its deformed one t'. We denote vertices of a tetrahedron t as **A**, **B**, **C**, and **D**. The vertices of the deformed tetrahedron t' are also described as **A′**, **B′**, **C′**, and **D′** (Fig. 3. A point **P**', which is inside of the deformed tetrahedron t', is represented by using four positional vectors **A′**, **B′**, **C′**, and **D′** and four real variables u, v, w, and x as

$$\mathbf{P}' = u\mathbf{A}' + v\mathbf{B}' + w\mathbf{C}' + x\mathbf{D}', \tag{4}$$

where u, v, w, and x satisfy

$$u + v + w + x = 1, \tag{5}$$
$$0 \leq u, v, w, x \leq 1. \tag{6}$$

By using Eqs. (4), (5), and (6), we can obtain actual values of u, v, w, and x. The point **P** of the tetrahedron t', which corresponds to **P′**, is also represented by using u, v, w, and x as

$$\mathbf{P} = u\mathbf{A} + v\mathbf{B} + w\mathbf{C} + x\mathbf{D}. \tag{7}$$

The CT value on the point **P′** is calculated from the CT value on **P** of the original image by the tri-linear interpolation. Consequently, we obtain the deformed CT image by calculating CT values on all grid points of the image.

2.6   Visualization

The deformed image is visualized by volume rendering method[7] for obtaining virtual laparoscopic image. It is possible to generate virtual laparoscopic view by putting a viewpoint of the virtual camera inside the virtually generated abdominal cavity. We can also color the liver, the kidney, and the descending aorta in virtual laparoscopic views by using the segmentation results of the organs.

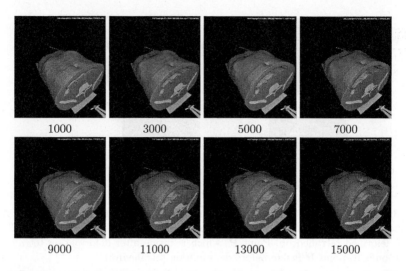

| 1000 | 3000 | 5000 | 7000 |

| 9000 | 11000 | 13000 | 15000 |

Fig. 4. Progress of abdominal wall elevation. Numbers of iterations in elastic deformation are shown below each figure. These figures show the abdominal wall is gradually elevated by our method.

3   Experiments

We have applied the proposed method to three cases of 3-D abdominal CT images and generated virtual laparoscopic images. Acquisition parameters of the CT images are: 512 × 512 pixels, 0.625 (Cases A and B) or 0.606 (Case C) mm / pixel, 489 (Case A), 171 (Case B), 229 (Case C) slices, 2.0 mm slice thickness, and 1.0 mm reconstruction interval. The parameter used in the experiments is adjusted experimentally so that the proposed method can generate appropriate virtual pneumoperitoneum images. Actual value of the parameter is set to $\Delta s = 0.3$. The abdominal wall regions are traced by one of the authors (Y. Hayashi).

The results of virtual pneumoperitoneum are shown in Fig. 4. This figure shows the progress of virtual pneumoperitoneum. It is clear that the abdominal wall is gradually lifted by the proposed method. An example of the deformed CT slices is shown in Fig. 5. Abdominal cavity is generated just above the stomach and the liver. Figure 6 shows a visualization of the liver, the descending aorta, the kidney, and the spleen, which were segmented by the method described in the reference[8] in the virtual laparoscopic image. A semi-translucent display technique was used. Figure 7 also shows a virtual laparoscopic view generated from the contrasted CT images (Case B). The liver and stomach regions are clearly visualized on these images. It took 75 minutes for the deformation process by a conventional PC that equips Intel Pentium III 933 MHz processor.

4   Discussion

As shown in Figs. 4-7, the proposed method can generate virtual laparoscopic views from abdominal CT images, which are taken before a real pneumoperi-

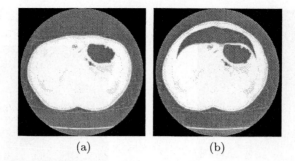

(a)   (b)

Fig. 5. Example of deformed slice images (Case A). (a) before deformation and (b) after deformation.

toneum process, by employing image deformation techniques based on the node-spring model. Virtual laparoscopic views depict the inside of the abdominal cavity and organs from arbitrary viewpoints view directions. Thus, a medical doctor can see the positional relation between lesions and the surrounding organs using these views before surgery. The virtual pneumoperitoneum proposed here can also be considered as a similation of pneumoperitoneum. A surgeon can intuitively determine the relation of each organ and where to insert instruments: a trocar, a laparoscope, and forceps. Therefore, virtual laparoscopic views generated by our method play an important role as images for surgical planning or as intraoperative reference images of laparoscopic surgery. We intend to use the generated virtual laparoscopic views in this paper as the reference images for making surgical plans before actual surgery, for understanding the relation of each organ, and for auxiliary views of a real laparoscope. The generated images are not used for surgical navigation that requires half a millimeter of guidance accuracy. We believe the simple elastic model employed here is enough for these purposes.

The elastic model in this paper is constructed only for abdominal wall regions. However, if we elevate the abdominal wall by inflating the abdominal cavity, the organ existing under the peritoneum also deforms because of air pressure. We ignored the deformation of organs here. As the future work, we need to develop a method that can simulate the deformation of abdominal organs and reduce the computation time. In addition, we need to improve a method that can clearly visualize organs existing inside the abdominal cavity, though the visibility of the segmented organs is improved by coloring the organs as shown in Fig. 6.

5   Conclusion

This paper proposed a method for virtual elevation of the abdominal wall for generating virtual laparoscopic views. Elastic modeling was used for simulating elevation. Virtual laparoscopic views were obtained from the image that is deformed by using the deformation results of the elastic model. Because CT images

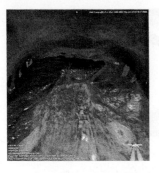

Fig. 6. Virtual laparoscopic view that visualizes the liver, the descending aorta, the kidney, and the spleen in the virtual laparoscopic image by employing semi-translucent display (Case A). The liver is colored in dark red, the kidney in yellow, the descending aorta in green, and the spleen in green.

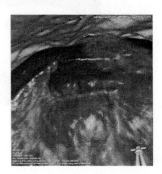

Fig. 7. Virtual laparoscopic view generated from contrasted CT images (Case B).

were taken before the elevation process, our method is quite useful for rendering virtual laparoscopic images from such images. Future work includes: (1) validation of the deformation results, (2) automated extraction of the abdominal wall, (3) application to many cases, and (4) reduction of the computation time.

Acknowledgments. The authors thank Dr. Shigeru Nawano of National Cancer Center East, Japan for providing CT images and foe his useful comments for the viewpoint of the medical field. The authors also thank our colleagues for their suggestions and advices. Parts of this research were supported by the Grant-In-Aid for Scientific Research from the Ministry of Education, the 21st century COE program, the Grant-In-Aid for Scientific Research from the Ministry of Education, Culture, Sports, Science, and Technology, Japan Society for Promotion of Science, and the Grant-In-Aid for Cancer Research from the Ministry of Health and Welfare.

References

1. N. Ayache, S. Cotin, H. Delingette et al., "Simulation of endoscopic surgery," Minimally Invasive therapy and Allied Technologies, vol. 7, no. 2, pp. 71–77, 1998
2. A. E. Kerdok, S. M. Cotin, M. P. Ottensmeyer et al., "Truth cube: Establishing physical standards for soft tissue simulation," Medical Image Analysis, vol. 6, no. 3, pp. 283–291, 2003
3. N. Suzuki and S. Suzuki, "Surgery simulation system with haptic sensation and modeling of elastic organ that reflect the patients' anatomy," Proc. of Surgery Simulation and Soft tissue Modeling, Lecture Notes in Computer Science, vol. 2673, pp. 155-164, 2003

4. M. A. Audette, A. Fuchs, O. Astley et al., "Towards patient-specific anatomical model generation for finite element-based surgical simulation," Proc. of Surgery Simulation and Soft tissue Modeling, Lecture Notes in Computer Science, vol. 2673, pp. 340-351, 2003
5. P. Rogalla, J.Terwisscha van Scheltinga, B. Hamm eds., "Virtual Endoscopy and Related 3D Techniques," Springer, Berlin, 2001
6. K. Mori, A. Urano, J. Hasegawa et al., "Virtualized endoscope system -An application of virtual reality technology to diagnostic aid," IEICE Trans. on Information and System, vol. E79-D, no. 6, pp. 809-819, 1996
7. K. Mori, Y. Suenaga and J. Toriwaki, "Fast software-based volume rendering using multimedia instructions on PC platforms and its application to virtual endoscopy," Medical Imaging 2003: Physiology and Function: Methods, Systems, and Application, Proceedings of SPIE, vol. 5031, pp. 111-122, 2003
8. K. Yokoyama, T. Kitasaka, K. Mori et al., "Liver region extraction from 3D abdominal X-ray CT images using distribution features of abdominal organs," Journal of Computer Aided Diagnosis of Medical Images, vol. 7, no. 4-3, 2003

Soft Tissue Resection for Prostatectomy Simulation

Miguel A. Padilla Castañeda and Fernando Arámbula Cosío

Image and Vision Lab.,
Centre of Applied Research and Technology (CCADET),
National Autonomous University of México (UNAM),
México, D.F., 04510
{arambula, padillac}@aleph.cinstrum.unam.mx

Abstract. In this paper we present a computer model of the prostate for prostatectomy simulation. Through the modification of the 3D mesh, the model is able to simulate resections of soft tissue produced by the user with a virtual resectoscope. At each resection the model shows deformations of the tissue surrounding the resection zone. A mass-spring 3D mesh is used to model tissue deformation due to the interaction with the surgical tool. Our model is designed to be the basis of a surgery training system for Transurethral Resection of the Prostate (TURP).

1 Introduction

The prostate is a chestnut sized gland located next to the bladder in human males. The urethra runs from the bladder neck through the prostate to the penile urethra. A frequent condition in men above 50 years old is the benign enlargement of the prostate known as Benign Prostatic Hyperplasia (BHP), which in some cases results in significant blockage of the urinary flow. The standard surgical procedure to treat a hypertrophied prostate gland is the Transurethral Resection of the Prostate (TURP). It essentially consists of the removal of the inner lobes of the prostate in order to relieve urinary outflow obstruction.

Less invasive surgical techniques such as Transuretral Incision of the Prostate, Microwave Therapy, Transurethral Needle Ablation, and High Frequency Focused Ultrasound, have been developed to treat BPH. However TURP remains the most commonly used surgical procedure to treat BPH [1]. During a TURP the surgeon inserts a cylindrical instrument called resectoscope - which carries in its interior a cylindrical lens and the resecting element - through the urethra of the patient up to the prostate. The surgeon then removes the lobes of the prostate by resection of small tissue chips. Mastering the TURP technique requires a highly developed hand–eye coordination which enables the surgeon to orientate inside the prostate, using only the monocular view of the lens of the resectoscope. Current training of TURP is mainly performed by example, with residents observing a large number of procedures performed by an experienced surgeon. Eventually, each resident is allowed to perform partial procedures under the supervision of the expert. Towards the end of the training period, the resident performs a full TURP under supervision. There are few practice

C. Barillot, D.R. Haynor, and P. Hellier (Eds.): MICCAI 2004, LNCS 3217, pp. 568–576, 2004.

opportunities available to the residents during the current training process. Practice is limited to the resection of artificial models which can be expensive, or potatoes which are unrealistic. Computers can help to improve TURP training through realistic simulation of prostate resections.

Realistic simulation of soft tissue cutting and deformation is one of the most important research topics in surgery simulation. The purpose is to manipulate 3D tissue models in real time with acceptable visual quality. Bro-Nielsen [2] reported an approach for surgery simulation based on a finite element method for real time deformations which uses a technique called condensation, in order to work only with the surface mesh elements, reducing in this way the time response of the model. Unfortunately this method is too slow for the simulation of tissue cutting operations even with simple mesh modifications. Bielser and Gross [3] reported an interactive simulation technique for surgical cuts that simulates cutting operations using a virtual scalpel. The cuts in their approach are made in a line like way, and they focus on the problem of refining the mesh along the cut line to produce continuous dissections. Gomes *et al.* [4] reported a computer assisted system for TURP based on real time optical tracking and a geometric model of the prostate, but which does not include a prostate model that simulates the physical behaviour of soft tissue. Ballaro *et al.* [5] reported a simulator for prostatic resection based on a magnetic tracker and a 3D model of the prostatic urethra which simulates deformation, resection and bleeding. The capsule of the prostate is not included in the model and therefore overall shape change of the prostate is not calculated. The paper focuses on the clinical aspects of the system and little technical detail of the model construction is provided.

In this work is reported a model for TURP simulation which incorporates tissue resection and deformation. The elastic behaviour of the whole prostate gland is modelled with the mass-spring method for deformable bodies. Resections are modelled through the removal of nodes and geometrical elements from the volumetric 3D mesh. The results show that the model is able to simulate deformations and resections performed by the user. This model is intended to be used in a surgery training system for TURP.

In the next section is described the construction of the geometric model of the prostate. In section 3 is described the use of the mass-spring method for simulation of deformations of the prostate model. In section 4 we report the tissue resection mechanism used for simulation. In section 5 we show a sequence of simulated prostate resections, and in section 6 we present the conclusions of the work reported.

2 Geometric Model of the Prostate

To reconstruct the three-dimensional shape of the prostate, the mesh generation method uses a set of transurethral, ultrasound images, separated by intervals of *5mm*. To acquire the images a lead screw mechanism, rigidly fixed to the operating table, was used to move the ultrasound probe along the urethra from the bladder neck to the *verumontanum* (Fig. 1).

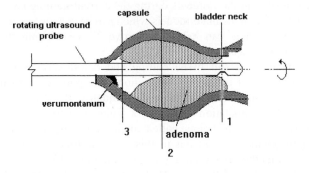

Fig. 1. Transurethral ultrasound scanning of the prostate

The lead screw mechanism maintains all the images parallel to each other and mostly transverse to the prostate. Some small distortion of the final prostate shape is likely to occur since the urethra has a natural slight bent at the middle and the ultrasound probe straightens it during image acquisition [6]. For a training simulator a slight distortion of the prostate model does not affect the usefulness of the system, as long as the final model still looks like a realistic prostate to a specialist. All the images acquired from a prostate are annotated by an expert in ultrasound (Fig. 2).

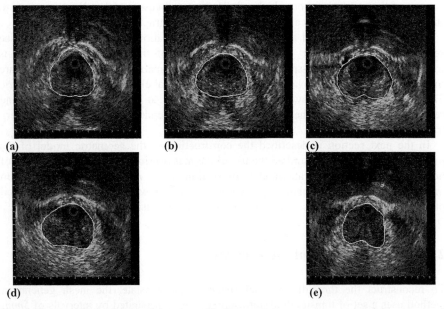

Fig. 2. Transurethral ultrasound images with the prostate contours annotated by an expert sonographer: **(a)** At *5mm* from the bladder neck; **(b)** At *10mm*; **(c)** At *15mm*; **(d)** At *20mm*; **(e)** At *25mm*

Each of the contours of the prostate capsule was sampled in a radial manner, taking as the origin the centre of the transurethral ultrasound transducer. The number of samples is determined by the size of the sampling angle α, which is the control parameter of the mesh generation method. The same procedure is applied to the contour of the prostatic urethra, forming a set of cross-sections C with both capsule and urethra samples. Since it is not possible to identify the prostatic urethra from ultrasound images, we drew an approximate urethra contour on each of the ultrasound images. In this manner, the sampled points of every cross-section cs_i (with the capsule and the urethra contours) in C, represent the control points of the prostate shape.

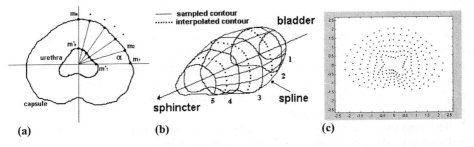

(a)   (b)   (c)

Fig. 3. (a) Radial sampling of a prostate cross-section with sampling angle α and n sample pairs ($n=360/\alpha$). (b) 3D surface mesh interpolated from the transurethral ultrasound cross-sections. (c) Internal points obtained from the capsule to the urethra with $\alpha = 10$ and $l = 0.187828$

In order to control the uniformity of the mesh, we calculated the average length (l) of all the segments m_{ij} and m'_{ij} in C, that join the control points m_i and m_j of the capsule, and the control point m'_i and m'_j of the urethra, respectively (Fig. 3.a). The next step is to transform the prostate shape C, typically composed by 5 to 12 cross-section images (separated at $5mm$), into the new shape C^* now composed by n target cross-sections separated by the average distance l, previously calculated. C^* is generated using cubic spline interpolation over the control points of C (Fig. 3.b). To model the prostate as a solid body, the algorithm also interpolates, for every cross-section cs_j in C^*, k internal sampled contours from the capsule to the urethra (Fig. 3.c). Again, the number of k inner contours depends on the l value. Finally, the last step is to arrange the solid body of the prostate as a mass-spring mesh of lattice form, where every node $v_{i,j,k}$ in the body is linked with at most 6 adjacent nodes ($v_{i+1,j,k}$, $v_{i,j+1,k}$, $v_{i,j,k+1}$, $v_{i+1,j+1,k}$, $v_{i+1,j+1,k+1}$ and $v_{i+1,j+1,k+1}$).

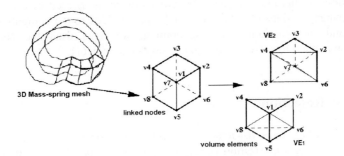

Fig. 4. Volume elements of the 3D mass-spring mesh of the prostate

Figure 4 illustrates the arrangement of the 3D prostate mesh. Additional geometric volume elements of the form of a pentahedron (VE_1 and VE_2) are constructed. As we will show in the next section, the form of these volume elements is useful for simulating tissue resection operations.

3 Physical Model of the Prostate

The behaviour of the prostate is modelled as a deformable body with physical characteristics like mass, stiffness and damping coefficients. These physical characteristics were adapted to the volumetric 3D mesh constructed before, to produce a viscoelastic 3D mesh. This was done using the spring-mass method [7, 8], where every node in the mesh represents a mass point that is interconnected with its neighbours by springs and which moves in a viscous medium, this method allows us to simulate real time deformations.

The dynamic behaviour of the system, formed by the spring-mass elements in the volumetric mesh, is based on the *Lagrange* equation of motion.

$$m_i \frac{d^2 \mathbf{x_i}}{dt^2} + \gamma_i \frac{d\, \mathbf{x_i}}{dt} + \mathbf{g_i}(t, \mathbf{x_i}) = \mathbf{f_i}(t, \mathbf{x_i}) \tag{1}$$

Where m_i is the mass of the node i in the mesh, at *Cartesian* coordinates $\mathbf{x}_i$; γ_i is the damping coefficient of the node (viscosity of the medium); $\mathbf{g}_i$ is the internal elastic force and $\mathbf{f}_i$ are the external forces acting on the node.

In this approach the internal elastic forces acting on the node i are given by the following linear equation:

$$g_i = \sum_{j \in N(i)} \mu_{i,j} \frac{\left(\left\| x_i - x_j \right\| - l^0_{i,j} \right) \left(x_i - x_j \right)}{\left\| x_i - x_j \right\|} \tag{2}$$

Where $N(i)$ is the set of neighbours of the node i; $\mu_{i,j}$ is the stiffness coefficient of the spring connecting the nodes i and j for every j in $N(i)$; and $l^0_{i,j}$ is the spring length at rest position. In this manner, the deformations occur as a result of the inner elastic energy change, produced by the spring deformation. Due to the computational speed needed and for simplicity of programming, we have used the Newton-Euler integration method to solve the dynamic systems equation (1).

4 Tissue Resection

During a TURP the basic tissue removal mechanisms consist of the resection (using a resection loop) or vaporization (using a vaporization roller) of small tissue chips. Tissue resection during TURP modifies significantly the shape of the prostate. The urologist produces a cavity inside the obstructed urethra, by resecting the adenomatous tissue until the capsule is reached.

Due to the shape of each cut during TURP, it is difficult to simulate tissue resections through geometric modifications of a tetrahedral mesh. Tetrahedral remeshing techniques are useful for tissue cutting produced by scalpels, but seem difficult to adapt for carving of small tissue chips, as it occurs during TURP. Instead, we use a simplified approach that takes advantage of the mass-spring mesh arrangement described in the previous section, based on pentahedral volume elements. Resection of tissue chips is simulated through the removal of volume elements around the resection zone, and the corresponding tissue deformation, as follows.

Let v_c be the node of the mesh where the collision between the prostate body and the resection element of the resectoscope, occurs; let c_r be the cutting radius of the resection element which controls the amount of tissue to be resected (typically *3mm* to *5mm*); let $\mathbf{fc_{ij}}$ be the force necessary to fully compress the spring that links the nodes i and j; let $\mathbf{fr_i}$ be the resection force exerted on the node i after a resection occurs (set initially to zero). Once a collision between the prostate and the resection element is detected, the closest surface node (v_c) to the resection element is calculated. Then, the algorithm determines the list L of volume elements on the vicinity of v_c, that are under the cutting radius c_r which must be removed from the mesh. After L is obtained, all the volume elements e in L and its mechanical elements -masses m in e, and springs s adjacent to m, must be removed from the mesh. During a TURP the prostate deforms and the capsule may slightly collapse as the surgery progresses. In order to simulate this change of size of the prostate, the algorithm deforms the mesh as a result of the energy produced by the internal force of the springs removed. As a result of this mesh modification procedure, tissue resections are produced.

The resection algorithm progressively removes the nodes inside the vicinity of c_r starting from the collision node v_c. The resection forces $\mathbf{fr_k}$ acting over the k nodes around c_r after the resection, must also be progressively determined. Initially $\mathbf{fr_n}$ is set to zero for the n nodes that form the original mesh.

After a spring ij is removed, the corresponding compressing force $\mathbf{fc_{ij}}$ needed to move the node i to the position of its j neighbour is calculated. The compressing force $\mathbf{fc_i}$ over i represents the resultant force needed to move i due to the contribution of $\mathbf{fc_{ij}}$ for every spring ij removed from the mesh. As the algorithm progresses if i must also be removed from the mesh (because there are no springs connected to i), its previously computed compressing force $\mathbf{fc_i}$ is added to the resection force $\mathbf{fr_k}$ of all its k neighbours. The algorithm continues until all the elements inside c_r are removed from the mesh. In this way, after a resection is performed, the $\mathbf{fr_m}$ forces acting on the resection zone around c_r, represent the resection forces acting on Eq. 1 for every node m adjacent to c_r that remains after the mesh modification. The local effect of resection is the deformation of the tissue surrounding the resection zone, as a result of the contribution of the resection forces of all the elements removed from the mesh. The global result of all resections and the corresponding local tissue deformations is the change of size of the prostatic capsule and the slight collapse of the remaining inner tissue.

5   Results

The model described was implemented in C using the OpenGL libraries for rendering, on a Sun-Solaris workstation (with one Sparc processor @ 1 Ghz), without graphics acceleration hardware. A display rate of 8 frames/s approx. was observed for a sampling angle of 8 deg., this is below the 10 frames/s recommended as the minimum for visual realism. However significantly higher frame rates should be possible with the use of graphics acceleration hardware, since the processing time of the model alone allows for more than 12 frames/s at a sampling angle of 8 deg. In addition, for the implementation of the simulator two computers may be used, one for processing of the user interface inputs and collision detection, and the other machine for model update and display.

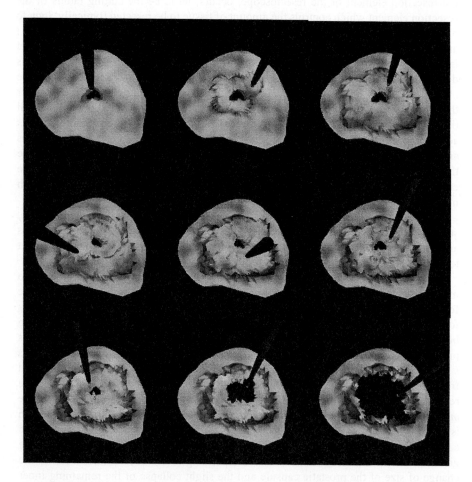

Fig. 5. Cavity produced near the urethra after some resections (from top-left to bottom-right). After every resection the tissue deforms, and after several tissue resections are performed a cavity is produced and the prostate slightly collapses

The slides on Fig. 5 show a simulated resection of the prostate model. The figure presents a prostate with a urethra, almost completely obstructed by the tissue that has grown in excess. The slides also show the removing process of the adenoma. It can be observed the cavity produced after several tissue resections from the obstructed urethra, and the progressive change of size of the prostate capsule.

6 Conclusions

This paper presents a computer model of the prostate that is the basis for the development of a real-time virtual reality simulator for TURP training. Details of the construction of the geometric model of the prostate, as well as the deformation and resection simulation schemes used, are reported.

The results show that the model is well suited for resection simulation that involves tissue resection and tissue deformation. During resection simulation, when collision with the virtual resectoscope is detected, appropriate mechanical and geometrical elements from the mesh are removed and the inner tissue of the prostate is exposed. The model is able to reproduce tissue resections of different sizes, depending on the cutting radius of the resectoscope. Along with resections, the model simulates in real-time tissue deformations and the global collapse of the prostate capsule as the resection of the adenoma progresses.

The user interface for the TURP simulator is currently being developed. As a first approximation a passive mechanism with 5 degrees of freedom, instrumented with position sensors will be used to provide positional feedback only. Force feedback is not considered at this stage since the forces felt by the user during resection are small due to the vaporization of tissue. A phantom of the prostate capsule will be used to limit the resection region. The suitability of using only positional feedback will be evaluated during clinical validation of the simulator.

References

1. Yang Q., Abrams P., Donovan J., Mulligan S., Williams G.: Transurethral resection or incision of the prostate and other therapies: a survey of treatments for benign prostatic obstruction in the UK. BJU International, **84**, (1999) 640-645.
2. Bro-Nielsen, M.: Finite Element Modeling in Surgery Simulation. Proceedings of the IEEE **86** No. 3 (1998) 490-503.
3. Bielser, D., Gross, M.: Interactive Simulation of surgical Cuts. Computer Graphics and Applications. Proceedings of the IEEE on The Eighth Pacific Conference, (2000) 116 – 442.
4. Gomes, M.P.S.F., Barret, A.R.W., Timoney, A.G., Davies, B.L.: A Computer Assisted Training/Monitoring System for TURP Structure and Design. IEEE Trans. On Information Technology in Biomed. **3** No. 4 (1999) 242-250.
5. Ballaro A., Briggs T., García-Montes F., MacDonald D., Emberton M., and Mundy A.R.: A Computer Generated Interactive Transurethral Prostatic Resection Simulator. Journal of Urology **162** (1999) 1633-1635.

6.   Nathan M.S., Mei Q., Seenivasagam K., Davies B., Wickham J.E.A. and Miller, R.A.,
      "Comparison of prostatic volume and dimensions by transrectal and transurethral
      ultrasonography", British Journal of Urology, **78**, pp.84-89, 1996.
7.   Güdükbay, U., Özgüç, B., Tokad, Y.: A spring force formulation for elastically
      deformable models. Computers & Graphics **21** No. 3 (1997) 335-346.
8.   Kühnapfel, U., Cakmak H.K., MaaB, H., "Endoscopic surgery training using virtual
      reality and deformable tissue simulation", Computers and Graphics, **24**, pp. 671-682, 2000

Precalibration Versus 2D-3D Registration for 3D Guide Wire Display in Endovascular Interventions

Shirley A.M. Baert, Graeme P. Penney, Theo van Walsum, and Wiro J. Niessen

Image Sciences Institute, University Medical Center Utrecht
Rm E 01.335, P.O.Box 85500, 3508 GA Utrecht, The Netherlands
{shirley,graeme,theo,wiro}@isi.uu.nl

Abstract. During endovascular interventions, the radiologist relies on 2D projection images to advance the guide wire, while often a pre-operative 3D image of the vasculature is available. To take full advantage of the 3D information, two different methods are proposed and compared for 3D guide wire reconstruction and visualization in the 3D vasculature. Upon tracking the guide wire in biplane fluoroscopy images, the first approach utilizes a precalibrated C-arm system to determine the guide wire position in the 3D coordinate system of the vasculature. In the second method the relation between the projection images and the 3D vascular data is determined using intensity based 2D-3D registration. Based on a study on an anthropomorphic phantom, it is shown that the calibration method is highly accurate, but that in case of imperfect geometry knowledge results rapidly degrade. For 2D-3D registration, similar accurate results were obtained with a 97.8 (84.2)% success rate if the registration starting position was within 4 (8) degrees rotation and 5 (10) mm translation of the reference position. The latter method has also been used to succesfully reconstruct a guide wire in a patient dataset.

1 Introduction

During endovascular interventions, it is important for the radiologist to accurately know the 3D position of the guide wire at any time during the procedure. Currently, 2D fluoroscopic projection images are used for navigation. Therefore, a mental reconstruction of the position and orientation of the guide wire in 3D has to be performed, which can be a difficult task. With the introduction of motorized calibrated X-ray angiography, a 3D reconstruction of the vasculature can be obtained immediately prior to the intervention. Visualizing the guide wire in the 3D vasculature could potentially be used as an additional navigation tool for the radiologist. One method is to track the guide wire in the biplanar fluoroscopic images to reconstruct its position in 3D.

In order to produce a 3D reconstruction of the guide wire and relate it to the 3D coordinate system of the 3D vascular data, accurate knowledge of the C-arm geometry is required. To this end, a wide range of calibration procedures have been proposed. In this paper two approaches are proposed and compared. In the

C. Barillot, D.R. Haynor, and P. Hellier (Eds.): MICCAI 2004, LNCS 3217, pp. 577–584, 2004.

first approach, the fact that the interventions are carried out on a fixed system with reproducible geometry is exploited. The system geometry is estimated in a precalibration step [1] that only has to be carried out once. The advantage of this approach is that it does not hamper intraoperative logistics or image quality, as no changes have to be made to the intraoperative situation. A disadvantage is that to maintain the relation between the 3D vascular data and the projection images, the patient should be stabilized or tracked during the intervention. In the second approach, anatomical information that is contained in the images is used to relate the 3D vascular data to projection images. There are various methods to achieve this, and in this paper intensity-based 2D-3D registration is considered.

2 Calibration Methods

2.1 Precalibration

For the precalibration, the calibration method of the 3D rotational angiography facility on the Philips Integris BV5000 is used (see [1]). In this calibration step the geometry of the system and the image distortions are determined for a reproducible 3D rotational run over 180 degrees of the C-arm. Two types of distortion are present, pincushion distortion caused by the curved input screen on the image intensifier and s-shaped distortion caused by interactions between the earth's magnetic field and electrons in the image intensifier. The distortion is measured using a Cartesian-grid phantom with equally spaced grid-points and is modelled using bivariate polynomials. Distortion correction is performed to subpixel accuracy. The projection geometry is measured for each projection angle using the same grids and a calibration phantom, since the isocenter position is not constant due to mechanical bending of the C-arm.

2.2 Image-Based Calibration

For the image-based calibration, a DSA sequence that is routinely made in cerebral interventions for both the frontal and lateral C-arm, is registered with the priorly obtained 3D volume of the vasculature. We have used an intensity based 2D-3D registration algorithm [2,3] to register the pre-operative 3DRA data to the interventional DSA images. The algorithm produces digitally reconstructed radiographs (DRR's) which are compared to the DSA image using a similarity measure (gradient difference). The geometry information is comprised of two sets of parameters, intrinsic parameters which define the projection geometry of the fluoroscopy set and extrinsic parameters (3 rotational and 3 translational) which define the pose and position of the 3D volume with respect to the fluoroscopy set. The algorithm assumes that the intrinsic parameters are known, and alters the extrinsic parameters, using a gradient descent type search strategy, in order to optimize the similarity measure. A circular region of interest is defined in the DSA images in order to limit the registration to a particular region of the image and to speed up the algorithm. Since in general there is also no knowledge of the relative position between the C-arms, the procedure is carried out for both biplane images separately, which means that a monoplane 2D-3D registration is performed twice and independently. A small modification has been made to the algorithm as presented in [2,3] in order to improve its capture range: a global search varying only in plane translations (up to 20 mm in steps of 2 mm) and rotations (up to 20 degrees in steps of 4 degrees) is carried out prior to the full six degree of freedom optimization. DRR's produced at different stages in the registration process and a target DSA image are shown in Figure 1.

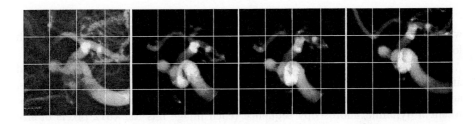

Fig. 1. Target DSA image (left) and three DRR's produced during the registration process; (from left to right) a DRR produced at the final registration position, after the initial in-plane registration, and at the starting position, respectively.

3   Experiments

After establishing the geometry information with either of the proposed methods, the 3D reconstruction of the guide wire is performed in three steps. Upon (i) tracking the guide wire in 2D biplane fluoroscopic images, the estimated geometry is used (ii) to determine corresponding points in both projections for guide wire reconstruction, and to (iii) show the guide wire together with the preoperatively acquired 3D vasculature. Information on the tracking method and 3D reconstruction method can be found in [4,5]. An accuracy study on a phantom and a feasibility study in a clinical case have been carried out.

3.1   Phantom Experiment

For all the experiments 3D runs over 180 degrees containing 100 projection images were made of an intracranial anthropomorphic vascular phantom using the rotational angiography facility of a Philips Integris BV5000 C-arm imaging system. Initially the phantom is filled with contrast to obtain a pre-operative 3D vasculature image ($256\times256\times256$ voxels of size $0.521\times0.521\times0.521$ mm^3), see Figure 2. After removing the contrast, a guide wire was advanced in 24 approximately equally spaced steps. After each advance a 3D reconstruction

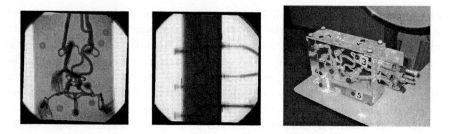

Fig. 2. Left and middle: two fluoroscopic images out of a 3D run showing the anthropomorphic vascular phantom (right) in frontal and lateral position.

was made. The extracted guide wire in these sequences servers as ground truth for the experiments.

From each 3DRA acquisition 19 of the 2D fluoroscopy images were extracted at 10 degree intervals between 0 and 180 degrees. Sets of fluoroscopy images, acquired at the same angle but at different time intervals, were used to represent a dynamic fluoroscopy sequence (each image has 512×512 pixels of size 0.527×0.527 mm^2). All images were corrected for distortion.

Experiments were carried out to determine the accuracy of the precalibartion based guide wire reconstruction as a function of the angle between the biplane images. Additionally, the influence of the accuracy of the precalibration was investigated.

Similar experiments were carried out for the image-based calibration. To estimate the capture range of the method, different starting positions were generated by altering the position of the 3D dataset from the precalibrated position using four different perturbations, consisting of ± 2°, ± 4°, ± 8°, ± 12° rotation and ± 2.5 mm, ± 5 mm, ± 10 mm, ± 15 mm translation, respectively. For each of these four perturbations, ten starting points were picked by randomly altering all of the six extrinsic parameters by either + or - the perturbation. In the experiments using image-based calibration, we used the distortion estimation from the precalibration method, to correct the images. If precalibration is only available in a number of C-arm positions, interpolation can be used, or other methods that have been proposed in the literature [6] can be applied.

3.2 Patient Experiment

Prior to a neuro-intervention a 3DRA image of the cerebral vasculature of the patient was made. At the beginning of the intervention, biplane DSA images were acquired for both C-arm positions, which were registered to the 3DRA volume (voxel size 0.385×0.385×0.385 mm^3) of the vasculature of the patient. During the intervention biplane fluoroscopy images were acquired (pixel size frontal images 0.278×0.278 mm^2 and pixel size lateral images 0.423×0.423 mm^2) while advancing the guide wire in the vasculature, on which the 2D guide wire tracking method was performed. An estimate of the source image distance, rotation and angulation of the C-arm system was obtained for both images from the C-arm system display. These values were used as a starting estimate for the registration algorithm.

4   Results

An example of the 3D reconstruction of the guide wire in the phantom images using precalibration is shown in Figure 3. Image-based calibration gives qualitatively similar results.

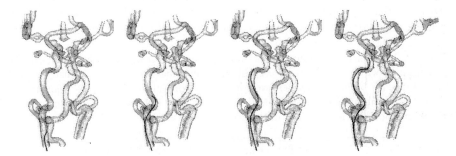

Fig. 3. Four frames (frame 2, 10, 16 and 24) out of a sequence of 24 frames, which gives an impression of the reconstruction results. The reconstructed guide wire position is within the vasculature in all cases.

4.1   Precalibration

The left graph in Figure 4 shows the mean distance between the estimated guide wire position and the reference position as a function of the angle between the biplane images and the errors in the precalibrated geometry. Using the precalibrated geometry, the mean distance is smaller than 0.5 mm and increases if the angle between the biplane images becomes very small (< 30 degrees) or very large (> 150 degrees). If an inaccuracy is introduced in the angulation, the error increases significantly. Table 1 presents the mean distance for all different combinations of inaccuracies in rotation and angulation, averaged over all experiments in the angular range from 30 to 150 degrees.

4.2   Image-Based Calibration

The right part of Figure 4 shows the mean errors in 3D guide wire reconstruction that are obtained with 2D-3D registration as image-based calibration method. Registration of the 2D DSA image with the 3DRA volume sometimes fails, especially when the starting position is located further away from the reference standard. If the distance between the estimated position of the focal spot after

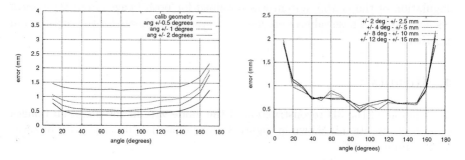

Fig. 4. Mean distance between the automatic reconstruction method and the manual 3DRA position segmentation for different angles between the biplane images (10-170 degrees) using precalibration (left) and image-based calibration (right).

Table 1. Distance in millimeters between the automatically and the manually obtained guide wire position using precalibration information. The mean distance and tip distance (in brackets) is taken over the angles from 30 to 150 degrees. The error is given if the calibrated geometry is used, and if errors (0.5, 1 and 2 degrees for rotation and angulation) in the accuracy of the geometry are introduced.

	Calibr. geom.	rot 0.5°	rot 1°	rot 2°
Calibr. geom.	0.42 [0.65]	0.60 [0.93]	0.79 [1.23]	1.37 [1.88]
ang 0.5°	0.62 [0.94]	0.75 [1.10]	0.99 [1.37]	1.57 [2.03]
ang 1°	0.85 [1.30]	0.96 [1.40]	1.17 [1.64]	1.74 [2.29]
ang 2°	1.31 [1.92]	1.43 [2.11]	1.62 [2.35]	2.12 [2.93]

registration and the focal spot position for the reference standard is larger than 3 centimeters, we define the registration to be unsuccessful. The unsuccessful registrations were not included in the calculation of the mean and tip distance of the 3D guide wire reconstruction. It can be observed that for small and large angles, the errors increase. Furthermore it can be observed that approximately the same minimum is found for all the successful registration regardless of the starting position.

Table 2 summarizes the mean and tip distances for the image-based calibration and lists the registration success rates. Values are averaged over 30 to 150 degrees angles, since the results are almost constant over this range. It can be observed from Table 2 that the geometry can be estimated using 2D-3D registration as accurately as by precalibration if a reasonable initialization is available. The success rate of the registrations falls off rapidly once the starting position exceeds 8° rotation and 10 mm translation from the reference standard.

Figure 5 shows the results if 2D-3D intensity based registration is used to determine the geometry information and the correspondence between the 2D

Table 2. Distance in millimeters between the automatically and the manually obtained guide wire position using image-based calibration. The mean distance and tip distance is taken over the angles from 30 to 150 degrees.

Starting position	Mean dist.	Tip dist.	Success rate
±2°-± 2.5 mm	0.42	0.71	100%
±4°-± 5 mm	0.39	0.69	97.9%
±8°-± 10 mm	0.40	0.70	84.2%
±12°-± 15 mm	0.42	0.67	55.8%

fluoroscopy images and the 3D volume in a clinical case. Owing to patient and table movement, which often occurs in our current clinical setup, only the image-based calibration procedure could be performed. It can be observed that the estimated position is within the vasculature. In the sixth image (lower right) a visualization is shown of a 3D reconstruction where the guide wire was manually outlined in the biplane projection images. Quantitative validation is not possible as no 3DRA image is acquired with the guide wire in the vasculature.

5   Discussion

3D information on the position of the guide wire with respect to the vasculature has the potential to improve the speed, accuracy and safety of endovascular interventions. Therefore, two methods for relating the projection images visualizing the guide wire to the preoperative obtained vasculature are described. The method based on precalibration requires that once the 3D vascular image is made, the patient should not move, or his motion should be tracked. The image-based registration method can be used if accurate precalibration information is not available or has become invalid due to patient and/or table movement.

Based on phantom experiments, it was concluded that for projection images with a relative angle in a large range (between 30 and 150 degrees) both methods achieved a mean distance error of approximately 0.4 mm and a tip distance of approximately 0.7 mm distance. For the precalibration method, the errors significantly increased if small inaccuracies in rotation and angulation were introduced, stressing the need for accurate calibration. For image-based calibration, the success rate depends on the initial starting positions. Byrne et al [7] have shown in a clinical setting for 10 patients, that patient movement between the 3D acquisition and the 2D intervention was within ± 4° rotation for 7 patients and within ± 8° rotation for the other 3 patients. In our experiments, for starting positions within 4° rotation and 5 mm translation in all directions, a success rate of 97.8% was obtained and for starting positions within 8° rotation and 10 mm translation, a success rate of greater than 84% could be obtained, which implies that image-based calibration could potentially be used in clinical practice.

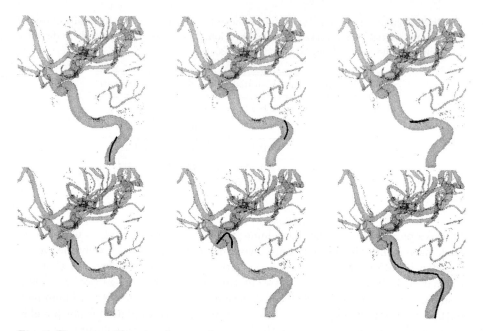

Fig. 5. Five non-subsequent frames of a patient image sequence. Only the tip is shown since in the 2D guide wire tracking only the proximal part of the guide wire is localized. The sixth image (lower right) is a 3D reconstruction from a manually outlined guide wire in the 2D projection images.

References

1. Koppe, R., Klotz, E., de Beek, J.O., Aerts, H.: 3D vessel reconstruction based on rotational angiography. In Lemke, H., Inamura, K., Jaffe, C., Vannier, M., eds.: Proceedings of CAR'95, Springer-Verlag, Berlin (1995) 101–107
2. Hipwell, J., Penney, G., Cox, T., Byrne, J., Hawkes, D.: 2D-3D intensity based registration of DSA and MRA - a comparison of similarity measures. In Dohi, T., Kikinis, R., eds.: Proceedings of MICCAI 2002, part II. Volume 2489 of Lecture Notes in Computer Science., Springer Verlag, Berlin (2002) 501–508
3. Penney, G., Batchelor, P., Hill, D., Hawkes, D., Weese, J.: Validation of a two- or three-dimensional registration algorithm for aligning preoperative CT images and intraoperative fluoroscopy images. Medical Physics **28** (2001) 1024–1032
4. Baert, S., Viergever, M., Niessen, W.: Guide wire tracking during endovascular interventions. IEEE Transactions on Medical Imaging **22** (2003) 965–972
5. Baert, S., van de Kraats, E., van Walsum, T., Viergever, M., Niessen, W.: 3D guide wire reconstruction from biplane image sequences for integrated display in 3D vasculature. IEEE Transactions on Medical Imaging **22** (2003) 1252–1258
6. Cañero, C., Vilariño, F., Mauri, J., Radeva, P.: Predictive (un)distortion model and 3-d reconstruction by biplane snakes. IEEE Transactions on Medical Imaging **21** (2002) 1188–1201
7. Byrne, J., Colominas, C., Hipwell, J., Cox, T., Noble, J., Penney, G., Hawkes, D.: An assessment of a technique for 2D-3D registration of cerebral intra-arterial angiography. British Journal of Radiology (2003)

Patient and Probe Tracking During Freehand Ultrasound

Giselle Flaccavento, Peter Lawrence, and Robert Rohling

Department of Electrical and Computer Engineering
University of British Columbia, Vancouver, Canada
{peterl,rohling}@ece.ubc.ca

Abstract. We present a system that measures the probe location with respect to the patient's body during an ultrasound exam. The system uses an inexpensive trinocular camera to track patches of points on a surface. The accuracy of the digital camera system is measured, using the Optotrak as a reference, and is less than ± 2 mm for a 20×20 mm patch. Fiducials, which can be seen in both the ultrasound images and the camera images, are used for a consistency test producing values with a standard deviation under 3.2 mm.

1 Introduction

The relative location of ultrasound images is often required for panoramic ultrasound, ultrasound assisted surgery, and freehand 3D ultrasound reconstruction [16]. The ultrasound probe is usually tracked with respect to a fixed coordinate system such as a bed or floor while the patient remains still. This stillness is achieved through the use of breath holds or restraining devices. Patient movement can be involuntary, due to respiration, or due to the force induced by the probe. In the dorsoventral direction, respiratory movement at the navel was recorded as 4.03 mm [4]. Probe force deformation as well as involuntary patient motion can cause much greater movement.

Although sometimes used to reduce the errors caused by respiration, breath holds and respiratory gating are not always feasible solutions as some people, especially young children [15], and sick patients would have difficulties holding their breath. Remaining still may be difficult due to arthritis in the neck, back, or shoulders [5]. Acquiring a set of data for a 3D ultrasound cardiac exam, can take up to 45 sec [11]. Maximum patient breath holds have been found to be 41 ± 20 sec [6]. Inconsistencies between breaths and respiratory drift after as little as 12 sec may also occur during a breath hold [9]. As the probe moves along the patient's skin, the tissue is displaced both globally and locally by the force of the probe [14].

In this paper, we present a probe and patient tracking system, shown in Figure 1, for use with both 3D and panoramic freehand ultrasound. We measure the probe location with respect to the patient's body by tracking both the probe and the patient. The goal is to produce a system with an accuracy better than

C. Barillot, D.R. Haynor, and P. Hellier (Eds.): MICCAI 2004, LNCS 3217, pp. 585–593, 2004.
© Springer-Verlag Berlin Heidelberg 2004

the motion incurred during the exam. The system we propose has the ability to track the motion of the area being examined during the ultrasound scan. Although we recognize that there is internal organ movement as well as external patient movement during the acquisition of images, this initial study aims to track only the external patient movement.

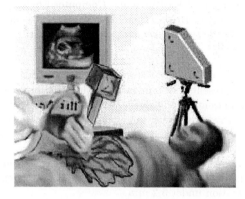

Fig. 1. Complete tracking system composed of both the digital camera and ultrasound tracking components.

Patient and probe motion compensation using external trackers during ultrasound have been previously investigated. In [1], an optical tracking system, with infra-red light emitting diode (IRED) markers, was used to track the probe along with one passive marker to track the navel. A single camera was used in [8] to track a rigid object with 4 known fiducial markers attached. Since only a few markers were used in both of these systems, the line of sight between the sensor and markers must be ensured throughout the procedure [10,13]. In [2], the patient motion is tracked using one magnetic sensor attached to the sternum. Magnetic position trackers are known to have reduced accuracy due to interference from ferromagnetic devices [7]. Instead of tracking the entire surface, these systems track only a small number of points on the patient or probe.

2   Methods

For our tracking system, we use a relatively inexpensive trinocular camera to track both the patient and the probe. A small object containing grayscale texture is attached to the probe in order to make tracking possible and more accurate. The number of features on the patient's skin is augmented with a painted grayscale texture as seen in Figure 1.

2.1 Digital Camera Tracking Component

The camera tracking component of our system uses a grayscale Digiclops trinocular stereo camera (Point Grey Research Inc., Vancouver, BC), with a field of view of 44°, a 6 mm focal length, and images of 1024 × 768 $pixels$. The accuracy of the digital camera system is computed in this paper through a series of experiments that track the location of two rigid objects, a calibration flat plate and a calibration sphere, which approximate a probe and the abdomen of a pregnant patient. We use the Optotrak 3020 positioning system (Northern Digital Inc., Waterloo, ON) as a reference standard to calculate the "true" location of our objects during tracking. Before the accuracy of the Digiclops can be calculated, it is first necessary to calculate the origin of the Digiclops coordinate system, C_D, which is located at the pinhole of one of the cameras, with respect to the Global Optotrak coordinate system, C_G. This is found by computing the transformation, T_G^D, shown in Figure 2, between C_D and C_G,

$$T_G^D = T_G^R T_R^P T_P^D = T_G^R T_R^P (T_D^P)^{-1} . \qquad (1)$$

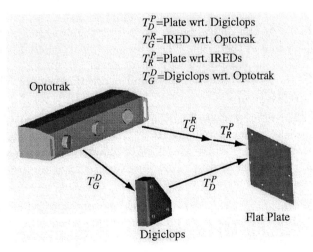

T_D^P=Plate wrt. Digiclops
T_G^R=IRED wrt. Optotrak
T_R^P=Plate wrt. IREDs
T_G^D=Digiclops wrt. Optotrak

Optotrak

T_G^R T_R^P

T_G^D T_D^P

Flat Plate

Digiclops

Fig. 2. Transformations used in determining the relationship between the Optotrak and Digiclops coordinate systems.

$\mathbf{T_D^P}$: The transformation between the plate and the Digiclops, T_D^P, is found using a grayscale texture with non-repeating features overlaid with 14 printed crosses and secured to the plate. The features are manually selected from the Digiclops images. Normalized correlation with subpixel interpolation is used to perform a template match between the two images. The 3D location of each feature point is found using triangulation. A plane and its normal are fitted to the 3D points using least squares minimization. The plate coordinate system,

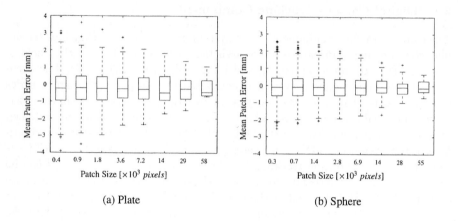

Fig. 3. Accuracy of tracking the surface of the flat plate and the sphere using various patch sizes. The standard deviation of the points for each test run is 0.9 mm to 1.6 mm for the plate and 0.6 mm to 1.1 mm for the sphere.

C_P, has a y direction that is computed by finding the direction vector between two chosen 3D points in the plane. The z direction is calculated parallel to the normal of the plane and passing through the origin of C_P. Finally, the x direction is calculated as the cross product of the y and z direction vectors. These vectors are then used to create T_D^P.

T_G^R: Six IREDs are attached to the surface of the plate enabling the Optotrak to also measure the plate's location. The transformation, T_G^R, from the IRED coordinate system, C_R, to C_G is next found. The geometry between 3 IREDs, secured to the back of the Digiclops case, is used to define C_G. Using the method described previously to find T_D^P, T_G^R is calculated.

T_R^P: The transformation, T_R^P, describes the offset between the location where the IREDs are attached to the plate and their recorded location based on the calibrated LED thickness.

T_G^D: Data is collected using various plate to Digiclops distances and angles. After calculating T_G^R, T_R^P, and T_D^P for each run, it is possible to calculate the unknowns in T_G^D using a least squares minimization to solve Equation 1.

The accuracy of the Digiclops system is next tested. A grayscale texture and 6 IREDs are attached to a flat test plate. The surface of a test sphere is painted with a grayscale texture and 12 IREDs are attached. The plate and sphere are placed at various locations ranging from 860 mm to 1050 mm from the Digiclops camera in order to mimic the workspace in a clinical setting. A Digiclops window of 360×160 $pixels$ for the plate images and 240×230 $pixels$ for the sphere images, records the 3D location of all detected features. The Optotrak records the IRED locations, P_G, which are next transformed from C_G to C_D using $(T_G^D)^{-1}$.

The error between the points calculated with the Digiclops and the true surface location for the plate and sphere are calculated as follows:

$$error_{plate} = \frac{A \cdot P_{D_x} + B \cdot P_{D_y} + C \cdot P_{D_z} + D}{\pm\sqrt{A^2 + B^2 + C^2}} \tag{2a}$$

$$error_{sphere} = \sqrt{(P_{D_x} - P_{D,cen_x})^2 + (P_{D_y} - P_{D,cen_y})^2 + (P_{D_z} - P_{D,cen_z})^2} - r_{true} \tag{2b}$$

where $P_D(P_{D_x}, P_{D_y}, P_{D_z})$ is each point recorded by the Digiclops, $Ax + By + Cz + D = 0$ is the true flat plate, and $P_D(P_{D,cen_x}, P_{D,cen_y}, P_{D,cen_z})$ and r_{true} are the true centre and radius of the sphere.

Our system obtains its accuracy by using the mean of a large number of point locations within each patch to calculate the surface location. The effect of accuracy on the size of each patch is therefore computed and the results are shown in Figure 3.

2.2   Image Based Consistency Test

The results found in subsection 2.1 show that using the Digiclops in our tracking system is feasible as it has sufficient accuracy for tracking large patient motion. An experiment is conducted to assess the consistency of the system when both probe and patient tracking are combined. A flat plate with a textured surface is attached to the probe, creating a surface with features that can be tracked by the Digiclops. The plate to the ultrasound imaging plane must also be located by calibration [12]. N-shaped fiducials are attached to the skin surface to assist in tracking. The components of this experiment create a mock scenario of the complete tracking system and are shown in Figure 4.

In this experiment, the patient is represented by one of two life-size tissue mimicking phantoms that approximate the acoustic properties of soft human tissue, while remaining rigid under the force of the probe. Two casts are first created from human models using plaster embedded gauze. One model is made from the torso of a 39 week pregnant female and the second from an adult male. A solution of distilled water and 8%($vol.$) glycerol, is mixed with 3%($mass$) cellulose particles, and 3%($mass$) agar. The mixture is heated to 85°C, cooled to 60°C, and poured into the torso casts.

Overlaid on the surface of the patient is an artificial skin made of latex and containing N-shaped fiducials. Latex was chosen as a matrix material as it does not alter the ultrasound image while the N fiducials produce small bright spots near the top of the ultrasound image. Using a similar approach to [3,12], the distance between the bright spots as well as their widths provide enough information to calculate the unique probe location with respect to each fiducial. For this experiment, only two N shaped fiducials are needed. In our experiment, one is visible to the Digiclops and the other in the ultrasound image. After extensive testing of different materials, soldered pieces of 1.24 mm diameter steel sewing needles were used to create the fiducials. The fiducials are placed

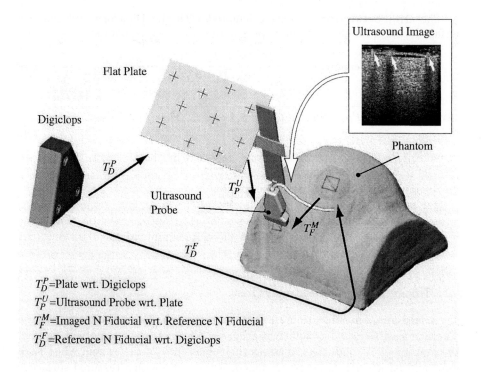

T_D^P=Plate wrt. Digiclops
T_P^U=Ultrasound Probe wrt. Plate
T_F^M=Imaged N Fiducial wrt. Reference N Fiducial
T_D^F=Reference N Fiducial wrt. Digiclops

Fig. 4. Relationship Between the Transformations used for the Tracking Experiment. An example ultrasound image is shown with arrows indicating the bright spots created by the N fiducial.

on moulds that have the form of each phantom. Several coats of latex rubber are applied to the surface of each mould, and then cured in a vacuum to remove any air bubbles.

In order to investigate the consistency of the results, data that describes the location of the ultrasound probe in C_D is calculated using two different sets of transformations. The points are transformed from the imaged fiducial coordinate system, C_M, and the ultrasound coordinate system, C_U,

$$P_{D_I} = T_D^F T_F^M P_M, \qquad P_{D_{II}} = T_D^P T_P^U P_U , \qquad (3)$$

and the error is calculated between the points, P_{D_I} and $P_{D_{II}}$, and is shown in Table 1.

P_M, P_U: The centre and diameter of each bright spot in the ultrasound image as seen in Figure 4 are manually located in C_U and a unique probe location is calculated within C_M. The chosen centres of the bright spots in C_U and calculated corresponding points in C_M, P_U and P_M, provide the starting points for the completion of the loop.

$\mathbf{T_P^U}$:   The probe is calibrated, providing the transformation between the ultrasound image and the plate, T_P^U, using a variation of the method presented in [12].

$\mathbf{T_D^F}, \mathbf{T_F^M}, \mathbf{T_D^P}$:   The Digiclops is used to find the transformation T_D^F, between the reference fiducial coordinate system, C_F, and C_D, using the same equations used to find T_D^P. The transformation T_F^M from C_M to C_F is made possible because the two N fiducials are fixed relative to each other during this experiment.

Table 1. Error between the points P_{D_I} and $P_{D_{II}}$ using 40 sets of probe locations on the phantom torso.

	$\mathbf{X_D}$ direction	$\mathbf{Y_D}$ direction	$\mathbf{Z_D}$ direction
Mean [mm]	-0.1	-0.3	-1.1
Maximum [mm]	6.7	8.3	2.4
Standard Deviation [mm]	2.9	3.2	1.7

3   Discussion

From Figure 3, we see that the Digiclops system is able to track a flat and spherical rigid object with mean errors less than ± 1.0 mm and ± 0.7 mm, respectively. Using the mean of 58000 $pixels$ for the plate and 55000 $pixels$ for the sphere, the standard deviations for the points are less than 1.6 mm and 1.1 mm for the plate and sphere, respectively. The location error for both the plate and the sphere tests remain under ± 2 mm as the patch size decreases to under 400 $pixels$. This is equivalent to an area of 20×20 mm on the surface of the patient's skin. At a distance of 1000 mm, the Digiclops is able to image an area of 600×800 mm. As a comparison of accuracies, the Fastrak® A/C magnetic tracker (Polhemus Inc., Colchester, VT) has an RMS accuracy of $0.762mm$, the Flock of Birds® D/C magnetic tracker (Ascension Technology Corp., Burlington, VT) has an RMS accuracy of $1.8mm$, and the Optotrak has an RMS accuracy of $0.15mm$. These systems track few points at a time as well as inhibit the ultrasound probe from passing over the area being tracked since the markers are protruding from the skin surface.

The consistency test reported a maximum mean error for each of the directions of less than 1.1 mm with a standard deviation under 3.2 mm. Errors during this second experiment are due to the variation in manual selection of the bright spots in the ultrasound image, feature mismatching between the stereo images, and probe calibration errors. As an approximation to the error introduced by the calibration procedure, a similar method, described in [12], resulted in a mean error of 0.23 mm with a standard deviation of 2.89 mm. Regardless of which external tracking system is used, a calibration between the probe and images is necessary and will introduce errors. For our system, this calibration error is included in our results. The consistency tests inspired ways to reduce this error.

We propose that the N fiducials be used to make corrections to the location measurements. We first estimate the location from the cameras and then correct this estimation using the 3 bright spots in the ultrasound image. This correction is made possible because the location of each fiducial is known relative to the grayscale surface. The main goal is to find the ultrasound image with respect to the skin. So, the incorporation of N fiducials into our tracking system could create on-the-fly correction of the ultrasound image location with respect to the skin.

We envision the camera and ultrasound components of our system working together to ameliorate the accuracy of the entire tracking system. In addition to improving accuracy, the complete system could be able to compensate for occlusions from the camera system. The camera tracking system is necessary to identify which particular fiducial is being imaged as well as to find the angles between the yaw and pitch of the probe. Unlike the feasibility experiment described in this paper, the complete system would be composed of many N fiducials. Although the surface is covered with fiducial marks, the width and material of the fiducials and matrix are such that a bright dot appears at the top of the ultrasound image but the anatomical information contained in the image is compromised very little. The complete system would also have a smaller object attached to the probe instead of the larger plate that we used in this experiment.

4   Conclusions

The accuracy of the inexpensive trinocular camera system that is used to track a patch of 20×20 mm is less than ± 2 mm. A plate was attached to the probe and a textured surface was placed on the skin surface. A consistency test of the complete system produced values with a standard deviation under 3.2 mm. These errors include all calibration steps required for a working system, and are sufficiently small to allow compensating of medium to large patient motion.

Future research with this tracking system will focus on implementing the error correction from multiple N fiducials to compensate for even smaller patient motion. Automation of bright spot detection in the ultrasound images as well as fiducial detection in the camera images must also be implemented. Studies into local deformation are also planned with camera tracking of small patch sizes.

References

1. D. Atkinson, M. Burcher, J. Declerck, and J. Noble. Respiratory motion compensation for 3-D freehand echocardiography. *Ultrasound Med Biol*, 27(12):1615–1620, 2001.
2. M. L. Chuang, M. G. Hibberd, R. A. Beaudin, M. G. Mooney, M. F. Riley, J. T. Fearnside, and P. S. Douglas. Patient motion compensation during transthoracic 3-D echocardiography. *Ultrasound Med Biol*, 27(2):203–209, 2001.

3. R. M. Comeau, A. F. Sadikot, A. Fenster, and T. M. Peters. Intraoperative ultrasound for guidance and tissue shift correction in image-guided neurosurgery. *Med Phys*, 27(4):787–800, 2000.

4. A. DeGroote, M. Wantier, G. Cheron, M. Estenne, and M.Paiva. Chest wall motion during tidal breathing. *J Appl Physiol*, 83(5):1531–1537, 1997.

5. D. D. Dershaw. Imaging guided biopsy: An alternative to surgical biopsy. *Breast J*, 6(5):294–298, 2000.

6. R. Groell, G. J. Schaffler, and S. Schloffer. Breath-hold times in patients undergoing radiological examinations: Comparison of expiration and inspiration with and without hyperventilation. *Radiol and Oncol*, 35(3):161–165, 2001.

7. A. Hartov, S. Eisner, M. David, W. Roberts, K. Paulsen, L. Platenik, and M. Miga. Error analysis for a free-hand three-dimensional ultrasound system for neuronavigation. *Neurosurg Focus*, 6(3), 1999.

8. M. Lee, N. Cardinal, and A. Fenster. Single-camera system for optically tracking freehand motion in 3D: Experimental implementation and evaluation. In *Proceedings SPIE Visualization, Display and Image-guided Procedures*, pages 109–120, 2001.

9. K. McLeish, D. L. Hill, D. Atkinson, J. M. Blackall, and R. Razavi. A study of the motion and deformation of the heart due to respiration. *IEEE T Med Imaging*, 21(9):1142–1150, 2002.

10. D. M. Muratore and J. Robert L. Galloway. Beam calibration without a phantom for creating a 3-D freehand ultrasound system. *Ultrasound Med Biol*, 27(11):1557–1566, 2001.

11. T. R. Nelson and D. H. Pretorius. Three-dimensional ultrasound imaging. *Ultrasound Med Biol*, 24(9):1243–1270, 1998.

12. N. Pagoulatos, D. R. Haunor, and Y. Kim. A fast calibration method for 3-d tacking of ultrasound images using a spatial localizer. *Ultrasound Med Biol*, 27(9):1219–1229, 2001.

13. G. Penney, J. Blackall, M. Hamady, T.Sabharwal, A.Adam, and D. Hawkes. Registration of freehand 3D ultrasound and magnetic resonance liver images. *Med Image Anal*, 8(1):81–91, 2004.

14. R. W. Prager, A. Gee, and L. Berman. Stradx: Real-time acquisition and visualization of freehand three-dimentional ultrasound. *Med Image Anal*, 3(2):129–140, 1998.

15. M. Riccabona, G. Fritz, and E. Ring. Potential applications of three-dimensional ultrasound in the pediatric urinary tract: Pictorial demonstration based on preliminary results. *Eur Radiol*, 13(12):2680–2687, 2003.

16. A. Roche, X. Pennec, G. Malandain, and N. Ayache. Rigid registration of 3-D ultrasound with mr images: A new approach combining intensity and gradient information. *IEEE T Med Imaging*, 20(10):1038–1049, 2001.

Real-Time 4D Tumor Tracking and Modeling from Internal and External Fiducials in Fluoroscopy

Johanna Brewer[1], Margrit Betke[1], David P. Gierga[2], and George T.Y. Chen[2]

[1] Computer Science Department, Boston University, Boston, MA 02215, USA
[2] Radiation Oncology, Massachusetts General Hospital, Boston, MA 02114, USA
johannab@cs.bu.edu, www.cs.bu.edu/groups/ivc

Abstract. Fluoroscopy is currently used in treatment planning for patients undergoing radiation therapy. Radiation oncologists would like to maximize the amount of dose the tumor receives and minimize the amount delivered to the surrounding tissues. During treatment, patients breathe freely and so the tumor location will not be fixed. This makes calculating the amount of dose delivered to the tumor, and verifying that the tumor actually receives that dose, difficult. We describe a correlation-based method of tracking the two-dimensional (2D) motion of internal markers (surgical clips) placed around the tumor. We established ground truth and evaluated the accuracy of the tracker for 10 data sets of 5 patients. The root mean squared error in estimating 2D marker position was 0.47 mm on average. We also developed a method to model the average and maximum three-dimensional (3D) motion of the clips given two orthogonal fluoroscopy videos of the same patients that were taken sequentially. On average, the error was 3.0 mm for four pairs of trajectories. If imaging is possible during treatment, such motion models may be used for beam guided radiation; otherwise, they may be correlated to a set of external markers for use in respiratory gating.

1 Introduction

Knowledge of tumor location is integral to radiation therapy. Fluoroscopy and computed tomography (CT) scans are typically used in the pre-treatment planning phase. Fluoroscopy is an imaging technique in which X-rays continually strike a fluorescent plate that is coupled to a video monitor. In a fluoroscopic image, tumors lack sufficient contrast with the surrounding tissue, so, in preparation for treatment, metal clips are often implanted around the tumor. Since these clips are radio opaque they are visible in fluoroscopy images and CT scans. In fluoroscopy, they provide a way to observe the tumor as it changes position due to various rigid and non-rigid body movements. For abdominal tumors, radiotherapy is particularly complicated by motion due to patient breathing. In order to compensate for this, the tissue volume that will be radiated, the planning target volume (PTV), is often expanded so that the tumor itself, the clinical target

C. Barillot, D.R. Haynor, and P. Hellier (Eds.): MICCAI 2004, LNCS 3217, pp. 594–601, 2004.

volume (CTV), will receive sufficient dose. This leads to undesirable radiation of healthy tissue surrounding the tumor.

Breath-hold techniques [9] have been introduced to reduce tumor movement. These techniques are not always feasible for the patient [6]. Gating methods seek to compensate for the motion by activating the radiation beam only when the tumor is at a predetermined position. The indirect gating method relies on the correlation between external markers or lung air flow and internal motion [5, 15]. Studies attested to the correlation of external marker motion with the 2D internal motion of the diaphragm [15,7] or internal markers [2]. However, for a given external marker, the ratio of internal to external marker motion can be relatively large [2].

Tumor position can also be directly detected by means of online fluoroscopic imaging of internal fiducial markers [12,13,14]. Due to large patient volume at treatment clinics, there is pressure to decrease the time of a treatment session, but this comes at the cost of increasing the size of the gating window (the time when the radiation beam is on) and thus more healthy tissue is irradiated. This is even more problematic in the typically longer sessions of intensity modulated radiation therapy (IMRT). Beam-guided radiation therapy seeks to address the problems of gating by moving the radiation beam in synchronization with the tumor. This was first introduced in robotic radiosurgery [10], and later adopted for motion-adaptive radiotherapy [13,4,8]. To accomplish the synchronization of motion, the accuracy and reliability of the tracking method is of paramount importance. While there has been significant work in the computer vision community on tracking [1], in particular in medical image analysis in the areas of fMRI, cardiac motion, and blood flow analysis (e.g. [3,11]), there have been only rudimentary efforts in applying tracking technology to measure abdominal tumor motion. The contribution of this paper is to address the problem of tumor tracking in a rigorous manner and provide methods to (1) accurately track internal and external fiducial markers in fluoroscopy, (2) compute trajectories of the average and worst-case motion based on two orthogonal fluoroscopy videos, and (3) establish the correlation of clip motion with external markers. Results are presented that use 10 sets of data from 5 patients.

2   Materials and Methods

Fluoroscopy imaging provides a two-dimensional projection of the density values of the imaged body. The surgically implanted clips can be detected and tracked in the fluoroscopy images since metal is radio opaque and has a higher density than the surrounding tissue. The surrounding tissue, however, may also appear dark or contain edges due to high-density bone structures such as the spine, and the images can become dark during inhalation (Fig. 2).

During treatment planning, radiation oncologists typically request fluoroscopy from two views, the Anterior-Posterior and the Lateral views. Because these views are orthogonal, we can combine the 2D tracking data to recover 3D information about the motion of the clips 1. The setup of the imaging system is

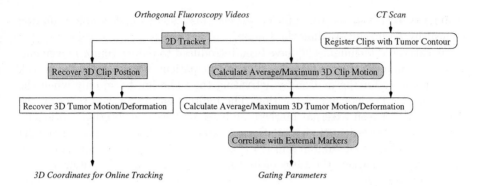

Fig. 1. Overview of method. Sharp-cornered boxes indicate online steps, and boxes with rounded corners offline steps. Methods in shaded boxes are implemented and results are presented here.

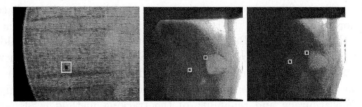

Fig. 2. Regions of fluoroscopic images containing surgical clips marked by white rectangles. Left: Spinal region with a clip and vertebrae edges with similar intensity values. Middle and Right: Two clips during inhalation and exhalation. The leftmost clip moved more significantly in the Cranio-Caudal direction than the rightmost clip. The image on the right is much darker.

such that the Anterior-Posterior and Lateral views share the y-axis of the respective images, which is the Cranio-Caudal axis of the patient, and the isocenter of the patient is at the center of the image.

To date, most hospitals do not have the capability to acquire two orthogonal views simultaneously. However, it is still possible to recover information about the tumor motion from two sequentially obtained orthogonal views. In simultaneous views, we can expect the Cranio-Caudal motion of a given internal marker to be the same in both images. In sequential views, this motion, although not exactly the same, is typically very similar because the fluoroscopy images are taken only minutes apart, during which the patient's breathing and anatomy do not change drastically. Because breathing is well described by a sinusoid, we use sine waves to approximate the average 3D motion and maximum range of the 3D motion in the two sequential views. These sine waves can be correlated with the motion of external markers for use in gating.

During treatment planning, tumors are also contoured manually on CT. This expert knowledge may be used to determine a relationship between the clips, which are visible in the scan, and the contour. With a sufficient number of clips, the motion and deformation of the tumor in 3D may be extrapolated from the 3D motion of the clips.

2.1 2D Clip Tracking

Initialization. The tracking method is initiated by manual selection of a rectangular region r containing each clip in an initial fluoroscopic image I. In order to find a minimal rectangle containing each clip, the largest "dark" connected component in each region is found by first binarizing the image according to an automatically computed "p-tile threshold" for the region. The rectangle is used as a grayscale template T of the clip. The dimensions of T are denoted by w and h. The locations of the templates in I provide the starting coordinates for tracking the clips in subsequent fluoroscopy frames.

Tracking Algorithm. The normalized correlation coefficient is used to find the position of the clip in subsequent image frames. The tracking algorithm searches for the best match of the clip template T with a region of the image I. This is done by shifting the template T through the image to various points (x', y') and correlating it with each $(w \times h)$ sub-image of I. The value of the normalized correlation coefficient at position (x', y') is

$$R_{I,T}(x', y') = \sum_{x,y} (I(x' + x, y' + y) - \bar{I}) \, (T(x,y) - \bar{T})/(\sigma_I \sigma_T), \qquad (1)$$

where $\bar{T}$ and $\bar{I}$ are the respective mean intensities within the template and image window, and σ_I and σ_T the respective standard deviations. The location (x', y') which maximizes $R_{I,T}$ is taken to be the new clip location.

Searching over all positions (x', y') in I is computationally expensive. Because we know that the clips do not move much from frame to frame, it is possible to restrict the size of the sub-region of I which will be searched. The apparent velocity of the clip's movement in the image is calculated to predict the clip location in the next frame. Velocity $(u, v) = (\frac{dx}{dt}, \frac{dy}{dt})$ is approximated in terms of the rate of change in x and y from the past frame to the current frame: $(u_{t+1}, v_{t+1}) = (x_t - x_{t-1}, y_t - y_{t-1})$. We assume that the velocity is constant, and use (u, v) as an offset from the current position to determine the center of a 5×5 region of interest to search over in the subsequent frame.

2.2 Calculation of Average and Maximum Range of 3D Clip Motion

Our 2D tracking method produces a set of time-indexed 2D coordinates for each view. Given these 2D trajectories, the average and maximum range of 2D motion is calculated for each view in the Cranio-Caudal direction as well as the Anterior-Posterior or Left-Right direction. To determine the maximum range of 2D motion, trajectories are first smoothed using a 1D Gaussian kernel with a support of 10 frames (or 1/3 second) and a standard deviation of one frame. This smoothing operation helps to identify the global maximum and minimum of each trajectory uniquely.

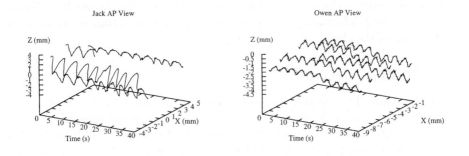

Fig. 3. 2D motion of clips of 2 patients in Anterior-Posterior Fluoroscopy.

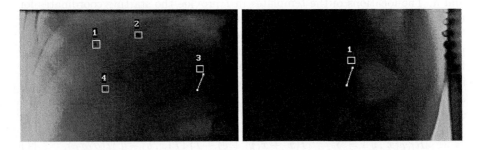

Fig. 4. Two subsections of fluoroscopic views (Anterior-Posterior on the left, Lateral on the right) taken during the peak of a breathing cycle. Clip 3 in the Lateral view and clip 1 in the AP view are the same clip. The white line is a projection of the 3D trajectory that models the average motion of this clip.

To compute an average 2D motion trajectory, first, the maxima and minima that correspond to full inspiration and expiration are located as follows. The difference in the Cranio-Caudal direction between the global maximum and minimum is scaled by 1.1. This scaled value is then used as a threshold during the search for the global maximum and minimum of each breathing cycle. In this search, if the most recently found optimum is a maximum, the distances between this maximum and subsequent points on the trajectory are aggregated until the threshold is reached. The global minimum of the breathing cycle is then determined among the set of points traversed. Similarly, the next maximum can be detected, and the process repeats until all breathing cycles are identified.

The set of minima and maxima is then used to compute amplitude a and frequency f of the 2D motion trajectory. The offset o is computed by averaging the values on the trajectory (1st coefficient of the Fourier Transform). We can then define the average 2D trajectory by sine wave $o + a\sin(2\pi ft)$, where t is time. Since two Cranio-Caudal motion trajectories are given, we average the parameters a, o, and f of these trajectories to obtain a single sine wave that describes average Cranio-Caudal motion. The average Anterior-Posterior

Table 1. Clip Localization Error

Patient	Direction of Motion	Root Mean Squared Error (RMS)		Max Error (mm)
		Mean (mm)	Std. Dev. (mm)	
Alice	Right-Left	0.61	0.58	2.31
Alice	Cranio-Caudal	1.21	0.58	2.00
Doug	Right-Left	0.40	0.15	0.74
Doug	Cranio-Caudal	0.39	0.38	1.50
Eve	Right-Left	0.25	0.25	0.74
Eve	Cranio-Caudal	0.23	0.26	1.00
Frank	Right-Left	0.25	0.23	0.74
Frank	Cranio-Caudal	0.41	0.33	1.00
Gary	Right-Left	0.48	0.32	1.48
Gary	Cranio-Caudal	0.47	0.24	1.00
Average		0.47	0.33	1.25

and Right-Left motions are described by sine waves with offset and amplitude parameters computed from the respective 2D trajectories. For convenience, the frequency parameter computed for the average Cranio-Caudal motion is also used to describe the Anterior-Posterior and Right-Left motions. The three sine waves together form a parametric description of the average motion of the clip in 3D.

3   Results

This study involved 7 patients (the names used here are fictitious). Fluoroscopy videos were collected with a Varian Ximatron radiotherapy simulator with a resolution of 640 × 480 pixels at 30 frames per second. The computer used to process the data was an Intel Xeon 1.7 GHz with 1 GB RAM and an ATI All-In-Wonder 9800 graphics card.

Ground truth was established for the motion of five clips, one per patient, using the Anterior-Posterior views. The centroid of each clip was manually recorded for every tenth frame of the video. The ground truth positions were then compared with the positions estimated by the proposed 2D-tracking method (Table 1). On average, the mean and standard deviation of the root mean squared (RMS) error in estimating the 10 motion trajectories are under 0.5 mm (< 1 pixel). We compared four pairs of trajectories to evaluate the accuracy of the average 3D motion trajectories in modeling clip motion (Table 2). The average RMS error is 3.0 mm. Fig. 4 shows a fluoroscopic image containing both internal and external markers. We found a high correlation between external and internal markers of two patients (0.88 on average).

Table 2. 3D Model Error

Patient	Direction of Motion	Root Mean Squared Error (RMS)		Max Error (cm)
		Mean (cm)	Std. Dev. (cm)	
Jack Lateral View	y-direction	0.01	0.02	0.24
Jack Lateral View	z-direction	0.07	0.11	0.58
Jack AP View	x-direction	0.02	0.03	0.14
Jack AP View	z-direction	0.25	0.31	1.87
Nancy Lateral View	y-direction	0.33	0.27	1.23
Nancy Lateral View	z-direction	1.49	1.22	5.43
Nancy AP View	x-direction	0.01	0.01	0.06
Nancy AP View	z-direction	0.27	0.38	2.37

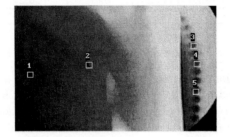

Fig. 5. Lateral fluoroscopic image with three external markers (beads), resting on the patient's abdomen (right), and two internal markers (clips).

4   Discussion and Conclusion

Estimating the location of a tumor accurately is crucial in providing effective and safe radiation therapy. The ground truth study of our tumor tracking system shows that the average RMS error is 0.47 mm, which is considerably smaller than the 1.5 mm error reported by Shirato et al. [14], given that the internal markers are typically only 5 mm long. Our method to model 3D tumor motion based on sequential fluoroscopy videos can be used in settings where the latest technology, i.e., simultaneous orthogonal fluoroscopy, is not available. Computing average tumor motion trajectories from fluoroscopy and CT data obtained in pre-treatment sessions may be helpful in estimating tumor position accurately during treatment.

Acknowledgments. Funding was provided by The Whitaker Foundation, the National Science Foundation (DGE-0221680, IIS-0093367, IIS-0308213 and EIA-0202067), and the Office of Naval Research (N000140110444).

References

1. D. A. Forsyth and J. Ponce. *Computer Vision, A Modern Approach*. Prentice Hall, NJ, 2003.
2. D. P. Gierga, G. Sharp, J. Brewer, M. Betke, C. Willett, and G. T. Y. Chen. Correlation between external and internal markers for abdominal tumors: Implications for respiratory gating. In *Proceedings of the 45th Annual Meeting of the American Society for Therapeutic Radiology and Oncology*, Salt Lake City, UT, October 2003. A journal version was submitted in May 2004.
3. I. Haber, D. N. Metaxas, and L. Axel. Using tagged MRI to reconstruct a 3D heartbeat. *Computing in Science and Engineering*, 2(5):18–30, 2000.
4. P. J. Keall, V. R. Kini, S. S. Vedam, and R. Mohan. Motion adaptive x-ray therapy: a feasibility study. *Phys Med Biol*, 46(1):1–10, 2001.
5. V. R. Kini, S. S. Vedam, P. J. Keall, S. Patil, C. Chen, and R. Mohan. Patient training in respiratory-gated radiotherapy. *Med Dosim*, 28(1):7–11, 2003.
6. H. D. Kubo, P. M. Len, S. Minohara, and H. Mostafavi. Breathing-synchronized radiotherapy program at the University of California Davis Cancer Center. *Med Phys*, 27(2):346–353, February 2000.
7. G. S. Mageras, E. Yorke, K. Rosenzweig, L. Braban, E. Keatley, E. Ford, S. Leibel, and C. Ling. Fluoroscopic evaluation of diaphragmatic motion reduction with a respiratory gated radiotherapy system. *J Appl Clin Med Phys*, 2(4):191–200, 2001.
8. T. Neicu, H. Shirato, Y. Seppenwoolde, and S. B. Jiang. Synchronized Moving Aperture Radiation Therapy (SMART): Average tumor trajectory for lung patients. *Phys Med Biol*, 48:587–598, March 2003.
9. K. E. Rosenzweig, J. Hanley, D. Mah, G. Mageras, M. Hunt, S. Toner, C. Burman, C. C. Ling, B. Mychalczak, Z. Fuks, and S. A. Leibel. The deep inspiration breath-hold technique in the treatment of inoperable non-small-cell lung cancer. *Int J Radiat Oncol Biol Phys*, 48(1):81–87, 2000.
10. A. Schweikard, G. Glosser, M. Bodduluri, M. J. Murphy, and J. R. Adler. Robotic motion compensation for respiratory movement during radiosurgery. *Comput Aided Surg*, 5(4):263–277, 2000.
11. A.M. Seifalian, D. J. Hawkes, C. R. Hardingham, A.C. Colchester, and J.F. Reidy. Validation of a quantitative radiographic technique to estimate pulsatile blood flow waveforms using digital subtraction angiographic data. *J Biomed Eng*, 3(3):225–233, May 1991.
12. Y. Seppenwoolde, H. Shirato, K. Kitamura, S. Shimizu, M. Van Herk, J. V. Lebesque, and K. Miyasaka. Precise and real-time measurement of 3d tumor motion in lung due to breathing and heartbeat, measured during radiotherapy. *Int J Radiat Oncol Biol Phys*, 53(4):822–834, 2002.
13. H. Shirato, S. Shimizu, K. Kitamura, T. Nishioka, K. Kagei, S. Hashimoto, H. Aoyama, T. Kunieda, N. Shinohara, H. Dosaka-Akita, and K. Miyasaka. Four-dimensional treatment planning and fluoroscopic real-time tumor tracking radiotherapy for moving tumor. *Int J Radiat Oncol Biol Phys*, 48(2):435–442, 2000.
14. H. Shirato, S. Shimizu, T. Kunieda, K. Kitamura, M. van Herk, K. Kagei, T. Nishioka, S. Hashimoto, K. Fujita, H. Aoyama, K. Tsuchiya, K. Kudo, and K. Miyasaka. Physical aspects of a real-time tumor-tracking system for gated radiotherapy. *Int J Radiat Oncol Biol Phys*, 48(4):1187–1195, November 2000.
15. S. S. Vedam, V. R. Kini, P. J. Keall, V. Ramakrishnan, H. Mostafavi, and R. Mohan. Quantifying the predictability of diaphragm motion during respiration with a noninvasive external marker. *Med Phys*, 30(4):505–513, April 2003.

Augmented Vessels for Pre-operative Preparation in Endovascular Treatments

Wilbur C.K. Wong[1], Albert C.S. Chung[1], and Simon C.H. Yu[2]

[1] Department of Computer Science,
The Hong Kong University of Science and Technology,
Clear Water Bay, Kowloon, HK
{cswilbur,achung}@cs.ust.hk
[2] Department of Diagnostic Radiology and Organ Imaging,
Prince of Wales Hospital, Shatin, NT, HK
simonyu@cuhk.edu.hk

Abstract. Three-dimensional rotational angiography is a very useful tool for accessing abnormal vascular structures related to a variety of vascular diseases. Quantitative study of the abnormalities could aid the radiologists to choose the appropriate apparatuses and endovascular treatments. Given a segmentation of an angiography, effective quantitation of the abnormalities is attainable if the abnormalities are detached from the normal vasculature. To achieve this, a novel method is presented, which allows the users to construct imaginary disease-free vessel lumens, namely *augmented vessels*, and demarcate the abnormalities on the fly interactively. The method has been tested on several synthetic images and clinical datasets. The experimental results have shown that it is capable of separating a variety of abnormalities, e.g., stenosis, saccular and fusiform aneurysms, from the normality.

1 Introduction

An endovascular treatment is a therapy performed inside vascular structures with the assistance of 2D angiography and micro-catheter. During the treatment, there is a few imaging technologies that can provide 3D vascular morphology. Three-dimensional rotational angiography (3D RA) is one of these technologies, which is capable of producing high resolution lumen images in isotropic voxels[1]. As such, 3D RA is a very useful tool for accessing abnormal vascular structures of a variety of pathologies. Given a vascular segmentation of a 3D RA image, it would be more effective to perform quantitation on the abnormalities if they are detached from the normal vasculature. This makes further processing exclusively on the abnormal structures possible. Therefore, this could allow interactive or automatic quantitative analysis of the abnormalities, and aid the radiologists to choose the appropriate apparatuses and treatments to cure the vascular diseases.

To the best of our knowledges, there is relatively little literature on separating abnormal vascular structures from the normal lumen in angiographies.

---

[1] We acquire the 3D RA images with a Philips Integris imager.

C. Barillot, D.R. Haynor, and P. Hellier (Eds.): MICCAI 2004, LNCS 3217, pp. 602–609, 2004.

Several researchers have suggested to detach a saccular aneurysm by defining the aneurysmal neck [1], [2] or by identifying the mesh covering the saccular aneurysm from the surface mesh of the vasculature [3]. Their algorithms, however, are restricted to a particular type of abnormality — saccular aneurysm.

In this paper, we present a novel approach to detaching a variety of vascular abnormalities, viz. stenosis, saccular and fusiform aneurysms, from the normal vasculature. We take a very different approach as compared with the published methodologies. Instead of manipulating the abnormal structures with sophisticated algorithms, we detach the abnormalities by explicitly modeling their opposite — normal vessels. Our method provides interactive tracking of imaginary disease-free vessel lumens, namely *augmented vessels*, and the demarcation of the abnormalities is performed on the fly. The method has been validated with synthetic images by comparing the results to a manual delineation of the abnormalities and tested on several clinical datasets.

2   Methods

In order to track the augmented vessels and detach the abnormalities from the normal vasculature, we have to preform the following tasks: (a) segment the vascular structures, (b) estimate the lumen diameters, (c) extract the centerline of the lumen, (d) track the augmented vessels and (e) detach the abnormalities.

2.1   Vascular Segmentation

In the image acquisition of 3D RA, the radiologist injects contrast agents in the vessel to fill the pathology of interest so as to image the vessel lumen in the angiography. Because of the application of the contrast agents, the blood vessel lumen is stood out on the background. This makes the segmentation of the lumen a less difficult task to accomplish. According to our experiments, a satisfactory 3D RA vascular segmentation can be produced by a global thresholding after the noisy angiography is smoothed with an edge-preserving filter. In this work, we applied the trilateral filter [4] to the angiography for denoising prior to the segmentation.

2.2   Lumen Diameter Estimation

In order to model the blood vessel lumen with a circular cross-sectional tube[2], we have to estimate the lumen diameter. We employ Saito and Toriwaki's Euclidean distance transformation algorithm [6] to calculate the Euclidean distance (ED) from each voxel inside the lumen to the nearest boundary of the lumen (aka ED map). Intuitively, the distance value approximates the radius of the largest sphere that can be completely enclosed within the lumen at the corresponding voxel. Therefore, the diameters of the vessel lumen can be estimated from the ED map and equal twice the EDs at the voxels along the vessel centerline.

---

[2] The assumption — blood vessel is a circular cross-sectional tubular object — is a commonly used hypothesis in medical image processing community [5].

2.3   Centerline Extraction

We use Palágyi et al. sequential 3D thinning algorithm [7] to extract voxels along the centerline of the blood vessel lumen. Their thinning algorithm iteratively reduces an object to produce an approximation to the object skeleton. The algorithm is simple and easy to implement, and, more importantly, the topology of the object is preserved in the skeleton. However, it may take several iterations to produce the skeleton if the object is large. Unfortunately, it is the case for the 3D RA images in a clinical environment — typically, the object of interest occupies $170,000$ voxels in a $256 \times 256 \times 256$ voxels volume with a 30 mm field of view in each dimension.

Providentially, in this work, we are not aiming at extracting the complete skeleton of the vessel. Indeed, our objective is to provide a few 3D points that are located at the centerline of the blood vessel to the user for the initialization of the tracking of the augmented vessel. As such, we can resample the binary image volume with a larger voxel size to reduce the computation of the thinning algorithm. In this work, a voxel size of $1 \times 1 \times 1 \, mm^3$ is used. This is because the diameter of the vessel of interest usually ranges from 2 mm to 10 mm. Therefore, in the resampled image volume, the diameter of the lumen is about $2-10$ voxels, and the object of interest occupies only 270 voxels. In general, the algorithm takes less than 1 sec. to extract the skeleton on a 2.6 GHz PC.

Once the skeleton points in the low resolution image volume are extracted, we can search for the 3D points that are located at the centerline of the lumen within a 3D spatial window of 1 mm in each dimension[3]. The centerline points are characterized by the local maxima in the ED map of the original binary image volume. In order to achieve subvoxel accuracy in the search of these points, we perform tricubic interpolation on the ED map and seek the position with the maximum ED within the spatial window at each skeleton point in a sampling space $1/8$ of the original voxel size.

2.4   Interactive Tracking of Augmented Vessel

After the centerline points are extracted, we present them together with the 3D surface mesh of the vessel lumen to the user[4]. Then the user has to select three centerline points at each end of the vessel of interest. The vessel of interest usually connects directly to the part of pathology of interest, such as an aneurysm or a stenosis, between the two vessel ends. The objective of the tracking task is to follow the trajectory of the augmented vessel. By tracking this imaginary trajectory, we can distinguish the abnormalities from the normal vasculature.

Instead of the conventional B-spline representation [2], [8], a cardinal spline[5] (with zero tension) is employed to approximate the vessel trajectory, because we desire the control points to be laid on the spline/vessel itself. This representation

---

[3] We assume that the skeleton points extracted are close to the vessel centerline.

[4] The Marching Cube algorithm is used to compose the surface mesh for visualization.

[5] Cardinal spline is a special type of the well-known TCB-spline (aka Kochanek-Bartels spline) with local tension control only [9].

is more intuitive in both the computation of the spline deformation and the presentation to the user.

The six points selected by the user are fixed throughout the deformation. They avoid high curvature at the ends of the deformed spline and allow a robust estimation of the lumen diameter[6]. The lumen diameter at one end can be approximated from the ED map and equals twice the average of the EDs at the corresponding three points. For the lumen diameters in between the two ends, linear interpolation is performed.

In addition to these fixed points, the user has to specify the number of movable points inserted in between the two ends of the spline. These non-fixed points characterize the degree of freedom of the trajectory approximation. In general, two to four movable points are sufficient for the approximation, since the desired imaginary trajectory is usually simple in practice.

Concerning the spline deformation, we apply Kass et al. active contour models (aka snakes) [10] with the dynamic programming implementation proposed in [11]. In this work, the energy functional to be minimized is defined as,

$$E^*_{snake} = \int_0^1 \Big(\beta \left| v_{ss}(s) \right|^2 + E_{image}(v(s)) \Big) ds, \tag{1}$$

where s is the parametric variable, $v(\cdot)$ denotes the cardinal spline, β defines the stiffness of the spline (equals 10 in this work) and $E_{image}(\cdot)$ defines the image forces. The term E_{image} plays an important role in driving the spline to follow the trajectory of the augmented vessel. It encourages the imaginary vessel to be confined within the imaged lumen. The image forces are expressed as,

$$E_{image}(v(s)) = \int \int \int_{G(v(s))} \Big(1 - f(x, y, z) \Big) dx\, dy\, dz, \tag{2}$$

where $G(v(s))$ denotes a sphere located at position $v(s)$ with its diameter equal to the lumen diameter approximated at $v(s)$. The function $f(\cdot)$ denotes the binary image volume, $f(x, y, z) = 1$ if the point (x, y, z) is laid inside the vascular structure; otherwise, $f(x, y, z) = 0$.

Figure 1(a) shows a synthetic object. Figure 1(b) shows the object in semi-transparent with a few points on the centerline of the object structures extracted as described in Section 2.3. The user-selected six fixed points are in darker color as highlighted by the arrows. Figure 1(c) shows the imaginary lumen before the spline deformation, whereas Figure 1(d) shows the lumen after the deformation. It is indicated that, with the proposed energy functional (see Equations 1 and 2), the cardinal spline (i.e. centerline of the imaginary lumen) deforms and follows the trajectory of the object structure. Moreover, the imaginary lumen is within the confines of the object (even in the high curvature region).

---

[6] It is assumed that the three points at each end are close to each other and are located at the centerline of the normal blood vessel lumen.

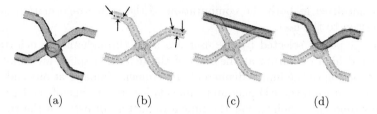

(a)	(b)	(c)	(d)

Fig. 1. Interactive tracking of a synthetic lumen. (a) 3D surface model of the object; (b) object in semi-transparent with a few centerline points presented, the user-selected six fixed points are in darker color as highlighted by the arrows; (c) imaginary lumen before the spline deformation; and (d) imaginary lumen after the deformation.

2.5   Formation of Augmented Vessel and Separation of Abnormalities

Once the imaginary lumen is tracked, the voxels that contribute to the abnormalities can be distinguished from the (imaginary) normal vascular voxels. The abnormal voxels can be picked up with a user-defined seed by applying a connectivity filter. As a consequence, the augmented vessel is obtained. In the case of an aneurysm, the abnormalities are the surplus vascular voxels that are attached to the augmented vessel. Whereas for the case of a stenosis, the abnormalities are the voxels that are absent from the augmented vessel.

3   Evaluation

The method is applied to three synthetic images for evaluation. We have also compared the accuracy of our methodology to a manual delineation of the abnormalities on one of the synthetic images. The design of the synthetic images takes several typical pathologies into consideration: cerebral aneurysm, abdominal aortic aneurysm and arterial stenosis. They are created to emulate the field of view of the region of interest $(30-100\,\text{mm})$ and the resolution $(256 \times 256 \times 256$ voxels) of typical 3D RA images.

Figure 2(a) shows the 3D surface model of the synthetic saccular cerebral aneurysm. Figure 2(b) shows the abnormalities (highlighted by the arrow) detached from the normal vascular structures with our method. Figure 2(c) shows the two imaginary vessel lumens (highlighted by the arrows) on top of the augmented vessel. While Figures 2(d)-(f) and Figures 2(g)-(i) show similar illustrations for the synthetic abdominal aortic aneurysm and arterial stenosis, respectively. It is evident that by constructing the imaginary normal lumen(s), we can separate the abnormalities from the normality with ease.

In a further study of the method, we have compared the accuracy of the abnormality estimation with our method to a manual delineation on the synthetic cerebral aneurysm image. The manual delineation is performed assuming the normal vessel lumen is a T-shape structure. To demonstrate the robustness of our method in handling object oriented at different angles, we have built the

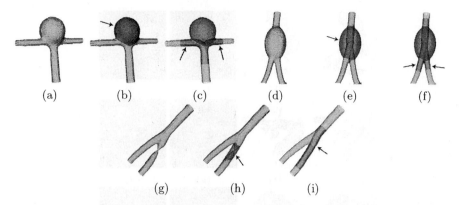

Fig. 2. Synthetic images of different typical pathologies: (a)-(c) cerebral aneurysm, (d)-(f) abdominal aortic aneurysm and (g)-(i) arterial stenosis. (a, d, g) 3D surface model of the pathology; (b, e, h) abnormalities, highlighted by the arrow, detached from the normal vasculature with our method; and (c, f, i) imaginary vessel lumen(s), highlighted by the arrow(s), on top of the augmented vessel.

augmented vessels in the image volumes with the synthetic cerebral aneurysm oriented at different angles ($0° - 90°$ with a step size of $15°$) around the axis perpendicular to the T-shape structure. It is found that the volumetric estimation of the synthetic aneurysm produced by our method (sensitivity: 99.32% and specificity: 99.42%) is, in general, more accurate than the manual delineation (sensitivity: 94.63% and specificity: 99.99%).

4   Results

We have applied our method to three 3D RA datasets. These datasets were acquired by a Philips Integris imager at the Department of Diagnostic Radiology and Organ Imaging, Prince of Wales Hospital, Hong Kong. The size of the image volume is $256 \times 256 \times 256$ voxels with the field of view ranges from $30 - 50\,\text{mm}$. The pathology of interest in the datasets is cerebral aneurysm with neck ranges from narrow ($\leq 4\,\text{mm}$) to wide ($> 4\,\text{mm}$) as classified in [12].

The first two columns of the images presented in Figure 3 show the results obtained by our method. The first column images show the vascular structures with the abnormalities in semi-transparent, highlighted by the arrows. While the second column images present the imaginary lumens, highlighted by the arrows, on top of the augmented vessels. The third and the forth column images show the scans before and after the embolizations, respectively. The Guglielmi detachable coils (GDC) are displayed as the brighter objects in the post-operative scans.

It is indicated that the GDC embolized volumes correspond to the abnormalities detached by our method in the pre-operative scans. One may find that there is an aneurysm left out in the embolization as observed in Figure 3(h), highlighted by the arrow. This is because the aneurysm is too small ($2.5\,\text{mm}^3$) to be treated in the endovascular treatment, according to the radiologist-in-charge.

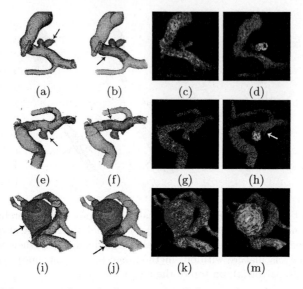

Fig. 3. Clinical datasets with cerebral aneurysms. Column 1 (a, e, i): vascular structures with the abnormalities in semi-transparent, highlighted by the arrows; Column 2 (b, f, j): imaginary lumens, highlighted by the arrows, on top of the augmented vessels; Column 3 (c, g, k): pre-operative scans; and Column 4 (d, h, m): post-operative scans.

Finally, for all the experiments conducted in this paper, the purposed method requires less than 15 sec. computation time[7] and only a few mouse clicks to build the augmented vessels and detach the abnormalities. It is also worth mentioning that our method is not restricted to separate abnormalities of pathology related to saccular aneurysm. We believe that our interactive tools can be applicable to other pathologies, for instance, fusiform aneurysm and stenosis, as illustrated with the synthetic images presented in Section 3.

5   Conclusions

A novel method that can allow users to separate a variety of vascular abnormalities from the normal vasculature is presented. By detaching the abnormalities, exclusive post-processing on the abnormal vascular structures becomes feasible. This allows effective quantitation of the structures and could aid the radiologists to choose the appropriate apparatuses and endovascular treatments to cure the vascular diseases that cause the abnormalities. Our method starts with vascular segmentation of 3D RA images, followed by lumen diameter estimation and centerline extraction. A few points on the lumen centerline and the surface mesh of the vasculature are then displayed to the user. The six user-selected fixed points at each end of the vessel of interest and the few inserted movable points

---

[7] The computation time does not include the time spent on filtering and segmentation, since they are not the foci of this work.

define a cardinal spline which deforms to follow the trajectory of the imaginary disease-free vessel lumen, namely *augmented vessel*. Once the augmented vessel is tracked, the abnormalities can be separated on the fly interactively.

The proposed method has been tested on several synthetic images and clinical datasets. It is validated with visual comparisons instead of other non-visual means. This is because in the clinical 3D RA datasets manual delineation of the abnormal structures from the vascular segmentations is not only difficult, if not impossible, but also inaccurate. Especially when the aneurysmal necks are out-of-plane with respect to the image slices, not to mention if the necks are wide and cannot be defined on planes. The experimental results have shown that the novel method is applicable for separating abnormalities of different kinds of pathologies, viz. stenosis, saccular and fusiform aneurysms.

Several analyses of the proposed method are of the current research interests. Experiments on clinical datasets that contains stenoses and abnormalities in much complex shape, for instance, saccular aneurysm that grows at the inner angle of a high curvature vessel lumen, are being conducted. Studies of the volumetric measurements of the detached abnormalities are being carried out.

References

1. van der Weide, R., Zuiderveld, K.J., Mali, W.P.T.M., Viergever, M.A.: CTA-based angle selection for diagnostic and interventional angiography of saccular intracranial aneurysms. IEEE TMI **17** (1998) 831–841
2. Wilson, D.L., Royston, D.D., Noble, J.A., Byrne, J.V.: Determining X-ray projections for coil treatments of intracranial aneurysms. IEEE TMI **18** (1999) 973–980
3. McLaughlin, R.A., Noble, J.A.: Demarcation of aneurysms using the seed and cull algorithm. In: MICCAI. Volume 2488 of LNCS., Springer-Verlag (2002) 419–426
4. Wong, W.C.K., Chung, A.C.S., Yu, S.C.H.: Trilateral filtering for biomedical images. In: IEEE ISBI. (2004) 820–823
5. Aylward, S., Bullitt, E.: Initialization, noise, singularities, and scale in height ridge traversal for tubular object centerline extraction. IEEE TMI **21** (2002) 61–75
6. Saito, T., Toriwaki, J.I.: New algorithms for Euclidean distance transformations of an n-dimensional digitized picture with applications. PR **27** (1994) 1551–1565
7. Palágyi, K., Sorantin, E., Balogh, E., Kuba, A., Halmai, C., Erdöhelyi, B., Hauseg-ger, K.: A sequential 3D thinning algorithm and its medical applications. In: IPMI. Volume 2082 of LNCS., Springer-Verlag (2001) 409–415
8. Frangi, A.F., Niessen, W.J., Hoogeveen, R.M., Walsum, T.V., Viergever, M.A.: Model-based quantitation of 3-D magnetic resonance angiographic images. IEEE TMI **18** (1999) 946–956
9. Kochanek, D., Bartels, R.: Interpolating splines with local tension, continuity and bias control. Comput. Graph. **18** (1984) 33–41
10. Kass, M., Witkin, A., Terzopoulos, D.: Snakes: Active contour models. IJCV **1** (1987) 321–331
11. Amini, A.A., Weymouth, T.E., Jain, R.C.: Using dynamic programming for solving variational problems in vision. IEEE PAMI **12** (1990) 855–867
12. Zubillaga, A.F., Guglielmi, G., Vinuela, F., Duckwiler, G.R.: Endovascular occlusion of intracranial aneurysms with electrically detachable coils: Correlation of aneurysm neck size and treatment results. AJNR **15** (1994) 815–820

A CT-Free Intraoperative Planning and Navigation System for High Tibial Dome Osteotomy

Gongli Wang[1], Guoyan Zheng[1], Paul Alfred Grützner[2], Jan von Recum[2], and Lutz-Peter Nolte[1]

[1]M.E. Müller Research Center for Orthopaedic Surgery, Institute for Surgical Technology and Biomechanics, University of Bern, Switzerland
{Gongli.Wang, Guoyan.Zheng, Lutz.Nolte}@MEMcenter.unibe.ch
http://www.MEMcenter.unibe.ch

[2]BG Trauma Center Ludwigshafen, University of Heidelberg, Germany
pa.gruetzner@urz.uni-heidelberg.de, recum@bgu-ludwigshafen.de

Abstract. High tibial dome osteotomy is a well accepted but technically demanding surgical procedure. Common complications include postoperative malalignment of either under- or over-correction, pin penetration of the tibial plateau, and damage to the tibial dorsal neurovascular structures. In order to address all these problems, we developed a CT-free intraoperative planning and navigation system based on SurgiGATE system (Praxim-Medivision, La Tronche, France). Following acquisition of fluoroscopic images and registration of anatomic landmarks, a patient specific coordinate system is established. The deformity is measured intraoperatively and the surgical procedure is planned interactively. The osteotomy and deformity correction are performed under navigational guidance. The system holds the promise to improve the accuracy, reliability, and safety of this surgical procedure.

1   Introduction

High tibial osteotomy is a proven treatment for uni-compartmental osteoarthritis of the knee and other proximal tibial deformities, particularly in young and active patients for whom total knee replacement is not advised [1]. Dome osteotomy introduced by Jackson [2] is a widely accepted technique particularly in European countries. With this technique, a series of closed pinholes equidistant from a rotational axis is drilled and connected each other by using a sharp osteotome. The deformity correction is accomplished as two separated cylindrical bone fragments slide on each other around the central rotational axis (Fig. 1). The advantage of this technique is to correct severe deformities without loss of metaphyseal bone or leg length. Additionally, it provides large bone-to-bone contact area thus enhances the postoperative stability and hastens the bone union. These advantages are not available with other techniques such as opening or closing wedge osteotomies [3], [4], [5].

However, dome osteotomy is generally recognized as technically demanding with a long learning curve. Conventional preoperative planning and surgical techniques have so far been inaccurate, and often resulted in postoperative malalignment of either under- or over-correction, which is the main reason of early failure or poor long-term

C. Barillot, D.R. Haynor, and P. Hellier (Eds.): MICCAI 2004, LNCS 3217, pp. 610–620, 2004.
© Springer-Verlag Berlin Heidelberg 2004

results [6].   With conventional techniques, it is difficult to achieve the clinical requirement of realigning the mechanical axis of the affected limb to within a narrow range of ±2° [7], [8]. An evaluation of recently reported clinical results (e.g., [9], [10], [11]) reveals that only 60% - 80% of postoperative axial alignments lie within this critical region even when operation is performed with jig systems. Moreover, an inaccurate drilling or bone cutting with conventional techniques may cause pin penetration of the tibial plateau, intercondylar fracture, or damage to the tibial dorsal neurovascular structures. They are also common complications of this surgical procedure [6].

Computer assisted surgery technologies can address these problems. As one of the main contributions of previous works, CT-based intraoperative guidance systems [12] and robot-assisted systems [13] have been developed for closing wedge osteotomy. However, despite the advantage of accurate removal a wedge from the bone, these systems have limitations of extra radiation exposure and the potential risk of infection caused by implanted fiducial markers. A more recently introduced CT-free hybrid computer-assisted navigation system [14] provides a reliable solution for opening wedge osteotomy, which uses fluoroscopic images in place of the CT scan, since they are already routinely used in operating rooms. However, to the authors' best knowledge, there has been to date no publication exploring a computer-assisted system for high tibial dome osteotomy.

In this paper, an intraoperative planning and navigation system is proposed for tibial dome osteotomy, which aims to address all the common intraoperative technical problems and to make this surgical procedure more accurate, safe, and reproducible. The system provides following advantages: (1) accurate measurement of the deformity, (2) interactive planning of the surgical procedure, (3) precise performance of the deformity correction under navigational guidance, (4) avoidance of the osteotomy failures such as intraarticular pin penetration or damage to the tibial dorsal neurovascular structures, (5) creation of a congruous cylindrical osteotomy surface that offers maximal postoperative bony contact, thus encouraging rapid bony union.

2   Materials and Methods

2.1   System Components

The system (Fig. 2) is developed based on SurgiGATE system (Praxim-Medivision, La Tronche, France). An optoelectronic infrared tracking localizer (OptoTrack 3020, Northern Digital Inc., Waterloo, Ontario, Canada), mounted on a movable stand, is used to track the position of optical targets equipped with infrared light-emitting diodes. These targets are attached to anatomical bodies, the image intensifier of the C-arm, and to other relevant surgical instruments.

A Sun ULTRA 10 workstation (Sun Microsystems Inc., Mountain View, Canada) is chosen for the image processing and visualization tasks. It is connected to the video output of the C-arm for acquisition of fluoroscopic images. The workstation communicates with the infrared tracking system through customized software using client/server architecture.

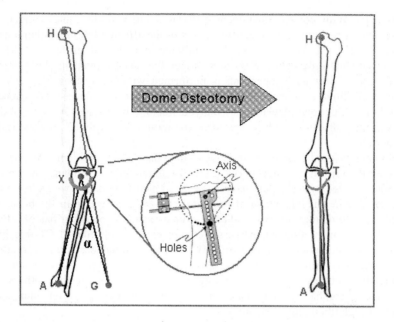

Fig. 1. Schematic of high tibial focal dome osteotomy. The goal of this surgical procedure is to realign the mechanical axis of the affected limb from the diseased compartment to the more healthy side. To accomplish this, a series of pinholes equidistant from a central rotational axis is drilled along anterior posterior direction with the help of a guiding tool (see close-up). The proximal and distal bone fragments are separated completely by connecting these pinholes each other with a sharp osteotome. The deformity is corrected as two cylindrical shaped bone fragments slide on each other rotating around the central axis under manual stress [3]. As shown in the image, H is the hip center, A is the ankle center, X is the rotational axis for deformity correction, T is the anticipated postoperative position of the weight bearing axis at the tibial plateau, G is the corresponding postoperative ankle center, and α is the necessary rotational angle to correct the deformity

The navigated instruments can be divided into three groups according to their functionalities. The first group includes a calibrated fluoroscopic C-arm, a tool for measuring the gravitational direction, an accuracy checker for the verification of system accuracy, and a pointing device (pointer) for percutaneous digitization and landmarks verification. This group of instruments is used for image acquisition and landmark registration. The next group consists of a navigated drill and a chisel. They are used for cutting the bone. The last group includes three dynamic reference bases (DRBs), which are affixed to the operated limb for tracking the motion of the corresponding anatomies during operation. All surgical instruments and DRBs can be gas or steam sterilized.

2.2   Landmark Registration and Deformity Measurement

Intraoperatively, after the surgeon affixes DRBs at the femur and the tibia of the affected limb, the fluoroscopic images (Fig. 3) are acquired and uploaded into navigation system at the beginning of operation, including knee AP (anterior-posterior), knee lateral, hip AP, hip lateral, ankle AP, and ankle lateral images.

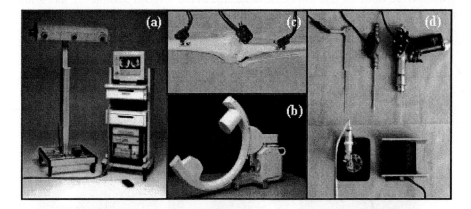

Fig. 2. System components consist of (a) optoelectric localizer and computer system, (b) registered fluoroscopic C-arm, (c) dynamical reference bases affixed to the affected limb, and (d) other navigated instruments, including navigated chisel, pointing device, navigated drill, gravitational direction measurement tool, and accuracy checker, shown in the image from top left to bottom right, respectively

Anatomic landmarks are then registered with a previous introduced hybrid concept [15], which involves kinematic pivoting movement [16], percutaneous digitization using a pointer [16], and bi-planar 3D (three-dimensional) point reconstruction based on multiple registered fluoroscopic images [17]. At the hip joint, the hip center is defined as the spherical center of the femoral head, and registered with bi-planar 3D point reconstruction using hip AP and hip lateral images. Alternatively, it can be registered through kinematic pivoting movement of the femur. At the ankle joint, the ankle center is defined as the center of the talus, and registered using ankle AP and ankle lateral images. Alternatively, it can be registered through percutaneous digitization using a palpable pointer and defined as the middle point of the transmalleolar axis formed by extreme points at lateral and medial malleoli. At the knee joint, the femoral posterior condylar axis, defined as the line between two most posterior aspects of the femoral condyles, and the tibial plateau, defined as a contour deformed with four points at the most lateral, medial, anterior and posterior edge of the tibial plateau, are registered using knee AP and knee lateral images. The knee center is defined as the geometric center of the tibial plateau.

Once the landmarks are registered, a patient specific coordinate system is established. For the mathematical description of the bone and joint geometry, each articulate joint component needs its own coordinate system. On the femoral side, the frontal plane is defined as the plane that passes through the hip and knee centers, and is parallel to the femoral posterior condyle axis; the sagittal plane passes through the hip and knee centers, and is perpendicular to the frontal plane. The transversal plane is orthogonal to both the frontal and sagittal planes. The coordinate systems of the proximal and distal fragments of the tibia are established with the knee, ankle centers, and affined lateral-medial direction, respectively. The affined lateral-medial direction is transferred from the femoral to the tibial side as the surgeon puts the leg into a fully extended neutral position.

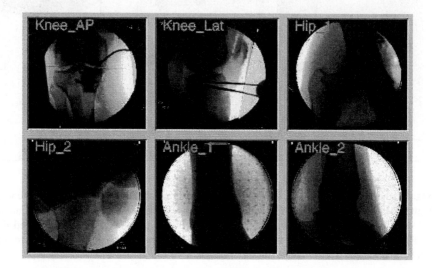

Fig. 3. Fluoroscopic images used for landmark registration and osteotomy navigation, which include knee AP, knee lateral, and optionally hip AP, hip lateral, ankle AP, and ankle lateral images

The functional parameters of the affected limb are measured intraoperatively, including varus/valgus angle, flexion/extension angle, tibial plateau slope, and joint lines orientation angle. These parameters are the basis of the surgical procedure, since only if the deformity is measured accurately, then it can be corrected correctly. We don't need any preoperative planning information derived from conventional full leg X-ray images because it is cumbersome and error prone.

2.3   Osteotomy Planning

The osteotomy is planned with the aid of fluoroscopic images. The cylindrical osteotomy plane is superimposed on the fluoroscopic images in order to help the surgeon make a decision based on clinical factors including severity of the deformity, type of the fixation, soft tissues coverage, and bone quality.

With the help of the knee AP image, the surgeon determines the position of the central rotational axis, the radius of the osteotomy arc, and the distance between pinholes (Fig. 4). A numerical scalar is superimposed to help the surgeon visually control the position of the cutting plane. With the help of knee lateral image, the surgeon determines the posterior slope of the osteotomy plane. Moreover, after the surgeon specifies the anticipated postoperative alignment of the affected limb, the necessary rotational angle and the corresponding increment of the leg length are calculated automatically.

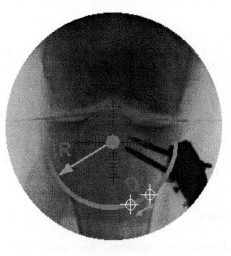

Fig. 4. Osteotomy plane is planed with the aid of fluoroscopic images. By default, the radius of the osteotomy plane (R) is 70 mm, the distance between rotational axis and the tibial plateau is 10 mm, and the distance between pinholes (D) is 5 mm. The surgeon can change these parameters according to clinical situation

2.4   Navigational Guidance

Bone Cutting

The accuracy of the osteotomy cannot be overemphasized. The creation of a congruous cylindrical osteotomy surface is essential in order to allow two fragments slide on each other and to provide a maximal, intimate contact between two cut surfaces, thus hastening the bone union. From the technical point of view, ideally, all drilled holes should be parallel in both the frontal and sagittal planes, and each bone cut with the osteotome should also follows the same direction. An inappropriate drilling or bone cutting, such as under-estimation of the drill depth, malorientation of the drill direction, or an excessive cut on the tibial dorsal side, may cause problems such as intercondylar fracture, pin penetration of the tibial plateau, or damage to the tibial neurovascular structures. Obviously, it is much more difficult to create such a cylindrical osteotomy surface than a straight cut.

Navigational guidance (Fig. 5) is therefore provided in order to address these technical problems. The navigated instruments used for bone cutting include a calibrated drill and a chisel. A rigid metal tube is used to prevent the bending of the drill bit during osteotomy. With virtual fluoroscopic technique, the surgeon is able to continuously monitor the position and orientation of the instruments in multiple fluoroscopic images simultaneously. Moreover, with real-time feedback of the deviation of the instrument to the planned cutting plane, the surgeon can minimize the risk of intraoperative technical pitfalls, and achieve a safe and accurate osteotomy.

Deformity Correction

The deformity correction is the most critical and difficult step, because once the alignment is achieved and the internal fixation implant is in place, little can be done to make further adjustments towards the ideal anticipated correction. Therefore, all the clinical relevant parameters are navigated, including three-dimensional axial alignment at the frontal, sagittal and transversal planes, the femorotibial rotational angle, the joint line orientation angle, the tibial plateau slope, and the weight-bearing axis position at the tibial plateau (Fig. 6). These parameters together can provide the surgeon with a comprehensive view of the clinical outcome, thus enabling him/her to perform the planned surgical procedure accurately.

2.5   Surgical Procedure

No preoperative planning is required for using the navigation system. Intraoperatively, the patient is placed on a radiolucent table as usual. Following standard exposure, two dynamical reference bases (DRB) are attached to the femur and the tibia using 2.8 mm Kirschner wires. After acquisition of fluoroscopic images and registration of anatomic landmarks, the deformity is measured intraoperatively and the osteotomy is planed interactively. After the surgeon is satisfied with the planning, a third DRB is affixed under navigational guidance at the proximal fragment of the tibia. The planned osteotomy and deformity correction are then performed under navigational guidance. The operation is finished in a conventional way after plate fixation.

3   Results

The concept of anatomic landmarks and functional parameters has been comprehensively validated in laboratory with a test bench, and the results are to be published separately [18]. It showed that the definitions of landmarks are appropriate and the algorithms for deformity measurement are accurate. With an entire leg model (RR0119, Synbone AG, Davos, Switzerland), the maximum inter-observer difference (five independent operators with identical experimental condition) was found to be 0.3° for varus/valgus angle, 0.6° for flexion/extension angle, and 1.0° for tibial plateau slope. For the intra-observer reproducibility, 25 pairs of fluoroscopic images were acquired at different C-arm poses (within 10° deviation from the well-aligned position), and the landmarks are registered accordingly. It showed that the mean deviation was 0.4° for varus/valgus angle, 0.4° for flexion/extension angle, and 1.0° for tibial plateau slope, with a standard deviation (95% confidence interval) of 0.6°, 0.8°, and 1.2°, respectively.

Following the encouraging laboratory evaluation, a clinical study on focal dome osteotomy has been launched recently. Meanwhile, the study is still going on therefore no statistical results are available.

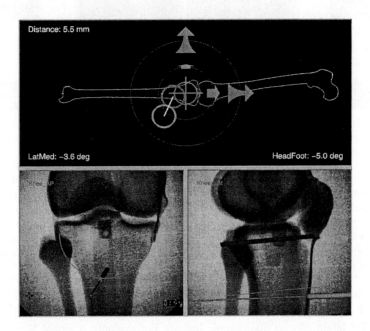

Fig. 5. The osteotomy is performed under navigational guidance. The deviation of the instrument is defined as the vector between instrument tip and current pinhole. The current active instrument, e.g., a drill, is the nearest tool to the patient. The current active pinhole, shown as the cross-circle in the figure, is the nearest pinhole on the osteotomy arc to the current active instrument. During osteotomy, the hinge axis, osteotomy arc, current pinhole, and navigated instrument are superimposed on knee AP and lateral images, in order to allow the surgeon to continually monitor the deviation and progress of the instrument. Moreover, the deviation of the instrument is intuitively displayed on the top of the window using "three circles", in which the red cross-circle is the target position, and two green circles are the tip and top of the current instrument. Four arrows are used to indicate the direction and amplitude of the further adjustment. The instrument is precisely aligned if three circles are overlapped each other

4   Discussion

High tibial dome osteotomy is generally recognized as complex and technical demanding. Success of such procedure depends on accurate deformity measurement, safe osteotomy with appropriate surgical technique, and precise correction of the existed deformity.

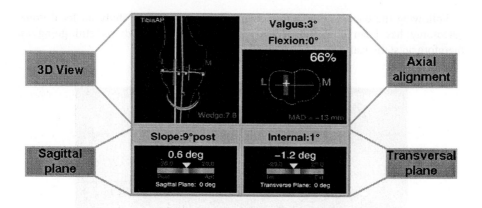

Fig. 6. The deformity is corrected under navigational guidance. The navigated parameters can be divided into three groups. The axial alignment includes varus/valgus angle (3° valgus shown in the image), extension/flexion angle (0° flexion), mechanical axis deviation (13 mm laterally), and the position of the weight-bearing axis at the tibial plateau (66%). The second group includes the tibial plateau slope (9° posterior) and the change of the slope due to osteotomy (0.6° toward anterior). The third group consists of femorotibial rotational angle (1° internal) and the angular change between the proximal and distal fragments of the tibia (1.2° internal) in the transversal plane

Accurate registration of anatomic landmarks is the key issues of the system. A variety of methods have been adopted to help the surgeon objectively and precisely identify the landmarks on fluoroscopic images. For example, a virtual Mose circle is used for identifying the circular center of the femoral head, and a virtual ruler is used for localizing the center of the talus. In our system, the knee center is defined as the geometric center of the tibial plateau, i.e., the middle point between lateral and medial edges of the tibial plateau in the frontal plane. Our laboratory evaluation showed that these edge points are more objective and reproducible than any other anatomical features, particularly if fluoroscopic images are misaligned from true AP or lateral direction.

From the technique point of view, the work presented here only supports high tibial dome osteotomy. However, we are already in the progress of extending the current software to a more generic one, aiming to support all common osteotomy techniques around the knee joint including opening wedge, closing wedge, dome osteotomies, and to enable surgeons to perform osteotomies at either high tibial or supracondylar femoral side.

5   Conclusions

A CT-free computer assisted navigation system for high tibial dome osteotomy has been developed and evaluated. Although clinical study is still underway, the first trials by a group of skilled surgeons have given very positive feedbacks. This system is substantially different from other computer assisted approaches for osteotomy planning or robotic preparation, as it does not require any preoperative procedure or alteration of the conventional surgical procedure; neither does it need any information derived from full leg X-ray images. It allows surgeons to accurately measure the deformity, interactively plan the surgical procedure, and precisely perform the osteotomy under navigational guidance. The system thus holds the promise to reduce the risk of intraoperative complications and consequently to improve the clinical outcome of this surgical procedure.

Acknowledgement. The financial support of the AO/ASIF Foundation, Davos, Switzerland, of the M.E. Müller Foundation, Bern, Switzerland, of the Swiss National Science Foundation (NCCR/CO-ME), and of Praxim-Medivision (previously Medivision AG), Bern, Switzerland, is gratefully acknowledged.

References

1. Phillips MJ, Krackow KA: High Tibial Osteotomy and Distal Femoral Osteotomy for Valgus or Varus Deformity Around the Knee. AAOS Instructional Course Lecture, Vol.47, 429-436
2. Jackson JP, Waugh W: The Techniques and Complications of Upper Tibial Osteotomy: a Review of 226 Operations. JBJS[Br] 56-B(1974)236-45
3. Paley D: Principles of Deformity Correction. With editorial assistance from Herzenberg J. ISBN 3-540-41665-X, Springer-Verlag, Berlin Heidelbery New York (2002)
4. Hankemeire S, Paley D, Pape HC, Zeichen J, Gosling T, Kretteck C: Die Kniegelenknahe Focal-dome-Osteotomie. Orthopäde 33(2004)170-177
5. Korn, M: A New Approach to Dome High Tibial Osteotomy. The American Journal of Knee Surgery 9(1996)13-21
6. Edgar GH, Morawski DR, Santore RF: Complications of High Tibial Osteotomy. In: Knee surgery, edited by Fu FH, Harner CD, and Vince KG. ISBN 0-683-03389-1 (1996)
7. Fujisawa Y, Masuhara R, Shiohi S: The Effect of High Tibial Osteotomy on Osteoarthritis of the Knee. Orthop Clin North Am. 10(1979)585-608
8. Noyes FR, Barber-Westin SD, TE Hewett: High Tibial Osteotomy and Ligament Reconstruction for Varus Angulated Anterior Cruciate Ligament-deficient Knees. The American J. of Sport Medicine 28-3(2000)282-293
9. Aydogdu S, Sur H: High Tibial Osteotomy for Varus Deformity of More Than 20 Degrees. Rev Chir Orthop Reparatrice Mot. 84(1997)439-46
10. Takahashi T, Wada Y, Tanaka M, Iwagawa M, Ikeuchi M, Hirose D, Yamamoto H: Dome-shaped Proximal Tibial Osteotomy Using Percutaneous Drilling for Osteoarthritis of the Knee. Arch Orthop Trauma Surg. 120(2000)32-37
11. Madan S, Ranjith, Fiddian NJ: Intermediate Follow-up of High Tibial Osteotomy: a Comparison of Two Techniques. Bull Hosp Jt Dis. 61(2002-2003)11-6
12. Ellis RE, Tso CY, Rudan JF, Harrison MM: A Surgical Planning and Guidance System for High Tibial Osteotomy. Computer Aided Surgery 4(1999)264-274
13. Phillips R, Hafez M, Mohsen A, Sheman K, Hewitt J, Browbank I, Bouazza-Marouf K: Computer and Robotic Assisted Osteotomy Around the Knee. In: MMVR 2000 - 8th Annual Medicine Meets Virtual Reality Conference, Newport Beach, January 27-30, 2000. pp 265-271
14. Wang G, Zheng G, C De Simoni, Staubli A, Schmucki D, Nolte LP: A Hybrid CT-free Computer Assisted System for High Tibial Osteotomy. In: Computer Assisted Orthopaedic Surgery, edited by Langlotz F, Davies BL and Bauer A, CAOS 2003, Marbella, Spina. p 394

15. Zheng G, Marx A, Langlotz U, Widmer K, Buttaro M, Nolte LP: A Hybrid CT-free Navigation System for Total Hip Arthroplasty. Computer Assisted Surgery 7(2002)129-145

16. Kunz M, Strsuss M, Langlotz F, Deuretzbacher G, Rüther W, Nolte LP: A non-CT Based Total Knee Arthroplasty System Featuring Complete Soft-tissues Balancing. In: Medical Image Computing and Computer-Assisted Intervention, 14-17 October 2001, Utrecht, Netherlands. p 409-415

17. Hofstetter R, Slomczykowski M, Krettek C, Koppen G, Sati M, Nolte LP: Fluoroscopy as an Imaging Means for Computer Assisted Surgical Navigation. Comp. Aided Surg. 4(1999)65-76

18. Wang G, Zheng G, Keppler P, Gebhard F, Staubli A, Müller U, Schmucki D, Flütsch S, Nolte LP: Implementation, Accuracy Evaluation, and Preliminary Clinical Trial of a CT-free Navigation System for High Tibial Opening Wedge Osteotomy. Submitted to Computer Assisted Surgery

A Phantom Based Approach to Fluoroscopic Navigation for Orthopaedic Surgery

Roger Phillips[1], Amr Mohsen[2], Warren Viant[1], Sabur Malek[1],
Qingde Li[1], Nasir Shah[2], Mike Bielby[1], and Kevin Sherman[2]

[1] Department of Computer Science, University of Hull, Hull, UK. HU6 7RX
{r.phillips,w.j.viant,s.a.malek,q.li,
m.s.bielby}@hull.ac.uk
http://www.dcs.hull.ac.uk/people/{rp}
[2] Hull Royal Infirmary, Hull and East Yorkshire Hospitals NHS Trust, Anlaby Road,
Hull, UK. HU3 2JZ
{amr.mohsen, kevin.sherman}@hey.nhs.uk

Abstract. The use of the C-arm fluoroscope for surgical navigation in various Computer Assisted Orthopaedic Surgery Systems (CAOS) has been an important success of research into CAOS technology. To use the fluoroscope for quantitative surgical navigation involves calibrating its 2D images and tracking the spatial position of the fluoroscope's image beam. This allows 3D reconstruction of anatomy from a series of 2D fluoroscopic images. This paper presents a new technique for determining the C-arm position and calibrating the image beam. This technique is based on a small imaging phantom that is placed close to the patient. This paper also briefly describes the CAOS system developed at Hull that uses this imaging phantom and reports on in vivo and in vitro studies.

1 Introduction

The C-arm fluoroscope is an indispensable intraoperative 2D imaging device for orthopaedic surgery but it does pose a radiation hazard to the theatre staff and patients. The fluoroscope is frequently used for surgical navigation in various Computer Assisted Orthopaedic Surgery Systems (CAOS).

The usual approach of using the C-arm fluoroscope for quantitative surgical navigation is by calibrating the 2D image to provide accurate 2D images. By tracking the position of the corresponding image beams, reconstruction can then give the 3D location of the anatomy at the operation site. The most common technical solution is to retrofit a device to the x-ray receptor end of the C-arm (e.g. Traxtal Technologies FluoroTrax). This device comprises a calibration grid and is surrounded by IREDs which are tracked by a camera system. C-arm fluoroscopes have now been developed that include tracking of a calibrated image beam, e.g. Medtronic Sofamor Danek's Fluoronav™ and SurgiGATE® (Medivision, Oberdorf, Switzerland).

The flexibility that the C-arm provides has led to intraoperative surgical navigation CAOS approaches for spine, total hip replacement, high tibial osteotomy, femoral

C. Barillot, D.R. Haynor, and P. Hellier (Eds.): MICCAI 2004, LNCS 3217, pp. 621–628, 2004.

neck fractures, distal locking of intramedullary nails, etc. The operating experience in fluoroscopic navigation and its use for the identification of anatomical landmarks, axes and planes has led to many CAOS navigation approaches that were previously based on preoperative CT surgical planning being replaced by CT-free CAOS approaches, e.g. spinal and pelvic surgery.

Another feature of having a quantified C-arm fluoroscope is its potential for virtual fluoroscopy (VF) [1]. Typically in VF a number of fluoroscopic images are taken of the patient during actual surgery. For each image, the position and geometry of the associated image beam is recorded. During surgery the position of the surgeon's instrument and bone(s) being operated upon are optically tracked by IREDs attached to them. This allows the computer to produce virtual fluoroscopic images by overlaying the projection of the instrument onto previously captured images.

The above approach to surgical navigation has a number of potential problems.
1. The calibration device attached to the C-arm camera reduces the useful imaging volume of the fluoroscope.
2. The optical tracking volume is large as the C-arm is often moved between the AP and lateral position, etc.
3. The calibration / registration zone is distant from the operation site and this may cause magnification of errors.
4. The markers of the calibration grid appear in the fluoroscopic image.

The authors have developed an alternative approach to calibrating and tracking the C-arm of the fluoroscope for surgical navigation for CAOS. This is based on a small tracked phantom that is placed in the C-arm image space close to the operating site. Section 2 presents this phantom based technique.

This phantom based approach is used in our Computer Assisted Orthopaedic Surgical System (CAOSS) for trauma surgery. This CAOSS has been used for over 4 years in preclinical trials and its navigation modules include implanting compression hip screws and locking of distal screws for intramedullary nails. Section 3 discusses the CAOSS and results from in vivo and in vitro studies. The paper concludes with a discussion that compares our tracked phantom to the explicitly tracked C-arm approach to surgical navigation.

2   Phantom-Based Approach to C-Arm Calibration and Tracking

To use fluoroscopic images for surgical navigation requires that, firstly, the 2D fluoroscopic images are accurately calibrated and, secondly, that the position of the corresponding fluoroscopic image beam is known accurately. The latter allows the partial 3D reconstruction of the operation site by projecting various 2D features extracted from 2D fluoroscopic images into 3D.

2.1 Preoperative Calibration of X-Ray Images

The fluoroscopic 2D images suffer from a number of distortion effects [2]. This image distortion has components which are static and dynamic. The latter is due partially to the influence of magnetic fields on the image intensification tube of the C-arm.

The calibration includes a preoperative step where an x-ray translucent plate containing an evenly spaced grid of 64 x 64 balls placed on the x-ray receptor cover of the C-arm is imaged. From this image, software calculates a distortion-undistortion map. Intraoperatively, all fluoroscopic images are then displayed with the distortion removed. Sufficient image accuracy is obtained by calibrating in just two positions, i.e. with the C-arm vertical and horizontal. This calibration is typically required once a month.

We have studied how dynamic distortion varies with the position of the C-arm. We observed the main effects are a twisting effect and a translation. Preoperative calibration in 2 positions considerably reduces the sizes of these effects. It should also be noted that the intraoperative C-arm tracking (see Section 2.2) in fact includes inherent calibration that further reduces dynamic distortion remaining after applying the preoperative calibration mapping.

2.2 Tracking the Fluoroscopic Image Beam Using a Small Imaging Phantom

Tracking the spatial position of the fluoroscope's image beam with an optical tracking system involves accurate localisation of the position of the x-ray source and the image plane of the C-arm. Our tracking approach involves placing a small registration phantom in the image space of the C-arm. This phantom consists of an H arrangement of 21 metal balls that measures approximately 2" x 2" by ½" (Fig. 1). The projection of these balls appears in a fluoroscopic image. The phantom is held by an end-effector and a lockable passive arm (Fig. 2). The position of the phantom is tracked by an optical camera tracking system. When a patient is imaged, software undistorts the image using the static calibration mapping and then automatically detects the position of the phantom in the image. Knowing the position of the phantom, an algorithm calculates the position of the C-arm in the coordinate space of the tracking system.

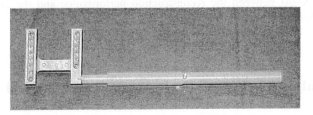

Fig. 1. Image phantom used for tracking the image space of the C-arm

Significant obscuration of the phantom frequently occurs in the image due to shadow of soft tissue, bone edges, retractors, etc. Furthermore, image contrast varies considerably between images and patients, and varies considerably within an image.

Software has been developed that is robust to such problems. The software comprises two distinct algorithms. The ball detection algorithm first detects a candidate set of metal ball projections from the image. The second, the phantom detector algorithm, selects a subset of these metal balls that provide a feasible projection of the phantom. The ball detection algorithm uses contrast gradient in two directions to initially select possible ball projections. It then applies a series of six filters to eliminate less promising projections. These filters include tests for size, shape, proximity, contrast and gradient variation. The robustness of the phantom detection algorithm is achieved by detection requiring a minimum of 14 balls.

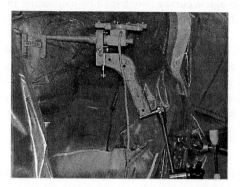

Fig. 2. Passive arm and end-effector for holding the imaging phantom in OR. The passive arm is clamped to horizontal bar of operating table. The position of the end-effector is tracked by 7 IREDS. There are two positions for the phantom used; one for AP and one for lateral imaging.

The software developed for the detection of the phantom from a fluoroscopic image has been extensively tested and fine-tuned using a database of over 200 fluoroscopic images obtained from early uses of the imaging phantom in the operating theatre.

Our tracking approach for the C-arm takes account of the C-arm flex both in terms of change in position of the x-ray source and change in direction of the x-ray beam. Also, as mentioned in Section 2.1 it caters for the dynamic distortion of images as it corrects for linear components of rotation and translation errors.

Extensive computer simulations were used to determine a phantom design that had the best trade-off between the reconstruction performance and the clinical need to make the phantom as unobtrusive as possible. In vitro tests have shown that a fluoroscopic image has a maximum calibration error of less than 0.5 mm.

3   Clinical Applications of the Phantom-Based Surgical Navigation

We have developed the Computer Assisted Orthopaedic Surgical System (CAOSS) for trauma orthopaedic surgery. This system uses intraoperative fluoroscopic navigation using the imaging phantom. The CAOSS comprises a trolley, an optical tracking system, an optically tracked end-effector attached to a lockable passive arm, the imaging phantom and various guiding cannulas. The CAOSS trolley houses a PC-based computer system, the optical tracking hardware, a monitor and a frame grabber with a video feed from the C-arm fluoroscope.

The camera array is mounted on the theatre laminar flow enclosure. This tracks the position of the end-effector via seven IREDs attached to it. The end-effector and passive arm are rigidly mounted to the side bar of the operating table (Fig. 2). The passive arm has three joints that are lockable via a single twist handle.

The end-effector is used by the surgeon to position the image phantom and to position the guiding cannulas. The guiding cannula has a sharp serrated end and this prevents whiplash and helps keep the guide wire straight.

The CAOSS currently has three surgical planning modules, namely: insertion of compression hip screw for femur neck fractures, distal locking of intramedullary nails for femur fractures and insertion of three cannulated screws for femur neck fractures [3]. Only the first two operations are described here. In addition we have developed a general purpose orthopaedic surgical navigation system using a virtual fluoroscopy approach that is based on the image phantom. It is currently being evaluated in vitro for unicompartmental knee replacement [4].

3.1 Insertion of Compression Hip Screw

The CAOSS for this operation was first used in the operating theatre in May 2000. Since then some 30 operations have been performed.

The computer-based planning for this operation requires an AP and a lateral fluoroscopic image of the fracture site. The anatomical features used for planning the surgery are the shaft of the proximal femur and the femoral neck and head. In the operating theatre these three anatomical features on the two images are marked with a mouse. The 2D projection of the femur shaft axis and the femoral neck and head centres is then determined. These 2D projections from the two views are reconstructed to create a 3D surgical plan.

The computer plans a trajectory for the guide wire of the compression hip screw by constructing a 3D line from a way point in the femoral head that intersects with the femoral shaft axis at the same angle as the hip screw and plate (typically 115° to 135°). The way point is taken to be one quarter distant along the 3D line joining the centre of the head with the centre of the neck. This trajectory is then overlaid on both AP and lateral images. The depth of the drill hole is also calculated. The surgeon reviews the suggested guide wire trajectory and, if necessary, modifies it by moving the entry point of the guide wire on the femur shaft or moving the waypoint.

3.1.1 In Vivo Study of Insertion of Compression Hip Screw
During 2002 and 3, a group of 10 patients underwent surgery using CAOSS for insertion of compression hip screw. There were 8 female and 2 male patients with ages ranging between 75 and 93 years (mean age 84.7 years). Mean follow up time was 11.5 months (9 to 21 months).

Fluoroscopic Images: Theoretically only four fluoroscopic images are required for insertion of a guide wire into the femoral neck when using CAOSS. An AP and lateral images is required for surgical navigation and another pair of images to confirm guide wire insertion. The average number of images required in this study was 6 with a range of 4 – 10. Three patients required the minimum of 4. Additional images were sometimes required because the imaging phantom was not fully in the image beam. A learning curve was observed with later cases requiring fewer images.

Time taken: this is the time taken just to plan the trajectory and then to insert the guide wire, under computer guidance, into the femoral neck of the patient. The average time taken to perform the procedure was 17.2 minutes (range 8 – 23 minutes). Again a learning curve was observed with times reducing with experience.

Position of the screw: Baumgaertner [5] describes the tip apex distance (TAD), which is the sum of the distances between the apex of the femoral head and the tip of the lag screw in the femoral head, both in anteroposterior and lateral views. They observed that cut out of implants had a TAD of more than 25 mm. We used TAD to confirm the position of the screw. Eight patients had TAD within the acceptable range of 25 mm with an average of 17.6 mm (range 6.7 - 20 mm). Two patients had a TAD of 31 mm. No cut out of the implant was seen during follow up.

3.2   Distal Locking of Intramedullary Nail

Many femur fractures are treated with intramedullary (IM) nails. To achieve stability, locking screws are used at both ends of the IM nail. The difficult part of the operation is inserting the distal locking screws.

The CAOSS surgical navigation module uses an AP and lateral image of the distal end of a nail. In the AP view, the IM nail and the long bone are identified by marking them with a mouse. In the lateral view, the nail is identified and each distal hole is identified by a surrounding square. CAOSS software then automatically determines the nail axis and recovers the geometry of both the distal holes from these images [6]; this provides the drilling axis of both holes and the length of screws needed for locking. An important feature is that the projection of the distal holes in the images need not be perfect circles. To drill each hole, the surgeon positions a guiding cannula using guidance displayed on the computer's monitor.

The conventional manual approach suffers from problems such as extended time required for distal locking, radiation risk to patient and staff and misplacement of the screw. CAOSS offers the opportunity to address these shortfalls.

3.2.1   In Vitro Study of Intraobserver Error in IM Nail Surgical Planning

We are part way through an extensive study of intraobserver error for surgical navigation in the distal locking of IM nails. This study will systematically vary the parameters that might affect the surgical planning result. Besides giving a fuller understanding of intraobserver variability, this study may also identify areas where the system can be tuned to improve performance. Examples of parameters being varied include:

1. The position of the nail with respect to the C-arm image beam in the three orthogonal directions.
2. The position of the image phantom in the image space in terms of its distance from the patient and its position within the image plane.

3. Rotating the nail position by up to 20° in both directions from its position where a perfect circle projection of the hole appears in the lateral image.
4. Using different end-effectors and imaging phantoms.

In vitro laboratory tests were performed using various IM nails and also using a 14 mm diameter hollow metal tube with two holes of 5 mm diameter that are 3 cm apart. A metal tube was used to provide a controlled environment for tests as it does not have any curves along its long axis. A screw-guide was designed with a 5 mm diameter solid cylinder at one end which fits into the nail holes precisely. By mounting the screw-guide in the end-effector, its position can be tracked by CAOSS. Thus when the screw guide is placed in a nail hole, the screw guide axis gives the true trajectory of this hole. This can be compared with the trajectory that the CAOSS software predicts.

In an initial series of 10 tests the nail position was varied with respect to the image space. The mean translation error for the planned drilling trajectory at the entry to the distal hole (of the distal hole pair) was 0.19 mm with a maximum error of 0.45 mm and a standard deviation of 0.12 mm. The mean angular error between the axis of the distal hole and the CAOSS predicted drilling trajectory was 0.18° with a max error of 0.42°. For the proximal hole the translation errors were 0.26, 0.44 and 0.10 mm respectively, and the rotational errors were 0.15° and 0.26°, respectively. The full set of intraobserver results is to be published shortly. These results indicated that these accuracy results are invariant to the position of the imaging phantom in the image space. It is also worth noting that accuracy of our approach depends on the relative error of the tracking system and not its absolute error. As the volume tracked is small, this relative error is very much smaller than the absolute error of the tracking system.

4 Discussion

Our small H-shaped phantom technique for the image calibration and the C-arm tracking of the fluoroscope has been used for over 36 months as part of our CAOSS preclinical trials for hip trauma surgery. Qualitative assessment of the complete system indicates satisfactory clinical performance in terms of accuracy. The laboratory tests of the phantom indicate a maximum calibration error of 0.5 mm of a fluoroscopic image. The phantom approach will work with any modern C-arm fluoroscope.

Our imaging phantom approach has advantages over existing fluoro navigation systems that use explicit C-arm tracking via an optically tracked grid attached to the C-arm's x-ray receptor. The key differences in the approaches are as follows.
1. The optically tracked volume for an imaging phantom is close to the operation site and it interferes very little with the set up in operating theatres. For C-arm tracked systems the tracked volume is very much larger as the x-ray receptor has to be tracked through a 90° vertical rotation of the C-arm and it is more likely to interfere with theatre set up, e.g. interference with vertical sterile drapes. The image phantom approach also suffers less from losing line of sight, as the tracked volume is very much smaller.
2. There is significantly less image obscuration with an imaging phantom. There are only 21 opaque markers of the phantom in the image. In C-arm tracking the whole

image is splattered by markers, however, some systems replace some markers in the image by their surrounding background which is undesirable.
3. The imaging phantom has to be manually placed in the image space. This is an extra step and multiple images may be required to achieve correct placement.

Another difference between the two approaches to fluoroscopic navigation is image calibration. In the phantom based approach, primary calibration occurs in two positions preoperatively but this is fine tuned by a secondary intraoperative calibration that is inherent in the phantom's design. In C-arm tracking the image is calibrated intraoperatively with every image. Our approach to calibration is more precise due to a denser calibration grid and calibration being closer to the operation site.

5 Conclusion

This paper presented a new approach for image calibration and image space tracking of a fluoroscope based on a small imaging phantom. This is an effective and viable alternative to the existing explicit C-arm tracking method of attaching a calibration grid and IREDs directly to the x-ray receptor of the C-arm. This approach is suitable for surgical navigation that requires interoperative fluoroscopic navigation. The imaging phantom has a number of ergonomic and efficacy advantages over the C-arm tracking approach. A study has shown that a surgical target can be reconstructed from a pair of fluoroscopic with a translation error of less than 0.5 mm. This imaging phantom has been used clinically in a Hull hospital for the past 4 years as part of CAOSS. Implementing a drilling trajectory under computer guidance by CAOSS provides a total system accuracy of less than 1.5 mm and an angular accuracy of less than 1°.

References

1. Hofstetter R, Slomyczykowski M, Sati M and Nolte L-P (1999). Fluoroscopy as an imaging means for computer-assisted surgical intervention. Computer Aided Surgery, 4, 65-76
2. Boone JM, Seibert JA and Blood W (1991). Analysis and correction of imperfections in the image intensifier TV-digitiser imaging chain. Medical Physics, 18, 236-42
3. Viant WJ, Phillips R and Mohsen A (1999). Computer assisted positioning of cannulated hip screw. in Lemke HU, Vannier MW, Inamura K and Farman AG (eds), CARS'99 Computer assisted radiology and surgery, Amsterdam, Elsevier, 751-5
4. Phillips R, Peter V, Faure G-E, Li Q, Sherman KP, Viant WJ, Bielby M, Mohsen AMMA (2002), A Virtual Fluoroscopy System based on a Small and Unobtrusive Registration / Calibration Phantom, Proceedings of Computer Assisted Radiology and Surgery, CARS 2002, 275-280, Springer Verlag, June 26-29,2002, Paris
5. Baumgaertner MR et al. (1995), The value of tip apex distance in predicting failure of fixation of peritrochanteric fractures of the hip. J Bone Joint Surg-Am; 77(7):1058 – 1064
6. Zhu Y, Phillips R, Griffiths JG, Viant WJ, Mohsen A, Bielby M (2002), Recovery of distal hole axis in intramedullary nail trajectory planning, IMechE Part H Journal of Engineering in Medicine, 216,(5),323-332

Real-Time Estimation of Hip Range of Motion for Total Hip Replacement Surgery

Yasuhiro Kawasaki[1], Fumihiko Ino[1], Yoshinobu Sato[2], Nobuhiko Sugano[2], Hideki Yoshikawa[2], Shinichi Tamura[2], and Kenichi Hagihara[1]

[1] Graduate School of Information Science and Technology
[2] Graduate School of Medicine
Osaka University
y-kawask@ist.osaka-u.ac.jp

Abstract. This paper presents the design and implementation of a range of motion estimation method that is capable of fine-grained estimation during total hip replacement (THR) surgery. Our method combines an adaptive refinement strategy with a high performance computing system in order to enable real-time estimation. The experimental results indicate that the implementation on a cluster of 64 PCs enables intraoperative estimation of $360 \times 360 \times 180$ stance configurations within a half minute, and thereby plays a key role in selecting and aligning the optimal combination of artificial joint components during THR surgery.

1 Introduction

Total hip replacement (THR) [1, 2] is a surgical procedure that relieves patients of hip pain and removes their difficulty in walking by replacing the hip joint with an artificial joint. The key issue in this surgery is to select and align the optimal combination of artificial joint components: the cup, head, neck, and stem components as illustrated in Fig. 1(a). These optimal selection and alignment are important for both the surgeon and patient because either inappropriate or malpositioned components increase the risk of clinical problems such as dislocation, wear, and loosening [2, 3].

In order to assist the surgeon in the selection and alignment, range of motion (ROM) estimation systems [1, 2, 4, 3, 5] have been developed in the past. Earlier systems are useful in developing preoperative surgical plans because they present the limitation of hip movement on three-dimensional (3-D) polygonal surface models reconstructed from patients' computed tomography (CT) images. However, the preoperative plans may need to be changed by unexpected conditions that reveal during surgery. For example, if the bone tissue around the preoperatively planned position is known to be fragile, another position has to be selected according to intraoperative circumstances. Thus, intraoperative estimation is essential to overcome such unexpected conditions.

One issue to develop intraoperative estimation systems is a large amount of computation due to collision detections (CDs) required for ROM estimation. For example, an earlier system [4] on a Sun Ultra 30 running at 300 MHz takes 0.05 seconds for detecting a collision for a stance configuration, so that it takes approximately 13 days when computing a 3-D ROM with $360 \times 180 \times 360 = 23\,328\,000$ configurations: $360°$, $180°$, and $360°$ for yaw (ϕ), pitch (θ), and role (ψ) angles, respectively, as illustrated

C. Barillot, D.R. Haynor, and P. Hellier (Eds.): MICCAI 2004, LNCS 3217, pp. 629–636, 2004.

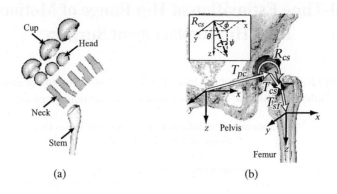

Fig. 1. (a) Components of artificial joint and (b) representation of hip joint motion.

in Fig. 1(b). Therefore, to achieve real-time estimation during surgery, earlier systems need to degrade the quality of estimations by limiting the area of estimations [1, 2] and by degrading the number of stance configurations [3] or the resolution of images [5].

In contrast to these coarse-grained estimations, the key contribution of this paper is to enable fine-grained estimations during surgery. To enable this, we have developed a real-time estimation system based on two key methods: 1) adaptive ROM refinement for computational complexity reduction and 2) parallelization for further acceleration. Our results indicate that the combination of the two methods is 11 times faster than a previous parallel system [6] without adaptive refinement.

The remainder of the paper is organized as follows. Section 2 summarizes an overview of ROM estimation while Section 3 gives the design and implementation of our method. Section 4 presents some experimental results. Section 5 concludes this paper.

2 Background: Range of Motion (ROM) Estimation

To describe the details of ROM estimation, we first show a brief representation of hip joint motion described in [3]. Let M_{pf} denote the transformation from the pelvis coordinate system (pelvis-CS) to the femur coordinate system (femur-CS). As illustrated in Fig. 1(b), the hip joint motion is given by:

$$M_{pf} = T_{pc}T_{cs}R_{cs}T_{sf},$$ (1)

where T_{pc} is a 4×4 transformation matrix representing the orientation of the cup in the pelvis-CS, T_{cs} is a fixed transformation matrix determined by the selected head and neck components, R_{cs} is a variable transformation matrix constrained to the rotational motion, and T_{sf} is a transformation matrix representing the reverse orientation of the stem in the femur-CS. Both T_{pc} and T_{sf} are determined by one of the following two methodologies. For preoperative assistances, the surgeon determines them by visualization and experience. For intraoperative assistances, optical 3-D position sensors give the

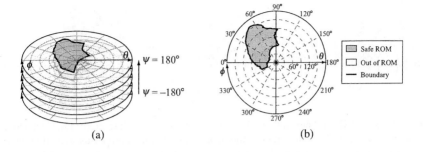

(a)   (b)

Fig. 2. (a) A 3-D ROM and (b) its slice, where $\psi = 0°$, given in polar coordinates. The entire region in the slice is separated into two pieces by a closed line. Enclosed region represents a safe ROM while the outside region represents an out of the ROM.

actual values of T_{pc} and T_{sf} by measuring implanted components. Thus, intraoperative estimations based on measured T_{pc} and T_{sf} are required to obtain precise ROMs.

Given T_{pc}, T_{cs}, and T_{sf}, the safe ROM is defined as a set of rotation transformation matrices, S, such that for all $R_{cs} \in S$, R_{cs} avoids any implant-implant, bone-implant, and bone-bone impingements. Fig. 2 shows an example of the safe ROM with two features: a closed line shapes the boundary between inside and outside the ROM, and the safe ROM does not always include the origin. Therefore, ROM estimation is a search problem that locates the boundary in a 3-D space. Since R_{cs} is defined in a 3-D space, ROM estimation is a compute-intensive application. In the following, we represent R_{cs} by the Euler angles, (ϕ, θ, ψ) $(0° \le \phi < 360°, 0° \le \theta < 180°, -180° \le \psi < 180°)$, as shown in Fig. 1(b).

To compute S, earlier systems investigate every stance configuration, (ϕ, θ, ψ), sampled at uniform intervals, whether it causes impingements. Therefore, the amount of computation increases with the number of stance configurations. Furthermore, it depends on the complexity of the CD algorithm employed for each stance configuration.

3   Real-Time ROM Estimation

This section describes the two key methods employed in our system.

3.1   Adaptive ROM Refinement

The key idea of adaptive ROM refinement, which aims to reduce the amount of computation, is to investigate in detail the stance configurations only close to the boundary between inside and outside the ROM. To realize this non-uniform refinement, our estimation algorithm employs the following two techniques.

1. Hierarchical refinement of sampling intervals.
2. Status control of each stance configuration.

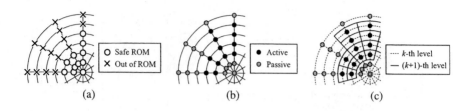

Fig. 3. Adaptive ROM refinement. (a) Given a safe ROM at the k-th level, (b) Eq. (2) determines the status of each stance configuration, and then (c) the algorithm refines the sampling intervals only around active configurations before advancing to the next $(k+1)$-th level.

Let i_k be the sampling interval for stance configurations at the k-th level of estimation hierarchy, where $k \geq 1$. To compute the safe ROM in a coarse-to-fine manner, the algorithm refines the interval when advancing the estimation level as follows: $i_{k+1} = i_k/2$, where $i_k \geq 1°$.

At each level, the algorithm associates each stance configuration with a status, $\mathcal{C}_{\phi,\theta,\psi} \in \{\text{active}, \text{passive}\}$. Then, it refines the sampling intervals only around active configurations and investigates the refined configurations whether they cause impingements. Refinement around the remaining passive configurations is omitted in order to reduce the amount of computation.

To enable this omission, the algorithm assumes that a stance configuration surrounded by others with impingements (or no impingements) also causes impingements (or no impingements). Based on this assumption, such surrounded configurations can be omitted. The status of each stance configuration is given by:

$$
\mathcal{C}_{\phi,\theta,\psi} =
\begin{cases}
\text{passive,} & \text{if } \forall p,q,r \in \{1,-1\} \mid (\phi+p, \theta+q, \psi+r) \in \mathcal{S} \\
& \quad \vee \; \forall p,q,r \in \{1,-1\} \mid (\phi+p, \theta+q, \psi+r) \notin \mathcal{S}, \\
\text{active,} & \text{otherwise.}
\end{cases}
\tag{2}
$$

In addition to the computational complexity reduction, our adaptive algorithm has another advantage compared to earlier algorithms without adaptive refinement. Since the algorithm refines the sampling intervals as it moves up the hierarchy, it enables progressive visualization of the safe ROM. Therefore, an outline of the safe ROM is visible in the early phase of estimation, allowing surgeons to immediately terminate the ongoing estimation when the outline is known to be obviously an unoptimal result.

3.2   Parallelization

In the presented algorithm, a CD for stance configuration (ϕ, θ, ψ) is independent of that for another configuration (ϕ', θ', ψ') if and only if status $\mathcal{C}_{\phi,\theta,\psi}$ determines whether to sample (ϕ', θ', ψ') or not at the refinement. That is, any two configurations without causal relation between them can be processed in parallel. Therefore, our method exploits task-level parallelism of the ROM estimation. Here, a task corresponds to CDs for a set of configurations in the same level and for that of configurations in different levels but with no causal relation among the configurations.

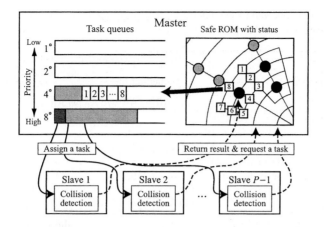

Fig. 4. Adaptive ROM estimation based on master/slave paradigm. Given P nodes, $P - 1$ slaves detect collisions for tasks assigned from a master while the master manages estimation results and task queues for each estimation level, and samples tasks $(1, 2, \ldots, 8)$ according to Eq. (2).

In order to exploit this parallelism, our method employs the master/slave (M/S) paradigm, where computing nodes are classified into two groups: a master and the remaining slaves. Fig. 4 shows an overview of the method. While the slaves detect collisions for tasks assigned from the master, the master manages estimation results, namely the safe ROM, and updates the status of each configuration. According to this status, the master determines which region need to be refined, and then samples stance configurations for the next level. These newly sampled configurations are enqueued as tasks to a queue prepared for each estimation level. Tasks are dequeued when assigning them to slaves. Since idle slaves are selected for this assignment, the M/S paradigm is capable of dynamic load balancing among slaves.

Note here that our method prevents synchronization among slaves when advancing the estimation level. This asynchronous behavior gives higher speedup but allows the master to simultaneously queue tasks sampled from different levels. Such tasks should be processed from the coarse-grained level because tasks in this level can generate many tasks due to the refinement. Therefore, each queue in the master has a priority to enable this coarse-to-fine processing.

4   Results

In this section, we evaluate the performance of our adaptive method by comparing it with the previous non-adaptive method [6] on a cluster of PCs. The cluster consists of 64 symmetric multiprocessor (SMP) nodes, each with two Pentium III 1-GHz CPUs and a Myrinet [7] and Fast Ethernet interconnects that provide bandwidth of 2 Gb/s and 100 Mb/s, respectively.

We have implemented our method using the C++ language and the MPICH-SCore library [8], a highly portable and efficient implementation of the Message Passing Interface (MPI) standard [9]. For each of CDs, we used the V-COLLIDE library [10, 11], which rapidly detects precise collisions at $O(n + m)$ time, where n and m denote the

Table 1. Execution time and its breakdown for fine-grained ROM estimation with $360 \times 180 \times 360$ stance configurations. AR denotes adaptive refinement.

Breakdown	Execution time (second)					
	Sequential		Parallel on 128 CPUs			
			Fast Ethernet		Myrinet	
	w/o AR	w/ AR	w/o AR	w/ AR	w/o AR	w/ AR
Initialization of V-COLLIDE			6.0			
Estimation at level 1 ($i_1 = 16°$)	—	6	—	0.1	—	0.1
level 2 ($i_2 = 8°$)	—	10	—	0.1	—	0.1
level 3 ($i_3 = 4°$)	—	43	—	0.8	—	0.5
level 4 ($i_4 = 2°$)	—	202	—	3.1	—	2.3
level 5 ($i_5 = 1°$)	16 318	996	191	16.8	135	10.7
Total	16 324	1263	197	26.8	141	19.6

number of polygonal objects and that of polygonal objects very close to each other, respectively.

The datasets of the pelvis and femur were composed of 116 270 and 30 821 polygons, respectively. See [3, 12, 6] for the detail explanation of how we generated them and utilized the system during surgery. The estimation hierarchy was composed of five levels with $i_1 = 16°$. The grain size of a task, namely the number of configurations that compose a task, was experimentally selected: 50 and 10 000 configurations for the adaptive and non-adaptive methods, respectively.

Table 1 shows the execution time for fine-grained ROM estimation with $360 \times 180 \times 360$ stance configurations. Compared to the parallel non-adaptive method, the parallel adaptive method reduces the execution time on Myrinet from 141 to 19.6 seconds and that on Fast Ethernet from 197 to 26.8 seconds. These timing results, below a half minute, are acceptable for intraoperative surgical planning. Since the sequential adaptive method takes 1263 seconds, parallelization as well as adaptive refinement is also a key method for intraoperative assistances.

In addition to this timing benefit, the adaptive method enables progressive visualization, as we mentioned in Section 3.1. For example, after 6.1, 6.1, 6.6, and 8.9 seconds on Myrinet, the system outlined the safe ROM with sampling intervals of $16°$, $8°$, $4°$, and $2°$, respectively. Here, even the initial coarsest level took 6.1 seconds. This is due to the initialization of V-COLLIDE, which takes 6 seconds to construct data structure from the input polygons for rapid CD. Thus, although V-COLLIDE requires pre-processing time for rapid CD, we think that progressive visualization is essential for intraoperative applications to report the progress of processing to surgeons.

Fig. 5 explains how the adaptive method reduces the amount of computation. It shows distribution maps of sampling intervals for the adaptive and non-adaptive methods. We can see that the adaptive method investigates in detail the stance configurations only around the boundary of the ROM. This reduces the number of investigated configurations from 23 328 000 to 1 594 816 configurations, and thereby the speedup to the non-adaptive method reaches a factor of 12.9 (=16 324/1263) on a single CPU machine.

Finally, to evaluate the scalability of our method, we measured its parallel speedup on different numbers of CPUs (Fig. 6). Here, the parallel speedup is the ratio of the sequential execution time to the parallel execution time. While the non-adaptive method

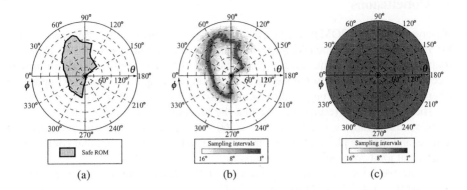

Fig. 5. (a) A slice of computed safe ROM, where $\psi = 0°$, and distribution maps of sampling intervals (b) for adaptive method and (c) for non-adaptive method.

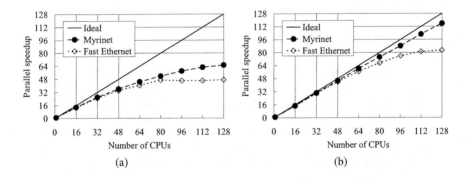

Fig. 6. (a) Parallel speedup of adaptive method and (b) that of non-adaptive method.

achieves linear speedup, the adaptive method seems to reach the peak performance as the number of CPUs increases. This is mainly due to the less parallelism of the adaptive method compared to that of the non-adaptive method. That is, although the adaptive method reduces the amount of computation, it loses the complete independence of tasks that the non-adaptive method has. Furthermore, the adaptive method needs the master to compute the status for each stance configuration. Thus, less parallelism and additional work decrease the parallel speedup of the adaptive method.

Note here that although the non-adaptive method offers better parallel speedup than the adaptive method, it takes approximately seven times longer execution time on 128 CPUs. Therefore, parallel speedup is not always a good measure for the evaluation of parallel methods.

5   Conclusions

We have presented a ROM estimation method that is capable of intraoperative estimation for THR surgery. Our method achieves real-time estimation based on two methods: adaptive ROM refinement strategy where the safe ROM is non-uniformly refined in a coarse-to-fine manner to reduce the computational complexity; and HPC approach where the safe ROM is computed in parallel to obtain further acceleration.

The experimental results indicate that the implementation on a cluster of 64 PCs enables intraoperative estimation of $360 \times 360 \times 180$ stance configurations within a half minute, and thereby plays a key role in selecting and aligning the optimal combination of artificial joint components during surgery.

Future work includes the parallelization of V-COLLIDE initialization in order to obtain further parallel speedup on many CPUs.

Acknowledgments. This work was partly supported by JSPS Grant-in-Aid for Young Scientists (B)(15700030) and Grant-in-Aid for Scientific Research on Priority Areas (16016254 and 16035209) by the Ministry of Education, Culture, Sports, Science and Technology of Japan.

References

1. DiGioia, A.M., et al.: Image guided navigation system to measure intraoperatively acetabular implant alignment. Clinical Orthopaedics and Related Research **355** (1998) 8–22
2. Jaramaz, B., et al.: Computer assisted measurement of cup placement in total hip replacement. Clinical Orthopaedics and Related Research **354** (1998) 70–81
3. Sato, Y., et al.: Intraoperative simulation and planning using a combined acetabular and femoral (CAF) navigation system for total hip replacement. In: Proc. 3rd Int'l Conf. Medical Image Computing and Computer-Assisted Intervention (MICCAI'00). (2000) 1114–1125
4. Richolt, J.A., et al.: Impingement simulation of the hip in SCFE using 3D models. Computer Aided Surgery **4** (1999) 144–151
5. Kang, M., et al.: Accurate simlation of hip joint range of motion. In: Proc. 15th Int'l Conf. Computer Animation (CA'02). (2002) 215–219
6. Kawasaki, Y., et al.: High-performance computing service over the Internet for intraoperative image processing. IEEE Trans. Information Technology in Biomedicine **8** (2004) 36–46
7. Boden, N.J., et al.: Myrinet: A gigabit-per-second local-area network. IEEE Micro **15** (1995) 29–36
8. O'Carroll, F., et al.: The design and implementation of zero copy MPI using commodity hardware with a high performance network. In: Proc. 12th ACM Int'l Conf. Supercomputing (ICS'98). (1998) 243–250
9. Message Passing Interface Forum: MPI: A message-passing interface standard. Int'l J. Supercomputer Applications and High Performance Computing **8** (1994) 159–416
10. Gottschalk, S., et al.: OBBTree: A hierarchical structure for rapid interference detection. Computer Graphics (Proc. ACM SIGGRAPH'96) **30** (1996) 171–180
11. Hudson, T.C., et al.: V-COLLIDE: Accelerated collision detection for VRML. In: Proc. 2nd Symp. Virtual Reality Modeling Language (VRML'97). (1997) 117–124
12. Sugano, N., et al.: Accuracy evaluation of surface-based registration methods in a computer navigation system for hip surgery performed through a posterolateral approach. Comput. Aided Surgery **6** (2001) 195–203

Correction of Accidental Patient Motion for Online Mr Thermometry

Baudouin Denis de Senneville[1,2,3], Pascal Desbarats[3], Rares Salomir[4],
Bruno Quesson[2], and Chrit T.W. Moonen[2]

[1] IMF, ERT CNRS/Université Bordeaux 2 - 146, rue Léo Saignat, F-33076 Bordeaux
[2] Image Guided Therapy SA - 2, allée du doyen George Brus, F-33600 Pessac
[3] LaBRI, UMR 5800 CNRS/Université Bordeaux 1 - 351, cours de la Libération,
F-33405 Talence
[4] U386 INSERM, France

Abstract. Magnetic Resonance (MR) temperature mapping can be used to monitor temperature changes in minimally invasive thermal therapies during the procedure. The proton resonance frequency (PRF) shift technique gives an estimate of the relative temperature variation, comparing contrast between dynamically acquired images and reference data sets. However, organ displacements due to physiological activity (heart and respiration) may induce important artifacts on computed temperature maps if no correction is applied. This paper summarizes existing classical methods and presents a new approach for correction of accidental motion in such MR images in order to increase robustness of temperature estimation using the PRF shift. The correction method described in this paper consists of using image registration techniques to estimate motion on anatomical images.

1 Introduction

Local hyperthermia can be used for a wide variety of medical interventions such as tumor ablation [1], treatment of heart arrhythmias [2], local drug delivery with thermosensitive microcarriers [3] and control of gene therapy using heat-sensitive promoters [4]. These interventions are usually monitored by CT scanner or ultrasound imaging (for the placement of the RF needle or the laser probe for example). However, MRI is the only technique that can provide on line quantitative thermometric information in addition to detailed anatomical information. It has been shown that tumor cell destruction occurs with a temperature increase included between 13^oC and 23^oC for a time treatment of several minutes [5]. The main principle of MRI is based on the detection of magnetic properties of the protons contained in the water molecules of the body [6]. The MR imaging system associates each volume unit of the target region of interest with a complex number $Me^{i\phi}$, where M is the magnitude and ϕ the phase. The corresponding graylevel of the anatomical image is proportional to M. ϕ is then used to construct a phase image (cf Fig. 1).

C. Barillot, D.R. Haynor, and P. Hellier (Eds.): MICCAI 2004, LNCS 3217, pp. 637–644, 2004.

Under well-controlled conditions, a difference of phase between two subsequent images is proportional to a difference of temperature [9], as shown in Fig. 2 (the arrow in the second phase of the figure highlights a phase contrast due to a local heating of the sample using a MR-compatible focused ultrasound (FUS) device). However as temperature maps result from phase differences, this technique is prone to motion artifact [7]. In addition, local magnetic susceptibility is generally not fully uniform and the resulting phase variation $\Delta\varphi$ can be described by the following equation [8] :

$$\Delta\varphi = \gamma.\alpha.B_0.\Delta T.T_E + \gamma.B_0.FT^{-1}\left[\left(\frac{1}{3} - \frac{K_z^2}{K^2}\right).FT(\Delta\chi)\right].T_E$$

where ΔT is the temperature difference, γ the gyromagnetic ratio ($\simeq 42.58$ MHz/T), α ($= 0.01 ppm/K$) the temperature coefficient, T_E the echo time, B_0 the main magnetic field, $K = (K_x, K_y, K_z)$ the position vector in the reciprocal space, and $\Delta\chi$ the modification of the susceptibility field. The first term of the sum is due to the PRF shift with temperature whereas the second term rises when an object motion occurs.

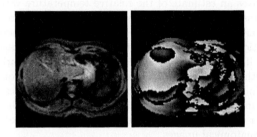

Fig. 1. Transverse magnitude and phase images of a human abdomen

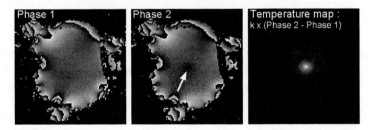

Fig. 2. Example of temperature map calculated on an ex-vivo muscle

Both PRF-shift with temperature and motion of the patient result in phase variation and it is not possible to separate these two contributions within a single phase image. Alternatively, it is possible to process magnitude images to extract and correct motion contribution to phase artifacts.

The case of uniform susceptibility object has already been studied [10]. However, modeling of inhomogeneous field of susceptibility in-vivo is difficult and this issue has to be addressed for clinical application. The approach described here allows to correct motion related errors in PRF based MR thermometry, avoiding explicit modeling of the susceptibility field.

For real time monitoring of temperature evolution, data treatment must be performed within the time duration between two successive acquisitions (i.e. in the range of 0.5s to 1s for a single 128x128 image for a standard thermometry sequence). Our test platform is an Athlon 2400MHz with 512Mo of RAM.

2   Physical Approaches

2.1   Respiratory Gating

Respiratory gating is a technique that allows reduction of artifacts due to respiration. The principle is to synchronize the acquisition of the images to a stable period of the respiratory cycle, usually at the end of expiration [11]. The major drawback of this method is that the temporal resolution depends on the respiration frequency. Moreover, artifacts due to irregular and/or deep respiration movements may induce erroneous temperature mapping.

2.2   Navigator Echoes

Navigator echoes uses an approach that consists of acquiring one or multiple lines of Fourier space including the center and applying an inverse Fourier transformation in order to obtain the profile of the object. Navigator echoes can be used in two different ways :

Synchronization. It is possible to synchronize the acquisition of the images to a stable period of the respiratory cycle by using the profile of the object provided by the navigator echo technique. This approach is more efficient than the respiratory gating because the synchronization is done by using directly the MR signal on the studied region. Irregular and/or deep respiration movements thus are not limitations. On the other hand, as for the respiratory gating technique, the temporal resolution depends on the respiration frequency.

Motion estimation and correction. The profile of the object given by the navigator echoes can also be used to estimate translation of the object [12]. This motion estimation is used to correct for temperature maps. If a motion occurs between t_{n-1} and t_n, the relative temperature map after motion will be erroneous. A simple method consists of detecting motion vector to correct phase and temperature maps . Then the phase image acquired at t_n (φ_n) is taken as new phase image reference, and the temperature mapping at t_i ($t_i \geq t_n$) is computed with :

$$\Delta T_i = \Delta T' + (\varphi_i - \varphi_n).k$$

where $\Delta T'$ is is the n-th temperature map after motion correction.

However, the use of navigator echoes is restricted to rigid body motion and may not be very efficient for complex organs displacements such as in the abdomen (liver, kidney). Thus, accidental patient motion can't be corrected efficiency with this technique.

2.3   Multi-baseline

A collection of multiple baseline images can be use to generate temperature maps [13]. Baseline selection can be made based on navigator echoes data [14].

3   Computational Approaches

Our approach consists of using image processing techniques to detect on line the displacements on the anatomic images in order to correct accidental patient motion. The objective is to relate the coordinate of each part of tissue in the image we want to register with the corresponding tissue in the reference image.

3.1   Motion Estimation Techniques

Methods based on a parameterized model of motion. The objective of this method is to determine a set of parameters for which a predetermined function of the parameters is minimized (or maximized). Optimum parameters can be calculated for example with the "Square Root Optimization" [15]).

"Block-matching" algorithm. This technique is used in the compression of videos in the MPEG format. The image to be registered is divided in blocks and the translation of each blocks in a research window is estimated [16]. It is supposed that the motion in the image is constant in a region.

Optical flow. This technique consists of extracting a displacement vector map from an image sequence assuming that intensity is conserved during displacement. Many methods can provide an estimation of the optical flow such as correlation methods (consists of establishing a correspondence between two images by localization of invariant markers [17]) and differential methods established by Horn and Schunck [18].

3.2   Choice of Motion Estimation Method

The most restrictive registration techniques are methods using parameterized models because the algorithm calculates a global transformation. The identification of the movement is done by the best possible adaptation of the parameters of the model (for example, there are six parameters to estimate in an affine model). The choice of the model requires to know the nature of the movement to obtain reliable results. The "Block-matching" technique is less restrictive because it corrects for local motion estimation. Therefore there is no limitation to the transformation that can be applied to the original image. The most permissive method is the calculation of the optical flow because the transformation is calculated on the vicinity of the pixels.

The choice of the registration method depends on which part of the body is observed [7]. In this article, motion of the kidney was shown to be correctly described using a global affine transformation and a "Square Root Optimization" algorithm.

3.3 Motion Correction

The correction technique is nearly the same as for navigator echoes (2.2) excepting that motion is directly estimated on anatomical image using image registration algorithms. The motion corrected temperature difference after the movement is added to temperature before movement. As an advantage, this technique is thus not limited to rigid body motion. Thus, this method is able to correct accidental patient motion and is complementary with periodic motion reduction techniques like respiratory gating.

3.4 Experimental Validation

Initial tests were performed on MR images acquired on a piece of an ex-vivo turkey muscle heated using a laser device (Dornier). 14 slices have been acquired each 15.3s by the MRI. The spatial resolution of those images was 128×128 pixels and the pixel size was 1×1 mm. During the heating process, a mechanical translation and rotation was applied.

A second experiment was performed on a healthy volunteer under free breathing. 3 slices have been acquired using respiratory gating (each 5s approximatively). The spatial resolution of those images was 128×128 pixels and the pixel size was 1.4×1.4 mm. In the middle of the acquisition, the volunteer was asked to make one body displacement and to stay in final position. The experiment consisted of measuring the stability of the thermometry baseline in the kidney of a healthy volunteer using our approach.

4 Results and Discussion

4.1 Motion Correction on an Ex-vivo Muscle Heated with a Laser Device

Figure 3 shows the anatomical image of the muscle (3. A) and the temperature mapping measured during the heating process when no movement occurs (3. B), when a movement occurs and no correction has been achieved (3. C), and with the same movement when our correction is applied (3. D). Motion was estimated with the "Square Root Optimization" algorithm using a global 3D rigid transformation and required 2.8s of computation time for the entire volume on our test platform. Figure 4 shows the temporal evolution of the temperature measured on a pixel situated on the heating zone of the muscle. A movement occurs after 250s and the heating process has been stopped after 350s.

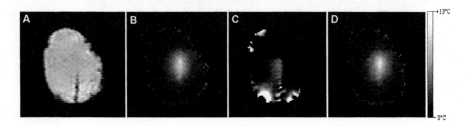

Fig. 3. Motion correction on an ex-vivo muscle

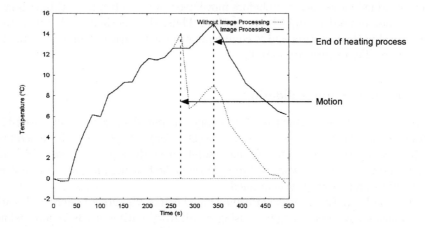

Fig. 4. Temporal evolution of the temperature on a pixel located in the heated zone

4.2   Motion Correction on a Healthy Volunteer

Figure 5 shows anatomical images obtained when no movement occurs (5. A) and when a movement occurs (5. B). Figure 5.C shows the temperature mapping measured when a movement occurs and no correction has been achieved. Motion is estimated with the "Square Root Optimization" algorithm using a global 2D affine transformation and required 1.9s of computation time for the 3 slices on our test platform. Figure 6 shows the temporal evolution of the temperature measured on a pixel situated on the kidney.

Experimental results demonstrated that this motion correction technique allowed a precise recovery of the temperature map.

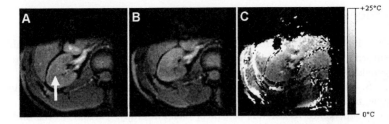

Fig. 5. Motion corrupted images in a healthy volunteer

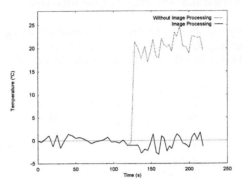

Fig. 6. Temporal evolution of the temperature on a pixel reported on Figure 5.A (white arrow)

4.3 Discussion

The implemented algorithm for image registration can be parameterized in order to perform on line temperature correction under these experimental conditions. Our approach allows to correct complex motion. This method must be combined to other techniques like respiratory gating to improve the stability of the thermometry.

Although this method can be used to correct for motion corrupted images during on line MR temperature mapping, several limitations remain. First, using this method information about temperature changes between the instant t_{n-1} and t_n is lost. Moreover, as mention in [12], noise in the temperature map increases with a number of motion artifacted images. In addition, uncertainty induced by the correction technique is reflected on all the images obtained after displacements. As a consequence, this technique can be applied when periodic motion has already been corrected with synchronization techniques. It has been demonstrated here that accidental displacement can be corrected in such cases. However, in the case of rapid MR acquisition without synchronization, added noise on phase images may dramatically hamper the quality of MR thermometry. This motion correction technique for accidental patient movements has a straightforward medical application in MR guided thermotherapies and further experiments are in progress including clinical cases.

References

1. Steiner P., Botnar R., Dubno B. et al. Radio-frequency induced thermoablation: monitoring with T1-weighted and proton frequency shift MR imaging in an interventional 0.5-T environment. Radiology 1998;206:803-810.
2. Levy S. Biophysical basis and cardiac lesions caused by different techniques of cardiac arrhythmia ablation. Arch. Mal. Coeur Vaiss. 1995;88:1465-1469.
3. Kim S. Liposomes as carriers of cancer chemotherapy: current status and future prospects. Drugs 1993;46:618-638.
4. Madio D.P., van Gelderen P., DesPres D., et al. On the feasibility of MRI-guided focused ultrasound for local induction of gene expression. J. Magn. Res. Imaging 1998;8:101-104.
5. Sapareto S. A., Dewey W. CL, Thermal dose determination in cancer therapy. Int. J. Radiation Oncology Biol. Phys. 10, 787-800. 1984.
6. Mansfield P. et Grannell P.K. NMR "diffraction" in solids?. J. Phys. C:Solid state phys 1973;6,L422-L426.
7. Denis de Senneville B., Desbarats P., Quesson B., Moonen C. T. W., Real-Time Artefact Corrections For Quantitative MR Temperature Mapping. Journal of WSCG, Vol.11, No.1.,ISSN 1213-6972. WSCG 2003, February 3-7,2003, Plzen, Czech Republic.
8. Salomir R., Denis de Senneville B., Moonen C. T. W., A fast calculation method for magnetic field inhomogeneity due to an arbitrary distribution of bulk susceptibility. Wiley InterScience. 7 July 2003.
9. Quesson B., de Zwart J. A., Moonen C. T. W., Magnetic Resonance Temperature Imaging for Guidance of Thermotherapy. Journal of Magnetic Resonance Imaging, 2000;12:523-533.
10. Vogel M. W., Suprijanto, Vos F.M., Vrooman H.A., Vossepoel A.M., Pattynama P.M.T., Towards motion-robust magnetic resonance thermometry. Miccai 2001.
11. Moricawa S, Inubushi T, Kurumi Y, Naka S, Seshan V, Tsukamoto T. Feasibility of simple respiratory triggering in MR-guided interventional procedures for liver tumors under general anesthesia.
12. de Zwart J. A., Vimeux F., Palussiére J., Salomir R., Quesson B., Delalande C., and Moonen C. T. W., On-Line Correction and Visualiszation of Motion During MRI-Controlled Hyperthermia. Magnetic Resonance in Medicine. 2001; 45:128-137.
13. Suprijanto, Vogel M.W., Vos F.M., Vrooman H.A., and Vossepoel A.M., Displacement Correction Scheme for MR-Guided Interstitial Laser Therapy, Medical Image Computing and Computer-Assisted Intervention. MICCAI 2003.
14. Vigen Karl K., Daniel Bruce L. , Pauly John M., Butts Kim, Triggered, navigated, multi-baseline method for proton resonance frequency temperature mapping with respiratory motion. Magn Reson Med 50:1003-1010, 2003.
15. Friston K.J., Ashburner J, Frith C.D., Poline J-B., Heather J.D. and Frackowiak R.S.J. Spatial registration and normalisation of images. Human Brain Mapping. 2:165-189. 1995.
16. Chen M.J. Chen L.G., Chiueh T.D. & Lee Y.P. A new block-matching criterion for motion estimation and its implementation. IEEE Transactions on Circuits and Sytems for Video Technology. 5:231-236. 1995.
17. Singh A., "An estimation-theoric framework for image-flow computation", Proc. 3rd Itern. Conf. Comput. Vis., Osaka, pp. 168-177, 1990.
18. Schunck B.G. Horn K.P. - Determining optical flow. *Artificial intelligence*, 17:pp. 185-203,1981.

Determining Malignancy of Brain Tumors by Analysis of Vessel Shape

Elizabeth Bullitt[1], Inkyung Jung[2], Keith Muller[2], Guido Gerig[3], Stephen Aylward[4], Sarang Joshi[5], Keith Smith[4], Weili Lin[4], and Matthew Ewend[1]

[1] Departments of Surgery,
[2] Biostatiscs,
[3] Computer Science,
[4] Radiology, and
[5] Radiation Oncology, University of North Carolina, Chapel Hill, NC, 27599, USA
{bullitt,jksmith,weili_lin,ewend}@med.unc.edu,
{keith_muller,aylward}@unc.edu,
{gerig,joshi}@cs.unc.edu

Abstract. Vessels supplying malignant tumors are abnormally shaped. This paper describes a blinded study that assessed tumor malignancy by analyzing vessel shape within MR images of 21 brain tumors prior to surgical resection. The program's assessment of malignancy was then compared to the final histological diagnosis. All tumors were classified correctly as benign or malignant. Of importance, malignancy-associated vessel abnormalities extend outside apparent tumor margins, thus allowing classification of even small or hemorrhagic tumors.

1 Introduction

Despite the development of new imaging techniques, noninvasive determination of tumor malignancy remains a difficult task [1], [2], [3], [4]. An intriguing observation made by those working from histological section is that blood vessels associated with malignant tumors exhibit characteristic shape abnormalities. As stated by Baish, such vessels display a "...a profound sort of tortuosity, with many smaller bends upon each larger bend" [5]. This abnormal tortuosity may be related to increases in nitrous oxide induced by VegF [6], and is found in many malignant tumors including those of the breast [7], brain [8], colon [9], and lung [10]. Moreover, changes in vessel tortuosity precede sprout formation, thus providing a potential marker for incipient malignancy [6]. Of equal importance, successful tumor treatment normalizes vessel shape [11]. All of the above observations were made from histological section. If one could quantify such vessel shape changes from *in vivo* medical images, the approach could offer a new and potentially powerful means of estimating tumor malignancy and of monitoring treatment response noninvasively. Indeed, indirect measurements of vessel tortuosity within *in vivo* images have already been described by Jackson et al., who note that variation in the recirculation characteristics of a contrast agent bolus is related to

C. Barillot, D.R. Haynor, and P. Hellier (Eds.): MICCAI 2004, LNCS 3217, pp. 645–653, 2004.

the tumor grade of gliomas, and may represent vascular tortuosity and hypoperfusion in areas of angiogenic neovascularization [12].

The current study originates from an accidental observation. Our group has focused upon the segmentation of vessels and tumors from magnetic resonance (MR) images. About two years ago, our vascular imaging protocols were upgraded to provide sub-millimeter voxel spacing. Shortly thereafter, we noticed that vessels segmented from the vicinity of malignant tumors appeared abnormally "wiggly". Since then, we have developed metrics to quantify the tortuosity of segmented vessels [13], and have performed a pilot study to define shape measures likely to be useful in characterizing vessels of malignancy [14].

This paper describes a blinded study that used measures of vessel shape to diagnose malignancy from images of twenty-one brain tumors in patients scheduled for tumor removal. The goal was to noninvasively discriminate malignant from benign tumors including cases difficult to classify by other imaging methods. Many "difficult" cases were included, such as hemorrhagic lesions, irradiated tumors, pinpoint abnormalities, and hypervascular benign lesions. For each tumor, the program's classification of benign or malignant was compared to the final pathological diagnosis. All twenty-one tumors were classified correctly. A surprising and significant finding was that the vessel shape changes associated with malignancy seem to extend well outside of apparent tumor margins. Although this report analyzes only MR images of the brain, the method is extensible to vascular images of any anatomical location.

2 Background

Detecting abnormal tortuosity within the intracerebral circulation is difficult because healthy intracerebral vessels are ordinarily tortuous. Most of the previous work on defining vessel tortuosity has been performed in 2D, focusing upon retinopathy of prematurity. The most common metric is the "Distance Metric" which provides the total path length of a vessel divided by distance between endpoints. Brey [15] extended this metric to 3D for analysis of vessels in histological section. A problem with the Distance Metric, however, is that it assigns a higher value to a healthy, long, "S" shaped vessel than to a short, abnormal vessel with tight coils. Baish [5] and Sabo [16] are attempting to stage tumor malignancy on the basis of vessel tortuosity within histological sections by using microvessal fractal dimension.

The current study takes a different approach, and assumes that the clinical assessment of "abnormal tortuosity" can refer to more than one type of shape abnormality. Webster's dictionary defines "tortuosity" as "full of twists, turns; crooked" [17]. However, what precisely is meant by "tortuosity" in a medical sense is unclear.

One can view "abnormal tortuosity" as comprising three different patterns [13]. Tortuosity type I occurs when a straight vessel elongates to form a "C" or "S", and occurs with retinopathy of prematurity, anemia, and hypertension. Tortuosity type II is characterized by a "bag of worms" configuration, and occurs within many hypervascular tumors and arteriovenous malformations. Tortuosity type III is characterized by high-frequency, low-amplitude coils or sine waves, and appears within malignant tumors.

We have previously described two 3D tortuosity metrics that act upon sets of segmented vessels [13]. The Inflection Count Metric (ICM) counts loci of minimum curvature along a 3D space curve, multiplies this number (plus 1) times the total path length of the curve, and divides by the distance between endpoints. The ICM detects abnormal tortuosity types I and II, but fails with type III. The second method, the Sum Of Angles Metric (SOAM), measures the curvature along a space curve and normalizes by total path length. The SOAM detects abnormal tortuosity type III, but fails with types I and II. Malignant tumor vessels, which exhibit "many smaller bends upon each larger bend" [5], tend to display a mix of tortuosity types II and III, and thus usually show increases in tortuosity as measured by both by SOAM and ICM. Figure 1 illustrates the typical tortuosity pattern of vessels within a malignant tumor.

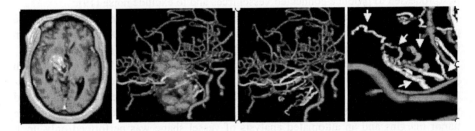

Fig. 1. Typical vessel shape changes with malignancy. Left: T1, gadolinium enhanced section of a glioblastoma. Central images: Vessels color-coded with relationship to the tumor surface and with the tumor shown at full and at no opacity. Right: Magnification of tumor vessels. Arrows point to abnormal, high-frequency wiggles (tortuosity type III, detectable by SOAM). Many of the vessels also have somewhat of a "bag of worms" appearance (tortuosity type II, detectable by ICM).

3   Methods

3.1   Patient Selection and Image Acquisition

Images of sixteen healthy subjects, ranging in age from twenty-two to fifty-four, were used to establish the healthy database. Tumor cases included twenty-one brain lesions in nineteen patients, each scheduled for total gross resection of their tumor or tumors.

Images were obtained upon a head-only 3T MR unit (Allegra, Siemens Medical Systems Inc., Germany) or upon a 1.5T MR unit (Sonata, Siemens Medical Systems Inc., Germany). A quadrature head coil was employed. T1, T2, and MRA sequences were performed on all subjects, with tumor patients additionally receiving a gadolinium enhanced T1 sequence.

Vascular images employed a 3D time-of-flight MRA sequence. Velocity compensation along both frequency and phase encoding directions was used to minimize signal dephasing induced by the flowing spins. In addition, a magnetization transfer pulse was employed to suppress signal from brain parenchyma while maintaining signal from flowing spins. Images were obtained at 512 x 512 x ~120. Voxel spacing was 0.5 x 0.5 x 0.8 mm^3 in the majority of cases (our current standard) but some early patients were scanned at 0.8 x 0.8 x 1.0 mm^3 or at 0.4 x 0.4 x 1.25 mm^3.

3.2 Image Processing

Vessel segmentation was done by Aylward's method [18]. Vessel extraction involves 3 steps: definition of a seed point, automatic extraction of an image intensity ridge representing the vessel's central skeleton, and automatic determination of vessel radius at each skeleton point. The output of the program provides sets of directed, 4-dimensional points indicating the (x,y,z) spatial position of each sequential vessel skeleton point and an associated radius at each point. Extracted vessels were then postprocessed to produce connected vessel trees and to exclude noise [19].

Tumor segmentation was performed using either a fully automated method [20] or a partially manual program that segments tumors via polygon drawing and filling on orthogonal cuts through an image volume (http://www.cs.unc.edu/~gerig/).

All images were registered via a mutual-information based, affine transformation [21], [22] into the coordinate system of the McConnell atlas [23] so that, via a combination of forward and backward mapping, the same region of interest could be defined within each image. For each tumor patient, vessels were automatically clipped to the tumor margins and an automated analysis of vessel shape was performed only upon those vessels lying within the tumor boundaries. This same region of interest was then mapped into the coordinate space of each healthy patient, and a similar, regional analysis was performed upon each healthy subject's vasculature.

Three vessel attributes of interest were defined during an earlier pilot study [14], and consist of one vessel density measure and the two tortuosity metrics discussed earlier. The terminal branch count (TBC) counts the number of vessels entirely contained within a region of interest. As described earlier, the SOAM is a tortuosity measure effective in detecting high frequency sine waves and tight coils, and the ICM is a tortuosity measure effective in detecting "bag of worms" tortuosity [13].

Tiny or hemorrhagic lesions may contain no vessels visualizable by MRA. Our approach requires some minimum number of vessels for analysis. We arbitrarily decided upon a minimum vessel number of 4. If an insufficient number of vessels were present within the tumor boundary as initially defined, we therefore expanded this boundary to include the edematous region around the tumor. For lesions without surrounding edema, the "tumor boundary" was dilated until it included 4 vessels. It takes 60-90 minutes to process each new case.

3.3 Blinded Study and Subsequent Discriminant Analysis

Nineteen patients with a total of twenty-one tumors were recruited, imaged by MR, and operated upon by a single surgeon. Image analysis was performed by a different individual who was blinded to the patient's history and histology until after the analysis was completed and reported to the surgeon. Each tumor was declared benign or malignant with results evaluated by comparison to the final histological diagnosis.

We entered into this study with the belief that high-frequency wiggles detectable by SOAM were likely to represent the single most important measure of vessel shape. Any tumor whose SOAM value was elevated by two or more standard deviations from the healthy mean was thus automatically defined as malignant. Any tumor whose SOAM value lay between one and two standard deviations above the healthy mean was viewed as suspicious, and the tumor was then declared malignant if the secondary ICM value lay more than two standard deviations above the healthy mean.

After study completion, a formal statistical analysis was conducted of the twenty-six tumors (five in the pilot study and twenty-one in the blinded study) to investigate whether a purely quantitative rule could be formulated that would automate diagnosis. Each score was standardized relative to the mean and standard deviation for values in the corresponding region of interest of the healthy subjects. The exploratory analysis led to concerns about assuming a Gaussian distribution or common covariance. A quadratic discriminant analysis and a nonparametric discriminant analysis were therefore performed.

4   Results

Of the twenty-one tumors, twelve were malignant and nine were benign. All cases were classified correctly during the blinded study. Potentially difficult cases such as a hypervascular benign tumor, a "pinpoint" metastatic lesion, a brain abscess felt preoperatively to be a malignant glioma, and a large intracerebral hemorrhage arising from an obliterated metastatic melanoma were properly labeled. Four benign and three malignant lesions had been treated by surgery and radiation therapy months or years earlier. History of prior irradiation therefore did not appear to disrupt vessel analysis. Figure 2 shows the vessels associated with two lesions, one benign and the second malignant, present in the same patient.

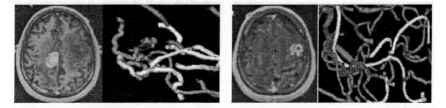

Fig. 2. Malignant tumor and associated vessels (left) and benign tumor with associated vessels (right) in the same patient. Note that the vessels associated with the malignant tumor have high-frequency wiggles, but that the vessels associated with the benign tumor are smooth.

The study contained one example of a grade III glioma. Such tumors are malignant, but do not display the vascular proliferation associated with tumors of higher malignancy. Vessel analysis appropriately noted the terminal branch count to be within healthy range in this case, but also accurately declared the tumor to be malignant by the two vessel tortuosity measurements. This tumor is of interest, as its vascular pattern fits Folkman's observation that increased vessel tortuosity precedes sprout formation during malignant tumor growth[6].

Although the majority of malignant tumors were hypervascular and the majority of benign tumors hypo- or normovascular, there was crossover in each group. Regardless of vessel density, malignancy was associated with vasculature bearing high-frequency tortuosity abnormalities detectable by SOAM. Tumors displaying these vascular changes included glioma grade IV, glioma grade III, lymphoma, metastatic melanoma, metastatic breast carcinoma, and pinealoblastoma.

Discriminant analysis, performed after completion of the prospective study, found the correlations between diagnosis (1 if malignant, 0 if benign) and the predictors to be {0.78 0.51, 0.30} for {SOAM, ICM, TBC}. Both quadratic and nonparametric discriminant rules classified all twenty-six patients correctly into the benign or malignant group using {SOAM, ICM, TBC}. More specifically, the quadratic discriminant function is $Y = .99*SOAM^2 + 3.58*ICM^2 + .36*TBC^2 - .95*SOAM*ICM + .20*SOAM*TBC - 2.26*ICM*TBC + .83*SOAM + 7.05*ICM -2.09*TBC$, with the tumor malignant for $Y > 4.04$ and benign otherwise. The scores of malignant and benign tumors are separated, as shown by Figure 3.

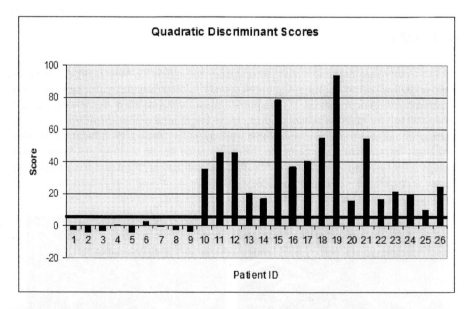

Fig. 3. Quadratic discriminant scores for 26 tumors. The first 9 tumors are benign and the remaining tumors are malignant. The thick black line is drawn through the cutoff point 4.04; all tumors with a lower score are benign and all tumors with a greater score are malignant.

5   Discussion

This report describes a new, noninvasive method of determining tumor malignancy from high-resolution 3D images using a computerized analysis of vessel shape. Potential advantages over other described methods include the capacity to deal with hemorrhagic lesions, resilience to the necrosis produced by prior surgery or radiation treatment, handling of small lesions, and ability to distinguish between malignancy and hypervascular benign lesions. The number of cases analyzed here is small, however, and the formal equation produced by the final discriminant analysis will require testing in a much larger series.

At the outset of this study we hypothesized that different tumor types might possess distinctive vascular patterns. If this were the case, vessel analysis might help make a specific diagnosis (glioma v metastasis, for example). The series is too small and contains too many different malignant tumor types to permit significant comparisons between malignant subtypes. However, comparison of the four metastatic lesions to the eleven malignant gliomas indicates no obvious difference in vessel shape or distribution. If this observation holds for a larger series, it would support the concept of a single shape that characterizes "vessels of malignancy".

An important and surprising finding is that abnormal vessel tortuosity is found not only within the enhancing margins of malignant tumors but also in the surrounding tissue. How distantly these morphological changes extend is unknown, and is a topic for future research. An advantage of these relatively widespread changes is that even tiny lesions can be classified as malignant or benign via examination of vessels in the surrounding tissue.

Another potentially important finding relates to Folkman's observation that vessel tortuosity abnormalities precede sprout formation during malignant tumor growth [6]. Our series contains one case of a non-enhancing glioma grade III, which exhibited abnormal vessel tortuosity but no significant neovascularity. It therefore seems possible that vessel analysis could provide a means of early detection of incipient cancers. A longitudinal study would be needed to test this hypothesis.

A limitation of the approach is the requirement for high quality, high resolution vascular images. The vessels of interest are small and contain high-frequency, low-amplitude wiggles. Extension of the method to anatomical regions such as the lung is thus likely to require imaging techniques adapted to prevent blurring of vessels by respiratory motion.

Acknowledgments. This work was supported by R01 EB000219 NIBIB and HL69808 NIH-HLB. Portions of the software are licensed to Medtronic Corp (Minn., Minn) and to R2 Technologies (Los Altos, CA). We are grateful to Daniel Rueckert for his registration software.

References

1. Benard F, Romsa J, Hustinx R: Imaging gliomas with positron emission tomography and single-photon emission computed tomography. Seminars Nuc. Med. 23: 148-162, 2003.
2. Burtscher LM, Holtas S: Proton magnetic resonance spectroscopy in brain tumors: clinical applications. Neuroradiology 43: 345-352, 2001.
3. Tosi MR, Fini G, Tinti A, Reggiani A, Tugnoli V: Molecular characterization of human healthy and neoplastic cerebral and renal tissues by in vitro ^{1}H NMR spectroscopy (Review). International Journal of Molecular Medicine 9: 299-310, 2002.
4. Law M, Yang S, Wang H, Babb JS, Johnson G, Cha S, Knopp EA, Zagzag D: Glioma Grading:Sensitivity, specificity, and predictive values of perfusion MR imaging and proton MR spectroscopic imaging compared with conventional MR imaging. AJNR 24:1989-1998, 2003.
5. Baish JS, Jain RK (2000) Fractals and cancer. Cancer Research 60:3683-3688, 2000.
6. Folkman J: Incipient Angiogenesis. Journal of the National Cancer Institute 92: 94-95, 2000.
7. Lau DH, Xue L, Young LJ, Burke PA, Cheung AT: Paclitaxel (Taxol): an inhibitor of angiogenesis in a highly vascularized transgenic breast cancer. Cancer Biother. Radiopharm. 14:31-6, 1999.
8. Burger PC, Scheithauer BW, Vogel FS.: Surgical Pathology of the Nervous System and its Coverings, Third Edition, Churchill Livingstone, New York (1991).
9. Siemann D: Vascular Targeting Agents. Horizons in Cancer Therapeutics 3:4-15, 2002.
10. Helmlinger G, Sckell A, Dellian M, Forbes NS, Jain RK: Acid production in glycolysis-impaired tumors provides new insights into tumor metabolism. Clinical Cancer Research 8:1284-1291, 2002.
11. Jain RK : Normalizing tumor vasculature with anti-angiogenic therapy: a new paradigm for combination therapy Nature Medicine 7: 987-98, 2001.
12. Jackson A, Kassner A, Annesley-Williams D, Reid H, Zhu X, Li K: Abnormalities in the recirculation phase of contrast agent bolus passage in cerebral gliomas: Comparison with relative blood volume and tumor grade. AJNR 23:7-14, 2002.
13. Bullitt E, Gerig G, Pizer S, Aylward SR: Measuring tortuosity of the intracerebral vasculature from MRA images. IEEE-TMI 22:1163-1171, 2003.
14. Bullitt E, Gerig G, Aylward S, Joshi S, Smith K, Ewend M, Lin W: Vascular Attributes and Malignant Brain Tumors. MICCAI 2003; Lecture Notes in Computer Science 2878:671-679, 2003.
15. Brey EM, King TW, Johnston C, McIntire LV, Reece GP, Patrick CW: A technique for quantitative three-dimensional analysis of microvascular structure. Microvascular Research 63:279-294, 2002.
16. Sabo E, Boltenko A, Sova Y, Stein A, Kleinhaus S, Resnick MB: Microscopic Analysis and Significance of Vascular Architectural Complexity in Renal Cell Carcinoma. Clinical Cancer Research 7:533-537, 2001.
17. Neufeld, V. Webster's New World Dictionary. New York: Warner Books, 1990, p. 623.
18. Aylward S, Bullitt E : Initialization, noise, singularities and scale in height ridge traversal for tubular object centerline extraction. IEEE-TMI 21:61-75, 2002.
19. Bullitt E, Aylward S, Smith K, Mukherji S, Jiroutek M, Muller K : Symbolic Description of Intracerebral Vessels Segmented from MRA and Evaluation by Comparison with X-Ray Angiograms. Medical Image Analysis 5:157-169, 2001.
20. Prastawa M, Bullitt E, Moon N, Van Leemput K, Gerig G: Automatic brain tumor segmentation by subject specific modification of atlas priors. Academic. Radiology 10:1341-1348, 2003.

21. Schnabel JA, Rueckert D, Quist M, Blackall JM, Castellano Smith AD, Hartkens T, Penney GP, Hall WA, Liu H, Truwit CL, Gerritsen FA, Hill DLG, and Hawkes JD: A generic framework for non-rigid registration based on non-uniform multi-level free-form deformations. MICCAI 2001; Lecture Notes in Computer Science 2208: 573-581, 2001.
22. Rueckert D (2002) "Rview". Available: www.doc.ic.ac.uk/~dr/software.
23. ICBM Atlas, McConnell Brain Imaging Centre, Montréal Neurological Institute, McGill University, Montréal, Canada.

Automatic Classification of SPECT Images of Alzheimer's Disease Patients and Control Subjects

Jonathan Stoeckel[1], Nicholas Ayache[1], Grégoire Malandain[1],
Pierre M. Koulibaly[2], Klaus P. Ebmeier[3], and Jacques Darcourt[2]

[1] EPIDAURE Project, INRIA,
2004 route des Lucioles, Sophia Antipolis 06902, France
Jonathan.Stoeckel@siemens.com, {na, greg}@sophia.inria.fr
http://www-sop.inria.fr/epidaure
[2] Service de Médecine Nucléaire - Centre Antoine Lacassagne
33 avenue de Valombrose, 06189 NICE cedex 2, France
[3] Royal Edinburgh Hospital, Morningside Park
Edinburgh EH10 5HF, United Kingdom

Abstract. In this article we study the use of SPECT perfusion imaging
for the diagnosis of Alzheimer's disease. We present a classifier based
approach that does not need any explicit knowledge about the pathology. We directly use the voxel intensities as features. This approach is
compared with three classical approaches: regions of interests, statistical parametric mapping and visual analysis which is the most commonly
used method. We tested our method both on simulated and on real data.
The realistic simulations give us total control about the ground truth.
On real data, our method was more sensitive than the human experts,
while having an acceptable specificity. We conclude that an automatic
method can be a useful help for clinicians.

1 Introduction

Alzheimer's disease (AD) is the most frequent type of dementia for elderly patients. Due to aging populations its occurrence will still increase. Even though
no definitive cure has been found for this disease, reliable diagnosis is useful for
excluding other dementias, choosing the right treatment and for the development
of new treatments.

AD is diagnosed using the criteria from the National Institute of Neurological
and Communicative Disorders and Stroke and Alzheimer's Disease and Related
Disorders Association (NINCDS-ADRDA) [1]. In practice the main tool for evaluating patients are neuro-psychologic tests, that test abilities like memory and
language. The Mini Mental State Examination (MMSE) is the most widely used
of these tests [2].

---

[1] JS is now with the CAD Solutions Group, Siemens Medical Solutions USA Inc.,
Malvern, PA

C. Barillot, D.R. Haynor, and P. Hellier (Eds.): MICCAI 2004, LNCS 3217, pp. 654–662, 2004.
© Springer-Verlag Berlin Heidelberg 2004

Brain images can provide some indication of AD. Magnetic resonance imaging (MRI) is used to study possible anatomical changes of the brain [3]. Images showing the local perfusion of the brain can be used for the diagnosis of AD because the perfusion pattern is affected by the disease. In this article we will look into the use of cerebral perfusion imaging acquired by single photon emitting computer tomography (SPECT) using Technetium-99m Hexamethyl Propylene Amine Oxime (HMPAO) as the tracer. Even though the perfusion pattern and its evolution are not the same for all patients some hypo-perfusion patterns seem to be typical for the disease. In the literature, three main regions are described as showing hypo-perfusion[4] signals, 1. the temporo-parietal region, 2. the posterior cingulate gyri and precunei, and 3. the medial temporal lobe. The first region is known as the predominant pattern for AD, however this region was not found for early AD [5]. The second region is probably more specific and more frequent in early AD [6]. Previous pathological studies have suggested that the third region is the first affected by the disease [7], however in practice it is only observed in more advanced stages of the disease [6].

There is not one single perfusion pattern that differentiates AD patients form healthy subjects. Thus it might be useful to have tools that could assist physicians in this difficult task. In this article we will present a method that does not need any explicit knowledge about the perfusion pattern of AD patients.

Some approaches for a computer aided diagnosis (CAD) system for the analysis of SPECT images for AD can be found in literature. The first family is based on the analysis of regions of interest. The mean values for these regions are analyzed using some discriminant functions (see e.g. [8][9]).

The second approach is statistical parametric mapping (SPM) and its numerous variants. Statistical parametric mapping is widely used in the neuro-sciences. Its framework was first developed for the analysis of SPECT and PET studies, but is now mainly used for the analysis of functional MRI data. It was not developed specifically to study a single image, but for comparing groups of images. One can use it for diagnostics by comparing the image under study to a group of normal images.

Statistical parametric mapping consists of doing a voxel-wise statistical test, in our case a t-test, comparing the values of the image under study to the mean values of the group of normal images. Subsequently the significant voxels are inferred by using the random field theory (see e.g. [10] for a full description of SPM). A largely used freely available implementation called SPM99 [11] has been developed and will be used in this article to compare our approach.

In this article we will propose another approach using as less a-priori information about the pathology as possible, by obtaining it implicitly from image databases. The other important aspect of our approach is the use of a global approach. This means that we will not provide the clinician with information about where the hypo-perfused areas are situated (e.g. as given by SPM) but we will only give a global answer to the question whether or not the image under study belongs to an AD patient. This has the advantage over a more local approach that all the information in the image can be used at once in contrast to the mono-variate methods like SPM. A multi-variate approach generally increases sensitivity at the price of loosing regional specificity (e.g. depicting local hypo-perfusion regions).

In [12] some very preliminary results were presented. In this article we present results on a large set of real data. This data comes from several centers to show the robustness of our method. However only limited knowledge about the perfusion pattern is available for real data. We only know if the perfusion pattern was that of an Alzheimer's subject or not. The locations of the hypo-perfused regions are not known, neither the amount of the hypo-perfusions. Therefore we chose to simulate images as to have complete local control, and thus knowledge of the ground truth.

The following section first discusses the pre-processing of the data, followed by the analysis of the data using classifiers. In section 3 we present the data we used for our experiments. We used both real data and simulated data. The results on the data are presented in section 4 and discussed in section 5.

2 Methods

Spatial Normalization. In the classifier based approach we need the assumption that the same position in the volume coordinate system within different volumes corresponds to the same anatomical position.

This means that we need to spatially register the volumes. Because of the limited anatomical information available in the volumes we chose to estimate affine transformations between the volumes. We used the correlation ratio as the similarity measure [13] that we minimized using Powell optimization [14]. To obtain a more robust result we used the following procedure. First of all, we registered all volumes to a single volume, this was done to obtain an average volume. This average volume was first put on the mid-sagittal plane by registering it with a flipped version (see [15]). Subsequently it was made to be symmetrical by taking the mean of itself with a flipped version around the mid-sagittal plane. Finally all volumes were matched to this symmetric average volume.

Intensity Normalization. HMPAO brain uptake is proportional to regional cerebral blood flow. However absolute measurement is not possible and only the relative distribution of the tracer can be studied. The cerebellum is usually not affected in AD and can therefore be chosen as reference area. We normalized the intensities by dividing by the summed intensity in the cerebellum. This was done automatically by using a template on the registered volumes.

Classification. Because the hypo-perfusion pattern for early AD is not very well defined we chose to develop a method where we did not use any explicit knowledge about the typical perfusion patterns. We used implicit knowledge about the perfusion patterns by using a database of images of AD patients and normal subjects.

To separate the images we used a classifier using the voxel intensities as features and this database to train the classifier. Using the voxel intensities as features makes it possible not to introduce any particular knowledge about the exact location of the hypo-perfusion area(s). Thus by using a database of images and the voxel intensities we circumvent the problem of the exact definition of the typical perfusion pattern for early AD.

In general the number of images available in the training databases is significantly smaller (< 100) than the number of voxels (> 1000). Thus the number of features (voxels) is much larger than the number of samples (training images). The number of samples is considered to be small if it is about the same or smaller than the number of dimensions. In this case we speak of almost empty spaces, the small sample size problem or the so called curse of dimensionality. In classical pattern recognition it was believed that no good generalization could be obtained for this cases. Generalization is the capacity of a classifier to rightly classify a sample never seen before.

Even though, traditionally it was thought that due to the curse of dimensionality it is necessary to fill the feature space with many more objects than its dimensionality in order to obtain a classifier that generalizes well. Recently it has become clear however, that there are several ways to construct classifiers in almost empty spaces (see the following review [16]).

We chose to use the pseudo-Fisher linear discriminant classifier (PFLDC) as it has already been applied to the small sample size problem for some non-medical applications [17][18][16]. We also did some experiments with the nearest mean classifier (NMC)[19].

All experiments carried out in this article (except noted otherwise) were carried out using the leave-one-out approach to have an independent test and training set, and thus this provides an unbiased estimate of the classification performance.

3   Materials

Simulations. We chose to use a so called photon simulator to generate simulated images. We used the freely available SimSET simulation package developed by the University of Washington Imaging Research Laboratory. More information about this package as well as further references can be found on its website[1].

The freely available Zubal phantom [20] was used to define the activities and the attenuation coefficients for each segmented region. Instead of using this phantom directly to generate volumes, we chose to deform it, to simulate the differences in morphology that exist between different subjects. To obtain realistic deformations we used the free-form deformation fields as generated by the Pasha algorithm (see [21] when registering the phantom with 23 MRI volumes of healthy subjects.

To simulate hypo-perfusion areas we lowered the activity by 20 % percent in the following areas: 1) internal temporal, 2) cingulum and precuneus, 3)

---

[1]   http://depts.washington.edu/~simset/html/simset_main.html

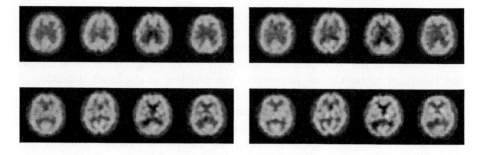

Fig. 1. Examples of four volumes from the Cologne center after intensity and spatial normalization. In each column the first two small images show two normal subjects, the last two images show slices of AD subjects. The sets of slices are ordered from left to right and from top to bottom. Strong hypo-perfusion can be seen for the first AD patient, whereas the hypo-perfusion is more subtle for the second patient.

temporal-parietal region. These regions were manually segmented in the Zubal atlas because the segmentation of the atlas was not fine enough. The three regions had respectively a volume of 72319 mm^3, 32010 mm^{3}and 18642 mm^3. For each simulated AD image, only one region was hypo-perfused.

We simulated 13 control volumes and 10 volumes per hypo-perfusion region and value (2 hypo-perfusion values times 3 regions times 10 images, gives 60 AD volumes). The volumes were reconstructed using filtered-back projection, without attenuation correction. The reconstructed volumes had a voxel size of 2.5 mm by 2.5 mm by 3.6 mm.

Real Data. The real images we used for our experiments were taken from a concurrent study investigating the use of SPECT as a diagnostic tool for the early onset of AD. A detailed description of this data can be found in [22]. Subjects of four different centers, Edinburgh (Scotland), Nice (France), Genoa (Italy), and Cologne (Germany) were included for this study. In total 158 subjects participated, including 99 patients with AD, 28 patients suffering from depression (not used in this article), and 31 healthy volunteers. An example of this data is seen in figure 1.

Applying the registration procedure as described above resulted in images of 128 by 128 by 89 voxels, with a voxelsize of 1.71 mm by 1.71 mm by 1.88 mm for all four centers.

Experts. All real images were rated in four categories(very probable, probably, probably not and very unlikely to have AD) by sixteen European expert nuclear medicine physicians .

To be able to compare the data from the experts with that of the automatic methods, we considered the first two ratings as positive and the other two as negative. The different observers turn out to have quite different sensitivities and specificities therefore we will also just show the results of the Nice experts.

4   Experiments

Simulated Data. We tested the nearest mean classifier (NMC) as well as the Fisher linear discriminant classifier (PFLDC) on the simulated data. The images were subsampled by a factor two in each dimension as to obtain a number of voxels that does not need excessive amounts of computing time and computer memory. This resulted in 9150 features.

The FLDC was able to classify the images with the following results per region 1: 90.0%, 84.6% 2: 70.0%, 76.9% 3: 80.0%, 84.6% sensitivity and specificity. The NMC classifer had slightly worse results. However SPM was not able to detect the hypo-perfusion areas at all, different significance levels were tried, at each level SPM showed approximately the same number of regions containing hypo-perfusions (true positives) as not containing hypo perfusions (false positives).

Real Data. Figure 2 shows the results on all the real data using the leave-one-out error estimate. The right side of the figure shows results when training on just data from one site and using the classifier for the remaining data. The FLDC ROI approach consisted of using a regions of interest approach (21 regions) similar to that found in literature [8][9] defined by the Zubal phantom and carrying out classification using the FLDC by using the mean intensities of those areas as features. In the SPM cluster approach we used SPM at a significance level of 0.1 at the cluster level. We considered each image where some significant clusters were found to be a positive result. The FLDC column shows the results for the Fisher linear classifier on the images after a subsampling of a factor two in each dimension resulting in 26950 features. All experts show the results of all 16 experts, whereas Nice experts show only the four experts from Nice.

On all the data the FLDC is statistically significantly more sensitive than the experts from all centers ($p<3.10^{-10}$), however the experts are significantly more specific than the FLDC ($p<0.05$). When training the FLDC on the data from Edinburgh and testing on the remaining data the FLDC is nearly significantly more specific ($p<0.07$) but there is no significant difference in sensitivity.

The difference in the results seen between the left and the right of figure 2 are due to the much smaller training set in the right case and also probably due to differences in the acquisition protocols between the different sites. However note that the classification approach still provides useful results even when using a small training set not acquired in exactly the same way. This shows that for clinical use larger databases are needed, however that classification of images with different acquisition parameters is possible.

5   Conclusion

Based on the experiments described in this article we conclude that automatic approaches to the classification of images perform at least as well as human observers. In general our automatic method is more sensitive while still being

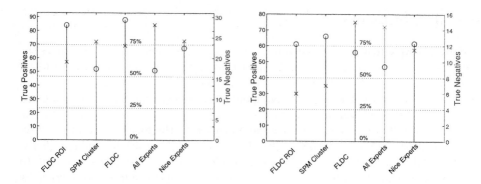

Fig. 2. Left: Graphical representation of the main results when using **all** the real data (AD: 93, normal: 31 cases), Right: results of testing on **all data except Edinburgh** (80 AD, 16 controls) when training on the data from the Edinburgh center only. The number of true positives is given by circles. The number of true negatives is given by crosses. Because the axes are scaled to the number of AD (93) and normal (31) images, sensitivity (circles) and specificity (crosses) are indicated by the dotted horizontal lines.

sufficiently specific. One would need more data, especially of control subjects to be able to state that automatic methods outperform human observers.

We have shown that classification of images using the voxel values as features equals or outperforms the other automatic methods. Thus classification without using any specific knowledge related to the pathology is shown to be possible.

The automatic methods used in this article, with the exception of SPM give only global information on the image. The best of them do outperform SPM. However only providing global information might not be sufficient for clinicians. Therefore in practice, results as those obtained by SPM might be used as additional information to the global classification.

For future work one might want to try the presented approach for differential diagnosis (e.g. AD versus Pick's disease) which might be an even more important clinical issue. ROC analysis of the classifier as well as of the experts will be useful to better compare performances, especially when observing the probable differences in position on the ROC curves (operating points) in the current study between the experts (see e.g. sensitivity differences between all the experts and a given group of experts only).

References

1. G. McKhann, D. Drachman, M. Folstein, R. Katzman, D. Price, and E.M. Stadlan. Mental and clinical diagnosis of Alzheimer's disease: report of the NINCDS-ADRDA Work Group under the auspices of the Department of Health and Human Services Task Force on Alzheimer's Disease. *Neurology*, 34(7):939–944, July 1984.
2. M.F. Folstein, S.E. Folstein, and P.R. McHugh. "Mini-Mental State": a practical method for grading the cognitive state of patients for the clinician. *Journal of Psychiatric Research*, 12(3):189–198, November 1975.

3. K.M. Gosche, J.A. Mortimer, C.D. Smith, W.R. Markesbery, and D.A. Snowdon. Hippocampal volume as an index of Alzheimer neuropathology: findings from the Nun Study. *Neurology*, 58(10):1476–1482, May 2002.

4. I. Goethals, C. van de Wiele, D. Slosman, and R. Dierckx. Brain SPET perfusion in early Alzheimer's disease: where to look? *European Journal of Nuclear Medicine*, 29(8):975–978, August 2002.

5. W.A. Van Gool, G.J. Walstra, S. Teunisse, F.M. Van der Zant, H.C. Weinstein, and E.A. Van Royen. Diagnosing Alzheimer's disease in elderly, mildly demented patients: the impact of routine single photon emission computed tomography. *Journal of Neurology*, 242(6):401–405, June 1995.

6. D. Kogure, H. Matsuda, T. Ohnishi, T. Asada, M. Uno, T. Kunihiro, S. Nakano, and M. Takasaki. Longitudinal evaluation of early Alzheimer's disease using brain perfusion SPECT. *Journal of Nuclear Medicine*, 41(7):1155–1162, July 2000.

7. H. Braak and E. Braak. Diagnostic criteria for neuropathologic assessment of Alzheimer's disease. *Neurobiology and Aging*, 18(4):S85–S88, July 1997.

8. M.R. Dawson, A. Dobbs, H.R. Hooper, A.J. McEwan, J. Triscott, and J. Cooney. Artificial neural networks that use single-photon emission tomography to identify patients with probable Alzheimer's disease. *European Journal of Nuclear Medicine*, 21(12):1303–1311, December 1994.

9. D. Hamilton, D. O'Mahony, J. Coffey, J. Murphy, N. O'Hare, P. Freyne, B. Walsh, and D. Coakley. Classification of mild Alzheimer's disease by artificial neural network analysis of SPET data. *Nuclear Medicine Communications*, 18(9):805–810, September 1997.

10. R.S.J. Frackowiak, K.J. Friston, C.D. Frith, and R. Dolan. *Human Brain Function*. Academic Press, 1997.

11. J. Ashburner, K. Friston, A. Holmes, and J.-B. Poline. Statistical Parametric Mapping, SPM'99. The Welcome Department of Cognitive Neurology. Institute of Neurology, University College London, 1999. Freely available at *http://www.fil.ion.ucl.ac.uk/spm*.

12. J. Stoeckel, G. Malandain, O. Migneco, P.M. Koulibaly, P. Robert, N. Ayache, and J. Darcourt. Classification of SPECT images of normal subjects versus images of Alzheimer's disease patients. In *Proc. MICCAI'01*, volume 2208 of *LNCS*, pages 666–674, October 2001.

13. A. Roche, G. Malandain, X. Pennec, and N. Ayache. The Correlation Ratio as a New Similarity Metric for Multimodal Image Registration. In W. M. Wells, A. C. F. Colchester, and S. Delp, editors, *Medical Image Computing and Computer-Assisted Intervention (MICCAI'98)*, volume 1496 of *Lecture Notes in Computer Science*, pages 1115–1124, Boston, USA, October 1998.

14. W. H. Press, S. A. Teukolsky, W. T. Vetterling, and B. P. Flannery. *Numerical Recipes. The Art of Scientific Computing*. Cambridge University Press, 2nd edition, 1997.

15. S. Prima, S. Ourselin, and N. Ayache. Computation of the mid-sagittal plane in 3D brain images. *IEEE Transaction on Medical Imaging*, 21(2):122–138, February 2002.

16. R.P.W. Duin. Classifiers in Almost Empty Spaces. In *Proceedings of the 15th International Conference on Pattern Recognition (ICPR'00)*, volume 2, pages 1–7, 2000.

17. J. Shürmann. *Polynomklassifikatoren für Zeichenerkennung*. R. Oldenburg Verlag, 1977.

18. S.J. Raudys and R.P.W. Duin. Expected classification error of the Fisher linear classifier with pseudo-inverse covariance matrix. *Pattern Recognition Letters*, 19:385–392, 1998.

19. R.O. Duda, P.E. Hart, and D.G. Stork. *Pattern Classification*. John Wiley & Sons, 2nd edition, 2001.

20. I.G. Zubal, C.R. Harrell, E.O. Smith, Z. Rattner, G. Gindi, and P.B. Hoffer. Computerized 3-Dimensional Segmented Human Anatomy. *Medical Physics*, 21(2):299–302, February 1994.

21. P. Cachier, E. Bardinet, D. Dormont, X. Pennec, and N. Ayache. Iconic Feature Based Nonrigid Registration: The PASHA Algorithm. *Computer Vision and Image Understanding*, 89(1-2), February 2003.

22. D. Soonawala, T. Amin, K.P. Ebmeier, J.D. Steele, N.J. Dougall, J. Best, O. Migneco, F. Nobili, and K. Scheidhauer. Statistical parametric mapping of (99m)Tc-HMPAO-SPECT images for the diagnosis of Alzheimer's disease: normalizing to cerebellar tracer uptake. *Neuroimage*, 17(3):1193–1202, November 2002.

Estimation of Anatomical Connectivity by Anisotropic Front Propagation and Diffusion Tensor Imaging

Marcel Jackowski[1], Chiu Yen Kao[3], Maolin Qiu[1], R. Todd Constable[2], and Lawrence H. Staib[2]

[1] Yale School of Medicine, Dept. of Diagnostic Radiology, New Haven CT 06520
[2] Yale School of Medicine, Dept. of Diagnostic Radiology and Biomedical Engineering, New Haven CT 06520
[3] University of California Los Angeles, Dept. of Mathematics, Los Angeles CA 90095

Abstract. Diffusion Tensor Magnetic Resonance Imaging (DT-MRI) allows one to capture the restricted diffusion of water molecules in fibrous tissues which can be used to infer their structural organization. In this paper, we propose a novel wavefront propagation method for estimating the connectivity in the white matter of the brain using DT-MRI. First, an anisotropic version of the static Hamilton-Jacobi equation is solved by a sweeping method in order to obtain accurate front arrival times and determine connectivity. Our wavefront then propagates using the diffusion tensor rather than its principal eigenvector, which is prone to misclassification in oblate tensor regions. Furthermore, we show that our method is robust to noise and can estimate connectivity pathways across regions where singularities, such as fiber crossings, are present. Preliminary connectivity results on synthetic data and on a normal human brain are illustrated and discussed.

1 Introduction

While the basic anatomy of white matter tracts in the human brain is generally known from anatomical dissection, much is unknown about its interconnections and its natural variations. Therefore, the characterization and quantitative measurement of its connections is of fundamental importance in understanding brain function. Diffusion Tensor Magnetic Resonance Imaging (DT-MRI) has emerged as a noninvasive imaging modality capable of providing this information in vivo, enabling the detailed study of white matter structure in the human brain.

Brain white matter, because of the long and fibrous nature of axons, exhibits higher restriction to water diffusion across the fibers than along them. This directional variation is measured in diffusivity rates and can be captured by diffusion-weighted MRI. By acquiring diffusion-weighted data in at least six non-collinear directions, it is possible to estimate a 3x3 symmetric matrix (i.e. diffusion tensor) which characterizes diffusion in anisotropic systems [2]. After tensor diagonalization, the eigenvector corresponding to the largest eigenvalue is considered to point along the direction of a fiber bundle.

C. Barillot, D.R. Haynor, and P. Hellier (Eds.): MICCAI 2004, LNCS 3217, pp. 663–670, 2004.
© Springer-Verlag Berlin Heidelberg 2004

Numerous connectivity studies relying on the straightforward integration of the principal tensor eigenvector have been described in the literature [4,3,9,8]. Several problems, however, affect their reliability. First, the diffusion images are subject to acquisition noise which can impede the ability to track fibers. Also, while it is true that the principal eigenvector provides an estimate of the microscopic fiber direction, because of partial voluming, signal contributions from multiple tissues can affect individual voxel measurements [1], resulting in a variation in the distribution of fiber directions. This problem becomes more severe when fiber tracts cross, branch or merge.

To account for these variations, level set methods [11] have been employed [12, 10,7]. These techniques model the evolution of an advancing front through the white matter tracts by following the local directionality provided by the diffusion tensor field. Such methods have been shown to be more robust to noise and singularities than classical streamlining methods. A tractography technique based on Tsitsiklis' fast marching method (FMM) was used by Parker *et al.* [12]. A front was evolved with a speed proportional to the colinearity between the front normal and the principal tensor eigenvector. A discrete approximation of front direction had to be used to drive the evolution through the eigenvector field, since the original FMM cannot handle propagation in oriented domains.

O'Donnell *et al.* [10] posed the connectivity problem in a Riemannian framework where the space is locally warped based on the three eigenvectors and the connectivity corresponds to the lengths of the underlying geodesic paths. Lenglet *et al.* [7] has similarly considered the white matter connectivity problem as one of finding minimal geodesics in the Riemannian space. Both methods employed a less efficient dynamic formulation for the problem, in which a narrow band was employed to constrain front propagation and reduce computation time.

We also propose a level set method to determine connectivity. Unlike other methods, we solve for the true anisotropic solutions of the static front propagation equation. Our sweeping method correctly computes the arrival times so that pathways can be determined. In addition, by using a static perspective of the level set equation, we avoid the localization and separate extraction of zero-level sets at different time steps of the dynamic formulation. Furthermore, the entire diffusion tensor is used to control propagation, avoiding possible biasing of its principal eigenvector in more isotropic regions. In the following, we first model the white matter connectivity problem as one of anisotropic wavefront evolution. We then proceed to describe our propagation equation and the method to solve it. Finally, we present our results on synthetic and real data and conclude.

2   Anatomical Pathways

White matter connectivity can be viewed as an instance of the minimum-cost path problem in an oriented weighted domain. Essentially, one would like to find a fiber path $P(s) : [0, \infty) \mapsto \mathbb{R}^3$ that minimizes some cumulative travel cost from a starting point A to some destination point B in the white matter.

Because of the directionality of the tensor field, the cost function, represented by τ or its reciprocal speed $F = 1/\tau$, is a function of both position $P(s)$ as well as direction $P'(s)$. Hence it is called anisotropic and the minimum cumulative cost at x is defined as:

$$T(x) = \min_P \int_0^L \tau(P(s), P'(s))\, ds. \tag{1}$$

where L is pathway length, and the starting and ending points are given by $P(0) = A$ and $P(L) = x$. A solution to (1) also satisfies the wave propagation equation:

$$\|\nabla T\| = \tau(x, \nabla T), \tag{2}$$

which describes a wavefront propagating with speed $1/\tau$ where $T(x)$ is the time of arrival of the front at point x. This equation typically arises in problems where a preferred direction of travel exists, such as propagating a front through a vector field. In continuous space, solutions to (2) are given by the Hamilton-Jacobi (HJ) equations. A classical solution to (2) may not exist, and therefore the viscosity solution is commonly sought. Numerical approximations of the viscosity solution can be found in [6,5,13].

Once the evolution equation (2) is solved for all points in the domain, one can use the obtained arrival times and find a solution for (1). The minimum-cost path between point A and an arbitrary point B in the white matter then becomes a solution to:

$$\frac{dX}{dt} = -\nabla T, \tag{3}$$

given $X(0) = B$. This optimal path can be constructed by integrating equation (3) at point B back to the seed point A using standard techniques. Next, we will elaborate on the front evolution equation that will be used to trace connectivity pathways in the white matter.

3 Front Propagation Model

We employ the entire tensor in our propagation model to avoid the possible misclassification of the principal eigenvector in oblate tensor regions, which may lead to wrong assignment of front arrival times. We rather design our wavefront to evolve from a seed point A, $T(A) = 0$, at a speed governed by a function of the diffusivity magnitude in the front normal direction $\boldsymbol{n}$:

$$d(\boldsymbol{n}) = \boldsymbol{n}^T D\, \boldsymbol{n}, \quad \boldsymbol{n} = \nabla T/\|\nabla T\|, \tag{4}$$

where D is the diffusion tensor. The motivation behind equation (4) is to let the speed vary locally according to the tensor profile, descriptive of the underlying tissue structure. In addition, we slow down the front more rapidly when diffusivity $d(\boldsymbol{n})$ decreases. Thus, we can write the propagation equation as follows:

$$\|\nabla T\| \cdot \alpha \cdot \exp(d(\boldsymbol{n})^\gamma) = 1, \tag{5}$$

where γ represents the slowing power based on the diffusivity response and α controls the final propagation speed. Since water diffusion measured in the ventricles and in the gray matter is more random than in the white matter, the resulting tensor profile tends to be spherical with eigenvalues $\lambda_1 \simeq \lambda_2 \simeq \lambda_3$. To prevent the propagation into these areas, we choose α to be a measure of diffusion tensor anisotropy. For that, we employed the well-known FA index [2] and after some experimentation, we chose $\alpha = FA^2$. Parameter γ was also empirically set and yielded smoother results when $\gamma = 2$ or 3.

Propagation equation (5) belongs to a family of static Hamilton-Jacobi equations described by:

$$\begin{cases} H(x, \nabla T) = V(x), & x \in \Omega \\ T(x) = q(x) \end{cases} \qquad (6)$$

where Ω is the domain in $\mathbb{R}^3$, $V(x) = 1$, and $q(x)$ is a function prescribing boundary condition values, $T(A) = q(A) = 0$. Therefore, we can rewrite (5) as the following Hamiltonian, after discarding the dependence of x on H:

$$H(p, q, r) = \alpha \sqrt{p^2 + q^2 + r^2} \cdot \exp\left\{ \left(\frac{p^2 d_{11} + q^2 d_{22} + r^2 d_{33} + 2pq d_{12} + 2pr d_{13} + 2qr d_{23}}{p^2 + q^2 + r^2} \right)^\gamma \right\}$$
$$(7)$$

where $p = \partial T/\partial x$, $q = \partial T/\partial y$, $r = \partial T/\partial z$ and d_{ij} are the tensor elements. While equation (5) can be reformulated as a time-dependent HJ equation and solved by recovering each zero-level set, it is more convenient and less computationally expensive to model it as a static problem and determine arrival times instead. In the following section, we will describe an iterative method that solves our static HJ equation (7) so that a viscosity solution can be obtained.

4   Front Propagation Method

Hamiltonians such as (7) cannot be correctly solved by isotropic propagation methods, such as the FMM. However, carefully crafted methods have been devised [6,5,13] to construct accurate solutions for anisotropic equations. We use a Lax-Friedrichs (LF) discretization of our Hamiltonian and employ a nonlinear Gauss-Seidel updating scheme [5] to solve the propagation equation. With the LF discretization, a solution at each grid point can be easily obtained in terms of its neighbors. Also, no minimization is required when updating an arrival time, and thus it is very easy to implement.

The Lax-Friedrichs Hamiltonian of equation (7) is defined as:

$$H^{LF} = H\left(\frac{p^+ + p^-}{2}, \frac{q^+ + q^-}{2}, \frac{r^+ + r^-}{2} \right) - \frac{\sigma_x}{2}(p^+ - p^-) - \frac{\sigma_y}{2}(q^+ - q^-) - \frac{\sigma_z}{2}(r^+ - r^-), \quad (8)$$

where $p^\pm$, $q^\pm$ and $r^\pm$ are the forward and backward difference approximations for ∇T, and σ_n is the artificial viscosity which depends on the partial derivative of H with respect to p, q and r.

In order to get a numerical approximation for (7), we solve for $H^{LF} = 1$ by sweeping the domain in the alternating directions $\pm x$, $\pm y$ and $\pm z$. Values from the previous sweeping step are used to make the approximation decreasing so that it updates an arrival time only if $T_{i,j,k}^{m+1} < T_{i,j,k}^{m}$. Because the LF method yields a solution utilizing all 6-connected neighbors, values for points outside the boundary of the domain are extrapolated to guarantee the outflow of the solution at the boundary. Sweeping is stopped when the convergence criterion $\|T_{i,j,k}^{m+1} - T_{i,j,k}^{m}\| \le \epsilon$ is met. Details on the algorithm, accuracy and convergence of LF sweeping (LFS) scheme can be found in Kao et $al.$ [5].

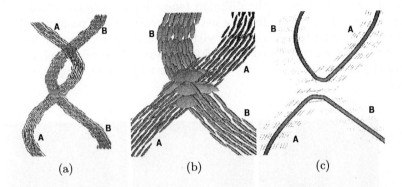

(a)   (b)   (c)

Fig. 1. (a) Synthetic tensor dataset containing two fiber bundles A, B with main diffusivities $\{1, 0.2, 0.1\}$ and $\{0.9, 0.2, 0.1\}$ mm^2/s, respectively. (b) Close-up look of the fiber-crossing location and resulting oblate tensors. (c). Result from streamline integration across the fiber-crossing region.

5   Results

Figure 1a shows our synthetic model consisting of two fiber bundles A, B oriented along helical paths which cross each other at their middle section (Fig. 1a). The background was filled with isotropic tensors (1 mm^2/s, not shown). Fig. 1b depicts a close-up view of the fiber-crossing region, where oblate tensors resulting from the crossing are found. Figure 1c depicts a failed attempt in reconstructing pathways from bundles A and B using the streamlining technique. The oblate tensors resulting from the fiber crossing region erroneously advect both pathways away from their true trajectories.

Using our method, we reconstructed the same pathways to demonstrate that it can handle the fiber crossing without deviating the fiber trajectories. First, diffusion-weighted images were created from our model, and increasing levels of Gaussian noise ($\sigma = 0.02$, 0.05 and 0.07) were added to them (Fig. 2a-c). The resulting SNRs were 7.62, 3.06 and 2.19, respectively. Then, a seed point A_1 was fixed at the bottom of bundle A (Fig. 2a) and our wavefront ($\gamma=2$) was propagated using the LFS method on the tensor images. Points A_2, B_1 and B_2 were fixed at the extreme ends of each bundle (Fig. 2a) and corresponding pathways A_2A_1, B_1A_1 and B_2A_1 were traced on ∇T images using a Runge-Kutta 4th-order integration.

Figures 2d, 2e, 2f illustrate the obtained connectivity pathways embedded in the arrival time images and corresponding arrival isocurves. Darker areas in the maps reveal earlier arrivals. The LFS method converged to a solution ($\epsilon = 10^{-4}$), after 40 iterations for all noise levels. As can be seen, the singularity region did not prevent pathways connecting different branches or the same branch (A_2A_1) from being recovered. To assess the variability of the extracted paths, we propagated the same front in the diffusion tensor image without added noise and then computed the mean distance between corresponding pathways. The mean distance for all paths under noise $\sigma=0.02$ was 0.07 voxels, for $\sigma=0.05$ the mean distance was 0.34 voxels and for $\sigma=0.07$, it was 0.64 voxels. Therefore, the recovered pathways remained very close to their trajectories, in spite of the added noise.

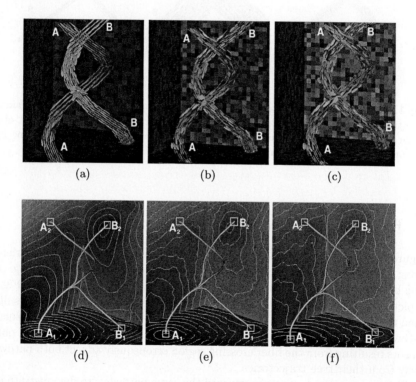

(a)   (b)   (c)

(d)   (e)   (f)

Fig. 2. (a-c) Tensor model with additive Gaussian noise ($\sigma = 0.02$, 0.05 and 0.07). (d-f) Times of arrival and connectivity pathways corresponding to images (a-c), respectively.

A diffusion-weighted image was acquired using a Siemens 3T Trio scanner with a standard coil. A single-shot EPI image of matrix size 128x128x40, resolution 2x2x3 mm^3, b-factors 0 and 1000 s/mm^{-2}, and 32 gradient directions uniformly sampled on a sphere was obtained. The diffusion tensor was calculated from a total of 12 averages to maximize signal to noise ratio. In this dataset, we fixed the seed point in the splenium of the corpus callosum (Fig. 3a). We then propagated our wavefront throughout the image using the LFS method. A total of 25 iterations were needed for convergence. Figure 3a depicts the resulting arrival time level sets between 0 and 500. In order to trace connectivity pathways to the splenium, we first obtained a rough boundary of the white matter according to the following procedure. The FA image was thresholded at 0.18, in order to obtain all points belonging to the white matter. Next, by using a morphological operator, we determined the inner boundary of the thresholded region. All pathways between points on this boundary and the point in the splenium were traced using the map of arrival times (Fig. 3b). Fig. 3c shows the resulting 20,817 pathways colored by the FA value at each point, where brighter points represent higher anisotropy. In Figures 3b and 3c, we can observe the main routes of connection between various brain regions and the splenium. Points leaving the genu of the corpus callosum (CC) connect to the splenium via the cingulum (CI) pathways, and points in the superior frontal lobe connect via the superior longitudinal fasciculi (SL) consistent with known anatomy.

Not all connections shown in figures 3b and 3c represent true anatomical pathways. A metric to rate their anatomical likelihood such as the co-linearity between pathway tangent and principal eigenvector as described by Parker *et al.* [12] will be investigated. In future work, we plan to propagate our wavefront from all points belonging to the white matter boundary and then trace all possible pathways back to corresponding seed points. By using geometric properties such as pathway length and tangent, as well as measures derived from diffusion images, we plan to design an automated system for brain fiber recovery.

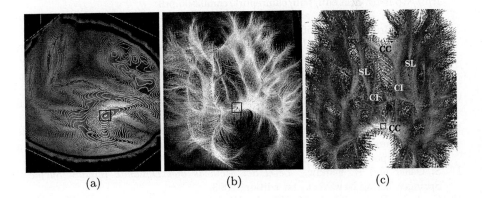

(a)   (b)   (c)

Fig. 3. (a) Level sets depicting arrival times between 0 and 500, after propagation using the LFS method. (b) 20,817 different pathways connecting white matter boundary to the splenium of the corpus callosum were extracted. (c) Close-up view of the main pathways connecting to the splenium.

6   Conclusions

An anisotropic front propagation method was described for determining connectivity pathways in the white matter. It successfully recovered pathways embedded in different levels of noise and was able to extract paths of connection across areas of singularities in the diffusion tensor, unlike streamlining techniques. The use of the static perspective of the level set equation allowed us to pose the problem so that front arrival times could be easily computed. Moreover, our formulation used the entire tensor for propagation, avoiding the possible biasing in the eigenvector classification. Finally, results on a real diffusion tensor dataset were presented where major fiber bundles were identified and were consistent with known anatomy.

References

1. A. L. Alexander, K. M. Hasan, M. Lazar, J. S. Tsuruda, and D. L. Parker. Analysis of partial volume effects in diffusion-tensor MRI. *Mag. Res. Medicine*, 45(5):770–780, May 2001.
2. P. J. Basser and C. Pierpaoli. Microstructural and physiological features of tissues elucidated by quantitative-diffusion-tensor MRI. *J. Mag. Res., Series B*, 111(3):209–219, Jun 1996.
3. P.J. Basser, S. Pajevic, C. PierPaoli, J. Duda, and A. Aldroubi. In-vivo fiber tractography using DT-MRI data. *Mag. Res. Medicine*, 44:625–632, 2000.
4. D. K. Jones, A. Simmons, S. C. Williams, and M. A. Horsfield. Noninvasive assessment of axonal fiber connectivity in the human brain via diffusion tensor MRI. *Mag. Res. Medicine*, 42:37–41, 1999.
5. C. Kao, S. Osher, and J. Qian. Lax-Friedrichs Sweeping scheme for static Hamilton-Jacobi equations. *Journal of Computational Physics*, in press, 2003.
6. C. Kao, S. Osher, and Y. Tsai. Fast Sweeping Methods for static Hamilton-Jacobi equations. Technical report, University of California Los Angeles, 2002. ftp://ftp.math.ucla.edu/pub/camreport/cam02-66.pdf.
7. C. Lenglet, R. Deriche, and O. Faugeras. Diffusion tensor magnetic resonance imaging: Brain connectivity mapping. Research Report 4983, INRIA, 2003.
8. N. F. Lori, E. Akbudak, J. S. Shimony, T. S. Cull, A. Z. Snyder, R. K. Guillory, and T. E. Conturo. Diffusion tensor fiber tracking of human brain connectivity: aquisition methods, reliability analysis and biological results. *NMR in Biomedicine*, 15(7-8):494–515, 2002.
9. S. Mori and P. C. M. van Zijl. Fiber tracking: principles and strategies - a technical review. *NMR in Biomedicine*, 15(7-8):468–480, 2002.
10. L. O'Donnell, S. Haker, and C.-F. Westin. New approaches to estimation of white matter connectivity in diffusion tensor MRI: Elliptic PDEs and geodesics in a tensor-warped space. *Proc. MICCAI*, pages 459–466, 2002.
11. S. Osher and R. Fedkiw. *Level Set Methods and Dynamic Implicit Surfaces*. Springer-Verlag New York, 1st edition, 2003.
12. G. J. M. Parker, C. A. M. Wheeler-Kingshott, and G. J. Barker. Estimating distributed anatomical connectivity using fast marching methods and diffusion tensor imaging. *IEEE Trans. Med. Imaging*, 21(5):505–512, 2002.
13. J. A. Sethian and A. Vladimirsky. Ordered Upwind Methods for static Hamilton-Jacobi equations. *PNAS*, 98(20), September 2001.

A Statistical Shape Model of Individual Fiber Tracts Extracted from Diffusion Tensor MRI

Isabelle Corouge[1,2], Sylvain Gouttard[2,3], and Guido Gerig[1,2]

[1] Department of Computer Science, gerig@cs.unc.edu
[2] Department of Psychiatry
University of North Carolina, Chapel Hill, USA
corouge@unc.edu
[3] ESCPE Lyon, France
sylvain.gouttard@cpe.fr [†]

Abstract. Diffusion Tensor MRI has become the preferred imaging modality to explore white matter structure and brain connectivity *in vivo*. Conventional region of interest analysis and voxel-based comparison does not make use of the geometric properties of fiber tracts. This paper explores shape modelling of major fiber bundles. We describe tracts, represented as clustered sets of curves of similar shape, by a shape prototype swept along a space trajectory. This approach can naturally describe white matter structures observed either as bundles dispersing towards the cortex or tracts defined as dense patterns of parallel fibers. Sets of streamline curves obtained from tractography are clustered, parametrized and aligned with a similarity transform. An average curve and eigenmodes of shape variation describe a compact statistical shape model. Reconstruction by sweeping the template along the trajectory results in a simplified model of a tract. Feasibility is demonstrated by modelling callosal and cortico-spinal fasciculi of two different subjects.

Keywords: Diffusion Tensor Imaging, statistical shape modelling.

1 Introduction

Diffusion Tensor Imaging (DTI) of brain structures measures diffusion properties by the local probability of self-motion of water molecules. A tensor field characterizes amount and locally preferred directions of local diffusivity. While diffusion can be considered isotropic in fluid it appears highly anisotropic along neural fiber tracts due to inhibition of free diffusion of intra- and extra-cellular fluid. DTI has become the preferred modality to explore white matter properties associated with brain connectivity *in vivo*. Most research work has been dedicated to the calculation of the tensor field, its regularization, its visualization

[†] This research is supported by the NIH-NIBIB grant P01 EB002779, the NIH Conte Center MH064065, and the Stanley Medical Research Institute. We acknowledge Matthieu Jomier and Julien Jomier, both UNC-Chapel Hill, for their precious help with software development.

C. Barillot, D.R. Haynor, and P. Hellier (Eds.): MICCAI 2004, LNCS 3217, pp. 671–679, 2004.

and subsequently to the design of fiber tracking algorithms [1], [2], [3], [4], [5], [6]. A few groups have investigated ways towards quantitative analysis of DT images. Alexander *et al.* discuss matching of tensor fields to characterize variations in white matter structure within subject populations [7]. Xu *et al.* combine tractography and spatial normalization to produce statistical maps of fiber occurrence [8]. Fillard *et al.* perform statistical analysis of diffusion properties along fibers [9] while Ding *et al.* quantify collective properties of an anatomical fiber bundle along its medial axis [10].

In this paper, we continue preliminary work in which we extracted fibers by tractography, clustered them into anatomical bundles and analyzed the variability of local shape properties (e.g. curvature and torsion) within bundles [11]. Here, we focus on the statistical shape modelling of individual white matter fiber tracts. Our approach estimates a prototype shape of the considered fiber tract, e.g. a mean shape, and characterizes statistical shape deviations from this template shape within the fiber tract. Ultimately, we aim at modelling fiber tracts not only by template shapes and statistical variation but also by a prototype and its space trajectory. This model would be particularly appropriate for fasciculi like dense callosal fibers, observed as a "sweeping" of a U-shaped template and which form a manifold. Such a model provides a simplified representation of a fiber tract and could be used in a wider framework handling inter-individual comparison or pathological changes, for example.

2   Preprocessing: Fiber Extraction and Filtering

The extraction of fiber tracts is performed with the fiber tracking tool described in [4]. The tensor field is computed from DTI data by solving the Stejskal-Tanner's diffusion equation system as described in [5]. Streamlines following the principal diffusion tensor directions between source and target regions of interest are then extracted by tractography under local continuity constraints [8]. Except at branching or crossing points, these 3D curves are assumed to represent the most likely pathways through the tensor field. Note that the term "fibers" is used for streamlines in the vector field which do not represent real anatomical fibers. The tracking is performed backwards and with sub-voxel precision. Since the robustness of fiber tracking remains limited at junctions and in noisy low-contrast regions, the extracted fiber set contains outlier curves. Also, the set of reconstructed fibers might contain curves that are part of other anatomical tracts. We developed an iterative algorithm to reject outliers and to cluster curves to fiber bundles based on pairwise distance metrics measuring position and shape similarity of pairs of fibers [11].

3   Shape Modelling of Individual Fiber Tracts

The individual fiber tract previously extracted and filtered acts as a training set from which we estimate a template shape, the mean shape, and statistical deviations by learning its inherent shape variability. The resulting model is related to what is commonly called a Point Distribution Model (PDM) [12]. Representation and matching of the training set relies on a data reparametrization and on the definition of a common origin from which we establish correspondences. Pose parameters are then estimated by a Procrustes analysis [13]. A principal component analysis is subsequently applied to characterize statistical shape variation. A simplified fiber tract model can finally be obtained by reconstruction based on the template shape and the set of individual pose parameters.

3.1 Parameterization and Correspondences

First, fibers represented as polylines are reparametrized by cubic B-spline curves. This ensures an equidistant sampling along each fiber as well as a consistent sampling for all fibers. We slightly oversample the observations in order to prevent any loss of shape information but also to avoid any undesirable increase of dimensionality. Second, for each fiber tract under analysis, we define a common origin which can be reliable identified across subjects. This is either a geometric criterion, e.g. a cross-section with minimal area, or anatomical information like intersection with the midsagittal plane. Points with the same curvilinear abscissæ along the fiber tract are defined as homologuous. This correspondence scheme handles fibers with different overall lengths in a simplified way. Only points with common curvilinear abscissae are matched; extreme pieces of individual fibers like the ones dispersing into various cortical regions for instance, are discarded. This explicit point to point matching has been proven relevant in [11] where we demonstrated that it properly aligns local shape features like curvature and torsion across all curves in a fiber bundle.

3.2 Pose Parameter Estimation: Procrustes Analysis

After establishing correspondence, we align all curves in a bundle by estimating pose parameters by Procrustes analysis.

Let $\mathcal{F} = \{\mathbf{F}_n, 1 \leq n \leq N, \mathbf{F}_n \in \mathcal{M}_{k,m}\}$ be a set of N fibers, each defined by a set of k corresponding points in $m = 3$ dimensions, and represented by a $k \times m$ matrix. For $N = 2$, an Ordinary Procrustes Analysis (OPA) gives the optimal similarity transformation parameters in a least squares sense by minimizing

$$d^2_{\text{OPA}}(\mathbf{F}_1, \mathbf{F}_2) = \| \mathbf{F}_2 - (s\mathbf{F}_1\mathbf{R} + \mathbf{1}_k\mathbf{t}^t) \|^2, \tag{1}$$

where $s \in \mathbb{R}^{+*}$ is a scaling parameter, $\mathbf{R} \in SO(m)$ is a rotation, $\mathbf{t}$ is a $m \times 1$ translation vector and $\mathbf{1}_k$ is a $k \times 1$ vector of ones. Minimization of (1) over the similarity group has an algebraic solution when shapes are centered, i.e $\mathbf{1}_k^t\mathbf{F} = 0$, and normalized to unit size, i.e. $\| \mathbf{F} \| = \sqrt{\text{trace}(\mathbf{F}^t\mathbf{F})} = 1$: $\mathbf{t} = 0$, $\mathbf{R} = \mathbf{U}\mathbf{V}^t$, $s = \text{trace}(\mathbf{D})$ where $\mathbf{V}\mathbf{D}\mathbf{U}^t = \mathbf{F}_2^t\mathbf{F}_1$ is the singular value decomposition of $\mathbf{F}_2^t\mathbf{F}_1$. In the actual case where $N > 2$, a Generalized Procrustes Analysis (GPA) estimates the similarity transformation parameters which minimize the sum of squared norms of pairwise differences

$$d_{\text{GPA}}^2(\mathbf{F}_1, \ldots, \mathbf{F}_N) = \frac{1}{N} \sum_{n=1}^{N} \sum_{p=n+1}^{N} \|(s_n \mathbf{F}_n \mathbf{R}_n + \mathbf{1}_k \mathbf{t}_n^t) - (s_p \mathbf{F}_p \mathbf{R}_p + \mathbf{1}_k \mathbf{t}_p^t)\|^2 .$$

(2)

The optimization is performed iteratively:

1. Translation. Fibers are centered with respect to their center of mass, $\mathbf{g}_n$:
   $\mathbf{F}_n^c = \mathbf{F}_n - \mathbf{g}_n$.
2. Scaling. Centered data is normalized to unit size: $\mathbf{F}_n^{cs} = \mathbf{F}_n^c / \|\mathbf{F}_n^c\|$.
3. Rotation. Let $\mathbf{F}_n^{\text{old}} = \mathbf{F}_n^{cs}$. The N shapes are rotated in turn. For each n,
   $1 \le n \le N$:
   a) $\bar{\mathbf{F}}_n = \frac{1}{N-1} \sum_{p \ne n} \mathbf{F}_p^{\text{old}}$,
   b) $s_n = 1$, $\mathbf{t}_n = 0$, $\mathbf{R}_n = \arg\min_{\mathbf{R}} d_{\text{OPA}}^2(\mathbf{F}_n^{\text{old}}, \bar{\mathbf{F}}_n)$,
   c) $\mathbf{F}_n^{\text{new}} = \mathbf{F}_n^{\text{old}} \mathbf{R}_n$ and $\mathbf{F}_n^{\text{old}} = \mathbf{F}_n^{\text{new}}$.

Step 3 is iterated until the Generalized Procrustes distance $d_{\text{GPA}}^2(\mathbf{F}_1^{\text{old}}, \ldots, \mathbf{F}_N^{\text{old}})$ can not be reduced further. The alignment of the training set is achieved by applying the estimated rotations to the centered but non unit-scaled initial shapes $\mathbf{F}_n^c$, resulting in the set of aligned fibers $\mathcal{F}^{\mathcal{A}} = \{\mathbf{F}_n^{\mathcal{A}}, 1 \le n \le N\}$. Indeed, the scaling is needed to optimally estimate the rotation but a size normalization is not desirable since the training fibers belong to the same individual fiber tract.

3.3   Estimation of the Mean Shape

Given the set of aligned shapes $\mathcal{F}^{\mathcal{A}}$, the estimated mean shape $\hat{\bar{\mathbf{F}}}$ is given by

$$\hat{\bar{\mathbf{F}}} = \frac{1}{N} \sum_{n=1}^{N} \mathbf{F}_n^{\mathcal{A}}.$$

(3)

3.4   Characterization of Shape Statistical Variability

We now perform a principal components analysis (PCA) on $\mathcal{F}^{\mathcal{A}}$. This linear analysis characterizes the variations within a given training population and extracts the principal modes of deformation relative to the mean shape. Briefly, PCA expresses the observations in a new orthogonal basis, with the mean fiber as the origin and eigenvectors or modes of the observations covariance matrix $\mathbf{C}$ as axes. In our case, an observation $\mathbf{f}$ is represented by the concatenation vector of the 3D fiber coordinates $\mathbf{f} = (x_1, y_1, z_1, \ldots, x_k, y_k, z_k)^t$ and the corresponding estimated mean fiber is denoted $\bar{\mathbf{f}}$. An approximation of these observations can be obtained by truncating certain number of modes. The reconstructed observation is then written as $\mathbf{f} = \bar{\mathbf{f}} + \Phi_m \mathbf{b}_m$ where m is the number of remaining modes, Φ_m the matrix of truncated modes and $\mathbf{b}_m = (b_i)_{i=1,\ldots,m}$ the m-dimensional vector representing the original observation in the truncated modal basis. Reconstruction quality can be measured by $\tau = \sum_{i=1}^{m} \lambda_i / \lambda_T$ where λ_i is the i th eigenvalue, in decreasing order, of matrix $\mathbf{C}$ and corresponds to the variance explained by the i th mode, and where λ_T is the total variance.

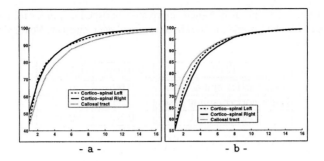

Fig. 1. Percentage τ_p of cumulative variance as a function of the number of modes for three fiber tracts (left and right cortico-spinal tract, callosal fiber tract) of two subjects (**a** and **b**); $\tau_p = \sum_{i=1}^m \lambda_i / \lambda_T \times 100$.

Under the assumption that the distribution of the elements of $\mathcal{F}^A$ is Gaussian, the variation of $b_{i,i=1,\dots,m}$ in an interval such as $[-3\sqrt{\lambda_i}, 3\sqrt{\lambda_i}]$ explains the variability of the set of objects. Calculating these statistics with a sufficient number of representative instances of shapes, these variations will cover the major variability of the population.

3.5   Fiber Tract Reconstruction

Qualitative views of 3D rendering suggest that sets of fibers might be described as a replication of a prototype curve along a space trajectory, simulating the sweeping of a space curve to form a manifold. In an initial attempt to test this hypothesis, we reconstruct an approximation to the initial fiber tract by applying the inverse rigid body transform per fiber to the template.

Let $\mathcal{T}$ be the set of transformations computed from the Procrustes analysis to align the training set, $\mathcal{T} = \{(-\mathbf{g}_n, \Gamma_n), 1 \le n \le N\}$ with $\mathbf{g}_n$ the translation vector defined by the center of mass of the nth fiber and Γ_n the resulting rotation for fiber n: $\Gamma_n = \Pi_i \mathbf{R}_n^{(i)}$, $\mathbf{R}_n^{(i)}$ being the rotation computed in the ith step 3 iteration of the Generalized Procrustes Analysis. The reconstructed fiber tract $\tilde{\mathcal{F}}$ is given by

$$\tilde{\mathcal{F}} = \{\tilde{\mathbf{F}}_n = \hat{\bar{\mathbf{F}}}\Gamma_n^t + \mathbf{g}_n, \ 1 \le n \le N\} \tag{4}$$

where $\hat{\bar{\mathbf{F}}}$ is the estimated mean fiber. The fiber set $\tilde{\mathcal{F}}$ is a simplified representation of the inital fiber tract defined as the template shape $\hat{\bar{\mathbf{F}}}$ and the set $\mathcal{T}^{-1} = \{(\mathbf{g}_n, \Gamma_n^t), 1 \le n \le N\}$ of inverse transformations. This model might have advantages for inter-subject matching and comparison since the template represents a robust estimate of the core shape whereas individual variability is encoded in the shape eigenmodes.

Table 1. Mean point to point distance (in voxels) between original and reconstructed fibers averaged over the bundle for the three tracts of each subject. Voxel size is $2 \times 2 \times 2$ mm^3.

Tract	Subject 1	Subject 2
Left cortico-spinal tract	0.60	0.71
Right cortico-spinal tract	0.66	0.63
Callosal tract	0.53	0.64

4   Experiments and Results

We selected two cases out of a 3Tesla high resolution ($2 \times 2 \times 2$ mm^3) DT MRI database of healthy controls and extracted three major fiber tracts. The first two represent the major projection tracts between the internal capsule and the upper cortex of the left and right hemisphere (see Fig. 2, left and Fig. 4, top left) while the third corresponds to a dense set of callosal fibers (see Fig. 3, top left and Fig. 4, bottom left). The common origin of all fibers for the cortico-spinal tracts is chosen as the location of minimal area cross-section between pons and internal capsule. For the callosal fiber bundle, a natural choice is the intersection with the midsagittal plane. For each tract, Figures 2, 3 and 4 present the set of aligned shapes and the estimated mean shape which defines the core shape of the tract. In addition to Fig. 1 which presents the percentage of cumulative variance as a function of the number of modes, Figures 2, 3 and 4 illustrate the variations around the mean fiber for the the first two modes. For all tracts and all subjects, less than 10 modes are needed to explain more than 90% of the variance. The figures also show the reconstructed fiber tract associated to each of the original data sets. The reconstructed tracts visually appear to be a very good approximation to the original data, representing the *major characteristics* of the bundle without small scale variability. This observation is corroborated by computing the mean point to point distance between original and reconstructed fiber tracts averaged over the bundle (see Table 1). We also observe that the results are quite consistent for both subjects, which suggests the processing scheme might achieve a good reproducibility of tract extraction and tract modelling. A quantitative validation of reproducibility and validity in 10 controls, including anatomical landmarking by clinical experts, is in progress.

5   Discussion and Perspectives

We propose a statistical shape model of individual white matter fiber tracts extracted from Diffusion Tensor MRI. Correspondences are derived from a reparametrization of the streamline curves and the definition of a common origin, and alignment is achieved by a Procrustes fit. Results obtained from two healthy control subjects seem consistent and suggest that these models might be reproducibly obtained for each subject. We currently test the new processing scheme on 10 healthy controls which got imaged with the best available DTI protocol on a new 3Tesla MRI scanner (Siemens Allegra head-only).

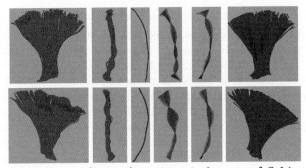

Fig. 2. Left (top) and right (bottom) cortico-spinal tracts of Subject 1. From left to right: original data sets (more than 600 fibers each); data sets after alignment; estimated mean fiber; variations around the mean shape according to first and second mode; reconstructed fiber tract.

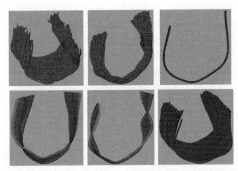

Fig. 3. Callosal fibers of Subject 1. From top left to bottom right: original data sets (363 fibers); data sets after alignment; estimated mean fiber; variations around the mean shape according to first and second mode; reconstructed fiber tract.

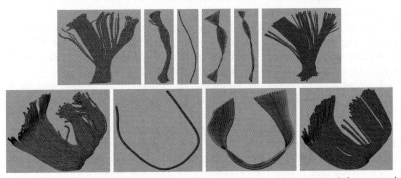

Fig. 4. Results for Subject 2. Top: left cortico-spinal tract with original data sets (more than 250 fibers); data sets after alignment; estimated mean fiber; variations around the mean shape according to first and second mode; reconstructed fiber tract. Bottom: callosal fiber tract with original data sets (128 fibers); estimated mean fiber; variations around the mean shape according to first mode; reconstructed fiber tract.

This paper focuses on the discussion of the calculation of the template and its major shape variation. Reconstructed bundles using the template $\hat{\mathbf{F}}$ and the inverse set of pose transformations $\mathcal{T}^{-1}$ closely represent the original bundle and suggest that this type of modelling might be a viable concept for the modelling of various major fiber tracts. The set of transformations $\mathcal{T}^{-1}$ is still unstructured with arbitrary ordering. The major focus of future research will be devoted to develop a concept for ordering the set of fibers and hence the transformations within the shape manifold and for describing this set as a continuous sweeping curve. Ultimately, each fiber tract would be characterized by the prototype and its sweeping along this curve. Preliminary results and our analysis of the major large and small tracts of interest (cortico-spinal, callosum, cingulum, uncinate, splenium and genu) suggest that modelling by "ribbon-cables" indeed might be an appropriate representation.

Modelling will potentially serve for improved inter-individual registration and comparison of diffusion tensor properties along and across fiber tracts. Clinical research is interested in a quantitative analysis which finally might lead to answer questions in regard to fiber integrity or fiber disruption and its effect on brain connectivity. Moreover, modelling of fiber tracts in healthy controls will help to study geometric and diffusion changes of white matter tracts in the presence of pathology, e.g. tumor and edema or white matter lesions.

References

1. P.J. Basser, S. Pajevic, C. Pierpaoli, and A. Aldroubi. Fiber tract following in the human brain using DT-MRI data. *IEICE Trans. on Information and Systems*, E85-D(1):15–21, 2002.
2. M. Björnemo, A. Brun, R. Kikinis, and C.-F. Westin. Regularized stochastic white matter tractography using diffusion tensor MRI. In *Proc. of MICCAI*, vol. 2488 of *LNCS*, pages 435–442, 2002.
3. O. Coulon, D.C. Alexander, and S.R. Arridge. A regularization scheme for diffusion tensor magnetic resonance images. In *Proc. of IPMI*, LNCS, pages 92–105, 2001.
4. P. Fillard and G. Gerig. Analysis tool for diffusion tensor MRI. In *Proc. of MICCAI*, vol. 2879 of *LNCS*, pages 967–968, 2003.
5. C.-F. Westin, S.E. Maier, H. Mamata, A. Nabavi, F.A. Jolesz, and R. Kikinis. Processing and visualization for diffusion tensor MRI. *Medical Image Analysis*, 6:93–108, 2002.
6. L. Zhukov and A.H. Barr. Oriented tensor reconstruction: tracing neural pathways from diffusion tensor MRI. In *Proc. IEEE Visualization*, 2002.
7. D.C. Alexander and J.C. Gee. Elastic matching of diffusion tensor images. *Computer Vision and Image Understanding*, 77:233–250, 2000.
8. D. Xu, S. Mori, M. Solaiyappan, P.C.M. van Zijl, and C. Davatzikos. A framework for callosal fiber distribution analysis. *NeuroImage*, 17:1131–1143, 2002.
9. P. Fillard, J. Gilmore, W. Lin, and G. Gerig. Quantitative analysis of white matter fiber properties along geodesic paths. In *Proc. of MICCAI*, vol. 2879 of *LNCS*, pages 16–23, 2003.
10. Z. Ding, J.C. Gore, and A.W. Anderson, Classification and quantification of neuronal fiber pathways using diffusion tensor MRI. *Magn. Res. Med.*, 49:716–721, 2003.

11. I. Corouge, S. Gouttard, and G. Gerig. Towards a shape model of white matter fiber bundles using diffusion tensor MRI. In *Proc. of IEEE ISBI*, pages 344–347, 2004.

12. T.F. Cootes, C.J. Taylor, D.H. Cooper, and J. Graham. Active shape models - their training and application. *Computer Vision and Image Understanding*, 61(1):38–59, 1995.

13. C. Goodall. Procrustes methods in the statistical analysis of shape. *J.R. Statist. Soc. B*, 53(2):285–239, 1991.

Co-analysis of Maps of Atrophy Rate and Atrophy State in Neurodegeneration

Valerie A. Cardenas and Colin Studholme

Department of Radiology, University of California, San Francisco and San Francisco
VA Medical Center

Abstract. The variability in atrophy rate in patients with neurodegenerative disease can be partially explained by disease stage. Since atrophy
state (baseline scan tissue volume) correlates with cognitive impairment
and disease stage, we use local atrophy state as a covariate in the analysis of local atrophy rate. A general linear model with a spatially varying
dependent variable was employed to study the effects of disease over the
brain. An efficient method of solving this spatially varying model was
developed, implemented, and applied to maps of atrophy state and rate
derived from serial MRI data of 13 Semantic Dementia (SD) and 13 control subjects. Our results demonstrate that group differences in atrophy
rate are affected by the inclusion of atrophy state in the model. Specifically, estimated contrasts in atrophy rate between controls and SD in
the left temporal lobe white matter increased when the local rate was
covaried for atrophy state.

1 Introduction

Spatial morphometric techniques such as voxel based morphometry (VBM) [1,2]
and deformation tensor morphometry [3,4] have been used to explore separately
both the patterns of atrophy state (amount of tissue lost) in neurodegenerative
disease and the atrophy rate (rate of tissue loss). These methods have added
significantly to the understanding of the progression of degenerative disease in
different regions of the brain.

From both manual region based measurements and spatial morphometric
approaches, significant brain atrophy in various anatomical structures has been
reported cross sectionally in patients compared to controls [5,6,7]. Many methods also exist for estimating atrophy rate from longitudinal structural images
[8,9,10]. These show more diagnostic promise than cross sectional tissue volume
measurements from a single subject because they remove the underlying variability in local tissue volume and focus simply on the change. There is evidence
that the rate of loss may increase with the progression of a disease [11,12], but
it is not clear how this relationship may vary for different regions in the brain.
Large clinical studies may include patients at a range of stages of the disease.
However, staging of a subject commonly depends only on imprecise clinical neurological testing. True differences in atrophy state and rate between patients and
controls may therefore be obscured if the stage of the disease is poorly defined,

C. Barillot, D.R. Haynor, and P. Hellier (Eds.): MICCAI 2004, LNCS 3217, pp. 680–687, 2004.

as illustrated by Fig 1. In this paper we therefore explore the use of local atrophy state as a covariate in the analysis of local atrophy rate, since atrophy state has been shown to be correlated with degree of cognitive impairment [13].

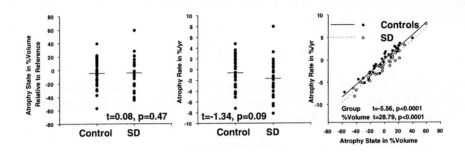

Fig. 1. On the left is a scatterplot of simulated atrophy states for controls and Semantic Dementia (SD) patients, showing a small, not significant difference in group means ($p = 0.47$). In the middle is a scatterplot of simulated atrophy rates, where the difference in rates nearly reaches statistical significance ($p = 0.09$). The right scatterplot shows atrophy state vs. atrophy rate. When the group comparison of atrophy rate is covaried for atrophy state, the group difference is highly significant ($p < 0.0001$)

Spatial Morphometric techniques such as deformation morphometry quantify differences between brains without a priori definition of ROIs, by fitting a fixed, common linear model to the deformation parameters and computing statistics at the voxel level. Covarying for atrophy state is complicated because the atrophy state varies spatially, so the linear model cannot be fixed. In this paper, we describe a linear model with a spatially varying dependent variable and present a technique for efficient solution of the model, and show the results of applying the model to patients with Semantic Dementia (SD).

2   Methods

2.1   Linear Model

We are going to use a general linear model [14,15] to analyze our maps of atrophy rate. Given n images that have been registered to a common coordinate system, we fit the following linear model at each voxel i in the image,

$$\mathbf{y}(\mathbf{v}_i) = \mathbf{A}\mathbf{x}(\mathbf{v}_i) \; , \tag{1}$$

where $\mathbf{v}_i = (v_{i1}, v_{i2}, v_{i3})$ denotes the location of voxel i in standard space, $\mathbf{y}(\mathbf{v}_i)$ is an n-vector of measurements (e.g., gray matter density, relative local contraction or expansion) at voxel $\mathbf{v}_i$, $\mathbf{x}(\mathbf{v}_i)$ is a p-vector of parameters (e.g., effect of disease, effect of age) to be estimated at voxel $\mathbf{v}_i$, and $\mathbf{A}$ is an $n \times p$ design matrix, where the p columns of $\mathbf{A}$ contain categorical or continuous variables for n subjects (e.g., column of subject diagnosis variables, column of subject ages). In this model, the independent variables that compose $\mathbf{A}$ are not dependent on spatial location within the image. For the usual case when $n > p$ and we have more equations than unknowns, we have a linear least-squares problem and can solve the reduced set of equations,

$$(\mathbf{A}^T \mathbf{A})\mathbf{x}(\mathbf{v}_i) = \mathbf{A}^T \mathbf{y}(\mathbf{v}_i) \ . \tag{2}$$

One method of solving these equations is to compute the Cholesky decomposition $\mathbf{LL}^T$ of $\mathbf{A}^T \mathbf{A}$, where $\mathbf{L}$ is lower triangular. The elements L_{kj} of $\mathbf{L}$ are computed from the elements A_{kj} of $\mathbf{A}$ as follows,

$$L_{kk} = \sqrt{A_{kk} - \sum_{m=1}^{k-1} L_{mk}^2} \quad \text{for } k = j, \tag{3}$$

$$L_{kj} = (A_{kj} - \sum_{m=1}^{j-1} L_{km}L_{jm})/L_{jj} \quad \text{for } k > j, \tag{4}$$

where k indexes rows and j indexes columns. We can then solve the trivial triangular systems $\mathbf{Lb}(\mathbf{v}_i) = \mathbf{A}^T \mathbf{y}(\mathbf{v}_i)$ and $\mathbf{b}(\mathbf{v}_i) = \mathbf{L}^T \mathbf{x}(\mathbf{v}_i)$. Because the design matrix $\mathbf{A}$ is fixed over the image, the Cholesky decomposition of $\mathbf{A}^T \mathbf{A}$ can be computed once, and parameter estimates $\mathbf{x}(\mathbf{v}_i)$ can be easily solved at each voxel by substituting a new $\mathbf{y}(\mathbf{v}_i)$.

The estimation of t-statistics for the parameter estimates requires the computation of the diagonal entries u_{jj} of $(\mathbf{A}^T \mathbf{A})^{-1}$, where j indexes columns. Because the inverse of a lower triangular matrix can be easily computed row by row, computation of u_{jj} is facilitated by using $(\mathbf{A}^T \mathbf{A})^{-1} = (\mathbf{L}^{-1})^T \mathbf{L}^{-1}$, then recognizing that $u_{jj} = l_j \cdot l_j$ where l_j are the columns of $\mathbf{L}^{-1}$.

If we want to compare the rate of atrophy between groups, while covarying for the spatially varying tissue volume at baseline, the linear model then becomes,

$$\mathbf{y}(\mathbf{v}_i) = \mathbf{A}(\mathbf{v}_i)\mathbf{x}(\mathbf{v}_i) \ , \tag{5}$$

where one column of the design matrix $\mathbf{A}(\mathbf{v}_i)$ is the tissue volume at baseline for voxel $\mathbf{v}_i$. Even though all other columns of $\mathbf{A}(\mathbf{v}_i)$ are fixed (e.g., diagnosis and age independent variables), the design matrix is no longer fixed over the image due to the inclusion of baseline tissue volumes at voxel $\mathbf{v}_i$, and subsequently the Cholesky decomposition will change at every voxel in the image. However, by choosing to make the tissue volume at voxel $\mathbf{v}_i$ the pth column of $\mathbf{A}(\mathbf{v}_i)$, we can avoid computing the full Cholesky decomposition of $\mathbf{A}(\mathbf{v}_i)^T \mathbf{A}(\mathbf{v}_i)$. Let $\mathbf{c}_j$ denote the jth column of $\mathbf{A}(\mathbf{v}_i)$, where only the last column $\mathbf{c}_p(\mathbf{v}_i)$ varies spatially, then

$$\mathbf{A}(\mathbf{v}_i)^T\mathbf{A}(\mathbf{v}_i) = \begin{bmatrix} \mathbf{c}_1 \cdot \mathbf{c}_1 & \mathbf{c}_1 \cdot \mathbf{c}_2 & \cdots & \mathbf{c}_1 \cdot \mathbf{c}_p(\mathbf{v}_i) \\ \mathbf{c}_1 \cdot \mathbf{c}_2 & \mathbf{c}_2 \cdot \mathbf{c}_2 & \cdots & \mathbf{c}_2 \cdot \mathbf{c}_p(\mathbf{v}_i) \\ \vdots & \vdots & \ddots & \vdots \\ \mathbf{c}_1 \cdot \mathbf{c}_p(\mathbf{v}_i) & \mathbf{c}_2 \cdot \mathbf{c}_p(\mathbf{v}_i) & \cdots & \mathbf{c}_p \cdot \mathbf{c}_p(\mathbf{v}_i) \end{bmatrix}, \qquad (6)$$

where $\mathbf{c}_i \cdot \mathbf{c}_j$ denotes the dot product of vectors $\mathbf{c}_i$ and $\mathbf{c}_j$. As shown in (6), only the last row and column of $\mathbf{A}(\mathbf{v}_i)^T\mathbf{A}(\mathbf{v}_i)$ change at each voxel, by Eq. (3,4) only the last row of the Cholesky factor $\mathbf{L}(\mathbf{v}_i)$ changes at each voxel, and in turn only the last row of $\mathbf{L}(\mathbf{v}_i)^{-1}$ changes at each voxel. Because of this, we can compute $\mathbf{L}(\mathbf{v}_1)$, then for each voxel update the last row of $\mathbf{L}(\mathbf{v}_i)$ using the last row of $\mathbf{A}(\mathbf{v}_i)^T\mathbf{A}(\mathbf{v}_i)$ and the previously computed $\mathbf{L}(\mathbf{v}_1)_{kj}$. Since the computational cost of the Cholesky decomposition is $p^3/3$ flops, computing only the last row of $\mathbf{L}(\mathbf{v}_i)$ saves $(p-1)^3/3$ flops at each voxel. We can also compute $\mathbf{L}(\mathbf{v}_1)^{-1}$, then simply update the last row of $\mathbf{L}(\mathbf{v}_i)^{-1}$ using the last row of $\mathbf{L}(\mathbf{v}_i)$ and the previously computed entries of $\mathbf{L}(\mathbf{v}_1)^{-1}$. Since the computational cost of computing a full inverse is p^3, computing only the last row of $\mathbf{L}(\mathbf{v}_i)^{-1}$ saves nearly $(p-1)^3$ flops. Computing only the last row of $\mathbf{A}(\mathbf{v}_i)^T\mathbf{A}(\mathbf{v}_i)$ provides an additional savings of about $(p-1)^2 n$ flops, which may actually be a greater savings for a large number of subjects n and small number of parameters p. For a typical analysis with approximately 1.5 million voxels, our implementation saves about $1.5 \times 10^6(p^3 + (p-1)^2 n)$ flops.

2.2 Application to Semantic Dementia

Subjects. Thirteen subjects (62 ± 7 yrs, 8 men) diagnosed with Semantic Dementia (SD) and 13 cognitively normal age and sex matched controls (64 ± 9 yrs, 8 men) were studied at least twice with a 3D gradient echo T1 weighted anatomical MPRAGE sequence (TR=10ms, TE=4ms). The images were reconstructed with a coronal slice plane at a voxel size of $1 \times 1 \times 1.5 mm^3$. The interval between images was 2.9 ± 1.2 yrs for controls and 1.0 ± 0.2 yrs for SD. These individuals were selected from a larger group of patients participating in research at the San Francisco VA hospital and the UCSF Memory and Aging Center.

Maps of Atrophy State and Rate. The scan from a single 72 year old cognitively normal female was used as the reference for this study, rather than a group average, in order to retain the finest anatomical structures in the target for accurate registration. An entropy driven B-Spline Free Form deformation algorithm [16,17] was used to register individual scans to the reference atlas. The Jacobian determinant of this transformation, giving the fractional volume contraction or expansion relative to the reference, was used to characterize the atrophy state $s(\mathbf{v}_i)$ at each voxel $\mathbf{v}_i$. Because both global (due to headsize differences between reference and subject) and local tissue changes are included in the estimate $s(\mathbf{v}_i)$, we computed the average atrophy state over the intracranial vault V as $\frac{1}{V}\sum_{i=1}^{V} s(\mathbf{v}_i)$, and we divided $s(\mathbf{v}_i)$ by this value to create a normalized atrophy state $s'(\mathbf{v}_i)$ that reflected only local changes relative to headsize. Detailed method descriptions are found in [18,19].

At higher resolution, the same general approach used to create maps of atrophy state can be used to register and model spatial changes within subject between multiple scans [20]. The previously estimated transformation between the initial time point of each subject and the reference anatomy then allows the spatial normalization of annualized pointwise volume change for each subject, yielding atrophy rate estimates $r(\mathbf{v}_i)$ at each voxel $\mathbf{v}_i$ in standard space.

Model of Atrophy Rate in Semantic Dementia. Linear models were fit to each voxel and t-statistics calculated to locate points where voxel level differences in the annualized rate of atrophy occurred. The effect of disease was initially examined using an ANCOVA analysis at each voxel with diagnosis (SD vs. control) as a categorical predictor while covarying for age. This is shown by

$$\mathbf{r}(\mathbf{v}_i) = x(\mathbf{v}_i)_1\iota + x(\mathbf{v}_i)_2\mathbf{d} + x(\mathbf{v}_i)_3\mathbf{a} \ , \tag{7}$$

where $\mathbf{r}(\mathbf{v}_i)$ is an vector of atrophy rates at voxel $\mathbf{v}_i$ from n subjects, $x(\mathbf{v}_i)_j$ are elements of the parameter vector $\mathbf{x}(\mathbf{v}_i)$, ι is an n-vector of ones to model an intercept, and $\mathbf{d}$ and $\mathbf{a}$ are n-vectors of subject diagnoses and ages. The effect of disease was then examined using a modified ANCOVA analysis, where atrophy state normalized by headsize was included as a covariate, as shown by

$$\mathbf{r}(\mathbf{v}_i) = x(\mathbf{v}_i)_1\iota + x(\mathbf{v}_i)_2\mathbf{d} + x(\mathbf{v}_i)_3\mathbf{a} + x(\mathbf{v}_i)_4\mathbf{s}'(\mathbf{v}_i) \ , \tag{8}$$

where $\mathbf{s}'(\mathbf{v}_i)$ is an n-vector of normalized atrophy state at voxel $\mathbf{v}_i$. For our analysis of 13 controls (coded 0) and 13 SD (coded 1), (8) can be written in matrix notation (as in (5))

$$\begin{bmatrix} r(\mathbf{v}_i)_1 \\ \vdots \\ r(\mathbf{v}_i)_{13} \\ r(\mathbf{v}_i)_{14} \\ \vdots \\ r(\mathbf{v}_i)_{26} \end{bmatrix} = \begin{bmatrix} 1 & 0 & 61 & s'(\mathbf{v}_i)_1 \\ \vdots & \vdots & \vdots & \vdots \\ 1 & 0 & 68 & s'(\mathbf{v}_i)_{13} \\ 1 & 1 & 68 & s'(\mathbf{v}_i)_{14} \\ \vdots & \vdots & \vdots & \vdots \\ 1 & 1 & 58 & s'(\mathbf{v}_i)_{26} \end{bmatrix} \begin{bmatrix} x(\mathbf{v}_i)_1 \\ x(\mathbf{v}_i)_2 \\ x(\mathbf{v}_i)_3 \\ x(\mathbf{v}_i)_4 \end{bmatrix} \tag{9}$$

3   Results

Fig 2 illustrates how covarying for atrophy state affects the estimation of atrophy rate differences between controls and SD. The middle panel of Fig 2 is the map of estimated $x(\mathbf{v}_i)_2$ from Eq 7. The bottom panel is the same map when atrophy state is included as a covariate (see Eq 8). Although both regions are statistically very significant ($p < 5.0 \times 10^{-6}$), the white matter of the left anterior temporal lobe is estimated to atrophy at a faster rate (white in bottom panel of Fig 2) in SD compared to controls when atrophy state is considered. This suggests that the rate of white matter loss in the anterior temporal lobe varies among our SD patients, and that the rate of white matter loss is related to white matter volume in the baseline scan. When only group differences are modeled, the variability in rates of white matter atrophy lead to a smaller group estimate (in the illustrated region, SDs atrophy about 1.57%/yr faster than controls). When atrophy state is included, the variability in rates of white matter atrophy are partially explained by white matter volume in the first scan, and a larger estimate of the group effect is obtained (1.84%/yr).

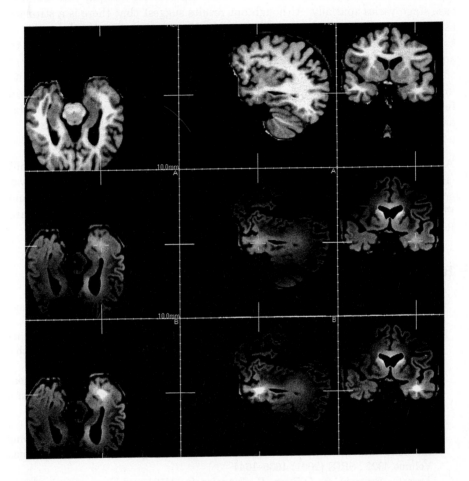

Fig. 2. Differences in atrophy rate between SD and controls when atrophy state is not included (middle panel) and is included (bottom panel) in the model, shown as a grey scale between 0.2% and 2% per year. Top row shows average MRI of the group after spatial normalization.

4 Discussion

The inclusion of atrophy state as a spatially varying independent variable in our general linear model resulted in the estimation of a larger group effect on the atrophy rate of white matter in the anterior temporal lobe. Including atrophy state had little effect on the estimation of group differences in the cortex or ventricular CSF, suggesting that the relationship between atrophy rate and disease stage varies spatially. Although our results suggest that there is a stronger association between cognition and rate of white matter atrophy than rate of cortical atrophy, our cohort of 13 SD patients may have simply been too few to adequately model the relationship in the cortex. We have shown the feasibility of the co-analysis of maps of atrophy rate and atrophy state, and demonstrated its importance using images from 13 SD patients and 13 controls. Future work will include expanding our SD group, examining other neurodegenerative diseases, and investigating permutation testing to correct for multiple comparisons.

Acknowledgements. This work was funded by a Whitaker foundation grant (RG-01-0115) and NIH grant MH65392-01. Image data used in this work was acquired as part of the NIH funded grants AG12435, AG10897, P01AG19724 and P01AA11493. The authors wish to thank Michael Weiner, Bruce Miller, Howard Rosen, and Helena Chui for access to data.

References

1. Ashburner, J., Friston, K.: Voxel-based morphometry-The methods. Neuroimage **11** (2000) 805–821
2. Davatzikos, C., Genc, A., Xu, D., Resnick, S.: Voxel-based morphometry using the RAVENS maps: Methods and validation using simulated longitudinal atrophy. Neuroimage **14** (2001) 1361–1369
3. Gaser, C., Nenadic, I., Buchsbaum, B., Hazlett, E., Buchsbaum, M.: Deformation-based morphometry and its relation to conventional volumetry of brain lateral ventricles in MRI. Neuroimage **13** (2001) 1140–1145
4. Pettey, D., Gee, J.: Using a linear diagnostic funcation and non-rigid registration to search for morphological differences between populations: An example involving the male and female corpus callosum. In: Proceedings SPIE Medical Imaging. Volume 4322., SPIE (2001) 1636–1644
5. Jack, C., Petersen, R., O'Brien, P., Tangalos, E.: MR-based hippocampal volumetry in the diagnosis of Alzheimer's disease. Neurology **42** (1992) 183–188
6. Rombouts, S., Barkhof, F., Witter, M., Scheltens, P.: Unbiased whole-brain analysis of gray matter loss in Alzheimer's disease. Neurosci Lett **285** (2000) 231–233
7. Tanabe, J., Amend, D., Schuff, N., DiSclafani, V., Ezekiel, F., Norman, D., Fein, G., Weiner, M.: Tissue segmentation of the brain in Alzheimer disease. Am J Neuroradiol **18** (1997) 115–123
8. Fox, N., Freebourough, P.: Brain atrophy progression measured from registered serial MRI: validation and application to Alzheimer's disease. J Mag Res Imaging **7** (1997) 1069–1075

9. Jack, C., Petersen, R., Xu, Y., O'Brien, P., Smith, G., Ivnik, R., Boeve, B., Tangalos, E., Kokmen, E.: Rates of hippocampal atrophy correlate with change in clinical status in aging and AD. Neurology **55** (2000) 484–489

10. Cardenas, V., Du, A., Hardin, D., Ezekiel, F., Weber, P., Jagust, W., Chui, H., Schuff, N., Weiner, M.: Comparison of methods for measuring longitudinal brain change in cognitive impairment and dementia. Neurobiology of Aging **24** (2003) 537–544

11. Fox, N., Scahill, R., Crum, W., Rossor, M.: Correlation between rates of brain atrophy and cognitive decline in AD. Neurology **52** (1999) 1687–1689

12. Chan, D., Janssen, J., Whitwell, J., Watt, H., Jenkins, R., Frost, C., Rossor, M., Fox, N.: Change in rates of cerebral atrophy over time in early-onset Alzheimer's disease: Longitudinal MRI study. Lancet **362** (2003) 1121–1122

13. Smith, C., Malcein, M., Meurer, K., Schmitt, F., Markesbery, W., Pettigrew, L.: MRI temporal lobe measures and neuropsychologic function in Alzheimer's disease. J Neuroimaging **9** (1999) 2–9

14. Worsley, K., Evans, A., Marrett, S., Neelin, P.: A three-dimensional statistical analysis for CBF activation studies in human brain. J Cereb Blood Flow Metab **12** (1992) 1040–1042

15. Friston, K., Holmes, A., Worsley, K., Poline, J., Frith, C., Frackowiak, R.: Statistical parametric maps in functional imaging: A general linear approach. Human Brain Mapping **2** (1995) 189–210

16. Studholme, C., Novotny, E., Zubal, I., Duncan, J.: Estimating tissue deformation between functional images induced by intracranial electrode implantation using anatomical MRI. Neuroimage **13** (2001) 561–576

17. Studholme, C., Constable, R., Duncan, J.: Accurate alignment of functional epi data to anatomical MRI using a physics based distortion model. IEEE Trans Med Imaging **19** (2000) 1115–1127

18. Studholme, C., Cardenas, V., Maudsley, A., Weiner, M.: An intensity consistent filtering approach to the analysis of deformation tensor derived maps of brain shape. Neuroimage **19** (2003) 1638–1649

19. Studholme, C., Cardenas, V., Blumenfeld, R., Schuff, N., Rosen, H., Miller, B., Weiner, M.: Deformation tensor morphometry of semantic dementia with quantitative validation. Neuroimage **21** (2004) 1387–1398

20. Studholme, C., Cardenas, V., Weiner, M.: Building whole brain maps of atrophy rate from multi-subject longitudinal studies using free-form deformations. In: Proceedings of the ISMRM, ISMRM (2001)

Regional Structural Characterization of the Brain of Schizophrenia Patients

Abraham Dubb, Paul Yushkevich, Zhiyong Xie, Ruben Gur, Raquel Gur, and James Gee

Departments of Psychiatry and Radiology
University of Pennsylvania
Philadelphia, PA, USA 19104
{adubb,pauly2,zxie}@grasp.cis.upenn.edu
{gur,raquel}@bbl.med.upenn.edu
gee@rad.upenn.edu

Abstract. Abnormal neuro-development and brain structure may play a role in the pathophysiology of schizophrenia. To study morphology and age-related changes in this disease, we started with a set of cranial MRI's of 46 schizophrenia patients and age/gender matched healthy controls. First, we deformed a template brain image to our set of subject images. The Jacobian fields of these deformations were then reduced to sets of 52 normalized region volumes for each subject using a neuro-anatomical atlas. The normalized regional volumes of the control and patient groups were compared using Student's t-test. In addition, the age correlation of each region volume was calculated for the two groups. All results were corrected for multiple comparisons using permutation testing. Finally, we used a classifier based on support vector machines and a feature selection method in order to determine our ability to discriminate brains of controls from those of patients. RESULTS: Analysis of the region-integrated Jacobians showed an enlargement of the third ventricle in patients. The age-correlation study demonstrated significant positive correlation in the third ventricle and right thalamus of controls, but not patients. Using an average of 6.5 features, our classifier was able to correctly identify 72% of patients and 70% of controls. CONCLUSIONS: In addition to enlargement of the third ventricle, the brains of schizophrenia patients demonstrate a different pattern of age-related changes.

1 Introduction

The study of schizophrenia has benefited from the advent of high resolution MRI and advanced morphometry techniques. Investigators have reported volumetric differences in multiple regions including the frontal and temporal lobes, ventricles, hippocampus and extra-pyramidal structures [1, 2, 3, 4, 5]. The existence of morphologic differences has motivated evaluation of the developmental course of neuroanatomic measures to assess whether abnormal neuro-development or neuro-degeneration play a role in schizophrenia. Several studies reported regional age-related changes of the brain [6, 7, 8]. While these studies have produced conflicting results, there is a growing consensus that brain plasticity is altered in schizophrenia, underscoring the importance of studying age-related changes in neuroanatomy [6].

C. Barillot, D.R. Haynor, and P. Hellier (Eds.): MICCAI 2004, LNCS 3217, pp. 688–695, 2004.
© Springer-Verlag Berlin Heidelberg 2004

A rigorous approach to brain volumetry must account for a number of factors. First, there is the issue of normalization: the sizes of internal brain structures are related to overall brain size, however this relationship may be quite variable. Second, discrepancies in the demographic factors of the study groups may have unforseen effects on the results. Finally, volumetric studies must account for multiple comparisons in calculating the significance of observed volumetric differences.

We attempt to address these concerns by using conservative statistical methods to analyze region-based volumes in a population of schizophrenia patients and a set of age/gender matched controls. We generate our region volumes by applying a high-resolution atlas to a set of spatially-registered brain MRI's. Although this approach precludes voxel-wise comparisons, region-based analysis reduces the dimensionality of our results, increases the robustness of our findings, and avoids thresholding issues in SPM-style cluster analysis. Finally, we implement a classification algorithm that uses feature selection in order to find that subset of structures which are most discriminating between patient and control groups.

2   Materials and Methods

2.1   Subjects and Data Acquisition

The Schizophrenia Research Center (SRC) at the University of Pennsylvania maintains a database containing hundreds of prospectively accrued cranial MRI's of psychiatric patients and healthy volunteers. The sample selection procedures have been detailed in Shtasel et al. [9], the MRI acquisition protocol has been described in detail in Gur et al. [10], and results of volumetric segmentation analysis for this sample have been reported [10]. SPGR scans were acquired on a 1.5 T scanner (Signa; General Electric Co., Milwaukee, WI) using the following parameters: flip angle of $35°$, repetition time of 35 ms, echo time of 6 ms, field of view of 24 cm, 1 repetition, 1 mm slice thickness and no interslice gaps. Transaxial images were in planes parallel to the orbitomeatal line, with resolution of 0.9375 x 0.9375 mm^2 [10].

To generate our dataset, we started by selecting the earliest cranial MRI scan of each schizophrenia patient. In order to eliminate the confounding effects of demographics, we chose a set of controls using bipartite graph matching, where each patient was matched to a single normal control of the same gender and of closest possible age. As a result of this matching, mean age, median age, age variance, as well as minimal and maximal ages were very similar in the two groups.

2.2   Brain Extraction

The skull, scalp, and other extra-cranial tissues were removed from each image using the Brain Surface Extraction Program, developed by Shattuck et al. [11] In most cases, the software performed perfectly and extracted the brain without error. In several cases, however, additional manual editing was required to remove retained extra-cranial tissue.

Table 1. Complete listing of all structures included in neuro-anatomical atlas.

corpus callosum	left middle temporal gyrus	right amygdala	right occipital lobe
left amygdala	left occipital lobe	right caudate	right occipitotemporal gyrus
left caudate	left occipitotemporal gyrus	right cerebellar hemisphere	right parahippocampal gyrus
left cerebellar hemisphere	left parahippocampal gyrus	right csf	right postcentral gyrus
left csf	left postcentral gyrus	right globus pallidus	right precentral gyrus
left globus pallidus	left precentral gyrus	right grey matter	right putamen
left grey matter	left putamen	right hippocampus	right superior frontal gyrus
left hippocampus	left superior frontam pdl gyrus	right inferior frontal gyrus	right superior parietal lobule
left inferior frontal gyrus	left superior parietal lobule	right inferior parietal lobule	right superior temporal gyrus
left inferior parietal lobule	left superior temporal gyrus	right inferior temporal gyrus	right supramarginal gyrus
left inferior temporal gyrus	left supramarginal gyrus	right lateral ventricle	right thalamus
left lateral ventricle	left thalamus	right middle frontal gyrus	right white matter
left middle frontal gyrus	left white matter	right middle temporal gyrus	third ventricle

2.3 Template Image and Atlas Creation

We obtained a simulated T1 1 mm isotropic brain MRI and accompanying tissue masks from the Brainweb website [1] [12,13] . This brain image served as our template image and was the basis for our atlas creation. We used a variety of methods to map out a total of 52 different regions on the brain. For the subcortical structures, we used a combination of manual slice-by-slice painting and automatic 3D level-set based segmentation facilities provided by the open source ITK–SNAP software [2]. In order to map out the cortical areas on the brain surface, we employed a three step method. First, a series of curves that separate the various regions of interest were drawn by an expert on the surface of the grey matter. Second, these curves were projected onto the surface of the white matter using a combination of Euclidean distance transform and Dijkstra's shortest path algorithm, resulting in series of ribbons that penetrate the grey matter hull. Finally, the ribbons were rasterized and automatic segmentation was used to fill in each region bounded by the ribbons. Figure 1 shows several projections of our atlas. Table 1 lists all structures included in the atlas.

2.4 Image Registration

The registration method we applied is a spline-based extension to Thirion's Demons technique [14]. It uses optical flow to determine the correspondence of voxels which exhibit sufficiently large intensity gradients. Based on the estimated, sparse correspondences, a B-spline function of the correspondences over the whole brain volume is determined using weighted scattered data approximation. This two-step algorithm is applied over multiple resolution levels in conventional coarse to fine fashion: both the resolution of the images and the number of spline control parameters are simultaneously adjusted. Specifically, starting with B-spline functions that have a small number of parameters, the algorithm is iterated to match the coarse features of the images. The result is used to initialize the registration at the next resolution level, where the number of spline parameters is increased to allow alignment of the finer features that are apparent in the higher resolution images. This strategy provides a way to incrementally refine the registration and improves the robustness of the method.

---

[1] Available from http://www.bic.mni.mcgill.ca/brainweb/

[2] Available from http://www.cognitica.com/snap

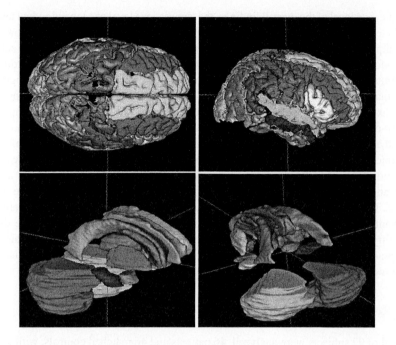

Fig. 1. Internal and external projections of the atlas used for our region-of-interest calculations.

This B-spline registration method has been validated on a separate labeled image set (unpublished data), and is capable of yielding overlap ratios of greater than 95% for lobar structures (frontal lobe, temporal lobe, etc) and close to 80% for small structures such as the amygdala and hippocampus. We used this registration method for the generation of our deformation fields and corresponding Jacobian images as described below.

2.5   Statistical Analysis of the Jacobian

We registered our template brain to each subject brain, generating a deformation field for each subject. The Jacobian of the deformation field was computed at each voxel, giving us a voxel-wise size comparison between subject and template. In each subject, the Jacobian was integrated over each region and normalized by total brain Jacobian, yielding a set of 52 normalized structure volumes. These structure volumes served as features in subsequent statistical studies.

Statistical analysis involved applying both hypothesis testing and classification in order to determine whether schizophrenia is associated with volumetric changes in the selected regions. In the hypothesis testing experiments we tested the equality of means for each feature using Student's t-test, as well as the within-group correlation with age, denoted R, using Fisher's one-sample z-test and inter-group difference in age correlation using the two-sample z-test. In order to account for the effect of multiple testing on the significance level of the overall findings, the significance level of each individual test was corrected using random permutations. In applying permutation testing we followed the techniques of Nichols and Holmes [15], repeatedly reassigning group labels to subjects at random, applying a given hypothesis test to each of the features, and recording the maximum value of the corresponding statistic (t or z). In the resulting histogram of maximal statistics, we found the fraction of random experiments, denoted p^*, for which the maximal value of the statistic exceeded the observed statistic for a given comparison.

To reinforce the results of hypothesis testing, we applied classification to gauge how well the region-based features can be used to correctly determine the group membership of subjects. We use a classifier based on support vector machines (SVM) and the feature selection method of Bradley and Mangasarian [16]. This classifier computes a linear separation boundary between the classes in a low-dimensional subspace of the feature space. This method has an added advantage of identifying the structures that are most relevant for classification. The method has one parameter that influences the dimensionality of the classification subspace, i.e. the number of stuctures used. We calculated the generalization ability of the classifier for 20 different parameter settings using the leave-one-out method.

3   Results

A total of 92 subjects were analyzed, 46 patients and 46 matched controls, with average ages of 30.8 ± 10.4 years and 31.0 ± 10.4 years, respectively. Both groups were composed of 30 males and 16 females. The ten most significant region volume comparisons are displayed in table 2. After correction for multiple comparisons, the third ventricle was the only structure which retained significance ($p^* = 0.065$), and it was larger in patients. Table 3 shows the five most significant correlations for controls and patients. The third ventricle and right thalamus were significantly positively correlated with age in controls ($p^* = 0.0124, 0.0191$, respectively). In patients, however, the most age-correlated region was the right cerebrospinal fluid volume (CSF) and had a p-value of only 0.1263. The CSF region is defined as the combination of the brain ventricles and the external fluid filling the cortical sulci. There were no significant findings for the two-sample Fisher's z comparison of age-correlations between the two groups.

Our SVM-based classifier achieved the lowest cross-validation error rate using a feature selection parameter that yielded an average of 6.5 features. Using this classifier, we correctly identified 72% of patients, and 70% of controls. The most frequently used structures in this classifier were the third ventricle (93% of experiments), left middle temporal gyrus (85%), and left superior parietal lobule (73%).

4   Discussion

We applied a neuro-anatomical atlas to a set of spatially registered images to study volumes and age-correlation of brain structures in schizophrenia. We validated our hierarchical non-rigid registration method on a separate expert-labeled dataset and found it to be superior to several other warping algorithms. Our study benefits from the quality of our atlas, which we created specifically for our template image. The cortical regions

Table 2. Partial listing of mean normalized region volume comparisons of patients vs. controls. p refers to uncorrected p-value for Student's t-test comparison. p^* denotes the p-value corrected for multiple comparisons through permutation testing.

Region	Controls	Patients	p	p^*
third ventricle	0.00067	0.00072	0.001	0.065
right middle frontal gyrus	0.01475	0.01416	0.014	0.454
left superior parietal lobule	0.00829	0.00794	0.016	0.485
right lateral ventricle	0.00555	0.00609	0.054	0.892
right thalamus	0.00319	0.00330	0.078	0.961
right superior parietal lobule	0.00886	0.00852	0.078	0.961
left caudate	0.00190	0.00198	0.083	0.968
right precentral gyrus	0.00544	0.00528	0.085	0.971
left postcentral gyrus	0.00687	0.00667	0.086	0.972
left lateral ventricle	0.00588	0.00639	0.088	0.974

Table 3. Partial listing of region volume-age correlation in controls (left) and patients (right). R refers to the Pearson correlation coefficient. p and p^* are the uncorrected and corrected scores for the Fisher's z statistic.

Controls:

Region	R	p	p^*
third ventricle	0.53	0.0001	0.0124
right thalamus	0.51	0.0002	0.0191
left thalamus	0.41	0.0046	0.2010
right white matter	-0.39	0.0074	0.2906
right hippocampus	0.33	0.0253	0.6525

Patients:

Region	R	p	p^*
right CSF	0.43	0.0025	0.1263
right inf. frontal gyrus	-0.42	0.0032	0.1577
third ventricle	0.42	0.0036	0.1732
right thalamus	0.33	0.0268	0.6836
right occipital lobe	-0.30	0.0438	0.8415

were generated from surface-drawn boundaries, rather than slice-by-slice painting. In addition, the use of 3D level-set segmentation for certain structures (e.g. ventricles) ensures high resolution and lack of inter-slice shift.

By using an atlas to define our features, we accomplish data-reduction in an anatomically meaningful way. Reducing each subject to a set of 52 region volumes allows us to apply permutation-based statistical techniques and classification algorithms that would otherwise be impractical. We employed rigorous and conservative statistical methods to avoid false positives and the confounding effects of subject demographics.

Our results showed a significance difference in only one region volume, the third ventricle. The lateral ventricles, which are generally believed to be larger in schizophrenia [17], are in the "top ten" of our results, but fail to achieve significance. Our methods can miss structural differences if they fall between regions defined by our atlas, or if such differences are averaged out by relatively large region sizes. Future work, therefore, includes development of a more detailed and hierarchical atlas. Correlations between age and volume in the two groups show no significant differences in the two-sample Fisher's z comparison, but suggest a different pattern of brain maturation; the third ventricle is highly age-correlated in controls, yet is smaller than in schizophrenia. The lack of age-correlation in schizophrenia of this structure suggests that this structure's age-related expansion occurred earlier in life and has plateaued, suggesting a neuro-developmental process.

The ability of our classification algorithm to achieve over 70% accuracy certainly suggests that morphologic differences exist between the subgroups, but that such differences are far from being robust enough to permit perfect discrimination. Interestingly, the left middle temporal gyrus was the second most frequently used feature, yet was ranked 12th in the direct volume comparison. This finding emphasizes the nature of schizophrenia as being a constellation of fairly slight morphologic changes.

The subtlety of our reported findings emphasize the need for high quality image analysis tools as well as a sufficient sample size. Further characterization of the neuro-degenerative versus neuro-developmental aspects of schizophrenia will aid in future diagnosis and treatment.

Acknowledgements. This work was supported in part by the USPHS under grants P30-NNC, LM-03504, MH-62100, MH60722, MH-19112, MO1RR0040, AG-15116, AG-17586, and DA-14418.

References

1. RE Gur, PE Cowell, A Latshaw, BI Turetsky, RI Grossman, SE Arnold, WB Bilker, and RC Gur. Reduced dorsal and orbital prefrontal gray matter volumes in schizophrenia. *Arch Gen Psychiatry*, 57(8):761–8, 2000.
2. RE Gur, BI Turetsky, PE Cowell, C Finkelman, V Maany, RI Grossman, SE Arnold, WB Bilker, and RC Gur. Temporolimbic volume reductions in schizophrenia. *Arch Gen Psychiatry*, 57(8):769–75, 2000.
3. W Cahn, HE Pol, M Bongers, HG Schnack, RC Mandl, NE Van Haren, S Durston, H Koning, JA Van Der Linden, and RS Kahn. Brain morphology in antipsychotic-naive schizophrenia: A study of multiple brain structures. *Br J Psychiatry – Suppl*, 43:s66–72, 2002.
4. RE Gur, V Maany, D Mozley, C Swanson, W Bilker, and RC Gur. Subcortical MRI volumes in neuroleptic-naive and treated patients with schizophrenia. *Am J Psychiatry*, 155:1711–1717, 1998.
5. MS Keshavan, D Rosenberg, JA Sweeney, and JW Pettegrew. Decreased caudate volume in neuroleptic-naive psychotic patients. *Am J Psychiatry*, 155(6):774–8, 1998.
6. LE Delisi. Regional brain volume change over the life-time course of schizophrenia. *J Psychiatr Res*, 33:535–541, 1999.
7. BT Woods, D Yurgelun-Todd, FM Benes, FR Frankenburg, Jr Pope HG, and J McSparren. Progressive ventricular enlargement in schizophrenia: comparison to bipolar affective disorder and correlation with clinical course. *Biol Psychiatry*, 27(3):341–52, 1990.
8. JL Rapoport, J Giedd, S Kumra, L Jacobsen, A Smith, P Lee, J Nelson, and S Hamburger. Childhood-onset schizophrenia progressive ventricular change during adolescence. *Arch Gen Psychiatry*, 54(10):897–903, 1997.
9. DL Shtasel, RE Gur, PD Mozley, J Richards, MM Taleff, C Heimberg, F Gallacher, and RC Gur. Volunteers for biomedical research: recruitment and screening of normal controls. *Arch Gen Psychiatry*, 48:1022–1025, 1991.
10. RC Gur, B I Turetsky, M Matsui, M Yan, W Bilker, P Hughett, and RE Gur. Sex differences in brain gray and white matter in healthy young adults. *J Neurosci*, 19:4065–4072, 1999.

11. DW Shattuck, SR Sandor-Leahy, KA Schaper, DA Rottenberg, and RM Leahy. Magnetic resonance image tissue classification using a partial volume model. *Neuroimage*, 13(5):856–76, 2001.

12. RK-S Kwan, AC Evans, and GB Pike. An extensible MRI simulator for post-processing evaluation. In *Visualization in Biomedical Computing*, volume 1131, pages 135–140. Springer-Verlag, Berlin, 1996.

13. DL Collins, AP Zijdenbos, V Kollokian, JG Sled, NJ Kabani, CJ Holmes, and AC Evans. Design and construction of a realistic digital brain phantom. *IEEE Transactions on Medical Imaging*, 17:463–468, 1998.

14. JP Thirion. Image matching as a diffusion process: an analogy with Maxwell's demons. *Med Image Anal*, 2(3):243–60, 1998.

15. TE Nichols and AP Holmes. Nonparametric analysis of pet functional neuroimaging experiments: A primer. *Human Brain Mapping*, 15:1–25, 2001.

16. PS Bradley, OL Mangasarian, and WN Street. Feature selection via mathematical programming. *INFORMS Journal on Computing*, 10:209–217, 1998.

17. R McCarley, C Wible, M Frumin, Y Hirayasu, J Levitt, I Fischer, and M Shenton. Mri anatomy of schizophrenia. *Biol. Psychiatry*, 45:1099–1119, 1999.

Temporal Lobe Epilepsy Surgical Outcome Prediction

Simon Duchesne, Neda Bernasconi, Andrea Bernasconi, and D. Louis Collins

Montréal Neurological Institute (MNI), McGill Univ., Montréal, Canada H3A 2B4
{duchesne,neda, andrea, louis}@bic.mni.mcgill.ca

Abstract. We wished to study pre-operative T1-weighted MRI of intractable temporal lobe epilepsy (TLE) patients who had undergone selective amygdala-hippocampectomy as part of their surgical treatment. We performed a voxel-based morphometry study of gray and white matter (GM,WM) concentration changes by comparing TLE patients with positive and negative surgical outcome. GM concentration changes were primarily located in the left lateral temporal neocortical region, while more extensive changes were found in left lateral temporal and occipital WM. Using those areas to define a region of interest, we showed that mean GM and WM concentration for all voxels within that region can be used to predict surgical outcome with 97% accuracy.

Keywords: Temporal Lobe Epilepsy, Surgical Outcome, Voxel-Based Morphometry, Grey Matter Atrophy, White Matter Atrophy, Linear Discriminant Analysis

1 Introduction

Predicting surgical outcome in the treatment of temporal lobe epilepsy (TLE) is an outstanding challenge. Some authors have attempted to find neuroimaging anatomical markers that can be used for that purpose, but no completely reliable indicator has been found to date.

The standard neurosurgical procedure in TLE consists in resection of the hippocampus and often parts of the neighboring structures, including portions of the amygdala and parahippocampal gyrus. Post-surgical outcome can be characterized as either positive (complete remission and disappearance of all seizures) or negative (all levels of complications). While the majority of patients undergoing surgery have positive outcome, it is impossible at present to determine a priori if the procedure will be successful.

It is now accepted that the hippocampus is not the only structure affected in TLE, as grey matter (GM) and white matter (WM) atrophy in temporal and extra temporal areas have been repeatedly demonstrated. Voxel-based morphometry (VBM) [1] analyses of T1-weighted (T1w) MRI in large groups of patients with TLE can reliably detect and localize regions of GM and WM atrophy associated with the disease [2] [3] [4].

C. Barillot, D.R. Haynor, and P. Hellier (Eds.): MICCAI 2004, LNCS 3217, pp. 696–702, 2004.

Our research hypothesis is that there exists areas that are linked to post-surgical outcome. The first step in our study was to identify those regions by comparing pre-operative MR volumes of patient cohorts having undergone surgery with positive and negative outcome. Our purpose is to explore whether surgical outcome is related to a pattern of GM or WM changes in TLE.

The second part of our work was an attempt at predicting surgical outcome based on simple image features. Our hypothesis is that in the regions of interest delineated by between-group analysis, there exists differences in GM or WM concentration, which can be used for classification purposes.

2 Subjects

The study population consisted of 39 consecutive patients with intractable, non-foreign-tissue TLE. Lateralization of seizure focus in TLE patients was determined by a comprehensive evaluation including prolonged video-electroencephalogram (EEG) telemetry. The EEG focus was defined as right or left if more than 70 % of seizures were recorded from one side. Manual MRI volumetry showed hippocampal atrophy ipsilateral to the seizure focus in all patients. Patients with left or right hippocampal atrophy were present in both groups.

Pre-operative T1w MR 3D images were acquired on a 1.5 T scanner using a T1-fast field echo sequence. All global MRI data were processed to correct for intensity non-uniformity due to scanner variations [5], linearly registered into stereotaxic space and resampled onto a $1mm$ isotropic grid [6].

All patients underwent selective amygdala-hippocampectomy. The post-operative follow-up was at least 12 months for all patients, on which basis they were consolidated in two outcome groups: seizure free (positive outcome, $n = 25$) or not seizure free (negative outcome, $n = 14$).

3 Methods

3.1 Detection of Atrophy Areas Related to Surgical Outcome

Our primary objective was to determine areas of GM and WM atrophy related to TLE surgical outcome. To this end we performed between-group VBM analyses of GM and WM density maps, comparing negative outcome TLE patients to positive outcome patients.

The density maps were obtained after classification of T1w MR volumes [7], linearly registered [6] to a common reference target of 152 young healthy volunteers (ICBM 152 symmetrical average [8]). GM or WM concentration maps were blurred using an isotropic Gaussian kernel of $5mm$ full-width at half-maximum. In those smoothed concentration maps, each voxel takes on a concentration value between $(0, 1)$ indicative of the presence or not of GM or WM in that voxel. T-statistics maps were obtained by estimating a generalized linear model at each voxel. Significant clusters, composed of a number or extent E of resels above a cluster threshold t-value, were obtained following the procedure developed by Worsley et al. [9] to correct for data nonuniformity.

3.2   Surgical Outcome Prediction

We used the results from the preceding VBM analysis to define as a region of interest the ensemble of significant clusters. Our hypothesis for predicting surgical outcome is that in this area there exists differences in GM or WM concentration, which can be exploited for classification purposes.

Two measures were developed to capture these differences for all subjects. The first measure was a straightforward calculation of the mean GM or WM concentration of all region-of-interest voxels j, where N_j is the number of such voxels. Thus, for subject i, with concentration map $[GM]_i$ for grey mater, the measure M_i was calculated as follows:

$$\mathbf{M_i} = \frac{\sum [GM]_{ij}}{N_j} \tag{1}$$

and a similar measure can be derived for the WM. For the second measure the t-value of the voxel in the between-group comparison volume was multiplied with the GM or WM concentration, thereby adding a weighting factor to the calculation. Thus, for subject i, the measure W_i was calculated as follows:

$$\mathbf{W_i} = \sum_j C_{ij} \times V_{ij} \tag{2}$$

where V_i is the between-group t-stat volume, C_i is the GM or WM concentration map for subject i, and each j is a voxel belonging to the ensemble of significant clusters determined in section 3.1.

For each of our four measures (GM/WM; mult/mean), linear discriminant analysis was used as a classifier for our two states, positive or negative outcome, using SYSTAT 10.2 (SSI, Point Richmond, CA).

4   Results

4.1   Atrophy Areas Related to Surgical Outcome

Figures 1 and 2 present the results of the between-group VBM analyses for GM and WM atrophy, respectively, for 14 negative outcome subjects compared to 25 positive outcome subjects. All voxels displayed are above the cluster threshold level of significance ($P < 0.05$, corrected for data nonisotropy and multiple comparisons) and shown using a glass-brain approach similar to SPM [1]. GM differences are detected primarily in the left lateral temporal neocortical areas. WM atrophy is more extensive, with contributions from left lateral temporal and occipital white matter.

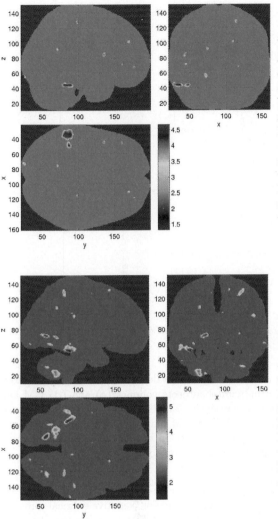

Fig. 1. GM atrophy for negative outcome group when compared to positive outcome group as determined by VBM, shown overlaid on a glass-brain. All voxels belong to significant clusters ($P < 0.05$, corrected for data nonisotropy and multiple corrections). The left lateral temporal neocortical area seems particularly particularly affected.

Fig. 2. WM atrophy map for negative outcome group when compared to positive outcome group as determined by VBM, shown overlaid on a glass-brain using the same parameters as Fig. 1. More areas seem related to surgical outcome, with predominance in the left lateral temporal and occipital white matter.

4.2   Predicting Surgical Outcome

Box plots of results for our two similarity measures are shown in Figure 3 (a) to (d). These show GM and WM measures taken for the average GM or WM concentration (mean) and t-stat weighted sum (mult).

Forward, stepwise jacknife classification scores based on linear discriminants (F-to-enter: 0.15) are shown in Table 1. The model retained two vectors out of four (GM and WM mean concentration) and achieved a 97 % accuracy.

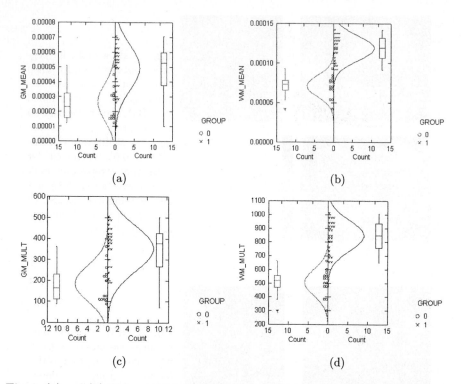

Fig. 3. (a) and (b) GM and WM mean concentration values, respectively, for all voxels belonging to regions of interest, in individual subjects volumes (c) and (d) GM and WM t-value weighted concentration, respectively, established by multiplying regions-of-interest voxels in individual subjects GM or WM maps with t-value in the corresponding voxel from the between-group comparison. In this figure group 0 represents negative outcome while group 1 represents positive outcome.

Table 1. Forward stepwise jacknife classification (F-to-enter = 0.15) gives best results to classify subjects as belonging to either Positive or Negative surgical outcome groups. True positive results on the Positive-Positive / Negative-Negative diagonal, shown in **bold**. The analysis reached near-perfect prediction using GM and WM mean concentration.

	Positive	Negative	% correct
Positive	**14**	0	100
Negative	1	**24**	96
Total	15	24	**97**

5   Discussion

We have been successful in identifying areas of GM and WM concentration differences that were related to surgical outcome in TLE patients having undergone selective amygdalo-hippocampectomy using a standard VBM approach. These areas could be refined if we were to use other approaches which improve the accuracy of VBM, such as modulation [10]; likewise, an increase in the number of patients would be required as many variables come to play in the post-surgical result. Nevertheless, the fact that there exists statistically significant areas of differences between the two groups is an indication that such information could be used for predictive purposes.

The accuracy of our classifier was excellent. This seems to reflect the straight-forward case that patients with poor surgical outcome are more affected by the disease in extra-hippocampal areas, including extra-temporal areas. Their average GM and WM concentration in selected regions of interest are lower than that of positive outcome patients as can be seen from Figure 3.

It should be noted that our first analysis is a between-group, voxel-by-voxel comparison of GM or WM concentration whereas the predictive results are individual, region-of-interest based measures. Hence, they do not represent the same information. Clearly, additional subjects, which we are in the process of recruiting, will be required for independent testing and before we can generalize this result in a clinical setting.

6   Conclusion

In this work we have set the basis for surgical outcome prediction for temporal lobe epilepsy patients undergoing selective amygdala-hippocampectomy, based on voxel-based morphometry analysis of pre-operative grey and white matter concentration maps. Regions of difference exist between positive and negative outcome patients, and can be used to predict surgical outcome with high accuracy.

Acknowledgments. The authors wish to acknowledge the financial contribution of the Fonds pour la Recherche en Santé du Québec.

References

1. J. Ashburner *et al.*, Voxel-Based Morphometry: The Methods. *NeuroImage*, 11:805-821, 2000.
2. N. Bernasconi *et al.*, Voxel-based statistical analysis of grey matter and white matter in patients with unilateral temporal lobe epilepsy. *NeuroImage*, 19(Suppl. 1): 575, 2003.
3. S.S. Keller *et al.*, Voxel-based morphometric comparison of hippocampal and extrahippocampal abnormalities in patients with left and right hippocampal atrophy. *NeuroImage*, 16(1):23-31, 2002.
4. K. Woermann *et al.*, Voxel-by-voxel comparison of automatically segmented cerebral gray matter - A rater-independent comparison of structural MRI in patients with epilepsy. *NeuroImage*, 10(4):373-384, 1999.
5. J. Sled *et al.*, A nonparametric method for automatic correction of intensity nonuniformity in MRI data. *IEEE TMI*, 17:87-97, 1998.

6. D. Collins *et al.*, ANIMAL: validation and applications of non-linear registration-based segmentation *IJPRAI*, 11:1271-1294, 1997.
7. A. Zijdenbos *et al.*, Morphometric analysis of white matter lesions in MR images: Method and Validation. *IEEE TMI*, 13: 716-724, 1994.
8. J. Mazziotta *et al.*, A probalistic atlas of the human brain: theory and rationale for its development. *NeuroImage*, 2:89-101, 1995.
9. K. Worsley *et al.*, Detecting changes in nonisotropic images *Human Brain Mapping*, 8: 98-101, 1999.
10. C.D. Good *et al.*, A voxel-based morphometric study of ageing in 465 normal adult human brains. *NeuroImage*, 14:21-36, 2001.

Exact MAP Activity Detection in *f*MRI Using a GLM with an Ising Spatial Prior

Eric R. Cosman, Jr.[1], John W. Fisher III[1], and William M. Wells III[1,2]

[1] Massachusetts Institute of Technology,
Computer Science and Artificial Intelligence Laboratory, Cambridge, MA, USA
ercosman@mit.edu, {fisher,sw}@csail.mit.edu
[2] Harvard Medical School, Brigham and Women's Hospital,
Department of Radiology, Boston, MA, USA

Abstract. Previous work [5] has shown how Ising spatial priors [1] can be incorported into *f*MRI analysis in a principled manner by using Mutual Information as a statistic for protocol-related activity. The activation image with maximum *a posteriori* (MAP) probability can then be computed exactly in polynomial time by reduction to a Min-Cut/Max-Flow Problem [4]. In this work, we show that an Ising prior can be applied in the same manner using a standard, linear activation model.

1 Introduction

The functional imaging literature contains a number of methods aimed at limiting false detection of protocol-related brain activity in *f*MRI by taking advantage of the well-known fact that adjacent regions of the brain are likely to act in unison. These methods involve one or more of the following approaches: noise reduction by spatial smoothing of the *f*MRI time-series to "average out" spatially-white noise [2,6,8], regularization of voxel-specific activation statistics [2,5], and/or adjustment of voxel-independent activation statistics to reflect the size of apparent, surrounding activity clusters [6]. Specifically, [5] introduces a Bayesian approach for regularizing voxel-specific, non-parametric activation statistics in which an Ising spatial prior on protocol-dependent activity is integrated with an information-theoretic activity detector. By reduction to a Min-Cut/Max-Flow Problem [4], the maximum *a posteriori* (MAP) estimate of activity over the whole brain can be computed *exactly* in polynomial time by the Ford-Fulkerson method. This integration hinges on the interpretation of Mutual Information as an approximation of the log-likelihood ratio of a hypothesis test that assesses the statistical independence of a BOLD signal and an experimental protocol.

In this paper, we show that standard activation statistics, such as F-statistics, are derived from the log-likelihood ratio of a subset hypothesis test under classical, linear models of the BOLD signal. Consequently, the same exact MAP activity detection mechanism can be used with such General Linear Models (GLMs), thereby controling false positive rates in a principled, Bayesian manner.

C. Barillot, D.R. Haynor, and P. Hellier (Eds.): MICCAI 2004, LNCS 3217, pp. 703–710, 2004.

2   The General Linear Model

An fMRI experiment produces a set of time series $\{y_i \in \Re^T : i = 1, \dots, V\}$, each of which measures the BOLD signal over T epochs in one of the V voxels comprising the imaged brain volume. Under the General Linear Model (GLM), it is assumed that the BOLD signal is a linear combination of protocol-dependent components (the columns of matrix $\boldsymbol{H}$), confounding signals due to cardio-pulmonary operations (the columns of matrix $\boldsymbol{D}$), and Gaussian noise [8]. For the special case of white noise, the GLM is written

$$\boldsymbol{y}_i = \boldsymbol{H}\boldsymbol{\eta}_i + \boldsymbol{D}\boldsymbol{\xi}_i + \boldsymbol{e}_i \qquad \boldsymbol{e}_i \sim \mathcal{N}(\boldsymbol{0}, \sigma^2\boldsymbol{I}) \text{ i.i.d.} \qquad i = 1, \dots, V \quad (1)$$

where $\boldsymbol{\eta}_i, \boldsymbol{\xi}_i$ are weight vectors on the columns of the *design matrix* $\boldsymbol{G} \equiv [\boldsymbol{H}\ \boldsymbol{D}]$. Under this model, classical activation statistics, such as the F statistic, can be derived from the log-likelihood ratio for a *two-sided, subset hypothesis test* $\{H_0 : \boldsymbol{\eta}_i = \boldsymbol{0},\ H_1 : \boldsymbol{\eta}_i \neq \boldsymbol{0}\}$, whereby we reject the null hypothesis (that there is no protocol-related neural activity) with an arbitrary threshold γ and the decision rule:

$$\lambda_i = \log \frac{\max_{\boldsymbol{\eta}_i, \boldsymbol{\xi}_i, \sigma^2} \mathcal{N}(\boldsymbol{y}_i; \boldsymbol{H}\boldsymbol{\eta}_i + \boldsymbol{D}\boldsymbol{\xi}_i, \sigma^2\boldsymbol{I})}{\max_{\boldsymbol{\xi}_i, \sigma^2} \mathcal{N}(\boldsymbol{y}_i; \boldsymbol{D}\boldsymbol{\xi}_i, \sigma^2\boldsymbol{I})} \overset{\text{``}H_1\text{''}}{\underset{}{>}} \gamma \quad (2)$$

$$\lambda_i - \gamma \overset{\text{``}H_1\text{''}}{\underset{}{>}} 0 \quad (3)$$

We optimize the numerator first, stacking $\boldsymbol{\eta}_i, \boldsymbol{\xi}_i$ into a single weight vector $\boldsymbol{\zeta}_i$:

$$
\begin{aligned}
0 &= \tfrac{d}{d\boldsymbol{\zeta}_i} \log \mathcal{N}(\boldsymbol{y}_i; \boldsymbol{G}\boldsymbol{\zeta}_i, \sigma^2\boldsymbol{I}) \\
0 &= \tfrac{d}{d\boldsymbol{\zeta}_i} \|\boldsymbol{y}_i - \boldsymbol{G}\boldsymbol{\zeta}_i\|^2 \\
0 &= \tfrac{d}{d\boldsymbol{\zeta}_i}(-2\boldsymbol{y}_i'\boldsymbol{G}\boldsymbol{\zeta}_i + \boldsymbol{\zeta}_i'\boldsymbol{G}'\boldsymbol{G}\boldsymbol{\zeta}_i) \\
0 &= -2\boldsymbol{G}'\boldsymbol{y}_i + (\boldsymbol{G}'\boldsymbol{G} + \boldsymbol{G}\boldsymbol{G}')\boldsymbol{\zeta}_i \\
\hat{\boldsymbol{\zeta}}_i &= (\boldsymbol{G}'\boldsymbol{G})^{-1}\boldsymbol{G}'\boldsymbol{y}
\end{aligned}
\qquad
\begin{aligned}
0 &= \tfrac{d}{d\sigma^2} \log \mathcal{N}(\boldsymbol{y}_i; \boldsymbol{G}\hat{\boldsymbol{\zeta}}_i, \sigma^2\boldsymbol{I}) \\
0 &= \tfrac{d}{d\sigma^2}\left(-\tfrac{1}{2}\log|\sigma^2\boldsymbol{I}| - \tfrac{\|\boldsymbol{y}_i - \boldsymbol{G}\hat{\boldsymbol{\zeta}}_i\|^2}{2\sigma^2}\right) \\
0 &= \tfrac{d}{d\sigma^2}\left(\tfrac{n}{2}\log\sigma^2 + \tfrac{\|\boldsymbol{y}_i - \boldsymbol{G}\hat{\boldsymbol{\zeta}}_i\|^2}{2\sigma^2}\right) \\
0 &= \tfrac{n}{2\sigma^2} - \tfrac{\|\boldsymbol{y}_i - \boldsymbol{G}\hat{\boldsymbol{\zeta}}_i\|^2}{2\sigma^4} \\
\hat{\sigma}^2 &= \tfrac{\|\boldsymbol{y}_i - \boldsymbol{G}\hat{\boldsymbol{\zeta}}_i\|^2}{n}
\end{aligned}
\quad (4)
$$

By analogous optimization of the denominator, we get the following expression for the log-likelihood ratio, in which $\boldsymbol{P}_{\boldsymbol{X}} \equiv \boldsymbol{X}(\boldsymbol{X}'\boldsymbol{X})^{-1}\boldsymbol{X}'$ (idempotent and symmetric) denotes a projection onto the column space of a matrix $\boldsymbol{X}$:

$$
\begin{aligned}
\lambda_i &= \log \frac{\mathcal{N}(\boldsymbol{y}_i; \boldsymbol{G}\hat{\boldsymbol{\zeta}}_i, \hat{\sigma}_1^2\boldsymbol{I})}{\mathcal{N}(\boldsymbol{y}_i; \boldsymbol{D}\hat{\boldsymbol{\xi}}_i, \hat{\sigma}_0^2\boldsymbol{I})} = \frac{(T/2\pi e)^{T/2}}{\|\boldsymbol{y}_i - \boldsymbol{G}\hat{\boldsymbol{\zeta}}_i\|^T} \bigg/ \frac{(T/2\pi e)^{T/2}}{\|\boldsymbol{y}_i - \boldsymbol{D}\hat{\boldsymbol{\xi}}_i\|^T} \\
&= \frac{T}{2}\log \frac{\boldsymbol{y}_i'(\boldsymbol{I} - \boldsymbol{P}_{\boldsymbol{D}})\boldsymbol{y}_i}{\boldsymbol{y}_i'(\boldsymbol{I} - \boldsymbol{P}_{\boldsymbol{G}})\boldsymbol{y}_i}
\end{aligned}
\quad (5)
$$

Since the F-statistic F_i typically used for this test is a monotonic function of λ_i, the likelihood ratio test and F-test are equivalent:

$$F_i = \frac{\boldsymbol{y}_i'(\boldsymbol{P_G} - \boldsymbol{P_D})\boldsymbol{y}_i/(g-d)}{\boldsymbol{y}_i'(\boldsymbol{I} - \boldsymbol{P_G})\boldsymbol{y}_i/(T-g)} \sim F_{g-d,T-g} \text{ under } H_0 \text{ [7]} \tag{6}$$

$$F_i = \left(\frac{T-g}{g-d}\right)\frac{-\boldsymbol{y}'(\boldsymbol{I} - \boldsymbol{P_G})\boldsymbol{y} + \boldsymbol{y}'(\boldsymbol{I} - \boldsymbol{P_D})\boldsymbol{y}}{\boldsymbol{y}'(\boldsymbol{I} - \boldsymbol{P_G})\boldsymbol{y}}$$

$$F_i = \frac{T-g}{g-d}\left(\exp\left\{\frac{2\lambda_i}{T}\right\} - 1\right) \tag{7}$$

$$\lambda_i = \frac{T}{2}\log\left(\frac{g-d}{T-g}F_i + 1\right) \tag{8}$$

where $g = \operatorname{rank}(\boldsymbol{G})$ and $d = \operatorname{rank}(\boldsymbol{D})$. We can use Equation 8 to compute the threshold γ_α on the log-likelihood ratio λ_i corresponding to a test of size α (or vice versa):

$$\gamma_\alpha = \frac{T}{2}\log\left(\frac{g-d}{T-g}F_{\alpha;g-d,T-g} + 1\right) \tag{9}$$

Furthermore, the threshold γ for the classical likelihood ratio test can be interpreted in a Bayesian framework as the prior log-odds of detection. Using a simple prior $p(H_0) = 1 - p(H_1)$ on the competing hypotheses, and assuming that parameters θ_k are fixed but unknown with flat priors $p(\theta_k \mid H_k) \propto c$, we get the following MAP decision rule:

$$\max_{\theta_1} p(\theta_1, H_1 \mid \boldsymbol{y}_i) \overset{\text{``}H_1\text{''}}{>} \max_{\theta_0} p(\theta_0, H_0 \mid \boldsymbol{y}_i) \tag{10}$$

$$\lambda_i = \log\frac{\max_{\theta_1} p(\boldsymbol{y}_i \mid \theta_1, H_1)}{\max_{\theta_0} p(\boldsymbol{y}_i \mid \theta_0, H_0)} \overset{\text{``}H_1\text{''}}{>} \log\frac{p(H_0)}{p(H_1)} \equiv \gamma \tag{11}$$

3   An Ising Model for Neural Activity

We are motivated to use an Ising Markov Random Field [1] as prior on assessments of neural activity, by the fact that neural activity and its sequel, the activity-dependent BOLD signal. We refer to $h \equiv h_1, \ldots, h_V$ as an *activation map*, where $h_i \in \{0, 1\}$ is the assessment of (in)activity at voxel i, such that $h_i = 0$ and $h_i = 1$ correspond to hypotheses H_0 and H_1, respectively, as defined using a GLM as in Section 2. An Ising prior on the activation map h quantifies the notion that adjacent voxels are likely to act in unison by assigning greater probability to configurations with a greater number of homogeneous second-order cliques (since adjacent voxels are defined to be neighboring). In this work, we augment the prior with singleton clique potentials that penalize the total number of voxels declared active:

$$p(h|\gamma, \beta) = \frac{1}{Z(\gamma, \beta)} \exp\left\{ -\gamma \sum_{i=1}^{V} h_i + \beta \sum_{i=1}^{V} \sum_{j\sim i} \delta(h_i - h_j) \right\} \tag{12}$$

$$= \frac{1}{Z(\gamma, \beta)} \exp\left\{ -\gamma \cdot \#\{h_i = 1\} + \beta \cdot \text{NHC}(h) \right\} \tag{13}$$

where $\text{NHC}(h)$ gives the number of homogeneous cliques in configuration h, $Z(\gamma, \beta)$ is the partition function, and $j \sim i$ denotes that voxel j is a neighbor of voxel i. Conditioned on the activation map, the BOLD signals $\boldsymbol{y}_i$ are mutually independent across voxels. Therefore, the likelihood of the data $\boldsymbol{y}$ is

$$p(\boldsymbol{y}|\theta_0, \theta_1, h) = \prod_{i=1}^{V} p(\boldsymbol{y}_i|\theta_{0i}, \theta_{1i}, h_i) = \prod_{i=1}^{V} \frac{p(\boldsymbol{y}_i|\theta_{1i}, h_i = 1)^{h_i}}{p(\boldsymbol{y}_i|\theta_{0i}, h_i = 0)^{h_i-1}} \tag{14}$$

Choosing a flat prior $p(\theta_0, \theta_1 \,|\, h) \propto c$ on the configuration of GLM parameters under each hypothesis, and taking γ and β as known hyperparameters, we get the following MAP estimation criteria:

$$\hat{h}, \hat{\theta}_0, \hat{\theta}_1 = \arg\max_{h, \theta_0, \theta_1} \log p(h, \theta_0, \theta_1 \,|\, \boldsymbol{y}, \gamma, \beta) \tag{15}$$

$$= \arg\max_{h, \theta_0, \theta_1} \log \prod_{i=1}^{V} \frac{p(\boldsymbol{y}_i \,|\, \theta_{1i}, h_i = 1)^{h_i}}{p(\boldsymbol{y}_i \,|\, \theta_{0i}, h_i = 0)^{h_i-1}} + \log p(h \,|\, \gamma, \beta) \tag{16}$$

Since h_i is binary-valued, it is clear from Equation 16 that the posterior is increased by maximizing θ_{0i} and θ_{1i} for each voxel independently. Therefore, $\hat{\theta}_0, \hat{\theta}_1$ are the maximum likelihood estimates derived as in Equation 4, and the MAP estimate for the activation map is given by

$$\hat{h} = \arg\max_h \sum_{i=1}^{V} \left(h_i \left(\log \frac{p(\boldsymbol{y}_i|\hat{\theta}_{1i}, h_i = 1)}{p(\boldsymbol{y}_i|\hat{\theta}_{0i}, h_i = 0)} - \gamma \right) + \beta \sum_{i\sim j} \delta(h_i - h_j) \right) \tag{17}$$

$$= \arg\max_h \sum_{i=1}^{V} \left(h_i (\lambda_i - \gamma) + \beta \sum_{i\sim j} \delta(h_i - h_j) \right) \tag{18}$$

4   Reduction to the Minimum-Cut Problem

Since the activation map h can assume 2^V values, direct search for the optimal configuration $\hat{h}$ is computationally intractible. However, Greig et al. [4] showed that the search can be reduced to the Minimum-Cut/Maximum-Flow Network Problem, which can be solved in polynomial time by the Ford-Fulkerson method (or Preflow Push algorithms). We review this reduction with minor modification. Construct a capacitated network with V+2 vertices, comprising i=1, ... ,V voxels, a source s, and a sink t. Let the graph have the following edges and corresponding capacities:

$$
\begin{array}{llll}
(s,i) & c_{si} = \lambda_i - \gamma & \text{if } \lambda_i - \gamma > 0 & \\
(i,t) & c_{it} = \gamma - \lambda_i & \text{if } \lambda_i - \gamma \le 0 & (19) \\
(i,j) \text{ and } (i,j) & c_{ij} = c_{ji} = \beta & \text{if } \quad i \sim j &
\end{array}
$$

For any activation map h, let $A = \{s\} \cup \{i : h_i = 1\}$ and $I = \{t\} \cup \{i : h_i = 0\}$ define a two-set partition of the network verticies. The set of edges with a vertex in A and a vertex in I is called a *cut*, and its *capacity* $C(h)$ can be written as follows:

$$
C(h) = \sum_{k \in A} \sum_{l \in I} c_{kl} \tag{20}
$$

$$
= \sum_{i=1}^{V} \left(h_i \max(0, \gamma - \lambda_i) + (1-h_i)\max(0, \lambda_i - \gamma) + \beta \sum_{i \sim j} 1 - \delta(h_i - h_j) \right) \tag{21}
$$

This expression differs from the log-posterior $\log p(h, \hat{\theta}_0, \hat{\theta}_1 | \boldsymbol{y}, \gamma, \beta)$ (Equation 18) by a term which does not depend on h. Therefore, the MAP esimation is equivalent to finding the minimum cut in the network. Voxels are active in MAP estimate if they are on the source size of the minimum cut. Otherwise, they are inactive.

5 Experiments

Figure 1 shows the effect of varying the strength β of the spatial prior, for a given threshold γ_α. Activation maps are shown overlaying two axial slices (at the level of the Sylvian fissure) from a word-association task, where the strength of a spatial prior $\beta = 0, 0.5, 1, 2, 3$ increases from left to right. A simple GLM was used in which $\boldsymbol{H}$ is an encoding of the protocol, and the confounder subspace is empty $\boldsymbol{D} = \boldsymbol{0}$. The equivalent test size for the threshold γ_α is $\alpha = 1 \times 10^{-7}$. For each β, voxels declared active in the MAP activation map are colored white. The fMRI data were not pre-processed or pre-smoothed, so that the effect of the spatial prior could be observed in isolation. Figures 2 and 3 show how the running time for MAP estimation varies with the hyperparameters. The estimation was performed with a MATLAB implementation of the Ford-Fulkerson method. Specifiically, we implemented the Edmonds-Karp algorithm, using depth-limited, depth-first search to find the shortest, feasible augmenting paths). The fMRI was aquired during a motor and auditory protocol and contains $V = 23187$ voxels.

Figure 2 shows how running time increases with the threshold γ, which we varied such that the number of above-threshold voxels $N = \text{size}(A) = 100, 250, 1000$ across runs. We also varied $\beta = 1, 2, 3$ for each setting of γ, which respectively corresponded to classical tests of size $\alpha = 6 \times 10^{-10}, 3 \times 10^{-7}, 6 \times$

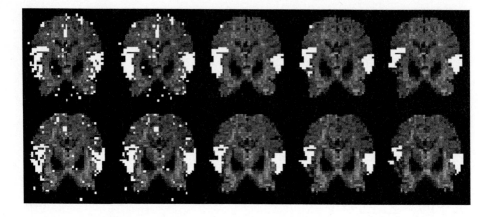

Fig. 1. Activation maps overlay two axial slices (at the level of the Sylvian fissure) from a word-association task, where the strength of a spatial prior $\beta = 0, 0.5, 1, 2, 3$ increases from left to right, and the equivalent test size for the threshold γ_α is $\alpha = 1 \times 10^{-7}$.

10^{-5}. For this and other datasets, the running time varied approximately linearly with N over this range. This is related to the fact that the Ford-Fulkerson method proceeds by sequentially augmenting *feasible paths* (i.e. those which can accomodate more flow) from the source s to the the sink t. Since the number of above-threshold voxels N (typically small relative to the total number of voxels) determines the number of edges emanating from the source s, the number of augmenting steps is roughly proportional to N.

Figure 3 shows that the same running time data varies roughly linearly as a function of $\beta = 1, 2, 3$. Again, this was typical over a number of fMRI datasets. Naturally, for increasing β, the network capacity increases monotonically, and with it, the number of long-range interactions and flow-augmenting steps.

6   Discussion

Inspection of the reduction in Section 4 clarifies the relationship between classical, voxel-independent fMRI analysis, and Bayesian analysis with an Ising prior. In both approaches, the log-likelihood ratio λ_i is computed at each voxel independently. Furthermore, in the Bayesian approach, voxels are initially partitioned into sets A and I (**A**ctive and **I**nactive) according to the decision rule $\lambda_i - \gamma > 0$, which is equivalent to that from the classical likelihood ratio test. Therefore, MAP estimation proceeds by first partitioning the data according to the classical, likelihood-ratio test, decision rule with threshold γ, and then adjusting the partition to account for the Ising prior. Moreover, the hyperparameter γ has a number of interpretations: (1) as a penalty for declaring a voxel active, (2) as corresponding to the size α of the classical, voxel-independent test, and (3) as the prior log-odds of detection in a simple, voxel-independent, Bayesian framework.

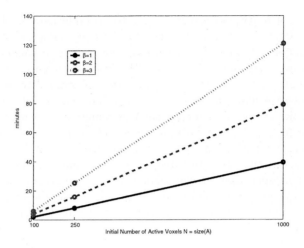

Fig. 2. Running Time as a function of the number of above-threshold voxels $N = \text{size}(A) = 100, 250, 1000$, for $\beta = 1, 2, 3$

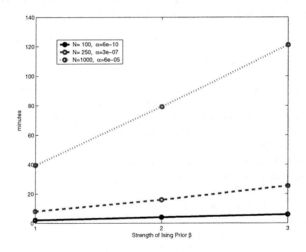

Fig. 3. Running Time as a function of strength of the Ising prior $\beta = 1, 2, 3$, for $N = \text{size}(A) = 100, 250, 1000$

The results of varying β (Figure 1) highlight the fact that the application of the Ising spatial prior is not simply a statistically-principled erosion operation. With increasing β, voxels which might be rejected at level α in a classical, voxel-independent test, may be declared active due to their proximity to other strongly active voxels. Of course, since the theshold typically exceeds the log-likelihood of most voxels, the primary effect of the Ising prior is to control the number of false detections by removing spatially-isolated activations.

Estimation of hyperparameters γ and β is complicated by the absence of ground truth activation maps. The MCMC-ML sampling approach of [3] could be adapted (in part) to find ML estimates of these hyperparameters using exact MAP estimates of the activation maps. However, the computational expense of such an approach is restrictive, as evaluation of optimality for each setting of (γ, β) involves running a min-cut computation and an MCMC simulation. Therefore, choice of optimal hyperparameters remains an open issue.

Finally, we note some possible extensions to this work. First, other classical activation statistics, such as the t-statistics, can also be derived from a likelihood ratio test and can thus be integrated into this framework. Furthermore, one can employ more specialized neighborhoods and clique potentials than we have shown. For instance, the coefficient β_{ij} might vary spatially according to prior beliefs about differences in regularity within and across anatomical boundaries derived from co-registered segmentations.

Acknowledgements. This research was supported in part by the grants NIH 5 P41 RR13218 and NCI 1 R21 CA89449-01. Further support was provided by FIRST BIRN, The Harvard Center for Neurodegeneration and Repair, and the NSF ERC grant, Johns Hopkins Agreement #8810274.

References

1. J. Besag. On the statistical analysis of dirty pictures. *Journal of the Royal Statistical Society. Series B (Methodological)*, 48:259–302, 1986.
2. X. Descombes, F. Kruggel, and D. Y. von Cramon. Spatio-temporal fmri analysis using markov random fields. *IEEE Transactions on Medical Imaging*, 17(6):1028–1039, December 1998.
3. X. Descombes, R. D. Morris, J. Zerubia, and M. Berthold. Estimation of markov random field prior parameters using markov chain monte carlo maximum likelihood. *IEEE Transactions of Image Processing*, 8(7), 1999.
4. D. M. Greig, B. T. Porteous, and A. H. Seheult. Exact maximum a posteriori estimation for binary images. *Journal of the Royal Statistical Society. Series B (Methodological)*, 51(2):271–279, 1989.
5. J. Kim, J. W. F. III, A. Tsai, C. Wible, A. Willsky, and W. M. W. III. Incorporating spatial priors into an information theoretic approach for fmri data analysis. *Third International Conference on Medical Image Computing and Computer-Assisted Intervention*, 1935:62–71, October 2000.
6. J.-B. Poline, K. J. Worsley, A. C. Evans, and K. J. Friston. Combining spatial extent and peak intensity to test for activations in functional imaging. *Neuroimage*, 5:83–96, 1997.
7. A. C. Rencher. *Methods of Multivariate Analysis*. Wiley, 2002.
8. K. J. Worsley and K. J. Friston. Analysis of fmri time series revisited – again. *Neuroimage*, 2:173–181, 1995.

Bias in Resampling-Based Thresholding of Statistical Maps in fMRI

Ola Friman and Carl-Fredrik Westin

Laboratory of Mathematics in Imaging, Department of Radiology
Brigham and Women's Hospital, Harvard Medical School

Abstract. Selecting a threshold for the statistical parameter maps in functional MRI (fMRI) is a delicate matter. The use of advanced test statistics and/or the complex dependence structure of the noise may preclude parametric statistical methods for finding appropriate thresholds. Non-parametric statistical methodology has been presented as a feasible alternative. In this paper we discuss resampling-based methods for finding thresholds and show that proposed non-parametric approaches can lead to severely biased results.

1 Introduction

Selecting a threshold for the statistical parameter maps in fMRI is a challenging and important problem. The challenge lies in the fact that employed test statistics and/or the dependence structure of fMRI noise may not conform with classical statistical procedures and assumptions. Nonetheless it is important to assess the statistical significance provided by a specific threshold. The statistical significance is customarily measured by the p-value, which in fMRI context translates to the probability of declaring voxels active when in fact they are not. In order to find a threshold that provides a desired p-value, knowledge about the null-distribution of test statistic used for forming the statistical maps is required, see Fig. 1. Under certain assumptions about the noise structure and for certain test statistics, an analytic expression for this distribution is known. Examples

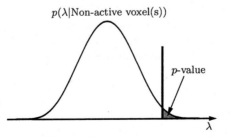

$p(\lambda|\text{Non-active voxel(s)})$

Fig. 1. The null-distribution is the distribution of a test statistic λ given that there is no activity in the examined voxel(s). The p-value is the probability of observing a value of the test statistic exceeding the threshold.

C. Barillot, D.R. Haynor, and P. Hellier (Eds.): MICCAI 2004, LNCS 3217, pp. 711–718, 2004.
© Springer-Verlag Berlin Heidelberg 2004

are the t and F statistics encountered in the widely employed General Linear Model analysis [1]. However, as soon as the test statistic or the dependence structure of the noise depart from those afforded by classical statistical theory, the analytic expression for the null-distribution is in general intractable. The difficulties in deriving analytic expressions for the test statistic's null-distribution have spawned a number of alternative non-parametric ways to finding thresholds for the statistical maps [2,3,4,5,6,7]. Instead of assuming a parameterized form of the null-distribution, non-parametric approaches estimate it by analyzing data sets synthesized to mimic real fMRI data. Since no distributional assumptions about the data are required, non-parametric thresholds can be more accurate than those found by parametric methods [8]. The accuracy of the non-parametric thresholds is, however, strongly dependent on our ability to generate data with characteristics similar to real fMRI data. For this purpose various resampling techniques, for example whitening resampling [3,5], Fourier resampling [9,7] and wavelet resampling [6], have been applied.

Even though non-parametric procedures assume less about the nature of the test statistic and noise dependence structure, there exist pitfalls which may lead to severely biased thresholds. In this paper we point on such pitfalls and show that Fourier and wavelet resampling methods are not suitable for finding thresholds for fMRI statistical parameter maps. In the following sections we present the data, methods and results that underpin this conclusion. Finally, under Discussion we provide a theoretical explanation of the results.

2   Material

To prove our point we make use of simulated and real fMRI data sets. The simulated data set consists of 500 Gaussian white noise time series, each 128 samples long. In 20 % of the time series a synthetic smooth blocked design Blood Oxygen Level Dependent (BOLD) response has been embedded, i.e. 20 % of the time series correspond to 'active' voxels. Even though this data do not have the same characteristic as real fMRI data, it serve an illustrative purpose since we will be able to compare estimated null-distributions with the theoretically correct null-distribution. The real fMRI data set is a blocked design mental calculation test acquired using a 1.5 T GE scanner with imaging parameters: TR 2 s, TE 60 ms, FOV 24 cm, slice thickness 3 mm, image size 128×128 voxels and 180 time points. The images were realigned and spatially smoothed with a 4 mm FWHM Gaussian filter prior to the analysis described below.

3   Methods

Our objective is to detect active voxels in the data sets described above with thresholds that provide prespecified p-values. Below we describe the procedures for calculating the statistical maps, resampling the data sets and finding suitable thresholds.

3.1   Statistical Maps

For analyzing the synthetic data set, we simply use the correlation coefficient between each time series and the known embedded BOLD response shape. In this simplified synthetic setting, we know that the correlation coefficient is the c optimal test statistic for detecting 'active' voxels [10]. In the the real data case we do not know the exact shape of the BOLD response. In a traditional GLM analysis fashion [1], we produce a BOLD response model by convolving the binary on/off paradigm with a canonical impulse response function, and augment this model with its temporal derivative in order to account for unknown delays. With this BOLD response model we calculate F-maps, i.e. statistical maps consisting of F-statistics [11].

3.2   Resampling

Resampling is the process of producing artificial null-data sets with a statistical dependence structure similar to an original data set. From such resampled data sets we can estimate the null-distribution of the employed test statistic and consequently find a threshold that provides the desired p-value. In its simplest form, resampling boils down to a random reshuffling or permutation of the samples in the fMRI time series [2,4]. However, since fMRI data are serially correlated [12], such an approach does not preserve the temporal dependence structure, leading to erroneous threshold estimates. Instead we need to transform the data to a domain where a reshuffling does not alter the statistical structure, randomly permute the data, and then apply an inverse transform. To this end, whitening, Fourier and wavelet transforms have been proposed for resampling fMRI data [3, 5,6,7]. The resampling schemes based on these transforms are described in more detail below.

Whitening resampling. By assuming a particular model for the serial correlation structure we can apply a whitening transform to the time series, after which a random reshuffling of the samples is allowed. AR(1) and ARMA noise models have been proposed for this purpose [3,5]. In this paper, the whitening resampling was implemented by first fitting an AR(1) noise model to each time series. The time series was then whitened and the samples in the resulting time series permuted. Lastly, the permuted time series was passed through the fitted AR(1) process in order to form a resampled time series.

Fourier resampling. The intrinsic whitening property of the Fourier transform makes it potentially useful for resampling. Fourier resampling was carried out by taking the Fourier transform of the time series, keeping the magnitude of each frequency but permuting the phase components, and then applying the inverse Fourier transform.

Wavelet resampling. The wavelet resampling works similarly to the Fourier resampling. As devised by Bullmore et al. [6], a 4:th order Daubechies wavelet was used for wavelet transforming the time series. The wavelet coefficients within each scale were then permuted before applying the inverse wavelet transform.

Since fMRI data sets are spatio-temporal, in addition to preserving the serial correlation, it is also important to preserve the spatial autocorrelation. This is easily accomplished by applying the same random permutation to every time series in the fMRI data set [7,9]. Finally, as will be evident in the Results section, resampling the original data set as it is or resampling the residual data set obtained after regressing out the BOLD response model (and other deterministic components such as drifts and trends) yield very different results. The standard way would be to resample the residual data, but here we examine both alternatives as it provides insight into the biases we are about to see.

3.3   Finding Thresholds

The inference in fMRI analysis is usually carried out either at a voxel-wise level or at a family-wise level. The former means that we have the probability of a single voxel falsely being declared active under control and the latter implies that we have the probability of seeing any false positive activations over an entire set of voxels under control [13,14]. By producing a large number of resampled data sets, both voxel-wise and family-wise thresholds can be found. Having a large number of observations of the test statistic, calculated using resampled data, it is an easy task to determine the threshold for the quantile implied by the p-value. A family-wise threshold is found in a similar manner, but instead using only the maximum statistics recorded from the resampled data sets. Hence, it is computationally more demanding to find family-wise thresholds compared to voxel-wise thresholds.

4   Results

Using the methods described above, the synthetic and real data sets were resampled 1000 times each. The estimated voxel-wise and family-wise null-distributions, together with the theoretically correct null-distribution for the correlation coefficient[1], obtained by resampling the synthetic data set are shown in Fig. 2. The important observation here is that the Fourier and wavelet methods produce null-distribution estimates far from the true null-distribution. While the threshold obtained by resampling original fMRI data is severely overestimated (Fig. 2ab), the threshold estimated by resampling residual data is severely underestimated (Fig. 2cd). The whitening resampling method produces null-distributions with less dramatic, though still significant, errors. The behavior of the different resampling methods applied to this simplified synthetic data set is

---

[1] $f(r) = \frac{1}{\sqrt{\pi}} \frac{\Gamma\left(\frac{N-1}{2}\right)}{\Gamma\left(\frac{N-2}{2}\right)} \left(1 - r^2\right)^{\frac{N-4}{2}}$, where N is the number of samples in the time series.

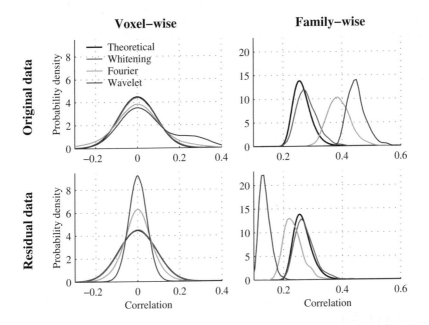

Fig. 2. Theoretical and estimated null-distributions for the correlation coefficient obtained by resampling the synthetic data set. Estimated voxel-wise and family-wise thresholds for a desired p-value can be determined from these distributions, cf. Fig. 1.

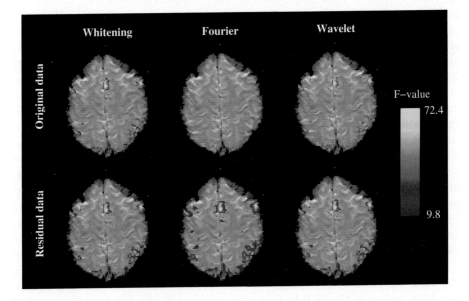

Fig. 3. A slice in the real fMRI data set subjected to the thresholds in Table 1. Note the difference between using the thresholds obtained by resampling original data and those obtained by resampling residual data.

the main result in this paper. However, before discussing the reasons underlying the biases seen in Fig. 2, we briefly show that similar results are obtained with real fMRI data too. In Table 1, the estimated family-wise thresholds for the real data set at $p = 0.05$ are listed. Note that while we cannot assess the accuracy of these thresholds, also here we observe substantially higher thresholds when resampling the original data set compared to the residual data set. Finally, in Fig. 3 the effect of the different thresholds are visualized.

Table 1. Estimated family-wise thresholds at significance level $p = 0.05$ for the F-maps calculated using the real data set.

	Whitening	Fourier	Wavelet
Original data	20.6	72.4	25.3
Residual data	16.9	9.8	17.0

5 Discussion

The results in the previous section show that Fourier- and wavelet-based resampling methods provide greatly biased thresholds while the whitening resampling approach seems to yield more accurate thresholds. There are two factors explaining this behavior. The first source of bias pertains to the fact that there are two classes of voxels in fMRI data, namely those containing a BOLD response and those who do not. In the blocked experimental design case, in original fMRI data voxels from these two classes have rather different spectra/autocorrelation functions, see top panel of Fig. 4. The second factor contributing to the bias is the number of degrees of freedom the resampling method has available for imitating the serial correlation structure in time series to be resampled. Both the Fourier and wavelet resampling schemes have large freedom in generating a time series with a spectrum matching that of the original time series. Therefore, when resampling original data with the Fourier and wavelet methods, if the time series is active also the resampled time series will have have a strong variation in pace with the BOLD response we are looking for. Hence, in the resampling process we will unproportionally often get time series that correlate well BOLD response model, leading to the biased null-distributions seen in Fig. 2a and Fig. 2c. If we try to circumvent this problem by removing the expected BOLD response from all voxels (i.e. create what we here denote residual data) prior to the resampling, we arrive in the situation shown in the bottom panel in Fig. 4. In this case the Fourier and wavelet methods produce resampled time series with too little power in the BOLD response frequencies. We will therefore instead find unproportionally small correlations between the BOLD response model and the resampled time series, as was seen in Fig. 2bd, leading to underestimated thresholds.

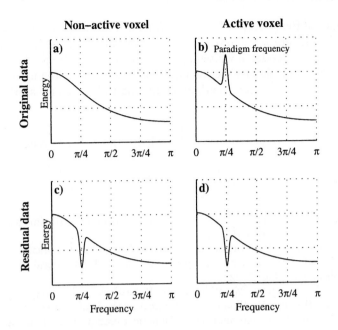

Fig. 4. Schematic spectra of time series in original and residual data (i.e. with a blocked BOLD response model removed from the time series).

In contrast to the Fourier and wavelet methods, the whitening resampling approach utilizes a specific model for the noise spectrum. In this paper an AR(1) model with only one degree of freedom is employed. When fitting this model to the observed spectrum of a time series, the absence or presence of power in the BOLD response frequencies has lesser impact on the resulting fit. Hence, the resampling process is regularized by the prior information provided by the noise model. Nevertheless, to some extent the presence of a BOLD response biases also the whitening approach, as was seen in Fig. 2b.

Hitherto, we have only discussed blocked experimental designs, as opposed to more rapid event-related designs. Due to the higher entropy, i.e. randomness, of event-related designs they tend to be more similar to noise when resampled. Thus, the bias effects discussed above are less pronounced, but still valid, when resampling fMRI data sets acquired during event-related experimental conditions.

6   Conclusions

Resampling-based methods based on Fourier and wavelet transforms have previously been proposed as appropriate for finding accurate thresholds for fMRI statistical maps. However, we have shown that even under simplified and controlled conditions, Fourier and wavelet resampling methods fail badly in this task. What ultimately makes Fourier and wavelet resampling unsuitable is the many degrees of freedom they have available for mimicking the serial correlation in the fMRI time series. We have also shown that due to the regularizing effect of a serial correlation model, a whitening resampling approach has the potential to provide accurate thresholds. We therefore conclude that whitening resampling is the preferred non-parametric method for finding thresholds for statistical maps in fMRI.

Acknowledgments. The authors acknowledge the NIH for research grant P41 RR 13218.

References

1. Friston, K., Jezzard, P., Turner, R.: Analysis of functional MRI time-series. Human Brain Mapping **1** (1994) 153–171
2. Holmes, A., Blair, R., Watson, J., Ford, I.: Nonparametric analysis of statistic images from functional mapping experiments. Journal of Cerebral Blood Flow and Metabolism **16** (1996) 7–22
3. Bullmore, E., Brammer, M., Williams, S., Rabe-Hesketh, S., Janot, N., David, A., Mellers, J., Howard, R., Sham, P.: Statistical methods of estimation and inference for functional MR image analysis. Magnetic Resonance in Medicine **35** (1996) 261–277
4. Brammer, M., Bullmore, E., Simmons, A., Williams, S., Grasby, P., Howard, R., Woodruff, P., Rabe-Hesketh, S.: Generic brain activation mapping in functional magnetic resonance imaging: A nonparametric approach. Magnetic Resonance Imaging **15** (1997) 763–770
5. Locascio, J., Jennings, P., Moore, C., Corkin, S.: Time series analysis in the time domain and resampling methods for studies of functional magnetic resonance brain imaging. Human Brain Mapping **5** (1997) 168–193
6. Bullmore, E., Long, C., Suckling, J., Fadili, J., Calvert, G., Zelaya, F., Carpenter, T., Brammer, M.: Colored noise and computational inference in neurophysiological (fMRI) time series analysis: resampling methods in time and wavelet domains. Human Brain Mapping **12** (2001) 61–78
7. Laird, A., Rogers, B., Meyerand, M.: Comparison of Fourier and wavelet resampling methods. Magnetic Resonance in Medicine **51** (2004) 418–422
8. Nichols, T., Holmes, A.: Nonparametric permutation tests for functional neuroimaging: A primer with examples. Human Brain Mapping **15** (2001) 1–25
9. Prichard, D., Theiler, J.: Generating surrogate data for time series with several simultaneously measured variables. Physical Review Letters **73** (1994) 951–954
10. van Trees, H.: Detection, Estimation, and Modulation Theory, Part I. John Wiley & Sons (1968)
11. Friston, K., Fletcher, P., Josephs, O., Holmes, A., Rugg, M., Turner, R.: Event-related fMRI: Characterizing differential responses. NeuroImage **7** (1998) 30–40
12. Woolrich, M., Ripley, B., Brady, M., Smith, S.: Temporal autocorrelation in univariate linear modeling of FMRI data. NeuroImage **14** (2001) 1370–1386
13. Worsley, K.: Local maxima and the expected Euler characteristic of excursion sets of χ^2, F and t fields. Advances in Applied Probability **26** (1994) 13–42
14. Nichols, T., Hayasaka, S., Wager, T.: Controlling the familywise error rate in functional neuroimaging: A comparative review. Statistical Methods in Medical Research **12** (2003) 419–446

Solving Incrementally the Fitting and Detection Problems in fMRI Time Series

Alexis Roche, Philippe Pinel, Stanislas Dehaene, and Jean-Baptiste Poline

CEA, Service Hospitalier Frédéric Joliot, Orsay, France
Institut d'Imagerie Neurofonctionnelle (IFR 49), Paris, France
roche@shfj.cea.fr

Abstract. We tackle the problem of real-time statistical analysis of functional magnetic resonance imaging (fMRI) data. In a recent paper, we proposed an incremental algorithm based on the extended Kalman filter (EKF) to fit fMRI time series in terms of a general linear model with autoregressive errors (GLM-AR model). We here improve the technique using a new Kalman filter variant specifically tailored to the GLM-AR fitting problem, the *Refined Kalman Filter* (RKF), that avoids both the estimation bias and initialization issues typical from the EKF, at the price of increased memory load. We then demonstrate the ability of the method to perform online analysis on a "functional calibration" event-related fMRI protocol.

1 Introduction

One of the current challenges in functional magnetic resonance imaging (fMRI) is to display reconstructed volumes and map brain activations in real time during an ongoing scan. This will make it possible to interact with fMRI experiments in a much more efficient way, either by monitoring acquisition parameters online depending on subject's performance, or by designing paradigms that incorporate neurophysiological feedback. To date, the feasibility of real-time fMRI processing has been limited by the computational cost of both the three-dimensional reconstruction of MR scans and their statistical analysis.

This paper addresses the latter item, and is therefore focused on the feasibility of online fMRI statistical analysis. In this context, our goal is to fit, on each scan time, the currently available fMRI time course in terms of an appropriate model of the BOLD response, and further test for brain regions that are significantly correlated with the model. We will focus here on general linear models (GLM) [1] as they are by far the most common in the fMRI processing community.

Although many detection algorithms have been proposed so far, most of them are intended to work offline in the sense that they process a complete fMRI sequence once at a time, with computational cost and memory load proportional to the sequence length. Applying such methods online would imply that the incremental computation time increases on each new scan, which is clearly a serious drawback when considering real-time constraints. To overcome this problem, some techniques were proposed that compute the correlation between the signal

C. Barillot, D.R. Haynor, and P. Hellier (Eds.): MICCAI 2004, LNCS 3217, pp. 719–726, 2004.

and the model, either in an incremental fashion [2], or by restricting computations to a sliding time window [3].

Such methods have the ability to process each new scan in a constant amount of time, but, being based on standard correlation, they work under the implicit assumption that the errors in the signal are temporally uncorrelated. Should this assumption be incorrect, the significance level of activation clusters may be substantially biased (over- or under-estimated). The importance of correcting inferences for temporal autocorrelations is widely recognized owing to the following facts: (i) errors may be found to be severely autocorrelated in some regions, especially when the model lacks flexibility; (ii) since autocorrelation is spatially dependent, it cannot be accounted for by a global threshold correction.

We recently advocated Kalman filtering techniques as good candidates for online fMRI analysis [4]. In its standard form, the Kalman filter is an incremental solver for ordinary least-square (OLS) regression problems, and is therefore well-suited for GLM fitting when assuming uncorrelated errors. In the more general case where the noise autocorrelation is unknown and is therefore to be estimated, the regression problem becomes nonlinear, a situation that may be handled using an extended Kalman filter (EKF) [4]. This technique's main drawback is that it requires parameter initialization to work; we observed from practical experience that good initialization is difficult to tune, and is very much machine-dependent.

To work around these issues, we design here a new Kalman filter variant to solve the GLM-AR fitting problem incrementally. Rather than using the linearization mechanism underlying the EKF, our basic idea is to rely on the standard Kalman filter to provide first parameter guesses on each iteration, and then refine the result using a simple optimization scheme. We will show that the algorithm outperforms the EKF in that it is insensitive to initialization, and provides asymptotically unbiased parameter estimates.

2   GLM-AR Model Fitting

Let us consider the time course vector $y = [y_1, \ldots, y_n]^t$ associated with a given voxel in an fMRI sequence, where the acquisition times are numbered from 1 to n. In the remainder, it will be assumed that each incoming scan is spatially aligned with the first scan, which may necessitate a realignment procedure. In our usual processing pipeline, no spatial filtering is applied to the original scans (this enables us to use a slice-specific model to account for slice timing effects).

2.1   The GLM-AR Model

The general linear model states that the measured time course is a linear combination of known signals $x_1, \ldots, x_p$ called regressors, up to an additive noise:

$$y = X\beta + \varepsilon,$$

where $X \equiv (x_1^t, \ldots, x_p^t)$ is a $n \times p$ matrix called the design matrix, which concatenates the different regressors columnwise, ε is the outcome of the noise, and β is the unknown $p \times 1$ vector of regression coefficients, or "effect" vector. The design matrix contains paradigm-related regressors obtained, e.g., by convolving the different stimulation onsets with a canonical hemodynamic response function [1], as well as regressors that model the low-frequency drift, hence enabling us to "detrend" the signal (we use polynomials up to order three). Notice that the design matrix can be assembled incrementally since it involves either causal convolutions, or pre-specified detrending functions.

In this work, we assume that ε is a stationary Gaussian zero-mean AR(1) random process, i.e. it is characterized by: $\varepsilon_i = a\varepsilon_{i-1} + n_i$, where a is the auto-correlation parameter, and n_i is a "generator" white noise, with instantaneous Gaussian distribution $N(0, \sigma^2)$. Notice that the condition $|a| < 1$ must hold for the AR noise to be stationary.

2.2   Offline Fitting

Solving the GLM-AR fitting problem means finding appropriate, somehow optimal, statistical estimators of the effect β, the noise autocorrelation a and scale parameter σ. A powerful estimation approach consists of maximizing the likelihood function or, equivalently, minimizing its negated logarithm given by [4]:

$$L(\beta, a, \sigma) = n \log \sqrt{2\pi}\sigma + \frac{1}{2}\log(1 - a^2) + \frac{1}{2\sigma^2}\left[(1 - a^2)r_1^2 + \sum_{i=2}^{n}(r_i - ar_{i-1})^2\right],$$
(1)

where $r_i \equiv y_i - x_i^t\beta$ denotes the residual at time i, and is a function of β only.

There is no closed-form solution to the minimization of equation (1), except when a is considered known beforehand, hence kept constant, in which case the problem boils down to traditional OLS regression. Based on this remark, maximum likelihood estimation may be implemented using an alternate optimization scheme, ensuring locally optimal parameter estimates [4]. However, because each iteration involves assembling and inverting a $p \times p$ matrix, it may be hopelessly time consuming when dealing with large models. Alternative estimation strategies include pre-coloring [1], pre-whitening [5], bias-corrected OLS estimation [6], restricted maximum likelihood [7], and variational Bayesian techniques [8].

2.3   Online Fitting: The Refined Kalman Filter

In real-time context, we aim to solve the fitting problem each time a new measurement is available, i.e., at time i, process the partial sequence $(y_1, y_2, \dots, y_i)$ as if it was the complete one. We discussed in section 1 the need for specific techniques to achieve such incremental analysis. We present here the refined Kalman filter (RKF) as an alternative to previous online fitting techniques [2,3,4].

The online estimation problem may be formulated in terms of maximizing the likelihood function (1) as applied to the sequence available at time i. For better computational tractability, we will however consider a slightly modified version of the likelihood criterion:

$$\tilde{L}_i(\boldsymbol{\beta}, a, \sigma) = i \log \sqrt{2\pi}\sigma + \frac{1}{\sigma^2} C_i(\boldsymbol{\beta}, a) \tag{2}$$

$$\text{with} \quad C_i(\boldsymbol{\beta}, a) = \underbrace{(1+a^2)\frac{1}{2}\sum_{k=1}^{i} r_k^2(\boldsymbol{\beta})}_{C_i^0(\boldsymbol{\beta})} - \underbrace{2\gamma_i a \frac{1}{2}\sum_{k=2}^{i} r_k(\boldsymbol{\beta}) r_{k-1}(\boldsymbol{\beta})}_{C_i^1(\boldsymbol{\beta})},$$

where we define $\gamma_i \equiv i/(i-1)$. It may be shown that this modified likelihood is asymptotically equivalent to the genuine likelihood in the sense that the average difference $(\tilde{L}_i - L_i)/i$ converges uniformly towards zero (on any bounded open set) as i approaches infinity. Therefore, the minimizers of (2) inherit the general maximum likelihood property of being asymptotically unbiased. Notice that for the parameter $\boldsymbol{\beta}$, the property holds not only asymptotically, but for any sample size. We introduce the correction factor γ_i to further reduce the estimation bias on a and σ. The RKF principles then arise from the following remarks:

• From equation (2), we observe that the estimation of σ may be completely decoupled from that of $(\boldsymbol{\beta}, a)$; clearly, the optimal scale is determined from the minimum of C_i by: $\sigma_i^2 = (2/i) \min_{\boldsymbol{\beta}, a} C_i(\boldsymbol{\beta}, a)$.

• The criterion $C_i(\boldsymbol{\beta}, a)$ is a weighted sum of two functions of $\boldsymbol{\beta}$ only, $C_i^0(\boldsymbol{\beta})$ and $C_i^1(\boldsymbol{\beta})$, the first of which is the classical OLS criterion, and may be calculated incrementally using a standard Kalman filter. A similar incremental calculation may be used for the second term $C_i^1(\boldsymbol{\beta})$ as it is also quadratic.

• From the calculation of both $C_i^0(\boldsymbol{\beta})$ and $C_i^1(\boldsymbol{\beta})$, an alternate minimization scheme similar to that described in section 2.2 can be used to iteratively estimate the autocorrelation a, and refine the OLS estimate of $\boldsymbol{\beta}$.

The RKF algorithm is detailed in table 1, and commented here below.

Standard Kalman iterations. The Kalman filter is used to incrementally update the OLS criterion C_i^0 defined in equation (2) so as to provide a starting guess of $\boldsymbol{\beta}$ on each scan time. One motivation for this strategy is that the OLS estimator is at least unbiased despite it is not optimal for the GLM-AR model [1,6]. On each scan time i, the Kalman filter updates the minimizer $\boldsymbol{\beta}_i^0$ of C_i^0, the minimum criterion value $c_i^0 \equiv C_i^0(\boldsymbol{\beta}_i)$, as well as its inverse Hessian $\boldsymbol{S}_i^0$. Since the Hessian $\boldsymbol{H}_i^0$ is later needed in the refinement loop, we also update its value recursively in order to avoid inverting $\boldsymbol{S}_i^0$.

Refinement loop. After performing one Kalman iteration, we update the "correction" function $C_i^1(\boldsymbol{\beta})$ involved in equation (2), which is quadratic, hence fully specified by its derivatives up to order two. Let $c_i^1 \equiv C_1^i(\boldsymbol{\beta}_i^0)$, $\boldsymbol{g}_i^1 \equiv \partial C_1^i/\partial\boldsymbol{\beta}(\boldsymbol{\beta}_i^0)$ and $\boldsymbol{H}_i^1 \equiv \partial^2 C_1^i/\partial\boldsymbol{\beta}^2$ denote respectively the function value, gradient and Hessian computed at the current OLS estimate $\boldsymbol{\beta}_i^0$. Those quantities are easily related to their previous values using equation (3) in table 1.

At the stage where both $C_i^0(\boldsymbol{\beta})$ and $C_i^1(\boldsymbol{\beta})$ are calculated, it becomes possible to minimize $C_i(\boldsymbol{\beta}, a)$ as defined in equation (2), which is the actual estimation criterion we are interested in. To that end, we perform an alternate minimization of $C_i(\boldsymbol{\beta}, a)$. When $\boldsymbol{\beta}_i$ is held fixed, the optimal autocorrelation is clearly given by $a_i = \gamma_i C_i^1(\boldsymbol{\beta}_i)/C_i^0(\boldsymbol{\beta}_i)$. On the other hand, when a_i is fixed, re-estimating $\boldsymbol{\beta}$ amounts to minimizing the sum of two quadratic functions, yielding a closed-form solution given by equation (4) in table 1. The formula involves $\boldsymbol{S}_i \equiv (\partial^2 C_i/\partial\boldsymbol{\beta}^2)^{-1}$, the inverse Hessian of $C_i(\boldsymbol{\beta}, a)$ w.r.t. $\boldsymbol{\beta}$, which is a function of a_i only as it is independent of $\boldsymbol{\beta}_i$. This matrix plays a key role at the detection stage as it closely relates to the covariance of $\boldsymbol{\beta}_i$ (see section 2.4).

Comparison with EKF. The key feature of the RKF is that its incremental updates do not involve any approximation, unlike the EKF [4] which proceeds by successive linearizations. This property is achieved exploiting the specific form of the estimation criterion (2), and jointly updating the two quadratic functions $C_i^0(\boldsymbol{\beta})$ and $C_i^1(\boldsymbol{\beta})$ exactly. Hence, the data information is fully preserved by the RKF, whereas it is unavoidably degraded across iterations using an EKF.

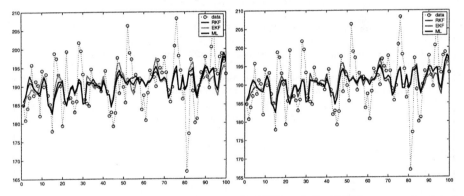

Fig. 1. Comparative fitting example using the RKF and the EKF in an event-related paradigm (see section 3). From left to right, RKF (dark curve) and EKF (bright curve) results using respectively 1 and 2 local iterations are compared with the maximum likelihood result (black curve) computed using the offline algorithm described in section 2.2. In this case, the model contains 15 regressors.

2.4 Online Detection

On each scan time i the RKF provides a current estimate $\boldsymbol{\beta}_i$ of the effect in each voxel. However, to test whether the effect is significant, we also need to evaluate some kind of measure of uncertainty on this estimate. Based on the remark that our estimation criterion is an asymptotically valid likelihood function (see section 2.3), its inverse "Fisher information" is a natural approximation of the variance matrix of $\boldsymbol{\beta}_i$: $\mathrm{Var}(\boldsymbol{\beta}_i) \approx (\frac{\partial^2 \tilde{L}_i}{\partial\boldsymbol{\beta}^2})^{-1} = \sigma_i^2 \boldsymbol{S}_i$, where σ_i is the current scale estimate, and $\boldsymbol{S}_i$ is the inverse Hessian defined in section 2.3.

Table 1. Refined Kalman Filter (RKF) synopsis.

Initialize with: $\boldsymbol{\beta}_0^0 = \mathbf{0}$, $\boldsymbol{H}_0^0 = \mathbf{0}_p$, $\boldsymbol{S}_0^0 = \lambda \boldsymbol{I}_p$, with λ large enough (e.g. $\lambda = 10^{10}$).
For $i \in \{1, 2, \ldots, n\}$,

1. Update the OLS estimate (standard Kalman iteration). Compute the auxiliary variables:
   $\rho_i = y_i - \boldsymbol{x}_i^t \boldsymbol{\beta}_{i-1}^0$, $\boldsymbol{k}_i = \boldsymbol{S}_{i-1}^0 \boldsymbol{x}_i$, $v_i = \boldsymbol{x}_i^t \boldsymbol{k}_i$, in order to perform the following recursion:

$$\boldsymbol{\beta}_i^0 = \boldsymbol{\beta}_{i-1}^0 + \Delta \boldsymbol{\beta}_i^0 \quad \text{with} \quad \Delta \boldsymbol{\beta}_i^0 = \frac{\rho_i}{v_i} \boldsymbol{k}_i$$

$$\boldsymbol{S}_i^0 = \boldsymbol{S}_{i-1}^0 - \frac{1}{v_i} \boldsymbol{k}_i \boldsymbol{k}_i^t$$

$$\boldsymbol{H}_i^0 = \boldsymbol{H}_{i-1}^0 + \boldsymbol{x}_i \boldsymbol{x}_i^t$$

$$c_i^0 = c_{i-1}^0 + \frac{\rho_i^2}{2 v_i}$$

2. Compute the value, gradient and Hessian of $C_i^1(\boldsymbol{\beta})$ at the new OLS estimate $\boldsymbol{\beta}_i^0$. Using the residuals $r_i = y_i - \boldsymbol{x}_i^t \boldsymbol{\beta}_i^0$ and $r_{i-1} = y_{i-1} - \boldsymbol{x}_{i-1}^t \boldsymbol{\beta}_i^0$, do:

$$c_i^1 = c_{i-1}^1 + (\boldsymbol{g}_{i-1}^1)^t \Delta \boldsymbol{\beta}_i^0 + \frac{1}{2} (\Delta \boldsymbol{\beta}_i^0)^t \boldsymbol{H}_{i-1}^1 \Delta \boldsymbol{\beta}_i^0 + \frac{1}{2} r_i r_{i-1}$$

$$\boldsymbol{g}_i^1 = \boldsymbol{g}_{i-1}^1 + \boldsymbol{H}_{i-1}^1 \Delta \boldsymbol{\beta}_i^0 - \frac{1}{2}(r_{i-1} \boldsymbol{x}_i + r_i \boldsymbol{x}_{i-1})$$

$$\boldsymbol{H}_i^1 = \boldsymbol{H}_{i-1}^1 + \frac{1}{2}(\boldsymbol{x}_i \boldsymbol{x}_{i-1}^t + \boldsymbol{x}_{i-1} \boldsymbol{x}_i^t) \tag{3}$$

3. Refinement loop. Initialize: $\boldsymbol{\beta}_i = \boldsymbol{\beta}_i^0$ and $\boldsymbol{S}_i = \boldsymbol{S}_i^0$, then repeat the following two-pass routine a fixed number of times:
   - Estimate the autocorrelation, using the values of $C_i^0(\boldsymbol{\beta})$ and $C_i^1(\boldsymbol{\beta})$ at the current estimate $\boldsymbol{\beta}_i$, and the deviation from the OLS estimate $\Delta \boldsymbol{\beta}_i = \boldsymbol{\beta}_i - \boldsymbol{\beta}_i^0$,

$$\tilde{c}_i^0 = c_i^0 + \frac{1}{2} \Delta \boldsymbol{\beta}_i^t \boldsymbol{H}_i^0 \Delta \boldsymbol{\beta}_i$$

$$\tilde{c}_i^1 = c_i^1 + (\boldsymbol{g}_i^1)^t \Delta \boldsymbol{\beta}_i + \frac{1}{2} \Delta \boldsymbol{\beta}_i^t \boldsymbol{H}_i^1 \Delta \boldsymbol{\beta}_i$$

$$a_i = \gamma_i \frac{\tilde{c}_i^1}{\tilde{c}_i^0}$$

   - Refine $\boldsymbol{\beta}_i$ and the inverse Hessian $\boldsymbol{S}_i$,

$$\boldsymbol{S}_i = \frac{1}{1 + a_i^2} (\boldsymbol{I}_p + \frac{2 \gamma_i a_i}{1 + a_i^2} \boldsymbol{S}_i^0 \boldsymbol{H}_i^1) \boldsymbol{S}_i^0$$

$$\boldsymbol{\beta}_i = \boldsymbol{\beta}_i^0 + 2 \gamma_i a_i \boldsymbol{S}_i \boldsymbol{g}_i^1 \tag{4}$$

4. Estimate the scale:

$$\sigma_i^2 = 2(1 - a_i^2) \frac{\tilde{c}_i^0}{i}$$

Given a contrast vector $\boldsymbol{c}$, we are interested in identifying the voxels that show a contrasted effect $\boldsymbol{c}^t \boldsymbol{\beta}$, for instance, significantly positive. As a first-order approximation, we may assume that the effect's estimate is normally distributed around the true, unknown effect $\boldsymbol{\beta}^*$, i.e. $\boldsymbol{\beta}_i \sim \mathrm{N}(\boldsymbol{\beta}^*, \sigma_i^2 \boldsymbol{S}_i)$. Hence, under the null hypothesis that $\boldsymbol{c}^t \boldsymbol{\beta}^* = 0$, the statistic:

$$z_i = \mathrm{Var}(\boldsymbol{c}^t \boldsymbol{\beta}_i)^{-\frac{1}{2}} \boldsymbol{c}^t \boldsymbol{\beta}_i = \sigma_i^{-1} (\boldsymbol{c}^t \boldsymbol{S}_i \boldsymbol{c})^{-\frac{1}{2}} \boldsymbol{c}^t \boldsymbol{\beta}_i,$$

defines a z-score. Testing for positive activations may thus be achieved at any time i by thresholding the image of z-scores. Notice that this approach may also be interpreted in a Bayesian perspective [4]. As is standard in practice, we apply some spatial Gaussian smoothing to the z-score image before thresholding to improve the localization power of detection [1]. We usually set the threshold so as to match an uncorrected p-value of 10^{-3}, although this should ideally be corrected for multiple comparisons.

3   Results

The method was tested *offline* on several fMRI datasets acquired on our site from both GE Signa 1.5T and Bruker 3T whole-body scanners, always providing final results consistent with SPM'99. For illustration, we present here a "functional calibration" protocol designed to localize the main brain functions in about five minutes. The experimental paradigm contains 11 different conditions (labelled as 'visual', 'motor', 'calculation' and 'language'), from which a total of 100 events are presented pseudo-randomly to the subject. The data was acquired on the Bruker 3T scanner using a 3s repetition time, for a total of 100 scans with $64 \times 64 \times 26$ voxels of size $3.75 \times 3.75 \times 4.5$ mm^3.

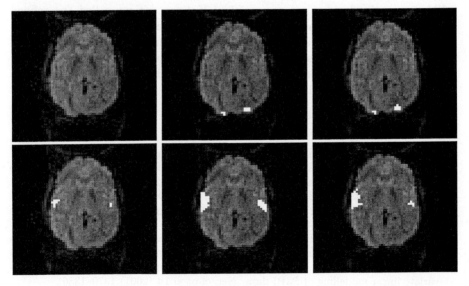

Fig. 2. Incremental detection of visual and auditory regions in a functional calibration paradigm. From left to right, activation maps after respectively 2'00", 3'30" and 5"00".

The RKF algorithm was applied *offline* to the fMRI sequence. One regressor was associated with each condition by convolving its onsets with a canonical hemodynamic response function [1]. Three additional polynomial regressors were used to model the low frequency drifts present in the signal. The number of iterations in the refinement loop was set to three. Using a C implementation, the computation time to process each time frame was about two tenth of second on a standard PC (1.80GHz processor).

The activation maps in figure 2 show in an axial slice the regions that were detected respectively after 40 (2'00"), 70 (3'30") and 100 (5'00"), for a contrast between visual and auditory sentences. As expected, positive effects are found laterally in the occipital lobe where is the visual cortex (top row), while negative effects are found in the temporal lobes (bottom row). After 2'00", no significant visual region is detected in this slice, whereas auditory regions are already appearing. Larger clusters are found after 3'30" without major changes until the end of the sequence. We notice a subtle loss of sensitivity in the right temporal lobe, which might be explained either by a late motion of the subject, or by a neuronal adaptation effect. Although rather qualitative, these results demonstrate the potential use of real-time fMRI, suggesting that functional regions may be detected significantly before the end of an experiment.

4   Conclusion

We have improved our previous incremental, EKF-based detection method for fMRI time series by designing an original Kalman variant called the refined Kalman filter (RKF). The new method achieves excellent statistical performances without requiring any initialization parameter unlike the EKF and classical variants such as the second-order EKF or the unscented Kalman filter [9]. The price to pay is essentially increased memory load, as the RKF tends to run even slightly faster than the EKF.

References

1. Friston, K.J.: 2. In: Human Brain Function. Academic Press (1997) 25–42
2. Cox, R., Jesmanowicz, A., Hyde, J.: Real-Time Functional Magnetic Resonance Imaging. Magnetic Resonance in Medicine **33** (1995) 230–236
3. Gembris, D., Taylor, J., Schor, S., Frings, W., Suter, D., Posse, S.: Functional Magnetic Resonance Imaging in Real Time (FIRE). Magnetic Resonance in Medicine **43** (2000) 259–268
4. Roche, A., Lahaye, P.J., Poline, J.B.: Incremental activation detection in fmri series using kalman filtering. In: Proc. 2st Proc. IEEE ISBI, Arlington, VA (2004) 376–379
5. Woolrich, M., Ripley, B., Brady, M., Smith, S.: Temporal autocorrelation in univariate linear modelling of fMRI data. Neuroimage **14** (2001) 1370–1386
6. Worsley, K., Liao, C., Aston, J., Petre, V., Duncan, G., Morales, F., Evans, A.: A general statistical analysis for fMRI data. Neuroimage **15** (2002) 1–15
7. Friston, K., Penny, W., Phillips, C., Kiebel, S., Hinton, G., Ashburner, J.: Classical and Bayesian Inference in Neuroimaging: Theory. NeuroImage **16** (2002) 465–483
8. Penny, W., Kiebel, S., Friston, K.: Variational Bayesian Inference for fMRI time series. NeuroImage (2003) In press.
9. Julier, S., Uhlmann, J.: A new extension of the kalman filter to nonlinear systems. In: Int. Symp. Aerospace/Defense Sensing, Simul. and Controls. (1997)

Extraction of Discriminative Functional MRI Activation Patterns and an Application to Alzheimer's Disease

Despina Kontos[1], Vasileios Megalooikonomou[1], Dragoljub Pokrajac[2],
Alexandar Lazarevic[3], Zoran Obradovic[1], Orest B. Boyko[4], James Ford[5],
Filia Makedon[5], and Andrew J. Saykin[6]

[1] Department of Computer and Information Sciences, Temple University, Philadelphia, PA
{dkontos,vasilis}@temple.edu, zoran@ist.temple.edu
[2] Department of Computer Science, Delaware State University, Dover, DE
dragoljub.pokrajac@verizon.net
[3] Department of Computer Science, University of Minnesota, Minneapolis, MN
alex@cs.umn.edu
[4] Department of Diagnostic Imaging, Temple University, Philadelphia, PA
oboyko@temple.edu
[5] Department of Computer Science, Dartmouth College, Hanover, NH
jford@cs.dartmouth.edu, makedon@cs.dartmouth.edu
[6] Brain Imaging Laboratory, Departments of Psychiatry & Radiology, Dartmouth Medical
School, Lebanon, NH
saykin@dartmouth.edu

Abstract. We propose a novel Dynamic Recursive Partitioning approach for discovering discriminative patterns of functional MRI activation. The goal is to efficiently identify spatial regions that are associated with non-spatial variables through adaptive recursive partitioning of the 3D space into a number of hyper-rectangles utilizing statistical tests. As a case study, we analyze fMRI datasets obtained from a study that explores neuroanatomical correlates of semantic processing in Alzheimer's disease. We seek to discover brain activation areas that discriminate controls from patients. We evaluate the results by presenting classification experiments that utilize information extracted from these regions. The discovered areas elucidated large hemispheric and lobar differences being consistent with prior findings. The overall classification accuracy based on activation patterns in these areas exceeded 90%. The proposed approach being general enough has great potential for elucidating structure-function relationships and can be valuable to human brain mapping.

1 Introduction

The detection of relationships between human brain structures and brain functions (i.e., human brain mapping) has been recognized as one of the main goals of the Human Brain Project [1]. Several approaches have been used in this problem domain [2]. One of the approaches used in functional brain mapping is to seek associations between brain activation patterns and tasks performed. A current obstacle in this type of analysis is the lack of methods to automatically classify such patterns (i.e., activation regions) and quantitatively measure levels of their similarity. In this paper, we focus

C. Barillot, D.R. Haynor, and P. Hellier (Eds.): MICCAI 2004, LNCS 3217, pp. 727–735, 2004.

on analyzing patterns of brain activity obtained using functional Magnetic Resonance Imaging (fMRI).

One of the most common approaches currently in use, *statistical parametric mapping* (SPM) [3] analyzes each voxel's changes independently of the others and builds a corresponding map of statistical values. The significance of each voxel is ascertained statistically by means of Student's t-test, F-test, correlation coefficient, or other univariate statistical parametric tests. The *multiple comparison problem*, which occurs when computing a statistic for many pairwise tests (introducing significant computational overhead), is usually handled by estimating corrected p-values for clusters.

Another approach to the problem is to model (estimate) the underlying distributions of the distinct classes (controls vs. patients) [4-5], utilizing parametric, nonparametric or semi-parametric techniques. EM and k-means algorithms [6] have been used in order to estimate the distribution densities. Statistical distance based methods are often used for distinguishing among distributions. The Mahalanobis distance [7] and the Kullback-Leibler divergence [6] are most often employed. The main problem of these techniques is that real data are not accurately modeled using a simple mixture of Gaussian components, since they correspond to highly non-uniform distributions.

In the proposed approach, we use an adaptive recursive partitioning approach on the 3D domain to discover highly informative 3D sub-regions with respect to the development of a disease. The method operates on brain activation maps generated by SPM when analyzing the subjects independently (post-analysis of activation maps has been shown to be very useful [8]). More specifically, we utilize *Dynamic Recursive Partitioning* (DRP) initially presented in [9] for the analysis of binary artificial and realistic data. Some initial attempts to apply the technique on brain images have been reported in [10]. Here, we present a detailed description of how we extended DRP in order to be applicable to real 3D functional activity data. We also present the results of a comprehensive study on a collection of datasets obtained from a series of semantic decision tasks designed to explore neuroanatomical correlates in Alzheimer's disease (AD) [11]. These results clearly demonstrate the ability of DRP to identify discriminative spatial patterns arising from functional imaging information, assisting in medical decision making. We also investigate the case of developing a classification model based on neural networks that utilizes information extracted from the subregions indicated by DRP to provide prediction and diagnosis.

2   Methodology

We seek to discover highly discriminative regions with respect to class membership (controls vs. patients). In the discussion that follows we present the method for a two-class problem although it can be easily extended to more than two classes. In order to evaluate the method we also seek to construct features (attributes) that can be used to develop and train a classification model for prediction and medical diagnosis.

The method is applied on activation maps that are the output of SPM (operating on individual subjects independently). SPM creates 3D activation maps of contrast and statistical significance values for pairs of conditions. The proposed algorithm treats the initial 3D volume of activation maps as a hyper rectangle and searches for infor-

> **Given**: Oct-tree T corresponding to the spatial domain D; Two sets $S_Y = \{S_{1,Y}, \ldots S_{n1,Y}\}$, $S_N = \{S_{1,N}, \ldots S_{n2,N}\}$ containing region data for samples belonging to classes Y and N respectively.
>
>   DYNAMIC RECURSIVE PARTITIONING (T,node, SY, SN)
>   *If* SPLITTING_CRITERION(T,node, SY, SN)=='yes'
> T=SPLIT(T,node)
>   *for* node_c *in* CHILDREN (T,node)
> T=DYNAMIC RECURSIVE PARTITIONING (T,node_c, SY, SN)
>   *Else*
>   ADD_TO_LEAF_LIST (node)
>   Return T

Fig. 1. The outline of the DRP algorithm in pseudocode

mative regions by partitioning the space into sub-regions (cuboids), in an adaptive way. We use the mean V_{mean} of all voxel values belonging to the cuboid under consideration as a measurement of activation/deactivation level. This measurement is treated as a candidate feature (attribute) for the corresponding sub-region. The adaptive partitioning of the 3D space continues in the following way: A hyper-rectangle is partitioned only if the corresponding attribute does not have a sufficient discriminative power to determine the class of samples. This is determined by the use of statistical tests, where a statistical significance threshold is employed (e.g. p-value < 0.001) as a stopping criterion for splitting. The procedure progresses recursively until all remaining sub-regions are discriminative or a sub-region becomes so small that it cannot be further partitioned. For this reason, the maximum number of partitioning steps (depth) that the partitioning can go through is also predefined. For the implementation of this procedure, efficient data representation and manipulation is accomplished using augmented oct-trees [12] and a dynamic array [13] to store pointers to the leaf nodes. If the splitting criterion is satisfied, the spatial sub-domain (or cuboid) corresponding to the node of the oct-tree is partitioned into 8 smaller sub-domains. The corresponding tree node becomes the parent of eight children nodes, each representing a new sub-domain. The new measurements V_{mean} corresponding to the children nodes become the new candidate attributes. Figure 1 shows the outline of the DRP algorithm.

As described above, the adaptive partitioning of the 3D space is guided by a statistics-based stopping criterion. Several statistical tests can be applied for this purpose. For example, the Pearson correlation coefficient [14] between the class label (considered as a binary numeric value) and the attribute value for each sample (V_{mean}) could be computed and an attribute considered significant if the correlation coefficient is larger than the pre-determined threshold. Another criterion is based on discretization of the candidate attribute and evaluation of the class/attribute contingency matrix using statistical tests (chi-square or the Fisher exact test [15]) with pre-determined maximal type I errors. A suitable value for the discretization threshold can be set ad-hoc or by using discretization techniques that maximize class/attribute mutual information [16]. Finally, the significance of a candidate attribute can be assessed by deciding whether the distributions of attribute values corresponding to the classes differ substantially using parametric (e.g. t-test [14]) or non-parametric tests (e.g. Wilcoxon rank sum [17]).

The proposed method effectively reduces the number of times a statistical test is applied due to the adaptive approach that is used. This is because the statistical tests are applied selectively on groups of voxels (cuboids), focusing only on certain potentially discriminative sub-regions. This is in contrast to the traditional voxel-wise application of statistical tests, such as in SPM [3], were repeated statistical tests on a voxel-wise basis introduce the *multiple comparison problem* (see Section 1).

3   Experimental Evaluation

3.1   The Dataset and Preprocessing

Our dataset consisted of 3D activation maps of 9 Alzheimer's disease patients and 9 elderly controls. The brain activation data were collected during a series of cognitive tests [11]. These tasks were selected to differentially probe semantic knowledge of categorical, functional, and phonological congruence between word pairs: (a) Category exemplar (catx): identify word pairs with correct category exemplar relationships from among incorrect ones, (b) Category function (catf): identify word pairs with correct category function relationships from among incorrect ones, (c) Nonsense pairs (nonpr): listen to nonsense pseudo-word pairs and decide if they are the same or different, and (d) Episodic recognition memory task (imprec): identify formerly heard words and pseudowords encountered in catx and catf tasks above versus new foils.

The word pairs were presented in groups of four at 7.0 second intervals, with each 28.0 second block of decision followed by a 10.5 second period of rest. Scans were conducted at 1.5 Tesla using a single shot, gradient echo, echo planar functional scan sequence (TR = 3500 ms, TE = 40 ms, interleaved, FOV = 24 cm, slice thickness = 6 mm, NEX = 1, flip angle= 90) on a General Electric Signa scanner with a multi-axial local gradient head coil system (Medical Advances, Inc., Milwaukee, WI). Scans consisted of 20–23 contiguous sagittal slices in a 64x64 matrix with in-plane resolution of $3.75mm^2$ (total slice acquisitions per run = 1920 scans) with anatomical reference images in the same slice locations using aT1-weighted spin-echo pulse sequence (TR = 450 ms; TE = 17 ms; interleaved; matrix = 256x192; NEX = 1; same FOV, slice thickness, and locations as the functional scans). All scans for each subject were acquired in the same session.

Prior to the application of the proposed technique, we applied preprocessing to bring homologous regions into spatial coincidence through spatial normalization. The spatial normalization of the scans to a standard template brain using the anatomical reference images was carried out in SPM99, resulting in resampling of the data to $2mm^3$ isotropic voxels. The resampled data were smoothed with a Gaussian filter (FWHM $15mm^3$). Each subject's task-related activation was analyzed individually versus the subject's rest condition, resulting in individual contrast maps giving a measurement of fMRI signal change at each voxel.

To reduce the effect of noise and sensor fluctuations in the original functional data we applied the following steps. First, we removed the effect of the background noise by subtracting the signal value measured in representative background voxels from all the voxels of the 3D volume. Second, we masked the data using a binary mask extracted from the T1 anatomical atlas used as the template the data were spatially registered to. Only signal within the binary mask was included in the analysis.

3.2   Experiments and Results

After preprocessing (see Section 3.1) we applied the DRP algorithm to the dataset to detect discriminative activation patterns. As splitting criterion, we considered two different statistical tests: t-test and non-parametric rank-sum test. The maximum allowed tree depth was set to 3 and 4. For the significance threshold value of the stopping criterion (min correlation or maximal p-value for statistical tests) we experimented with the values of 0.05 and 0.01. The majority of the results elucidated large hemispheric and lobar differences between Alzheimer's patients and controls for all semantic decision tasks. In particular, for CATX (semantic memory) major differences were seen in the right posterior parietal and temporal lobe regions. A more focal left inferior prefrontal region was also present. For CATF (semantic memory) group differences appeared primarily in the right frontal and distributed posterior regions including the left inferior temporal lobe. The NONPR (phonological discrimination) task showed differences in a highly dispersed set of regions including bilateral frontotemporal, parietal and subcortical sites which were more pronounced for the right than left hemisphere. Finally, in IMPREC (episodic memory), a distributed network of differences in memory associated regions including the right frontal and medial temporal regions and the left fronto-temporal neocortex was demonstrated.

The neuropathology of early AD is relatively diffuse with atrophy in widespread cortical and subcortical areas, including the medial temporal lobes and temporal parietal and frontal cortical regions [18]. On functional neuroimaging studies (fMRI and PET) patients with very early AD manifest as Mild Cognitive Impairment (MCI) often show compensatory activations outside of areas typically used by healthy elderly controls [19]. This is thought to represent the brain's recruitment of proximal and possibly distal neural units in an attempt to maintain performance in the face of progressive pathology. Therefore, the findings of multiple distributed regions that differentiate patients and controls, as detected by the DRP, may be consistent with a distributed reorganization of networks subserving the semantic memory task [11]. Due to space limitations, Figure 2 illustrates some of these regions (overlayed on the T1 atlas).

To evaluate the predictive power and association of the indicated ROIs with the disease, we proceeded with classification experiments. The goal is, given an fMRI image of a new subject, to determine the group to which it belongs, i.e., control vs. patient. For the classification model we used Neural Networks. As inputs to the classifier we used the attributes V_{mean} of the detected discriminative regions, standardized to have zero mean and unit standard deviation. As output we used a binary class label indicating the class of the samples. To avoid overfitting due to a small training dataset we applied one-layer perceptron networks trained by the Pocket algorithm [20]. The leave-one-out approach was employed to evaluate out of sample classification [6-7]. More specifically, the training set consisted of patients and controls with indices $1,2,3,\ldots,i-1,i+1,\ldots9$ and the method was tested on patient and control with an index i, where $i=1,\ldots,9$. Taking into consideration the stochastic nature of the Pocket algo-

rithm, we repeated the process of training and testing the model in each of the leave-
one-out loops for 5 times and averaged the percentage of the correct predictions to
obtain the reported accuracy. Table 1 shows the most characteristic classification results obtained for control and patient samples separately as well as the *total* classification

Table 1. Classification accuracy based on discriminative regions detected by DRP for different
experimental settings and cognitive task dataset

Cognitive Test	Statistical Test	Threshold	Tree Depth	Accuracy		
				Controls	Patients	Total
CATX	t-test	0.05	4	84.44 %	100 %	92.22 %
CATF	t-test	0.05	4	82.22 %	97.78 %	90.00 %
IMPREC	t-test	0.05	4	93.33 %	93.33 %	93.33 %
NONPR	t-test	0.05	4	86.67 %	95.56 %	91.11 %
CATF	ranksum	0.01	4	88.89 %	100 %	94.44 %
NONPR	ranksum	0.01	4	91.11 %	100 %	95.56 %

Table 2. Comparative classification accuracy using distributional distance-based approaches
and static partitioning of the volume for the *CATX* set

Alternative Method	Accuracy		
	Controls	Patients	Total
Maximum Likelihood - EM	77.04	67.04	72.04
Kullback-Leibler - EM	79.26	57.04	68.15
Static partitioning	57.78%	78.89%	68.33%

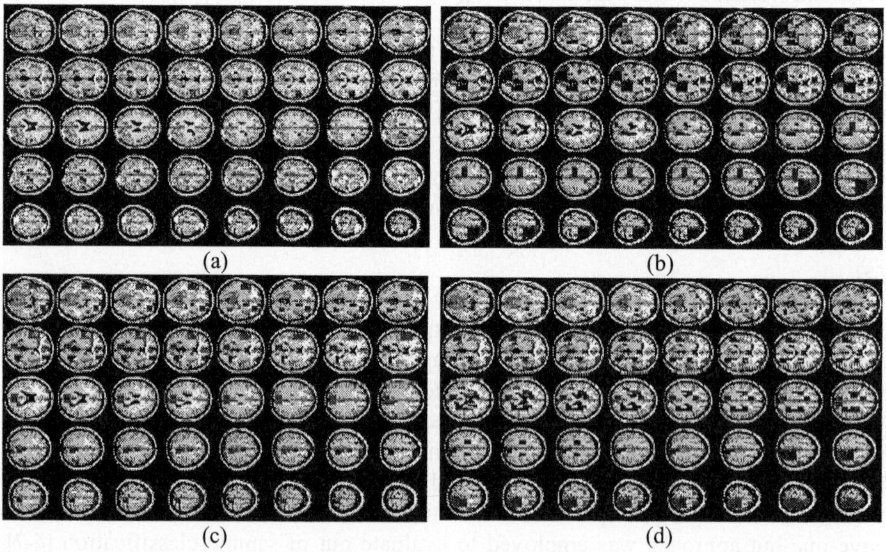

(a)   (b)

(c)   (d)

Fig. 2. The areas discovered by DRP when applied with t-test, significance threshold 0.05 and
maximum tree depth 4 for (a) CATX, (b) CATF, (c) IMPREC and (d) NONPR tasks

accuracy for each experiment; the accuracy achieved was 90% or more. As Table 2 shows, *DRP* outperforms other methods, such as distributional distance-based methods [4-5] and static partitioning where each dimension is split into 3 equal length bins, resulting in 27 cuboids that span the entire 3D space (best obtained results). DRP also outperformed a Fisher linear discriminant classifier approach [21]. Finally the results support the argument that the regions discovered by DRP in the specific study are indeed discriminative for AD and may be useful in assisting early detection of AD.

4   Conclusions and Future Work

We proposed and evaluated methods for the analysis of brain activation scans potentially suitable for the effective discovery of spatial activation patterns that are discriminative among different groups of subjects. The methods are applied on activation maps that are the output of SPM (operating on individual subjects independently). We replace the typical "second level" of SPM analysis (group model) by a *Dynamic Recursive Partitioning* (DRP) procedure that utilizes statistical tests to guide the recursive splitting of the spatial domain. We applied DRP to discover discriminative activation patterns associated with Alzheimer's disease (AD). DRP identified large hemispheric and lobar differences between Alzheimer patients and controls. It was not surprising that a broadly distributed set of sites emerged in the results. AD begins with microscopic cell loss and pathology in the medial temporal region which then spreads to broad posterior lobar areas, as reflected in the numerous reports of posterior hypometabolism seen in PET studies. Most of the sites showing classification differences are related to networks involved in human memory processes tapped by one or more of the fMRI tasks. Although there is some variation in the discovered areas related to the cognitive test that was performed to generate the datasets, the choice of the statistical test and other parameters, the most significant regions persist in all examined cases. Experiments demonstrated the ability of the indicated regions to provide efficient classification and discriminative information, improving on previous work [21] using the Fisher linear discriminant classifier. The proposed technique considers groups of voxels (spatial sub-domains) and effectively reduces the computational cost of repeated statistical tests. Experiments demonstrated that this technique outperforms other approaches, such as distributional distance-based methods, static partitioning and Fisher linear discriminant classifier. It is also more robust than methods performing voxel-wise analysis that are more prone to registration errors and variability of individual voxel values across runs, subjects and analysis techniques.

Acknowledgements. This work was supported in part by NSF (IIS-0083423, IIS-0237921), NIH R01 MH68066-01A1 (funded by NIMH, NINDS, and NIA), Alzheimer's Association, Delaware State University PDF fund, and NIA AG19771.

References

1. Koslow, S.H., Huerta, M.F., NeuroInformatics: an Overview of the Human Brain project, Mahway, NJ, Lawrence Erlbaum, (1997)
2. Megalooikonomou, V., Ford, J., Shen, L., Makedon, F., Saykin, F.: Data mining in brain imaging, Statistical Methods in Medical Research, 9 (2000) 359-394
3. Friston, KJ., Holmes, AP., Worsley, KJ., Poline, JP., Frith, CD., Frackowiak, RSJ.: Statistical parametric maps in functional imaging: a general linear approach. Human Brain Mapping (1995) 189–210
4. Lazarevic, A., Pokrajac, D., Megalooikonomou, V., Obradovic, Z.: Distinguishing Among 3-D Distributions for Brain Image Data Classification, in Proceedings of the 4th International Conference on Neural Networks and Expert Systems in Medicine and Healthcare, Milos Island, Greece (2001) 359-394
5. Pokrajac, D., Lazarevic, A., Megalooikonomou, V., Obradovic, Z.: Classification of brain image data using meaasures of distributional distance, 7th Annual Meeting of the Organization for Human Brain Mapping (OHBM01), Brighton, UK (2001)
6. Duda, R., Hart, P., Stork, D.: Pattern Classification, John Wiley and Sons, NY (2000)
7. Fukunaga, K.: Introduction to Statistical Pattern Recognition, Academic Press, San Diego (1990)
8. Coulon, O., Mangin, J.-F., Poline, J.-B., Zilbovicius, M., Roumenov, D., Samson, Y., Frouin, V., Bloch, I.: Structural group analysis of functional maps, NeuroImage, 11(6) (2000) 767-782
9. Megalooikonomou, V., Pokrajac, D., Lazarevic, A., V., Obradovic, Z.: Effective classification of 3-D image data using partitioning methods, in Proc. of the SPIE 14th Annual Symposium in Electronic Imaging: Conference on Visualization and Data Analysis San Jose, CA, Jan. (2002)
10. Megalooikonomou, V., Kontos, D., Pokrajac, D., Lazarevic, A., Obradovic, Z., Boyko, O., Saykin, A., Ford, J., Makedon, F.:Classification and Mining of Brain Image Data Using Adaptive Recursive Partitioning Methods: Application to Alzheimer Disease and Brain Activation Patterns, Human Brain Mapping Conf. (OHBM'03), New York, NY (2003) also in NeuroImage, 19 (2) S48 (2003)
11. Saykin, A.J., Flashman, L.A., Frutiger, S.A., Johnson, S.C., Mamourian, A.C., Moritz, C.H., O'Jile, J.R., Riordan, H.J., Santulli, R.B., Smith, C.A., Weaver, J.B.: Neuroanatomic substrates of semantic memory impairment in Alzheimer's disease: Patterns of functional MRI activation, Journal of the International Neuropsychological Society, 5 (1999) 377-392
12. Fujimura, K. , Toriya, H., Yamaguchi, K., Kunii, T. L.: Oct-tree algorithms for solid modeling, in Computer Graphics, Theory and Applications, T. L. Kunii ed., Springer Verlag, (1983) 96-110
13. Cormen, T. H., Leadsperson, C. E., Rivest, R. L.: Introduction to Algorithms, 2nd edn., MIT Press, Cambridge (2001)
14. Devore, J.L.: Probability and Statistics for Engineering and the Sciences, 5th edn., International Thomson Publishing Company, Belmont (2000)
15. Agresti, A.: An Introduction to Categorical Data Analysis, Wiley, New York (1996)
16. Ching, J., Wong, A.: Class-dependent discretisation for inductive learning from continuous and mixed-mode data, IEEE Trans. Pattern Analysis and Machine Inteligence, 17 (1995) 641-651
17. Conover, W.J.: Practical Nonparametric Statistics, Wiley, New York (1999)
18. Flashman, L.A., Wishart, H.A., Saykin, A.J.: Boundaries Between Normal Aging and Dementia: Perspectives from Neuropsychological and Neuroimaging Investigations, in: Emory VOB and Oxman TE, editors. Dementia: Presentations, Differential Diagnosis and Nosology. Baltimore: Johns Hopkins University Press (2003) 3-30

19. Saykin A.J., Wishart H.A.: Mild cognitive impairment: Conceptual issues and structural and functional brain correlates. Seminars in Clinical Neuropsychiatry, 8 (2003) 12-30
20. Gallant, S.I.: Perceptron-Based Learning Algorithms, in IEEE Transactions on Neural Networks, 1 (1990) 179-191
21. Ford, J., Farid, H., Makedon, F., Flashman, L.A., McAllister, T.W., Megalooikonomou, V., Saykin, A.J.: Patient Classification of fMRI Activation Maps, in Proc. of the 6th Annual International Conference on Medical Image Computing and Computer Assisted Intervention (MICCAI'03), Montreal, Canada, Lecture Notes in Computer Science 2879 (2003) 58-65

Functional Brain Image Analysis Using Joint Function-Structure Priors

Jing Yang[1], Xenophon Papademetris[2], Lawrence H. Staib[1,2],
Robert T. Schultz[3], and James S. Duncan[1,2]

[1] Departments of Electrical Engineering
[2] Diagnostic Radiology
[3] Child Study Center
Yale University, P.O. Box 208042, New Haven CT 06520-8042, USA,
j.yang@yale.edu

Abstract. We propose a new method for context-driven analysis of
functional magnetic resonance images (fMRI) that incorporates spatial relationships between functional parameter clusters and anatomical
structure directly for the first time. We design a parametric scheme that
relates functional and structural spatially-compact regions in a single
unified manner. Our method is motivated by the fact that the fMRI and
anatomical MRI (aMRI) have consistent relations that provide configurations and context that aid in fMRI analysis. We develop a statistical
decision-making strategy to estimate new fMRI parameter images (based
on a General Linear Model-GLM) and spatially-clustered zones within
these images. The analysis is based on the time-series data and contextual information related to appropriate spatial grouping of parameters in
the functional data and the relationship of this grouping to relevant gray
matter structure from the anatomical data. We introduce a representation for the joint prior of the functional and structural information, and
define a joint probability distribution over the variations of functional
clusters and the related structure contained in a set of training images.
We estimate the Maximum A Posteriori (MAP) functional parameters,
formulating the function-structure model in terms of level set functions.
Results from 3D fMRI and aMRI show that this context-driven analysis potentially extracts more meaningful information than the standard
GLM approach.

1 Introduction

Functional magnetic resonance images (fMRI) has revolutionized the study of
normal and pathological brain function. Its ability to localize brain function
has become crucial in neuroscience for characterizing and understanding brain
function.

General Linear Model (GLM) [1] was introduced to functional imaging to
generalize the simple t-test approach to activation detection and allow the incorporation of more specific modeling. These ideas can be written as an estimation problem, where one has a set of data at one voxel over time written as a

C. Barillot, D.R. Haynor, and P. Hellier (Eds.): MICCAI 2004, LNCS 3217, pp. 736–744, 2004.
© Springer-Verlag Berlin Heidelberg 2004

column vector, $\mathbf{v}$, a design matrix B made up of column vectors representing different temporal aspects of the modeling, including the functional paradigm, cardiac motion, etc., and a set of coefficients $\mathbf{y}$ also written as a column vector. One estimates an optimal set of coefficients by solving: $\hat{\mathbf{y}} = \arg\max_{\mathbf{y}} \|\mathbf{v} - B\mathbf{y}\|$. Then, for each component of $\mathbf{y}$, one can observe the variation over many data sets or spatial voxels and test for differences under different conditions.

In order to improve the detection of activated areas, spatial smoothing is used. However, smoothing may produce a biased estimate by displacing activation peaks and underestimating their height. Spatial modeling has been proposed to begin to take the spatial activation pattern into consideration using, for example, Markov random field approaches [2] which model the activation with spatial smoothing priors. Others incorporate local spatial context with probabilistic models of the signal [3]. Woolrich et al. [4] use an autoregressive spatio-temporal model of the noise. Solo et al. [5] proposed incorporating spatial information without smoothing using spatio-temporal system identification. A spatiotemporal linear regression method for fMRI activation detection [6] has also been developed. Friston and Penny [7] use a hierarchical model with an expectation-maximization (EM) framework to estimate spatial covariances that will help determine statistical priors for a voxel-wise estimation of the GLM parameters. Other work formulates fMRI signal reconstruction using support vector regression [8].

Contextual information can be incorporated using clustering methods for fMRI data analysis. Statistical clustering offers a relatively unsupervised approach for partitioning data into self-similar groups without prior knowledge of the form of the fMRI response [9]. These techniques are primarily concerned with temporal features, although spatial context is sometimes considered. Salli et al. use clustering in conjunction with an MRF model [10]. The contextual information here is primarily limited to agreement with local neighborhoods. Kiebel et al. [11] have incorporated anatomic basis functions based on Gaussian-blurred flattened gray matter surfaces. However, the surface-based representation limits the expressiveness of the approach. Penny and Friston [12] use EM for a kind of spatio-temporal clustering based on a GLM model using mixtures of Gaussians.

It is our goal in this paper to develop a framework where coherent information in a single registered function/structure space can be reasoned about in a unified way to obtain more contextually-informed functional and structural quantitative parametric information about the human brain. We intend to incorporate context not simply in terms of local neighborhoods but in terms of anatomic regions. The study of normal and Autism Spectrum Disorders (ASD) subjects with fMRI using face/object recognition tasks designed based on the deficits associated with ASD, yielded significant functional activation differences between groups in the area of the fusiform gyrus and the amygdala. We endeavor to incorporate both function and structure in order to gain more sensitivity and apply them into ASD study.

2   Integration for Functional/Structural Analysis

2.1   MAP Framework with Function-Structure Joint Prior

Local spatial continuity of functional activation parameters (e.g. regularizing, or smoothing, assumptions on components of $\mathbf{Y}$) as well as proper anatomical location (e.g. is the functional information in gray matter or not?) each are separately useful as constraints for more sensitively detecting activation. Here, we propose to combine these two ideas with GLM in order to find improved estimates of GLM-like parameters $\mathbf{Y}'$ that: agree with the functional data $\mathbf{V}$, are spatially-coherent over individual voxels at spatial position and are roughly constrained (accounting for image resolution) to lie within particular regions. Assume a level set [13] representation of the underlying gray matter structure of interest $\mathbf{S}$ and the activation clusters image that is related to this structure $\mathbf{I_A}$, we can maximize $p(\mathbf{I_A}, \mathbf{Y}'|\mathbf{V}, \mathbf{S})$ using the following MAP equation (including simplification via multiple applications of Bayes rule and taking logarithms):

$$\hat{\mathbf{I}}_\mathbf{A}, \hat{\mathbf{Y}}' = \arg\max_{\mathbf{I_A}, \mathbf{Y}'} \left[\ln p(\mathbf{V}|\mathbf{I_A}, \mathbf{Y}', \mathbf{S} = \tilde{\mathbf{S}}) + \ln p(\mathbf{Y}'|\mathbf{I_A}, \mathbf{S} = \tilde{\mathbf{S}}) + \ln p(\mathbf{I_A}, \mathbf{S} = \tilde{\mathbf{S}}) \right] \quad (1)$$

While the joint prior $p(\mathbf{I_A}, \mathbf{S})$ will be found from training data, the segmented structure in each aMRI test image $\tilde{\mathbf{S}}$ will limit the search space for each problem (i.e. $\mathbf{S} = \tilde{\mathbf{S}}$).

The first term requires that the new GLM-like parameter values $\mathbf{Y}'$ agree with the fMRI data $\mathbf{V}$. For our initial design, this term essentially reduces to GLM with design matrix B:

$$\ln p(\mathbf{V}|\mathbf{I_A}, \mathbf{Y}', \mathbf{S} = \tilde{\mathbf{S}}) \propto -\|\mathbf{V} - B\mathbf{Y}'\| \quad (2)$$

The second term relates to the gathering of similar-valued $\mathbf{Y}'(\mathbf{x})$'s over spatial voxels $\mathbf{x}$ in the fMRI image. This term will push the estimation towards functional clusters containing $\mathbf{Y}'(\mathbf{x})$ values that are relatively homogeneous and separated in value from the $\mathbf{Y}'(\mathbf{x})$ values that are just outside it, while at the same time requiring that the clusters be near an anatomical structure $\mathbf{S}$. Since the most basic and common approach to activation detection from fMRI data is to separate different $\mathbf{Y}'$ values for two different conditions(task vs. baseline or task vs. task), we can approximate the second term by:

$$\ln p(\mathbf{Y}'|\mathbf{I_A}, \mathbf{S} = \tilde{\mathbf{S}}) \propto -\{T(\mathbf{Y}') \cdot [H(T(\mathbf{Y}') - t_1) - H(T(\mathbf{Y}') - t_2)] - \mathbf{I_A}\}^2 \quad (3)$$

$T(\mathbf{Y}')$ gives the difference of the $\mathbf{Y}'$ with respect to a reference $\mathbf{Y_{ref}}$ obtained from some reference task. H is the Heaviside function: $H(z) = 1, if z \geq 0; H(z) = 0, if z < 0$. t_1 and t_2 are the low and high thresholds to suppress the noise. The computation $T(\mathbf{Y}')$ is a key component of any statistical test that would be used to detect activations (e.g. t-test). Improvements in $T(\mathbf{Y}')$ will directly result in more significant statistics. Construction of appropriate statistical significance tests for this methodology is in ongoing work.

The third term is the joint prior between $\mathbf{I_A}$ and $\mathbf{S}$. It contains the functional prior information, the related structural prior information, as well as their relationship.

2.2   Function-Structure Joint Prior Model

We use level set [13] as our representation to build a model for the function-structure joint prior, and then define the joint probability density function used in Equation 1.

Consider a training set of $2n$ aligned structural and functional images from n subjects, with a shape of interest in each of the n structural images and the coherent activation regions in each of the n functional images $I_{A1}, I_{A2}, ..., I_{An}$. The registration between structural and functional images was done with a rigid linear intensity based method [14]. The surfaces of each of the n shapes in the training set are embedded as the zero level set of n separate higher dimensional level sets $\{S_1, S_2, ..., S_n\}$ with negative distances inside and positive distances outside the object. Using techniques developed previously [15], each of the I_{Ai} and S_i is placed as a column vector with N^3 elements, where N^3 is the number of voxels of each functional image or number of samples of each level set function. We can use vector $[I_{Ai}^T, S_i^T]^T$ as the representation of the activation image and the anatomical structure. Thus, the corresponding training set is $\{[I_{A1}^T, S_1^T]^T, [I_{A2}^T, S_2^T]^T, ..., [I_{An}^T, S_n^T]^T\}$. Our goal is to build a function-structure model over the distribution of the level set function and activation intensity pair.

The mean and variance of the function-structure pair can be analyzed using Principal Component Analysis(PCA) [15]. The mean function-structure pair, $\overline{[I_A^T, S^T]^T} = \frac{1}{n}\sum_{i=1}^{n}[I_{Ai}^T, S_i^T]^T$, is subtracted from each $[I_{Ai}^T, S_i^T]^T$ to create the deviation from the mean. Each such deviation is placed as a column vector in a $2N^3 \times n$ dimensional matrix Q. Using Singular Value Decomposition(SVD), $Q = U\Sigma W^T$. U is a matrix whose column vectors represent the set of orthogonal modes of function-structure variation and Σ is a diagonal matrix of corresponding singular values. An estimate of the function-structure pair $[I_A^T, S^T]^T$ can be represented by k principal components and a k dimensional vector of coefficients(where $k < n$), α[15]: $\begin{bmatrix} \widetilde{I_A} \\ S \end{bmatrix} = \begin{bmatrix} \overline{I_A} \\ S \end{bmatrix} + U_k\alpha.$

Under the assumption of a Gaussian distribution of function-structure pair represented by α, the joint probability of a certain shape S and the related activation image intensity I_A, $p(I_A, S)$, can be represented by:

$$p(\alpha) = \frac{1}{\sqrt{(2\pi)^k |\Sigma_k|}} \exp[-\frac{1}{2}\alpha^T \Sigma_k^{-1} \alpha] \tag{4}$$

Figure 1 shows a training set of fusiform gyri(FG) in 2 out of 9 MR brain images in our sample and the coherent functional activation images generated by $T(\hat{Y}_{GLM}) \cdot [H(T(\hat{Y}_{GLM}) - t_1) - H(T(\hat{Y}_{GLM}) - t_2)]$ (where $\hat{Y}_{GLM}$ is the GLM based estimation) for a face recognition task. Using PCA, we can build a model of the function-structure profile of the FG. Figure 2 illustrates zero level sets and the associated activation intensities corresponding to the mean and two primary modes of variance of the distribution of the profile of the FG. The mean function-structure pair and primary modes are representative of the shapes and activation regions being learned. The shape varies correspondingly as the associated functional intensities vary, and vice versa.

Fusiform Gyri   Functional Activation Clusters

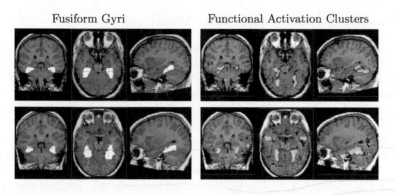

Fig. 1. Training set:fusiform gyri (left) and functional activation clusters (right) from 2 out of 9 subjects overlaid on the anatomical MR brain images.

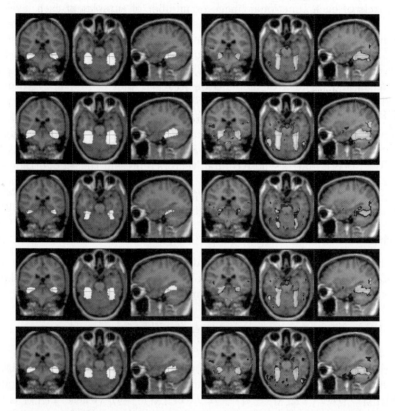

Fig. 2. The two primary modes of variance of the fusiform gyrus (left) and the functional activation clusters (right) overlaid on the mean aMRI. 1st row: The mean; 2nd, 3rd row: $\pm\sigma$ variance of the 1st primary mode; 4th, 5th row: $\pm\sigma$ variance of the 2nd primary mode.

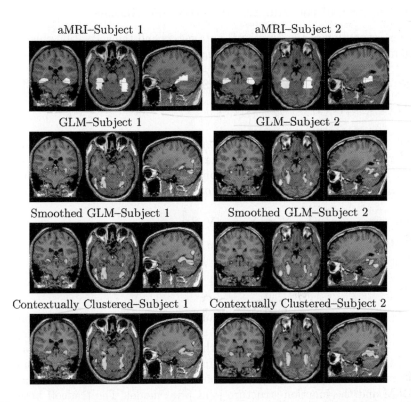

Fig. 3. Contextual fMRI result for two subjects (left and right). Three orthogonal slices of functional clusters overlaid on the aMRI showing functional activation computed using our integrated estimation method (bottom – labeled as contextually clustered) compared with standard GLM (row 2) and smoothed GLM (row 3). $\lambda 1 = \lambda 2 = 0.5$.

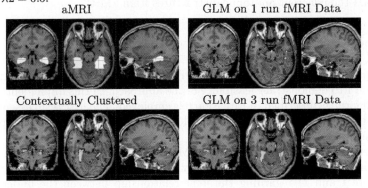

Fig. 4. Contextual fMRI result on 1 run fMRI data. Three orthogonal slices of functional clusters overlaid on the aMRI showing functional activation computed using our integrated estimation method (labeled as contextually clustered) compared with standard GLM on 1 run data and GLM on 3 run data. $\lambda 1 = 0.3$, $\lambda 2 = 0.7$.

2.3   Estimation of the Functional Activation Clusters

The MAP estimation of the functional parameters and the activation clusters in Equation 1 can be expressed by combining Equations 2, 3, and 4.

$$
\begin{aligned}
\hat{\mathbf{I}}_{\mathbf{A}}, \hat{\mathbf{Y}}' &= \arg\min_{\mathbf{I}_{\mathbf{A}}, \mathbf{Y}'} -\ln\Big[p(\mathbf{I}_{\mathbf{A}}, \mathbf{Y}'|\mathbf{V}, \mathbf{S})\Big] = \arg\min_{\mathbf{I}_{\mathbf{A}}, \mathbf{Y}'}\Big[\lambda\|\mathbf{V} - B\mathbf{Y}'\| \\
&\quad + \lambda_1\{T(\mathbf{Y}') \cdot [H(T(\mathbf{Y}') - t_1) - H(T(\mathbf{Y}') - t_2)] - \mathbf{I}_{\mathbf{A}}\}^2 + \lambda_2\alpha^T \Sigma_k^{-1}\alpha\Big]
\end{aligned}
\tag{5}
$$

While we can pose the MAP estimation of both $\hat{\mathbf{Y}}'$ and $\hat{\mathbf{I}}_{\mathbf{A}}$ from the time-series data $\mathbf{V}$ and structural aMRI data $\mathbf{I}$ in this integrated framework, we are more intereted in the estimation of functional activation clusters. Assuming $\hat{\mathbf{Y}}' \approx \hat{\mathbf{Y}}_{\mathbf{GLM}}$, we simplify the estimation of the activation $\hat{\mathbf{I}}_{\mathbf{A}}$:

$$
\begin{aligned}
\hat{\mathbf{I}}_{\mathbf{A}} &= \arg\min_{\mathbf{I}_{\mathbf{A}}} -\ln\Big[p(\mathbf{I}_{\mathbf{A}}, \mathbf{Y}' \approx \hat{\mathbf{Y}}_{\mathbf{GLM}}|\mathbf{V}, \mathbf{S})\Big] \\
&= \arg\min_{\mathbf{I}_{\mathbf{A}}} \lambda_1\{T(\hat{\mathbf{Y}}_{\mathbf{GLM}}) \cdot [H_\varepsilon(T(\hat{\mathbf{Y}}_{\mathbf{GLM}}) - t_1) - H_\varepsilon(T(\hat{\mathbf{Y}}_{\mathbf{GLM}}) - t_2)] - \mathbf{I}_{\mathbf{A}}\}^2 \\
&\quad + \lambda_2\left(\begin{bmatrix} G(\mathbf{I}_{\mathbf{A}}) \\ S \end{bmatrix} - \overline{\begin{bmatrix} I_A \\ S \end{bmatrix}}\right)^T U_k \Sigma_k^{-1} U_k^T \left(\begin{bmatrix} G(\mathbf{I}_{\mathbf{A}}) \\ S \end{bmatrix} - \overline{\begin{bmatrix} I_A \\ S \end{bmatrix}}\right)
\end{aligned}
\tag{6}
$$

where $G(\cdot)$ is an operator to form a column vector from a matrix by column scanning. We use a regularized version of the Heaviside function H, denoted by $H_\varepsilon(z) = \frac{1}{2}[1 + \frac{2}{\pi}\arctan(\frac{z}{\varepsilon})]$ [15]. Thus, the MAP functional activation can be estimated at each evolving step using simple gradient descent on Equation 6.

The parameters λ_1 and λ_2 are used to balance the influence of the estimation from GLM and the function-structure joint prior model. The tradeoff between GLM estimation and function-structure information depends on how much faith one has in the function-structure joint prior model and the functional data for a given application. We set these parameters empirically for particular functional tasks, given the general fMRI quality and the relations between the activation clusters and the coherent anatomical structures from aMRI.

3   Experimental Results

We have implemented this new context-driven fMRI analysis strategy described in Equation 1 to demonstrate feasibility of the approach. In this implementation, a modified form as described in Equation 6 is employed. The first term essentially pushes the new $\hat{\mathbf{I}}_{\mathbf{A}}$ values towards the values constrained by the pre-computed GLM-based values $\hat{\mathbf{Y}}_{\mathbf{GLM}}$.

An example result based on 3 run fMRI data for a face recognition task is shown in Figure 2.2, using n=9 normal controls to form the prior informa-tion (Figure 1 and 2) regarding the joint relationship between the underlying shape/size of the fusiform gyrus (FG) and the typical functional parameter vari-ation in response to this task. Basically, the solution provides a tradeoff between pure GLM data-driven results and prior model-based information. As seen in Figure 2.2, for this test example, the new approach improves the expected ho-mogeneity of object-related activation bilaterally in and around the FG, while suppressing unexpected activations outside these regions, in comparison to standard GLM. The improvement is more evident in the case of the left FG where activations are generally weaker (shown on the right in the images). The results are encouraging, and show that the context-driven analysis potentially extracts more meaningful information than the standard GLM approach.

Next, we test our estimation method comparing the analysis of a single run of data using our method with standard GLM using one and three runs (Using the same task and same subjects as above). As shown in Figure 4, our estimation greatly improves the homogeneity of the activations in the FG and suppresses activations outside these regions. The improvement is very evident for 1 run data, where activations are generally weaker. Furthermore, our 1 run data based estimation results in activation clusters close to the 3 run GLM results. Although a task or stimulus can be repeated over and over again, there are limits due to time constraints, habituation, etc. The results show that our method achieves greater similarity in the detection and characterization of functional activity.

4   Conclusions

The use of context in the analysis of fMRI data that incorporates spatial relationships between functional parameter clusters and anatomical structure has the potential to improve sensitivity. We present a Bayesian MAP formulation using joint prior information of function and anatomy, along with information derived from the input fMRI and aMRI. Our results show that this context-driven analysis potentially extracts information more sensitively and more coherently than the standard GLM approach.

Acknowledgement. The authors would like to thank Andrea P. Jackowski and Pawel Skudlarski for their help with data processing.

References

1. K. J. Friston, A. P. Holmes, K. J. Worsley, J. P. Poline, C. D. Frith, and R. S. J. Frackowiak: Statistical Parametric Maps in Functional Imaging: A General Linear Approach. Human Brain Mapping, 2:189-210, 1995.
2. X. Descombes, F. Kruggel, and D. Y. von Cramon: Spatio-temporal fMRI Analysis Using Markov Random Fields. IEEE TMI, Vol.17, No.6:1028-1039, 1998.
3. Hartvig, N. V. and Jensen, J. L.: Spatial mixture modeling of fMRI data. Human Brain Mapping, 11:233-248 ,2000.
4. M. W. Woolrich, M. Jenkinson, J. M. Brady, and S. M. Smith: Fully Bayesian Spatio-Temporal Modeling of FMRI Data. IEEE TMI, 23(2):213–231, 2004.
5. V. Solo, P. Purdon, R. Weisskoff, and E. Brown: A Signal Estimation Approach to fMRI. IEEE TMI, 20(1):26-35, 2001.
6. Katanoda, K., Matsuda, Y., and Sugishita, M.: A spatio-temporal regression model for the analysis of functional MRI data. NeuroImage, 17:1415-1428, 2002.
7. K. Friston and W. Penny: Posterior Probability maps and SPMs. NeuroImage, 19(3):1240-1249, 2003.

8. Y. Wang, R. Schultz, R. T. Constable, and L. H. Staib: Nonlinear Estimation and Modeling of fMRI data using Spatio-temporal Support Vector Regression. Information Processing in Medical Imaging(IPMI), 647-659, 2003.
9. Goutte, C., Toft, P., Rostrup, E., Nielsin, F., and Hansen, L.: On clustering fMRI time series. NeuroImage, 9:298-310, 1999.
10. E. Salli, H. Aronen, S. Savolainen, A. Korvenoja, and A. Visa: Contextual Clustering for Analysis of Functional MRI Data. IEEE TMI, 20(5):403-414, 2001.
11. S. Kiebel, R. Goebel, and K. Friston: Anatomically Informed Basis Functions. NeuroImage, 11:656-667, 2000.
12. W. D. Penny and K. J. Friston: Mixtures of General Linear Models for Functional Neuroimaging. IEEE TMI, 22(4):504-514, 2003.
13. S. Osher and J. A. Sethian: Fronts propagating with curvature-dependent speed: Algorithms based on Hamilton-Jacobi Formulation. J. Comp. Phy., **79** (1988) 12–49.
14. C. Studholme, D. Hill, D. Hawkes: Automated Three-Dimensional Registration of Magnetic Resonance and Positron Emission Tomography Brain Images by Multiresolution Optimisation of Voxel Similarity Measures. Med. Phys., 24(1):25-35, 1997.
15. J. Yang and J. Duncan: 3D Image Segmentation of Deformable Objects with Shape-Appearance Joint Prior Models. MICCAI, vol.1 (2003) 573-580, 2003.

Improved Motion Correction in fMRI by Joint Mapping of Slices into an Anatomical Volume

Hyunjin Park, Charles R. Meyer, and Boklye Kim

Department of Radiology, University of Michigan Medical School, MI 48109, USA
{hyunjinp, cmeyer, boklyek}@umich.edu
http://www.med.umich.edu/dipl

Abstract. Motion correction in fMRI time series is essential for accurate statistical analyses. Typically motion correction is applied in a rigid fashion between time series volumes. Such corrections assume no relative motion between slices. An improved motion correction scheme, map-slice-to-volume (MSV), was developed previously using mutual information (MI) to register individual fMRI slices onto an anatomical volume to account for inter-slice motion [6]. As each slice's orientation represents a statistically independent sampling of the patient's motion at multiple intervals throughout the acquisition, a smoothed estimate of the patient's trajectory in time can be computed by jointly estimating each slice's orientation while minimizing the implied acceleration of the patient's head subject to applying *a priori,* slice-related weights based on known registration reliabilities. The results of this joint mapping of slices into a volume (JMSV) show further substantial improvement in slice registration and subsequent motion estimation.

1 Introduction

Subject head motion is a major obstacle in accurate measurements of voxel intensity changes in fMRI. A widely used method is to register each EPI (echo planar imaging) volume (i.e., a stack EPI slices) in an fMRI time series onto a reference EPI volume volumetrically [4, 5]. This method assumes that there is no inter-slice motion, i.e. individual slices within a volume do not move independently in the subject's frame of reference. This assumption is valid only when there is very little motion as might occur with the subject's head wedged into the head coil with MRI-compatible packing materials during finger tapping. However, in the presence of frank motion as might occur in a verbalized speech individually acquired slices are no longer parallel in the subject's frame of reference. During the acquisitions of sequential slices in an interleaved acquisition, sequential slices may have significantly different motion trajectories relative to the geometric reference frame of the subject. Previously a new motion correction scheme, MSV (Map Slice to Volume), that can account for inter-slice relative motion was developed and demonstrated an improved capability in correcting image shifts due to the rigid head motion [6]. It allows individual slices within a volume to be mapped onto the subject's anatomic volume reference before statistical testing for activation is performed. Use of the MSV method shows improved sensitivity and specificity in locating activated regions compared to other widely used, parallel slice-stack based methods, e.g. statistical parametric mapping (SPM).

The MSV method uses mutual information as the objective function in the automatic image registration process. For the most part, the estimated position parameters

C. Barillot, D.R. Haynor, and P. Hellier (Eds.): MICCAI 2004, LNCS 3217, pp. 745–751, 2004.
© Springer-Verlag Berlin Heidelberg 2004

from the middle slices of the brain are accurate since there is sufficient information from a large region of support to drive the registration. The reliability of the estimated position parameters for the end cap slices, however, is reduced due to lower information content created by smaller regions of support. Our goal is to improve not only the accuracy of the registration of the end cap slices but the accuracy of the middle slices as well by imposing the condition that the motion trajectory of the subject's head as measured by the resulting time series of slice orientations is acceleration limited, i.e. smooth. In MSV we estimated the position of each slice independently of others. Here we present a method of jointly estimating the position of multiple slices in the time series using MI subject to simultaneously minimizing the associated acceleration in the motion trajectory of the subject. This new motion correction method is referred as the Joint Mapping of Slices into Volume (JMSV) method.

2   Motion Correction Methods

The goal of an fMRI experiment is to localize regions of activation in response to certain stimuli. Typically a time series of low resolution fMRI data are acquired using GRE (gradient recalled echo) -EPI sequence at the rate of 2 to 3 seconds per volume. The image matrix size is typically 128x128 or 64x64. In a block design, alternating phases of activation and rest are repeated. A *high resolution anatomical reference* volume is acquired following the fMRI session. Statistical difference in image intensities between the activation and rest images is used to determine whether the region is active or not. The statistical analysis assumes that the EPI scans are all aligned to a chosen reference scan. Thus, at a given location in the reference scan, it is comparing MR signals coming from the same location over different EPI volumes. An accurate motion correction that guarantees consistent voxel location is essential for accurate statistical analysis. Whereas the commonly used SPM method based on a volumetric rigid registration of EPI volumes works only for cases of limited motion, MSV can correct more complex motion by allowing slices within a volume to move independently and provide an effective localization capability [6]. Here we improve on the results of the MSV method by jointly registering multiple slices onto the subject's anatomical volume.

2.1   Motion Correction by Map Slice to Volume (MSV)

The registration process in MSV is inter-modality, since it registers the T_2^*-weighted EPI slices with the T_1-weighted anatomical scan. MSV uses mutual information (MI) as the similarity measure and 6 DOF rigid transform for the geometric model. MI is an effective similarity measure for inter-modality registrations [2, 3]. The MI used here is the classical Shannon MI where all PDFs, both marginal and joint PDFs, are estimated by a histogram with an appropriately chosen number of bins [2]. The optimizer is the Nelder-Mead simplex optimizer. The following equation (1) is the formulation of the MSV method. The motion correction capabilities of MSV provide improved sensitivity and specificity in localizing activated regions compared to the widely used volume registration methods where the volume is assumed to consist of a set of parallel stack of slices.

$$\hat{\theta}_i = \arg\max_{\theta} MI(S_i(\theta), V_{ref}) \quad i = 0,.., NM - 1 \tag{1}$$

$\theta = (t_x, t_y, t_z, rot_x, rot_y, rot_z)$; rigid motion param.

$\hat{\theta}_i$; estimated motion param. for i-th EPI slice

S_i; i-th EPI slice V_{ref}; anatomical volume

N;No. of EPI scans M; No. of slices per EPI scan

2.2   Joint Mapping of Slices into Volume (JMSV) Method

Sometimes the estimated motion parameters for sequentially acquired slices in a volume using the MSV method can be noisy; at one slice the estimated rotation about z axis could be at 2 degrees and then change to -5 degrees at the subsequently acquired slice. This kind of abrupt change in the motion parameters implies very unlikely motion, since it requires a sudden, large acceleration. This abnormality in the motion parameters typically occurs either at the top or the bottom slices of the EPI head scan. The MSV method provides accurate estimations in motion parameters for slices with sufficient information, i.e., enough detail and no severe geometric distortion. Towards the top slice of the brain, however, slices contain less information (i.e. less textured area and more background) than the slices from the mid-brain region and may not have enough information for the stable estimation of slice position. In the regions near the bottom of the head, slices contain significant geometric distortion, especially where air/tissue interface occurs [7], and this in turn negatively affects the reliability of the motion parameter estimates. Here we implement a joint estimation of the registration of slices while penalizing the implied acceleration. The formulation of the new motion correction method, referred as Jointly Mapping Slices into a Volume (JMSV) method, follows.

$$\hat{\theta} = \arg\max_{\theta} \left\{ \sum_{i=0}^{K-1} w_i MI(S_i(\theta_i), V_{ref}) - \beta R(\theta) \right\} \tag{2}$$

$$= \arg\max_{\theta} \left\{ \sum_{i=0}^{K-1} (w_i MI(S_i(\theta_i), V_{ref}) - \beta((\theta_i - \theta_{i-1}) - (\theta_{i+1} - \theta_i))^2) \right\}$$

θ_i; motion param. for i-th EPI slice

$\theta = (\theta_0,.., \theta_{K-1})$; collection of motion param. over K slices

$\hat{\theta}$; estimated motion param. for K slices

S_i; i-th EPI slice V_{ref}; anatomical volume

w_i; weight associated with MI value of the i-th slice

$R(\theta)$; roughness penalty β; weight for roughness penalty

Motion parameters for K slices are jointly estimated by maximizing the objective function in equation (2). The number K, the number of jointly registered slices, may be as small as 3 or as large as the number of slices in the entire time series. Smoothness of the motion parameters is implemented through a roughness penalty term $R(\theta)$ in the objective function. We have chosen a discrete 2nd order difference roughness penalty. This roughness penalty encourages the motion parameters of sequentially acquired slices to have constant angular and translational velocities. As noted before, some slices may lead to less reliable motion parameter estimations, thus the MI values of those slices should be weighted less than the MI values from more reliable slices in the objective function. For example, we know *a priori* that the top slice and the bottom slice of the brain should be weighted less than the slices in between. In this paper, we used both a flat weighting that does not account for the less reliable slices and a linear weighting that starts at 1 for the middle slice and decreases to 0.05 for both the top slice and the bottom slice. The linear weighting has a triangular waveform when plotted with respect to the location of the slice. Additional computational effort is required to perform the JMSV method since it is jointly estimating the motion parameters for multiple slices rather than estimating the motion parameters for one slice at a time as in MSV. Also it is worthy to note that in case of no roughness penalty (i.e. $\beta=0$) and a flat weighting for MI values (i.e. $w_i=1$), the JMSV method reduces to the MSV method.

3   Experiments

A data set for typical fMRI time series were acquired using GRE-EPI sequence on a GE Signa system operating at field strength of 1.5 Tesla. The acquisition parameters were: 6mm slice thickness with no gaps, FOV= 24x24 cm in 128x128 matrix. A T_1-weighted *high resolution anatomical reference* volume was acquired following the fMRI session using 3D spoiled GRASS (SPGR) sequence where the slice thickness = 1.5mm, and the FOV= 24x24 cm in a 256x256 matrix. For an experiment to test the algorithm, an EPI volume, that was believed to be almost motionless, acquired with no activation, i.e. a dry run, was used. Figure 1 shows a corresponding pair of slices from the EPI dry run and T_1 weighted anatomical volume.

We have applied a series of synthetic rigid motion to individual slices of the dry run to create simulated EPI volumes where the ground truth for the motion is established. The series of synthetic motion was applied in the order of the slice acquisition, not the order of physical stacking of the slices as in figure 2. The synthetic motion was only applied as in-plane rotation about z axis; the direction of inferior/superior. The applied motion is $rot\{z(j)\} = 3\sin(j/4.7746)$, where j is the index of the slice acquisition order and $rot\{z\}$ is the value of rotation about z axis. Two synthetic EPI volumes were created by letting j vary from 0 to 31. Both the MSV and JMSV methods have been applied to recover the motion. For the JMSV method, the flat and triangular weighting, as described earlier, were applied in separate runs and compared. Root mean squared (RMS) errors between the estimated and true motions are reported in Table 1. As shown in table 1, the error is the largest for MSV; the error is reduced using JMSV with uniform weighting, and finally the error is smallest using JMSV with triangular weighting. Figure 3 shows the recovered motion parameters for all the motion correction methods. Typically EPI slices are acquired in an interleaving fashion as in Figure 2. Thus the top two slices occur at the slice acquisition indices 0 and 8, and the bottom two slices at 7 and 15. For the second EPI volume of 16 slices, the top two slices occur at the acquisition indices 16 and 24 and the bottom two occur at 23 and 31. In Figure 3, MSV shows abrupt changes on the slice acquisition indices, 0, 8, 15, and 24, all of which belong to either the top two or the bottom two slices. Improvement is noticeable just by exploiting the correlation of the motion parameters. The RMS error decreased from 1.06 to 0.59 by going from MSV to JMSV with the flat weights. Additional improvement was achieved by incorporating a smart weighting; the RMS error decreased to 0.47 for the JMSV method with the triangular weights.

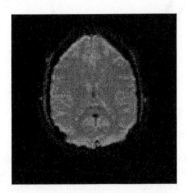 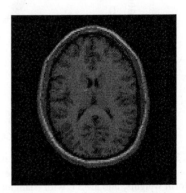

Fig. 1. A corresponding pair of slices from the EPI and anatomical data sets selected from the 3D data sets. The left is the EPI slice and the right is the anatomical T_1 slice. The slices are located in about mid brain.

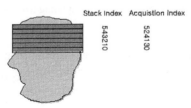

Fig. 2. Comparison of slice acquisition index and slice stacking index of an EPI scan.

4 Summary

Our previous work with MSV demonstrated an effective rigid motion correction by allowing individual slices to move independently as each slice is subject to different motion [6]. Improvement in registration noise reduction is desirable since the registration accuracies were less reliable for slices from the extreme locations of the brain. In this paper, we propose to improve our MSV method by minimizing the implied acceleration for sequentially acquired slices and adopting a slice-based weighting for

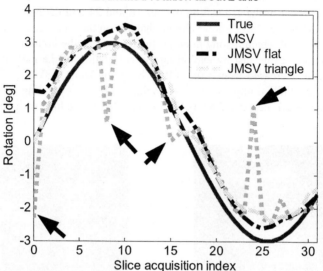

Fig. 3. Recovered motion parameters for different motion correction methods. The true motion parameters are shown in solid red. The estimated motion parameters from MSV, JMSV with uniform weights, and JMSV with triangular weights are in dotted green, dash dotted blue, and dashed yellow respectively. For the MSV method abrupt changes in motion parameters can be observed at the acquisition index 0, 8, 15, and 24 (i.e. marked with arrows). These abrupt changes are smoothed using the JMSV method. There is a substantial improvement by using JMSV instead of MSV. Within the JMSV method, imposing a slice-based weighting related to the variance of the MSV estimate (i.e. triangular weights) further reduces the error as shown in table 1, but this improvement is less noticeable than going from MSV to JMSV.

Table 1. Root Mean Squre (RMS) error associated with different motion correction methods.

Methods	RMS Error [degrees]
MSV	1.06
JMSV with uniform weights	0.59
JMSV with triangular weights	0.47

the similarity measure. Although motion correction methods (i.e. MSV, JMSV with uniform and triangular weights) have been performed on a simulated data set, we believe the error reduction between the methods proves to be meaningful. Future work will include multiple runs of the motion correction methods to establish statistical comparisons. Also, we used triangular weighting to account for *a priori* knowledge of the reliability of the estimated motion parameters. This simple weighting can be further improved by using appropriately estimated variance measures for the registration accuracy of each slice position across subjects. While the JMSV method requires additional computation to implement the joint registration of multiple slices, we believe that the accuracy gained by improved motion correction warrants such costs.

References

1. Jenkinson, M., Smith, S.: The role of registration in functional magnetic resonance imaging. In: Hajnal, J. V., Hill, D. L. G., Hawkes, D. J.(eds.): Medical image registration. CRC press, 2001 183-198.
2. Hill, D. L. G., Batchelor, P. G., Holden, M., Hawkes, D. J.: Medical image registration. Physics in medicine and biology 46 (2001) r1-r45.
3. Meyer, C. R., Boes, J. L., Kim, B., Bland, P. H.: Demonstration of accuracy and clinical versatility of mutual information for automatic multimodality image fusion using affine and thin plate spline warped geometric deformations. Medical image analysis 3 (1997) 195-206.
4. Friston, K. J., Williams, S. R., Howard, R., Frackowiak, R. S. J., Turner, R.: Movement related effects in fMRI time-series. Magnetic resonance in medicine 35 (1996) 346-355.
5. Hajnal, J. V., Myers, R., Oatridge, A., Schwieso, J. E., Young, I. R., Bydder, G. M.: Artefacts due to stimulus correlated motion in functional imaging of the brain. Magnetic resonance in medicine 31 (1994) 283-291.
6. Kim, B., Boes, J. L., Bland, P. H., Chenervert, T. L., Meyer, C. R.: Motion correction in fMRI via registration of individual slices into an anatomical volume. Magnetic resonance in medicine 41 (1999) 964-972.
7. Jezzard, B., Balaban, R. S.: Correction for geometric distortion in echo planar images from B0 field variations. Magnetic resonance in medicine 34 (1995) 65-73.

Motion Correction in fMRI by Mapping Slice-to-Volume with Concurrent Field-Inhomogeneity Correction

Desmond T.B. Yeo[1,2] , Jeffery A. Fessler[2], and Boklye Kim[1]

[1] Department of Radiology, University of Michigan Medical School, MI 48109, USA
{tbyeo,boklyek}@umich.edu
[2] Department of Electrical Engineering and Computer Science, University of Michigan, MI 48109, USA
fessler@umich.edu

Abstract. Head motion is the major source of error in measuring intensity changes related to given stimuli in fMRI. The effects of head motion are image shifts and field inhomogeneity variations which cause local changes in geometric distortions. The previously developed motion correction method, mapping slice-to-volume (MSV), retrospectively remaps slices that are shifted by head motion to their spatially correct locations in an anatomical reference. Images exhibiting spatially varying geometric distortions require non-linear mapping solutions. An accurate field map can be used for the correction of such spatial distortions. However, field-map changes with head motion and, in practice, only one field-map is available typically. This work evaluates the improved motion correction capability of MSV with *concurrent* iterative field-corrected reconstruction using only an initial field-map. The results from simulated motion data show effective convergence and accuracy in image registration for the correction of image artifacts complicated by the motion induced field effects.

1 Introduction

In fMRI, the voxel intensity differences of echo-planar imaging (EPI) data from the stimulus and rest images, typically in the range of 1% to 4%, are used to generate an activation map. A major source of signal variation that has adverse effect in accurate measurements of the voxel intensity changes is rigid head motion. EPI technique is sensitive to magnetic susceptibility-induced geometric distortions, especially in the mid to lower brain images. The effect of head motion is not only the artificial linear spatial shifts in the image intensities, but the subsequent local changes in geometric distortions caused by the field inhomogeneity variations induced by the head rotation. Such effects cause the inconsistency of the voxel positions between the images and, consequently, the inaccuracy in statistical testing of the signal changes in response to the given tasks in activation studies.

In multi-slice EPI data, each slice is subject to different motion. Previously, in our group, a realistic motion-correction scheme, mapping a slice to volume (MSV),

C. Barillot, D.R. Haynor, and P. Hellier (Eds.): MICCAI 2004, LNCS 3217, pp. 752–760, 2004.

that accounts for inter-slice motion, was developed [1]. It allows individual slices within a volume to be mapped onto an anatomically correct volume reference. The MSV method using rigid-body function has demonstrated a capability to accurately correct image shifts due to the rigid head motion and improved sensitivity and specificity in locating activated regions as compared to the widely used, volume-to-volume registration of EPI volumes which assumes no inter-slice motion, i.e., incorrectly stacked EPI slices [1]. While the rigid-body transform function is sufficient for localizing activations in the sensorimotor cortex, spatial distortions in EPI slices acquired from the mid to lower structures of the brain cause difficulty in localizing activations, i.e., language. Consequently, MSV was expanded to include a non-linear warping function for the studies involving activations in mid brain regions [2][3], however, at a computational cost of longer optimization process associated with higher degrees of freedom (DOF) in registration.

Geometric distortion can be corrected by an accurate field-map which quantifies the deviation of the magnetic field induced by the position of an object in the applied field. Since the head movement causes change in a field map, an accurate geometric distortion correction requires multiple real time field-maps to track the temporal changes in the field-inhomogeneity. This may require modified acquisition sequences to collect field maps simultaneously with each EPI slice by collecting additional k-space data, which may not be available in most scanners, with the increased acquisition time to obtain an adequate resolution in field maps.

In this work, a concurrent motion and field-inhomogeneity correction using a quadratic penalized least squares reconstruction is introduced as an enhancement to the MSV process [1][4]. The method requires only the acquisition of an initial field-map. At each iteration, the field map is updated using the motion parameters obtained from MSV. The result demonstrates an improved accuracy in MSV with rigid-body function by incorporating changes in field map to correct image distortions.

2 Background

2.1 EPI Susceptibility-Induced Geometric Distortion

Geometric distortion is readily observed in the area where local magnetic field-inhomogeneity is observed, typically at the boundary of two tissues with significant magnetic susceptibility difference. *Changing the orientation of the tissue boundary with B_0 (i.e., out-of-plane rotations) may change the field-map drastically. Translations and in-plane rotations are less likely to change the susceptibility-induced component of the field-map.* In EPI, field-inhomogeneity causes pixels to shift mainly in the phase-encode, i.e., PE, direction [5]. The shift in PE direction, which causes the local geometric distortion, depends on the EPI readout time $T_{readout}$ and the point field-inhomogeneity $\Delta B(x_i,y)$ as shown in the impulse response

$$h(x_i, y) = \delta\left(x_i, y - \gamma \Delta B(x_i, y_1) T_{readout} \Delta y\right) \tag{1}$$

where γ is the gyromagnetic ratio, y is the voxel length in the PE direction and $\delta(x_i,y)$ is the input impulse location before distortion.

2.2 Map Slice-to-Volume (MSV) Registration

Statistical analysis of brain activations in fMRI relies on the intensity variation at consistent image voxel locations throughout the time series data. The voxel displacements, in-plane and out-of-plane, associated with the patient's head motion is corrected retrospectively by mapping a slice image onto an anatomically correct reference volume (i.e. map-slice-to-volume, MSV) [1]. The MSV method in this paper allows each slice to have its own six DOF, i.e., rigid-body transform. Automated 3D registration of a slice into an anatomical volume is accomplished by optimizing the mutual information metric. The transformation that gives the lowest MI metric in the iterative optimization scheme is used to compute the final position of a slice in the spatial reference.

2.3 Iterative Field-Corrected Reconstruction

Most geometric distortion correction methods assume a smooth field-map [5][6]. We use an iterative field-corrected reconstruction method that does *not* assume a smooth field-map [4]. The continuous object f and field-map $\Delta\omega$ are parameterized into a sum of weighted rect functions $b(\vec{r} - \vec{r}_n)$. Ignoring spin relaxation and assuming uniform receiver coil sensitivity, the parameterized MR signal equation for a slice is

$$s(t_i) \approx B(\vec{k}(t_i)) \sum_{n=0}^{n_p-1} f_n e^{-j\Delta\omega_n t_i} e^{-j2\pi(\vec{k}(t_i)\bullet\vec{r}_n)} \qquad (2)$$

where $s(t_i)$ is the baseband signal sample at time t_i during readout, $B(\vec{k}(t_i))$ is the Fourier transform of $b(\vec{r} - \vec{r}_n)$, f_n and $\Delta\omega_n$ are the object intensity and field-inhomogeneity, respectively, at $\vec{r}_n$. The dominant noise in MRI is conventionally modeled as a white Gaussian noise [7]. In matrix form, the sampled signal vector is

$$y = \mathbf{A}f + \varepsilon \qquad (3)$$

where f and ε are the column-wise stacked vector of the parameterized object and noise, respectively, y is the k-space data vector and $\mathbf{A}$ is the system-object matrix with elements $a_{m,n} = B(\vec{k}(t_m))e^{-j\Delta\omega_n t_m} e^{-j2\pi(\vec{k}(t_m)\bullet\vec{r}_n)}$. The object f is estimated directly from the k-space data y by minimizing a quadratic penalized least squares (QPLS) cost function using the conjugate gradient optimization algorithm in conjunction with time-segmentation and min-max interpolation. The cost function and estimator are

$$\psi_1(f) = \frac{1}{2}\|y - \mathbf{A}f\|^2 + \frac{1}{2}\beta f^T \mathbf{C}^T \mathbf{C} f \qquad (4)$$

$$\hat{f}_{QPLS} = \arg\min_f \psi_1(f) = [A^*A + \beta R]^{-1} A^*[Af + \varepsilon] \qquad (5)$$

where $\mathbf{C}$ is a $n_p\text{-}1 \times n_p$ second order differencing matrix.

3   Methods

3.1   Concurrent Motion and Field-Inhomogeneity Correction Scheme

The concurrent correction scheme is summarized in Fig. 1. The key idea is to use the rigid-body motion parameter estimates from the MSV process to transform the *original* field-map into an updated field-map volume. This new field-map is then used to reconstruct the *original* EPI slices using the iterative QPLS method. The reconstructed EPI slices are registered with rigid-body MSV to obtain a new set of motion parameters. The algorithm repeats until good estimates are obtained. Estimation error propagation is minimized by using the *original* data in each cycle.

A set of geometrically distorted EPI images with motion are simulated from a T_2-weighted volume from the International Consortium of Brain Mapping (ICBM) such that ground truths exist for each slice's motion parameters and its non-distorted form. A simulated field-map is used for the forward distortion. The concurrent correction scheme is then applied to the simulated EPI images and evaluated in terms of its ability to recover the true motion parameters and the true non-distorted images.

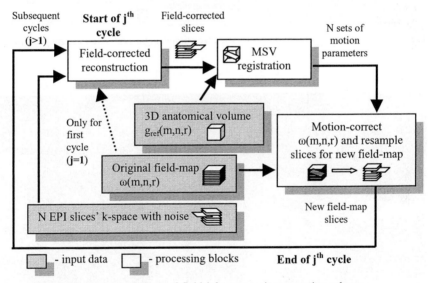

Fig. 1. Concurrent motion and field-inhomogeneity correction scheme.

3.2   Motion and Distortion Simulation

Two anatomically correct T_1- and T_2-weighted image datasets from the ICBM are used for this motion correction experiment. The two volumes, in 256x256x181 matrix with a voxel size of 1 mm^3, are originally in perfect registration. The T_2-w volume is used to simulate the geometrically distorted EPI data with motion as shown in Fig. 2. The ICBM T_2-w volume is resampled in the slice direction to make the slice thickness 5mm; EPI slices are typically 3mm to 6mm thick. For simplicity, only the rigid body motion parameters t_x, t_y, t_z (translation) and θ_z (in-plane rotation) are applied to the T_2-w volume.

The field-inhomogeneity is simulated at a level comparable to realistic values. The maximum simulated field-inhomogeneity is 8 ppm at 1.5T, which is close to the air-tissue field-inhomogeneity range of $\approx$ 9 ppm. The range of applied motion was intentionally large with maximum values of 7.85mm, 7.85mm, 10.2mm and 7.85° for t_x, t_y, t_z and θ_z, respectively. The motion applied is smooth with respect to time as the head does not typically make sudden movements. Rotation about the z-axis and all translations do not change the orientation of the air-tissue interface with respect to B_0 and thus is unlikely to change the field-map except for the respective linear translation or in-plane rotation. Thus, forward distorting the T_2 volume with the rotated-translated field-map is reasonable as long as out-of-plane rotations θ_x and θ_y are not applied.

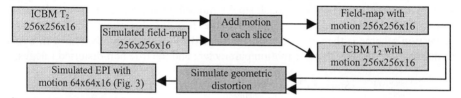

Fig. 2. Simulating the motion and geometric distortion using a synthetic field map applied to the T_2-w ICBM images.

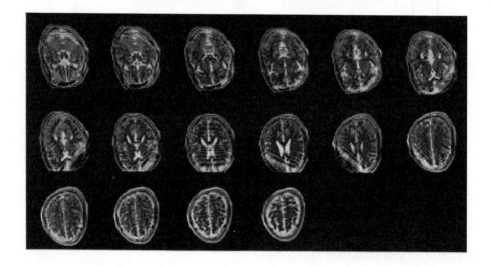

Fig. 3. Simulated images with geometric distortion representing EPI data with motion artifacts.

3.3 Field-Map Update

The set of MSV-recovered registration parameters for each slice is applied to the field-map which is then resampled at the appropriate slice locations to obtain the updated field-map for the next cycle. In the first cycle, field-corrected reconstruction uses the original field-map, which is inaccurate because the head has moved since the time of acquisition. *It is hypothesized that not all the 6 motion parameters should be used in the initial cycle(s) to compute the updated field-map as some are unreliable estimates when the field-map is initially not correct.* Since any error in the field-map will likely manifest itself as a larger MSV registration error in the phase-encoded direction, t_y is not a reliable parameter for updating the field-map in the initial cycle(s). The out-of-plane rotation parameters θ_x and θ_y may change the field-map significantly and thus are also not deemed to be reliable in the early cycles. *In the first cycle, only t_x, t_z and θ_z are used to update the field-map.* In the second and third cycles, t_x, t_y, t_z and θ_z are used to update the field-map.

4   Results

Figure 4 shows the absolute error or $|\theta_l - \theta_{l,\text{round truth}}|$ at different stages in the proposed correction scheme. θ_l is the MSV-recovered rigid-body motion parameter vector for slice l and $\theta_{l,\text{round truth}}$ is the applied ground truth motion parameter vector. Table 1 lists the RMS error of the data plotted in Fig. 4. In cycle one, the inaccurate original field-map was used to perform the initial field-corrected reconstructions. These cycle1-reconstructed images yield lower RMS in recovery error for all motion parameters compared to the distorted simulated EPI volume. Upon updating the field-map with the cycle1 MSV rigid motion parameters, t_x, t_z and θ_z, and performing the field-corrected reconstructions again, the RMS MSV-recovery error for the second cycle is further reduced to a level that is comparable to the experimental ground truth. A third cycle of the proposed scheme is then performed using *all* the MSV motion parameters from cycle two (except θ_x and θ_y) to update the field-map. The RMSE values for the third cycle remain close to the experimental ground truth, which suggests that convergence has occurred experimentally for the proposed scheme under the applied conditions. The experimental ground truth is the RMS error obtained when registering the T_2-w volume with simulated motion without geometric distortion to the T_1 anatomical volume. *The first cycle RMS error can be viewed as the performance of the MSV with rigid-body transform function and field-inhomogeneity scheme where the two problems are corrected separately.* Nevertheless, the RMS errors in the third cycle in table 1 shows improved average performance of over 3 mm for translations and over 4 degrees for rotations.

Next, the reconstructed image quality at various stages of the proposed correction scheme is compared. Figure 5 shows plots of the normalized RMS error (NRMSE) for each slice using the non-distorted ground truth images with motion as reference images. Compared to the first cycle, the images reconstructed in the second and third cycles have much lower NRMSE values for almost all slices. To provide a performance benchmark, reconstruction is performed using the actual field-map that was used to forward distort the T_2-w volume. Theoretically, these reconstructed images should have the lowest NRMSE values compared to all the previously corrected images. However, *due to reconstruction errors*, they serve only as an estimate of the best image quality performance achievable. The NRMSE values for the second and third cycles are comparable to each other and to the benchmark, which again suggests that the proposed scheme is experimentally stable under the applied conditions. In summary, the proposed scheme improves both the rigid motion parameters estimates as well as the final reconstructed image quality.

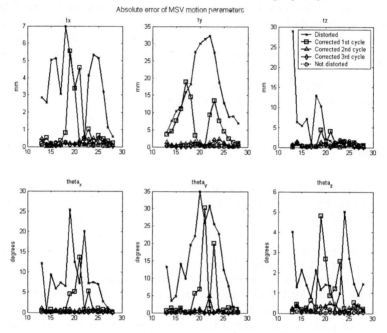

Fig. 4. MSV motion parameters absolute error at different stages in concurrent correction

Table 1. RMS error of MSV-recovered motion parameters over all slices. The ground truth is obtained from registering the T_2-w slices with simulated motion without geometric distortion to the T_1 anatomical volume.

Dataset	\multicolumn{6}{c}{RMS error over all slices}					
	t_x(mm)	t_y(mm)	t_z(mm)	θ_x(°)	θ_y(°)	θ_z(°)
Distorted EPI with motion	3.95	19.48	8.80	10.61	18.75	2.14
Corrected 1st cycle	2.04	8.48	1.63	4.08	9.38	1.59
Corrected 2nd cycle	0.24	1.08	0.63	0.45	1.32	0.25
Corrected 3rd cycle	0.28	0.74	0.78	0.42	0.38	0.19
Ground truth	0.17	0.20	0.89	0.23	0.29	0.14

5 Discussion and Conclusions

A field inhomogeneity correction method using an iterative quadratic penalized least squares reconstruction technique was implemented as a part of MSV motion correction. The motion induced field variation is updated concurrently with the MSV rigid-body transform vectors. The convergence and performance of the concurrent method were evaluated using simulated data to determine the accuracy in registration. Applying the method to motion simulated synthetic phantom data warrants the accurate evaluation of the mapping results with the known ground truths. The results in Table 1, Figs. 4 and 5 demonstrate the effective corrections of the motion artifacts that are complicated by the field effects induced by rigid head motion. The ground truth NRMSE in Fig. 5 is non-zero because of reconstruction errors. Future work will include a study of the tolerance in the range of out-of-plane motion for the correction of human EPI data as well as the validation of the robustness with a phantom.

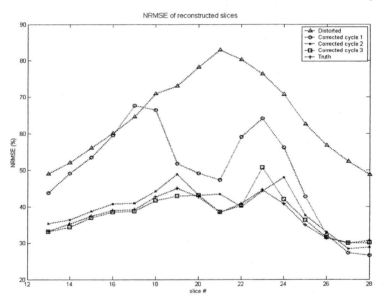

Fig. 5. Normalized RMS error (NRMSE) of each slice

References

1. Kim, B., J.L. Boes, P.H. Bland, T.L. Chenevert, C.R. Meyer, Motion correction in fMRI via registration of individual slices into an anatomical volume, Magnetic Resonance in Medicine, 41(4), 964-972, 1999
2. Kim, B., P.H. Bland, C.R. Meyer, Correction of local deformations in fMRI by 3D non-linear warping in map-slice-to-volume approach, Proc. Seventh Annual Meeting of ISMRM, p. 1765, 2000
3. Kim, B, Chenevert, TL, Meyer, CR, Motion correction with a non-linear warping solution for activations in temporal region, Proc. Tenth Annual Meeting of ISMRM, p. 2304, 2002

4. Bradley P. Sutton, Douglas C. Noll, Jeffrey A. Fessler, Fast, iterative image reconstruction for MRI in the presence of field inhomogeneities, IEEE Transactions on Medical Imaging, Vol. 22, No.2, 178-188, February 2003
5. Peter Jezzard, Robert S. Balaban, Correction for geometric distortion in echo planar images from B0 field variations, Magnetic Resonance in Medicine, 34, 65-73, 1995
6. Rhodri Cusack, Matthew Brett, Katja Osswald, An evaluation of the use of magnetic field maps to undistort echo-planar images, Neuroimage, 18, 127-142, 2003
7. E.M. Haacke, R.W. Brown, M.R. Thomson, R. Venkatesan, Magnetic resonance imaging: physical principles and sequence design, New York, 1999, John Wiley and Sons

Towards Optical Biopsies with an Integrated Fibered Confocal Fluorescence Microscope

Georges Le Goualher, Aymeric Perchant, Magalie Genet, Charlotte Cavé,
Bertrand Viellerobe, Fredéric Berier, Benjamin Abrat, and Nicholas Ayache

Mauna Kea Technologies, 9, Rue d'Enghien,
75010 Paris, France
{georges,aymeric}@maunakeatech.com
http://www.maunakeatech.com

Abstract. This paper presents an integrated endoscope-compatible
Fibered Confocal Fluorescence Microscope (FCFM) for medical imaging, the F-400. *In situ* high resolution images can be obtained thanks to
a set of flexible miniaturized optical probes of 0.5 to 1.5 mm diameter
that can be inserted through the working channel of an endoscope. We
briefly present in this paper the FCFM system, with a particular focus
on the image formation and the design of a dedicated image processing
software allowing for drastically reduce the inherent artifacts occurring
when imaging through an image bundle. The goal of the FCFM is to
perform *optical biopsy* (i.e. *in vivo* and *in situ* observations of thin sections of biological tissues at the cellular level). As a first step towards
this goal, we present here results of a clinical trial assessing the ability of
the F-400 to perform rapid morphologic examination in the endoscopy
room of medical specimens (polypectomy).

1 Introduction

In the very first step of epithelial cancer, abnormal cell proliferation first starts
just above a specific tissue layer: the basal membrane, which is located at
approximately 100 μm deep from the tissue surface for malpighian epithelium
(cervix epithelium for example) and 300 μm for glandular epithelium (tissue
that contains secretion glands: colon, pancreas, thyroid are examples of organs
composed of glandular tissue). For such epithelial cancers (most cancers
affecting solid organs), the medical procedure is to take a tissue sample (a
biopsy) and to have it examined under the microscope of a pathologist. Most of
these biopsy procedures are performed via endoscopy. However, an endoscope
provides only a visualization of the surface of the tissue at a macroscopic level.
It can neither see below the surface of the tissue nor provide a microscopic
view of the tissue. Therefore, in a number of cases the best area to biopsy
is difficult to assess. In order to improve the capability of an endoscope to
perform early cancer detection, there is a need for an instrument that could
provide a local sub-surfacic and high-resolution vision of the tissue, in other
words to perform *optical biopsy, i.e.* non invasive optical sectioning within a

C. Barillot, D.R. Haynor, and P. Hellier (Eds.): MICCAI 2004, LNCS 3217, pp. 761–768, 2004.
© Springer-Verlag Berlin Heidelberg 2004

thick transparent or translucent tissue with high resolution. Several systems are today under study to reach the ultimate goal of performing *in vivo* and *in situ* optical biopsies. Let's first mention fluorescence spectroscopy where dysplasia and early carcinoma are detected based on the analysis of fluorescence spectra [1]. Drawback of fluorescence spectroscopy lies in the lack of morphological information (i.e. no cell architecture is available from this modality) and the important rate of false positives due to inflammatory processes. High magnification chromoscopic endoscopy (chromoendoscopy) has been introduced recently providing *in vivo* micro-architecture [2]. Magnification colonoscopic techniques when combined with colonic chromoscopy (dye spraying of the colon) permit *in vivo* assessments of lesions at a magnification and resolution similar to a stereoendoscope. In particular *in vivo* prediction of histological characteristics by crypt or pit pattern analysis can be performed using high magnification chromoendoscopy [3]. One drawback of this technique is that it cannot provide at the same time the macroscopic view (for global localization) and the zoomed image (for optical biopsy). We present here an integrated endoscope-compatible Fibered Confocal Fluorescence Microscope (FCFM) (we refer the reader to [4,5] for other fibered systems). The confocal nature of the system makes it possible to observe sub-surfacic cellular structure (optical section parallel to the tissue surface at a depth from 0 to 100 μm), which is of particular interest for early detection of cancer. *In situ* imaging (typical lateral resolution of the images presented in this study are of 5 μm, axial resolution of 15 μm and field of view of 400x280 μm) can be obtained thanks to a set of flexible miniaturized optical probes of 0.5 to 1.5 mm diameter that can be inserted through the working channel of an endoscope. Note that, as the FCFM is used in conjunction with an endoscope, both macroscopic (endoscope image) as well as microscopic view (FCFM optical probe image) can be obtained at the same time, facilitating the selection of the area to be biopsied. As a first step towards the goal of *in vivo* and *in situ* optical biopsy, we present a related application which is the rapid morphologic examination in the endoscopy room of medical specimens, freshly excised, of colonoscopic polypectomy. First images acquired with the F-400 are presented showing that visual inspection of images may allow an expert to classify the pathology from the cell architecture.

2   Fibered Confocal Fluorescence Microscopy System

A FCFM is based on the principle of confocal microscopy which is the ability to reject light from out-of-focus planes and provide a clear in-focus image of a thin section within the sample. This optical sectioning property is what makes the confocal microscope ideal for imaging thick biological samples. Schematically, the adaptation of a confocal microscope for *in situ* and *in vivo* imaging in the context of endoscopy can be viewed as replacing a microscope's objective by a probe of length and diameter compatible with the working channel of an endoscope in order to be able to perform *in situ* imaging. For such purpose, we used an image bundle is as the link between the scanning device and the microscope objective (see figure 1).

2.1   Image Formation

A laser scanning unit, based on a laser at 488 nm, compatible with fluorescent dyes usable *in vivo* in clinical application, is scanned by two mirrors on the proximal surface of an optical image bundle. Horizontal line scanning is performed using a 4 kHz oscillating mirror while a galvanometric mirror performs frame scanning at 12 Hz. A custom synchronization hardware controls the mirrors and digitizes, synchronously with the scanning, the fluorescent signal using a mono-pixel photodetector. When organized according to the scanning, the output of the FCFM can be viewed as a raw image (see figure 3, left). Scanning amplitude and signal sampling frequency have been adjusted to perform a spatial over-sampling of the image bundle, this is clearly visible on the previous raw image where one can see individual fibers composing the bundle. Optical probes are composed of a connector, an image bundle and an optical head. The typical image bundle we use is composed of 30,000 optical fibers, with a fiber inter-core distance $d_{ic} = 3.3$ μm, and a fiber core diameter of 1.9 μm.

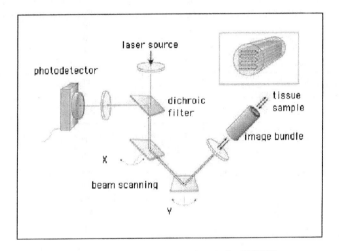

Fig. 1. Schematic principle of the FCFM

Critical elements in the image formation process lie in the correct spatial sampling of the image bundle by the scanning unit to avoid aliasing and the adjustment of the probe's optical head resolution (PSF) with this image bundle spatial sampling. In fact, when analyzing the probe's resolution with the sampling theory, we can consider that the optical resolution of the head corresponds to a low pass filter, and the image bundle to the sampling grid. The sampling Nyquist frequency of the image bundle is given by $2 * (1/d_{ic})$, which becomes $2 * (M/d_{ic})$ at the tissue focal plane, with M the magnification of the optical head (typical values of M goes from 1.0 to 2.5 depending on the probe's micro-optical head). The optical resolution of the head must therefore satisfy this frequency (as a rule of thumb the FWHM of the optical head's PSF should be no larger that one-half of the minimal spatial period T_{min} of a sine wave that can be resolved given the

Nyquist frequency ([6], page 373): $FWHM \approx 0.5 * T_{min} = 0.5 * (d_{ic}/M)$). The resulting lateral resolution of such a system is then: d_{ic}/M (*i.e.* the system has the ability to resolve a sine wave of period d_{ic}/M).

2.2   Image Processing

To represent the raw data measured from a given optical fiber composing the image bundle, we propose the following model:

$$I = I_0 * \left(a * \tau_{inj} * \tau_{col} * \alpha_{fluo} + b * \tau_{inj} * \alpha_{autofluo} \right) \qquad (1)$$

where a and b are constants[1], τ_{inj} and τ_{col} are injection rate, and collection rate of the fiber, $\alpha_{autofluo}$ is the intrinsic auto-fluorescence of the fiber, and α_{fluo} is the biological sample fluorescence we want to measure; I_0 is the intensity of the laser source. The task of the processing module is to restore the true physical measurement by removing the image bundle modulation (*i.e.* to estimate the biological sample fluorescence α_{fluo} given the raw data measured by each fiber I). Figure 2 presents the image processing sequence that was designed for this purpose.

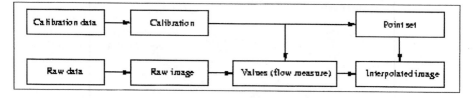

Fig. 2. Schematic principle of the image processing

Calibration – The image calibration process follows the top line of figure 2. As a preliminary step, we build a mapping between the FCFM raw image and the fibers composing the image bundle. Once the mapping between the raw data and each individual fiber is obtained, characteristics of each fiber are estimated. For this purpose, a non-fluorescent sample is imaged ($\alpha_{fluo} = 0$), followed by a sample of constant fluorescence ($\alpha_{fluo} = cst$). We note respectively I_b and I_s the associated measurements. The other output of the calibration is a point set representing the exact position of the fibers of the bundle.

Restoration – The image restoration process follows the bottom line of figure 2. The raw FCFM data is organized as a raw 2D image. Given the raw image to image bundle mapping, the fiber intensity I can be used in conjunction with the calibration data, to estimate the true physical measure (α_{fluo}), using the following equation:

---

[1] Note that more complicated intensity models can be proposed, i.e. where a and b are spatially variant, but we will not address them here

$$I_{restored} = \frac{I - I_b}{I_s - I_b} = K * \alpha_{fluo} \quad (K \; is \; a \; constant). \tag{2}$$

Reconstruction – At this step, we have a restored intensity: $I_{restored}$ for each fiber composing the image bundle. The final process is the interpolation of this point set into a numerical image on a square grid. The simplest method is the construction of a mosaic where all the pixels within the area of one fiber have a constant value. Other interpolation methods includes linear ($\mathcal{C}^0$ reconstruction), or cubic interpolation built from point set triangulation. For instance, the Clough-Tocher method allows a $\mathcal{C}^1$ reconstruction [7]. Considering that $\mathcal{C}^1$ reconstruction methods still present artifacts in particular for further image processing, $\mathcal{C}^2$ interpolations were also tested. Radial basis functions [8] allow such interpolation but at a high computational cost. We found that a B-spline iterative approximation, proposed by [9], was a good compromise between spatial continuity($\mathcal{C}^2$) and computational cost. In fact this method has a linear complexity in the number of points, and offers the possibility to control the reconstruction precision.

Results – A constant fluorescence solution (FITC) of controlled concentration to avoid detector saturation was imaged using the FCFM (see figure 3). If the true physical measurement was retrieved from the FCFM, the image should be constant (observed sample: $\alpha_{fluo} = cst$). The image on the left hand side of figure 3 represents the raw FCFM image. Note that individual fiber composing the image bundle are visible on this raw image, illustrating the correct spatial oversampling of the image bundle as well as the the interaction between each optical fiber and the laser spot transmission as a modulation of the true sample response. The image in the middle represents the reconstructed image using B-spline iterative approximation without any calibration step. The signal to noise ratio of this reconstructed image is 16 dB. Signal variations in this image are related to differences between individual fiber composing the image bundle. Given that the image bundle is made of fibers of different diameters and shapes, the transmission changes from one fiber to the other. The right image represents the reconstructed image using B-spline iterative approximation after restoration step was applied. The measured SNR in this image is now 32 dB. Residual noise on this image comes mainly from the electronic.

Finally, figure 4 is a comparison of a histologic section of a colonic tissue obtained by the pathologist with a restored and reconstructed image of a FCFM acquisition performed *in vivo* on a mouse [10]. Note that, on this normal tissue colonic crypts have the apearance of gun barrels. Typical size of such a colonic crypt on a mouse is 50 μm while it is 200 μm on humans.

2.3 Challenges

One of the main challenges for the design of the FCFM was to obtain a high laser coupling efficiency in a micron-sized fiber optic. For that purpose, a specific opto-mechanical connector has been designed to connect the probe to the scanning

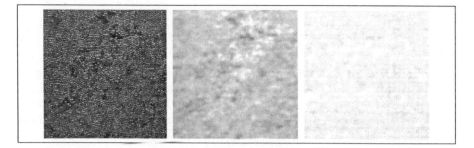

Fig. 3. From left to right: raw image of a constant signal, reconstruction without signal level calibration, and reconstruction using signal level calibration from equation 2. Uncalibrated image has a signal to noise ratio (SNR) of 16 dB, calibrated image of 32 dB.

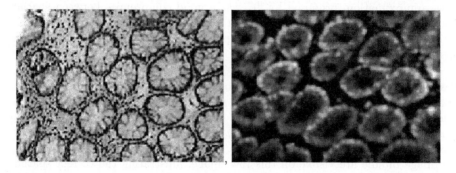

Fig. 4. Colonic tissue. Left: histologic section (http://pathweb.uchc.edu) ; Right: FCFM processed image (restored and reconstructed). FOV: 400x280 μm (image courtesy of Igor Charvet, CMU, Geneva, Switzerland)

unit. The connector gives a high repeatability in the focus position, as well as the optimal injection along the whole image field. Finally, the optical wave front error of the scanning beam has been optimized to ensure that only one fiber is injected at a time. When dealing with signal processing, the challenge resides here in the correct modeling of the data transmission and acquisition process has well and the real-time constraint on image processing (12 Hz).

3   Optical Biopsies of Freshly Excised Colonoscopic Polypectomy

In this section, we present the first images obtained by the FCFM on freshly human excised colonoscopic polypectomy. The protocol was the following: during a colonoscopy, polyps on the wall of the colon were localized using the macroscopic view provided by the endoscope. Before resection of a polyp, a catheter containing a vital dye commonly used in chromoendoscopy (cresyl violet) was inserted within the working channel of the endoscope. Cresyl violet offers con-

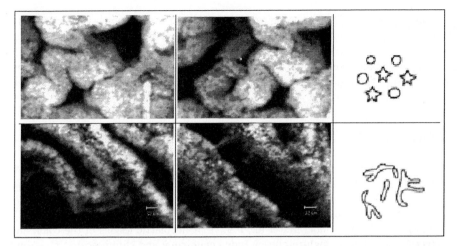

Fig. 5. Freshly excised specimens observed using the FCFM. Lateral resolution is about 5 μm, axial resolution is about 15 μm, Field of view is 400x280 μm. Top: hyperplastic polyp. Bottom: tubulo-villous adenoma with low grade dysplasia. Right column: schematic representation taken from the classification of Kudo ([3])

trast by accentuating the morphological landscape of tissues and is commonly used for chromoendoscopy of the colon. A very important property of cresyl violet is that, eventhough it is not considered to be a fluorescent dye but a vital dye (therefore not toxic for cells) it becomes fluorescent when excited at 488 nm allowing imaging to be performed by the FCFM. In fact, cresyl violet was successfully tested as a fluorophore for histopathology with confocal laser scanning microscope (CLSM) [11]. Once the polyp is resected, the FCFM is used to image the freshly excised sample. Figure 5 represents a sample of acquired images. Note that the micro-architecture of the tissue sample is clearly visible on these images. Using the Kudo "Pit Pattern" classification ([3]), visual inspection of the two images in the top raw on figure 5 suggest hyperplastic polyps (*type II* in the Kudo nomenclature) since the shape and size of the colonic crypts are similar to those associated with the corresponding Kudo diagram (right image). Note in particular *star-like* shape of the colonic cript in the inferior part of the image. Using the same methodology, sizes and shapes of colonic crypts as observed on the bottom raw, suggest tubulo-villous adenoma with low grade dysplasia (*type IIIL* in the Kudo classification).These assumptions were confirmed by a pathologist after histology.

4   Conclusion

An integrated fibered confocal system for *in vivo* and *in situ* fluorescence imaging has been presented. As a first step towards *in vivo* and *in situ* optical biopsy, we have presented here first images obtained on freshly excised surgical specimens. On reconstructed images, micro-architecture is clearly visible (colonic crypt organization) suggesting that these images could be used by an expert to detect and classify underlying pathologies. A clinical trial is currently under way to study the capability of the FCFM to provide biopsy guidance which will be of particular interest for the analysis of flat adenomas (*i.e.* adenomas very difficult to localize at the macroscopic scale) and assessment of tumor margins. Future works include the study of micro-optic designs in order to get an improved cellular resolution.

References

1. Bourg-Heckly, G., Blais, J., Padila, J.J., Bourdon, O., Etienne, J., Guillemin, F., Lafay, L.: Endoscopic ultraviolet-induced autofluorescence spectroscopy of the esophagus : tissue characterization and potential for early cancer diagnosis. Endocopy **32** (2000) 756–765
2. Jaramillo, E., Watanabe, M., et al., P.S.: Flat neoplastic lesions of the colon and rectum detected by high-resolution video endoscopy and chromoscopy. Gastrointestinal Endoscopy **42** (1995) 114–122
3. Kudo, S., Rubio, C., Teixeira, C., Kashida, H., Kogure, E.: Pit pattern in colorectal neoplasia: endoscopic magnifying view. Endoscopy **33** (2001) 367–373
4. Sabharwal, Y., Rouse, A., Donaldson, L., Hopkins, M., Gmitro, A.: Slit-canning confocal microendoscope for high-resolution in vivo imaging. Applied optics **38** (1999) 7133–7144 classeur confocal fibré - 049.
5. Sung, K., Liang, C., Descour, M., Collier, T., Follen, M., Richard-kortum, R.: Fiber optic reflectance for in vivo imaging of human tissues. IEEE Transactions on biomedical engineering **49** (2002) 1168–1172
6. Castleman, K.R.: Digital Image Processing. Prentice Hall (1996) ISBN 0-13-211467-4.
7. Amidror, I.: Scattered data interpolation methods for electronic imaging systems: a survey. Journal of Electronic Imaging **11** (2002) 157–176
8. Carr, J.C., Beatson, R.K., Cherrie, J., Mitchell, T.J., Fright, W.R., McCallum, B.C., Evans, T.R.: Reconstruction and representation of 3D objects with radial basis functions. In: ACM SIGGRAPH, Los Angeles (2001) 67–76
9. Lee, S., Wolberg, G., Shin, S.Y.: Scattered data interpolation with multilevel B-splines. IEEE Transactions on Visualization and Computer Graphics **3** (1997) 228–244
10. Perchant, A., Le Goualher, G., Genet, M., Viellerobe, B., Berier, F.: An integrated device for *in vivo* and *in situ* fluorescence confocal microscopy for endoscopic images in small animals. In: IEEE International Symposium on Biomedical Imaging: From Nano to Macro. (2004) to appear.
11. Meining, G.M.: Cresyl violet as a fluorophore in confocal laser scanning microscopy for future in vivo histopathology. Endoscopy **35** (2003) 585–589

A Prospective Multi-institutional Study of the Reproducibility of fMRI: A Preliminary Report from the Biomedical Informatics Research Network

Kelly H. Zou[1,2,6], Douglas N. Greve[3,6], Meng Wang[1,6],
Steven D. Pieper[1,6], Simon K. Warfield[1,4,5,6], Nathan S. White[3,6],
Mark G. Vangel[3,6], Ron Kikinis[1,6], William M. Wells[1,4,6], and
First Birn[6]

[1] Surgical Planning Laboratory, Brigham and Women's Hospital,
[2] Department of Health Care Policy, Harvard Medical School,
[3] Athinoula A. Martinos Center for Biomedical Imaging, Massachusetts General Hospital,
[4] Computer Science and Artificial Intelligence Laboratory,
Massachusetts Institute of Technology,
[5] Computational Radiology Laboratory, Brigham and Women's Hospital,
[6] Functional Imaging Research of Schizophrenia Testbed (FIRST),
Biomedical Informatics Research Network (BIRN)

{zou,mwang,pieper,warfield,kikinis,sw}@bwh.harvard.edu,
{greve,nwhite,vangel}@nmr.mgh.harvard.edu

Abstract. Functional magnetic resonance imaging (fMRI) has significantly contributed to understanding both normal and diseased human brains. Variability often exists in the magnitude, spatial distribution, and statistical significance of the resulting fMRI maps due to differences in equipment and other site-specific differences. In addition, because of costly imaging, demanding tasks, and analytical burden, understanding the effect of these differences may help develop an efficient pooling and comparison mechanism.

Prospective multi-institutional repeated fMRI data were acquired recently in the first phase of the extensive Functional Imaging Research of Schizophrenia Testbed study, sponsored by the Biomedical Informatics Research Network (BIRN) in the US. Five "human phantoms," who were right-handed healthy males, were included in the study. These subjects repeatedly performed the same sensory-motor task over 10 of the 11 study sites on 2 separate visits per site.

The effects of factors such as subject, study site, field strength, vendor, K-space, visit, and repeated run on the fMRI reproducibility were evaluated. Over 4 repeated runs per visit at each site, at a given binarizing activation threshold, we first calculated a three-dimensional (3D) brain activation map via an intial expectation and maximization (EM) algorithm. Site-to-site differences were then assessed based on a second-level hiearchical EM. Against the estimated gold standard of the 3D activation map, activation percentage, sensitivity, specificity, and receiver operating characteristic curves were then estimated using voxel counts. A statistical regression model was used to assess the significance of accuracy predictors with p-values generated in order to explain those factors contributing towards the variability in repeated brain activation maps.

C. Barillot, D.R. Haynor, and P. Hellier (Eds.): MICCAI 2004, LNCS 3217, pp. 769–776, 2004.
© Springer-Verlag Berlin Heidelberg 2004

1   Introduction

Functional MRI (fMRI) has significantly contributed to studies of both the normal and diseased human brain. Unfortunately, variability may exist in the magnitude, spatial distribution, and statistical significance of resultant fMRI maps. The reasons for such variability are multi-factorial and are important to study [1-7].

Recently, in the US, the functional subsection of the Biomedical Informatics Research Network (BIRN; http://nbirn.net) aimed at comparing and calibrating the fMRI signals in order to determine whether the inter-relation of fMRI maps from different sites was meaningful. This is an initial extensive effort prior to collecting prospective fMRI data of the Schizophrenic versus control subjects in the next phase of this large multi-institutional prospective study.

In this prospective study with 5 healthy "human phantoms" performing the same tasks during two visits at each of the 11 sites, we investigated the effects of factors such as study site, field strength, vendor, visit, repeated run on the reproducibility of the performance of a sensory-motor (SM) task by these healthy human phantoms in a prospective multi-institutional study. The main goal of our analysis was to characterize the variability seen in a sensory-motor task across runs and sites.

2   Methods

2.1   Study Subjects

A total of 11 sites formed the functional BIRN component of the study. Data were collected from 10 of these 11 sites (five 1.5T, four 3T scanners, and one 4T scanner). Five healthy right-handed male subjects were scanned at each site in two visits on separate days, with 10 task runs per visit. In addition, 3 of those had extra scans in a total of 4 visits only at one of the 10 sites.

2.2   Sensory-Motor (SM) Task

The SM task was performed for 4 out of these 10 fMRI runs during each visit. A block design was used with 15-second epochs of alternating baseline (fixation) and task for a total of 85 (plus the first 2 initally used to reach equalibrum and thus discarded) acquisitions per run. Subjects were instructed to perform bilateral finger tapping on button boxes (1 dummy button box and 1 actual) in time with a 3Hz audio cue and a reversing checkerboard. The subjects pressed buttons 1 through 4 in consecutive order and then back again using both hands, simultaneously and in sync.

2.3   Data Acquisition

Anatomical T2W images were acquired at all sites with FSE/TSE or equivalent RARE: oblique axial, FOV 22 cm, 35 slices, 4 mm, TR/TE 4000 ms/68 ms, train length 12, 256×192 matrix, scan time 2:24 min. In addition, 3DSPGR was acquired at 1 site: axial, FOV 22×16.5 cm, 124-128 slices, 1.2 mm, TR/TE/FA 9.8 ms/min/15 deg, T1 300 ms, 256×192 matrix, BW $\pm$ 15.625 khz, NEX 2, scan time 9:02 min.

Table 1. A list of variables examined in the funcational BIRN study

No	Variable	Value	No	Variable	Value
1	Subject	1, ..., 5	5	Strength	1.5T, 3T, 4T
2	Site	1, ..., 10	6	Vendor	Siemens, GE, Picker
3	Visit	1, 2 (all); 1, ...,4 (3 subjects at 1 site)	7	K-space	Raster, Spiral,
4	Run	1, ..., 4/Visit			Dual-Echo Raster

Functional images were acquired with block-design EPI or spiral GRE: oblique axial, FOV 22cm, 35 slices, 4 mm, TR 3000 ms, TE 30 ms (3T; 4T) 40 ms (1.5T), FA 90 deg, BW> ± 100 khz, 64 × 64 matrix, 1 shot, 2 dummy frames. The pulse sequences were allowed to vary the K-space trajectory by site. A bite bar was used to minimize head movement.

2.4 Per-voxel fMRI Analysis

Motion correction at each run was applied to middle time point using AFNI (http://afni.nimh.nih.gov/afni). Smoothing was based on FWHM 5mm. Fourier model was used to conduct an F-test to compute the statistical significance at each voxel.

Subject-specific registration was performed over the repeated runs and across the sites in FreeSurfer (http://surfer.nmr.mgh.harvard.edu). Image registration of the anatomical volume with the functional volume was conducted to convert the subject's anatomical volume to the corresponding functional space.

2.5 Statistical Methods

We examined the factors impacting the activation patterns. These included subject ($n = 5$), site ($n = 10$), visit ($n = 2$ or 4), run ($n = 4$), field strength ($n = 3$), vendor ($n = 3$), and K-space ($n = 3$) (Table 1).

Task-related significance (Y) at each voxel was computed using an F-test on the Fourier componant of the task fundamental frequency. At each fixed voxel significance threshold (γ), an estimation-maximization algorithm, developed previously, called the Simultaneous Truth and Performance Level Estimation (STAPLE) [8,9], was applied across the 4 runs to optimally derive a composite 3D gold standard activation map, under a Level 1 STAPLE EM. This algorithm combined all of the factors and enabled visualization of the gold standard in the software, 3D Slicer (http://slicer.org) [10].

Furthermore, a Level 2 STAPLE EM was applied to compare site-to-site differences (see the hiearchical EM-algorithm illustrated in Fig. 1).

Following the Level 1 EM, voxel fractions in the whole brain were used to compute the sensitivity and specificity, for fixed γ, defined respectively as follows:

$$\text{Sensitivity} = \text{True Activation Fraction}$$
$$= \Pr(Y > \gamma \mid \text{Gold Standard=Activated Voxel}),$$
$$\text{Specificity} = \text{True Non-Activation Fraction}$$
$$= \Pr(Y \leq \gamma \mid \text{Gold Standard=Non-Activated Voxel}).$$

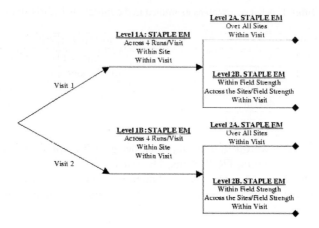

Fig. 1. Subject-specific flowchart of a hierarchical scheme to apply the STAPLE EM algorithm, stratified by visit; *Level 1*: within-site EM was performed, and *Level 2*: between-site EM was performed to generate 3D gold standard activation maps

Following the Level 2 EM, site-specific bi-normal parametric receiver operating characteristic (ROC) curves, a plot of sensitivity vs. (1−specificity), were generated from the activation data on a continuous scale. The area under each ROC curve (AUC) represented the overall classification accuracy, where $\text{AUC} = \Phi\left(\alpha/\sqrt{1+\beta^2}\right)$, (α, β) are the bi-normal ROC parameters based on their maximum likelihood estimates [11-16], and $\Phi(\cdot)$ is the cumulative distribution function of a standard normal.

Linear models were used to compute the p-values for assessing the significance of the factors. Analytic software used included Matlab (http://www.mathworks.com) and S-Plus (http://www.insightful.com).

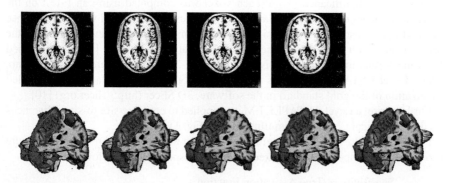

Fig. 2. Registered activation maps on anatomical data of Subject 3 during Visit 1 at one site with a 3T scanner: *top 4 panels*: Runs 1 to 4 in 2D; *bottom left 4 panels*: Runs 1 to 4 in 3D over 35 slices, and *bottom right panel*: the estimated 3D gold standard activation map derived by Level 1 STAPLE EM

Table 2. P-values indicating the significance of the factors on sensitivity and specificity, respectively, based on Level 1 STAPLE EM and regression analysis

Variable	n	p-Value on Sensitivity	p-Value on Specificity
Subject	5	**0.01**	**0.04**
Site	10	0.66	0.47
Strength	3	0.26	0.57
Vendor	3	0.79	0.85
K-space	3	0.93	0.40
Visit	{2; 4}	0.38	0.91
Run	4	0.35	**0.04**

Table 3. Mean activation percentage of all voxels in the brain, sensitivity, and specificity by field strength and subject, based on Level 1 STAPLE EM and regression analysis

Strength	Subject	Activation Percentage	Sensitivity	Specificity
1.5T	1	0.0922	0.5548	0.9997
	2	0.1777	0.6845	0.9996
	3	0.2468	0.5691	0.9992
	4	0.0626	0.5544	0.9998
	5	0.0606	0.4185	0.9498
3T	1	0.7484	0.6558	0.9981
	2	1.2848	0.7543	0.9982
	3	3.0342	0.6199	0.9883
	4	0.8781	0.5792	0.9967
	5	1.1136	0.6834	0.9970
4T	1	0.7550	0.5694	0.9977
	2	1.9181	0.7972	0.9973
	3	1.7149	0.6268	0.9946
	4	0.4274	0.4365	0.9979
	5	0.8185	0.6727	0.9986

3 Results

Of all scanners, 5 were 1.5T; 4 were 3T; 1 was 4T. Significant factors for sensitivity included subject (p=0.01) and for specificity included subject (p=0.04) and run (p=0.04) (Table 2). Registered data for a subject and site were provided in Fig. 2.

At the threshold of $\gamma = 10^{-9}$ to minimize false discovery rates [17], the mean activation percentage of all voxels in the brain, sensitivity, and specificity are presented (Table 3 and Fig. 3). At 3T, the mean sensitivity per subject ranged $0.58 - 0.76$ while the mean specificity ranged $0.99 - 1.00$. At 4T, available at only one study site, the mean sensitivity per subject ranged $0.44 - 0.80$ while the mean specificity ranged $0.99 - 1.00$. At 1.5T, however, the mean sensitivity only ranged $0.42 - 0.69$ while the mean specificity ranged $0.95 - 1.00$.

The ROC curves and their AUCs (Table 4 and Fig. 4) demonstrated moderate to high classification accuracy, which was generally higher at 3T (AUC ranged $0.69 - 0.92$) and 4T (AUC ranged $0.77 - 0.96$), than at 1.5T (AUC ranged $0.52 - 0.77$).

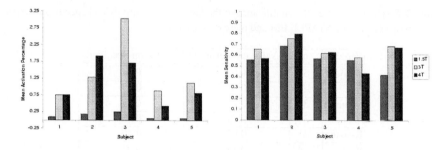

Fig. 3. *Left panel*: mean activation percentage and *right panel*: mean sensitivity, by subject and field strength using Level 1 EM; *left to right bins*: 1.5T, 3T, and 4T for each subject. See Table 3 for actual values, with specificities all close to 1.

Table 4. Estimated ROC parameters (α, β) and the corresponding areas under the ROC curves, AUC, based on Level 2 STAPLE EM

Strength	Site	Vendor	K-space	Visit 1			Visit 2		
				α	β	AUC	α	β	AUC
1.5T	1	Siemens	Raster	9.1029	12.3057	0.7695	4.1368	8.6258	0.6831
	2	Siemens	Raster	0.2703	1.7500	0.5533	3.5568	6.6278	0.7022
	3	GE	Raster	2.3450	4.0026	0.7151	2.5243	5.0277	0.6888
	4	GE	Spiral	3.8472	6.5266	0.7199	5.6221	7.5293	0.7704
	5	Picker	Raster	0.0621	0.7772	0.5195	0.0772	0.9449	0.5224
3T	6	Siemens	Dual-Echo Raster	3.9681	4.0588	0.8288	4.1202	4.1097	0.8350
	7	Siemens	Raster	9.4499	6.7944	0.9156	6.4577	5.7678	0.8650
	8	GE	Spiral	1.6394	2.3350	0.7407	2.3597	2.8091	0.7856
	9	GE	Raster	4.1490	6.0816	0.7496	1.9062	3.6907	0.6909
4T	10	GE	Spiral	5.5703	2.9369	0.9637	2.4119	3.1739	0.7657

4   Conclusions

In this unique multi-institutional prospective fMRI reproducibility study, we discovered the effects of the following factors in terms of the estimated mean activation percentage, sensitivity, specificity, and AUC:

The effect of individual subjects: There was a significant between-subject variability; however calibration may be feasible as part of the pooling mechanism of different cohorts.

The effect of field strengths: Both 3T and 4T were better than 1.5T, yielding more activation and less variability in terms of sensitivity and specificity.

The effect of repeated runs: The activation patterns were variable over the runs after the rest and task periods.

The effect of site vs. subject: The variability across subjects appeared greater than that across sites. This finding may help develop a calibration plan to minimize the variability introduced by the sites themselves, ultimately enabling us to pool independent functional data of normal and diseased subjects across different institutions.

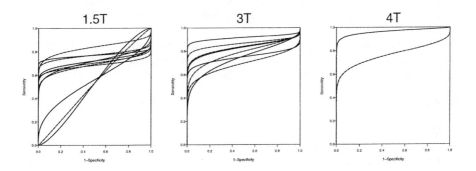

Fig. 4. ROC Curves for Subject 2, by field strength and visit using Level 2 EM; *left panel*: 1.5T, *middle panel*: 3T, and *right panel*: 4T; in each panel, *solid lines*: Visit 1 and *dashed lines*: Visit 2

The effect of visit on different days: Less activation was observed and more robust and systematic activation under different thresholds for the second vs. the first visit. For those three subjects who participated in 4 visits at one site only, less activation was observed for the latter two days. However, there was higher specificity and less variability on these days. A learning effect was not apprarent.

Acknowledgement. The funding for the BIRN study was provided by Grant NCRR P41RR13218. The authors are partially supported by NIH R01LM007861-01A1, R03HS013234-01, CA89449-01, R21MH67054, the Harvard Center for Neurodegeneration and Repair, and the Whitaker Foundation.
We acknowledge with thanks constructive comments from investigators and collaborators from all of the 11 participating institutions in the US, particularly the members of the functional BIRN "calibration" group.

References

1. Brannen JH, Badie B, Moritz CH, Quigley M, Meyerand ME, and Haughton VM: Reliability of functional MR imaging with word-generation tasks for mapping Broca's area. American Journal of Neuroradiology 22 (2001) 1711-1718.
2. Machielsen WCM, Rombouts SARB, Barkhof F, Scheltens P, and Witter MP: fMRI of visual encoding: reproducibility of activation. Human Brain Mapping 9 (2000) 156-164.
3. Le TH and Hu X: Methods for assessing accuracy and reliability in functional MRI. NMR in Biomedicine 10 (1997) 160-164.
4. Genovese CR, Noll, DC and Eddy, WF: Estimating test-retest reliability in fMRI I: statistical methodology. Magnetic Resonance in Medicine 38 (1997) 497-507.
5. Maitra R, Roys SR, and Gullapalli RP: Test-retest reliability estimation of functional MRI Data. Magnetic Resonance in Medicine 48 (2002) 62-70.
6. Casey BJ, Cohen JD, O'Craven K, Davidson RJ, Irwin W, Nelson CA, Noll DC, Hu X, Lowe MJ, Rosen BR, Truwitt CL, Turski PA. Reproducibility of fMRI results across four institutions using a spatial working memory task. NeuroImage 8 (1998) 249-261

7. Wei XC, Yoo S-S, Dickey CC, Zou KH, Guttmann CRG, Panych LP. Functional MRI of auditory verbal working memory: long-term reproducibility analysis. NeuroImage 21 (2004) 1000-1008.

8. Warfield SK, Zou KH, Wells WM III: Validation of image segmentation and expert quality with an expectation-maximization algorithm. Medical Image Computing and Computer-Assisted Intervention-MICCAI, Lecture Notes in Computer Science 2488, Tokyo, Japan (2002) 290-297.

9. Warfield SK, Zou KH, Wells WM III: Simultaneous Truth and Performance Level Estimation (STAPLE): An Algorithm for the Validation of Image Segmentation. IEEE Transactions on Medical Imaging (2004) In Press.

10. Gering DT, Nabavi A, Kikinis R, Hata N, O'Donnell LJ, Grimson WE, Jolesz FA, Black PM, Wells MW III: An integrated visualization system for surgical planning and guidance using image fusion and an open MR. Journal of Magnetic Resonance Imaging 13 (2001) 967-975.

11. Metz CE, Merman BA, Shen JH. Maximum likelihood estimation of receiver operating characteristic (ROC) curves from continuously-distributed data. Statistics in Medicine 17 (1998) 1033-1053.

12. Zou KH, Warfield SK, Bharatha A, Tempany CMC, Kaus M, Haker S, Wells WM III, Jolesz FA, Kikinis R: Statistical validation of imagage segmentation quality based on a spatial overlap index. Academic Radiology 11 (2004) 178-189.

13. Zou KH, Warfield SK, Fielding JR, Tempany CM, Wells MW III, Kaus MR, Jolesz FA, Kikinis R: Statistical validation based on parametric receiver operating characteristic analysis of continuous classification data. Academic Radiology 10 (2003) 1359-1368.

14. Zou KH, Wells WM, Kaus MR, Kikinis R, Jolesz FA, Warfield SK. Statistical validation of automated probabilistic segmentation against composite latent expert ground truth in MR imaging of brain tumors. Medical Image Computing and Computer-Assisted Intervention-MICCAI, Lecture Notes in Computer Science 2488, Tokyo, Japan (2002) 315-322.

15. Zou KH, Wells MW III, Kikinis R, Warfield: Three validation metrics for automated probabilistic image segmentation of brain tumors. Statistics in Medicine (2004) In Press.

16. Zou KH, Hall WJ, Shapiro DE: Smooth non-parametric receiver operating characteristic (ROC) curves for continuous diagnostic tests. Statistics in Medicine 16 (1997) 2143-2156.

17. Genovese CR, Lazar NA, and Nichols T: Thresholding of statistical maps in functional neuroimaging using the false discovery rate. NeuroImage 15 (2002) 870-878.

Real-Time Multi-model Tracking of Myocardium in Echocardiography Using Robust Information Fusion

Bogdan Georgescu[1], Xiang Sean Zhou[1], Dorin Comaniciu[1], and Bharat Rao[2]

[1] Real-Time Vision and Modeling Department, Siemens Corporate Research
755 College Road East, Princeton, NJ 08540, USA
bogdan.georgescu, xiang.zhou, dorin.comaniciu@scr.siemens.com
[2] Siemens Medical Solutions
51 Valley Stream Parkway, Malvern, PA 19355, USA
bharat.rao@siemens.com

Abstract. Automatic myocardial wall motion tracking in ultrasound images is an important step in analysis of the heart function. Existing methods for Myocardial Wall Tracking are not robust to artifacts induced by signal dropout, significant appearance or gain control changes. We present a unified framework for tracking the myocardium wall motion in real time with uncertainty handling and robust information fusion. Our method is robust in two aspects, firstly robust information fusion is used for combining matching results from multiple appearance models and secondly fusion is performed in the shape space to combine information from measurement and prior knowledge and models. Our approach fully exploits uncertainties from the measurement, shape priors, motion dynamics, and matching process based on multiple appearance models. Experiments illustrate the advantages of our approach validating the theory and showing the potential of very accurate wall motion measurements.

1 Introduction

Accurate analysis of the myocardial wall motion of the left ventricle is crucial for the evaluation of the heart function. This task is difficult due to the fast motion of the heart muscle and respiratory interferences. It is even worse when ultrasound image sequences are used since ultrasound is the noisiest among common medical image modalities such as MRI or CT. Figure 1 illustrates the difficulties of the tracking task due to signal drop-out, poor signal to noise ratio or significant appearance changes.

Several methods have been proposed for myocardial wall tracking. Model-based deformable templates [1,2], Markov random fields [3], optical flow methods [4,5,6], or combinations of above, have been applied for tracking left ventricle (LV) from 2-D image sequences. Jacob et al. provided a brief recent review in [7]. Other related work focuses on the tracking, segmentation, or registration in 3D, 2D+T (spatial + time) or 4-D space [8], [9], [10].

One of the main problems of visual tracking is to maintain a representation of target appearance that is robust enough to cope with inherent changes due to target movement and/or imaging device movement. Methods based on template matching have to adapt the model template in order to successfully track the target. Without adaptation, tracking

C. Barillot, D.R. Haynor, and P. Hellier (Eds.): MICCAI 2004, LNCS 3217, pp. 777–785, 2004.
© Springer-Verlag Berlin Heidelberg 2004

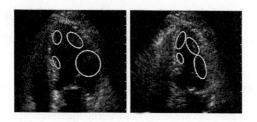

Fig. 1. Echocardiography images with area of acoustic drop-out, low signal to noise ratio and significant appearance changes. Local wall motion estimation has covariances (depicted by the solid ellipses) that reflect heteroscedastic noise.

is reliable only over short periods of time when the appearance does not change significantly. However, in most applications, for long time periods the target appearance undergoes considerable changes in structure. When the model is adapted to the previous frame accumulated motion error and rapid visual changes make the model to drift away from the target. Tracking performance can be improved by maintaining a statistical representation of the model. Using only a normal distribution, where the mean represents the most likely template, will however, not capture the full range of the appearance variability.

It is a common practice to impose model constraints in a shape tracking framework. In most cases, a subspace model is suitable for shape tracking, since the number of modes capturing the major shape variations is limited and usually much smaller than the original number of feature components used to describe the shape. A straightforward treatment is to project tracked shapes into a PCA subspace [1]. However, this approach cannot take advantage of the measurement uncertainty and is therefore not complete: In most real-world scenarios, measurement noise is heteroscedastic in nature (i.e., both anisotropic and inhomogeneous). Alternatively, one could directly incorporate a PCA shape space constraint into a Kalman filter-based tracker. In [11,12] it is suggested to set the system noise covariance matrix to be the covariance of a PCA shape model. However it does not provide a systematic and complete fusion of the model information because, for example, the model mean is discarded and it mixes the uncertainty from system dynamics with the uncertainty from the statistical shape constraint.

In this paper we introduce a unified framework for *fusing motion estimates from multiple appearance models* and *fusing a subspace shape model with the system dynamics and measurements with heteroscedastic noise*. The appearance variability is modeled by maintaining several models over time. This amounts for a nonparametric representation of the probability density function that characterizes the object appearance. Tracking is performed by obtaining independently from each model a motion estimate and its uncertainty through optical flow. A recently proposed robust fusion technique [13] is used to compute the final estimate for each component. The method, named Variable-Bandwidth Density-based Fusion (VBDF), manages the multiple data sources and outliers in the motion estimates. To obtain the final shape estimate we specifically address the issue of heteroscedastic measurement noise and its influence during the fusion with other information sources. When measurement noise is anisotropic and inhomogeneous, joint fusion of all information sources becomes critical for achieving superior performance.

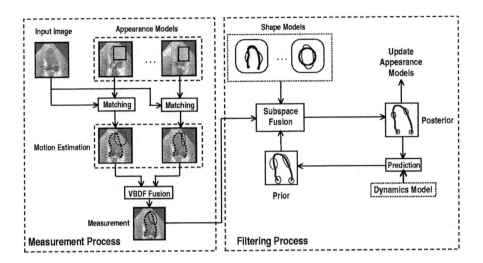

Fig. 2. The block diagram of the robust tracker with the measurement and filtering processes.

In this paper we demonstrate the advantages of the proposed framework for ultrasound heart sequences.

2 Multi-model Tracker with Robust Information Fusion

The diagram of the proposed robust tracking is illustrated in Figure 2. Our approach is robust in two aspects: in the *measurement process*, VBDF fusion is used for combining matching results from multiple appearance models and in the *filtering process*, fusion is performed in the shape space to combine information from measurement, prior knowledge and models while taking advantage of the heteroscedastic nature of the noise.

To model the changes during tracking we propose to maintain several exemplars of the object appearance over time which is equivalent to a nonparametric representation of the appearance distribution. Figure 2 illustrates the *appearance models*, i.e. the current exemplars in the model set, each having associated a set of overlapping components. Throughout this paper, we represent shapes by control or landmark points (components). These points are fitted by splines before shown to the user. A component-based approach is more robust that a global representation, being less sensitive to structural changes thus being able to deal with nonrigid shape deformations.

Each component is processed independently, its location and covariance matrix is estimated in the current image with respect to all of the model templates. For example, one of the components is illustrated by the rectangle in Figure 2 and its location and uncertainty with respect to each model is shown in the motion estimation stage. The VBDF robust fusion procedure is applied to determine the most dominant motion (mode) with the associated uncertainty.

The location of the components in the current frame is further adapted by imposing subspace shape constraints using pre-trained *shape models*. Robust shape tracking is achieved by optimally resolving uncertainties from the system dynamics, heteroscedastic measurements noise and subspace shape model. By using the estimated confidence in each component location reliable components contribute more to the global shape motion estimation. The current frame is added to the model set if the residual error to the reference appearances is relatively low.

3   Measurement Process

Consider that we have n models $M_0, M_1, \ldots, M_n$. For each image we maintain c components with their location denoted by x_{ij}, $i = 1 \ldots n$, $j = 1 \ldots c$. When a new image is available we estimate the location and the uncertainty for each component and for each model. We adopt for this step the robust optical flow technique proposed in [13] which is also an application of the VBDF technique. The result is the motion estimate $\hat{x}_{ij}$ for each component and its uncertainty $\hat{C}_{ij}$. Thus $\hat{x}_{ij}$ represents the location estimate of component j with respect to model i. The scale of the covariance matrix is also estimated from the matching residual errors.

The VDBF estimator is based on nonparametric density estimation with adaptive kernel bandwidths [13]. The choice of the VDBF estimator is motivated by its good performance in the presence of outliers in the input data when compared to previous methods such as Covariance Intersection or BLUE estimation assuming single source, statistically independent data. The VDBF estimator is defined as the *location of the most significant mode* of a density function. The mode computation is based on the variable-bandwidth mean shift technique in a multiscale optimization framework.

Let $\hat{x}_i \in \mathbb{R}^d$, $i = 1 \ldots n$ be the available d-dimensional estimates, each having an associated uncertainty given by the covariance matrix $\hat{C}_i$ (we drop the component index j for now). A bandwidth matrix $\hat{H}_i = \hat{C}_i + \alpha^2 I$ is associated with each point $\hat{x}_i$, where I is the identity matrix and the parameter α determines the scale of the analysis. The sample point density estimator at location $\hat{x}$ is defined by

$$\hat{f}(x) = \frac{1}{n(2\pi)^{d/2}} \sum_{i=1}^{n} exp\left(-\frac{1}{2}(x - \hat{x}_i)^\top \hat{H}_i^{-1}(x - \hat{x}_i)\right). \tag{1}$$

The variable bandwidth mean shift vector at location x is given by

$$m(x) = H_h(x) \sum_{i=1}^{n} \omega_i(x) \hat{H}_i^{-1} \hat{x}_i - x \quad \text{where} \quad H_h(x) = \left(\sum_{i=1}^{n} \omega_i(x) \hat{H}_i^{-1}\right)^{-1}. \tag{2}$$

H_h represents the harmonic mean of the bandwidth matrices weighted by the data-dependent weights $\omega_i(x)$ computed at the current location x

$$\omega_i(x) = \frac{\frac{1}{|\hat{H}_i|^{1/2}} exp\left(-\frac{1}{2}(x - \hat{x}_i)^\top \hat{H}_i^{-1}(x - \hat{x}_i)\right)}{\sum_{i=1}^{n} \frac{1}{|\hat{H}_i|^{1/2}} exp\left(-\frac{1}{2}(x - \hat{x}_i)^\top \hat{H}_i^{-1}(x - \hat{x}_i)\right)}. \tag{3}$$

Updating iteratively the current location using the mean shift vector yields a hill-climbing procedure which converges to a stationary point of the underlying density. The

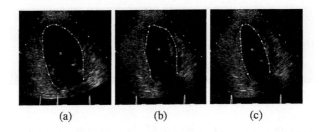

(a)   (b)   (c)

Fig. 3. Multiple models versus single model. (a) initial contour; (b) 17th contour tracked using a single appearance model (c) 17th contour tracked using multiple appearance models.

VBDF estimator finds the most important mode by iteratively applying the mean shift procedure at several scales. It starts from a large scale by choosing the parameter α large with respect to the spread of the points. In this case the density surface is unimodal and the determined mode will correspond to the globally densest region. The procedure is repeated while reducing the value of the parameter α and starting the the mean shift iterations from the mode determined at the previous scale. In the final step the bandwidth matrix associated to each point is equal to the covariance matrix, ($\hat{H}_i = \hat{C}_i$).

The VBDF estimator is a powerful tool for information fusion with the ability to deal with multiple source models. This is important for motion estimation as points in a local neighborhood may exhibit multiple motions. The most significant mode corresponds to the most relevant motion. The VBDF robust fusion technique is applied to determine the most relevant location $\hat{x}_j$ for component j in the current frame. The mode tracking across scales results in

$$\hat{x}_j = C(\hat{x}_j) \sum_{i=1}^{n} \omega_i(\hat{x}_j)\hat{C}_{ij}^{-1}\hat{x}_{ij} \quad \text{and} \quad C(\hat{x}_j) = \left(\sum_{i=1}^{n} \omega_i(\hat{x}_j)\hat{C}_{ij}^{-1} \right)^{-1}. \quad (4)$$

Figure 3 shows the advantage of using multiple appearance models. The initial frame with the associated contour is shown in Figure 3a. Using a single model yields an incorrect tracking results (Figure 3b) and the multiple model approach correctly copes with the appearance changes (Figure 3c).

4   Filtering Process

The analysis is based on vectors formed by concatenating the coordinates of all control points [7,1]. A typical tracking framework fuses information from the prediction defined by a dynamic process and from noisy measurements. For shape tracking additional *global* constraints are necessary to stabilize the overall shape in a feasible range.

Let us now turn our attention to the problem of information fusion with one of the sources in a subspace. Given two noisy measurements of the same n-dimensional variable x, each characterized by a multidimensional Gaussian distribution, $\mathcal{N}(x_1, C_1)$ and $\mathcal{N}(x_2, C_2)$, the maximum likelihood estimate of x is the point with the minimal sum of Mahalanobis distances to the two centroids. Now, assume that one of the Gaussians

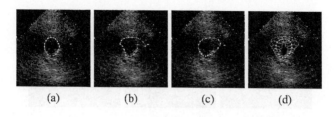

(a)   (b)   (c)   (d)

Fig. 4. Orthogonal projection versus our proposed fusion approach. (a) expert-drawn contour; (b) un-constrained flow results; (c) constrained flow using orthogonal projection; (d) contour obtained by our fusion framework with uncertainty ellipses.

is in a subspace of dimension p, e.g., C_2 is singular. With the singular value decomposition of $C_2 = U\Lambda U^T$, where $U = [u_1, u_2, \ldots, u_n]$, with u_i's orthonormal and $\Lambda = diag\{\lambda_1, \lambda_2, \ldots, \lambda_p, 0, \ldots, 0\}$. The distance to be minimized becomes:

$$d^2 = (U_p y - x_1)^T C_1^{-1} (U_p y - x_1) + (U_p y - x_2)^T C_2^+ (U_p y - x_2) \tag{5}$$

where $U_p = [u_1, u_2, \ldots, u_p]$ represents the subspace basis and y the value in this subspace. Taking derivative with respect to y yields the fusion estimator for the subspace:

$$y^* = C_{y^*} U_p^T (C_1^{-1} x_1 + C_2^+ x_2) \quad \text{where} \quad C_{y^*} = [U_p^T (C_1^{-1} + C_2^+) U_p]^{-1} . \tag{6}$$

Equivalent expressions can be obtained in the original space:

$$x^* = U_p y^* = C_{x^*} (C_1^{-1} x_1 + C_2^+ x_2) \quad \text{where} \quad C_{x^*} = U_p C_{y^*} U_p^T . \tag{7}$$

It can be shown that C_{x^*} and C_{y^*} are the covariance matrices for x^* and y^* (see [14]).

To complete the shape tracking method, the subspace fusion with shape models is integrated into a Kalman filtering framework [15]. Kalman filtering with subspace constraints provides a unified fusion of the system dynamics, a subspace model, and measurement noise information. For details please see [14].

For endocardium tracking what we theoretically need is *the statistical shape model of the current heart* instead of a generic heart. Therefore we apply a strongly-adapted-PCA (SA-PCA) model by assuming that the PCA model and the initialized contour *jointly* represent the variations of the current case [14]. With SA-PCA, our framework now incorporates four information sources: the system dynamic, measurement, subspace model, and the initial contour.

An example is shown in Figure 4 for comparison between our approach and orthogonal projection. The fusion will not correct the error completely, but note that this correction step is accumulative so that the overall effect at a later frame in a long sequence can be very significant.

5 Experiments

In this section we will apply and evaluate the new framework to track heart contours using very noisy echocardiography data. The tracker was implemented in C++ and is running

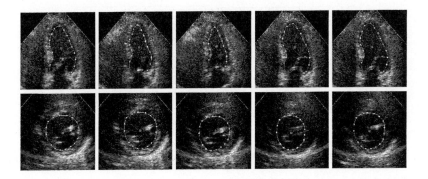

Fig. 5. Two tracking examples in rows, with 5 snapshots per sequence.

at about 20 frames per second on a single 2GHz Pentium 4 PC. Our data were selected by a cardiologist to represent normals as well as various types of cardiomyopathies, with sequences varying in length from 18 frames to 90 frames. Both training and test data were traced by experts, and confirmed by one cardiologist. We used both apical two- or four-chamber views (open contour with 17 control points) and parasternal short axis views (closed contour with 18 control points) for training and testing. PCA is performed and the original dimensionality of 34 and 36 is reduced to 7 and 8, respectively. For the appearance models we maintain 20 templates to capture the appearance variability. For systematic evaluation, we use a set of 32 echocardiogram sequences outside of the training set for testing, with 18 parasternal short-axis views and 14 apical two- or four-chamber views, all with expert-annotated ground-truth contours.

Figure 5 shows snapshots from two tracked sequences. Notice that the endocardium is not always on the strongest edge. Sometimes it manifests itself only by a faint line; sometimes it is completely invisible or buried in heavy noise; sometimes it will cut through the root of the papillary muscles where no edge is present. To compare performance of different methods, we used the Mean Sum of Squared Distance (MSSD) (*cf.* [16]) and a Mean Absolute Distance (MAD) (*cf.* [17]). Our proposed method ("Proposed") is compared with a tracking algorithm without shape constraint ("Flow") or with the same tracker with orthogonal PCA shape space constraints ("FlowShapeSpace"). Figure 6 and Table 1 show the comparison using the two distance measures. Our proposed method ("Proposed") significantly outperforms others, with lower average distances and lower standard deviations for such distances.

It should be noted that our results are not indicative for *border localization* accuracies, but rather for *motion tracking* performances given an initial contour. We have set our goal to track control points on the endocardium, with anisotropic confidence estimated at each point at any given time step by using multiple appearance models, and exploit this information when consulting a prior shape model as a constraint. Our framework is general and can be applied to other modalities. Future potential applications include tracking in MR, perfusion, and extensions to tracking in 3-D or 4-D.

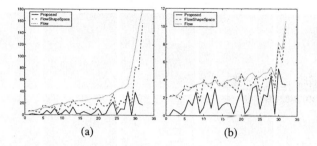

(a)   (b)

Fig. 6. Mean distances ((a) $MSSD_i$, (b) MAD_i) between tracked points and the ground truth.

Table 1. Error analysis ("Most Difficult Cases" are the last three cases in Figure 6a).

Methods	All Cases				Most Difficult Cases			
	$MSSD$	$\bar{\sigma}_{MSSD}$	MAD	$\bar{\sigma}_{MAD}$	$MSSD$	$\bar{\sigma}_{MSSD}$	MAD	$\bar{\sigma}_{MAD}$
Flow	38.1	82.9	4.3	3.6	147.9	325.0	8.8	8.2
FlowShapeSpace	24.7	35.5	3.8	2.4	106.0	181.2	7.9	6.3
Proposed	8.3	14.3	1.7	1.6	25.8	34.8	4.1	2.8

Acknowledgment. We would like to thank Dr. Alan Katz from St. Francis Hospital for fruitful interactions and guidance. We are grateful for the inspiring discussions and generous support from Alok Gupta and Sriram Krishnan of Siemens Medical Solutions.

References

1. Cootes, T., Taylor, C.: Statistical models of appearance for medical image analysis and computer vision. In: Proc. SPIE Medical Imaging. (2001) 236–248
2. Chalana, V., Linker, D.T., Haynor, D.R., Kim, Y.: A multiple active contour model for cardiac boundary detection on echocardiographic sequences. IEEE Trans. Medical Imaging **15** (1996) 290–298
3. Mignotte, M., Meunier, J., Tardif, J.C.: Endocardial boundary estimation and tracking in echocardiographic images using deformable templates and markov random fields. Pattern Analysis and Applications **4** (2001) 256–271
4. Mailloux, G.E., Langlois, F., Simard, P.Y., Bertrand, M.: Restoration of the velocity field of the heart from two-dimensional echocardiograms. IEEE Trans. Medical Imaging **8** (1989) 143–153
5. Adam, D., Hareuveni, O., Sideman, S.: Semiautomated border tracking of cine echocardiographic ventricular images. IEEE Trans. Medical Imaging **6** (1987) 266–271
6. Baraldi, P., Sarti, A., Lamberti, C., Prandini, A., Sgal-lari, F.: Semiautomated border tracking of cine echocardiographic ventricular images. IEEE Trans. Biomedical Eng. (1986) 259–272
7. Jacob, G., Noble, J., Behrenbruch, C., Kelion, A., Banning, A.: A shape-space-based approach to tracking myocardial borders and quantifying regional left-ventricular function applied in echocardiography. IEEE Trans. Medical Imaging **21** (2002) 226–238
8. Roche, A., Pennec, X., Malandain, G., Ayache, N.: Rigid registration of 3d ultrasound with mr images: a new approach combining intensity and gradient information. IEEE Trans. Medical Imaging **20** (2001) 1038–1049

9. Montillo, A., Metaxas, D., Axel, L.: Automated segmentation of the left and right ventricles in 4d cardiac spamm images. In: Proc. of Medical. Image Computing and Computer Assisted Intervention (MICCAI), Tokyo, Japan. (2002) 620–633
10. Hellier, P., Barillot, C.: Coupling dense and landmark-based approaches for non rigid registration. IEEE Trans. Medical Imaging **22** (2003) 217–227
11. Jacob, G., Noble, A., Blake, A.: Robust contour tracking in echocardiographic sequence. In: Proc. Intl. Conf. on Computer Vision, Bombay, India. (1998) 408–413
12. Blake, A., Isard, M., Reynard, D.: Learning to track the visual motion of contours. Artificial Intelligence **78** (1995) 101–133
13. Comaniciu, D.: Nonparametric information fusion for motion estimation. In: Proc. IEEE Conf. on Computer Vision and Pattern Recognition, Madison, Wisconsin. (2003) 59–66
14. Comaniciu, D., Zhou, X.S., Krishnan, S.: Robust real-time myocardial border tracking for echocardiography: An information fusion approach. In: IEEE Trans. Medical Imaging. (2004) to appear
15. Grewal, M.S., Andrews, A.P.: Kalman Filtering: Theory and Practice. Prentice Hall (1993)
16. Akgul, Y., Kambhamettu, C.: A coarse-to-fine deformable contour optimization framework. IEEE Trans. Pattern Anal. Machine Intell. **25** (2003) 174–186
17. Mikić, I., Krucinski, S., Thomas, J.D.: Segmentation and tracking in echocardiographic sequences: Active contours guided by optical flow estimates. IEEE Trans. Medical Imaging **17** (1998) 274–284

Simulation of the Electromechanical Activity of the Heart Using XMR Interventional Imaging

Maxime Sermesant[1], Kawal Rhode[1], Angela Anjorin[1], Sanjeet Hegde[1],
Gerardo Sanchez-Ortiz[2], Daniel Rueckert[2], Pier Lambiase[3], Clifford Bucknall[3],
Derek Hill[1], and Reza Razavi[1]

[1] Division of Imaging Sciences, Guy's, King's & St Thomas' School of Medicine,
King's College London, 5th Floor Thomas Guy House, Guy's Hospital, London, UK
[2] Department of Computing, Imperial College London
[3] Department of Cardiology, St Thomas' Hospital, London

Abstract. Simulating cardiac electromechanical activity is of great interest for a better understanding of pathologies and therapy planning. Design and validation of such models is difficult due to the lack of clinical data. XMR systems are a new type of interventional facility in which patients can be rapidly transferred between x-ray and MR systems. Our goal is to design and validate an electromechanical model of the myocardium, using this XMR system. The proposed model is computationally fast and uses clinically observable parameters. We present the integration of anatomy, electrophysiology, and motion from patients. Pathologies are introduced in the model and the simulations are compared to measured data. Initial qualitative comparison is encouraging. Quantitative local validation is in progress. Once validated, these models will make it possible to simulate different interventional strategies.

1 Introduction

Simulation of normal and pathological electromechanical activity in the heart is of great current interest [6]. The validation of such models is extremely difficult, especially in the case of human pathology. In this paper we describe an electromechanical model of the heart that is designed to simulate the behaviour of the heart during normal and abnormal heart rhythms. The long term aim of this work is to devise a technique to make electrophysiology studies (EPS) to correct abnormal heart rhythms less invasive and more successful. We use a catherisation lab incorporating both MRI and conventional fluoroscopy (XMR) to enable us to collect data from patients about cardiac anatomy, motion and electrical activity during their catherisation. This data is integrated into a common coordinate system using device tracking and registration. A sub-set of this data can be used to initialise the model, and simulate the observed pathology. The modelled behaviour can then be validated using the rest of the collected data. This approach is applied to two patients, one with a ventricular tachycardia, and the second with left bundle branch block.

C. Barillot, D.R. Haynor, and P. Hellier (Eds.): MICCAI 2004, LNCS 3217, pp. 786–794, 2004.
© Springer-Verlag Berlin Heidelberg 2004

Modelling the Cardiac Electromechanical Activity. Combination of medical image analysis and organ simulation opens new perspectives in clinical applications. The integration of knowledge from biology, physics and computer science makes it possible to combine *in vivo* observations, *in vitro* experiments and *in silico* simulations. During recent decades, there have been great advances in the knowledge of heart function, from the nanoscopic to the mesoscopic scale. A global integrative model of this organ becomes conceivable.

Understanding and modelling cardiac electrophysiology, studying the inverse problem from body surface potentials and direct measurement of heart potentials are active research areas. Moreover, many constitutive laws have been proposed in the literature for the mechanical modelling of the myocardium [12].

All these models need rich electromechanical data for validation. Macroscopic measures of the electrical and mechanical activities on the same heart are now available [7]. However, these measures are difficult to obtain and very invasive. Only animal data is available this way. None of these models have been validated against *in vivo* human data.

The presented work makes possible the validation of an electromechanical model of the human myocardium, due to integration of electrical and mechanical clinical data. The modelling choices are guided by both the nature of the measures (e.g. only the extracellular potential is available for electrophysiology) and their resolution (e.g. spatial and temporal resolution of MR). This model can help to make the most of these measurements, as well as allow simulation of different pathologies and interventional strategies.

Electrophysiological Pathologies and Interventions. Cardiac arrhythmias are the cause of considerable morbidity and even occasional mortality. Tachyarrhythmias (fast heart rhythms) can originate from ectopic foci of electrical depolarisation or from abnormal conduction pathways in the myocardium. The treatment of choice for patients with tachyarrhythmias is radio-frequency ablation (RFA), where the abnormal electrical focus or pathway is ablated by applying radio-frequency energy. For patients with heart failure associated with ventricular asynchrony, the treatment of choice is biventricular pacing through a pacing device.

An electrophysiology study (EPS) is performed prior to these interventions: an electrical measurement catheter is inserted into the appropriate chamber of the heart and the electrical activity on the endocardial surface is measured.

Two Cardiac Electrophysiology Mapping Systems Used. The contact mapping system employs the Constellation catheter from Boston Scientific, a multi-electrode basket catheter. The basket adapts to the endocardial surface and deforms so that contact is maintained through the cardiac cycle.

The non-contact mapping system Ensite from Endocardial Solutions employs a catheter containing a flexible balloon made from a wire mesh. The balloon floats inside the desired cardiac chamber and does not contact the endocardial surface. A second catheter (roving catheter) is inserted and emits a radio-frequency signal from its tip that is detected by the balloon. It is used to map the endocardium. The electrical activity measured by the balloon is then extrapolated to this surface.

XMR Interventional Imaging. The XMR interventional suite at King's College London (Guy's Hospital Campus) comprises a 1.5 T MR scanner (Philips Intera I/T) and a mobile cardiac x-ray set (Philips BV Pulsera). The patient can be easily moved between the two systems using a specially modified sliding MR table top that docks with and transfers patients to a specially modified x-ray table. The docking and transfer takes less than 60 seconds.

Although it is possible to acquire MR images and x-ray images of the same patient during a procedure, the XMR system has no inherent ability to register these images. We have previously described the validation of a novel XMR registration technique that is applicable to the sliding table XMR configuration [9].

2   Clinical Cases

Clinical Case 1: Contact Mapping System. Patient 1, male aged 15, had an intermittent ventricular tachycardia that was to be treated by EPS and RFA. Initially, MR imaging was performed, using SSFP three-dimensional multiphase sequence and myocardial motion imaging was performed in both short axis (SA) and long axis (LA) views using SPAMM tagged imaging. The patient was then transferred to the x-ray system. Dynamic biplane tracked x-ray images were acquired with the catheters in place and at the same time the electrical activity was recorded from the Constellation catheter during two ventricular ectopic beats. The patient then underwent a successful RFA.

Clinical Case 2: Non-Contact Mapping System. Patient 2, male, aged 68, had poor left ventricular function following a myocardial infarction. The patient was to undergo EPS and programmed pacing to assess the optimal location of pacing wires for biventricular pacing. Initially, MR imaging was performed using SSFP 3D multiphase sequence and myocardial motion imaging was performed in both SA and LA views using CSPAMM spiral tagged imaging sequence. The patient was then transferred to the x-ray system and the myocardial electrical activity was measured. Dynamic biplane tracked x-ray images were acquired with the catheters in place. The patient then underwent programmed pacing and had a successful pace maker implantation at a later date.

3   Integration of the Electromechanical Data

For each of these cases, we have access to different types of information: anatomy from MR 3D volume images, motion with multislice tagged MR images, invasive electrophysiology with the mapping system, position of the mapping system with x-ray images and XMR registration technology.

MR images were segmented to isolate the anatomy of interest using the Analyze software package (Mayo Clinic, Minnesota, USA). And the myocardial motion was extracted by analysis of the tagged MR images with a non-rigid registration approach [4].

The combination of these data provide a very rich material for modelling the myocardium. Before using these data for a model, we have to integrate all the different information in the same coordinate system (fig. 3).

3.1   Mapping Electromechanical Data to Patient Anatomy

The XMR registration technique aligns the MRI and electrophysiology data to an accuracy of 4-10 mm. There are residual errors due primarily to respiratory motion and errors in the surface location from the EP system (fig. 4).

Clinical Case 1: Rigid Registration. We correct for residual mis-registration with a surface to image registration technique based on the Iterative Closest Point algorithm [8]. For each vertex of the basket mesh, we computed the corresponding boundary voxel in the MR image by looking along the normal for a boundary point, defined from gradient value and direction. Then from all the matched vertex/boundary point pairs we estimated the best rigid body transformation, and iterate until convergence.

Clinical Case 2: Non-Rigid Registration. The EnSite system produces a surface representation of the left ventricle. This surface is estimated with the roving catheter, considering the furthest position as end-diastolic. When registered to the segmented MR anatomy with the XMR registration technology, it appears that its shape do not exactly match the left ventricular MR anatomy.

We correct this using a deformable surface, which evolves like a snake method under the influence of an external energy computed from the gradient of the image and adjusting the surface to the image boundaries and an internal energy keeping the surface regular from [5]. For each vertex of the surface, a force is applied on the vertex, proportional to the distance to the closest boundary point.

These transformations make it possible to have the anatomy, motion an electrophysiology information in the same coordinate space (see fig. 3).

4   Modelling the Cardiac Electromechanical Activity

Simulation of the Cardiac Electrophysiology. Simulation of the cardiac electrophysiology is usually done using either the *Luo-Rudy* type of models or the *FitzHugh-Nagumo* type. The former is based on the simulation of all the different ions present in a cardiac cell along with the different channels. The latter is based on a more global scale, only modelling the potential difference between the intracellular and the extracellular space (the action potential).

As we are more interested in the timing of the wave propagation than in what is happening at the ion scale, and we intend to interpret it in terms of local conductivity, we use a *FitzHugh-Nagumo* type of model. Moreover, *Luo-Rudy* variables are not observable *in vivo*, and much too numerous to be adjusted from such data. We use the adapted version for cardiac cells of the FitzHugh-Nagumo equations proposed by [1], in a simplified form:

$$\partial_t u = \text{div}\,(D\,\nabla u) + ku(1-u)(u-a) - uz$$
$$\partial_t z = -\varepsilon(ku(u-a-1)+z)) \tag{1}$$

u: normalised action potential, z: repolarisation variable, k, ε: repolarisation parameters, a: reaction parameter. We can solve these equations on a volumetric tetrahedral mesh (3D Finite Element Method) if we want to compute a whole myocardium propagation or only on triangulated surfaces (2D Finite Element Method), if we want to simulate the propagation on the endocardium. We can also introduce the muscle fibre directions in the computation, through the diffusion tensor D, as they intervene in the propagation speed. More details about the electrical model can be found in [11].

Simulation of the Myocardium Contraction. The action potential controls the mechanical contraction of the myocardium. To simulate this phenomenon, the constitutive law for the myocardium must include an active element, responding to an action potential by developing a contraction stress. We use a model based on the one presented in [10], derived from a multi-scale modelling of the myocardium detailed in [3]. This model is a combination of a (transverse anisotropic, piecewise) linear visco-elastic passive constitutive law, with an active element creating a contraction stress tensor controlled by the action potential.

$$M \frac{d^2U}{dt^2} + C \frac{dU}{dt} + KU = F_e + F_c \qquad (2)$$

where M is the mass matrix, C the damping matrix, K the stiffness matrix, U the displacement vector, F_e the external forces vector and F_c the contraction vector. This model makes it possible to simulate the cardiac cycle, by using different boundary conditions depending on the current phase (filling, isovolumetric contraction, ejection, isovolumetric relaxation). The transition from one phase to another is automatically controlled by the pressure and the flow in the simulated model.

5   Simulation Results

The model described in section 4 has been applied to simulate the electrical activity and motion in the two clinical cases, and compare this simulated behaviour to the measured electrical and mechanical behaviour.

Clinical Case 1: Simulation of an Ectopic Focus. An ectopic focus can be simulated by introducing an additional depolarising area in the model, located from the measured position with the Constellation catheter, and starting at the time given by the electrical recordings (fig. 5).

The electromechanical model of the myocardium has been registered with the anatomical MR to obtain the patient geometry. Then, the vertices corresponding to the ectopic focus were determined, looking for the closest vertices to the Constellation electrodes where this focus was observed.

The timing of the ectopic beat was deduced from the observation of the electrical recordings, which also comprise several ECG derivations. Then an ectopic beat was simulated, the ectopic excitation taking place during the P wave, before the normal QRS complex.

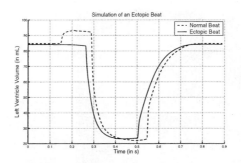

Fig. 1. Consequences on cardiac function parameters: comparison between the simulated normal (dashed) and the simulated ectopic (solid) left ventricle volume.

We can observe in the simulation that the early contraction of the myocardium prevents the atrial contraction from filling the ventricles completely. The ejected volume drops from 71 mL to 61 mL.

Moreover, the simulation of several ectopic beats leads to an even greater difference, with a smaller end diastolic volume for the ectopic heart. Thus the consequences of arrhythmia on simulated cardiac function are well represented.

Clinical Case 2: Simulation of a Scar with a Left Branch Block. This patient has a scar which can be clearly observed in the late enhancement MR image acquired. This scar led to a left branch block, which is observable in the electrophysiological measures: the excitation in the left ventricle only comes from the septum area, without any other Purkinje excitation.

A myocardial scar can be simulated by modifying the local conductivity and/or contractility parameters of the model. The branch block can be simulated with no excitation from the Purkinje network in the left ventricle (fig. 6).

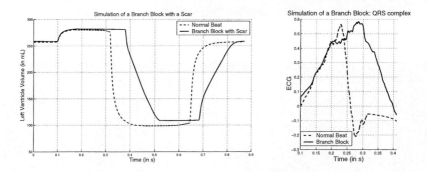

Fig. 2. Simulated left ventricle volume (left) and ECG (right) for a normal heart (dashed) and with a left branch block and a scar (solid).

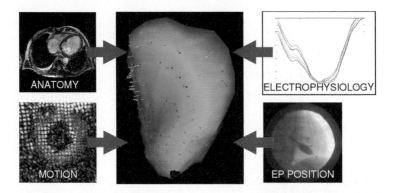

Fig. 3. Integration of the electromechanical data in the same coordinate space.

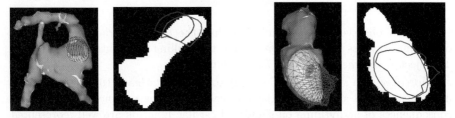

Fig. 4. Final registration between electrophysiology measures and anatomy from MRI.

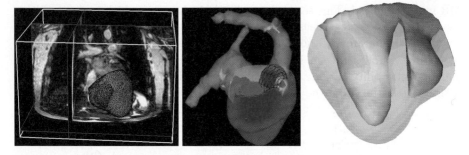

Fig. 5. Simulation of an ectopic focus from XMR measures.

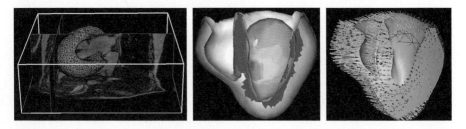

Fig. 6. Simulation of a Left Bundle Branch Block and scar from XMR measures.

The simulated isochrones compare well with the measured ones. The simulated ECG (precordial lead, simulated with an infinite conductivity thorax [2]) shows the characteristics of a left branch block, with a larger "M" shaped QRS complex.

Moreover, the contraction is less efficient, so it needs a higher pre-load to guarantee a cardiac output high enough, which is observed *in vivo*.

6   Conclusion

In this paper we have presented a patient-specific electromechanical model of the heart. Using an XMR system, we have collected registered information about cardiac anatomy, motion and electrical activity from two patients with heart rhythm abnormalities. We have used this patient information to initialise the models, and validate the results they produce. Initial results show good agreement, and further, more quantitative validation is underway. We believe this is the first time that an electromechanical model of the heart has been clinically validated using the combination of anatomy, motion and invasive electrophysiology measurements. This validation process will lead to refinement of the model, and also enable us to identify the information required to initialise the models. Our long term aim is to use the model to devise less invasive techniques for EPS that could transform the clinical applicability and effectiveness of these procedures.

Figures Legends

Fig. 4: (left) Rigid registration of Constellation catheter surface with segmented MR. (right) Non-rigid registration of EnSite surface with segmented MR. Visualisation of initial (blue) and final (red) position and intersection with segmented MR (white).

Fig. 5: (left) Model adjusted to patient anatomy with MR. (middle) visualisation of Constellation catheter (meshed sphere), segmented anatomy (transparent), and bi-ventricular myocardium model. Colour: electrical potential when ectopic beat starts. (right) Isochrones of the simulation of the ectopic beat (red to green: 0 to 200 ms).

Fig. 6:(left) Model adjusted to patient anatomy with MR. (middle) scar introduced in the model (red zone) from late enhancement MR and visualisation of the registered Ensite surface with measured isochrones. (right) end-systolic simulated contraction.

Acknowledgements. The authors acknowledge the UK-EPSRC (Grant JR/R41019/1), the UK Medical Imaging and Signals IRC, the UK JREI, Philips Medical Systems and the Charitable Foundation of Guy's & St Thomas' Hospitals for funding. The authors acknowledge the contributions of Dr. E. Rosenthal, Dr. C. Bucknall, Dr. P. Lambiase, D. Elliott, ESI and the use of the MIPS software from the Epidaure project, INRIA, France.

References

1. R. Aliev and A. Panfilov. A simple two-variable model of cardiac excitation. *Chaos, Solitons & Fractals*, 7(3):293–301, 1996.
2. O. Berenfeld and J. Jalife. Purkinje-muscle reentry as a mechanism of polymorphic ventricular arrhythmias in a 3-dimensional model of the ventricles. *Circulation Research*, 82(10):1063–1077, 1998.
3. J. Bestel, F. Clément, and M. Sorine. A biomechanical model of muscle contraction. In *MICCAI'01*, volume 2208 of *LNCS*, pages 1159–1161. Springer, 2001.
4. R. Chandrashekara, R. H. Mohiaddin, and D. Rueckert. Analysis of myocardial motion in tagged MR images using non-rigid image registration. In *SPIE Medical Imaging*, volume 4684, pages 1168–1179, 2002.
5. M. Desbrun, M. Meyer, P. Schröder, and A. Barr. Implicit fairing of arbitrary meshes using diffusion and curvature flow. In *Siggraph'99*, pages 317–324. 1999.
6. P. Hunter, A. Pullan, and B. Smaill. Modeling total heart function. *Annual Review of Biomedical Engineering*, 5:147–177, 2003.
7. E. McVeigh, O. Faris, D. Ennis, P. Helm, and F. Evans. Measurement of ventricular wall motion, epicardial electrical mapping, and myocardial fiber angles in the same heart. In *FIMH'01*, number 2230 in LNCS, pages 76–82. Springer, 2001.
8. J. Montagnat and H. Delingette. Globally constrained deformable models for 3D object reconstruction. *Signal Processing*, 71(2):173–186, 1998.
9. K. S. Rhode, D. L. Hill, P. J. Edwards, J. Hipwell, D. Rueckert, G. Sanchez-Ortiz, S. Hegde, V. Rahunathan, and R. Razavi. Registration and tracking to integrate X-ray and MR images in an XMR facility. *IEEE Transactions on Medical Imaging*, 22(11):1369–78, 2003.
10. M. Sermesant, Y. Coudière, H. Delingette, and N. Ayache. Progress towards an electro-mechanical model of the heart for cardiac image analysis. In *IEEE International Symposium on Biomedical Imaging (ISBI'02)*, 2002.
11. M. Sermesant, O. Faris, F. Evans, E. McVeigh, Y. Coudière, H. Delingette, and N. Ayache. Preliminary validation using *in vivo* measures of a macroscopic electrical model of the heart. In *IS4TM'03*, number 2230 in LNCS. Springer, 2003.
12. N. Virag, O. Blanc, and L. Kappenberger, editors. *Computer Simulation and Experimental Assessment of Cardiac Electrophysiology*. Futura Publishing, 2001.

Needle Insertion in CT Scanner with Image Overlay – Cadaver Studies

Gabor Fichtinger[1], Anton Deguet[1], Ken Masamune[2], Emese Balogh[1],
Gregory Fischer[1], Herve Mathieu[1], Russell H. Taylor[1], Laura M. Fayad[1], and
S. James Zinreich[1]

[1]Johns Hopkins University, Baltimore, MD, USA
[2]Tokyo Denki University, Japan
contact email: gabor@cs.jhu.edu

Abstract. An image overlay system is presented to assist needle placement in conventional CT scanners. The device consists of a flat LCD display and a half mirror and is mounted on the gantry. Looking at the patient through the mirror, the CT image appears to be floating inside the patient with correct size and position, thereby providing the physician with two-dimensional "X-ray vision" to guide needle placement procedures. The physician inserts the needle following the optimal path identified in the CT image that is rendered on the LCD and thereby reflected in the mirror. The system promises to increase needle placement accuracy and also to reduce X-ray dose, patient discomfort, and procedure time by eliminating faulty insertion attempts. We report cadaver experiments in several clinical applications with a clinically applicable device.

1   Introduction

Numerous studies have demonstrated the potential efficacy of CT-guided percutaneous needle-based therapy and biopsy in a wide variety of medical problems. Contemporary practice, however, is limited by the freehand technique, which requires mental registration of the patient's anatomy to the CT image in targeting and precise hand-eye coordination in inserting the needle. This often leads to faulty needle placement attempts followed by repeated CT scans and adjustments, increasing the discomfort and radiation exposure of the patient and lengthening the procedure. Practitioners generally agree that, given enough time and opportunity for intermittent CT imaging and adjustments, the target usually can be reached with appropriate accuracy. The important question is, however, whether the same objective could be achieved with just one attempt, because each correction requires taking an extra CT image (or even series of images) and reinsertion of the needle, which in turn increases the risk of post-procedure complication, discomfort, and radiation exposure to the patient. Therefore, eliminating faulty needle insertion attempts is a prime objective of our research.

A variety of tracked navigation systems and surgical robots have been investigated; all resulting in systems that are prohibitively complex and/or expensive for routine clinical use. Head-mounted displays [1,2], video projections [3], and volumetric image overlay systems [4] have been tried out. Unfortunately, all such methods require

C. Barillot, D.R. Haynor, and P. Hellier (Eds.): MICCAI 2004, LNCS 3217, pp. 795–803, 2004.
© Springer-Verlag Berlin Heidelberg 2004

elaborate calibration, registration, and spatial tracking of all actors and components; a rather complex and expensive engineering entourage. In the pursuit of simpler image overlay systems, our group [5,6] and concurrently Stetten [7,8] have been investigating 2D image reflection produced in a semitransparent mirror. This technique provides an optically stable 2D reflection image without auxiliary tracking, requiring only a simple pre-operative alignment. As the majority of needle placement procedures are executed "in-plane" (i.e. when the needle is completely contained a single CT slice), giving up 3D rendering for engineering simplicity and low cost appears to be a reasonable tradeoff. This paper describes a clinically deployable embodiment of the Masamune-Stetten concept, optimized for needle placement procedures in conventional CT scanners. In particular, we report new hardware, display software, and the results of phantom and human cadaver studies. Approval is being sought to begin human trials.

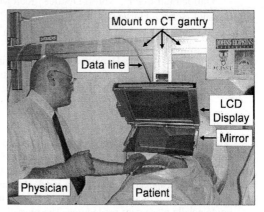

Fig. 1. Spinal needle insertion in human cadaver

2   System Design

A flat LCD display and a semi-transparent mirror are mounted on the gantry of a CT scanner (Figure 1) A CT slice is acquired and rendered on the display. The display is positioned with respect to the mirror so that the reflection of the CT image in the mirror coincides with the patient's body behind the mirror (Figure 2), as was described previously in [6]. The overlay is mounted on the gantry, so it tilts with it, if necessary. In many needle placement procedures, after the entry point is selected with the use of skin fiducial markers, three degrees-of-freedom (DOF) motion of the needle need to be controlled. The physician uses the overlay image to control the in-plane insertion angle (1st DOF), while holding the needle in the axial plane marked by the gantry's laser light (2nd DOF). The insertion depth (3rd DOF) is marked on the overlay image. In our proof-of-concept prototype [6], the overlay image was created in the imaging plane of the scanner, which allowed for rapid imaging update, but it prohibitively constrained the workspace. The

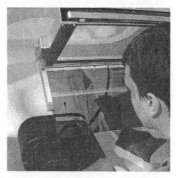

Fig. 2. Needle insertion in phantom. The CT image appears to be floating inside the body with correct alignment and magnification.

new device uses the outer laser plane of the scanner. While this arrangement provides a conveniently large workspace, it also requires moving the table between imaging and insertion.

The procedural workflow is as follows. The patient is externally marked with IZI CT Biopsy Strip (IZI Corporation, Baltimore, MD). We acquire a CT volume (Siemens Somatom-4), with a slice thickness appropriate for the given application. The plane of insertion is identified and the slice of interest is transferred to the plan-

ning and display software running on a Windows-XP laptop. The entry and target points are picked in the CT image, a visual needle guide is displayed, and the scene is pushed to the overlay display as it will be seen later in the left panels of Figure 7. The CT table is translated out by the known offset between the slice of interest and plane of the overlay. The physician places the needle tip at the entry point and lines it up with the visual insertion guide seen in the mirror, while holding the needle in the plane of the laser (Figure 1.) The skin fiducials are visible on both the patient and in the overlay image and coincidence between the corresponding marks indicates correct alignment. This feature is particularly useful when

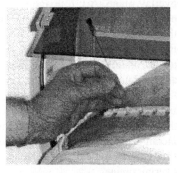

Fig. 3. Needle insertion with single stroke with the assistance of virtual needle guide

the target anatomy is prone to motion due to respiration or mechanical force. (This was not found to be a limiting factor in cadaver studies, however.) Usually, a confirmation image is acquired after insertion, as we show later in Figures 6,7, and 8.

3 Display Software and Registration

Pre-operative calibration, insertion planning, and display image generation are performed on the stand-alone laptop. The CT image containing the target is transferred from the scanner a DICOM receiver client running on the laptop. The laptop concurrently drives the flat panel LCD display of the overlay device, for which the image is flipped horizontally so that the mirror would flip the image back to normal lateral polarity. The insertion planning component is kept simple and intuitive to speed up the process. We refrain from 3D scenes altogether. In the interactive display, the physician can select a sub-image of interest, for which the magnification, display, and level can be adjusted. The target and entry points are assigned by two mouse-clicks. A visual needle guide and depth-gauge automatically appear on the screen. The computer flips the scene, and after ensuring correct magnification and orientation, pushes the image to the overlay display. The physician holds the needle at the entry point behind the mirror and adjusts the needle to match with the virtual guide. This posture allows the physician to insert the needle with a single stroke along to the marked trajectory, without overdriving (Figure 3.)

After mounting, the display, mirror, and scanner must be aligned. The angle of the display and mirror are fixed with respect to one another and an adjustable arm is used to set up the display-mirror unit with respect to the CT laser. For the in-plane registration a phantom made of a 10 mm thick acrylic board containing an asymmetric set of 5 mm diameter aluminum pegs is mounted in the overlay plane. A CT image of the pegs is acquired and rendered on the overlay display as seen in Figure 4. The magnification, in-plane rotation, and translation are

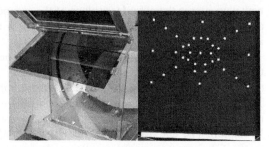

Fig. 4. Calibration phantom and its CT image

adjusted until each aluminum peg coincides with its mark in the CT image.

Calibration has a decisive impact on the system's performance; thus this step must be robust to algorithmic and human errors, while still simple and fast. The marks of the aluminum pegs are auto-segmented in the phantom's CT image and then the technician leans over the mirror and selects the points where the pegs appear in the mirror. From these we calculate the in-plane translation and rotation and then correct the overlay image.

We analyzed the combined effects of human and optical errors on synthetic data, with the objective to determine the optimal number, distribution, and selection order of registration points. We artificially misaligned the two sets of points (i.e. the pegs and their respective image coordinates) by applying a known transformation on each pair and adding noise to each data point, as explained in Figure 5a. Let Q and R be the corresponding points to register in CT and real space. To simulate the error induced by the user and the physical property of the semi-transparent glass, we added some "noise" to the position of R, obtaining point P. We registered P to Q getting a rigid-body transformation T_{reg}. Using this transformation, we transformed R obtaining S. Therefore, the system error was the distance between points S and Q. We simulated human error by adding a random value (±2 pixels) to the position of the point to be registered. Parallax error from the mirror may induce a significantly large error. At d=4 mm thickness and α=30° view angle and using the formulas derived in Figure 5b, the parallax error was about x=1.28 mm, the effect of which fortunately can be substantially reduced by altering the view points during the calibration process. We also concluded that iterative re-registration more favorable than collecting all registration points first and then calculating a single global registration. This observation was true

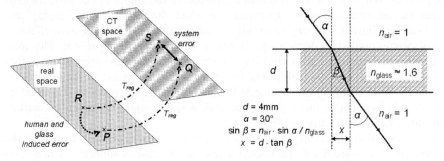

Fig. 5. Definition of registration error (a) and the calculation of parallax error (b)

across the range of practically relevant amplitudes and distributions of noise and number of registration points. The best strategy was found to be the following: (1) Pick a peg near the area of interest in the vicinity of expected target and entry. Let the computer calculate translation and readjust the overlay image. (2) Pick a peg far out from the previous one. Let the computer calculate rotation and readjust the overlay image. (3) Pick a new peg again relatively close to area of interest to adjust transla-tion. (4) Pick another peg to adjust rotation, far out and in 90° from the previous one. (5) Repeat the pair-wise process until sufficient registration is observed between the phantom and its CT image. It is particularly important to compensate for the parallax error by altering the viewpoint. The registration error, using four pairs of registration points and assuming ±2 pixel human error was 1.23 mm (STD=0.31) at 30° view angle and 0.74 mm (STD=0.21) at perpendicular view (α=0°). This performance appears to be sufficiently accurate for most CT-guided needle placement procedures.

4   Experiments and Results

Body Phantoms: A male body phantom was fabricated by attaching three cm-thick tissue-equivalent bolus material (Harpell Associates Inc., Oakville, ON, Canada) on the back of a plastic male torso and placing 1.5 mm diameter metal balls in the bolus at various depths. This phantom represented a male upper body in prone position, with hard fat/muscle layer with mechanical targets in the back, spine, and shoulder. The objectives were to (1) demonstrate accurate needle placement at the pre-marked targets and (2) assess the ergonomics of the system. Experienced and novice inter-ventionalists each executed four needle insertions with 18G diamond needles. The accuracy of needle placement was assessed in post-insertion CT, with 1 mm slice thickness. The experienced and novice users alike approached the implanted targets within 2 mm, in every attempt. The device had excellent ergonomics: there was no interference in the workspace and all targets were conveniently accessible. The ergo-nomics of the system was also tested on a commercial interventional phantom (CIRS,

Norfolk, VA) shown in Fig-ure 2, resulting in essentially the same outcome. Also importantly, the reproduction error of the CT gantry mount, without any adjust-ment, was consistently below 2 mm (which is less than the width of the laser), tested in 10 trials.

Cadaver   Experiments: The objective of human cadaver experiments was to demonstrate the ability clini-cally adequate needle place-ment to various anatomical

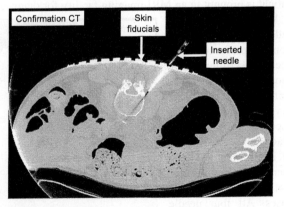

Fig. 6. CT of confirmation of needle placement for spinal pain management

targets, in several potential clinical applications. The accuracy of needle placement was assessed in post-insertion CT. The slice thickness was 1.0-3.0 mm, which was clinically adequate for the procedures in our study.

Spinal Nerve Blocks and Facet Joint Injections are demanding because the interventional team must perform these bilateral injections under 10 minutes. We positioned the cadaver in prone position for nerve root and facet joint injections in the lumbar spine area in the setup seen in Figure 1. We performed four needle insertions with standard 22G beveled needles at the L4 and L5. Contrast and therapeutic substances were not injected. All four spinal nerve block and facet joint needle placements produced clinically adequate results, the needle tip landed within 3 mm from the selected target, without overdriving. One of the confirmation CT images is shown in

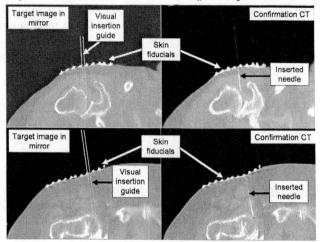

Fig. 7. Target and confirmation CT for arthography of shoulder (top) and hip joint (bottom)

Figure 6, where the needle tip touches the correct anatomical target. The needle is completely included in the confirmation image, indicating that the physician managed to keep the needle exactly in the gantry's laser plane.

Shoulder and Hip Arthographies are diagnostic procedures frequently applied for assessment of joint injury. Typically, some MRI contrast agent is injected percutaneously into the injured joint under CT or X-ray fluoroscopy guidance and then the patient is brought to an MRI imaging facility for diagnostic scanning.

We fixed a female cadaver in supine position and performed four needle insertions to the shoulder and hip joint, using standard 22G beveled needles. The accuracy of needle placement was assessed in intermittent CT and then contrast substance was also injected in two cases. All four needle placements for joint arthography of the

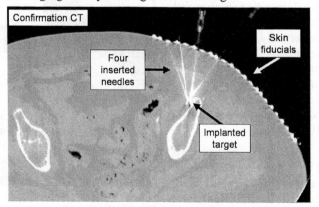

Fig. 8. Confirmation CT of pilot needle insertion in bone biopsy

shoulder and hip were clinically successful, as the needles landed in the targeted joint space. Two cases are shown in Figure 7. Each needle enters the body in the selected entry point, proceeds along the marked trajectory, and touches the selected anatomical target point in the joint space. Contrast material (not shown in the figures) was very hard to inject into the stiffened joint of the cadaver and it did not distribute as evenly as in live patients.

Pilot Needle for Bone Biopsy: Bone biopsies are demanding procedures because the needle must make contact with the bone in some predefined angle that is often very difficult to achieve freehand. One must also avoid sensitive structures (like nerves and blood vessels) in the path. As we almost always operate on damaged bone, faulty placement and misalignment of the large needle or drill may cause structural damage to the already weakened bone; in fact, fracture is not an insignificant intra-operative risk. Many patients have preexisting micro-fractures, a condition that may develop into a full fracture if the instrument is accidentally wedged in the fracture line. Altogether, unassisted freehand planning of the skin entry, trajectory, bone entry, and cortical target can become exceedingly difficult.

We fixed a female cadaver in supine position and performed four needle insertions to the pelvis, using standard 22G beveled needles. A 1.5 mm metal ball marker was implanted percutaneously into the right lateral wall of the left pelvis, and then this location was targeted from several directions from different entry points. All four the pilot needle insertions for pelvic bone biopsy were clinically successful. A confirmation CT is shown in Figure 8. Unfortunately, the artifact caused by the needles suppresses the signal of the implanted metal target, but the needles converge in a confined area, indicating adequate accuracy for bone biopsy. Three of the four needles are completely included in the image slice, while the fourth one is slightly deflected from the image plane.

5 Discussion

In our previous prototype the image overlay device was mounted in the inner laser plane of the scanner, the physician's workspace was often restricted and several targets were not accessible [6]. Therefore, the unanimous decision of the participating physicians was to use the outer laser plane of the scanner, even though it required translation of the CT table between imaging and needle insertion. Needle insertion was more accurate in phantoms than in human cadavers, for several reasons. First, the phantom tissue was softer and more homogeneous than human cadavers. Also, in phantoms we used 18G diamond tip needles that barely deflected during insertion, while in the human cadavers we used 22G beveled needles that had a tendency to deflect in the hard and inhomogeneous tissues. Less experienced users had difficulty in holding the needle in the plane of the laser. Although this presently does not seem to be a clinically significant impediment, we consider applying some form of mechanical constraint to aid the physician with holding the needle in the laser plane.

Although respiration could not be simulated in the passive phantoms and cadavers, the IZI Biopsy Strip fiducials placed on the patient around the insertion point are expected to provide robust real-time indication of any patient motion, in which case the insertion can be halted till the patient's body is correctly re-registered. Alternatively, the fiducials can be used for re-registration of the patient, in the same manner as the calibration fixture is registered.

We have encountered several minor issues that could prove to be significant as our efforts are gearing up toward clinical trials. For example, it is inconvenient to have the planning laptop in the scanner room and its wire connection may also disrupt normal traffic. (In the clinical device, the laptop will be situated next to the console and apply wireless communication to the mouse used for calibration. Also, slight changes in backlight and glare on the display frame have also caused difficulties.)

Adequate needle placement was confirmed in post-insertion CT imaging in all insertion attempts, without needing re-insertion and intermittent CT. The workflow and instrumentation have not been optimized for time and the ergonomics of the system still need to improve. Nevertheless, the system was found to be adequate for initial human trials in several needle placement applications and the cadaver studies were predicative of good clinical performance. Presently, IRB approval is being sought to commence human trials while software and hardware refinements will continue.

Acknowledgements. Funding was available from NSF EEC-9731478, Siemens Corporate Research (Princeton, NJ), and Japanese Ministry of Education, Science, Sports and Culture, Grant-in-Aid for Young Scientists #14702071. We are grateful to Beatrice Mudge, RTT for her help throughout the experiments and Frank Sauer, PhD (Siemens) for his advice.

References

1. Sauer F, Khamene A, Vogt S: An Augmented Reality Navigation System with a Single-Camera Tracker: System Design and Needle Biopsy Phantom Trial. *Fifth International Conference on Medical Image Computing and Computer-Assisted Intervention, Lecture Notes in Computer Science 2489*, pp 116-124, Springer, 2002.
2. Birkfellner, W. Figl, M. Huber, K. Watzinger, F. Wanschitz, F. Hummel, J. Hanel, R. Greimel, W. Homolka, P. Ewers, R. Bergmann, H: A head-mounted operating binocular for augmented reality visualization in medicine - design and initial evaluation, *IEEE Transactions on Medical Imaging*, Volume: 21, No. 8, pp 991-7, 2002.
3. Grimson WEL, Lozano-Perez L, Wells WM, Ettinger GJ, White SJ, Kikinis R: An Automatic Registration Method for Frameless Stereotaxy, *Image Guided Surgery, and Enhanced Reality Visualization, IEEE Trans. Med. Imag.* Vol.15, No.2, 1996.
4. Blackwell M, Nikou C, DiGioia AM, Kanade T: An Image Overlay System for Medical Data Visualization, *First International Conference on Medical Image Computing and Computer-Assisted Intervention, Lecture Notes in Computer Science 1496*, pp.232-240, Springer, 1998.
5. Masamune K, Masutani Y, Nakajima S, Sakuma I, Dohi T, Iseki H, Takakura K: Three-dimensional Slice Image Overlay System with Accurate Depth Perception for Surgery, *Third International Conference on Medical Image Computing and Computer-Assisted Intervention, Lecture Notes in Computer Science 1935*, pp.395-402, Springer, 2000.
6. Masamune K, Fichtinger G, Deguet A, Matsuka D, Taylor RH: An Image Overlay System with Enhanced Reality for Percutaneous Therapy Performed Inside CT Scanner, *Fifth International Conference on Medical Image Computing and Computer-Assisted Intervention, Lecture Notes in Computer Science 2488*, Part 2, pp 77-84, Springer, 2002.

7. Stetten G, Chib V: Magnified Real-Time Tomographic Reflection, *Fourth International Conference on Medical Image Computing and Computer-Assisted Intervention, Lecture Notes in Computer Science 2208*, pp.683-690, Springer, 2001.
8. Stetten GD, Cois A, Chang W, Shelton D, Tamburo RJ, Castellucci J, von Ramm O: C-Mode Real Time Tomographic Reflection for a Matrix Array Ultrasound Sonic Flashlight. *Sixth International Conference on Medical Image Computing and Computer-Assisted Intervention, Lecture Notes in Computer Science 2879*, pp 336-343, Springer, 2003.

Computer Aided Detection in CT Colonography, via Spin Images

Gabriel Kiss, Johan Van Cleynenbreugel, Guy Marchal, and Paul Suetens

Faculties of Medicine & Engineering
Medical Image Computing (Radiology - ESAT/PSI)
University Hospital Gasthuisberg
Herestraat 49, B3000 Leuven, BELGIUM
Gabriel.Kiss@uz.kuleuven.ac.be

Abstract. A technique for Computer Aided Detection (CAD) of colonic polyps, in Computed Tomographic (CT) Colonography is presented. Following the segmentation of the colonic wall, normal wall is identified using a fast geometric scheme able to approximate local curvature. The remaining structures are modeled using spin images and then compared to a set of existing polypoid models. Locations with the highest probability of being colonic polyps are labeled as final candidates. Models are computed by an unsupervised learning technique, using a leave one out technique on a study group of 50 datasets. True positive and false positive findings were determined, employing fiber optic colonoscopy as standard of reference. The detection rate for polyps larger than 6mm was above 85%, with an average false positive detection rate of 2.75 per case. The overall computation time for the method is approximately 6 minutes. Initial results show that Computer Aided Detection is feasible and that our method holds potential for screening purposes.

1 Introduction

Alongside lung cancer in males and breast cancer in females colorectal cancer is one of the most frequent causes of cancer related deaths in the industrialized world. Studies [1] show that it has a mortality rate of 20-25 cases/10^5/year. The typical sequence is from adenoma to carcinoma and the evolution includes in 95% of the cases the appearance of adenomatous polyps [2]. Luckily, this process is a lengthy one taking from 5 up to 10 years. Furthermore, the survival rate after 5 years is 92%, when early treatment is received and polyps are removed endoscopically [3]. The lasting prophylactic effects of polyp removal make screening for adenomatous polyps a viable alternative to reduce mortality rate due to colorectal cancer.

Numerous methods are available for colonic polyps detection, well-known methods include: fecal occult blood testing (FOBT), barium enema examinations, sigmoidoscopy and conventional colonoscopy. When looking for the most effective methods for polyp detection the choice is between conventional colonoscopy and barium enema examinations. It has been proven that conventional colonoscopy has the highest accuracy in detecting polyps and furthermore,

C. Barillot, D.R. Haynor, and P. Hellier (Eds.): MICCAI 2004, LNCS 3217, pp. 804–812, 2004.
© Springer-Verlag Berlin Heidelberg 2004

once found polyps can be immediately removed. Although, considered as the gold standard conventional colonoscopy has its pitfalls, when patient screening is taken into consideration. It is quite invasive, there is a small risk of wall perforation and in some cases the examination of the entire colon is not attainable.

That is why lately other methods usable for screening were investigated. Among these FOBT is the only one used for clinical screening. Although, safe and inexpensive it has a low sensitivity and thus effectiveness. Lately, CT colonography has emerged as an alternative for screening. Introduced in 1994 by Vining et. al. [4], it is a method for exploring the colonic area hinging on CT data. When over 1000 axial slices have to be interpreted it is not difficult to see that perceptual errors will have a negative effect on the performance of CT colonography. To overcome this problem computer aided detection (CAD) methods have been developed; they automate the process of finding polypoid structures.

In the literature some methods have been proposed [5] [6] [7]. All of the cited methods use shape properties of the colonic wall while trying to identify polyps. Polyps are viewed as spherical or semi-spherical structures protruding inwards into the colonic lumen. The mathematical description of polyps differs from author to author. While some choose curvature as their shape descriptor, others use information given by the local normals to differentiate between polyps, colonic wall and haustral folds (the main structures contained in the colon).

The remaining of the paper is organized as follows: first our method for CAD is explained, followed by results on 50 colonoscopic data-sets. The advantages and pitfalls of the method are presented in the discussion section. Finally, some conclusions on the future of CAD are given.

2   Method

Since it is well know that over 90% of the colonic surface represents normal wall, this has to be identified and disregarded as quickly as possible. That is why most of CAD algorithms contain two steps a generation step (colonic wall is identified) and a filtering step (final polyp candidates are selected from the remaining structures). The novelty of our method is twofold, first it introduces a fast method for wall identification and second, it models polyps using spin images. The following sections will present the method in detail. A brief overview of our segmentation is given, followed by the colonic wall identification process. Finally the filtering step and the algorithm for building polypoid models are detailed.

Segmentation. During segmentation the colonic wall is determined. A classic region growing algorithm [8], with multiple seed points (to overcome collapsed regions) is used. The threshold value is determined automatically, using the cumulative Laplacian histogram of the volume [9]. A detailed description of the segmentation process can be found in [7]. Figure 3 (left) illustrates the normal and the Laplacian histograms for abdominal images. As depicted in the figure

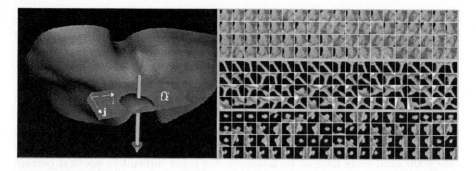

Fig. 1. Part of the colonic surface intersected with the rectangle α. On the right the resulting intersection patterns for colonic wall, haustral folds and colonic polyps.

the optimal threshold value for the transition between colonic air and tissue can be easily identified using the cumulative Laplacian histogram.

The final result of the segmentation algorithm is a set of disjunctive regions representing voxels on the colonic wall. It has to be mentioned that some voxels represent in fact colonic fluid.

Normal colonic wall identification. When detecting voxels belonging to the colonic wall we take advantage of its concavity. The principle of our method is presented in figure 1 (left). For each voxel, the colonic wall is intersected with the rectangle α, perpendicular to the local surface normal and situated at a distance d inside the surface of the wall. The resulting patterns of intersection can be seen in figure 1 (right). As highlighted in the figure the colonic wall gives completely filled planes while polyps and folds give a smaller number of voxels in the rectangle.

Thus, to identify colonic wall a thresholding method based on the number of voxels in the reformatted rectangle (in fact in a squared region of n pixels) can be used. The size of the rectangle is taken as $n = 12mm$ and the distance from the surface is $d = 1.5mm$. A voxel is classified as normal colonic wall if the number of pixels, N_{plane} situated in the rectangle α and having a CT value higher than the segmentation threshold (expressed as a percentage of n^2) is higher than $T_{plane} = 70\%$. The relation between n, d and the radius of detectable polyps (r_p) is given by equation 1, while the number of the voxels N_{plane}, in the worst-case scenario, is given by equation 2. With the selected parameter values the theoretical range of detectable polyp diameters $(r_p * 2)$ is from 5 mm up to 18.16 mm.

$$r_p = \frac{(\frac{n-2}{2})^2 + d^2}{2d} \quad (1) \qquad\qquad N_{plane} = \frac{\pi d(2r_p - d)}{2} + \frac{n^2}{2} \quad (2)$$

Spin images. The voxels remaining after colonic wall identification are modeled using spin images. Spin images were introduced by A.E. Johnson et al. [10] as a way of matching 3D surfaces. They are a local description of the global shape of the object, invariant to rigid transformations. Given a basis $(P, \overrightarrow{G_1})$, P a 3D point and $\overrightarrow{G_1}$ the image gradient in P, a spin map $S_{(P,\overrightarrow{G_1})}$ that projects 3D points T to 2D coordinates (α, β) can be defined as follows, considering that $\bullet$ is the scalar product:

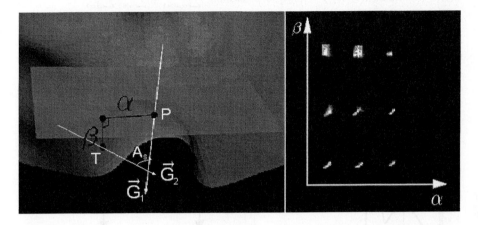

Fig. 2. On the left the process of spin image generation is depicted, on the right some example spin images are given. The first row corresponds to haustral folds, the second to real colonic polys, the last row represents the spin images given by perfect spheres of diameters 10, 8, and 6 mm respectively

$$S_{(P,\overrightarrow{G_1})} : \Re^3 \to \Re^2$$

$$S_{(P,\overrightarrow{G_1})}(T) \to (\alpha, \beta) = (\sqrt{\| T - P \|^2 - (\overrightarrow{G_1} \bullet \overrightarrow{T-P})^2}, \overrightarrow{G_1} \bullet \overrightarrow{T-P}) \quad (3)$$

Supposing that $\overrightarrow{G_2}$ is the image gradient in T, a support angle is introduced as:

$$A_s = acos(\overrightarrow{G_1} \bullet \overrightarrow{G_2})$$

Given a basis $(P, \overrightarrow{G_1})$ a spin image I, with N bins is generated as follows:

$$foreach \ (T, \overrightarrow{G_2}), \ T \neq P, \ distance(P,T) < N \ and \ A_s < T_{support} :$$
$$compute \ (\alpha, \beta) \ as \ indicated \ by \ (3)$$
$$I(\alpha, \beta) = I(\alpha, \beta) + 1$$

The distance between two spin images $I_1(\alpha, \beta)$, $I_2(\alpha, \beta)$, each having N bins, is computed using the confidence C of the normalized correlation coefficient $R(I_1, I_2)$. Their analytical formulas are:

$$R(I_1, I_2) =$$

$$= \frac{N^2 \sum_{\alpha,\beta=1}^{N} I_1(\alpha,\beta).I_2(\alpha,\beta) - \sum_{\alpha,\beta=1}^{N} I_1(\alpha,\beta). \sum_{\alpha,\beta=1}^{N} I_2(\alpha,\beta)}{\sqrt{\left(N^2 \sum_{\alpha,\beta=1}^{N} I_1(\alpha,\beta)^2 - \left(\sum_{\alpha,\beta=1}^{N} I_1(\alpha,\beta)\right)^2\right)\left(N^2 \sum_{\alpha,\beta=1}^{N} I_2(\alpha,\beta)^2 - \left(\sum_{\alpha,\beta=1}^{N} I_2(\alpha,\beta)\right)^2\right)}}$$

$$C(I_1, I_2) = (atanh(R(I_1,I_2)))^2 - \lambda \frac{1}{N-3}; \quad \lambda = constant; \quad \sum_{\alpha,\beta=1}^{N} \equiv \sum_{\alpha=1}^{N}\sum_{\beta=1}^{N}$$

Polyp labeling using spin images. For each remaining voxel (after the normal colonic wall was identified) its spin image is generated. The spin image has a number of bins $N = 12$, equal to the size of the reformatted rectangle used during the generation step. To limit the negative effects of surrounding wall the support angle of the spin image is limited to values below $T_{support} = 90°$.

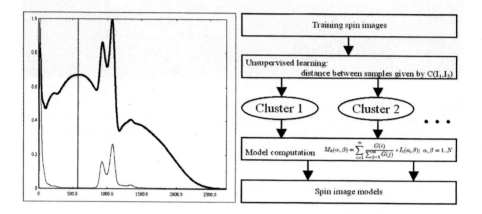

Fig. 3. The cumulative Laplacian histogram for abdominal images. The vertical line corresponds to the threshold used during region growing. On the right, the process of generating spin image models starting from a set of unlabeled samples.

Once a spin image $I(\alpha, \beta)$ is generated it is compared to a set of learned model spin images $M_k(\alpha, \beta), k = 1...N_m$, N_m the number of models. The models are representative spin images for polyps, haustral folds and remaining wall structures; their generation is described in chapter 3. The similarity measure between a spin image and a model is the confidence $C(I, M_k)$. The current voxel is labeled with the class of the closest model.

Finally, clusters of polyp labeled positions are identified using a connected component extraction algorithm. The connectedness is not limited to first order neighbors but to all neighbors situated at a distance $d_{neighbor} < T_{neighbor}$, where $T_{neighbor} = 2$ is a defined constant. The mean position of the elements belonging to large clusters (having a number of components higher than $T_{component} = 40$) is returned as a polyp candidate. The corresponding axial and 3D volume rendered positions are presented to the reading radiologist.

3   Polyp Models

In this section the process of obtaining model spin images is described, figure 3 (right). The model-building algorithm receives as input all the locations present in the training data, which were not labeled as normal colonic wall. It is not feasible to label each position (approximately 7000/case) as polyp, fold, colonic fluid or wall and thus a supervised classifier is not a valid choice. Instead an unsupervised learning algorithm is employed to cluster the input spin images and the resulting clusters are labeled. The method of Hutchinson [11] is the current classifier. The method can be seen as a statistical clustering since it is based on numerical similarity (given by the confidence C) within object descriptors (spin images $I(\alpha, \beta)$). The classifier provides as output a set of clusters, containing similar spin images.

Inside a cluster, the most representative spin image is considered to be the one for which the average correlation coefficient C, towards all the remaining elements of the cluster is the smallest. This spin image will have the highest contribution to the cluster's model. The weight of an element is computed in a gaussian manner as given by equation 4. Finally, the model for a given cluster is built using equation 5. Let's consider m the number of samples in the current cluster and N the number of bins in the spin image. The following notations can be introduced:

$$avgDist(i) = \tfrac{1}{m}\sum_{j=1}^{m} C(I_i, I_j); \quad minDist = min(avgDist(i)), \quad i = 1..m$$

$$\sigma^2 = \tfrac{1}{m}\sum_{i=1}^{m}(avgDist(i) - minDist)^2$$

The Gaussian weights $G(i)$ for each sample and the model M_k representing the current cluster are computed as:

$$G(i) = \frac{1}{\sigma.\sqrt{2\pi}}e^{-\frac{(avgDist(i)-minDist)^2}{2\sigma^2}}; \quad i = 1..m \qquad (4)$$

$$M_k(\alpha, \beta) = \sum_{i=1}^{m} \frac{G(i)}{\sum_{j=1}^{m} G(j)} * I_i(\alpha, \beta); \quad for\ each\ \alpha, \beta = 1..N \quad (5)$$

Due to computational limitations the previous scheme was modified to have a hierarchical behavior, as described in [12].

4   Patient Data and Results

Fifty data-sets belonging to 26 patients, 25 normal and 25 with 40 polyps of various sizes (Table 1) were considered as input for our CAD scheme. Seven polyps were submerged under residual fluid and were not considered as false negative cases, since our method was not designed to detect them. All patients underwent CT colonography prior to conventional colonoscopy. Informed consent was

obtained from all patients. The patient preparation consisted in the oral administration of 3 to 5 liter of precolon, an in-house developed tagging agent. In some
cases the use of polyethylene glycol electrolyte solution was preferred. Immediately before CT colonography a bowel relaxant was injected intravenously. CO_2
was insufflated using a bag system.

Table 1. Polyp distribution and detection results. (No = total number of polyps, TP
= true positives)

Type	Submerged	Detectable	TP	Sensitivity
Flat	1	5	3	60.00%
< 5 mm	2	6	2	33.33%
6-9 mm	3	7	6	85.70%
> 9 mm	1	11	10	90.90%
Tumor	0	4	4	100.00%
Total	7	33	25	75.75%

CT colonography was performed on a multi-detector CT (Multi Slice Helical CT; Volume Zoom, Siemens, Erlangen, Germany) using 4x1 mm detector
configuration, 7 mm table feed per 0.5 s tube rotation, 0.8 mm reconstruction
increment as well as 60 effective mAs and 120 keV. Patients were scanned in
both supine and prone positions, in breath holds of 20 to 30 seconds.

The CAD process was carried out as follows: after the CT data was transferred to an offline workstation (Intel Pentium 2.4 GHz system), seed points
were selected manually to ensure complete colonic segmentation. For the model
building step a leave one patient out technique was employed. The reason for
it was that the same polyp in prone and supine positions could be considered
similar. Using the remaining data-sets as training data models were generated.
These models are then used when running the CAD as described in section 2.
This process is repeated for each of the 26 patients.

Using conventional colonoscopy, as standard of reference, true positive (TP)
and false positive (FP) findings were determined. The detection rate differentiated on polyp size is presented in Table 1. The average computation time for
the whole CAD process (excepting seed point selection) as well as for different
steps is shown in Table 2 (left). The total number of false positives was 137,
which gives us a mean value of 2.74 false positive findings per data-set. The
main causes for false positives are presented in Table 2 (right)

5   Discussion

In this paper a fast yet robust method for CAD in CT colonography is presented.
Using spin images the complexity of the colonic wall is reduced to a 2D space,
while preserving 3D clues. The method gives better classification results (especially on flat lesions) than our earlier experiments [12] involving slope density
functions (SDF). This we believe is due to the fact that spin images contain

Table 2. Average times for completing the CAD algorithm (left). Main causes of false positives, both number and percent (right).

Step	Average time	Cause	Number	Percent
Segmentation	0:11	Haustral fold	75	54.74 %
CAD	5:46	Colonic wall	34	24.82 %
Polyp extraction	0:07	Stool or fluid	13	9.49 %
		Insuflation tube	9	6.57 %
		Ileocecal valve	6	4.38 %
Overall	6:04		137	

information coming from different depths, while SDF's were built at a fixed depth. However, the improvements come at the expense of some computation time, although 6 minutes/data-set is still a clinically acceptable time.

Intrinsic improvements due to the use of newer scanners (e.g. Somatom Sensation 16) are expected. Other advantages of the new scanner relate to the possibility of quicker scan times thus reducing motion artifacts and to low-dose scanning, with or without the use of edge preserving filters. Initial experiments with the new scanner are underway.

Looking at the drawbacks of the method one can observe that polyps are only geometrically modeled. The reason is patient preparation and more explicitly fluid tagging. Some of our polyps are close to tagged colonic fluid or even semi-submerged and thus missed by schemes taking into account intensity values.

A possible debate point is the choice of the unsupervised learning algorithm for clustering the training space. However, we feel that due to the large number of training points (on average 7000/polyp) it is not feasible to label each position apriori, that is why we prefer to label the generated models. The effects of different support angles on the outcome of our method are currently evaluated.

Compared with other CAD methods, this method is faster due to the colonic wall identification step. Opposed to other methods [5],[6] our technique employs a simple method for identifying the wall and then applies more elaborated (computationally costly) modeling. The presented results are comparable with the ones present in the literature and they can be considered very good when looking at clinically relevant polyps (polyps of 6 mm or larger).

To conclude, if our early results are proven on a larger data-base, the method can become clinically useful and can be considered as a "second reader", helping to improve the accuracy and efficiency of the reading process.

Acknowledgement. This work is part of the GOA/99/05 project: "Variability in Human Shape and Speech", financed by the Research Fund, K.U. Leuven, BELGIUM. We would like to thank Maarten Thomeer for his involvement in the project and Dirk Vandermeulen for his idea of using spin images.

References

1. Tumori Aparato Gastroenterico, Dati per la pianificazione dell'assistenza Edited by CPO Piemonte, May 1998
2. Morson, B.C.: Factors Influencing the Prognosis of Early Cancer in the Rectum. Proc R Soc Med (1966) 59:607-8
3. Colorectal cancer - Oncology Channel. http:// www.oncologychannel.com /colon-cancer/
4. Vining, D.J., et al.: Virtual colonoscopy. Radiology (1994) 193:446 (abstract)
5. Summers, R.M., et al.: An Automated Polyp Detector for CT Colonography - Feasibility Study. Radiology (2000) 284-290
6. Yoshida, H., Nappi, J.: 3-D Computer-Aided Diagnosis Scheme for Detection of Colonic Polyps. IEEE Transactions on Medical Imaging (2001) 1261-1274
7. Kiss, G., et al.: Computer Aided Detection of Colonic Polyps via Geometric Features Classification. Proceedings 7th International Workshop on Vision, Modeling, and Visualization (2002) 27-34
8. Ballard, D.M., Brown, C.M.: Computer Vision. Prentice Hall (1982) 123-166
9. Wiemker R., Pekar, V.: Fast Computation of Isosurface Contour Spectra for Volume Visualization. Proceedings Computer Assisted Radiology and Surgery CARS (2001)
10. Andrew J.: Spin-Images: A Representation for 3-D Surface Matching. Ph.D. thesis, Carnegie Mellon University, Pittsburgh, PA, Aug. 1997.
11. Unsupervised learning http://www.cs.mdx.ac.uk /staffpages /serengul /ML /unsupervised.html
12. Kiss, G., et al.: Computer Aided Detection in CT Colonography. MICCAI (2003) 746-753

Foveal Algorithm for the Detection of Microcalcification Clusters: A FROC Analysis

Marius George Linguraru[1,2], Michael Brady[1], and Ruth English[3]

[1]Medical Vision Laboratory, University of Oxford,
Ewert House, Ewert Place, Summertown, Oxford OX2 7BZ, UK
[2]EPIDAURE Research Project, INRIA,
2004 route des Lucioles, B.P. 93, 06902 Sophia Antipolis Cedex, France
Marius.Linguraru@sophia.inria.fr
[3]Breast Care Unit, the Churchill Hospital, Oxford OX3 9DU, UK

Abstract. Clusters of microcalcifications are often the earliest signs of breast cancer and their early detection is a primary consideration of screening programmes. We have previously presented a method to detect microcalcifications based on normalised images in standard mammogram form (SMF) using a foveal segmentation algorithm. In this paper, we discuss the selection and computation of parameters, which is a key issue in automatic detection methods. Deriving the parameters of our algorithm from image characteristics makes the method robust and essentially removes its dependence on parameters. We carry out a FROC analysis to study the behaviour of the algorithm on images prior to normalisation, as well as the contribution of the stages employed by our method. We report results from two different image databases.

1 Methodology

Our method of microcalcification detection relies on using a normalised representation of breast tissue, for example the standard mammogram form (SMF) [3] Having an SMF image as input, the first objective is the removal of curvilinear structures (CLS), which turn out to be an important consideration in the specificity but whose computation is itself a major challenge. This is performed using the local energy model for feature detection of Kovesi [4] and is presented in [1].

The SMF model accounts for the majority of imaging artefacts (scatter, glare, anode heel, extra-focal, quantum mottle, film grain). Inevitably, however, there are imperfections arising from deconvolution and model simplifications that are intrinsic to the SMF (or any similar) generation process [3,9]. These possible sources of errors leave residual high-frequency noise in mammographic images. Digitiser noise, also of high frequency, adds to it. We employ an anisotropic diffusion filter to smooth the remaining high-frequency noise [4]. A priori, this is a reasonable thing to attempt, as anisotropic diffusion smoothes the image, reduces noise (hence increases signal to noise, which is generally poor for mammographic images), and preserves image structure.

C. Barillot, D.R. Haynor, and P. Hellier (Eds.): MICCAI 2004, LNCS 3217, pp. 813–820, 2004.

Unfortunately, the substantial number of parameters required for anisotropic diffusion makes the results of this process highly dependent on fine-tuning of its input parameters. In practice, the more complex and variable the images in a dataset, the more problematical it is to choose a single set of values for the parameters that works well for the entire dataset. To address this problem, we propose using image characteristics to set the diffusion parameters for each individual image in the dataset.

It should be noted from the outset that although they may be important early indicators of breast cancer, microcalcifications generally occupy only a tiny percentage of the pixels of a mammogram image. Typically, they are very small and present in about a quarter of the total number of screening mammograms.

For these reasons, we consider that at most five percent of the total number of mammogram pixels suffices to account for the entire population of calcium salts. Since the x-ray attenuation of calcium is far larger than that of normal tissue, microcalcifications are expected to appear bright in a mammogram, indeed to be amongst the brightest/highest pixels of the mammogram, though the brightness can be reduced by scattering of x-ray photons. As made explicit in equation (1), we compute the contrast k as a measure of the gradient, where $K_\sigma(I)$ is a Gaussian blurring of the image I. k becomes a value with well-defined physical meaning that discriminates between these brightest structures and the background; more precisely, we select the 4.4% structures with highest contrast.

The second parameter to be set is σ, the standard deviation of the Gaussian filter used to smooth the image. We need to choose a value for σ such that, on the one hand, it removes high-frequency noise; but, on the other, preserves microcalcifications. We compute σ according to (2), where S is the maximal size of features to be smoothed and R the image resolution.

The number of iterations t of the anisotropic diffusion process is related to the spatial width of the Gaussian kernel [8]. To blur features of the kernel order ($n*\sigma$, n=ct.) t is computed according to (3), which gives excellent noise reduction results while preserving microcalcifications.

$$M = |K_\sigma{}'(I)|, \quad g_i = M_i - \frac{1}{N}\sum_{j\in\delta_i} M_j, \quad k = 2*\text{std}(g) \tag{1}$$

$$\sigma = S / R \tag{2}$$

$$t = (n*\sigma)^2 / 2 \tag{3}$$

The process is completed by applying what we call a foveal algorithm to segment microcalcifications; the name derives from a model of the adaptability of the human eye to detect features in textured images [6]. The eye's ability to perceive luminance gradients is controlled by the w factor in (4), where μ_N is the weighted mean of the neighbourhood of the object to segment and μ_B the mean value of the image background. w is a suitable weight (between 0 and 1) which controls the amount of background used in the computation of contrast, which gives a global measure to the locally adapted contrast. Once more, the parameters are computed from the image characteristics, as seen in (5), where C_{min} is the adapted threshold used to segment microcalcifications and b a constant.

$$\mu_A = w + (1-w)\,\mu_B \tag{4}$$

$$C_{min} = \frac{c_w}{\mu_N}\left(b + \sqrt{\frac{\mu_N^2}{\mu_A}}\right)^2 , \; c_w = \sqrt{k}\,/\,200 \tag{5}$$

The detection method is described in greater detail in [6].

2   FROC Analysis

In this section we present comparative Free-response Receiver Operating Characteristic (FROC) curves to test the outcome of our method with variations in algorithm and input images. We plot the true positive (TP) ratio against the number of false positives (FP) per image. We used a database of 102 samples of digital SMF images: 78 of them contain between 1 and 3 clusters per image, while 24 are normal mammogram samples. There are a total of 98 microcalcification clusters annotated in the database. All images were digitised at a resolution of 50 μm and have sizes at most 1500x1500 pixels. A cluster is detected if it contains at least three microcalcifications, where a distance of maximum 0.5 cm connects each calcification to the rest of cluster. In Figure 1 we note the impact of CLS removal, image smoothing and image normalisation (SMF images) on detecting microcalcification clusters. The results are clearly superior when the detection algorithm uses all of the stages in the algorithm, though they are not very different when the algorithm is applied to intensity (not normalised) images.

In the previous section, we noted the significance of w in setting the minimal perceivable contrast for obtaining the best detection results when our algorithm is applied. The literature proposes 7.7% of the adaptive luminance to be due to the background luminance 1, which gives a value of 0.923 to our weight w. We ran parallel tests to test the consistency of our conclusion to use the value 0.923 for w, by varying the value of w over 5-10%. Figure 2 shows the comparative detection results with the variation of w.

The results used in building the FROC curves in Figures 1 and 2 are based on processing cropped samples of mammograms. To illustrate results on whole mammograms, we used a total number of 83 mammograms in SMF format from the Oxford Screening Database: 59 of them contain between 1 and 5 clusters/image, adding the total number of clusters to 85, while 24 mammograms have no sign of abnormality. The pooled opinions of the clinicians at the Oxford Breast Care Unit, Churchill Hospital were used as ground truth. The breast margin is detected in SMF, thus a threshold above 0 removes the background. Now we can compute the value of k (see Methodology) for the inner area of the breast. The detection results are accurate and similar to those achieved on the mammogram samples (see Figure 3). The most challenging cluster to detect is located in the breast margin. The presence of CLS remains the main source of FP, or more precisely their imperfect removal. A few isolated calcifications were also depicted, but they were not labelled as microcalcification clusters.

The ultimate goal of any CAD algorithm is to work reliably on any given similar database, no matter where it comes from. As is acknowledged by many authors, without image normalisation this is hard to achieve. The SMF generation algorithm is designed precisely to cater for this situation; but excepting the Oxford database, no other image collections have mammograms in SMF format. Our detection algorithm, through its parametrical relation to the image attributes, facilitates the generalisation of detection standards, but without the use of a normalisation algorithm (a corner stone in our reasoning), the results are not ideal.

We used for comparison a collection of images from the University of South Florida Digital Database for Screening Mammography (DDSM). The new database consists of 82 image samples, of which 58 show abnormalities in the form of microcalcification clusters and 24 are normal. The abnormal images contain between 1 and 4 clusters/image and the total number of clusters is 82. All images are intensity images (using the earlier terminology) so the FROC curve shown in Figure 4 compares the performance of the microcalcification detection algorithm between the Oxford Screening Database in intensity form and the DDSM collection.

As expected, the algorithm performs better on the Oxford Screening database, on which the parameters were originally trained. Nevertheless, the detection results on the two databases converge at about 0.5 FP/image and they both achieve 100% TP fraction in the vicinity of 2 FP/image. A more appropriate test of the detection algorithm on the DDSM database will be done when images will be available in SMF form.

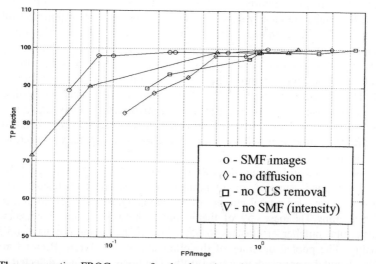

Fig. 1. The comparative FROC curves for the detection of microcalcifications. o - represents the detection on SMF images; ◊ - are the results without noise removal by anisotropic diffusion; □ - are the results without CLS removal; ∇ - shows results on intensity images, when no SMF generation is present. All algorithms reach 100% TP fraction with a clear better performance on SMF images that were de-noised and CLS-removed

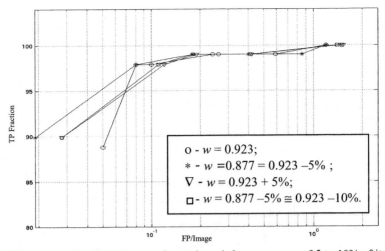

Fig. 2. The comparative FROC curve when *w* is varied over a range of 5 to 10% of its default value of 0.923. The difference in detection results is quite small and all four algorithms converge smoothly to 100% TP ratio.

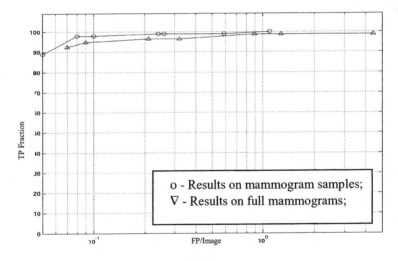

Fig. 3. The comparative FROC curve of the detection of microcalcifications when mammogram samples are used versus full mammograms. The behaviour of the algorithm is similar and robust with the image size.

Finally, this section compares three algorithms to detect microcalcification clusters that operate upon the SMF representation of mammograms. The first has been described previously in this paper and is addressed as the "foveal algorithm"; the second one is Yam *et al.*'s physics based approach that was described in 9. The third is a variation of the statistical analysis introduced in Methodology, here addressed as the "statistical approach", and is presented in [6]. Using FROC analysis, we demonstrate the superiority of the foveal algorithm in Figure 5.

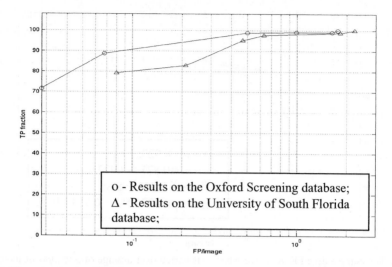

Fig. 4. The comparative FROC curve between the detection results on intensity images from the Oxford Screening Database and the University of South Florida Digital Database for Screening Mammography.

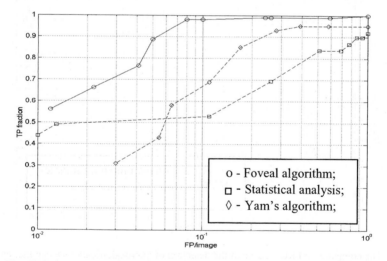

Fig. 5. The FROC curves of the three microcalcification-detection methods on SMF images, where we notice the better performance of the Foveal Approach.

3 Discussion

From a combination of solutions to partial differential equations (PDE), wavelet methods and statistics, the developed technique presents the user with a map of detected microcalcifications. In the first original step of our method, we presented a working example of tuning the parameters of anisotropic diffusion to an application. In a more general framework, anisotropic diffusion is a feature detector, namely an edge detector. The contrast k, being closely related to the gradient in the image, can be derived according to the percentage of features that we desire to enhance in an image. σ gives a measure of scale and must be set according to the size of searched features at the image resolution (multiscale analysis may be performed). The number of iterations t can be expressed as a function of σ, which can be well related to noise removing, but may be more difficult to combine with feature enhancement for some applications. With the automatic tuning of parameters that we propose, anisotropic diffusion may be used in a way that has minimal dependence on preset parameters and which uses some limited, but essential, a-priori knowledge. Potentially, this is more widely applicable in diffusion, a method that has attracted criticism for its parametrical dependency.

The second original step is the development of a method for adaptively thresholding the filtered results in order to segment microcalcifications. The combination of filters, statistical analysis and adaptive thresholding adds to the novelty of our technique. We compare detection methods on SMF images as well as the outcome of our algorithm on both SMF and intensity images. An example of microcalcification detection is shown in Figure 6.

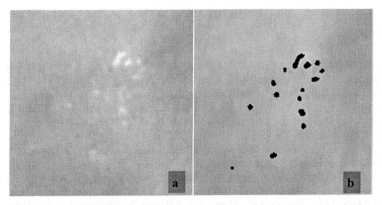

Fig. 6. An example of microcalcification detection. On the left (a) we present the input image in SMF format with a microcalcification cluster, while on the right (b) we note the result of our detection method.

The subsequent filters (SMF related, diffusion) model and correct for specific image analysis problems, rather than trying to amalgamate into a single (linear or nonlinear) filter that attempts to do everything. Separating them should make things clearer for the developer of such a filter, even if, for the end user, it is all reduced to a "black-box" that detects microcalcifications. Hence, we have a collection of blurring/low-pass and deblurring/high-pass filters.

Many methods to detect microcalcifications attempt to tune the variety of parameters used in the implementation of the algorithm to best suit the studied cases. The consistency and reproducibility of results becomes highly dependant on the operators and their capability to find the best parametrical configuration for the detection. We propose a fully automated non-parametric method to detect microcalcifications using the SMF normalised representation of the breast.

4 Conclusion

In this paper we presented a FROC analysis of an algorithm for the detection of microcalcification clusters mammography. The robustness of the algorithm has been demonstrated by the FROC analysis performed over a range of parameters. The method converged in each case to 100% TP ratio. Similar results were obtained on intensity images, although for the lower scale of FP/image there is a more significant difference in results. We also compared the performance of our algorithm on data from different databases with good detection results.

Adding adaptive contrast segmentation based on characteristics of the human visual system significantly enhances the detection of microcalcifications. The parameters are set according to the image attributes and the method is fully automated. In future work, we aim to develop the algorithm by incorporating additional knowledge of X-ray attenuation.

References

1. Evans, C.J. Yates, K. Brady, J.M.: Statistical Characterisation of Normal Curvilinear Structures in Mammograms. In: Digital Mammography, Lecture Notes in Computer Science, Springer-Verlag, Berlin Heidelberg New York (2002) 285-291
2. Heucke, L. Knaak, M. Orglmeister, R.: A New Image Segmentation Method Based on Human Brightness Perception and Foveal Adaptation. In: IEEE Signal Processing Letters, Vol. 7, No. 6 (2000) 129-131
3. Highnam, R.P. Brady, J.M.: Mammographic Image Analysis. Kluwer Academic Publishers, Dordrecht Boston London (1999)
4. Kovesi, P.: Image Features from Phase Congruency. In: Videre: Journal of Computer Vision Research, Vol. 1 (1999) 1-26
5. Linguraru, M.G. Brady, J.M. Yam, M.: Filtering h_{int} Images for the Detection of Microcalcifications. In Niessen, W. Viergever, M. (eds.): Medical Image Computing and Computer-Assisted Intervention 2001, Lecture Notes in Computer Science, Vol. 2208. Springer-Verlag, Berlin Heidelberg New York (2001) 629-636
6. Linguraru, M.: Feature Detection in Mammographic Image Analysis. Ph.D Thesis, University of Oxford (2002)
7. Linguraru, M.G. Brady, J.M.: A Non-Parametric Approach to Detecting Microcalcifications. In: Digital Mammography, Lecture Notes in Computer Science, Springer-Verlag, Berlin Heidelberg New York (2002) 339-341
8. Weickert, J.: Anisotropic Diffusion in Image Processing. B.G. Teubner, Stuttgart (1998)
9. Yam, M. Brady, J.M. Highnam, R.P. English, R.: Denoising h_{int} Surfaces: a Physics-based Approach. In: Taylor, C. Colchester, A. (eds.): Medical Image Computing and Computer-Assisted Intervention, Springer-Verlag, Berlin Heidelberg New York (1999) 227-234
10. Yam, M., Brady, J.M. Highnam, R.P. Behrenbruch, C.P. English, R. Kita, Y.: Three-dimensional Reconstruction of Microcalcification Clusters from Two Mammographic Views. In: IEEE Trans Med Imaging, Vol. 20 No. 6 (2001) 479-489

Pulmonary Micronodule Detection
from 3D Chest CT

Sukmoon Chang[1,2], Hirosh Emoto[3], Dimitris N. Metaxas[1], and Leon Axel[4]

[1] Center for CBIM, Rutgers University, Piscataway, NJ, USA
{sukmoon,dnm}@cs.rutgers.edu
[2] Computer Science, Penn State Capital College, Middletown, PA, USA
[3] National Institute of Information and Communications Technology, Tokyo, Japan
jiang@nict.go.jp
[4] Department of Radiology, New York University, New York, NY, USA
leon.axel@med.nyu.edu

Abstract. Computed Tomography (CT) is one of the most sensitive medical imaging modalities for detecting pulmonary nodules. Its high contrast resolution allows the detection of small nodules and thus lung cancer at a very early stage. In this paper, we propose a method for automating nodule detection from high-resolution chest CT images. Our method focuses on the detection of discrete types of granulomatous nodules less than 5mm in size using a series of 3D filters. Pulmonary nodules can be anywhere inside the lung, e.g., on lung walls, near vessels, or they may even be penetrated by vessels. For this reason, we first develop a new cylinder filter to suppress vessels and noise. Although nodules usually have higher intensity values than surrounding regions, many malignant nodules are of low contrast. In order not to ignore low contrast nodules, we develop a spherical filter to further enhance nodule intensity values, which is a novel 3D extension of Variable N-Quoit filter. As with most automatic nodule detection methods, our method generates false positive nodules. To address this, we also develop a filter for false positive elimination. Finally, we present promising results of applying our method to various clinical chest CT datasets with over 90% detection rate.

1 Introduction

Early detection of lung cancer is critical to improving chances of survival. The five-year survival rate of lung cancer patients is nearly 50% if lung cancer is found at a localized state (i.e., before it has spread to other organs) and can reach 85% if it is diagnosed in an early stage and surgery is possible [1,2]. Once the cancer has spread to other organs, the survival rates decline dramatically— 20% at regional stage and 2.2% at distant stage. Nevertheless, only 15% of lung cancer cases are found at the localized early stage. For early diagnosis of lung cancer, it is critical to detect nodules less than 5mm in size.

Various computational methods have been developed and considerable efforts have been made on automating nodule detection from chest radiographs [16].

C. Barillot, D.R. Haynor, and P. Hellier (Eds.): MICCAI 2004, LNCS 3217, pp. 821–828, 2004.
© Springer-Verlag Berlin Heidelberg 2004

However, the low sensitivity of chest radiographs to small nodules restricts current systems to the detection of nodules larger than 1cm in diameter. Newer medical imaging modalities such as low-dose helical CT allow the detection of pulmonary nodules smaller than those from conventional radiographs. With its high contrast resolution, CT makes it possible to detect nodules of small size or low-contrast that are hard to be seen on conventional radiographs [8].

In this paper, we propose a method for automating nodule detection from high-resolution chest CT images. Our method focuses on the detection of discrete types of granulomatous nodules less than 5mm in size using a series of 3D filters. Since pulmonary nodules can be anywhere inside lung, we first develop a new cylinder filter to suppress vessels and noise. Moreover, noting that many malignant nodules are of low contrast, we develop a spherical filter to further enhance nodule intensity values. Finally, we develop a new filter for false positive elimination. We also present promising results of applying our method to various clinical chest CT datasets.

2   Previous Work

Pulmonary nodule detection is one of the most challenging tasks in medical imaging. Various factors can hinder the automatic detection of nodules. Some factors are related to nodule properties, while others are related to the complex lung geometry. Most frequently used properties of nodules in automatic detection are the shape, size, and intensity profile. Template matching techniques were used to explore these features in automated detection of nodules. For example, spherical models with Gaussian distribution in intensity were used as base nodular models for template matching [10]. Takizawa et. al. also used cylindrical vascular models along with spherical nodular models in template matching [15]. Various pattern recognition techniques have also been used such as fuzzy clustering [7], a linear discriminant classifier [3,9], rule-based classification [4], and patient-specific a priori model [5].

A filtering technique called *Quoit filter* has shown promising results [17]. The filter is designed to produce strong response to an isolated circular area. However, it fails when nodules do not match with the filter in size or when nodules are not sufficiently isolated from nearby or penetrating vessels. To remedy the deficiencies of the Quoit filter, Miwa et. al. developed the *Variable N-Quoit filter* [12]. However, their system for nodule detection using the new filter dramatically increased the number of false positives. In addition, their system is overly complicated involving two 2D Quoit filtering and a 3D Quoit filtering processes.

In this paper, we propose a novel and efficient method for automatic detection of granulomatous nodules less than 5mm in size from chest CT images. Since nodules can be anywhere inside lung, the automatic nodule detection may be hindered by other structures such as lung walls, nearby vessels, or even penetrating vessels. For this, we first develop a new cylinder filter to suppress vessels and other structures. Although granulomatous nodules frequently have higher

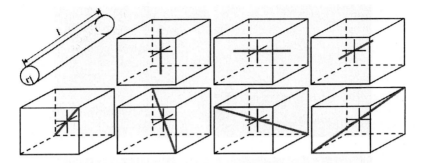

Fig. 1. Bar filter and its orientations.

intensity values than surrounding regions due to extensive calcification, most malignant nodules are noncalcified and, thus, of lower contrast. In order to detect low-contrast noncalcified nodules, we develop a spherical filter to further enhance nodule intensity values. The spherical filter is a novel and straightforward 3D extension of the Variable N-Quoit filter [12]. As with most nodule detection methods, our method generates many false positive nodules. Thus, we also develop a new filter for false positive elimination that performs a sphericity test for each candidate nodule. We finally report promising preliminary results of our method applied to clinical chest CT images.

3   Method

In this section, we develop a series of 3D filters for automatic micronodule detection from chest CT images. Our primary focus is the detection of discrete types of granulomatous nodules less than 5mm in size. Although granulomas usually appear brighter than surrounding regions due to their extensive calcification resulting in a higher X-ray absorption rate, most malignant nodules are noncalcified and, thus, of lower contrast. Our approach to micronodule detection can cope with the aforementioned nodule properties and targets both calcified and noncalcified nodules.

3.1   Cylinder Filter for Vessel and Noise Suppression

Nodules can be anywhere inside lung. For example, they can be adjacent to lung walls or fissures, near vessels, or they even can be penetrated by vessels. The performance of any nodule detection method may be hindered by various structures inside lung. To address this difficulty, we first develop a cylinder filter. The cylinder filter is used to suppress intensity values of vessels and other elongated structures inside the lung, while maintaining nodule intensity values intact.

The cylinder filter F_{cyl} is defined as:

$$F_{\mathrm{cyl}}(\boldsymbol{x}) = \max_{\theta} \left(\min_{\boldsymbol{y} \in \Omega_{\theta}^{\boldsymbol{x}}} I(\boldsymbol{y}) \right) \tag{1}$$

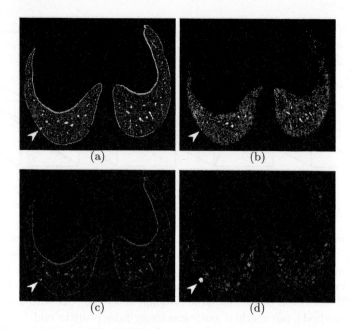

Fig. 2. Filtered images. (a) Original image (I), (b) Image filtered with F_{cyl}, (c) Image filtered with $I - F_{cyl}$, and (d) Final image filtered with F_{sph}. The arrow in each image points to the location of a nodule.

where, Ω_θ^x is the domain of the cylinder filter centered at x with orientation θ. F_{cyl} is a hybrid maxmin neighborhood filter that produces strong responses to cylindrical elongated regions (i.e., vessels). In this paper, we have selected the parameters of F_{cyl} empirically and used a cylinder with radius of 2 voxels and length of 7 voxels at 7 different orientations, as shown in Fig 1.

To suppress vessel intensity values using F_{cyl}, we use

$$I'(x) = I(x) - F_{cyl}(x) \qquad (2)$$

Applying F_{cyl} as in (2), the vessel intensity values are effectively suppressed while the nodule intensity values remain almost intact. Fig. 2(b) illustrates the result of applying F_{cyl} to a dataset containing the original image in (a) Note that F_{cyl} responded strongly to vessels but weakly to the nodule. By subtracting the two images in (a) and (b) using (2), we obtain a new image shown in (c). In this figure, we can see that vessels and noise are effectively suppressed while the nodule intensity remains intact.

3.2   Spherical Filter for Nodule Enhancement

Feature-based approaches for pulmonary nodule detection have shown promising results. The features most widely used are the size, shape, and intensity of nodules [3,4,17]. Granular nodules tend to be spherical with higher intensity than surrounding regions. However, many malignant nodules are of relatively

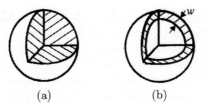

(a)   (b)

Fig. 3. Sphere filters. (a) Filled sphere filter F_{fill} and (b) Hollow sphere filter, F_{hollow}. Domains (Ω_{fill} and Ω_{hollow}) of the filters are shaded in the figure.

low contrast. In order not to miss low contrast nodules, we develop a spherical filter that enhances the intensity values of nodule areas (i.e., spherical regions with relatively high intensity compared to surrounding regions). To achieve this, we develop a non-linear spherical filter F_{sph} with two component filters F_{fill} and F_{hollow}. Let $I(\boldsymbol{x})$ be a 3D image and $S_r(\boldsymbol{x})$ a solid sphere with radius r centered at $\boldsymbol{x}$. Then, the response of the filter F_{sph} at a point $\boldsymbol{x}$ is

$$F_{\text{sph}}(\boldsymbol{x}) = F_{\text{fill}}(\boldsymbol{x}) - F_{\text{hollow}}(\boldsymbol{x}) = \max_{\boldsymbol{y} \in \Omega_{\text{fill}}^{\boldsymbol{x}}} I(\boldsymbol{y}) - \max_{\boldsymbol{y} \in \Omega_{\text{hollow}}^{\boldsymbol{x}}} I(\boldsymbol{y}) \tag{3}$$

where, $\Omega_{\text{fill}}^{\boldsymbol{x}}$ and $\Omega_{\text{hollow}}^{\boldsymbol{x}}$ are the domains of the filters F_{fill} and F_{hollow} centered at $\boldsymbol{x}$, respectively. In other words, as illustrated in Fig. 3,

$$\Omega_{\text{fill}}^{\boldsymbol{x}} = S_r(\boldsymbol{x}) \quad \text{and} \quad \Omega_{\text{hollow}}^{\boldsymbol{x}} = S_r(\boldsymbol{x}) - S_{r'}(\boldsymbol{x}), \quad r > r' \tag{4}$$

F_{sph} responds strongly to isolated spherical nodules and weakly to cylindrical vessels. The large differences of the filter responses between nodules and vessel areas allows the automatic detection of pulmonary nodules by a simple thresholding operation. Note that F_{sph} fails to produce strong responses to nodules when the size of a nodule does not match with the size of F_{sph}. The size of nodules to be detected is determined by the size of F_{sph}. If the filter size is smaller than a nodule, F_{hollow} is embedded inside the nodule and produces a strong response, weakening the overall response of F_{sph} from (3). On the other hand, if the filter size is too large, F_{hollow} may again produce a strong response due to nearby vessels if there are any. To avoid such difficulties, we follow the approach in [12] and employ the adaptive F_{sph} whose size is optimally adjusted by

$$r(\boldsymbol{x}) = r'(\boldsymbol{x}) + w \quad \text{and} \quad r'(\boldsymbol{x}) = \min_{\pi \in \Pi(\boldsymbol{x})} (|\pi|) \tag{5}$$

where, $\Pi(\boldsymbol{x})$ is the set of all paths from $\boldsymbol{x}$ to the background, $|\pi|$ is the length of a path π, and w is the width of F_{hollow} as in Fig. 3. The result of F_{sph} applied to a cylinder-filtered image is shown in Fig. 2(d). As expected, only the nodule produced strong response to F_{sph}.

3.3 False Positive Elimination

The challenging problem for any automatic nodule detection system is to keep the false positive detection rate low while maintaining high sensitivity. Various methods have been developed to reduce the false positive detection rates, including feature analysis [3,11] and template matching [6,10,15]. In this paper, we use a sphericity test for each candidate nodules detected by F_{sph}. Note that the detected nodules have already been through the sphericity test in 3D as well as the peak-valley ratio test in the intensity histogram by F_{sph}. Thus, the sphericity test for false positive elimination is performed in a 2D context.

Let C be a cube surrounding a suspicious nodule area. The intensity values inside C are projected onto C along x, y, and z-axes by applying MIP [14], generating three 2D images, C_i, $i = 1, 2, 3$. The suspicious nodule area in each of these images is extracted separately by thresholding. In order not to affect the degree of automation, the three threshold values are automatically computed using a threshold selection method such as [13]. The sphericity test is then applied to the three segmented nodule areas. Let A_i and L_i be the area and the border length of C_i, respectively. Then, the sphericity of the area is tested using

$$F_e^i = \frac{4\pi A_i}{L_i^2} \tag{6}$$

Note that F_e^i is 1 for a circle and the more elongated the area, the weaker the response of F_e^i. The suspicious nodules are classified as false positives and eliminated if any of the three segmented nodule areas fails to pass the test.

4   Experiments

We applied the method to twelve clinical CT datasets. Each dataset was digitally resliced to ensure cubic voxels and the lung areas were extracted. F_{cyl} was then applied to each dataset to suppress vessels and noise. We have selected the parameters of F_{cyl} empirically and used a cylinder with radius of 2 voxels and length of 7 voxels at 7 orientations. The results were filtered again with F_{sph} to enhance nodule intensities. Then, suspicious nodule regions were extracted by thresholding. Each of the candidate nodules was further processed with F_e^i for the sphericity test. Our method reported 69 nodules in all the datasets. An experienced radiologist verified that all the 62 nodules present in the datasets were correctly identified and confirmed that they were less than 5mm in diameter. The results are summarized in Table 1. Although our method detected all the 62 nodules present in the datasets, it also reported 7 false positive nodules. These cases were caused by abrupt intensity changes in small regions of vessels, which are very similar to nodules penetrated by vessels.

Fig. 4 shows typical cases of the detected nodules. In each pair of images in this figure, the processed image is shown on the left and the original image on

Table 1. Results.

Datasets	Nodules(Rad.)	Nodules(F_{sph})	Nodules(F_e^i)	TP	FP	FN
8	62	127	69	62	7	0

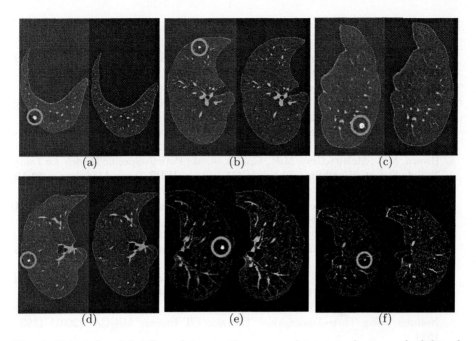

Fig. 4. Detected nodules. In each image, the processed image is shown on the left and the original image on the right.

the right. The method successfully detected nodules that are close to lung walls (Fig. 4 (a)), sufficiently isolated nodules (Fig. 4 (b)), nodules with nearby vessels (Fig. 4 (c)), nodules with penetrating vessels (Fig. 4 (d) and (e)), and nodules adjacent to a fissure (Fig. 4 (f)).

5 Conclusions

We have introduced a series of filters for automated micronodule detection from 3D chest CT. These include a cylinder filter for vessel suppression, which generates sufficient gaps in intensities between nodule and vessel regions for further processing. Then, the sphere filters were introduced for nodule enhancement, which were natural 3D extensions of 2D quoit filters. Finally, we proposed a filter for sphericity test for false positive elimination.

We conducted a preliminary set of experiments with the filters on twelve clinical CT datasets. The experiments confirmed that the proposed method was able to detect various nodules including those with nearby vessels or even penetrating vessels and fissures. The datasets contained 62 nodules with size less than 5mm and the method detected all of them. However, it also reported 7 false positive cases. These cases result from the abrupt intensity changes on small regions of vessels, which is very hard to differentiate from nodules with penetrating vessels. With the promising preliminary results, we plan to further our experiments in the future to obtain statistically useful validation.

References

1. Alliance for Lung Cancer Advocacy, Support, and Education: Early Detection and Diagnostic Imaging (2001)
2. American Cancer Society: Cancer Facts and Figures (2003)
3. Armato, S.G., Giger, M.L., Moran, et. al.: Computerized Detection of Pulmonary Nodules on CT Scans. Radiographics **19** (1999) 1303–1311
4. Betke, M., Ko, J.P.: Detection of Pulmonary Nodules on CT and Volumetric Assessment of Change over Time. MICCAI (1999) 245–252
5. Brown, M.S., McNitt-Gray, M.F., Goldin, et. al.: Patient-Specific Models for Lung Nodule Detection and Surveillance in CT Images. IEEE Trans. Med. Imag. **20:12** (2001) 1242–1250
6. Hara, T., Fujita, H., Goto, S., et. al.: Pattern Recognition Technique for Chest CAD System. Computer-Aided Diagnosis in Medical Imaging (1999) 57–61
7. Kanazawa, K., Kawata, Y., Niki, N., et. al.: Computer-Aided Diagnosis for Pulmonary Nodules based on Helical CT Images. Comput. Med. Imag. Graph. **22:2** (1998) 157–167
8. Kaneko, M., Eguchi, K., et. al.: Peripheral Lung Cancer: Screening and Detection with Low-Dose Spiral CT versus Radiography. Radiology **201** (1996) 798–802
9. Kawata, Y., Niki, N., Ohmatsu, H., et. al: Computer-Aided Diagnosis of Pulmonary Nodules Using Three-Dimensional Thoracic CT Images. MICCAI (2001) 1393–1394
10. Lee, Y., Hara, T., Fujita, H, Itoh, S., Ishigaki, T.: Automated Detection of Pulmonary Nodules in Helical CT Images Based on an Improved Template-Matching Technique. IEEE Trans. Med. Imag. **20:7** (2001) 595–604
11. McNitt-Gray, M.F., Wyckoff, E., Hart, M., et. al.: Computer Aided Techniques to Characterize Solitary Pulmonary Nodules Imaged on CT. Computer-Aided Diagnosis in Medical Imaging, (1999) 101–106
12. Miwa, T., Kako, J., et. al.: Automatic Detection of Lung Cancers in Chest CT Images by the Variable N-Quoit Filter. Syst. Comput. Jpn. **33:1** (2002) 53–63
13. Otsu, N.: A Threshold Selection Method from Gray-Level Histograms. IEEE Trans. Syst. Man and Cybern. **9:1** (1979) 62–66
14. Sato, Y., Shiraga, N., Nakajima, S., Tamura, S., Kikinis, R.: LMIP: Local Maximum Intensity Projection–A New Rendering Method for Vascular Visualization. J. Comput. Assist. Tomogr. **22:6** (1998) 912–917
15. Takizawa, H., Shigemoto, K., Yamamoto, S.: A Recognition Method of Lung Nodule Shadows in X-Ray CT Images Using 3D Object Models. IJIG **3:4** (2003) 533–545
16. van Ginneken, B., ter Haar Romeny, B.M., Viergever, M.A.: Computer-Aided Diagnosis in Chest Radiography: A Survey. IEEE Trans. Med. Imag. **20:12** (2001) 1228–1241
17. Yamamoto, S., Matsumoto, M., Tateno, Y., et. al.: Quoit Filter: A New Filter Based on Mathematical Morphology to Extract the Isolated Shadow, and Its Application to Automatic Detection of Lung Cancer in X-ray CT. ICPR **2** (1996) 3–7

SVM Optimization for Hyperspectral Colon Tissue Cell Classification

Kashif Rajpoot[1] and Nasir Rajpoot[2]

[1] Faculty of Computer Science & Engineering, GIK Institute, Pakistan
[2] Department of Computer Science, University of Warwick, UK
kmr@giki.edu.pk, nasir@dcs.warwick.ac.uk

Abstract. The classification of normal and malginant colon tissue cells is crucial to the diagnosis of colon cancer in humans. Given the right set of feature vectors, Support Vector Machines (SVMs) have been shown to perform reasonably well for the classification [4,13]. In this paper, we address the following question: how does the choice of a kernel function and its parameters affect the SVM classification performance in such a system? We show that the Gaussian kernel function combined with an optimal choice of parameters can produce high classification accuracy.

1 Introduction

Bowel cancer is the third most commonly diagnosed cancer in the UK after lung and breast cancer. It is the second most common cause of cancer death after lung cancer accounting for over ten percent of all cancer deaths. In the UK alone, there were over 35,000 colorectal cancer (a combined term for colon/rectum cancer) cases in the year 1999 and more than 16,000 deaths from bowel cancer in year 2000 [1]. The limited availability of specialist pathological staff and the huge amount of information provided by hyperspectral sensors means that user fatigue is a significant obstruction in the examination of these images and the identification of colon cancer in early stages. It is estimated that 80% of the deaths can be avoided if the cancer can be caught at its early stage. New improved screening and diagnosis methods could potentially save thousands of lives each year.

Hyperspectral imaging captures tens to hundreds of spectral bands at varying wavelengths in response to an image scene. The availability of this large amount of information can potentially help in the analysis of a scene. The use of hyperspectral images is widespread in remote sensing and related applications. The coupling of hyperspectral imaging with microscopy [10] has found its way into biomedical applications, such as the classification of colon tissue cells [4,13] into normal and malignant cells. Figure 1 shows selected bands from two hyperspectral colon tissue cell image cubes containing normal and malignant cells. In [4], Davis et al. proposed a completely supervised system for both segmentation and classification and achieved an accuracy of 86%. In our previous work [13], unsupervised segmentation and supervised classification were employed, with an

C. Barillot, D.R. Haynor, and P. Hellier (Eds.): MICCAI 2004, LNCS 3217, pp. 829–837, 2004.
© Springer-Verlag Berlin Heidelberg 2004

increased potential of operating without significant human intervention, achieving an accuracy of 87%. Unfortunately, for both cases, the classification accuracy is not as high as desired in a real-world application of these algorithms.

In this paper, we present our work on improvement of the classification performance of the algorithm in [13]. Assuming that the right set of feature vectors were used to train and test the SVM classifier, we focus our attention in this paper on finding optimal parameters for three kernel functions: linear, Gaussian, and polynomial. A grid-search based method is employed in order to find an optimal set of parameters for each of the kernels. Our experiments show that the Gaussian kernel is most efficient in approximating the non-linear decision boundary between the two cell classes. Classification accuracy of over 99% was achieved using optimal parameters for the Gaussian kernel on a limited data set.

In the next section, a brief description of the classification algorithm of [13] is presented. Section 3 presents succint details of the SVM classifier optimization procedure. Experimental results are provided in Section 4, and the paper concludes with remarks on the effect of parameter selection on the classifier performance and some future directions.

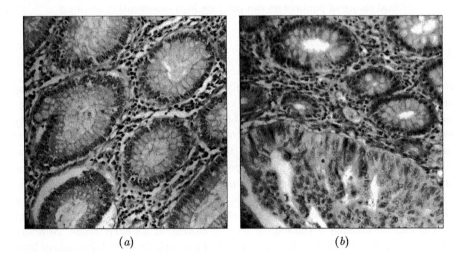

(a)   (b)

Fig. 1. Selected bands from hyperspectral colon tissue imagery. Two colon tissue sample images at 490nm; images contain (a) normal cells and (b) normal and malignant (towards the bottom-left) cells.

2   Materials and Methods

Microscopic level image data cubes of normal and malignant (adenocarcinoma) human colon tissue were acquired from archival H & E (hematoxylin & eosin) stained micro-array tissue sections. The dimensions of each data cube were $1024 \times 1024 \times 20$, where 20 spectral bands in the wavelength interval 450–640nm were used. The challenge is the automated analysis of hyperspectral colon tissue images to classify between normal and malignant tissue sections with a reasonable accuracy. This will lead to a method that can be used without significant human intervention, once the machine is trained, and may be adopted as an assistance tool for the pathologists. Such a tool can be potentially helpful in evaluating the proportions of normal and malignant parts in an input colon image. A tissue cell classification problem can typically be approached through a traditional pattern recognition methodology. This involves: (i) segmentation, (ii) feature extraction, and (iii) classification. In hyperspectral imagery, a preprocessing step of dimensionality reduction may be included before the segmentation process. This approach is dissimilar to the one normally employed in the remote sensing field for classification problems, which merely exploits spectral signature for a direct classification task [11,6]. In this section, we give a very brief description of the classification method proposed previously by the authors. A more detailed treatment can be found in [13].

2.1 Segmentation

The segmentation of hyperspectral colon tissue images into four constituent parts of the human colon tissue cell (ie, nuclei, cytoplasm, lamina propria, and lumen) at the microscopic level was performed as follows. Independent Component Analysis (ICA) was employed to extract statistically independent components from the high-dimensional data. A preprocessing step of high-emphasis preceded the FlexICA variant [5] of ICA, which was used to achieve dimensionality reduction. The objective of this preprocessing was to force the data distribution towards heavy-tailedness, which is further exploited by the FlexICA algorithm, that is sensitive to kurtosis (4th order statistic). The extracted independent components (with reduced dimensionality in the spectral dimension) were fed into an unsupervised nearest-centroid (k-means) clustering algorithm, which resulted in a 1024×1024 labelled image for each hyperspectral image cube.

2.2 Feature Extraction

The segmented image was used to extract discriminant features which were subsequently utilized during the SVM classifier training stage. Multiscale morphological features (area, eccentricity, equivalent diameter, Euler number, extent, orientation, solidity, major axis length, minor axis length) were collected to extract the structural characteristics corresponding to each distinct 16×16 size patch of the segmented image. In almost all our experiments, morphological features performed better than statistical features mainly due to the fact that these were gathered from the segmented tissue cell image. The features associated with each patch were those for the patch itself and all of its parent resolutions up to a resolution of 256×256 (doubling the resolution each time) in order to exploit both local as well as global characteristics. This formed a 180-dimensional multiscale feature vector (36 features for each resolution) for every 16×16 patch of the image, yielding $4,096$ feature vectors for each hyperspectral image cube.

2.3 Classification

A total of $45,056$ such feature vectors were gathered through eleven hyperspectral image cubes. During the training stage of the SVM, about two-thirds $(30,000)$ of the feature vectors were used as training set while the rest $(15,056)$ were kept for a future testing stage. The algorithm achieved a classification accuracy of 87% on the unknown test data set using the Gaussian kernel. The need to improve the accuracy was one of the motivating factors for the investigation of SVM kernel optimization studied in this paper.

3 SVM Optimization

SVM [15] is an emerging area of research in the fields of machine learning and pattern recognition. SVM performs particularly well with high dimensional feature vectors and in case of lack of training data, two factors which may significantly limit the performance of most neural networks. Its true potential is highlighted when the classification of non-linearly separable data becomes possible with the use of a kernel function, which maps the input space into a possibly higher dimensional feature space in order to transform the non-linear decision boundary into a linear one. There exists a range of kernel functions, where a particular function may perform better for certain applications. The kernel functions can sometimes be categorized as *local* kernels (Gaussian, KMOD) and *global* kernels (linear, polynomial, sigmoidal) where local kernels attempt to measure the proximity of data samples and are based on a distance function rather than dot-product based global kernels. Table 1 lists the kernel expressions and corresponding parameters. Note that $< x, y >$ represents dotproduct, where x and y denote two arbitrary feature vectors. The process of determining the decision boundary is greatly influenced by the selection of kernel. In addition, each of the kernel functions have varying number of *free* parameters which can be selected by the *teacher*. As can be seen from Table 1, the performance of an SVM using linear, Gaussian, or polynomial kernels is dependent upon one, two, and four parameters respectively. All the kernels share one common parameter C, the constant of constraint violation which observes the occurring of a data sample on the wrong side of the decision boundary. Parameter γ of the Gaussian kernel denotes the width of the Gaussian radial basis function. For the polynomial kernel, d, γ, a respectively denote degree of the polynomial, coefficient of the polynomial function, and the coaddaptive constant. For a given application, it is hard to determine in advance which kernel function or set of respective kernel parameters will produce the best results. Selection of optimal parameters is currently a research issue in itself and is also known as the parameter or model selection problem. Another research direction is to make the parameter estimation process internal to the SVM classifier, with some researchers focusing on how to incorporate the process as an internal task to the SVM classifier, like finding optimal decision and margin boundaries.

Parameter (model) selection is essentially the search for optimal parameters for a particular kernel function. A simple way of doing so is the gride-search [7] procedure which is not always an exhaustive method (depending on the grid resolution). Other automatic methods, such as [14,2,9], exist but are iterative and can be computationally expensive too. Some other techniques which can be used to possibly improve the classification performance are: (i) *feature selection* [16]: to discard irrelevant features which may not be helpful for the classification process, (ii) *kernel selection*: choice of a kernel function for SVM for the mapping procedure, (iii) *data reduction* [12]: to discard irrelevant training samples as only samples near to the decision/margin boundary are important to the SVM; this is normally done by using a grid-search, (iv) *cross-validation*: splitting the data set into subsets to avoid overfitting and to improve on its general performance, (v) *marginal boundary determination*: finding an optimal boundary such that opposite class samples are well-separated, and (vi) *SVM classifier ensemble*: grouping or fusion of various SVM classifiers with different parameter settings.

4   Experimental Results and Discussion

Our experiments focussed on the selection of optimal parameters for each of the kernel functions. In order to avoid overfitting and to estimate the generalized performance, a 4-fold cross-validation exercise was conducted, where the whole feature data set was divided into four subsets such that one subset was iteratively tested using the classifier trained on the remaining data subsets. Table 2 shows classification accuracy results for all three kernels for different cross-validation trials. The parameter values used for these trials are: $C = 1, \gamma = 1, d = 3, a = 1$. As can be seen from the table, for a given kernel function, the classification accuracy does not vary significantly among different trials. This indicates that the optimal parameters are fairly generic in their application to classification of the unseen data. The search for optimal set of parameters can normally be carried out through an extensive experimentation process known as grid-search [7], which is the testing of different parameter values for the SVM kernels. This may

Table 1. Commonly used SVM kernel functions and their parameters

Kernel	Expression $K(x_i, x_j)$	Parameters
Linear	$< x_i, x_j >$	C
Gaussian	$e^{-\gamma \|x_i - x_j\|^2}$	γ, C
Polynomial	$(\gamma < x_i, x_j > + a)^d$	γ, C, d, a

Table 2. Classification accuracy (%) with 4-fold cross-validation

Trial#	Linear	Gaussian	Polynomial
1	82.2	86.9	83.1
2	81.5	87.8	83.2
3	81.5	86.7	83.9
4	82.0	87.1	83.7

Results of cross-validation with fixed parameters for all three kernels while the data was divided into four subsets and classification trials were carried out with the SVM trained on three subsets and tested on the fourth subset.

sometimes be preceded by a data reduction [12] preprocessing step to discard irrelevant data items, which are far away from the decision/margin boundary, in order to reduce the computational time involved in the search process. We omitted the data reduction stage since only one quarter of the total data samples were used for training and a coarse resolution grid-search based method was employed.

The feature data were divided into a training set (11,000 samples) and a test set (34,056 samples) and the search for optimal set of parameters was conducted using a grid-based method for all three kernel functions. Although Hsu et al. [7] suggest a grid range and grid steps of their choice for performing the grid-search, there is no hard and fast rule on this. Figure 2 shows progressive results of optimal parameter search for linear, Gaussian, and polynomial kernels. It can be seen from the Figure that a change in the value of parameter C, the penalty parameter common to all the kernels, does not have significant effect on the classification accuracy for any of the kernels, provided the remaining parameters are kept constant. It can also be observed from Figure 2(b) that the classification performance of the SVM using a Gaussian kernel approaches 99% for $\gamma = 17$ and $C = 1$. Results of classification are shown in Figure 3, where high contrast points to malignant sections and low contrast to normal sections. Quantitative results for this particular configuration of the SVM, ie using a Gaussian kernel function with optimal parameter values, are shown in Table 3. These results show the promise exhibited by the SVM classifier and highlight the importance of selecting the right kernel and optimal set of kernel parameters.

Table 3. Classification results (%) with optimal parameters for Gaussian kernel

Classification Accuracy	True +ve	True -ve	Sensitivity (Recall)	Specificity
99.72	99.62	99.82	99.82	99.62

According to [8], the hold-out testing (by distributing the available data into training and test sets) and quantified measures of Table 3 are a good way to estimate the generalization performance, though not totally unbiased, of the trained machine. The fact that a Gaussian kernel outperforms linear and polynomial kernel settings may be due to a number of reasons: (i) it can determine a non-linear decision boundary (not possible for a linear kernel), (ii) it has fewer parameters than the polynomial kernel and is consequently simpler to tune, and (iii) it faces less numerical difficulties (polynomial kernel value may go to infinity).

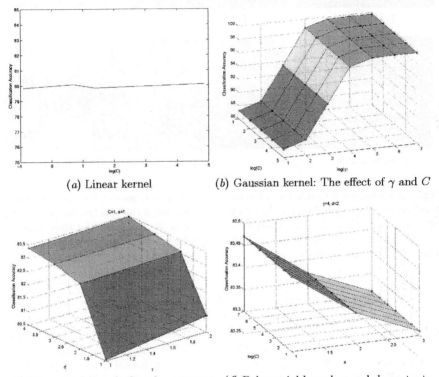

(a) Linear kernel   (b) Gaussian kernel: The effect of γ and C

(c) Polynomial kernel: C and a constant   (d) Polynomial kernel: γ and d constant

Fig. 2. Grid-search results for kernel parameters. The effect of varying the values of kernel parameters on the classification performance: (a) accuracy vs. parameter C for linear kernel, (b) surface of accuracy parameterized by C and γ for Gaussian kernel, surface of accuracy for polynomial kernel parameterized by (c) d and γ while keeping C and a constant, and (d) C and a while keeping d and γ constant. Where used, log is to the base 2.

5   Conclusions

In this paper, we studied parameter selection procedure to optimize the SVM classifier performance for a hyperspectral colon tissue cell classification system

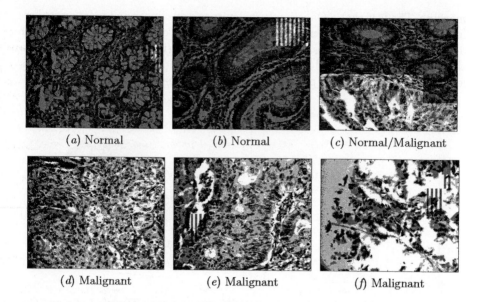

(a) Normal   (b) Normal   (c) Normal/Malignant

(d) Malignant   (e) Malignant   (f) Malignant

Fig. 3. Experimental results for colon tissue cell images. Classification results for some colon tissue images overlaid on the original image (one of the spectral bands) showing 16×16 patches of cell areas classified as *normal* in *low* contrast and those classified as *malignant* in *high* contrast; on-off type of patchy artifacts can be observed in areas where the classifier perhaps does not have enough information.

[13]. It was shown that considerably high classification accuracy can be achieved for our tissue cell classification system by selecting optimal set of parameters for the Gaussian kernel. These results are in conformance with the recent findings [3] that the Gaussian kernel function is close to the natural diffusion kernel which produces the best mapping results. Gaussian kernel is also more efficient compared to the other two kernels, since it is a local distance-based kernel. One of the limitations of our optimization approach is that it is rather exhaustive. Our future work will look into efficient methods for the automatic selection of optimal kernel parameters for the Gaussian kernel and validation of our results on a larger data set.

Acknowledgements. The authors gratefully acknowledge obtaining hyperspectral imagery data used in this work from and having fruitful discussions with Ronald Coifman and Mauro Maggioni of the Applied Mathematics Department of Yale University. We also thank Abhir Bhalerao, Roland Wilson, and anonymous reviewers for their useful suggestions to improve the quality of this paper.

References

1. Bowel cancer factsheet, April 2003. Cancer Research UK.
2. O. Chapelle and V. Vapnik. Model selection for support vector machines. In *Proc. Advances in Neural Information Processing Systems (NIPS)*, 1999.
3. R. Coifman and S. Lafon. Geometric harmonics. Technical report, Department of Applied Mathematics, Yale University, 2003.
4. G. Davis, M. Maggioni, R. Coifman, D. Rimm, and R. Levenson. Spectral/spatial analysis of colon carcinoma. In *United States and Canadian Academy of Pathology Meeting, Washington DC*, March 2003.
5. R. Everson and S. Roberts. Independent component analysis: A flexible non-linearity and decorrelating manifold approach. In *Proc. IEEE NNSP*, 1998.
6. J.A. Gualtieri and R.F. Cromp. Support vector machines for hyperspectral remote sensing classification. In *Proc. SPIE Workshop, Advances in Computer Assisted Recognition (ACAR)*, October 1998.
7. C.W. Hsu, C.C. Chang, and C.J. Lin. A practical guide to support vector machines. Technical report, Department of Computer Science & Information Engineering, National Taiwan University, July 2003.
8. J. Joachims. Estimating the generalization performance of a svm efficiently. In *Proc. Intl. Conf. on Machine Learning*. Morgan Kaufmann, 2000.
9. J.H. Lee and C.J. Lin. Automatic model selection for SVM. Technical report, Department of Computer Science & Information Engineering, National Taiwan University, November 2000.
10. R. Levenson and C. Hoyt. Spectral imaging & microscopy. *American Laboratory*, pages 26–33, November 2000.
11. G. Mercier and M. Lennon. Support vector machines for hyperspectral image classification with spectral based kernels. In *Proc. IEEE Intl. Geoscience & Remote Sensing Symposium (IGARSS)*, 2003.
12. Y.Y. Ou, C.Y. Chen, S.C. Hwang, and Y. J. Oyang. Expediting model selection for SVM based on data reduction. In *Proc. Intl. Conf. on Systems, Man, and Cybernetics (ICSMC)*, October 2003.
13. K.M. Rajpoot and N.M. Rajpoot. Hyperspectral colon tissue cell classification. In *SPIE Medical Imaging (MI)*, February 2004.
14. C. Staelin. Parameter selection for support vector machines. Technical report, HP Labs, Israel, 2002.
15. V. Vapnik. *The Nature of Statistical Learning Theory*. Springer-Verlag, New York, 1995.
16. J. Weston, S. Mukherjee, O. Chapelle, M. Pontil, T. Poggio, and V. Vapnik. Feature selection for SVMs. In *Proc. Advances in Neural Information Processing Systems (NIPS)*, 2000.

Pulmonary Nodule Classification Based on Nodule Retrieval from 3-D Thoracic CT Image Database

Yoshiki Kawata[1], Noboru Niki[1], Hironobu Ohmatsu[2], Masahiko Kusumoto[3],
Ryutaro Kakinuma[3], Kouzo Yamada[4], Kiyoshi Mori[5], Hiroyuki Nishiyama[6],
Kenji Eguchi[7], Masahiro Kaneko[3] , and N. Moriyama[3]

[1] Dept. of Optical Science, Univ. of Tokushima, Tokushima
{kawata, niki}@tokushima-u.ac.jp
[2] National Cancer Center Hospital East,
[3] National Cancer Center Hospital
[4] Kanagawa Cancer Center,
[5] Tochigi Cancer Center,
[6] The Social Health Insurance Medical Center,
[7] Univ. of Tokai

Abstract. The purpose of this study is to develop an image-guided decision support system that assists decision-making in clinical differential diagnosis of pulmonary nodules. This approach retrieves and displays nodules that exhibit morphological and internal profiles consistent to the nodule in question. It uses a three-dimensional (3-D) CT image database of pulmonary nodules for which diagnosis is known. In order to build the system, there are following issues that should be solved, (1) to categorize the nodule database with respect to morphological and internal features, (2) to quickly search nodule images similar to an indeterminate nodule from a large database, and (3) to reveal malignancy likelihood computed by using similar nodule images. Especially, the first problem influences the design of other issues. The successful categorization of nodule pattern might lead physicians to find important cues that characterize benign and malignant nodules. This paper focuses on an approach to categorize the nodule database with respect to nodule shape and CT density patterns inside nodule.

1 Introduction

Lung cancer is a leading cause of death among men in Japan [1]. Early detection of lung cancer by means of screening thoracic CT images is considered as an effective way to reduce the mortality rate of resulting lung cancer. Physicians' diagnosis, however, becomes more difficult in correctly classifying all lesions detected at three-dimensional (3-D) thoracic CT images into benign or malignant cases as the detection rate of pulmonary lesions with smaller diameter increases. Computer-aided diagnosis (CAD) has been investigated to provide physicians with quantitative information, such as estimates of the malignancy likelihood, to aid in the classification of abnormalities detected at screening [2-5]. These conventional CAD techniques provide only potential malignancies. Physicians often compare an indeterminate nodule with nodules diagnosed in the past. In order to get interpretable CAD results, it is required to relate

C. Barillot, D.R. Haynor, and P. Hellier (Eds.): MICCAI 2004, LNCS 3217, pp. 838–846, 2004.

an indeterminate nodule to similar nodules stored in a nodule database. The purpose of this study is to explore an image-guided decision support system to assist physician's decision-making of the clinical differential diagnosis of pulmonary nodules.

Some works have been done to address the problem of lesion detection and classification using similar images [6-9]. The interpretation of the pulmonary nodule images often involves the matching features extracted from a database of the nodules with associated clinical information. When the matching procedure performs well, the database provides physicians with more diagnosis and prognosis information of the queried nodule. Moreover, the corresponding structures retrieved from the database might help to design the CAD scheme for the distinction between benign and malignant nodules.

In our own recent study [9], we developed an example-based assisting approach for the nodule classification. The approach formulates the classification problem of the indeterminate nodule as one of learning to recognize nodule patterns from examples of similar nodule images. The central module makes possible analysis of the query nodule image and extraction of the features of interest: shape, surrounding structure, and internal structure of the nodules. The malignant likelihood is estimated by the difference between the representation patterns of the query case and the retrieved lesions. In order to build a decision support system using similar nodule images, there are following issues that should be solved, categorization of the nodule database with respect to morphological and internal features, quick search of nodule images similar to an indeterminate nodule from a large database, and computation of malignancy likelihood based on similar nodule images. The first problem influences the design of other issues and the successful categorization of nodule pattern might lead physicians to find important cues that characterize benign and malignant nodules. In this paper, we focus on an approach to categorize the nodule database with respect to nodule shape and CT density patterns inside nodule, and we introduce the approach to our retrieval method.

2 Methods

The nodule database used here is provided by the National Cancer Center East in Japan. The malignant cases were diagnosed by histological diagnosis and benign nodules were confirmed by surgery or diagnostic follow-up examinations. Additionally, the malignant cases have information of the stage of lesion prognosis. The database contains nodule images with known diagnosis result and consists of two elements, such as text-based and image-based elements. The text-based elements of the database are as follows: ID number, measurement conditions, gender, age, and diagnosis result. The image-based elements consist of following seven elements; (a) thin-section CT images, (b) the 3-D ROI image with a nodule of interest, (c) the segmented nodule image by a deformable surface model, (d) shape features, (e) pattern of CT density histogram, (f) the histogram-based representation using CT density value inside nodule, and (g) the histogram-based representation using curvature indexes of internal nodule. Each step is described in the following sections.

2.1　3-D Thoracic CT Images

The 3-D thoracic images used in this paper were reconstructed from thin-section CT images obtained by a multislice helical CT scanner (Toshiba Aquilion; Toshiba Medical Systems, Japan). The thin-section CT images were measured under the following conditions; beam width: 0.5mm, table pitch: 3, scan time: 0.5 sec, tube voltage: 120kV, tube current: 300mA. For the scan duration, patients held their breath at full inspiration. The slice images at 0.2 mm intervals were obtained to observe whole nodule region and its surroundings. The number of slices per patient ranges from 200 to 300 slices. The range of pixel size in each square slice of 512 pixels was between 0.3×0.3 mm^2 and 0.5×0.5 mm^2, and the slice contains an extended region of the lung area. The 3-D thoracic image was reconstructed from the thin-section CT images by a cubic B-spline interpolation technique to make each voxel isotropic [10]. The data set in this study included 174 3-D thoracic images. Of the 174 cases, 98 contained malignant nodules, and 76 contained benign nodules. Whole malignant nodules were histologically diagnosed. In benign cases lesions showed no change or decreased in size over a 2-year period were considered benign nodules.

2.2　Extraction of Nodule Region

The segmentation of the 3D pulmonary nodule image consists of three steps [3] ; 1)extraction of lung area, 2) selection of the region of interest (ROI) including the nodule region, and 3) nodule segmentation based on a geometric approach. The lung area extraction step plays an essential role when the part of a nodule in the peripheral lung area touches the chest wall. The ROI including the nodule was selected interactively. A pulmonary nodule was segmented from the selected ROI image by the geometric approach. Attachments of the nodule such as vessels were eliminated by morphological filtering approach.

2.3　Feature Extraction

2.3.1　Shape Feature
In order to characterize the shape of the 3-D nodule image, we compute the direction of principal axes of the 3-D nodule image and obtain the lengths along these directions [9]. Additionally, to measure the irregularity of the segmented nodule surface we compute the compactness that is obtained by volume and surface area of tnodule. Using theses values, we classify nodule shapes into six categories as shown in Fig. 1.

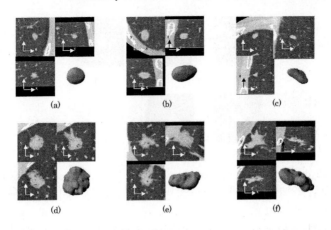

Fig. 1. Shape types. (a) Round shape with smooth surface. (b) Elongated shape with smooth surface. (c) Flat shape with smooth surface. (d) Round shape with irregular surface. (e) Elongated shape with irregular surface. (f) Flat shape with irregular surface.

2.3.2 Pattern Classification of CT Density Histogram Inside Nodule

Recent advantages of CT technology enable analysis of internal density patterns of small pulmonary nodules. From visual assessment of the presence of ground-glass opacities within nodule, internal density patterns are classified into solid, part-solid, and nonsolid nodules [11]. Associating internal density patterns with malignant status attracts researchers' interests. Quantification of internal density patterns is required for assisting physicians in decision of adequate treatments. In our own recent study, we investigated numerical criteria for classifying nodule density patterns that provides information with respect to nodule status [12]. The pattern classification approach of CT density distribution inside nodule might provide a nodule categorization method to let physicians estimate malignancy status. Therefore, we introduced the pattern classification approach into image-guided decision support scheme.

The pattern classification approach categorizes nodule density patterns into five types that are named as Type A, B, C, D, and E. Slice images of typical types are shown in Fig.2. The approach consists of three steps. The nodule region is volumetrically separated into two parts such as core and marginal part using distance value from the nodule surface. Then, a CT density histogram for each region is computed. These CT density histograms are named as two layers histogram. Finally, nodule density patterns are classified by using the characteristics of two layers histogram. The characterizations are based on position and shape of two layers histogram pattern. The first characterization is computed by average of each layer histogram. The second characterization is performed by the standard deviation, skewness, and kurtoisis of each layer histogram. Observing those characteristics, classification rules were designed. The two layers histograms of the nodules shown in Fig. 2 are demonstrated in Fig. 3.

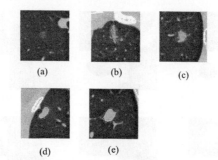

(a)   (b)   (c)

(d)   (e)

Fig. 2. Typical CT density patterns of pulmonary nodules. The nodule contours extracted automatically are superimposed nodule slice images. (a) Type *A*. (b) Type *B*. (c) Type *C*. (d) Type *D*. (e) Type *F*.

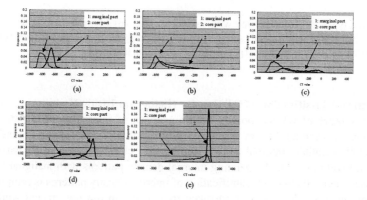

(a)   (b)   (c)

(d)   (e)

Fig. 3. Two layers histogram of nodule presented In Fig.2. (a) Type *A*. (b) Type *B*. (c) Type *C*. (d) Type *D*. (e) Type *F*.

2.3.3 Computation of Curvature Indexes

Each voxel in the region of interest (ROI) including the pulmonary nodule was locally represented by two curvature indexes that represented the shape index and the curvedness [5]. By assuming that each voxel in the ROI lies on the surface which has the normal corresponding to the 3-D gradient at the voxel, we computed directly the curvatures on each voxel from the first and the second derivatives of the gray level image of the ROI.

2.4 Joint Histogram-Based Representation

In order to characterize the distribution pattern of the CT density and the shape index inside nodule, we compute two joint histograms using the distance value from the nodule center [9]. Since the distance value depends on nodule size, the first type is directly derived from the distance value and used to search similar lesions. Once obtained similar lesions, the variation of internal structure provides more important information to classify nodule patterns rather than nodule size. Therefore, the second type is derived from the normalized distance value which ranges between zero and one value and used to evaluate the likelihood of the malignancy. Statistically, the normalized joint histogram denotes a joint probability of CT density value and distance value. It measures how the CT density value distributes inside nodule with respect to the distance from the nodule center. The similar equation of joint histogram of shape index and distance values was obtained.

2.5 Searching Similar Nodule Images

We classify nodules in databases into several categories with respect to the nodule shape, pattern of CT density histogram ,and histogram-based representations. The shape categories used here are round shape, elongated shape, flat shape, round shape with irregular surface, elongated shape with irregular surface, and flat shape with irregular surface. The patterns of CT density histogram are type A, B, C, D, and E as shown in Fig. 3. It is a possible way to directly apply a similarity measure to the 3-D nodule image. However, this approach requires solving the registration between two images. In this study, we apply a simple similarity measure, which is the correlation coefficient (CC) to the nodule representation based on the joint histogram. At the first glance of a given nodule image, it is thought of that the nodule size and nodule density are important indexes for the visual assessment. First, we select the shape category and the pattern of CT density histogram to which the query case belongs. Then, the features with respect to the local intensity structure are examined in detail to search similar patterns. In this study, we generate the list of similar nodule image by the searching process based on the similarity.

2.6 Classification of Benign and Malignant Nodules

We select respectively the M examples from each list of the malignant and benign similar pattern to construct local two malignant and benign classes that are similar to the indeterminate case concerning the CT density distribution pattern and the nodule size. The second type of joint-histogram is used to model the distributions of retrieved malignant and benign examples. Each malignant and benign example is represented by joint histogram of shape index. The Mahalanobis distance is used as a distance measure between the query nodule and each class. The query case is classified into the cluster with small Mahalanobis distance. The Mahalanobis distance from the retrieved benign and malignant classes are represented by MDB and MDM, respectively. A decision index (DI) is formulated by MDB/MDM. When DI is larger than 1, the query nodule is classified into malignant class. While the query case having smaller DI than one has less malignancy likelihood.

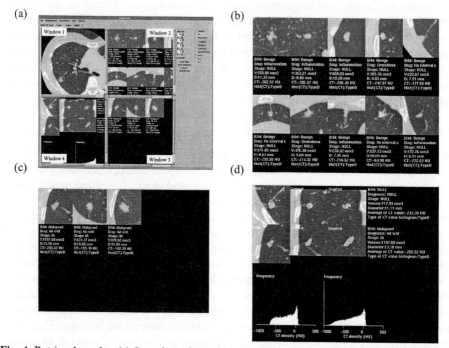

Fig. 4. Retrieval results. (a) Snapshot of searching similar nodule cases from our data set. (b) Expansion of window 2. (c) Expansion of window 3. (d) Expansion of window 4.

3 Experimental Results

Fig. 4 presents a snapshot of searching similar nodule cases from our data set. The window 1 shows a slice image of a query nodule. The window 2 and 3 show retrieval results of benign and malignant cases, respectively. These similar cases were selected from the same shape type and CT density histogram pattern as those of the query case. The retrieved cases are sorted in the order of the CC value. The diagnosis results of the similar cases are presented simultaneously. The window 4 presents slices of region of interests including the query nodule and a malignant case selected from the retrieval result. This window also presents CT density histograms of them. The shape index distribution and histogram can be presented in the same window 4.

In order to compare with retrieval results based on combination with shape type, CT density histogram pattern, and CC value, retrieval results were obtained by other combinations. From visual assessment, it is found that the lack of shape type or CT density histogram pattern from similarity criterion results in retrieving the dissimilar. To evaluate the categorization of data set quantitatively, it is though that an evaluation of DI from similar cases obtained from each categorization may be one of approaches.

We computed *DI* values for the following five categorizations: shape type alone, pattern of CT density histogram alone, *CC* value alone, combination with shape type and *CC* value, combination with pattern of CT density histogram and CC value, and combination with whole categories. These results of *DI* computation of the query cases presented in Fig. 4 were 0.87, 1.1, 0.91, 2.0, 2.3, and 2.3, respectively. Since the query case is a malignant nodule, the correct classification is that the query case has *DI* value larger than 1. In this case, it is found that the combination of categorizations provides better classification performance. More researches using a large data set will be required to conclude in detail. Still, the preliminary experimental result encourages us to develop an image-guided decision support scheme combining the nodule categorization techniques.

4 Conclusion

We have explored a nodule categorization approach to develop an image-guided decision support system of pulmonary nodules. The main idea is to give representations of nodule internal density patterns by introducing a two layers histogram. We presented application results of searching similar images for a query nodule. We believe that the proposed approach might be considered as one of important technique for that image-guided decision support system. The proposed approach could be expanded to include prognosis of lung cancer and build a model showing a likelihood of patient's disease-free survival.

References

1. Kaneko M., Eguchi K., Ohmatsu H., Kakinuma R., Naruke T., Suemasu K., Moriyama N.: Peripheral lung cancer: Screening and detection with low-dose spiral CT versus radiography. Radiology. 201 (1996) 798-802
2. Cavouras D., Prassopoulos P. and Pantelidis N.: Image analysis methods for solitary pulmonary nodule characterization by computed tomography. European Journal of Radiology, 14. (1992) 169-172
3. Kawata Y., Niki N., Ohmatsu H., Kakinuma R., Eguchi K., Kaneko M., Moriyama N.: Quantitative surface characterization of pulmonary nodules based on thin-section CT images. IEEE Trans. Nuclear Science. 45 (1998) 2132-2138
4. McNitt-Gray M. F., Hart E. M., Wyckoff N. Sayre J. W., Goldin J. G., and Aberle D. R. : A pattern classification approach to characterizing solitary pulmonary nodules imaged on high resolution CT: Preliminary results. Medical Physics. 26 (1999) 880-888
5. Kawata Y., Niki N., Ohmatsu H.: Curvature based internal structure analysis of pulmonary nodules using thoracic 3-D CT images. Trans IEICE, J83-DII (2000) 209-218
6. Giger M. L., Huo Z., Lan L., Vyborny C. J.: Intelligent search workstation for computer-aided diagnosis. Proc. Computer Assisted Radiology and Surgery. (2000) 822-827

846   Y. Kawata et al.

7. Kawata Y., Niki N., Ohmatsu H., Kakinuma R., Mori K., Eguchi K., Kaneko M., Mori-yama N. : Three-dimensional CT image retrieval in a database of pulmonary nodules. Proc. IEEE International Conference on Image Processing. vol. III (2002) 149-152

8. Li Q., Aoyama M., Li F., Sone S., MacMahon H. M., Doi K.: Potential clinical usefulness of an intelligent computer-aided diagnostic scheme for distinction between benign and malignant pulmonary nodules in low-dose CT scans. RSNA 2002 Scientific Program (2002) 534-535

9. Kawata Y., Niki N., Ohmatsu H., Moriyama N.: Example-based assisting approach for pulmonary nodule classification in three-dimensional thoracic computed tomography images. Academic Radiology. 10 (2003) 1402-1415

10. Unser M., Aldroubi A., and Eden M.: B-spline signal processing: Part II: Efficient design and applications. IEEE Trans. Signal Processing. 41 (1993) 834-848

11. Henschke C. I., Yankelevitz D. F., Mirtcheva R., McGuinness G., McCauley D., Mietti-nen O. S.: CT screening for lung cancer: Frequency and significance of part-solid and nonsolid nodules. American Journal Roentgenology. 178 (2002) 1053-1057

12. Kawata Y., Niki N., Ohmatsu H., Kakinuma R., Kaneko M., Moriyama N. : A classifica-tion method of pulmonary nodules using 3-D CT images. 89th Scientific Assembly and Annual Meeting of the Radiological Society of North America (RSNA). (2003) 648

Physics Based Contrast Marking and Inpainting Based Local Texture Comparison for Clustered Microcalcification Detection

Xin Yuan[1,2] and Pengcheng Shi[2]

[1] College of Computer Science
Zhejiang University, Hangzhou, China
[2] Department of Electrical and Electronic Engineering
Hong Kong University of Science and Technology
Clear Water Bay, Kowloon, Hong Kong
{eeyxxy, eeship}@ust.hk

Abstract. As important early signs of breast cancers, microcalcifications (MCs) are still very difficult to be reliably detected by either radiologists or computer-aided diagnosis systems. In general, global, regional, and local properties of the mammogram should all be considered in the analysis process. In our effort, we incorporate the physical nature of the imaging process with the image analysis techniques to detect the clustered microcalcifications based on local contrast marking and self-repaired texture comparison. Suspicious areas are first obtained from a simplified X-ray imaging model where the MC contrast is a nonlinear function of local intensity. Following a removal and repair (R&R) procedure of the suspicious areas from their surrounding background textures, pre- and post- R&R local characteristic features of these areas are extracted and compared. A modified AdaBoost algorithm is then used to train the classifier for detecting individual microcalcification, followed by a clustering process to obtain the clustered MCs. Experiments on the MIAS database have shown promising results.

1 Introduction

In many parts of the world, breast cancer remains the leading cause of death for women. The most effective technique for early detection is screening mammography, followed by diagnostic mammography if necessary, a low-dose x-ray procedure that can detect tiny tumors and breast abnormalities. Microcalcifications (MCs) are the earliest signs of breast cancer [2], appearing as tiny (0.05–1mm in diameter) bright spots embedded within non-stationary backgrounds [4]. MC detection has been sofar an extremely difficult task because of the projection nature of mammogram, the low image contrast in high tissue density regions, the varying shapes of the MC clusters, the blurred margins of the MCs, and the different types of noises caused by the x-ray imaging and digitization processes.

A typical MC detection algorithm can be divided into three steps: the enhancement of mammographic features, the localization of suspicious areas, and

C. Barillot, D.R. Haynor, and P. Hellier (Eds.): MICCAI 2004, LNCS 3217, pp. 847–855, 2004.

the classification of these areas [7]. Treating the microcalcifications as high frequency signals, various multi-scale filtering techniques have been widely used in recent studies of suspicious area localization [3,13,14]. Although these methods have shown some effectiveness in MC detection, they often miss significant numbers of microcalcifications in high tissue density regions and produce false positives caused by interferences from normal breast tissues, blood vessels, and fat. Effort thus has been devoted to employ local signal-dependent thresholds which take into account background intensity information [16]. Once the suspicious regions are localized, texture features are extracted from these areas, and various training and classification techniques have been used [5,8,20].

Without prior knowledge on imaging parameters, we believe that the detection of suspicious areas must incorporate imaging-physics knowledge. Because the MC contrast is a nonlinear function of its local image intensity, as previously shown that intensity contrast of a MC of a given size increase then decrease as its surrounding background intensity increases [17], a *particle analysis* (PA) scheme, which regards image as a series of scan lines consisting of several peak-valley intervals, is developed to mark suspicious pixels from background [1]. Corresponding suspicious areas, or *blobs*, are then formed through morphological operations.

Further, we hypothesize that the *local* characteristic features of the tissues surrounding microcalcifications are of particularly great importance for MC detection, and it motivates us to make *direct* texture comparison between a suspicious area and its localized neighborhood through a texture removal and repair (R&R) process. The so-called *virtual biopsy* (VB) procedure, which aims to extract unbiased, classifiable features from the suspicious areas, removes the blobs to form empty holes and then fills them up with texture inpainting techniques. Local characteristic features of these blobs can then be extracted and compared before and after the R&R process. A modified AdaBoost algorithm is used to classify the feature space into normal and abnormal categories, where blobs belonging to the abnormal category are regarded as individual MCs. A clustering process is finally performed to obtain the clustered MCs.

2   Methodology

In this paper, we are focusing on our contributions in terms of physics-based marking of the suspicious pixels and recognition of the individual microcalcifications using localized texture comparison.

---

[1] We have recently noticed that in [18], mammogram intensity is plotted as a function of the pixel location in 2D, and flagpole-like blobs are detected within a given local range. For computational considerations, we have independently developed the 1D particle analysis along 4 scan lines instead of the 2D analysis. For all our experiments sofar, we have not missed any suspicious MCs using the 1D analysis.

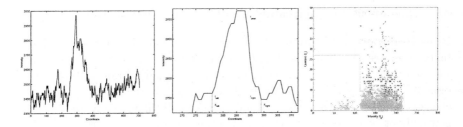

Fig. 1. A intensity scanline (left), the corresponding particle analysis curve (middle, slightly enlarged), and the feature distribution and nonlinear threshold function (right).

2.1   Physics-Based Marking of Suspicious Pixels: Particle Analysis

It has been observed from mammographic images that pixel contrast is an important sign in discriminating suspicious pixels from background tissues. Further, we notice that, typically, the MC contrast in darker area is actually larger than that in brighter area. This inspires us to think that the lower bound of MC contrast could be a function of background intensity, i.e. $I_c = f(I_b)$. Limited by the available space, readers are referred to [19] for detailed analysis of the *much simplified* physical nature of the mammographic imaging process.

To effectively detect the suspicious MC pixel from mammogram, we use the profiles of the multi-orientation (horizontal, vertical, diagonal, and anti-diagonal) image scanlines to obtain the particle contrast, which is evaluated as the minimum of two difference values from peak to the left and right valleys. A particle consists of pixels within an interval that contains a peak I_{peak} and is bounded by two nearest valleys I_{left} and I_{right}. The particle contrast is then $I_c = \min(I_{peak} - I_{left}, I_{peak} - I_{right})$ and the particle intensity is $I_b = \max(I_{left}, I_{right})$. Fig. 1 shows a scanline and the associated particle contrast analysis diagram.

After marking all MC particles of the training images, feature vectors $\mathbf{V}_p = (I_c, I_b, s)$ are formed where $s = +1$ if p is a microcalcification and $s = -1$ if p is normal. The nonlinear threshold function $I_{th} = f(I_b)$ is obtained through a training process, which is posed as an optimization problem on an empirical risk function, $R(I_c, I_b, s) = \sum_{i=1}^{l} \theta[1 - s_i(I_{c_i} - f(I_{b_i}))]$ with l the number of samples, to maximize the number of positive samples, minimize the number of false positive samples, and maximize the margin between the nearest positive and negative samples. Detailed algorithm can be found in [19]. The right figure of Fig. 1 shows the feature distribution of the training set, as well as the obtained nonlinear threshold function.

Once the suspicious pixels are marked, a region growing procedure is used to obtain the blobs. The blobs are discarded if their size is larger than $W_m \times W_m$ with W_m the maximum width of microcalcification, 1mm in our implementation.

2.2   Recognition of Individual Calcification: Virtual Biopsy

Blob Removal and Repair. Assuming that normal tissues have continuous texture properties, then mislabeled normal blobs can be *recovered* from their surrounding tissues. If we remove a blob from the mammogram and use texture inpainting techniques to *repair* the void, we can get direct measure on the difference between the blob and its surrounding tissues. If the blob is a true MC, then it would not be reasonably recovered by its surrounding normal tissues, and the pre- and post- R&R difference would be substantially different from the cases where the blob is actually normal tissue.

Since the breast tissues have relatively high local variations, typical inpainting techniques based on total variation [6] or texture [11] cannot obtain the desirable results in our experience. Instead, we have developed a new texture-like inpainting approach based on wavelet diffusion. Since the variation of the image intensity reflects the changes of tissue types and thickness, we regard these signals as the linear combination of some basis functions. The texture-like inpainting now becomes a diffusion process of these basis functions. Because wavelet theory is well suited to analyze local scale phenomena [12], we use the diffusion of the wavelet subbands to realize our texture-like inpainting.

In our implementation, an image is decomposed into four subbands (smoothing, horizontal, vertical, and diagonal), denoted by W_{LL}, W_{HL}, W_{LH}, and W_{HH}, which represent responses of different orientations. With $I_i, (1 \leq i \leq N)$, denoting the neighboring subblocks of blob I which is being repaired, and $d(I_i, I)$ denoting the distance between I_i and I, we use the following weighted average of subbands to estimate the blob's wavelet subbands, and reconstruct the inpainted blob $I_{inpaint}$ by inverse wavelet transform:

$$W_{LL}(x,y) = \frac{1}{C} \sum_{i=1}^{N} e^{-d(I_i,I)} W_{LL}^i(x,y), \ W_{HL}(x,y) = \frac{1}{C} \sum_{i=1}^{N} e^{-d(I_i,I)} W_{HL}^i(x,y)$$

$$W_{LH}(x,y) = \frac{1}{C} \sum_{i=1}^{N} e^{-d(I_i,I)} W_{LH}^i(x,y), \ W_{HH}(x,y) = \frac{1}{C} \sum_{i=1}^{N} e^{-d(I_i,I)} W_{HH}^i(x,y)$$

and $C = \sum_{i=1}^{N} e^{-d(I_i,I)}$. The advantage of this inpainting scheme is that, in theory, local structure can be *recovered* after repairing. Visual appearance of the repaired voids is actually not important here, because we only care for the blob's texture features extracted from pre- and post-inpainting process. Hence, the appearance continuity between the blob and its background is not necessary achieved. Nevertheless, visually plausible inpainting results are often obtained and an example is shown in Fig. 2.

Local Feature Extraction. The following local features from the pre- (I) and post-repairing $(I_{inpaint})$ blob are extracted:

- M_s: the post-inpainting mean intensity of the *support domain* of the blob, which includes the blob and its surrounding subblocks I_i;

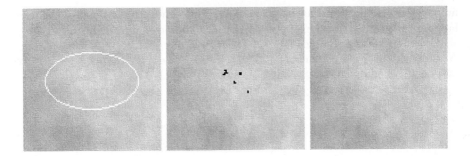

Fig. 2. Effectiveness of image inpainting: pre-inpainting (left), blob removal (middle), and post-inpainting (right).

- S_I: area of the blob;
- N_s: number of suspicious blobs within the support domain of blob I;
- post-inpainting average energies of the detailed subbands of the blob support domain, which reflect texture information of the support domain:

$$E_{HL} = \frac{1}{M_{HL} \times N_{HL}} \sum_{i=1}^{M_{HL}} \sum_{j=1}^{N_{HL}} |W_{HL}(i,j)|,$$

$$E_{LH} = \frac{1}{M_{LH} \times N_{LH}} \sum_{i=1}^{M_{LH}} \sum_{j=1}^{N_{LH}} |W_{LH}(i,j)|$$

$$E_{HH} = \frac{1}{M_{HH} \times N_{HH}} \sum_{i=1}^{M_{HH}} \sum_{j=1}^{N_{HH}} |W_{HH}(i,j)|$$

where M_{HL}, M_{LH}, and M_{HH} are widths, N_{HL}, N_{LH} and N_{HH} are heights of the wavelet subbands, and W_{HL}, W_{HL} and W_{HL} are wavelet coefficients;
- ΔM_s: difference between the pre- and post-inpainting mean intensity values of the blob support domain;
- $\Delta \sigma_s$: difference between the pre- and post-inpainting intensity standard deviations of the blob support domain;
- ΔV_{max}: difference between the pre- and post-inpainting maximum intensity values of the blob support domain;
- ΔE_{HL}, ΔE_{LH}, and ΔE_{HH}: differences between the pre- and post-inpainting average energies of the detailed subbands of the blob support domain.

We note that these particular features, in one way or another, have actually been used in many earlier efforts. We do want to point out that the *localized comparison* of these features is, as far as we know, the completely novel idea.

Training and Classification. In the training step, we have adopted and modified the AdaBoosting algorithm [9,15], which boosts a series of weak classifiers into a strong classifier. The rationale is that the AdaBoosting allows a certain number of false positives for each classifier, thus conceptually handles the overlapping feature distributions between the normal and microcalcification tissues.

Given l training samples $(\mathbf{x}_1, s_1), (\mathbf{x}_2, s_2), \ldots, (\mathbf{x}_l, s_l)$, $\mathbf{x}_i \in \mathbf{X}$ where $\mathbf{X}$ is a N-dimensional feature space, $s_i \in \mathbf{S} = \{-1, +1\}$ where $\mathbf{S}$ are labels for positive and negative samples, and weights C^+ and C^-:

1. Let $t = 1$, initialize:

$$
\omega_i^{(1)} = \begin{cases} \frac{C^+}{C^+ + C^-} \cdot \frac{1}{m^+} & if \ s_i = +1 \\ \frac{C^-}{C^+ + C^-} \cdot \frac{1}{m^-} & if \ s_i = -1 \end{cases}
$$
$$
i = 1, 2, \ldots, l
$$

where m^+ and m^- are the numbers of positive and negative samples, with $m^+ + m^- = l$;

2. Train a weak classifier $h_t(\mathbf{x}) = sign(x_t - h_t)$ using distribution $\omega_i^{(t)}$, i.e. minimize $R_{emp}(\mathbf{x}) = -\sum_{i=1}^{l} \omega_i^{(t)} s_i h_t(\mathbf{x}_i)$, where x_t is an element of the feature vector, and h_t is a threshold value of the element decided by this step;

3. Calculate the training error $\epsilon_t = \sum_{h_t(\mathbf{x}_i) \neq s_i} \omega_i^{(t)}$;

4. Choose $\alpha_t = \frac{1}{2} \ln \frac{1-\epsilon_t}{\epsilon_t}$;

5. Update $\omega_i^{t+1} = \omega_i^t e^{[-\alpha_t s_i h_t(\mathbf{x}_i)]}$, $i = 1, 2, \ldots, l$;

6. Normalize $\omega_i^{t+1} = \dfrac{\omega_i^{t+1}}{\sum\limits_{i=1}^{l} \omega_i^{t+1}}$, $i = 1, 2, \ldots, l$;

7. Let $t = t + 1$, if $t < T$ where T is the maximum number of weak classifiers, goto step 2; otherwise, stop.

Hence, the final decision function becomes:

$$
H(\mathbf{x}) = sign \left[\sum_{t=1}^{T} \alpha_t h_t(\mathbf{x}) \right] \tag{1}
$$

We have used a simple threshold function as the weak classifier for each dimension of the feature space, with $T = N$ and $h_i(\mathbf{x}) = sign(x_i - h_i)$, and where x_i is one element of the feature vector and h_i is a threshold value of the corresponding element.

2.3   Clustering of Microcalcifications

Clustered MCs, which is typically defined to have at least 2 to 3 MCs within a $1cm^2$ region [10], provide useful diagnosis information. We have used a simple clustering method, similar to the dynamic clustering algorithm, to generate the MC clusters. Each blob is added to certain cluster with the distance from blob to the center of cluster less than D_I, otherwise create a new cluster and add this blob to it. If the distance between two centers of clusters is less than D_c, they would be merged. Finally clusters are removed if the number of blobs in them is less than N_c. The user-specified parameters D_I, D_c, and N_c are dependent on the image resolution under study.

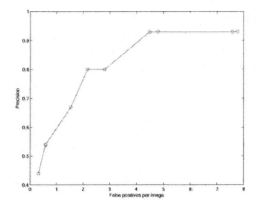

Fig. 3. FROC curve on the MIAS database.

3   Experiment and Discussion

To evaluate our method for clustered microcalcification detection, we have used the digital mammography dataset provided by the Mammographic Image Analysis Society (MIAS) [1] (the reduced resolution version). This particular database contains 322 images with medio-lateral oblique (MLO) view representing 161 bilateral mammogram pairs, among them 24 images contains 29 microcalcification clusters. Each image has 200 micron pixel edge and the size is 1024 × 1024 pixels with 8-bit grayscale. It also includes radiologist's truth-markings on the locations of any abnormalities that may be present. These images has no information about x-ray imaging parameters, so they are uncalibrated mammograms.

We have selected 11 images containing 14 clusters as the training set, and other 311 images as the testing set. Contrast marking was done manually on those ROIs which contain microcalcifications, extracted from the training set with four orientations. 1915 samples were collected for training the nonlinear threshold function $f(I_b)$. After applying this threshold function to all mammograms of the training set and doing blob generation with $W_m = 5$, we obtained 471 blobs totally. In the virtual biopsy step, we have used 4th order Deubechies wavelets (DB4) to decompose the image blocks for only one level. The size of the support domain was selected as 10×10. The left figure on Fig. 2 gives subimage around a ROI from image mdb209 before inpainting, after blob removal, and post inpainting. The appearance of the post-repairing blob region is very similar to normal tissues. Blob classifier based on feature space was trained by $C^+ = 0.7, C^- = 0.3$. Clustering process was carried out with $D_I = 50$ (10mm), $D_c = 25$ (5mm), and $N_c = 3$.

All 311 test images were processed by the same flow. Fig. 3 shows the FROC curve through changing C^+ and C^-. Overall, it seems that we can achieve the best detection result at 93.3% precision and 4.8 false positives per image. It is, however, not easy to compare the effectiveness of our method to other studies since different work has used different databases or different numbers of mammographic images from the MIAS dataset. Among them, Gulsrud used optimal filters to detect MCs on the MIAS images [10]. But he only tested on 43 images and achieved a true positive (TP) rate of 100% with 2.3 false positives per image, or alternatively TP 100% with one FP cluster per image.

Our initial results on the MIAS dataset suggest that our method could extract clustered microcalcifications effectively and our algorithm is a promising idea for detecting abnormalities on projection medical images. However, the false positive rate is relatively high for practical purposes and has become our current research focus, including the possibilities of introducing image and feature space normalization.

This work is supported in part by HKRGC under HKUST-DAG02/03.EG45.

References

1. Digital mammography database of the mammographic image analysis society. http://www.wiau.man.ac.uk/services/MIAS/MIASweb.html.
2. S. Astley, I. Hutt, et al. Automation in mammography: Computer vision and human perception. In *State of The Art in Digital Mammographic Image Analysis*, pages 1–25. World Scientific, 1994.
3. T. Bhangale, U.B. Desai, and U. Sharma. An unsupervised scheme for detection of microcalcifications on mammograms. In *IEEE ICIP*, pages 184–187, 2000.
4. G. Boccignone, A. Chianese, and A. Picariello. Using Renyi's information and wavelets for target detection: An application to mammograms. 3:303–313, 2000.
5. H.P. Chan, S.C. B. Lo, B. Sahiner, K.L. Lam, and M.A. Helvie. Computer-aided detection of mammographic microcalcifications: Pattern recognition with an artificial neural network. *Medical Physics*, 22(10):1555–1567, 1995.
6. T.F. Chan and J. Shen. Inpainting based on nonlinear transport and diffusion. In *Inverse problems, image analysis, and medical imaging*, pages 53–65. 2002.
7. Y. Chitre, A.P. Dhawan, and M. MoskoWitz. Artificial neural network based classification of mammographic microcalcifications using image structure features. In *State of The Art in Digital Mammographic Image Analysis*, pages 167–197. World Scientific, 1994.
8. I. El-Naqa, Y. Yang, M.N. Wernick, N.P. Galatsanos, and R. Nishikawa. A support vector machine approach for detetcion of microcalcifications in mammograms. In *IEEE ICIP*, pages 201–204, 2002.
9. Y. Freund and R.E. Schapire. Experiments with a new boosting algorithm. In *International Conference on Machine Learning*, pages 148–156, 1996.
10. T.O. Gulsrud, J.H. Husøy, and H. Stavanger. Optimal filter for detection of clustered microcalcifications. In *ICPR*, volume 1, pages 508–511, 2000.
11. J. Jia and C.K. Tang. Image repairing: robust image synthesis by adaptive *n*d tensor voting. In *IEEE CVPR*, pages 643–650, 2003.
12. S. Mallat. *A Wavelet Tour of Signal Processing*. Academic Press, 1998.
13. T. Netsch. Detection of micro calcification clusters in digital mammograms: A scale space approach. In *IWDM*, 1996.
14. R.N. Strickland and H.I. Hahn. Wavelet transforms for detecting microcalcifications in mammograms. *IEEE TMI*, 15(2):218–229, 1996.
15. V.N. Vapnik. *The Nature of Statistical Learning Theory*. Springer, 2000.

16. W.J.H. Veldkamp and N. Karssemeijer. Accurate segmentation and contrast measurement of mcs in mammograms: a phantom study. *Medical Physics*, 25(7):1102–1110, 1998.
17. W.J.H. Veldkamp and N. Karssemeijer. Normalization of local contrast in mammograms. *IEEE TMI*, 19(7):731–738, 2000.
18. Margaret Yam. *Detection and Analysis of Microcalcification Clusters in X-ray Mammograms Using the hint Representation*. PhD thesis, University of Oxford, 2001.
19. X. Yuan and P.C. Shi. The physical nature of mammographic image processing. Technical report, Biomedical Research Laboratory, Department of Electrical and Electronic Engineering, Hong Kong University of Science and Technology, 2003.
20. O.R. Zaïane, M.-L. Antonie, and A. Coman. Mammography classification by an association rule-based classifier. In *ACM SIGKDD: International Workshop on Multimedia Data Mining*, pages 62–69, 2002.

Automatic Detection and Recognition of Lung Abnormalities in Helical CT Images Using Deformable Templates

Aly Farag[1], Ayman El-Baz[1], Georgy G. Gimel'farb[2], Robert Falk[3], and Stephen G. Hushek[4]

[1] Computer Vision and Image Processing Laboratory
University of Louisville, Louisville, KY 40292, USA.
{farag, elbaz}@cvip.Louisville.edu, http://www.cvip.louisville.edu
[2] Department of Computer Science, Tamaki Campus
University of Auckland, Auckland, New Zealand.
[3] Director, Medical Imaging Division, Jewish Hospital, Louisville, KY, USA.
[4] Technical Director, iMRI Department, Norton Hospital, Louisville, KY, USA.

Abstract. Automatic detection of lung nodules is an important problem in computer analysis of chest radiographs. In this paper we propose a novel algorithm for isolating lung nodules from spiral CT scans. The proposed algorithm is based on using four different types of deformable templates describing typical geometry and gray level distribution of lung nodules. These four types are (*i*) solid spherical model of large-size calcified and non-calcified nodules appearing in several successive slices; (*ii*) hollow spherical model of large lung cavity nodules; (*iii*) circular model of small nodules appearing in only a single slice; and (*iv*) semicircular model of lung wall nodules. Each template has a specific gray level pattern which is analytically estimated in order to fit the available empirical data. The detection combines the normalized cross-correlation template matching by genetic optimization and Bayesian post-classification. This approach allows for isolating abnormalities which spread over several adjacent CT slices. Experiments with 200 patients' CT scans show that the developed techniques detect lung nodules more accurately than other known algorithms.

1 Introduction

Automatic detection of lung nodules is an important problem in computer analysis of chest radiographs. One in every 18 women and every 12 men develop lung cancer, making it the leading cause of cancer deaths. Early detection of lung tumors (visible on the chest film as nodules) may increase the patient's chance of survival [2].

At present, low-dose spiral computed tomography (LDCT) is of prime interest for screening (high risk) groups for early detection of lung cancer [2]. The LDCT provides chest scans with very high spatial, temporal, and contrast resolution of anatomic structures and is able to gather a complete 3D volume of a human thorax in a single breath-hold [3]. The automatic screening typically involves

C. Barillot, D.R. Haynor, and P. Hellier (Eds.): MICCAI 2004, LNCS 3217, pp. 856–864, 2004.
© Springer-Verlag Berlin Heidelberg 2004

two-stage detection of lung abnormalities (nodules). First, the initial candidate nodules are selected and then the false candidates, called false positive nodules (FPNs) are partially eliminated while preserving the true ones (TPNs).

At the first stage, conformal nodule filtering [4] or unsharp masking [5] can enhance nodules and suppress other structures to separate the candidates from the background by simple thresholding (to improve the separation, background trend is corrected in [6] within image regions of interest). Circular nodule candidates can be detected by template matching [5] or Hough transform [7]. Other methods detect lung nodules by using morphological operators such as the algorithm proposed in [8]. The drawbacks of this algorithm are it fails to detect cavity lung nodules and has difficulties in detecting lung wall nodules.

The FPNs are excluded at the second stage by feature extraction and classification [6,9]. Such features as circularity, size, contrast [6], or local curvature [9] are extracted by morphological techniques, and artificial neural networks (ANN) are frequently used as post-classifiers [10]. The critical issue is to adequately discriminate between the nodules and non-nodules.

In this paper nodule types are modelled with four central-symmetric deformable templates:(*i*) solid spherical model of large-size (above 10 mm) calcified and non-calcified nodules appearing in several successive slices; (*ii*) hollow spherical model of large lung cavity nodules; (*iii*) circular model of small nodules appearing in only a single slice; and (*iv*) semicircular model of lung wall nodules. This approach allows for isolating abnormalities which spread over several adjacent CT slices.

Each template has a specific gray level pattern which is analytically estimated in order to fit the available empirical data. Normalized cross-correlation is used for template matching. The 3D or 2D position, size, and gray level pattern of each template is adjusted to the most similar part of the segmented veins, arteries, and lung abnormalities by a genetic optimization technique [11]. After all the candidates are detected, a supervised Bayesian classification of geometric and textural features of the candidate nodules partially excludes the FPNs.

2   Deformable Templates of Abnormalities

Our detection of lung nodules begins with two segmentation stages which considerably reduce the search space. At the first stage shown in Fig. 1(a) and Fig. 1(b), lung tissues are separated from the surrounding anatomical structures, e.g., ribs, liver, and other organs, appearing in the chest CT scans. The second stage extracts arteries, veins, bronchi, and lung abnormalities (see Fig. 1(c)) from the already segmented lung tissues. Segmentation algorithms are based on representing each CT slice as a sample of a Markov–Gibbs random field of region labels and gray levels. Details of the algorithms are presented in [1], and in this paper we focus only on the third stage of detecting and classifying the nodules among the extracted objects. Figure 2(a) shows the empirical gray level distribution over the extracted regions in Fig. 1(c). Both the nodules and normal tissues such as arteries, veins, and bronchi, have almost the same gray level distributions, so abnormality detection must include their geometrical shape. Four basic classes of lung abnormalities are: small calcified; large calcified; non-calcified; and cavity nodules. The first three classes tend to have solid spherical shapes, whereas the cavity nodules are hollow spheres. Generally, the smaller nodules

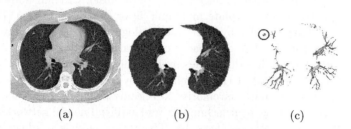

(a)   (b)   (c)

Fig. 1. First two segmentation steps.

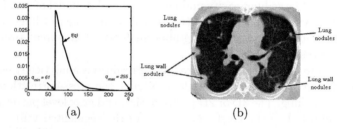

(a)   (b)

Fig. 2. (a) The empirical gray level distribution over the extracted regions in Fig. 1(c) (b) Nodule positions and shapes.

appear only in a single 2D slice like in Fig. 2(b), whereas the larger ones spread over a 3D volume represented by several successive slices. The lung wall nodules may also appear in one or more slices, depending on their size. However, they are semicircular in shape as shown in Fig. 2(b). Our analysis of 2D CT slices suggests that spatial changes of gray levels across the central cross-section of a solid-shape 3D nodule or across a solid-shape 2D nodule can be approximated with a central-symmetric Gaussian-like template $q(r) = q_{max} \exp\left(-(r/\rho)^2\right)$; $0 \leq r \leq R$. Here, r is the radius from the template's center and $q(r)$ is the gray level in a template point with Cartesian coordinates (ξ, η) with respect to the center (i.e., $r^2 = \xi^2 + \eta^2$), q_{max} denotes the maximum gray level for the template, R is the template radius depending on the minimum gray level $q_{min} = q(R)$, and the parameter ρ specifies how fast the signals decrease across the template.

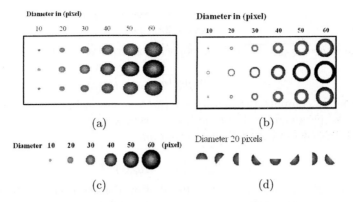

Fig. 3. Examples of the deformed templates for GA template matching process. (a) Solid spherical models consisting of three slices to detect large calcified and non-calcified nodules. (b) Hollow spherical models consisting of three slices to detect thick cavity nodules. (c) Circular models to detect small nodules. (d) Semicircular models to detect lung wall nodules.

3   Genetic Algorithm(GA) Template Matching

GA template matching is used to effectively search for the location of lung nodules scattered within the lung areas. In this method, the genetic algorithm is used to determine the target position in an observed image and to select a suitable radius to generate a template model for the template matching process. Details of the GA process are described below.

3.1   Template Identification

The CT slices in our study have in-plane spatial resolution of 0.4 mm per pixel so that the radius range for all lung nodules is $R = 5$–30 pixels. Because the third spatial axis has lower resolution, for large solid and hollow lung nodules we use the 3-layer template. Thin lung nodules appearing only in a single slice have the circular templates. The lung wall nodules are of semicircular shape. We assume that the template deformations, other than translations are restricted to different scales (radii) of all the templates and also different (orientation) angles of the semicircular templates. Examples of the deformed templates are presented in Fig. 3. In order to get better matching between the template model and the lung nodules we have to generate a template which has a density close to the density of the segmented veins, arteries, and lung abnormalities which are shown in Fig. 2(a). Gray level distribution density over the 2D Gaussian template can be found as follows:

$$\psi(q) = 2\pi r(q) \tag{1}$$

since $r(q) = \rho\sqrt{lnq_{max} - lnq}$, then $\psi(q)$ can be expressed as follows:

$$\psi(q) = 2\pi\rho\sqrt{lnq_{max} - lnq} \tag{2}$$

In order to compute the density for the template using Eq.(2), we need to estimate the parameter ρ. For a template which has radius R, the parameter ρ can be estimated from the following equation:

$$\rho = R\left(\ln q_{max} - \ln q_{min}\right)^{-\frac{1}{2}} \tag{3}$$

By using Eq.(3), the gray level distribution density over the 2D Gaussian template can be expressed in the following closed form:

$$\psi(q|q_{min}, q_{max}) = 2\pi R\sqrt{\frac{lnq_{max} - lnq}{lnq_{max} - lnq_{min}}} \tag{4}$$

This relationship allows us to roughly estimate the template parameters q_{max} and q_{min} from the empirical density in Fig. 2(a) (in this particular case $q_{max} = 255$ and $q_{min} = 61$). In particular, for the circular templates of the radii $R = 5$ and 30, the estimated $\rho = 4.18$ and 25.08, respectively. Figure 4 demonstrates how close the empirical gray level distribution for the objects in Fig. 1(c) are to the estimated distribution for the above two templates under its discretization.

In the case of the 3D solid spherical templates, the 2D template is first identified for the central cross-section. Then the upper and lower cross-sections are specified by the same parameters in the following equation ($q_t(r) = q_{max}\exp(-(r^2 + t^2)/\rho^2)$) where t is the slice thickness in pixels ($t = 7$ in our experiments below). The radius of upper and lower circles is specified by the relationship $q_t(R) = q_{min}$.

The hollow spherical templates to detect cavity lung nodules are obtained in a similar way by removing the central part of the solid templates up to 75% of the radius R.

3.2   The GA Template Matching Process

As mentioned above GA is used to determine the target position in an observed image and select a suitable radius to generate a template model. In this paper we use the genetic algorithm with the following structure (for more details about GA see [11]).

- *Chromosome*: Each chromosome has 28 bits, of which 23 determine the target position. The 23 position bits are divided into 9-, 9-, and 5-bit sets corresponding to the coordinates (x, y, z) respectively. The last 5 bits determine the radius of the generated templates R. Once we know R, q_{min}, and q_{max} we calculate ρ from Eq. 3. By using ρ, and q_{max} we generate the corresponding template. Then similarities between the cut image and the generated template are calculated.

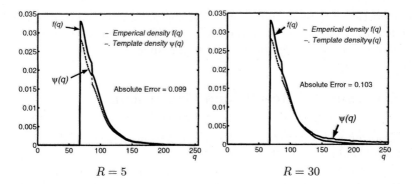

Fig. 4. Estimated template gray level distributions ($\psi(q)$) w.r.t. the empirical density ($f(q)$).

– **Fitness**: We define the fitness of an individual template as the "similarity" calculated by the normalized cross-correlation of two images a, and b [12], as

$$Similarity_{a,b} = \frac{\sum_{i=1}^{n}\sum_{j=1}^{n}(a_{ij} - m_a)(b_{ij} - m_b)}{\sqrt{\sum_{i=1}^{n}\sum_{j=1}^{n}(a_{ij} - m_a)^2}\sqrt{\sum_{i=1}^{n}\sum_{j=1}^{n}(b_{ij} - m_b)^2}}$$

where $m_a = \frac{1}{n}\sum_{i=1}^{n}\sum_{j=1}^{n} a_{ij}$, $m_b = \frac{1}{n}\sum_{i=1}^{n}\sum_{j=1}^{n} b_{ij}$, the values a and b signify the images for comparison. The a_{ij} is the value of a pixel at site (i, j) in image a, similarly b_{ij}.

The matching algorithm runs separately for each type of lung abnormality (Note that for semicircular template model we add another part in the chromosome that represent the angle). All spatial locations where the similarity score is greater than a certain threshold (in our experiments 0.8) are extracted as candidate nodules.

4   Post-classification of Nodule Features

Because actual lung nodules are not exactly spherical, circular, or semicircular, some true nodules can be missed. A number of false positive nodules (FPNs) can also be encountered during the initial extraction of the candidates. To reduce the error rate, post-classification of the candidate nodules is performed with three textural and geometric features of each detected nodule: (i) radial non-uniformity $U = \max_{\theta}(d(\theta)) - \min_{\theta}(d(\theta))$ of its borders (here, $d(\theta)$ is the distance at the angle θ between the center of the template and the border of the segmented object in Fig. 1(c)); (ii) mean gray level (q_{ave}) over the 3D or 2D nodular template, and (iii) the 10%-tile gray level for the marginal gray level distribution over the 3D or 2D nodular template. To distinguish between the FPNs and true positive nodules(TPNs), we use Bayesian supervised classifier learning statistical characteristics of these features from a training set of false and true nodules. All three features (*i*)–(*iii*) are used to classify the FPNs in lung, while only the last two features can be applied to the lung wall nodules.

5   Experimental Results and Conclusions

The algorithm was tested on the CT scans of 200 subjects enrolled to the screening study. Among them, 21 subjects had abnormalities in their CT scans and 179 subjects were normal (this classification validated by a radiologist). At stage one, the template matching extracted 110 true candidates (out of the true 130 nodules) and 49 FPNs.

The classification at stage two reduced the number of the FPNs to 12 but simultaneously rejected three true nodules. Thus the final number of the TPNs became 107 out of 130 giving the overall correct detection rate of 82.3% with the FPNs rate of 9.2%. Table 1 presents the numbers of TPNs and FPNs before and after the post-classification stage.

Table 1. Detection rate for different types of abnormalities (TPNs : the nodules determined by a radiologist).

Type of Lung Nodules	True detecting nodules before removing FPNs	False detecting nodules before removing FPNs	True detecting nodules after removing FPNs	False detecting nodules after removing FPNs
Lung wall	28 : 29	8	27 : 29	2
Calcified	46 : 49	4	46 : 49	1
Non-calcified	12 : 18	5	12 : 18	3
Cavity	8 : 11	7	8 : 11	1
Small	17 : 23	25	15 : 23	5

Table 2. Detection rate for different types of abnormalities by using the algorithm proposed in [12] (TPNs : the nodules determined by a radiologist).

Type of Lung Nodules	True detecting nodules before removing FPNs	False detecting nodules before removing FPNs	True detecting nodules after removing FPNs	False detecting nodules after removing FPNs
Lung wall	14 : 29	86	13 : 29	17
Calcified	31 : 49	35	31 : 49	9
Non-calcified	14 : 18	25	14 : 18	14
Cavity	-	-	-	-
Small	10 : 23	34	9 : 23	12

To illustrate the efficiency of the proposed algorithm we compare the results obtained by the proposed algorithm with the results obtained by other algorithms. To the best of our knowledge, there is only one related work [12] that detects lung nodules from spiral CT scan by using a template matching method. The proposed algorithm by Lee [12] detects only **three types** of nodules: large lung nodules, small lung nodules, and lung wall nodules by using fixed templates and the parameters for each template are selected **manually** from the given data set. We ran Lee's algorithm on the same data sets. The algorithm detects at stage one, 69 true candidates (out of the true 130 nodules) and 180 FPNs. The classification at stage two reduced the number of FPNs to 52 but simultaneously rejected two true nodules. Thus the final number of TPNs became 67 out of 130 giving the overall correct detection rate of 51.5% with the FPNs rate of 40%. Table 2 presents the details of the results obtained by the algorithm proposed in [12]. It is clear from Table 2 that this algorithm fails to detect large numbers of true nodules because this algorithm used fixed size templates and these templates sometimes give low correlation between the template and the true nodules. They estimate the parameters that determine the gray levels manually, and they use them for the whole volume. At times this is not the best estimation because the distribution for the gray level can change from one slice to another (depends on the cross section that scanned it, and the organs that appear in that cross section). In our proposed algorithm we estimate these parameters analytically using Eq. (3) for each CT slice.

Our experiments show that the proposed adaptive deformable templates, with analytical parameter estimation, allow for detection of more than 80% of the true lung abnormalities. The number of simultaneously detected false nodules can be considerably reduced by accounting for simple geometrical and textural features of the candidate nodules.

Acknowledgement. This research has been supported by grants from the Jewish Hospital Foundation and the Kentucky Lung Cancer Program.

References

1. Aly A. Farag, Ayman El-Baz, G.L.Gimel'farb, "Precise Image Segmentation by Iterative EM-Based Approxiation of Empirical Grey Level Distributions with Linear Combinations of Gaussions", *IEEE Workshop on Learning in Computer Vision and Pattern Recognition*, Washington, DC, June, 2004
2. P. M. Boiselle and C. S. White (Eds.) *New Techniques in Thoracic Imaging.* M. Dekker, New York, 2002.
3. L. Quekel, A.Kessels, R. Goei, and J. V. Engelshoven, "Miss rate of lung cancer on the chest radiograph in clinical practice," *Chest*, Vol. 115, no. 3, pp. 720–724, 1999.
4. S.-C. B. Lo, M. T. Freedman, J.-S. Lin, and S. K. Mun, "Automatic lung nodule detection using profile matching and back-propagation neural network techniques," *J. Digital Imaging*, Vol. 6, no. 1, pp. 48–54, 1993.

5. F. Mao, W. Qian, J. Gaviria, and L. Clarke, "Fragmentary window filtering for multiscale lung nodule detection," *Academic Radiology*, Vol. 5, no. 4, pp. 306–311, 1998.
6. X. Xu, S. Katsuragawa, K. Ashizawa,H. MacMahon, and K. Doi, "Analysis of image features of histograms of edge gradient for false positive reduction in lung nodule detection in chest radiographs," *Proc. SPIE*, Vol. 3338, pp. 318–326, 1998.
7. W. Lampeter, "ANDS-V1 computer detection of lung nodules," *Proc. SPIE*, Vol. 555, pp. 253–261, 1985.
8. Catalin I. Fetita, Francoise Preteux, Catherine Beigelman-Aubry, and Philippe Grenier, "3D Automated Lung Nodule segmentation in HRCT," *Proc. MICCAI*, LNCS 2878, pp. 626-634, November 2003.
9. M. J. Carreira, D. Cabello, M. G. Penedo,and J. M. Pardo, "Computer aided lung nodule detection in chest radiography," in R. T. Chin et al. (Eds.) *Image Analysis Applications and Computer Graphics*, (*Lecture Notes in Computer Science* 1024), Springer, Berlin, pp. 331–338, 1995.
10. S-C. B. Lo, S.-L. A. Lou, J.-S. Lin, M. T. Freedman, M. V. Chien, and S. K. Mun, "Artificial convolution neural network techniques and applications for lung nodule detection," *IEEE Trans. Med. Imaging*, Vol. 14, pp. 711–718, August 1995.
11. D. E. Goldberg, *Genetic Algorithms in Search, Optimization and Machine Learning*. Addison-Wesley, Reading, Mass., 1989.
12. Y. Lee, T. Hara, H. Fujita, S. Itoh, and T. Ishigaki, "Automated Detection of Pulmonary Nodules in Helical CT Images Based on an Improved Template-Matching Technique," *IEEE Tran. Med. Imaging*, Vol. 20, pp. 595–604, July 2001.

A Multi-resolution CLS Detection Algorithm for Mammographic Image Analysis

Lionel C.C. Wai, Matthew Mellor, and Michael Brady

Medical Vision Laboratory, Robotics Research Group, University of Oxford.
Ewert House, Summertown, Oxford OX2 7DD, United Kingdom.
{lwai,matt,jmb}@robots.ox.ac.uk

Abstract. Curvilinear structures (CLS) are locally one-dimensional, relatively thin objects which complicate analysis of a mammogram. They comprise a number of anatomical features, most especially connective tissue, blood vessels, and milk ducts. The segmentation, identification and removal of such structures potentially facilitate a wide range of mammographic image processing applications, such as mass detection and temporal registration. In this paper, we present a novel CLS detection algorithm which is based on the monogenic signal afforced by a CLS physical model. The strength of the proposed model-based CLS detector is that it is able to identify even low contrast CLS. In addition, a noise suppression approach, based on local energy thresholding, is proposed to further improve the quality of segmentation. A local energy (LE)-based junction detection method which utilises the orientation information provided by the monogenic signal is also presented. Experiments demonstrate that the proposed CLS detection framework is capable of producing well-localized, highly noise-tolerated responses as well as robust performances as compared to classical orientation-sampling approach.

1 Introduction

Mammographic image processing aims primarily to detect, classify, and measure anatomical features such as masses and microcalcifications, and to monitor the development of such features over time, view, and bilaterally. Amongst the anatomical features that can be seen in mammograms, curvilinear structures (CLS) are often the most pervasive but the most complex feature to segment. They correspond to relatively dense connective stroma, milk ducts, and blood vessels, and appear locally linear and thin. The detection of CLS is often difficult because of their low contrast, variable widths, and the often noisy parenchymal background against which the feature has to be detected. The projective nature of mammography further complicates detection. The detection and segmentation of CLS has been studied in various applications such as the validation of calcification detectors and registration [1,2]. Identifying the CLS is often a key step in distinguishing tumour spicules from overlying CLS. Some previous researchers have tackled the problem of detecting and removing the CLS. For example, Cerneaz [3] proposed a CLS detector based on spatial second dimensional derivative operators. Zwiggelaar et. al. [4] suggested an

C. Barillot, D.R. Haynor, and P. Hellier (Eds.): MICCAI 2004, LNCS 3217, pp. 865–872, 2004.

nonlinear line strength operator to detect the linear structures in mammograms. In this study, we extended the work of Schenk [5] on local energy (LE) feature detection which is based on a steerable filter framework.

From the perspective of low-level feature detection, the CLS segmentation problem can be regarded as a ridge detection task. However, most previous work on feature detection has been focused on the edge detection, of which has the sudden intensity change or higher local energy than the corresponding ridge. Kovesi's [6] Phase Congruency algorithm (based on previous work by Morrone and Owens) *defines* a feature as an image location for which the local phase remains relatively constant across a sufficient range of bandpass filters. Kovesi's approach is intrinsically one-dimensional, requiring a framework such as steerable filters to extend it to images. More recently, coupled with the Reisz transform, Felsberg [7] has developed the construction of a two or more dimensional feature detection scheme. This has significant advantages over steerable filtering both in terms of the robustness and speed of execution and isotropicity of filter responses. This paper adapts the monogenic signal to the task of CLS detection and removal.

In the remaining of this paper, the framework and the algorithms of the CLS detector are introduced. Subsequently, the effect of noise and the responses of the algorithm of CLS with different widths are showed and its performance is discussed. Finally, segmentation results on real mammographic images are presented.

2 Segmentation Methodologies

In this section, we introduce the CLS model, which approximates the intensity profile of a CLS feature in a digitized image, and the multi-resolution ridge detection algorithm based on the monogenic signal.

2.1 The Digitized Intensity Profile Model of CLS

The CLS model employed in our detection framework is adapted from the work of Cerneaz, which introduced a two medium model that estimates the intensity profile of the CLS. In this model, the CLS are assumed to have circular cross section when the breast is not compressed. Since the CLS cannot be assumed orthogonal to the beam, the cross section for mammography will be elliptical. To simplify the analysis, though not the detection process, the x-ray beam is assumed to be monogenic, with no scatter.

Imagine that an x-ray beam goes through a compressed breast of thickness H and a CLS with an elliptic cross-section area which is of radii a and b, in which radii a is parallel to the film surface. Thus the x-ray path that transverses through the cross section of the CLS can be represented by the function $h(x)$:

$$h(x) = \frac{2b}{a}\sqrt{a^2 - x^2}, \quad -a \leq x \leq a. \tag{1}$$

Thus the net beam attenuation of the two medium model will be

$$E(x) = \begin{cases} E_o e^{-\mu_1(H-h(x))} e^{-\mu_2 h(x)} & -a \le x \le a \\ E_o e^{-\mu_1 H} & otherwise \end{cases}, \tag{2}$$

where E_o is the energy of the monoenergetic incident beam, μ_1 and μ_2 are the x-ray attenuation coefficients of the parenchyma and the CLS respectively. The basic model is depicted in Fig. 1. By a linear approximation of the film characteristic curve, we arrive at a film density function D:

$$D = \gamma \log_{10}(\beta E), \tag{3}$$

where β is the film speed and γ is the film gradient.

Based on this relationship, the pixel intensity profile on a digitised image can be modeled, depending on which of two main categories of digitisation method is used: film density and transmitted-light. For film density direct digitisation, the pixel intensity profile is well approximated by P_d:

$$P_d(x) = \frac{m\gamma}{\ln 10} \left[\ln(\beta\phi X_c \varepsilon_p) - \mu_1 H - (\mu_2 - \mu_1)\frac{2b}{a}\sqrt{a^2 - x^2} \right] + q \quad, -a \le x \le a. \tag{4}$$

Correspondingly, for transmitted-light, the profile is calculated by the equation P_l which is showed below:

$$P_l(x) = \frac{al_l}{\left(\beta\phi X_c \varepsilon_p\right)^\gamma} \exp\left[\gamma\mu_1 H + \gamma(\mu_2 - \mu_1)\frac{2b}{a}\sqrt{a^2 - x^2} \right] + \lambda \quad, -a \le x \le a. \tag{5}$$

In the two equations above, γ represents the film gradient, ε_p is the photon density, m and q are the gradient and offset of the linear approximation of the film density digitalisation curve respectively, and $\beta\phi X_c \varepsilon_p$ are the imaging parameters which are functions of H and μ_1. And in this study, 0.6 D 3.0, 0 P 255, $\gamma=3$, $\varepsilon_p=17.4$, $\mu_1=0.558$, $\mu_2=1.028$, $H=3.5$.

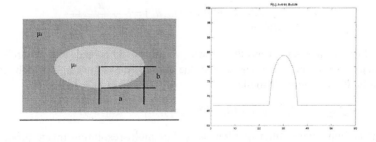

Fig. 1. The cross section of a CLS and its intensity profile. Left: The CLS model parameters as described in section 2.1. Right: An example of the intensity profile generated by the model, which is through transmitted-light digitalisation. The maximum pixel intensity is set to be 256.

2.2   The Multi-resolution Ridge Detector

A multi-resolution approach is opted for because of the variable widths of vascular structures. The CLS in mammogram are composed of large connective stroma, arteries and veins as well as narrow capillaries and milk ducts, which covers a set of vessels with width ranges from 1800 microns to 5 microns. However, in view of current limits on sampling and signal-to-noise, we are only interested in detecting the structures of widths between 1800 microns to 180 microns. This specification is enough to cover most vascular structures in mammograms sampled at as fine as 50 microns per pixel.

From the model described in section 2.1 and visualized in Fig. 1, the response of the filter should be localised at the ridges of CLS in order to get the "skeleton" extracted. In this study, we adopt the notion of phase congruency (PC) in detecting features [6]. This is a measure of the phase similarity of the Fourier components of a point. Phase congruency of a point with spatial coordinate given by x can be defined as follows:

$$PC(x) = \underset{\theta \in (0, 2\pi)}{Max} \frac{\int_{-\infty}^{\infty} a_\omega \cos(\omega x + \phi_\omega - \theta) d\omega}{\int_{-\infty}^{\infty} a_\omega d\omega}. \tag{6}$$

In order to compute PC, the local phase of the pixel must be estimated from the analytical signal. In previous work, including that by Schenk [5], a set of steerable filters are designed to estimate the local phase by analysing one dimensional cross sections of the image at each point in several different orientations. This intrinsically computationally intensive approach stems from the fact that the analytic signal, the basis for local phase of a signal, is only defined for one dimension signals. However, by using vector filters as suggested by Felsberg [7], a quadrature filter triple for the image can be obtained. The odd filter is based on the Reisz transform $H(u_1, u_2) = (H_1, H_2)$, in which

$$H_1(u_1, u_2) = i \frac{u_1}{\sqrt{u_1^2 + u_2^2}} \quad \text{and} \quad H_2(u_1, u_2) = i \frac{u_2}{\sqrt{u_1^2 + u_2^2}}. \tag{7}$$

In this expression u_1 and u_2 are the Fourier variables. This leads to a generalization of the analytical signal, which is called the monogenic signal and which can be described by the following formula:

$$f_M(x_1, x_2) = (f(x_1, x_2), (h_1 * f)(x_1, x_2), (h_2 * f)(x_1, x_2)), \tag{8}$$

where f is an appropriate filter or filter bank. For multi-resolution image processing, those filters constitute a family which tries to analyse the image from different perspective. One of the most common filter sets is the difference of two Gaussian kernels, which has the advantage of effective analysis in both one- and two-dimensional domains.

Based on the idea of ridge detection which is built on the support of monogenic signal and phase congruency, the degree of scale span of the multiresolution filters are designed based on the tuning on a set of CLS with certain widths. For example, if the

CLS identified are then removed, the CLS width range should be as wide as possible. On the other hand, if CLS segmentation is for registration purposes, only salient and large vessels are needed so that the CLS detector should be biased towards CLS in the higher scale. Thus the CLS model can improve the specificity and selectivity of the detector under different applications.

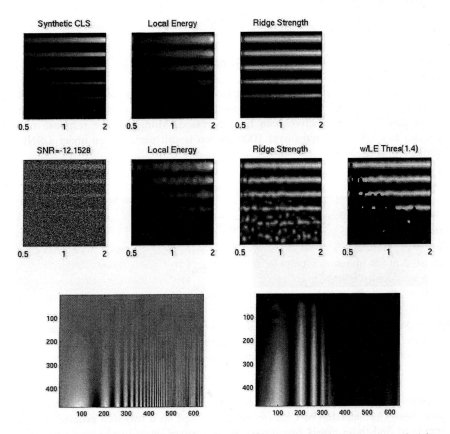

Fig. 2. Performance of the CLS detector evaluation. Upper graph: The ridge strength (phase congruency and the phase angle compound measure) of the 50 micron detector against 6 synthetic CLS with widths 180, 504, 828, 1152, 1476 and 1800 microns. The contrast on each individual synthetic CLS is varied by the *a-b ratio*: the ratio of the horizontal and vertical radii of the CLS shown in both Fig. 1 and Eq. 1. The a-b ratio ranges from 0.5 to 2 as depicted. Middle graph: The performance of the detector against same synthetic CLS as upper graph with noise added, and the performance of the detector with noise suppression by local energy (LE) thresholding strategy. Lower graph: The performance of the detector compare with that of human visual system. The left image is the original CSF image, and the response of the CLS detector is shown on the right.

3 Noise Suppression and Junction Detection

Another problem is noise. As CLS are typically low contrast and poor signal-to-noise can badly affect the performance of the CLS detector, as one can see in Fig. 2. In the proposed framework, we use local energy (LE) thresholding [8] to suppress the undesirable response from noise. The local energy is related to phase congruency, in discrete terms, as follows:

$$LE(x) = PC(x)\sum_n A_n \,, \tag{9}$$

where A_n is the amplitude of the nth bandpass filter. The performance of LE thresholding is showed in Fig. 2.

It is well-known that phase congruency is sensitive to noise as it is the trade-off of its high sensitivity of features of low contrast. However, by thresholding LE, it is found that the false positives can be suppressed. Moreover, the response of the detector to CLS with widths over 1000 micron is still perfect even under a SNR as low as -12. (Fig. 2)

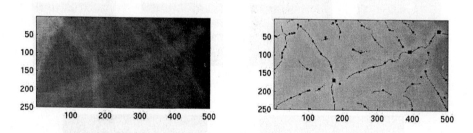

Fig. 3. Sample output of the junction detection algorithm. Larger marks are the affirmed junctions, which are inferred based on the neighbourhood orientation information and local energy. The smaller ones are rejected candidates (i.e. number of branches <= 2).

Apart from noise removal, the local energy is also used to determine CLS junctions. The detection of CLS junctions is based on a two-step process. The first step is to find those pixels which have a *local maximum* of local energy, based on a notion that the convergence, or intersection, of ridges will result in a point with high local energy. In other words, we try to find junctions that are more "salient" than their branches. In our approach, we search the CLS skeletons to find the local maxima of LE, this will end up with a set of candidate points. In the second step, these candidate points are then searched through a neighbourhood of radius r, where $r=kLE(x)$. We search inside the neighbourhood to find any CLS (branches) that point towards that candidate point, by comparing the orientation of the CLS and the vector pointing to the branch from the junction point. The orientation information can be computed from the monogenic signal. A junction is detected if the number of branches is more than 2. Some typical results of junction detection are shown in Fig. 3.

4   Performance Evaluation

We have applied our CLS detector to a set of mammograms and some of the results are shown in Fig. 4. In our tests, we have used mammograms digitised at resolutions of 50 microns/pixel and 300 microns/pixel.

In addition, we are interested in comparing the capability of our CLS detector with the capability of human vision (Fig. 2). A Contrast Sensitivity Function (CSF) test image, which was originally a tool to study how the human visual system responds to different contrast and spatial frequency [9], is used to test the responses of our feature detector. Two findings can be derived from the test. Firstly, the dome-shaped response resembles the human visual system. Secondly, the sensitivity of the detector in low contrast regions in specific spectra is comparable to that of the human visual system and may even surpass it. This facts further support that appropriate usage of such a segmentation algorithm might enhance the ease of feature detection tasks for radiologists.

Some of the sample results carried out on real images are displayed in Fig. 4. As can be seen, the detector gives well-localized and contrast-insensitive responses on most of the weak ridges of the CLS and is not sensitive to two-dimensional structures, for example, masses. As shown in the figure, the CLS detector does not give false responses to the edges of the mass and the boundary of the pectoral muscle. Also, in regions with rapidly varying contrasts, for example, across the pectoral muscle and near the breast boundary, the response of the detector is still strong and well-localized. Some discontinuities can be observed from the response, which can be solved by applying further processing techniques like Hough transform or by morphological operations.

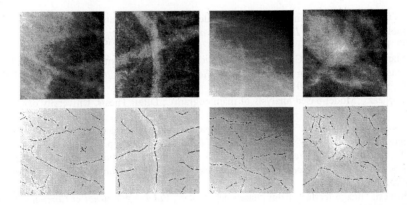

Fig. 4. Some results of the CLS detector on mammograms (digitized at a resolution of 50 micron per pixel). Here shows the response of the CLS detector in different parts of the mammogram. From left to right: 1. a CLS crossing between the parenchyma and the pectoral muscle; 2. a typical X-junction; 3. a region near the breast boundary; 4. a region around a mass. All the parameters of the CLS detector is identical for these response demonstrated.

5 Conclusions

We have proposed a CLS ridge detection algorithm in this paper. Departing from previous approaches, this algorithm is based on the monogenic signal. As the segmentation is phase-based, the algorithm is able to detect CLS in low-contrast. When equipped with LE noise suppression, it has proven to be highly effective in noise removal. A CLS intensity profile model has been incorporated into the design to provide utilities for scale tuning and performance evaluation. In addition, the performance of the CLS detector is compared with the capability of human vision system by using a CSF image, which shows comparable performance of our design with the naked eye. Overall, we showed that our novel CLS detection strategy is superior in aiding or enhancing the potential, or current, CLS detection and segmentation tasks in the industry, such as employing CLS junctions as landmarks in mammogram registration, enhancing the reliability of mass detection by CLS removal, or reduction of the false positives in microcalcifications detection (in which most false positives are indeed intersections of capillaries). Moreover, as one-dimensional vascular structures (e.g. blood vessels, lymph nodes) are pervasive anatomical entities itself, we hope that our algorithm can be applied to linear structure identification in other x-ray image processing and even to other modalities.

Acknowledgements. Lionel C. C. Wai is supported by the Croucher Foundation, Hong Kong; Matthew Mellor is supported by the MIAS Interdisciplinary Research Consortium funded by the EPSRC and MRC.

References

1. N. Vujovic, "Establishing the correspondence between control points in pairs of mammographic images," *IEEE Transactions on Image Processing,* vol 6, no. 10, ppl 1388-1399, 1997.
2. R. Marti, R. Zwiggelaar, C. Rubin, "Automatic registration of mammograms based on linear structures", in *Information Processing in Medical Imaging (IPMI 2001),* pp. 162-168, LNCS 2082, Spinger-Verlag, 2001.
3. N. Cerneaz, "Model-based analysis of mammograms", DPhil Thesis, University of Oxford, 1994.
4. R. Zwiggelaar, T. Parr, C. Taylor, "Finding orientated line patterns in digital mammographic images", in *Proceedings 7th British Machine Vision Conference,* pp. 715-724, 1996.
5. V. U. B. Schenk, M. Brady, "Finding CLS using multiresolution oriented local energy feature detection," in *Proceedings 6th International Workshop on Digital Mammography (IWDM 2002),* June 2002.
6. P. Kovesi, "Image features from phase congruency", *Videre: A Journal of Computer Vision Research,* Vol.1, No.3, 1999.
7. M. Felsberg, G. Sommer, "A new extension of linear signal processing for estimating local properties and detecting features", in *Proceedings of DAGM Symposium,* Spinger-Verlag, pp. 195-202, 2002.
8. V. U. B. Schenk, "Visual identification of fine surface incisions", DPhil Thesis, University of Oxford, 2001.
9. F. W. Campbell, J. B. Robson, "Application of Fourier analysis to the visibility of gratings", *Journal of Physiology, vol. 197, pp. 551-566, 1968.*

Cervical Cancer Detection Using SVM Based Feature Screening*

Jiayong Zhang and Yanxi Liu

The Robotics Institute, Carnegie Mellon University
{zhangjy,yanxi}@cs.cmu.edu

Abstract. We present a novel feature screening algorithm by deriving relevance measures from the decision boundary of Support Vector Machines. It alleviates the "independence" assumption of traditional screening methods, e.g. those based on Information Gain and Augmented Variance Ratio, without sacrificing computational efficiency. We applied the proposed method to a bottom-up approach for automatic cervical cancer detection in multispectral microscopic thin PAP smear images. An initial set of around 4,000 multispectral texture features is effectively reduced to a computationally manageable size. The experimental results show significant improvements in pixel-level classification accuracy compared to traditional screening methods.

1 Introduction

Finding abnormal cells in PAP smear images (Fig. 1) is a "needle in a haystack" type of problem, which is tedious, labor-intensive and error-prone. It is therefore desirable to have an automatic screening tool such that human experts are only called for when complicated and subtle cases arise. Most researches on automatic cervical screening extract morphometric/photometric features at the cellular level in accordance with the "Bethesda System" rules [1]. However, accurate segmentations of cytoplasm and nucleus on cancer images are rather difficult due to the presence of blood, inflammatory cells, or thick cell clumps.

Using a micro-interferometric spectral imaging setup, we have obtained a set of multispectral Pap smear images. The wavelengths range from 400 nm to 690 nm, evenly divided into 52 bands. In [2], we propose a bottom-up approach to automatically detect cancerous regions in such images without the requirement of accurate segmentation. Our approach takes advantage of both the local multispectral and textural properties by learning a spatially-homogeneous discriminative filter. Cancerous regions are then detected from the filter output through a relatively simple procedure.

There are two critical issues that must be addressed in such a scheme: (1) what features should be extracted from multispectral images, and (2) how to remove irrelevant and/or redundant features from a pool of thousands of potential features to locate a feature subset that is well balanced between performance

---

* This research was supported in part by NIH award N01-CO-07119 and PA-DOH grant ME01-738.

C. Barillot, D.R. Haynor, and P. Hellier (Eds.): MICCAI 2004, LNCS 3217, pp. 873–880, 2004.
© Springer-Verlag Berlin Heidelberg 2004

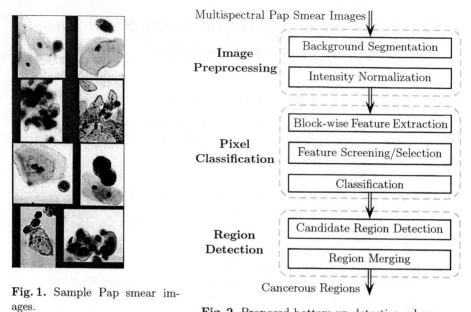

Multispectral Pap Smear Images

Image Preprocessing
- Background Segmentation
- Intensity Normalization

Pixel Classification
- Block-wise Feature Extraction
- Feature Screening/Selection
- Classification

Region Detection
- Candidate Region Detection
- Region Merging

Cancerous Regions

Fig. 1. Sample Pap smear images.

Fig. 2. Proposed bottom-up detection scheme.

and compactness. For the first issue, we have identified a feasible feature space of about 4,000 dimensions that well captures local multispectral and texture information. For the second issue, given that 4,000 dimensions is still intractable for traditional feature selection methods, we have employed two simple screening measures, i.e. Information Gain (IG) and Augmented Variance Ratio (AVR), to rule out irrelevant features. However, as each feature is evaluated independently, such screening methods may fail to capture all highly discriminative feature subsets, which are composed of individually less discriminative features.

In this paper, we present a novel feature screening algorithm by deriving relevance measures from the decision boundary of Support Vector Machines [3]. The proposed relevance measures have several advantages: 1) As derived simultaneously for all dimensions, they do not only focus on single dimension as most existing measures do; 2) As the maximum margin boundary of SVM has been proven to be optimal in a structural risk minimization sense, they may better indicate the discriminative power of features; 3) As efficient routines for SVM training are available that can readily deal with huge number of features and samples, they do not sacrifice in computational cost. Our experimental results show significant improvements in pixel-level classification accuracy by using the proposed method.

2   Detection System Overview

A flowchart of the proposed bottom-up detection scheme is given in Figure 2. Here we summarize the main steps.

Preprocessing. We first segment cells from the background, which is much easier than traditional nuclei/cytoplasm segmentation. Then we normalize all band images by subtracting the spectral signature of the image background.

Feature Extraction. For each pixel, we extract various types of image features including: 1) Statistics of pixel intensity; 2) Daubechies 2 and Daubechies 16 asymmetric orthogonal wavelets; 3) Biorthogonal wavelet; and 4) Gabor wavelet. This procedure is applied to every band, resulting in a very high dimensional multispectral image feature set.

Feature Screening. The initial feature set is pruned by the proposed SVM based screening algorithm to remove those features irrelevant to the detection task. This is the main focus of the paper, and will be discussed in detail in Section 3. To further eliminate feature redundancy, Sequential Backward Selection (SBS) is applied to the surviving features of the screening procedure.

Discriminative Filtering. Let x be the final n-dimensional feature vector of a pixel after SBS selection. For each class (cancerous or normal), a modified version of quadratic discriminant is defined as

$$g(x) = \sum_{i=1}^{k} \frac{1}{\lambda_i} \left[\varphi_i^T (x - \mu) \right]^2 + \sum_{i=k+1}^{n} \frac{1}{\beta^2} \left[\varphi_i^T (x - \mu) \right]^2 + \ln \left[\beta^{2(n-k)} \prod_{i=1}^{k} \lambda_i \right] \quad (1)$$

where μ is the class mean, $\{\lambda_i, \varphi_i\}$ are the i-th eigenvalue and eigenvector of covariance matrix Σ, $\lambda_1 \geq \lambda_2 \geq \cdots \geq \lambda_n$, and β is a positive constant. The discriminative filter output is then computed as $h(x) = g_{normal}(x) - g_{cancer}(x)$.

Region Detection. Based on the continuous output surface $h(x)$ from discriminative filtering, cancerous regions can be located by a relatively simple procedure (see Fig. 3 for example): 1) Smooth $H = \{h(x)\}$ with a Gaussian filter; 2) Find all local maxima m_i in H, and their corresponding effective regions R_i, defined as the points immediately around m_i with values above a fixed fraction (0.5) of $h(m_i)$; 3) For each R_i extract a geometric feature $G = C/L$, where C is the circumference of R_i, L is the distance from m_i to the boundary. Prune those R_i if $h(m_i) < 0.5 \max_i h(m_i)$ or $G < 2$, and generate the candidate region set; 4) Merge candidate regions that are overlapping.

3   SVM Based Feature Screening

Given a set of features in a classification problem, a basic question in many learning tasks is: what is the best feature subset for classification purpose? Although many feature subset selection methods have been proposed [4,5], few of them can be directly applied to domains with more than 100 dimensions. The huge feature dimension (near 4,000) and sample complexity (over 100,000) in our task make them computationally prohibitive. Alternatively, we present a new feature screening algorithm by deriving relevance measures from the decision boundary of Support Vector Machine. Features are ranked according to these measures, and a subset is then selected via some statistical significance test.

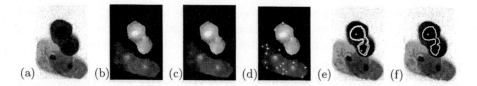

Fig. 3. An example of cancerous region detection. (a) Original image. (b) Scaled output surface from discriminative filtering. (c) Gaussian smoothing of (b). (d) Local maxima points found in (c). (e) Contours of candidate cancerous regions. (f) Merged result.

The SVM decision function of a two-class problem can be written as

$$h(x) = w \cdot \Phi(x) + b = \sum_{i=1}^{n} \alpha_i y_i K(x, x_i) + b \qquad (2)$$

where $x_i \in \mathbb{R}^d$ is the training sample, and $y_i \in \{\pm 1\}$ is the class label of x_i. A transformation $\Phi(\cdot)$ maps the data points x of the input space $\mathbb{R}^d$ into a higher dimensional feature space $\mathbb{R}^D, (D \geq d)$. The mapping is performed by a kernel function $K(\cdot, \cdot)$ which defines an inner product in $\mathbb{R}^D$. The parameters $\alpha_i \geq 0$ are optimized by finding the hyperplane in feature space with maximum distance to the closest image $\Phi(x_i)$ from the training set, which reduces to solving a linearly constrained convex quadratic program. In the general case of nonlinear mapping Φ, SVM generates a nonlinear boundary $h(x) = 0$ in the input space.

Given any two points $z_1, z_2 \in \mathbb{R}^d$ such that $h(z_1) h(z_2) < 0$, a surface point $s = \alpha z_1 + (1 - \alpha) z_2, \alpha \in [0, 1]$, can be found by solving the following equation with respect to α:

$$h(s) = h(\alpha z_1 + (1 - \alpha) z_2) = 0 \qquad (3)$$

The unit normal vector $N(s)$ at the boundary point s is then given by

$$N(s) = \nabla h(s) / \|\nabla h(s)\| \qquad (4)$$

where $\nabla h(s) = \partial h(s)/\partial s = \sum_{i=1}^{n} \alpha_i y_i \, \partial K(s, x_i)/\partial s$. $N(s)$ identifies the orientation in the input space along which the projected training data are well separated locally around the neighborhood of s. Therefore, the orientation difference between $N(s)$ and any direction u can be used to measure the local discriminative relevance for that direction at s. Formally, we measure this difference by $|u^T N(s)|$, or equivalently $u^T N(s) N(s)^T u$. To summarize all the local feature relevance information, we compute the decision boundary scatter matrix as

$$M = \int_{\mathcal{B}} N(s) N^T(s) p(s) \, ds \qquad (5)$$

and a global relevance measure for direction u as $u^T M u$. When sample-size is finite, M can be replaced by the sample estimate $\hat{M} = \sum_{i=1}^{l} \hat{N}(\hat{s}_i) \, \hat{N}(\hat{s}_i)^T / l$, where $\hat{s}_i$ are l points sampled from the estimated decision boundary. This global relevance measure can be readily extended to multi-category problems by repeating the procedure in either one-vs-all or pairwise mode. Now we summarize the SVM based feature screening algorithm as follows.

Input: n sample pairs $\{(x_i, y_i)\}_{i=1}^{n}$, where $x_i \in \mathbb{R}^d$ and $y_i \in \{k\}_{k=1}^{Q}$.
Output: d nested feature subsets $\mathcal{S}_1 \subset \mathcal{S}_2 \subset \ldots \subset \mathcal{S}_d$ such that $\dim(\mathcal{S}_m) = m$.
Algorithm:

S1 For $k = 1$ to Q

S2 Divide the n samples into two subsets $T^+ = \{x_i | y_i = k\}$ and $T^- = \{x_i | y_i \neq k\}$. Learn a SVM decision function $h(x)$ using T^+ and T^-.

S3 Sort the n samples in ascending order by the absolute function output values $|h(x_i)|$. Denote the subset consisting of the first r samples as T'.

S4 Select l pairs of points $\{(z_1^j, z_2^j)\}_{j=1}^{l}$ from T' randomly such that $h(z_1^j)\,h(z_2^j) < 0$. For each pair solve equation (3) to an accuracy of ϵ, and thus get l estimated boundary points $\{\hat{s}_j\}_{j=1}^{l}$.

S5 Compute the unit surface norm $\hat{N}(\hat{s}_j)$ at $\hat{s}_j$ according to equation (4), and estimate the decision boundary scatter matrix as $\hat{M}_k = \sum_{j=1}^{l} \hat{N}(\hat{s}_j)\hat{N}(\hat{s}_j)^T$.

S6 End (For $k = 1$ to Q)

S7 Compute $\hat{M} = \sum_{k=1}^{Q} \hat{M}_k / Q$, and denote its diagonal value as $\{\hat{\lambda}_j\}_{j=1}^{d}$.

S8 Sort feature directions $\{u_j\}_{j=1}^{d}$ descendingly by $\{\hat{\lambda}_j\}_{j=1}^{d}$. Let $\mathcal{S}_m = \{u_j^{sort}\}_{j=1}^{m}$.

Note that first, we prune those training samples far away from the decision boundary in locating the boundary points. This helps to reduce computational cost and suppress the negative influence of outliers. Second, we adopt the one-vs-all approach for solving Q-class problems with SVMs. Totally Q classifiers need to be trained, each of which separates a single class from all remaining classes. Third, the complexity of the algorithm can be controlled by several parameters including l, the number of boundary points to be sampled, and ϵ, the accuracy of the root to equation (3). Our experience suggests that the algorithm is not very sensitive to the choice of these parameters. Finally, we have used p-degree polynomial kernels in our experiments, where $p = 2$.

It can be proven that a feature u is irrelevant if and only if $u^T M u$ equals zero. In theory we can prune all irrelevant features via this screening method. However, inherent uncertainty in our estimation prevent us from doing so. A more practical reason is that, features' contribution to discrimination may be unevenly distributed that the subset dimension can be significantly reduced while achieving *almost* the same accuracy. Therefore model selection technique is required in order to decide an appropriate subset. This problem will not be discussed in this paper, but we want to point out that nested subsets generated by SVM based screening can easily facilitate such explorations.

4 Experiments and Analysis

We evaluated the proposed SVM based screening algorithm and the resultant cervical cancer detection system on a multispectral PAP smear image database containing 40 images (each has 52 spectral bands) with a total of 149 cells (41 cancerous and 108 normal). The image size ranges from 93x64 to 300x227. First, all images are preprocessed to remove the background and normalize intensity by setting background spectral signature to zero. Then for each pixel to be

	DB2	DB16	Bio2.2	Gabor	Combined
Original Dim.	800	800	900	1200	3700
After Screening	48	42	52	30	68

Table 1. Various dimensions before and after SVM based feature screening.

classified, various image features are extracted in a 16×16 block (the block size is chosen via cross-validation) around it in each band, as described in section 2. Thus a very high dimensional multispectral texture feature vector is associated with each pixel. At pixel level, we collect a total of 156,732 sample vectors (26,064 positive and 132,063 negative) from all 40 images. As samples from the same image are often highly correlated, they are always kept as a whole when partitioning training and test sets in all the following experiments.

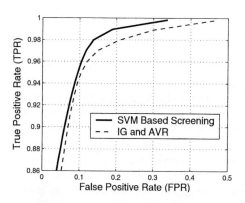

We evaluated the selected 68 features on the original full sample set using the modified quadratic discriminant. The ROC curve is plotted in Figure 4 against the ROC curve of IG+AVR screening depicted for comparison. It is easy to observe that SVM based screening outperforms IG+AVR, especially when the True Positive Rate (TPR) is high.

Fig. 4. Comparison between SVM and IG+AVR based screenings.

Pixel Classification. We investigated the effect on pixel-level classification by replacing IG and AVR feature screening [2] with the proposed method. In order to reduce the training complexity, a total of 29,487 samples were randomly selected (13,022 positive and 16,465 negative). SVM based feature screening method with p-degree polynomial kernels was applied to each of four types of wavelet features respectively. For each type of wavelet, images were randomly divided into training set (32 images) and test set (8 images) for a number of times. Each time we record False Positive Rate (FPR) on the test set versus subset dimension. Then we averaged these FPR curves, based on which a proper feature dimension m was manually selected. After that we collected all features ever appeared among the top m features in each image partition, and regarded them as the selected features for that wavelet type. Then we put together all the selected features from four types of wavelets, and applied the SVM based feature screening algorithm. Again we did random partition of training and test images, and selected a proper dimension m' based on the average FPR curve. Various dimensions before and after feature screening are summarized in Table 1.

Finally, we applied Sequential Backward Selection (SBS) to the 68 survivals of SVM based screening to investigate their redundancy. 8-fold cross validation error on the training set was chosen as the evaluation function in SBS. The aver-

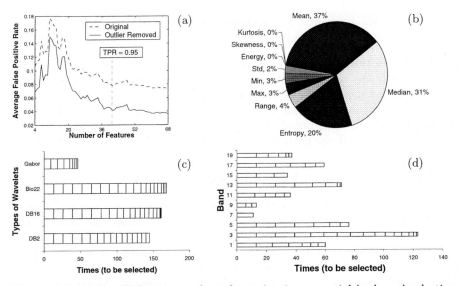

Fig. 5. (a) Average FPR versus subset dimension in sequential backward selection. Analysis of the selected feature subsets with respect to their feature type and spectral band distribution is also provided for us to gain some insight of the selected features. Plots shown are frequency histograms of selected statistics (b), wavelet features (c), and spectral bands (d). Each short segment in (c-d) corresponds to a particular feature.

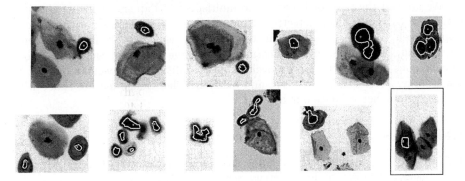

Fig. 6. Example cancerous cell detection results. All images contain one or more cancerous cells except the last one (with frame), which is a false positive case.

age accuracy over 13 test runs is depicted in Fig 5(a). It is observed that feature dimension can be consistently reduced below 40 with little loss of accuracy. We analyzed those features that rank among the top 40 in any of the 13 runs with respect to their feature type and spectral band distribution, and the results are summarized in Figure 5(b-d). Note that distributions of discriminative features are not uniform. For instance, 86.9% features are from 3 out of 10 types of statistics (mean 36.5%, median 30.8%, entropy 19.6%). Over 15 features are selected from spectral band 3 while only 1 from band 7.

Region Detection. As the number of available images is small, we evaluate the performance of the complete detection system by leave-one-out cross validation method. Each time 39 images are used to train the pixel classifier, and one image is reserved for test. Some typical detection results are shown in Figure 6. Among the 149 cells distributed in 40 images, one cancerous cell is missed (TPR $= 40/41 \approx 98\%$), and one normal cell is falsely detected (FPR $= 1/108 \approx 1\%$).

5   Related Work and Conclusion

In this paper, we presented a novel SVM-based feature screening method. Guyon et al. [6] proposed a feature ranking scheme by linear SVMs. The basic idea is to use the magnitude of the weights of a linear discriminant classifier as an indicator of feature relevance. Our method can be considered as a nonlinear extension of this linear scheme. SVM boundary has also been used in locally adaptive metric techniques to improve k-NN performance [7]. Measures of local feature relevance are computed by the surface normal near the query, from which a local full-rank transformation is derived. Such local methods need to perform k-NN procedure multiple times in the original high-dimensional space. On the contrary, our method tries to globally characterize the discriminative information embedded in the SVM decision boundary. It generates global feature relevance measures, and thus is computationally more efficient.

We applied the proposed method to multispectral Pap smear image classification for cervical cancer detection. Comparative experiments show significant improvements on pixel-level classification accuracy using the new feature screening method. We have shown the effectiveness of image feature screening/selection in cancerous cell detection on a novel image modality (multispectral image). A much larger PAP smear image set and an even richer image feature space will be used to further validate our method.

References

1. Kurman, R., Solomon, D.: The Bethesda System for Reporting Cervical/Vaginal Cytologic Diagnoses. Springer-Verlag, New York (1994)
2. Liu, Y., Zhao, T., Zhang, J.: Learning multispectral texture features for cervical cancer detection. In: Proc. Int. Symp. Biomedical Imaging. (2002) 169–172
3. Cristianini, N., Shawe-Taylor, J.: An Introduction to Support Vector Machines. Cambridge University Press, Cambridge, UK (2000)
4. Blum, A., Langley, P.: Selection of relevant features and examples in machine learning. Artificial Intelligence **97** (1997) 245–271
5. John, G., Kohavi, R., Pfleger, K.: Irrelevant features and the subset selection problem. In: Proc. 11th Int. Conf. Machine Learning. (1994) 121–129
6. Guyon, I., Weston, J., Barnhill, S., Vapnik, V.: Gene selection for cancer classification using support vector machines. Machine Learning **46** (2002) 389–422
7. Domeniconi, C., Gunopulos, D.: Adaptive nearest neighbor classification using support vector machines. In: Advances in NIPS 14, MIT Press (2001)

Robust 3D Segmentation of Pulmonary Nodules in Multislice CT Images

Kazunori Okada[1], Dorin Comaniciu[1], and Arun Krishnan[2]

[1] Siemens Corporate Research, Inc.
755 College Road East, Princeton, NJ 08540, USA
[2] Siemens Medical Solutions USA, Inc.
51 Valley Stream Parkway, Malvern, PA 19355, USA

Abstract. We propose a robust and accurate algorithm for segmenting the 3D pulmonary nodules in multislice CT scans. The solution unifies i) the parametric Gaussian model fitting of the volumetric data evaluated in Gaussian scale-space and ii) non-parametric 3D segmentation based on normalized gradient (mean shift) ascent defining the basin of attraction of the target tumor in the 4D spatial-intensity joint space. This realizes the 3D segmentation according to both spatial and intensity proximities simultaneously. Experimental results show that the system reliably segments a variety of nodules including part- or non-solid nodules which poses difficulty for the existing solutions. The system also processes a 32x32x32-voxel volume-of-interest efficiently by six seconds on average.

1 Introduction

One of the major goals of the computer-assisted diagnosis with the chest CT scans (chest CAD [1]) is reliable volumetric measurement of the pulmonary nodules [2,3,4]. Tumor change quantification based on such volume measurements plays an integral part of the cancer therapy monitoring and post-surgical examinations [5]. There are a number of previous studies addressing the computer-assisted volume measurement of nodules (e.g., Zhao et al. [6], Kostis et al. [5]). In these studies, the 2D or 3D tumor segmentation based on voxel intensity thresholding is used as the foundation of their solutions. Although such solutions are sufficient to delineate the well-defined solid nodules with the similar average intensity, they provide unreliable segmentations for the part- or non-solid nodules, as shown in Fig.1. A recent clinical study [7] has revealed that such nodules occur frequently and have a higher tendency to be malignant, motivating the development of the robust solution for these technically challenging cases.

This article proposes a novel 3D tumor segmentation method addressing the above issue. Our solution consists of two successive steps: i) 3D nodule center and spread estimation by fitting the anisotropic Gaussian intensity model in the Gaussian scale-space and ii) an iterative 3D nodule segmentation based on the basin of attraction in the 4D spatial-intensity joint space. The former step provides the reliable parametric estimation of the nodule's anisotropic structure by robustly fitting a Gaussian intensity model in the Gaussian scale-space of the

C. Barillot, D.R. Haynor, and P. Hellier (Eds.): MICCAI 2004, LNCS 3217, pp. 881–889, 2004.

given data [8,9]. The latter step provides the non-parametric 3D nodule segmentation, according to both spatial and intensity proximities simultaneously, by using the normalized gradient ascent-based data segmentation in the 4D joint space. The results from the first step is interpreted as a normal prior and used to determine the analysis bandwidth of the latter step, resulting in an efficient segmentation solution. The joint-space segmentation that exploits the basin of attraction has provided a robust solution for the general image segmentation problem [10]. However, the method has not been considered in the medical imaging domain and provides an alternative segmentation principle to the intensity thresholding.

This article is organized as follows. Sec.2 and Sec.3 describe the first and the second step of our segmentation method, respectively. Sec.4 presents the results of our validation. This article is concluded by discussing our future work in Sec.5.

2   3D Tumor Center and Anisotropic Spread Estimation by Robust Scale-Space Analysis

This section presents a robust estimation method for 3D tumor center location and anisotropic spread as the first reliable step towards the tumor segmentation. We assume that a marker $\mathbf{x}_p$, indicating the rough location of the target tumor, is given *a priori*. Such markers can be provided from an automatic tumor detection system (e.g., [11]) or the screening results of radiologists and do not need to be accurate. Our solution is based on the anisotropic 3D Gaussian intensity model fitting in the Gaussian scale-space proposed in [8]. The following briefly describes this solution.

The volumetric CT data is formalized as a continuous positive function $I : \mathcal{R}_+^3 \rightarrow \mathcal{R}_+$ over the data space $\mathbf{x} = (x_1, x_2, x_3)$. A local region of $I(\mathbf{x})$ around a spatial extremum $\mathbf{u}$, expressing a pulmonary tumor, is modeled by the anisotropic 3D Gaussian intensity model,

$$I(\mathbf{x}) \simeq \alpha \times \Phi(\mathbf{x}; \mathbf{u}, \boldsymbol{\Sigma})|_{\mathbf{x} \in \mathcal{S}}, \tag{1}$$

$$\Phi(\mathbf{x}; \mathbf{u}, \boldsymbol{\Sigma}) = (2\pi)^{-d/2} |\boldsymbol{\Sigma}|^{-1/2} \exp(-\frac{1}{2}(\mathbf{x} - \mathbf{u})^t \boldsymbol{\Sigma}^{-1}(\mathbf{x} - \mathbf{u})) \tag{2}$$

where α is an amplitude parameter, $\boldsymbol{\Sigma}$ is a fully-parameterized 3×3 symmetric positive definite covariance matrix, and $\mathcal{S}$ is a set of data points in the neighborhood of $\mathbf{u}$, belonging to the basin of attraction of $\mathbf{u}$. The mean $\mathbf{u}$ and covariance $\boldsymbol{\Sigma}$ of Φ describes the tumor location and spread, respectively. Thus the problem of our interest can be understood as parametric model fitting or robust estimation of $(\mathbf{u}, \boldsymbol{\Sigma})$ given $I(\mathbf{x})$. Anisotropy of the tumor can only be described by considering the estimation of the fully-parameterized covariance.

Multi-scale analysis is employed for this estimation, given a set of ordered and densely sampled *analysis scales* $\{h_k | k = 1, .., K\}$. The model mean and covariance are robustly estimated, by the method described below, for each analysis scale h_k, resulting in a set of successive estimates $\{(\mathbf{u}_k, \boldsymbol{\Sigma}_k)\}$. The final result

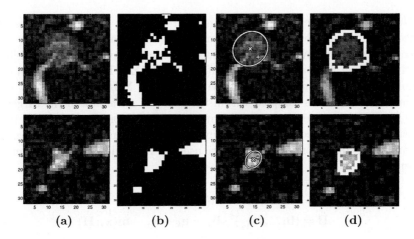

(a)   (b)   (c)   (d)

Fig. 1. 2D examples of the pulmonary nodule segmentation. From left to right, (a): 2D profile of two nodule examples, (b): segmentation results by the FWHM intensity thresholding, (c): center ($\times$) and anisotropic spread (ellipse) estimated by our method ($+$ indicates the marker location $\mathbf{x}_p$ described in Sec. 2), (d): nodule segmentation result by our method without any geometrical post-processings. The first row is an example of the part- and non-solid nodules while the second row is of the solid nodules. Both methods provides similar segmentation results for the solid case, however, the intensity thresholding method fails for the non-solid case. The maximum intensity for (b) was computed using the prior information shown in (c).

is given by finding the most stable estimate using a divergence-based stability test. The most stable estimate $(\mathbf{u}^*, \mathbf{\Sigma}^*)$ is defined as the estimate with the scale h^* that assumes a local minimum of the modified Jensen-Shannon divergence profile over the scales [12,8] At each scale h_k, the divergence is computed over three neighboring scales.

For each analysis bandwidth h_k, $(\mathbf{u}_k, \mathbf{\Sigma}_k)$ are estimated by *scale-space mean shift analysis* together with the robust estimation technique based on the basin of attraction. *Gaussian scale-space* of $I(\mathbf{x})$, or the solution of the diffusion equation $\partial_h I = \frac{1}{2}\nabla^2 I$, is defined by a convolution of $I(\mathbf{x})$ with a set of Gaussian kernels with the analysis scales $\{h > 0\}$, $L(\mathbf{x}; \mathbf{H}) = f(\mathbf{x}) * \Phi(\mathbf{x}; \mathbf{0}, \mathbf{H})$, where $\mathbf{H}$ is an isotropic bandwidth matrix of a form $\mathbf{H} = h\mathbf{I}$. Its gradient vector is given by,

$$\nabla L(\mathbf{x}; \mathbf{H}) = I(\mathbf{x}) * \nabla\Phi(\mathbf{x}; \mathbf{0}, \mathbf{H}) = \mathbf{H}^{-1}L(\mathbf{x}; \mathbf{H})\mathbf{m}(\mathbf{x}; \mathbf{H}) \qquad (3)$$

$$\mathbf{m}(\mathbf{x}; \mathbf{H}) \equiv \frac{\int \mathbf{x}'\Phi(\mathbf{x} - \mathbf{x}'; \mathbf{H})f(\mathbf{x}')d\mathbf{x}'}{\int \Phi(\mathbf{x} - \mathbf{x}'; \mathbf{H})f(\mathbf{x}')d\mathbf{x}'} - \mathbf{x} = \mathbf{H}\frac{\nabla L(\mathbf{x}; \mathbf{H})}{L(\mathbf{x}; \mathbf{H})} \qquad (4)$$

The vector $\mathbf{m}(\mathbf{x})$ is called *scale-space mean shift vector* and proportional to the gradient vector $\nabla L(\mathbf{x}; \mathbf{H})$. A convergent iterative algorithm [12] for the normalized gradient ascent in the scale-space, $\mathbf{x}_{k+1} = \mathbf{m}(\mathbf{x}_k) + \mathbf{x}_k$, is used to estimate the tumor center $\mathbf{u}_k$, to which the given marker $\mathbf{x}_p$ converges. To increase the robustness, a set of the gradient ascents are performed from different initial points sampled uniformly around $\mathbf{x}_p$. The convergence point of the majority of the initial points defines the center estimate $\mathbf{u}_k$.

Next, given the center estimate, the corresponding covariance Σ_k is estimated. Substituting the Gaussian tumor model (1) to the definition of the scale-space mean shift (4) reveals that the mean shift can be expressed as a quasi-linear matrix equation after some algebra, $\mathbf{m}(\mathbf{x};\mathbf{H}) = \mathbf{H}(\Sigma + \mathbf{H})^{-1}(\mathbf{u} - \mathbf{x})$. An overcomplete set of the linear equations with unknown Σ is constructed by using the mean shift vectors sampled within the *basin of attraction* of the target tumor. For this, we perform a set of the mean shift iterations from different initial points that are sampled uniformly around the center estimate $\mathbf{u}_k$. N_u mean shift vectors along convergent trajectories are used for constructing the overcomplete system,

$$\mathbf{A}\Sigma = \mathbf{B}, \ \Sigma \in \mathcal{SPD} \tag{5}$$

$$\mathbf{A} = (\mathbf{m}(\mathbf{x}_1;\mathbf{H}), .., \mathbf{m}(\mathbf{x}_{N_u};\mathbf{H}))^t \mathbf{H}^{-t} \tag{6}$$

$$\mathbf{B} = (\mathbf{b}_1, .., \mathbf{b}_{N_u})^t, \ \mathbf{b}_j = \mathbf{u}_k - \mathbf{x}_j - \mathbf{m}(\mathbf{x}_j;\mathbf{H}) \tag{7}$$

where $\mathcal{SPD}$ denotes a set of all symmetric positive definite matrices in $\mathcal{R}^{3\times3}$. A closed-form solution of this constrained system is given by minimizing an area criterion $\|\mathbf{AY} - \mathbf{BY}^{-t}\|_F^2$ where $\mathbf{Y}$ is Cholesky factorization of $\Sigma = \mathbf{YY}^t$ and $\|\cdot\|_F$ is the Frobenius matrix norm. The solution is expressed by a function of symmetric Schur decompositions of $\mathbf{P} \equiv \mathbf{A}^t\mathbf{A}$ and $\tilde{\mathbf{Q}} \equiv \Sigma_P \mathbf{U}_P^t \mathbf{Q} \mathbf{U}_P \Sigma_P$ given $\mathbf{Q} \equiv \mathbf{B}^t\mathbf{B}$,

$$\Sigma_k = \mathbf{U}_P \Sigma_P^{-1} \mathbf{U}_{\tilde{Q}} \Sigma_{\tilde{Q}} \mathbf{U}_{\tilde{Q}}^t \Sigma_P^{-1} \mathbf{U}_P^t \tag{8}$$

$$\mathbf{P} = \mathbf{U}_P \Sigma_P^2 \mathbf{U}_P^t, \tag{9}$$

$$\tilde{\mathbf{Q}} = \mathbf{U}_{\tilde{Q}} \Sigma_{\tilde{Q}}^2 \mathbf{U}_{\tilde{Q}}^t \tag{10}$$

The robustness of the solution is endowed by using the information only within the basin of attraction, which effectively suppresses outliers.

This parametric estimation step yields the estimates of the 3D tumor center and tumor spread in the form of 3D mean vector $\mathbf{u}^*$ and 3×3 covariance matrix Σ^* in (1). Also provided is the bandwidth h^* that yields the above estimates which are most stable among others. The center and spread estimates can be interpreted as the normal probability distribution $g(\mathbf{x})$ of the center estimate,

$$g(\mathbf{x}) = \mathcal{N}(\mathbf{x}; \mathbf{u}^*, \Sigma^*) = \frac{1}{|2\pi\Sigma^*|^{1/2}} \exp(-\frac{1}{2}(\mathbf{x} - \mathbf{u}^*)^t \Sigma^{*-1}(\mathbf{x} - \mathbf{u}^*)) \tag{11}$$

3   3D Tumor Segmentation Based on Basin of Attraction in 4D Spatial-Intensity Joint Space

This section presents our solution for the non-parametric 3D nodule segmentation based on defining the basin of attraction of the target nodule in the 4D spatial-intensity joint space. The solution exploits the normal prior from the previous step, improving the efficiency of the original method proposed in [10].

The spatial-intensity joint space is conceived by interpreting the 3D function as a set of data points in a 4D space. This is achieved by introducing, to the 3D data space $\mathbf{x} \in \mathcal{R}_+^3$, another orthogonal dimension for the distribution of the function responses, resulting in the joint space $\mathbf{y} \equiv (\mathbf{x}, I(\mathbf{x})) \in \mathcal{R}_+^4$. A volumetric CT data is a discretization of the function $I(\mathbf{x})$ over a 3D regular lattice, resulting N data locations $\{\mathbf{x}_i \in \mathcal{Z}_+^3 | i = 1, .., N\}$ where $N = \prod_{d=1}^3 N_d$ and N_d is the number of voxels along the dimension d. Therefore, in the spatial-intensity joint space, the discretized samples $\{I(\mathbf{x}_i)\}$ is interpreted as a set of 4D data points $\{\mathbf{y}_i \equiv (\mathbf{x}_i, I(\mathbf{x}_i)\}$. The sample density estimate with normal kernel with a 4×4 bandwidth matrix $\mathbf{H}$ is given at a data point $\mathbf{y}$ by,

$$f(\mathbf{y}) = \frac{1}{N|2\pi\mathbf{H}|^{1/2}} \sum_{i=1}^{N} \exp(-\frac{1}{2}(\mathbf{y} - \mathbf{y}_i)^t \mathbf{H}^{-1}(\mathbf{y} - \mathbf{y}_i)) \tag{12}$$

Consequently, the gradient of the density $f(\mathbf{y})$ is given by,

$$\nabla f(\mathbf{y}) = \frac{1}{N|2\pi\mathbf{H}|^{1/2}} \sum_{i=1}^{N} \mathbf{H}^{-1}(\mathbf{y}_i - \mathbf{y}) \exp(-\frac{1}{2}(\mathbf{y} - \mathbf{y}_i)^t \mathbf{H}^{-1}(\mathbf{y} - \mathbf{y}_i)) \tag{13}$$

$$= \mathbf{H}^{-1} f(\mathbf{y})\mathbf{m}(\mathbf{y}) \tag{14}$$

$$\mathbf{m}(\mathbf{y}) \equiv \frac{\sum_{i=1}^{N} \mathbf{y}_i \exp(-\frac{1}{2}(\mathbf{y} - \mathbf{y}_i)^t \mathbf{H}^{-1}(\mathbf{y} - \mathbf{y}_i))}{\sum_{i=1}^{N} \exp(-\frac{1}{2}(\mathbf{y} - \mathbf{y}_i)^t \mathbf{H}^{-1}(\mathbf{y} - \mathbf{y}_i))} - \mathbf{y} = \mathbf{H}\frac{\nabla f(\mathbf{y})}{f(\mathbf{y})} \tag{15}$$

The vector $\mathbf{m}(\mathbf{y})$ is the density mean shift in the 4D joint space. A convergent iterative algorithm for the normalized density gradient ascent is obtained by,

$$\mathbf{y}_{k+1} = \mathbf{m}(\mathbf{y}_k) + \mathbf{y}_k \tag{16}$$

The iterator (16) is employed to cluster the data points according to both spatial and intensity proximities simultaneously. The points belonging to the basin of attraction of the target nodule are detected by applying (16) from a set of initial points, sampled according to the normal prior in (11), until convergence at $\nabla f(\mathbf{y}) = 0$. Initial points are sampled within a confidence interval of the 3D normal distribution between p_{lo} and p_{up} percentiles. The points that converge to the vicinity of $(\mathbf{u}^*, m_I)$ are merged into a cluster which defines the target nodule. The points with the probability above p_{up} are also considered to be a part of the nodule. For each point $\mathbf{y}_i$ in the joint space, there is only one corresponding point $\mathbf{x}_i$ in the 3D data space. Thus, the cluster membership of $\mathbf{y}_i$ is directly associated with the data point $\mathbf{x}_i$, resulting in the segmentation of the tumor and background in the data space $\mathbf{x}$.

The advantages of this method include i) robust segmentation without intensity thresholding and ii) its insensitivity to variation of the intensity range, in comparison with the global threshold-based approach. However, for achieving the robustness in the segmentation results, it is crucial that the kernel bandwidth $\mathbf{H}$ is set appropriately for a given data $\{I(\mathbf{x}_i)\}$. Our solution determines $\mathbf{H}$ by exploiting the normal prior. $\mathbf{H}$ is formed as a diagonal matrix with the most stable bandwidth h^* and the variance estimate of the intensities σ_I^2,

$$\mathbf{H} = \text{diag}(h^*, h^*, h^*, \sigma_I^2) \tag{17}$$

where σ_I^2 is given by the sample variance of the intensity values within a q-percentile confidence ellipsoid of the normal distribution $g(\mathbf{x})$,

$$\sigma_I^2 = \frac{1}{N_\sigma} \sum_{i=1}^{N_\sigma} (I(\mathbf{x}_i) - m_I)^2 \big|_{\mathbf{x}_i \in \{\mathbf{x}_i | (\mathbf{x}_i - \mathbf{u}^*)^t \boldsymbol{\Sigma}^{*-1}(\mathbf{x}_i - \mathbf{u}^*) < c\}} \tag{18}$$

The sample mean of the set of the intensity values and the number of voxels within the confidence ellipsoid are denoted by m_I and N_σ, respectively. The parameter c is directly derived from the specific choice of the percentile q. The segmentation procedure using (16) is carried out using the mean shift vectors computed with the resulting bandwidth matrix.

4   Experimental Results

The proposed segmentation method is evaluated with a database of clinical multislice chest CT scans with $1mm^2 \times 1.5mm$ slice thickness, containing 77 nodules of 14 patients. The size of the nodules ranges between $3mm$ to $25mm$ in diameter. The data is also provided with the markers $\mathbf{x}_p$ and the classification labels for the part- or non-solid nodules given by radiologists. The database includes i) 6 cases of the part- or non-solid nodules, ii) 28 cases of small nodules whose size is less than $5mm$, iii) 20 cases of nodules attached to the pleural surface, iv) 12 cases of largely non-spherical (anisotropic) nodules. An implementation of the above method is instantiated with the following settings. For the scale-space anisotropic intensity model fitting, a set of 25 analysis scales $h = \{0.5^2, 0.75^2, .., 6.5^2\}$ are used. For the 4D joint space segmentation, the confidence limits for sampling the initial points and for estimating the sample intensity variance are set to $p_{lo} = 25\%$, $p_{up} = 75\%$, and $q = 75\%$, respectively.

The performance evaluation of the system resulted in the correct parametric fits and non-parametric segmentations for 69 nodules by experts inspections. The 8 failures were due to i) very small nodules attached to pleural surface (6 cases), ii) very small vascularized nodule (1 case), iii) extremely elongated nodule (1 case). All the part- or non-solid and solitary small nodules were correctly estimated and segmented. The rejection criterion based on chi-square residual analysis [8] is applied, resulting successful rejection of all the failure cases attached to pleural surfaces. Fig. illustrates examples of the results. Each image is a 2D dissection of the target volume intersecting the estimated nodule center. The estimation results from the first step are visualized as an intersection of 50%-confidence ellipsoid of the normal prior (11). More results can be found at http://www.scr.siemens.com/anisotropic/. The system's sensitivity to the initial marker locations is studies by randomly perturbing the markers within the 50%-confidence limit range, using 36 nodules. The average error of the mean and covariance estimates from total average of the perturbation were 1.12 voxel and 8.21 Frobenius matrix norm, respectively. The results show the robustness of our method against the uncertainty of the marker locations.

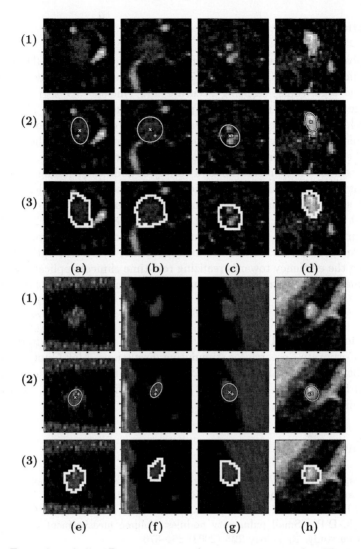

Fig. 2. Examples of the 3D estimation and segmentation results. The results are projected to a 2D plane for visualization. (1): 2D profile of input nodules, (2): parametric fitting results ("+": $\mathbf{x}_p$, "×": $\mathbf{u}^*$, ellipse: $\mathbf{\Sigma}^*$). (3): non-parametric segmentation results. (a)-(b): non-solid, (c): part-solid, (d)-(f): anisotropic, (g)-(h): pleural attachments. Our method flexibly refines the nodule shape approximated by a Gaussian in (2) to the non-parametric segmentation in (3) (see cases (d-g)). The method provides reliable segmentation even in the presence of neighboring structures (see cases (b), (d), (g-h)).

5   Conclusions

We proposed a robust and accurate method for segmenting the 3D pulmonary nodules in multislice CT scans. Our solution unifies the parametric and non-parametric algorithms, realizing accurate and efficient 3D segmentation according to both spatial and intensity proximities simultaneously. The parametric model fitting in the first step realizes robust characterization of tumor's anisotropic structures, while the non-parametric segmentation in the second step refines the results for finding more accurate 3D tumor boundary. The method provides reliable 3D segmentation of a variety of nodules including the clinically significant small and part- or non-solid nodules. The system implemented in C language segments the nodules efficiently. It processes a 32-voxel cubic volume-of-interest 6 seconds on average using an off-the-shelf PC with a 2.4 GHz Intel CPU. Our future work includes i) further validation of the proposed method with more data and for volumetric measurements, ii) system optimization for enhancing the efficiency towards realizing real-time clinical applications, and iii) improvement of the segmentation results by accounting for the partial volume effect.

Acknowledgments. The authors wish to thank Visvanathan Ramesh from Siemens Corporate Research for stimulating discussions, Alok Gupta from CAD group, Siemens Medical Solutions, for his support and encouragement, and Jonathan Stoeckel from CAD group, Siemens Medical Solutions, for his valuable technical supports.

References

1. Reeves, A.P., Kostis, W.J.: Computer-aided diagnosis of small pulmonary nodules. Seminars in Ultrasound, CT, and MRI **21** (2000) 116–128
2. Ko, J.P., Rusinek, H., Jacobs, E.L., Babb, J.S., Betke, M., McGuinness, G., Naidich, D.P.: Small pulmonary nodules: Volume measurement at chest CT - phantom study. Radiology **228** (2003) 864–870
3. Ko, J.P., Naidich, D.P.: Lung nodule detection and characterization with multislice CT. Radiol. Clin. N. Am. **41** (2003) 575–597
4. Wormanns, D., Kohl, G., Kotz, E., Marheine, A., Beyer, F., Heindel, W., Diederich, S.: Volumetric measurements of pulmonary nodules at multi-row detector CT : in vivo reproducibility. Eur. Radiol. **14** (2004) 86–92
5. Kostis, W.J., Reeves, A.P., Yankelevitz, D.F., Henschke, C.I.: Three-dimensional segmentation and growth-rate estimation of small pulmonary nodules in helical CT images. IEEE Trans. Medical Imaging **22** (2003) 1259–1274
6. Zhao, B., Yankelevitz, D., Reeves, A., Henschke, C.: Two-dimensional multi-criterion segmentation of pulmonary nodules on helical CT images. IEEE Trans. Medical Imaging **22** (2003) 1259–1274
7. Henschke, C.I., Yankelevitz, D.F., Mirtcheva, R., McGuinness, G., McCauley, D., Miettinen, O.S.: CT screening for lung cancer: frequency and significance of part-solid and non-solid nodules. AJR Am. J. Roentgenol. **178** (2002) 1053–1057

8. Okada, K., Comaniciu, D., Dalal, N., Krishnan, A.: A robust algorithm for characterizing anisotropic local structures. In: Euro. Conf. Computer Vision. (2004)
9. Okada, K., Comaniciu, D., Krishnan, A.: Scale selection for anisotropic scale-space: Application to volumetric tumor characterization. In: IEEE Conf. Computer Vision and Pattern Recognition. (2004)
10. Comaniciu, D., Meer, P.: Mean shift analysis and applications. In: Int. Conf. Computer Vision. (1999) 1197–1203
11. Lee, Y., Hara, T., Fujita, H., Itoh, S., Ishigaki, T.: Automated detection of pulmonary nodules in helical CT images based on an improved template-matching technique. IEEE Trans. Medical Imaging **20** (2001) 595–604
12. Comaniciu, D.: An algorithm for data-driven bandwidth selection. IEEE Trans. Pattern Anal. Machine Intell. **25** (2003) 281–288

The Automatic Identification of Hibernating Myocardium

Nicholas M.I. Noble[1], Derek L.G. Hill[1], Marcel Breeuwer[2], and Reza Razavi[1]

[1] Computer Imaging Science Group, Guy's Hospital, Kings College London, UK
{Nicholas.Noble,Derek.Hill,Reza.Razavi}@kcl.ac.uk
[2] Philips Medical Systems, Medical Imaging Information Technology - Advanced Development
Marcel.Breeuwer@philips.com

Abstract. Delayed enhancement imaging is a recently described technique that enables for the first time, the direct observation of areas of myocardium that have scarred following infarction. When this information is combined with information about myocardial contraction, areas that are neither dead, nor contracting can be identified. Such areas will resume contraction following revascularisation (hibernating myocardium). The identification of such areas is consequently of great interest to clinicians. This paper describes how registration can be used to align the images prior to the identification of areas that will benefit from revascularisation. Patient data is used to demonstrate image alignment and image-derived information combination. This is then mapped onto patient-specific 2D and 3D representations of the heart.

1 Introduction

It has recently been observed that gadolinium-based contrast agents have substantially different uptake characteristics in regions of scarred myocardium as opposed to in living areas [1]. Whereas these contrast agents wash into and out of the vascular system of living myocardium in a few heart beats, in areas of scarring, dead cardiomyocytes are replaced by a matrix of collagenous fibres —scarred myocardium— into which contrast agent accumulates 15-20 minutes post-injection. Called delayed enhancement imaging, this technique enables for the first time, the direct non-invasive observation of scarred myocardium. When information about areas of scarred myocardium is combined with knowledge of local myocardial contraction or perfusion, areas of myocardium that are neither dead nor contracting —*hibernating myocardium*— can be distinguished. Hibernating myocardium has the potential to resume contracting if revascularised [2]. Its location is thus of considerable importance to clinicians planning revascularisation.

Currently, to identify areas of myocardial scar, clinicians use either Positron Emission Tomography (PET), or Single Photon Emission Computed Tomography (SPECT). Scar size measurements using delayed enhancement imaging have been shown to correlate closely with those measured using PET [3]. In addition MR has been shown to systematically detect small sub-endocardial infarcts that were not identified using SPECT [4]. The higher voxel resolution and non-ionising nature of MR make it well suited for the identification of hibernating myocardium. An emergent technology that is competing

C. Barillot, D.R. Haynor, and P. Hellier (Eds.): MICCAI 2004, LNCS 3217, pp. 890–898, 2004.

with delayed enhancement is contrast enhanced echocardiography. It remains to be seen which technique emerges as the clinical method of choice.

The identification of hibernating myocardium from MR images can be performed in two ways. The first entails finding areas that demonstrate both perfusion defects in first-pass perfusion images, and an absence of scar in delayed enhancement images. Recently, Breeuwer *et al.* investigated aligning such images [5]. The second approach involves finding areas of myocardium that exhibit reduced contraction in cine anatomical images, and are not scarred in the delayed enhancement image. To identify such regions the images need to be aligned, this is normally performed mentally by the observer. Differences in the position of the heart due to inter-image motion and inconsistent breath-hold positions confound this already difficult task. This paper will investigate the alignment of cine anatomical images with delayed enhancement images, before identifying areas of hibernating myocardium.

2 Data

Short axis ECG triggered steady state free precession images with SENSE factor 2 were obtained in 3 patients undergoing cardiac MRI for the investigation of coronary artery disease. Eight contiguous slices, taken in up to three breath-holds, were imaged with: slice thickness 8 - 10 mm, field of view 350×344 - 390×390 mm, acquisition matrix 192×192 with 120% phase encode direction sampling, reconstructed to 256×256 giving a resolution of 1.8 mm $\times$ 1.8 mm $- 2 \times 2$ mm, with 20 phases in the cardiac cycle, flip angle 50 - 55°, TE 1.56 - 1.68 ms and TR 3.11 - 3.37 ms. A 0.4 mmol/kg body weight bolus of gadolinium DPTA was then administered intravenously. Fifteen minutes post-injection, a single end diastolic image was acquired. The images were acquired on a Philips Gyroscan Intera 1.5 T with master gradients, using a 5 element cardiac synergy coil and vector ECG.

3 Methods

Before information about contraction and scarring can be combined, misalignment of the heart between the cine anatomical and delayed enhancement images, due to inter-scan motion and breath-hold inconsistencies, must be compensated for. Both the delayed enhancement and cine anatomical images are acquired using ECG gating, the delayed enhancement image should consequently be at the same point in the cardiac cycle as the end diastolic cine anatomical image. A rigid registration should hence suffice to align the heart, however, rigid registration of the entire image will only recover differences in bodily position and not those attributable to inconsistent diaphragm position. The registration of a Region Of Interest (ROI) in the delayed enhancement image —defined by manually segmenting the epicardial surface— overcomes this problem. The end diastolic cine anatomical image was thus rigidly registered to the ROI of the delayed enhancement image (both images were preblurred with an isotropic in-plane Gaussian kernel of 2.5mm scale). Normalised mutual information [6] was chosen as the similarity measure because of its ability to align areas that include contrast in one image but not the other. The transformation produced by the registration may well result in some degree

Patient 1   Patient 2   Patient 3

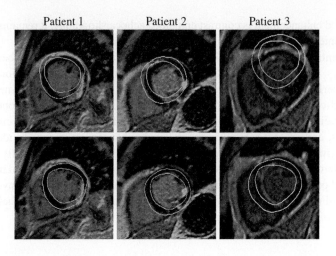

Fig. 1. Manually created end diastolic anatomical contours overlaid onto the delayed enhancement images prior to registration (*top row*), and following registration (*bottom row*).

of through-plane motion, because of the massive voxel anisotropy inherent in these images, a smooth 3D contour must hence be created prior to its transformation. Shape-based interpolation [7] of binary volumes produced by segmentation of anatomical end diastolic epicardial and endocardial surfaces provides approximately isotropic voxels. Isotropic Gaussian blurring of the interpolated binary volume with $\sigma = 1mm$ followed by the marching cubes algorithm [8], then extracted a smooth 3D surface. Figure 1 shows sections through these contours overlaid on the delayed enhancement image both prior to registration and following registration and transformation. To enable the later assessment of wall thickening, end systolic epicardial and endocardial segmentations were also prepared as described above and transformed by the same transformation. The end systolic image should be correctly aligned with the end diastolic image because it is acquired with the same breath-holds, there is thus no need for alignment of the end diastolic images to the end systolic cine images.

To combine information about contraction and scarring, areas of scarring must first be identified. In the literature, techniques have typically employed intensity thresholding to distinguish areas of scar. Intensity thresholds have been identified manually [5], from manually identified non-scar areas [9], using properties of the histogram [10], using k-means clustering [11] and also fuzzy k-means clustering [12]. In a comparison of these different thresholding techniques with manually identified areas of scar, fuzzy k-means clustering produced the best results [13]. To demonstrate this technique, the amount of identified scar, expressed as a percentage of the wall thickness —the *transmurality* of the infarct— was plotted on a bullseye representation of the heart —as is frequently employed in cardiac image analysis packages— Fig. 5, first column. However, as can be seen from the adjacent plots of transmurality following manual identification of areas of scar, fuzzy k-means clustering mis-classifies large amounts of myocardium.

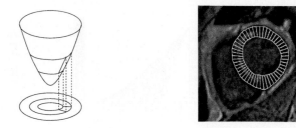

Fig. 2. Illustration of how the three-dimensional location of myocardial segments are mapped onto the 2D bullseye plot (*left*). Parameters for each segment of the bullseye plot were measured in-slice at equi-spaced angular locations about the in-slice centroid of the delayed enhancement endocardial contour (*right*).

A bullseye plot is a series of contiguous concentric rings, segments of each ring are colour coded according to the parameter calculated for corresponding segments of myocardium. Each of the concentric rings in the plot represents information originating from a particular slice, the slice nearest the apex representing the innermost ring, and the outermost ring information from the slice nearest the base —Fig. 2. The in-plane angular location of the information determines the angular location at which it is positioned in the bullseye plot. In this case, parameters for each segment of the bullseye plot were measured in-slice at equi-spaced angular locations about the in-slice centroid of the delayed enhancement endocardial surface —Fig. 2.

However, thresholding by itself as a means of identifying scar tissue is unsatisfactory in two respects. Firstly, the probability density functions of healthy myocardium and enhanced areas often overlap. In the absence of any spatial continuity constraints, this leads to voxel mis-classification. Secondly, microvascular obstruction in areas of scarring can sometimes totally prevent the entrance of any contrast agent whatsoever, resulting in areas of scar with 'dark cores' [14]. The sole exception to the employment of thresholding for the purpose of scar identification is O'Donnell *et al.*'s work [15], they employ support vector machines [16,17] to identify the hyper-surface in parameter space that separates scarred from unscarred tissue, this technique requires a large amount of training data which prevented our investigation of it. Although not explicitly stated in the paper, this technique may be able to correctly classify dark core areas.

Given the high incidence of mis-classification when using fuzzy k-means clustering, the general flaws associated with thresholding techniques, and our inability to assess O'Donnell's technique due to the number of data sets required for training, areas of scar were identified manually and the transmurality plotted on a bullseye —Fig. 5, second column. The percentage wall thickening (a metric routinely employed in echocardiography) was then calculated from the transformed end diastolic and end systolic contours, and mapped onto bullseyes —Fig. 5, third column. Because the contours have been aligned prior to being mapped onto the bullseye plots, for the purposes of data combination, it will be sufficient to combine the information associated with the segments of the bullseye plots.

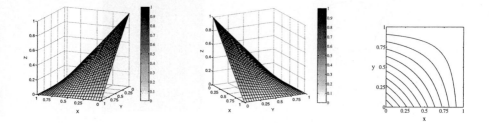

Fig. 3. Two different views of the revascularisation candidacy surface as described by $z = (1 - x)(1 - y)$ where x and y represent the transmurality and wall thickening values (*left and middle*) and a contour map of the surface (*right*).

To combine the information from the two bullseye plots, a function of the wall thickening (x) and transmurality (y) needs to be defined. This function should be maximum in areas of low thickening and low scarring, indicating the likely location of hibernating myocardium —candidate areas for revascularisation. The function should in addition be minimum in areas of maximal thickening and also in areas of maximal transmurality —areas, the revascularisation of which, will not benefit the patient. One such candidacy function can be described by $z = (1 - x)(1 - y)$, Fig. 3. This function was used to combine the wall thickening and transmurality information on bullseye plots for each patient —Fig. 5, fourth column. It should be noted that although this function has the desired features as described above, its behaviour away from these points is a somewhat arbitrary estimation of the benefit associated with the revascularisation of such areas. The true revascularisation candidacy function, can only be determined experimentally by the assessment of both pre- and post-revascularisation images.

Although the bullseye plot permits two-dimensional observation of the location of three-dimensional data, it is somewhat abstract. An easier to interpret representation would be if the combined information were visualised on a 3D representation of the myocardium. To thus represent the combined wall thickening and transmurality information, a coordinate system that can be used to translate between the bullseye plot and the surface must be defined. Segments in the bullseye plot can be easily identified using a polar representation, on the surface this corresponds to a (z, θ) coordinate system —as opposed to an (r, θ) system on the bullseye plot. The location of the centroid of any of the 3D surface's facets on the bullseye can be identified from its z-position and its theta value calculated with respect to its in-slice centroid. This is a continuous coordinate system and the resulting location in the bullseye plot may consequently be at a non-integer position. To enable interpolation of intermediate values from the bullseye plot, it was unwrapped (see Fig. 4). Cubic b-spline interpolation —wrapped around at the image edges to account for radial continuity— then enabled smooth $C2$ interpolation of the bullseye plot. Examples of the bullseye plots for transmurality, wall thickening and the combined function are shown mapped onto prepared segmentations of the delayed enhancement epicardial surface in Fig. 6.

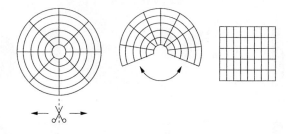

Fig. 4. The unwrapping of the bullseye plot into a rectangular image.

4   Results

The contour overlays in Fig. 1 clearly demonstrate that for patients 1 and 2, the registration has aligned the hearts very well. For patient 3 however, there is a substantial registration error. It would seem that the registration algorithm has aligned the enhanced region with the blood pool in the cine anatomical image. As can also be seen from Fig. 1, patient 3's delayed enhancement image is of poor quality when compared to patient 1 and 2's images. Experimental investigation of the mis-registration concluded that it was due to poor contrast because of inappropriate TI selection during imaging [13]. Despite this poor result, it was decided to continue with the analysis of patient 3 for the purpose of illustrating the technique.

Figure 5 shows bullseye plots of transmurality, wall thickening and candidate areas for revascularisation for all three patients. It can be seen that patient 1 has a sizable amount of scar tissue in the basal and mid anterior segments of the heart, a corresponding area of reduced thickening can be seen in the wall thickening plot. The combined plot does not indicate any substantial areas with high revascularisation candidacy, although a small region may be seen in the basal septal areas. This is nicely illustrated in Fig. 6, where for the first two positions, one can clearly see the reduced wall thickening in areas of scar.

Patient 2 has two small areas of scar in the basal anterior segments, the wall thickening bullseye plot shows reduced thickening in this area and also in the septal segments. When combined, it can be seen that there is a large candidate area for revascularisation in the basal and mid septal segments. This is also seen in Fig. 6.

The bullseye plot for patient 3 —Fig. 5, demonstrates a large septal area of scarring in the mid slices, the transmurality is around 50% for most of the scarred tissue. Reduced wall thickening is correspondingly seen in the wall thickening plot. The combined plot is patchy, not distinctly indicating any large areas suitable for revascularisation, however the septal side of the heart does have seem to have slightly higher candidacy values.

5   Discussion and Conclusion

This paper has addressed the task of automatically combining information from cine anatomical and delayed enhancement images and, to the author's knowledge, is the first paper to attempt this. Rigid registration using normalised mutual information of a

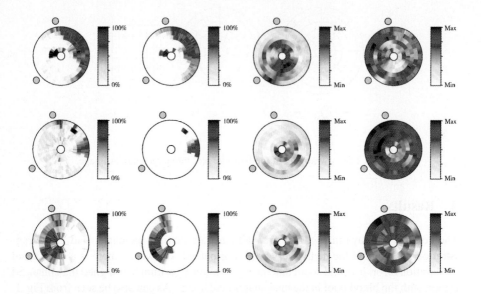

Fig. 5. Bullseye plots showing; transmurality determined using fuzzy k-means clustering [12] (*first column*), transmurality determined manually (*second column*), wall thickening (*third column*), and candidate areas for revascularisation (*fourth column*), for patients 1, 2 and 3 (*top, middle and bottom rows*). Dots indicate the location of the conjunction of the left and right ventricles.

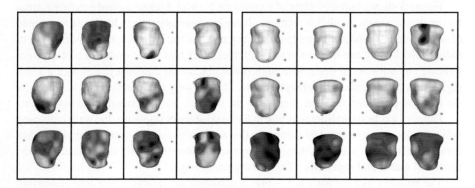

Fig. 6. Mappings of transmurality (*top row*), wall thickening (*middle row*) and candidate areas for revascularisation (*bottom row*) for patients 1 (*left*) and 2 (*right*). Spheres indicate the location of the conjunction of the left and right ventricles.

region of interest was shown be to sufficient to compensate for both inter-scan patient movement and inconsistent breath-hold positions. Following registration, the location of manually identified areas of scarring was then combined with manually determined wall thickening information using a combination function. Although at this stage the combination function is rather arbitrary, it enables candidate areas for revascularisation to be highlighted for the first time. The results of the information combination were shown on both 2D bullseye representations of the heart, and on 3D representations of the myocardial surface. Future work required to make this technique clinically employable would be the empirical identification of a revascularisation candidacy function, this will require a substantial set of both pre- and post-revascularisation images. Following this, the technique could be validated by comparison with results derived from PET—the current gold standard.

Acknowledgements. We are grateful to Philips Medical Systems Nederland B.V. Medical Imaging Information Technology - Advanced Development for funding this work, and to Professor Hawkes and all those at the Computer Imaging Sciences Group for their assistance.

References

1. R.J. Kim, D.S. Fieno, T.B. Parrish, K. Harris, E. Chen, O. Simonetti, Bundy J., J.P. Finn, F.J. Klocke, and R.M. Judd. Relationship of MRI Delayed Contrast Enhancement to Irreversible Injury, Infarct age, and Contractile Function. *Circulation*, 100:1992–2002, 1999.
2. S. Rahimtoola. The Hibernating Myocardium. *Am. Heart J.*, 117(1):211–230, 1989.
3. C. Klein, S.G. Nekolla, F.M. Bengel, M. Momose, A. Sammer, F. Haas, B. Schnackenburg, W. Wolfram Delius, H. Mudra, D. Wolfram, and M. Schwaiger. Assessment of myocardial viability with contrast enhanced magnetic resonance imaging: comparison with positron emission tomography. *Circulation*, 105(2):162–167, 2002.
4. A. Wagner, H. Mahrholdt, T.A. Holly, M.D. Elliott, M. Regenfus, M. Parker, F. Klocke, R.O. Bonow, R.J. Kim, and R.M. Judd. Contrast-enhanced mri and routine single photon emission computed tomography (SPECT) perfusion imaging for detection of subendocardial myocardial infarcts: an imaging study. *Lancet*, 361:374–379, 2003.
5. M. Breeuwer, R. Muthupillai, S. Flamm, E. Nagel, I. Paetsch, J. Ridgeway, and S. Plein. Combining first-pass and late-enhancement myocardial perfusion analysis. In *Proc. Society of Cardiovascular Magentic Resonance*, 2003.
6. C. Studholme, D.L.G. Hill, and D.J. Hawkes. An Overlap Invariant Entropy Measure of 3D Medical Image Alignment. *Pattern Recognition*, 32:71–86, 1999.
7. G.T. Herman, J. Zheng, and C.A. Bucholtz. Shape-Based Interpolation. *IEEE Comput. Graph. Appl.*, pages 69–79, 1992.
8. W.E. Lorensen and H.E. Cline. Marching Cubes: A High Resolution 3D Surface Reconstruction Algorithm. *Comput. Graph.*, 21(4):163–169, 1987.
9. B.L. Gerber, C.E. Rochitte, D.A. Bluemke, J.A. Melin, P. Crosille, L.C. Becker, and J.A.C. Lima. Relation between Gd-DTPA contrast enhancement and regional inotropic response in the periphery and center of myocardial infarction. *Circulation*, 104:998–1004, 2001.
10. A. Kolipake, G.P. Chatzimavroudis, R.D. White, and R.M. Setser. Segmentation of non-viable myocardium in delayed enhancement magnetic resonance images. In *ISMRM*, 2003.
11. P. Madhav, V. Mai, M. Zhang, and Q. Chen. An Automated Segmentation Method for Assesing Myocardial Infarct Size Using K-Means Algorithm. In *ISMRM*, 2003.
12. V. Positano, A. Pingitore, M.F. Santarelli, M. Lombardi, L. Landini, and A. Benassi. Quantitative 3D assessment of myocardial viability with MRI delayed contrast enhancement. In *Computers in Cardiology*, Thessalonika, Greece, 2003.

13. N.M.I. Noble. *Information alignment and extraction from cardiac magnetic resonance images*. PhD thesis, University of London, 2004. Publication pending.
14. A.S. John and D.J. Pennell. Cardiovascular magnetic resonance imaging of dysfunctional myocardial tissue in ischemic heart disease. *Heart Metab.*, 20:19–22, 2003.
15. T. O'Donnell, N. Xu, R. Setser, and R.D. White. Semi automatic segmentation of non-viable cardiac tissue using cine and delayed enhancement magnetic resonance images. In *Proc. SPIE medical imaging*, volume 5031, pages 242–251, 2003.
16. C. Burgess. A tutorial on support vector machines for pattern recognition. *Data Mining and Knowledge Discovery*, 2(2):1–43, 1998.
17. N. Christiani. *An introduction to support vector machines and other kernal-based learning methods*. Cambridge university press, 2000.

A Spatio-temporal Analysis of Contrast Ultrasound Image Sequences for Assessment of Tissue Perfusion

Quentin R. Williams and J. Alison Noble

Medical Vision Laboratory, University of Oxford, UK
{quentin,noble}@robots.ox.ac.uk

Abstract. The evaluation of tissue perfusion in various parenchymatous organs is important in the diagnosis and determination of the severity of ischemic disease. Contrast ultrasound perfusion imaging can be used for this purpose. This paper describes a method that identifies different areas of perfusion in a contrast ultrasound perfusion study. Pixels in an image sequence are automatically classified into different classes, by analysing their distinct temporal relationships. A novel method is presented that uses a Bayesian Factor Analysis Model set in a Markov Random Field framework; utilising both the temporal and spatial characteristics of the pixels for classification. Preliminary results are demonstrated for simulated data, and a myocardial perfusion in-vivo dataset.

1 Introduction

Tissue perfusion imaging is becoming an increasingly employed method to assess internal organ blood supply and flow in clinical applications. For example the assessment of tissue viability through perfusion imaging, has many clinical applications which include: detection of coronary artery disease (CAD) in asymptomatic and symptomatic patients; estimation of the severity of CAD; risk stratification for coronary events, and analysis of disease state in other organs such as the liver, kidneys and the brain. Tissue perfusion has been traditionally analysed by nuclear medicine imaging procedures, like T1-SPECT, which measure cell membrane integrity, or more recently by PET-FDG, which shows metabolism and blood flow rates. Limitations of these techniques are low spatial resolution and the use of ionising radiation.

The availability, low cost and non-invasiveness of echocardiography have fostered an increasing interest in the use of this modality to provide an accurate and quantitative diagnosis of tissue perfusion. The intravenous injection of contrast agents (microbubbles) has allowed the visualisation of blood flow information and regional perfusion. The contrast agents submerged in blood, increase the echo-backscatter of perfused tissues and blood pool in cavities, and are ideal as they remain intravascular and have a particle size similar to red blood cells [1]. However, interpretation of the results is very difficult, and doctors must often rely on visual assessment, which is subjective and results in various discrepancies [2]. Techniques have been proposed to quantify the dynamics of perfusion by evaluating the signal intensities with time in the ultrasound images. For instance, Mor-Avi et al. [3] proposed methods for quantifying both regional blood flow distribution and transit time, by frequency domain

C. Barillot, D.R. Haynor, and P. Hellier (Eds.): MICCAI 2004, LNCS 3217, pp. 899–906, 2004.
© Springer-Verlag Berlin Heidelberg 2004

analysis of regional time curves. Wei et al. [4] introduced the 'negative bolus indicator dilution technique' which is based on high power ultrasound induced destruction of microbubbles and the assessment of their replenishment during a constant venous infusion of a contrast agent. The replenishment (wash-in) curves, showing the refilling of microbubbles, were then fitted to exponential models to extract parameters involving the microbubble velocity and myocardial blood volume. These pixel-based techniques all suffer from ad hoc smoothing in space and time, and the loss of temporal information that is available by analysing the correlation between pixels. Noise present in the images can also greatly influence the shape of the intensity-time curves, while registration has mostly been ignored in these methods. Factor Analysis of Dynamic Studies (FADS) has also been suggested to analyse perfusion curves. Much of the work on FADS has been carried out on dynamic nuclear medicine studies [5], as well as MRI [6]. These methods attempt to rotate the final factor solution in such a way that it satisfies certain constraints (e.g. the positivity constraint) that endeavor to make the results more interpretable. These constraints are however subjective and often not sufficient on their own to produce a unique solution.

In this paper a method is presented to assess myocardial perfusion by automatically classifying the ultrasound images into different regions of perfusion, using a novel spatio-temporal technique. This is done in a global manner by analysing the temporal pattern of relationships between pixels, using a Bayesian Factor Analysis model, and incorporating spatial information through a Markov Random Field. In this manner pixels can be classified into particular types of perfusion (from which quantitative parameters can be obtained if necessary), and the nature and structure of any perfusion study can be examined. This probabilistic view of factor analysis allows a unique solution to be found automatically, without the use of subjective constraints, and has to our knowledge not before been applied to tissue perfusion studies. An interesting and novel way of interlinking the Bayesian Factor Analysis with a Markov Random Field is also presented in this paper. Although not limited to these applications, results are shown for a myocardial perfusion study.

2 Methods

2.1 Bayesian Classification Using a Markov Random Field Prior Model

In this paper classification is treated as a statistical problem, which involves assigning to each pixel a class label taking a value from the set $L = \{1,2,...,l\}$. The pixels are indexed by a two-dimensional rectangular lattice $S = \{1,2,...,n\}$ and each pixel is characterised by a p-variate vector of intensity values $\mathbf{y}_i = (y_{i1},..., y_{ip})$, $i \in S$. In this case each observation vector $\mathbf{y}_i$ represents an intensity-time curve for a single pixel location (i.e. there are p images), where each intensity value is taken from the same image location in consecutive timeframes in the image sequence.

A labelling of S will be denoted $\mathbf{x}$, where $x_i, i \in S$ is the corresponding class label of pixel i. The true but unknown labelling configuration, $\mathbf{x}^*$, and the configuration estimate, $\hat{\mathbf{x}}$, are both interpreted as particular realisations of a random field X. The p-

variate observation vectors on n pixels are then, $\mathbf{Y}' = (\mathbf{y}_1,\ldots,\mathbf{y}_n)$, which is also a realisation of a random variable, Y. The problem of classification is to estimate $\mathbf{x}^*$, given the observed intensity time vectors $\mathbf{Y}$. In particular, the maximum a posteriori (MAP) estimate of $\mathbf{x}$ is used:

$$\hat{\mathbf{x}} = \arg\max{}_{\mathbf{x} \in X} \{P(\mathbf{Y} \mid \mathbf{x})P(\mathbf{x})\}. \tag{1}$$

The right-hand side of the above equation contains two parts: $P(\mathbf{Y} \mid \mathbf{x})$ and $P(\mathbf{x})$, which are defined below as a Bayesian Factor Analysis likelihood distribution and a Markov Random Field prior distribution, respectively.

2.2 Bayesian Factor Analysis Model

In the Bayesian Factor Analysis model it is assumed that the correlation between individual pixel intensity-time curves can be explained in terms of a small number of underlying hidden factors [8]. A generative latent variable model is constructed,

$$(\mathbf{y}_i \mid \mu, \Lambda, \mathbf{f}_i) = \mu + \Lambda\mathbf{f}_i + \varepsilon_i, \tag{2}$$

for each observation vector $\mathbf{y}_i$ ($i=1,\ldots,n$), where μ is the overall population mean, Λ is a matrix of constants called the factor loading matrix; $\mathbf{f}_i = (f_{i1},\ldots,f_{il})$, $l \in L$, is the factor score vector for pixel i; and the ε_i's are assumed to be mutually uncorrelated and Normally distributed $N(0,\Psi)$ variables. The factor loading matrix, Λ, expresses how each hidden factor loads onto the observed variables, therefore giving an indication of how the hidden factors might look. In the case of a perfusion study, each column in the factor loading matrix will represent an intensity-time curve associated with each different type of perfusion present in the dataset. The factor scores give the estimated value ("weight") of the observations on the hidden factors. Therefore, if each hidden factor represents a class, the factor score vector gives an indication of how much an observation belongs to each class. Since the parameters μ, Λ, the $\mathbf{f}_i$'s, and Ψ are all unobservable, a Normal likelihood distribution for each $\mathbf{y}_i$ is assumed, and written as:

$$p(\mathbf{y}_i \mid \mu, \Lambda, \mathbf{f}_i, \Psi) = (2\pi)^{-\frac{p}{2}}\left|\Psi\right|^{-\frac{1}{2}} e^{-\frac{1}{2}(\mathbf{y}_i - \mu - \Lambda\mathbf{f}_i)'\Psi^{-1}(\mathbf{y}_i - \mu - \Lambda\mathbf{f}_i)}. \tag{3}$$

Assuming independence between the observations, the joint likelihood becomes:

$$p(\mathbf{Y} \mid \mu, \Lambda, \mathbf{f}_i, \Psi) = (2\pi)^{-\frac{np}{2}}\left|\Psi\right|^{-\frac{n}{2}} e^{-\frac{1}{2}\sum_{i=1}^{n}(\mathbf{y}_i - \mu - \Lambda\mathbf{f}_i)'\Psi^{-1}(\mathbf{y}_i - \mu - \Lambda\mathbf{f}_i)}. \tag{4}$$

2.3 Markov Random Field

Markov Random Field (MRF) theory provides a convenient and consistent way to model the spatial relationships of context-dependent entities such as image pixels. In an MRF, only neighbouring sites have direct interactions with each other and they tend to have the same class labels. The probability of an MRF realisation, $\mathbf{x}$, is given by the Gibbs distribution:

$$P(\mathbf{x}) = Z^{-1} e^{(-\omega U(\mathbf{x}))},$$ (5)

where
$$U(\mathbf{x}) = \sum_{c \in C} V_c(\mathbf{x}),$$ (6)

is the energy function which is a sum of *clique potentials* $V_c(\mathbf{x})$ over all possible cliques C. Z is a normalisation term and ω is a positive constant which controls the size of clustering(*). A *clique c* is defined as a subset of sites in S in which every pair of distinct sites are neighbours, except for single-site cliques. In this paper, only cliques of size two are counted. The clique potential is then of the form:

$$V_c(x_i) = -\delta_{x_i = x_{i'}}.$$ (7)

This is the same potential function as used by Xiao et al. [7] where $\delta_{x_i = x_{i'}} = 1$, if $x_i = x_{i'}$, and 0 otherwise. It is easy to show from Eqns. (1), (4), (6) and (7) that the MAP estimate of the classification is found by

$$\hat{\mathbf{x}} = \arg\min_{\mathbf{x} \in X} \{U(\mathbf{x} \mid \mathbf{Y})\},$$ (8)

where the posterior energy $U(\mathbf{x}|\mathbf{Y})$ is given by

$$U(\mathbf{x} \mid \mathbf{Y}) = \sum_{i=1}^{n} \tfrac{1}{2}[(\mathbf{y}_i - \mu - \Lambda\mathbf{f}_i)'\Psi^{-1}(\mathbf{y}_i - \mu - \Lambda\mathbf{f}_i) + \log|\Psi|] - \omega \sum_{c \in C} \delta_{x_i = x_{i'}}.$$ (9)

MAP estimation is then computed using the iterated conditional modes (ICM) algorithm suggested in [7].

2.4 Connection Between Factors Scores and the Classification

It has been noted that the factor score vector indicates how much an observation belongs to a particular class. It is therefore assumed that the prior probability of the factor scores matrix, $\mathbf{F}' = (\mathbf{f}_1, \ldots, \mathbf{f}_n)$, follows the same prior probability of the classification configuration, $\mathbf{x}$, and in fact that the factor score for each hidden factor (or class) is equivalent to the posterior probability of the class label. For every $l \in L$ and $i \in S$

$$f_{il} = P(\mathbf{y}_i \mid l)P(x_i = l).$$ (10)

Using the prior probability and the likelihood function with respect to x_i and f_{il} gives

$$f_{il} = Z^{-1} e^{(-\omega U(x_i))} \times (2\pi)^{-\frac{p}{2}} |\Psi|^{-\frac{1}{2}} e^{-\frac{1}{2}(\mathbf{y}_i - \mu - \Lambda_l f_{il})'\Psi^{-1}(\mathbf{y}_i - \mu - \Lambda_l f_{il})}.$$ (11)

Therefore the posterior probability values obtained through the MRF-MAP classification can directly be used as the factor scores.

---

* ω is used to avoid confusion with the replenishment curve blood velocity, β, in Eqn. 21.

2.5 μ, Λ, Ψ Estimation

The parameters μ, Λ, and Ψ are still unknown and thus require estimation. Rowe [8] proposed using an ICM MAP estimation procedure that maximises the posterior conditional distributions of the unknown parameters by cycling through their modes. The approach is summarised here, and the reader is referred to [8] for more detail.

In [8] it is assumed that the parameters μ, Λ, and Ψ are random variables with generalised natural conjugate prior distributions:

$$p(\mu) \propto |\Gamma|^{-1/2} e^{-\frac{1}{2}(\mu-\mu_0)'\Gamma^{-1}(\mu-\mu_0)} , \tag{12}$$

$$p(\Lambda) \propto |\Delta|^{-1/2} e^{-\frac{1}{2}tr(\Lambda-\Lambda_0)'\Delta^{-1}(\Lambda-\Lambda_0)} , \tag{13}$$

$$\text{and } p(\Psi) \propto |\Psi|^{-\nu/2} e^{-\frac{1}{2}tr\Psi^{-1}B} , \tag{14}$$

with $\Gamma, \Delta, B, \Psi > 0$ and B a diagonal matrix. ν is set as described in [8].

The posterior distributions are then obtained through Bayes rule giving:

$$p(\mu \mid F, \Lambda, \Psi, Y) \propto e^{-\frac{1}{2}(\mu-\tilde{\mu})'[(n\Gamma)^{-1}+\Psi^{-1}](\mu-\tilde{\mu})} , \tag{15}$$

$$p(\Lambda \mid \mu, F, \Psi, Y) \propto e^{-\frac{1}{2}tr(\Lambda-\tilde{\Lambda})[\Delta^{-1}+\Psi^{-1}\otimes F'F](\Lambda-\tilde{\Lambda})'} , \tag{16}$$

$$p(\Psi \mid \mu, y, \Lambda, Y) \propto |\Psi|^{-\frac{(n+\nu)}{2}} e^{-\frac{1}{2}tr\Psi^{-1}[(Y-e_n\otimes\mu'-F\Lambda')'(Y-e_n\otimes\mu'-F\Lambda')+B]} , \tag{17}$$

where

$$\tilde{\mu} = [(n\Gamma)^{-1} + \Psi^{-1}]^{-1}[(n\Gamma)^{-1}\mu_0 + \Psi^{-1}(\bar{y} - \Lambda\bar{f})] , \tag{18}$$

$$\tilde{\Lambda} = [\Delta^{-1} + \Psi^{-1} \otimes F'F]^{-1}[\Delta^{-1}\Lambda_0 + (\Psi^{-1} \otimes F'F)((F'F)^{-1}F'(Y - e_n \otimes \tilde{\mu}'))'] . \tag{19}$$

The ICM procedure is then used to estimate the parameters by cycling through their modes $\tilde{\mu}$, $\tilde{\Lambda}$ (as defined above), and

$$\tilde{\Psi} = \frac{(Y - e_n \otimes \mu' - F\Lambda')'(Y - e_n \otimes \mu' - F\Lambda') + B}{n + \nu} , \tag{20}$$

respectively. The Kroneker product is denoted by $\otimes$ and $\mathbf{e}_n$ is a vector of ones with length n.

Thus, the strategy underlying this algorithm can be summarised as follows: (1) Estimate the labelling configuration, $\hat{\mathbf{x}}$, using the current estimate of the parameters; (2) use it to specify the factor scores matrix, $\mathbf{F}$; (3) and estimate new values for the parameters, μ, Λ, and Ψ, using the ICM approach outlined above. These steps are iteratively followed until suitable convergence is reached.

3   Experimental Analysis

Examples of applying the method to both simulated and in-vivo data are given in this section. In-vivo results are shown for a myocardial perfusion study.

3.1   Results in Simulated Data Sets

In order to illustrate the method, a simple experiment was constructed. Figure 1(a) shows 3 intensity time-curves generated using the exponential curve model:

$$\mathbf{y}_i = A(1 - e^{-\beta t}). \tag{21}$$

According to myocardial perfusion literature [1], [4]; the replenishment curves can be successfully modelled using the above equation. In this experiment, A was kept constant at a maximum intensity value of $A = 204$, while β was selected as 0.2, 0.6 and 1, respectively, to represent 3 different classes. A classification image template (Fig. 1(b)), showing various random regions classified into 3 different classes, was used to give the original classification of each pixel based on its location in the image template. Image sequences, each consisting of 14 different images ($t = \{0,1,\ldots,13\}$) could then be generated, where each image was created by selecting an intensity value for every pixel using Eqn. 21 and adding Gaussian noise with mean $= 0$ and varying standard deviation. The pixel class determined which β value to use in the equation. Therefore each pixel had an intensity time profile (with added Gaussian noise), similar to the replenishment curve of the class that the pixel belonged to. Figure 2(a)-(c), illustrates a perfect image sequence (noise $= 0$). It can be seen that pixel intensities in each class region, goes from black (intensity values close to zero), to almost white (intensity values close to 204), in different ways depending on the replenishment curve of their class. Since classes 2 and 3, reach the same level of intensity after the 8th timeframe, it can be seen that they overlap in later images in the sequence. In this experiment 3 such image sequences were simulated, where the standard deviation of the Gaussian noise, was 10% (20.4), 15% (30.6) and 45% (91.8) of the maximum intensity value of 204, respectively. Figure 3(a), (b) and (d) show the classification obtained from applying the BFA-MRF method on these image sequences, while (c) shows the BFA model applied without the MRF (noise $= 15\%$). The misclassification ratio (*MCR*) is also shown. From the figures it can be seen that the method performed reasonably well and correct classification was obtained despite the random shapes of the regions. Overlaps and high misclassification ratios, were only seen at very high levels of noise ($> 25\%$), which is as expected. For the BFA model alone, overlaps were already seen at a noise level of 15%, and without the MRF, a much higher misclassification ratio was obtained. Figure 3(d), (noise $= 45\%$), shows that most of the misclassification occurs between regions of classes 2 and 3, while regions of class 1 was correctly classified. The reason for this is the similarity between the 2 classes, as can be seen from their intensity-time profiles in Fig. 1(a). This was deliberately done to test the sensitivity of the method. These results show that the BFA-MRF method can be successfully used to classify perfusion data, even in the presence of noise, and despite certain similarity of classes.

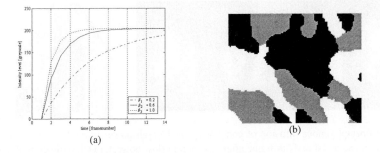

(a)

(b)

Fig. 1. The three simulated classes represented as (a) 3 replenishment curves; and (b) the classification template where the 3 classes are black ($\beta_1 = 0.2$), grey ($\beta_2 = 0.6$) and white ($\beta_3 = 1$).

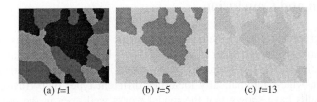

(a) $t=1$ (b) $t=5$ (c) $t=13$

Fig. 2. Changing of intensities in the image sequence from very dark (a) to very bright (c).

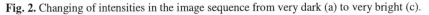

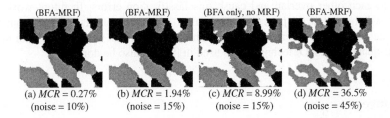

(BFA-MRF)   (BFA-MRF)   (BFA only, no MRF)   (BFA-MRF)

(a) $MCR = 0.27\%$ (b) $MCR = 1.94\%$ (c) $MCR = 8.99\%$ (d) $MCR = 36.5\%$
(noise = 10%)   (noise = 15%)   (noise = 15%)   (noise = 45%)

Fig. 3. Classification results for the BFA-MRF method, along with the misclassification ratio for 3 different noise levels where noise = (a) 10%, (b) 15%, (c) 15% (with the BFA model applied without MRF) and (d) 45% (BFA-MRF again), respectively.

3.2 In Vivo Dataset

A myocardial perfusion study was obtained for a healthy patient, using contrast echocardiography and the Power Pulse Inversion (PPI) technique described in [1]. The dataset consisted of 14 images, acquired in 2-chamber apical view and ECG-triggered. Only the left ventricle was of interest in the classification task. Figure 4(a)-(d) shows 4 images taken from the study, while Fig. 4(e) shows the classification results obtained. Visually, the classification appears good, showing that 3 different regions of perfusion were found. The 3 regions was correctly classified as the myocardium where normal replenishment occurs (grey), the left ventricular cavity where no replenishment occurs (dark grey), and the lateral segments where ultrasound attenuation occurred (black).

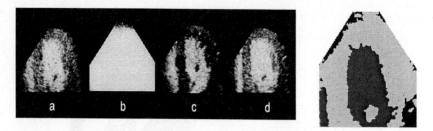

Fig. 4. a) Constant venous infusion of contrast agent. b) high power frame to destroy the microbubbles. c) and d) 1st and 5th frame after destruction (low power). e) Classification obtained showing 3 different types of perfusion present.

4   Discussion and Conclusion

This paper has presented a novel method for automatic classification of tissue perfusion ultrasound images. In particular it has been shown how both the spatial and temporal characteristics of the pixels can be incorporated into a single statistical model for classification, which automatically identifies different types of perfusion. Initial experimental results have shown that the model works well even in the presence of high-levels of noise. The preliminary results on in-vivo data are encouraging, showing plausible classification results. There are still problems where classes that are very similar to each other overlap and cause misclassification errors. In future work the method will be tested on patients with proven coronary stenosis to show that the method detects regions where an infarct might have occurred. Comparison with manual semi-quantitative ROI techniques as used in [9] will also be done.

References

1.   H. Becher and P. Burns. *Handbook of Contrast Echocardiography.* Springer Verlag, 2000.
2.   B.P. Paelinck and J.D. Kasprzak. Contrast-enhanced echocardiography: review and current role. *Acta Cardiol*, vol. 54:195-201, 1999.
3.   V. Mor-Avi, S. Akselrod, D. David, L. Keselbrener, and Y. Bitton. Myocardial transit time of the echocardiographic contrast media. *Ultrasound Med Biol*, vol. 19:635-48, 1993.
4.   K. Wei, et al. Quantification of myocardial blood flow with US induced destruction of microbubbles administered as a constant venous infusion. *Circulation*, vol. 97:473-83, 1998.
5.   D.G. Pavel, et al. FA of dynamic renal studies in urology, *J. Nucl. Med*, 29:P816, 1988
6.   A. Martel, A.R. Moody, et al. Extracting parametric images from dynamic contrast enhanced MRI studies of the brain using factor analysis. *Med Image Anal*, vol. 5:29-39, 2002.
7.   G. Xiao, J.M. Brady, J.A. Noble, and Y. Zhang. Intensity Inhomogeneity Correction and Segmentation of Ultrasound Images, *IEEE Trans. Medical Imaging*, vol. 21(1):48-57, 2002.
8.   Daniel Rowe. A Bayesian Factor Analysis Model with generalized Prior information. *Social science working paper 1099*, California institute of technology, August 2000.
9.   A.Z. Linka, J. Sklenar, K. Wei, et al. Assessment of transmural distribution of myocardial perfusion with contrast echo. *Circulation*, vol. 18:1912-20, 1998.

Detecting Functional Connectivity of the Cerebellum Using Low Frequency Fluctuations (LFFs)

Yong He, Yufeng Zang, Tianzi Jiang, Meng Liang, and Gaolang Gong

National Laboratory of Pattern Recognition, Institute of Automation, Chinese Academy of
Sciences, 100080, Beijing, P. R. China
{yhe, yfzang, jiangtz}@nlpr.ia.ac.cn

Abstract. So far, resting state functional connectivity (RSFC) has been performed mainly by seed correlation analysis (SCA) on functional MRI (fMRI)
studies. In previous studies, the seeds are usually selected on the basis of prior
anatomical information or previously performed activation maps. In this paper,
we proposed a novel way to select the desired seeds by taking the natures of
resting state data into account. The proposed approach is based on the measurement of regional homogeneity (ReHo) of brain regions. Using this technique,
2 locations showing higher ReHo in the cerebellum (i.e. the bilateral anterior
inferior cerebellum, AICb) were identified and used as the seeds for RSFC patterns studies. We found that the bilateral AICb show significant functional connectivity with the bilateral thalamus, the bilateral hippocampus, the precuneus,
the temporal lobe and the prefrontal lobe. Further, the differences of RSFC patterns between the bilateral AICb were ascertained by a random effect paired t-
test. These findings may improve our understanding of cerebellar involvement
in motor and a variety of non-motor functions.

1 Introduction

Functional connectivity in the context of functional brain imaging has been considered
as a descriptive measure of spatiotemporal correlations between spatially distinct brain
regions [1]. Functional connectivity in the human brain has traditionally focused on
characterizing neuronal interactions between activated regions in a given experiment
task [2]. Such task-specific functional connectivity (TSFC) may reflect coactivations
resulting from the task itself and therefore strongly depend on the performance of the
task. Recently, increasing attention has been focused on exploring functional depend-
encies between brain regions in no specific cognitive task, defined as resting state
functional connectivity (RSFC). Some convincing evidence from functional MRI
(fMRI) studies has demonstrated that there exists very low frequency fluctuations
(LFFs) (< 0.08 Hz) in MR signals measured in the resting brain [3-6]. In functionally
related regions of the brain, these fluctuations are synchronous and exhibit high temporal coherence, even in those regions located remotely, which implies the existence
of neuronal connectivity coordinating activity in the human brain. Thus, RSFC based
on the LFFs may offer a more direct measure of functional interactions between brain
regions since it is task-free.

C. Barillot, D.R. Haynor, and P. Hellier (Eds.): MICCAI 2004, LNCS 3217, pp. 907–915, 2004.
© Springer-Verlag Berlin Heidelberg 2004

So far, RSFC has been studied in the motor cortex [3, 4], visual cortex [3, 4], language regions [5], and also in the subcortical regions, such as the thalamus [6] and the hippocampus [6, 7]. Moreover, recent studies in patients have suggested that it would also be of specific clinical interest [8, 9].

Despite these studies, RSFC patterns in the cerebellum have not been reported in detail so far. As one of important subcortical structures in the brain, many investigations have indicated that the cerebellum not only contributes to the control of coordinated movement [10], but also may be involved in a variety of non-motor functions, including sensory discrimination [11], working memory [12] and emotional modulation [13]. It therefore would be very meaningful to ascertain which brain regions show significant functional connectivity with the cerebellum during rest. The investigation of RSFC patterns in the cerebellum may improve our understanding of cerebellar involvement in various functions.

One popular way for RSFC studies is seed correlation analysis (SCA), i.e. by selecting a predefined seed region of interest (ROI) as a reference and cross-correlating the time course of the seed with that of all other voxels in the whole brain to produce a functional network. In these studies, the seed ROIs are usually selected on the basis of prior anatomical information [6] or previously performed activation maps [3, 14]. However, such investigator-dependent selections may not be optimal for evaluating RSFC since the bias resulting from external effects (e.g. different experimental tasks) may make the connectivity patterns show completely different features. Intuitively, one should make full use of the information inferred from resting state data to select a relevant seed while evaluating RSFC using a SCA technique.

In this study, we propose a novel way to define the desired seed ROIs by taking into account the natures of resting state data. This approach is based on the measurement of regional homogeneity (ReHo) of brain areas. The ReHo may better represent the characteristics of brain areas in activity, as described by Zang et al. [15].

The paper is organized as follows: An experimental protocol in fMRI was first described. Then, the ReHo was reviewed and performed on resting state data; 2 locations showing higher ReHo in the cerebellum were identified and used as the seed leading to further RSFC analysis. Finally, a summary was provided.

2   Methods

2.1   Data Acquisition

FMRI studies of 34 healthy, right-handed volunteers (25 males; age range 22-40, mean 26.2) were performed with a 1.5-Tesla GE Signa scanner. Each subject was scanned for 400 sec in a resting state. Functional images were acquired axially by using an EPI sequence with the following parameters: 2000/40 ms (TR/TE), 20 slices, 64×64 matrix, $90°$ FA, 24-cm FOV, 5-mm thickness, and 1-mm gap.

2.2   Data Preprocessing

The first 10 time points of the resting state were discarded because of the instability of the initial MRI signal leaving 190 time points. The data were first preprocessed (slice timing, realignment, spatially normalization and re-sampled at 3 mm^3) using SPM2 (www.fil.ion.ucl.ac.uk/spm). Then, in the AFNI package [17], linear drift was removed and the data were spatially smoothed using a 4-mm FWHM Gaussian kernel. After these, a low-pass frequency filter (f <0.08 Hz) was applied to remove physiological high frequency noise [3]. The resulting LFFs were further analyzed.

2.3 Regions of Interest (ROIs)

In our previous study, the ReHo has been used to differentiate brain regions showing changes in activity between different states [15]. In this study, it was extended to define the seed ROIs located in the cerebellum. The description in detail is as follows:

Basic ReHo algorithm. In the context of the ReHo, it seems to be reasonable to assume that the voxels within a functional cluster have higher temporal homogeneity than that within a general cluster [15]. The ReHo of a cluster is measured using Kendall's coefficient of concordance (*KCC*) [18]:

$$W = \frac{\sum (R_i)^2 - n(\overline{R})^2}{\frac{1}{12} K^2 (n^3 - n)} \tag{1}$$

where *W* is the *KCC* of a cluster, ranged from 0 to 1; $R_i = \sum_{j=1}^{k} r_{ij}$, where r_{ij} is the rank of the *i*-th time point in the *j*-th voxel; $\overline{R} = (n+1)k/2$; *n* is the number of time points of each voxel time series (here *n* = 190); *k* is the number of voxels in the cluster, (here *k* = 27, for selecting the number of voxels, see ref [15]). Individual *KCC* maps were obtained on a voxel by voxel basis for each subject data set and further used to define the desired seed ROIs.

Definition of ROIs. The seed ROIs located in the cerebellum are defined as follows. First, a random effect one-sample t test [19] against 0.5 (i.e., H$_0$: *KCC* = 0.5, d.f. = 33) was performed on the *KCC* maps above. Voxels with t > 15.52 (*P* < 1 × 10^{-16}, uncorrected) and clusters volume (CV) > 540 mm^3 were superimposed on high-resolution anatomical images (Fig.1). The resulting t-map shows higher ReHo in the bilateral anterior inferior cerebellum (AICb), the posterior cingulate cortex (PCC, Brodmann's area [BA] 23 and 31), etc. Here, we are just concerned about the bilateral AICb. Thus, anatomical location of peak voxel (i.e. highest t value) within them was identified (Talairach coordinates: the left AICb [-26 -47 -32] and the right AICb [27 -47 -32]. Since the normalization of the data was performed in SPM2, we have transformed the coordinates of brain areas from the MNI space into the Talairach space using an algorithm proposed by http://www.mrc-cbu.cam.ac.uk/Imaging/Common/mnispace.shtml). Finally, each peak voxel obtained above and its nearest 26 neighbors were defined as a group ROI. Subject-specific ROIs were precisely consistent with the group ROIs anatomically. According to the above strategy, 2 subject-specific AICb ROIs for each subject were obtained leading to further RSFC analyses.

2.4 Functional Connectivity Analyses

RSFC patterns of the cerebellum were explored by a SCA approach on the basis of the seed ROIs above. Time series were first extracted for each subject-specific AICb

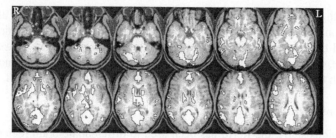

Fig. 1. A group t-map based on the individual KCC maps. The arrows indicate the locations of the bilateral AICb respectively. Z-axis from Z = −36 to Z = +19 in Talairach and Tournoux (TT) coordinates [16]. L indicates the left hemisphere of the brain. For other details, see *Methods*.

ROIs by averaging the time series of all the 27 voxels in the ROI. Then, the resulting time series was used as a reference for cross-correlation analysis (i.e. SCA). These correlation coefficients were further normalized using Fisher's z transformation [20]:

$$z = 0.5 \log \left(\frac{1 + r}{1 - r} \right) \tag{2}$$

where r is the Pearson correlation coefficient at each voxel. The resulting z values is approximately normal distribution with mean and

$$\mu = 0.5 \left[\log \left(\frac{1 + r_{true}}{1 - r_{true}} \right) + \frac{r_{true}}{n - 1} \right] \tag{3}$$

standard deviation $\sigma \approx 1/\sqrt{n - 3}$. Finally, the individual z-maps entered into a random effect one-sample t-test [19] to determine brain regions showing significant functional connectivity across subjects. According to the above processing, 2 RSFC t-maps were obtained respectively. Voxels with t > 9.917 (d.f. = 33, $P < 1 \times 10^{-11}$, uncorrected) and CV>540 mm^3 were superimposed on high-resolution anatomical images (Fig.2). The differences of RSFC patterns between the bilateral AICb was further ascertained by a random effect paired t-test performed on the z-maps above. Voxels with |t| > 2.036 (d.f. = 33, $P < 0.05$, uncorrected) and CV > 540 mm^3 were considered as significantly different between the RSFC patterns of the bilateral AICb.

The above procedures were coded in MATLAB (The MathWorks, Inc., Natick, MA) or processed in the AFNI package [17].

3   Results

Brain areas Showing Higher ReHo During Rest. Fig. 1 shows brain areas having higher ReHo during the rest, including the bilateral AICb, the bilateral superior cerebellum (SCb), the PCC (BA 23 and 31) and the anterior cingulate cortex (ACC, BA 32). Here, we just focused on exploring the AICb as detailed in *Methods*.

RSFC Patterns of the Bilateral AICb. The right AICb showed significant RSFC with the following brain areas: the left AICb, the bilateral SCb, the bilateral thalamus (Th), the bilateral hippocampus (Hi), the left medial prefrontal cortex (MPFC, BA11), the

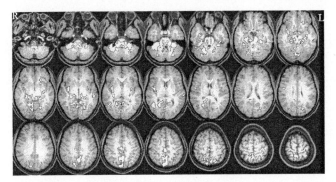

Fig. 2. RSFC t-map for the right AICb. The arrow indicates the location of the right AICb. Z-axis from Z = –44 to Z = +60 in TT coordinates. For other details, see *Methods*.

precuneus (PCu, BA 7) and the temporal lobe (BA21, 37 and 42) (Fig.2). The left AICb showed significant RSFC with the following brain regions: the right AICb, the bilateral SCb, the bilateral Th, the bilateral Hi, the PCC (BA 23), the PCu (BA 7) and the supplement motor area (SMA, BA 6) (The figure is not given here).

The Differences of RSFC Patterns Between the Bilateral AICb. Fig.3 shows the differences of RSFC patterns for the bilateral AICb detected by a paired t-test. Of 29 brain regions with significant differences, 14 showed higher connectivity with the right AICb, compared with the left AICb. Further details regarding these brain regions were presented in Table 1.

4 Discussion

In this study, we used a novel way, the ReHo, to define the desired seed ROIs while exploring RSFC patterns of brain regions using a SCA method. As compared to other methods used for the selection of the seed in the resting state, e.g., anatomically knowledge-based or task activation-based methods, the main advantage of ReHo is that it makes full use of the nature of the resting state data. Using this technique, we identified the seed ROIs located in the bilateral AICb and ascertained their connectivity patterns during rest. Results demonstrate that the bilateral AICb show significant functional connectivity with a distinct set of brain regions during rest, thus providing insight into understanding functional pathways related to the cerebellum.

A large body of evidences has shown that the cerebellum not only participates in motor control, but also may be involved in a variety of non-motor functions. The explorations about functional pathways related to the cerebellum would be very significant for understanding of how the cerebellum works. However, these studies so far have usually focused on exploring TSFC patterns related to the cerebellum [23, 26]. Obviously, such patterns strongly depend on the performance of the tasks. In contrast, RSFC analysis based on the LFFs may provide a more direct measure for neural circuitry. To probe the possibility, we mapped the connectivity patterns for the bilateral AICb during rest respectively. Results show that the right AICb has significant functional connectivity with the left AICb, the bilateral Th, the bilateral Hi, the

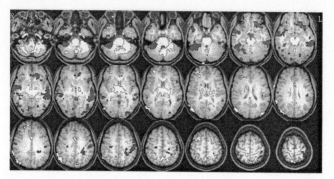

Fig. 3. Paired t-test for the differences of RSFC patterns between the bilateral AICb. Z-axis from Z = −44 to Z = +60 in TT coordinates. White cluster: the left AICb > the right AICb. Grey cluster: the right AICb > the left AICb. For other details, see *Methods* and Table 1.

Table 1. Paired t-test for the difference of RSFC patterns between the bilateral AICb.

Left < Right						Left > Right					
k	x	y	z	t	Regions, BA	k	x	y	z	t	Regions, BA
1306	27	-47	-32	-26.8	R.AICb	1227	-24	-49	-32	27.4	L.AICb
352	-21	28	-9	-4.39	L.MPFC, 10	46	-40	-92	17	5.20	L.OL, 19
601	-55	-32	-13	-4.19	L.MTG, 20	711	9	-23	8	4.26	R.Th
23	25	31	-10	-3.67	R.MPFC, 11		-11	-14	6	4.09	L.Th
108	-24	-92	-1	-3.65	L.OL, 18	418	58	-48	24	4.06	R.IPC, 40
300	-21	-44	30	-3.64	L.WM	118	21	-72	-42	3.91	R.PICb
32	26	-35	39	-3.44	R.WM	28	22	35	22	3.38	R.SFG, 10
102	-42	-33	41	-3.40	L.M1, 4	62	1	2	35	3.28	R.CG, 24
48	58	-15	34	-3.19	R.PrCG, 6	176	2	-60	51	2.93	R.PCu, 7
48	-27	-92	-21	-3.14	L.SCb	57	19	0	55	2.91	R.MFG, 6
48	26	-90	-2	-3.04	R.OL, 18	27	10	46	35	2.86	R.SFG, 9
31	7	-78	-5	-2.94	R.PCC, 18	26	-8	-84	33	2.85	L.Cu, 19
55	-45	-6	45	-2.91	L.PrCG, 6	89	27	48	12	2.82	R.MFG, 10
36	-45	13	10	-2.70	L.IFG, 44	29	-26	-59	6	2.70	L.WM
						27	16	13	31	2.58	R.ACC, 32

Left part: results showing more significant RSFC with the right AICb. Right part: results showing more significant RSFC with the left AICb. k, cluster size in voxels; BA, Brodmann's area; x, y, z, coordinates of TT. Abbreviations: AICb, anterior inferior cerebellum; MPFC, medial prefrontal cortex; MTG, middle temporal gyrus; MFG, middle frontal gyrus; OL, occipital lobe; M1, primary motor cortex; PrCG, precentral gyrus; SCb, superior cerebellum; PCC, postulate cingulate cortex; IFG, inferior frontal gyrus; Th, thalamus; IPC, inferior parietal cortex; PICb, posterior inferior cerebellum; WM, white matter; SFG, superior frontal gyrus; CG, cingulate gyrus; PCu, Precuneus; ACC, anterior cingulate cortex.

PCu, the left MPFC and the temporal lobe (Fig. 2). Moreover, RSFC pattern of the left AICb was very similar to that of the right AICb. The findings were strongly supported by quite a few previous studies. First, of the regions above, the bilateral Th and the Hi have been shown significant RSFC with the cerebellum while they are selected as the seeds respectively leading to a SCA [6]. Second, Middleton and Strick's study of using transneuronal tracing methods in monkeys has indicated there are ipsi- and contra-lateral connections between cerebellum and prefrontal cortex related by the mediodorsal (and other) thalamic nuclei [24]. Third, in the "cognitive dysmetria" model, the cerebellum has been considered as a key structure in a cerebellar-thalamic-prefrontal circuit [25]. Our findings may provide a new insight to understand the cerebellar involvement in motor control and cognitive functions.

Despite the similarity for the bilateral AICb RSFC maps and the similar symmetry in anatomical locations, paired t-test still demonstrates that there exist significant differences in a widely variety of brain regions (Fig. 3, Table 1). Of 29 brain regions with significant differences, 14 showed higher connectivity with the right AICb, compared with the left AICb. Interestingly, we found that the left M1 shows more significant functional connectivity with the right AICb than that with the left AICb, however, we did not observe similar phenomenon for the right M1. In addition, the temporal lobe and the prefrontal lobe were observed significant connectivity with the right AICb, but the bilateral Th and the right SFG show more with the left AICb.

Although we have mapped connectivity patterns in the AICb during rest, brain's functional connectivity is highly flexible and can be modulated for a given changing environment. Our recent study has indicated that functional connectivity of the cerebellum varies from the resting state to the motor task [21]. The modulation is very important for the brain to execute different function in different brain states. In addition, recent evidence from TSFC studies has indicated that altered functional pathways related to the cerebellum appear in the schizophrenia [23, 26]. As an alternative to TSFC analysis, our methods may show more powerful ability in clinical studies, especially for those patients with progressed state of the disease since it is task-free.

It is important to emphasize that, in this study, the connectivity patterns of the AICb during rest were explored by combining the SCA and the ReHo. Besides the AICb, our finding that the PCC may be very active (higher ReHo) is consistent with a recent study that the PCC is considered as a critical node during rest [14]. It may provide a powerful support for the validity of our methods. Anyway, the selection of the seed based on the ReHo seems to be more reasonable, compared with conventional methods. The present study could also be generalized to ascertain RSFC patterns of other brain regions, and especially to explore altered functional connectivity between the patients and the controls.

Acknowledgment. This work was partially supported by the Hundred Talents Programs of the Chinese Academy of Sciences, the Natural Science Foundation of China, Grant No. 60172056 and 60121302.

References

1. Friston KJ, Frith CD, Liddle PF, Frackowiak RS: Functional connectivity: the principal component analysis of large (PET) data sets. J Cereb Blood Flow Metab 13 (1993) 5–14.
2. Homae F, Yahata N, Sakai KL: Selective enhancement of functional connectivity in the left prefrontal cortex during sentence processing. NeuroImage 20 (2003) 578–586.

3. Biswal B, Yetkin FZ, Haughton VM, Hyde JS: Functional connectivity in the motor cortex of resting human brain using echo-planar MRI. Magn Reson Med 34 (1995) 537–541.
4. Lowe MJ, Mock BJ, Sorenson JA: Functional connectivity in single and multislice echoplanar imaging using resting state fluctuations. Neuroimage 7 (1998) 119–132.
5. Hampson M, Peterson BS, Skudlarski P, Gatenby JC, Gore JC: Detection of functional connectivity using temporal correlations in MR images.Hum Brain Mapp 15(2002)247-262.
6. Stein T, Moritz C, Quigley M, et al. Functional connectivity in the thalamus and hippocampus studied with fMRI. Am J Neuroradiol 21 (2000) 1397–1401.
7. Rombouts SA, Stam CJ, Kuijer JP, Scheltens P, Barkhof F: Identifying confounds to increase specificity during a "no task condition". Evidence for hippocampal connectivity using fMRI. Neuroimage 20 (2003) 1236–1245.
8. Lowe MJ, Phillips MD, Lurito JT, Mattson D, Dzemidzic M, Mathews VP: Multiple sclerosis: low-frequency temporal blood oxygen level-dependent fluctuations indicate reduced functional connectivity—initial results. Radiology 224 (2002) 184–192.
9. Li SJ, Biswal B, Li Z, Risinger R, Rainey C, Cho JK, Salmeron BJ, Stein EA: Cocaine administration decreases functional connectivity in human primary visual and motor cortex as detected by functional MRI. Magn Reson Med 43 (2000) 45–51.
10. Thach WT, Goodkin HP, Keating JG: The cerebellum and the adaptive coordination of movement. Annu Rev Neurosci. 15 (1992) 403–442.
11. Gao JH, Parsons LM, Bower JM, Xiong J, Li J, Fox PT: Cerebellum implicated in sensory acquisition and discrimination rather than motor control. Science 272 (1996) 545–547.
12. Klingberg T, Kawashima R, Roland PE: Activation of multi-modal cortical areas underlies short-term memory. Eur J Neurosci 8 (1996) 1965–1971.
13. George MS, Ketter TA, Parekh PI, Horwitz B, Herscovitch P, Post RM: Brain activity during transient sadness and happy in healthy women. Am J Psychiatry 152(1995)341–351.
14. Greicius MD, Krasnow B, Reiss AL, Menon V: Functional connectivity in the resting brain: A network analysis of the default mode hypothesis, Proc Natl Acad Sci 100(2003) 253–258.
15. Zang YF, Jiang TZ, Lu YL, He Y, Tian LX: Regional homogeneity approach to fMRI data analysis. NeuroImage 22(2004) 394–400.
16. Talairach J, Tournoux PA: Coplanar stereotactic atlas of the human brain, Thieme, (1988).
17. Cox, RW: AFNI software for analysis and visualization of functional magnetic resonance neuroimages. Comput Biomed Res 29 (1996) 162–173.
18. Kendall M, Gibbons JDR: Correlation methods. Oxford: Oxford University Press (1990).
19. Holmes AP, Friston KJ: Generalisability, random effects & population inference. NeuroImage 7 (1998) 754.
20. Press WH, Teukolsky SA, Vetterling WT, Flannery BP (1992): Numerical recipes in C, 2 ed. U.K. Cambridge Univ. Press.
21. Jiang TZ, He Y, Zang YF, Weng XC: Modulation of functional connectivity during the resting state and the motor task. Hum Brain Mapp 22 (2004) 63-71.
22. Schmahmann JD: From movement to thought: anatomic substrates of the cerebellar contribution to cognitive processing. Hum Brain Mapp 4 (1996) 174–198.
23. Stephan KE, et al. Effects of olanzapine on cerebellar functional connectivity in schizophrenia measured by fMRI during a simple motor task. Psychol Med.31 (2001) 1065-1078.
24. Middleton FA, Strick PL: Anatomical evidence for cerebellar and basal ganglia involvement in higher cognitive function. Science 266 (1994) 458-461.

25. Andreasen NC, O'leary DS, Cizadlo T, Arndt S, Rezai K, Ponto LL, Watkins GL, Hichwa RD: Schizophrenia and cognitive dysmetria: A positron-emission tomography study of dysfunctional prefrontal-thalamic-cerebellar circuitry. Proc Natl Acad Sci 93(1996) 9985-9990.
26. Schlosser R, Gesierich T, Kaufmann B, Vucurevic G, Hunsche S, Gawehn J, Stoeter P: Altered effective connectivity during working memory performance in schizophrenia: a study with fMRI and structural equation modeling. Neuroimage 19 (2003) 751-763.

Independent Component Analysis of Four-Phase Abdominal CT Images

Xuebin Hu[1], Akinobu Shimizu[1], Hidefumi Kobatake[1], and Shigeru Nawano[2]

[1]Graduate School of Bio-Applications and Systems Engineering,
Tokyo University of Agriculture & Technology
2-24-16 Naka-cho, Koganei-shi, Tokyo, 184-8588 Japan
{huxb, simiz, kobatake}@cc.tuat.ac.jp
[2]National Cancer Center Hospital East
6-5-1 Kasiwanoha, Kasiwa-shi, Chiba, 277-8577 Japan
snawano@east.ncc.go.jp

Abstract. This paper presents a new analysis result of two-dimensional four-phase abdominal CT images using variational Bayesian mixture of ICA. The four-phase CT images are modeled as being produced by a mixture of data generators, where each data generator consists of a set of independent components and is responsible for generating a particular cluster. ICA results show that the CT images could be divided into a set of clinically and anatomically meaningful components. Initial analysis of the independent components shows its promising prospect in medical image processing and computer-aided diagnosis.

1 Introduction

Independent component analysis (ICA), as one of the most powerful tool in multivariate analysis, has attracted a great of interests in medical signal and image processing. Examples include in EEG, ECG de-noising, removing artifacts and signal analysis, coloring multi-channel MR imaging data, extracting blood vessel-related component from dynamic brain PET images, and analysis of functional magnetic resonance imaging (fMRI) data etc. In this paper, we attempt to use the recently developed variational Bayesian mixture of ICA (vbmoICA) [1], to analyze four-phase abdominal CT images for finding the latent meaningful components.

ICA mixture model was first formulated by Lee et al. in [2], in which it is defined as that the observed data are categorized into several mutually exclusive classes, and the data in each class are modeled as being generated by a linear combination of independent sources. It relaxes the assumption of standard ICA that the sources must be independent, and shows improved performance in data classification problems [3]. Lee et al. use the extended Infomax algorithm [4] to switch the source model between sub-Gaussian and super-Gaussian regimes, and learn parameters of the model using gradient ascent to maximize a log-likelihood function. The variational Bayesian

C. Barillot, D.R. Haynor, and P. Hellier (Eds.): MICCAI 2004, LNCS 3217, pp. 916–924, 2004.
© Springer-Verlag Berlin Heidelberg 2004

mixture of ICA used in this paper differs from the Lee's method mainly in two aspects. The first is that, instead of a predefined density model, vbmoICA uses a fully adaptable mixture of Gaussians as the ICA source model, allowing complex and potentially multi-model distributions to be modeled. The second difference is that the mixtures of ICA model are trained using variational Bayesian method, which is carried through to the mixture model. This allows model comparison, incorporation of prior knowledge, control of model complexity thus avoiding over-fitting.

Four-phase abdominal CT images are taken at different phases before and after the contrast material injected. It is often used as an effective measure for tumor detection. The four-phase CT images are modeled as being produced by a mixture of data generators, where each data generator consists of a set of independent components and is responsible for generating a particular cluster. ICA mixture analysis results show that the CT images could be divided into a set of clinically and anatomically meaningful components. Initial analysis of the independent components shows the promising prospect of ICA mixture analysis in medical image processing and computer-aided diagnosis.

In the subsequent pages of this paper, the variational Bayesian mixture of ICA is briefly introduced in section 2. Section 3 presents the meaningful ICA result. In section 4, we discuss its applications with some preliminary analysis. At the last is the conclusion.

2   Variational Bayesian Mixture of ICA

2.1   ICA Mixture Model

Assume that the data $X = \{x^n, n = 1, \cdots, N\}$ are drawn independently and generated by a mixture density model. N is the total number of data vectors and each data vector x^n is of S-dimension. The probability of generating a data vector x^n from a C-component mixture model given assumptions M is given by [1]:

$$p(x^n | M) = \sum_{c=1}^{C} p(c | M_0) p(x^n | M_c, c) \tag{1}$$

A data vector x^n is generated by choosing one of the C components stochastically under $p(c | M_0)$ and then drawing from $p(x^n | M_c, c)$. $M = \{M_0, M_1, \cdots, M_C\}$ is the vector of component model assumption, M_c, and assumption about the mixture process, M_0. The variable c indicates which component of the mixture model is chosen to generate a given data vector x^n. $p(c | M_0)$ is a vector of probabilities. $p(x^n | M_c, c)$ is the component densities and assumed to be non-Gaussian. The mixture density $p(x^n | M)$ is known as the evidence for model M and quantifies the likelihood of the observed data under model M [1].

In the C-component (cluster) mixture model, the observed variables, x, within each cluster are assumed to be generated by linearly transforming an unobserved source vector s_c, of dimension L_c with added Gaussian noise e_c [1],

$$x = A_c s_c + y_c + e_c \tag{2}$$

where y_c is an S-dimensional bias vector, e_c is S-dimensional additive noise and c represents the c-th ICA model (component). In signal processing nomenclature, S is the number of sensors and L_c is the number of latent sources. Equation (2) acts as a complete description for cluster c in the data density. The bias vector, y_c, defines the position of the cluster in the S-dimensional data space, A_c describes its orientation and s_c describes the underlying manifold. The noise, e_c, is assumed to be zero-mean Gaussian and isotropic with precision $\lambda_c I$. The probability of observing data vector x^n under component c is given by [1]

$$p(x^n | \theta_c, c) = \left(\frac{\lambda_c}{2\pi}\right)^{\frac{S}{2}} \exp[-E_c] \tag{3}$$

where $\theta_c = \{A_c, s_c^n, \lambda_c, y_c\}$ and

$$E_c = \frac{\lambda_c}{2}(x^n - A_c s_c^n - y_c)^T (x^n - A_c s_c^n - y_c) \tag{4}$$

Since the sources $s_c = \{s_{c,1}, \cdots, s_{c,i}, \cdots s_{c,L_c}\}$ are by definition mutually independent, the distribution over s_c for data point n can be written as [1]

$$p(s_c^n | M_{S_c}, c) = \prod_{i=1}^{L_c} p(s_{c,i}^n | M_{S_c,i}, c) \tag{5}$$

where the product runs over the L_c sources of component c, and M_{S_c} is the vector of source model assumptions.

In equation (5), $p(s_c^n | M_{S_c}, c)$ is the source model for ICA component c. It is a factorized mixture of 1-dimensional Gaussians with L_c factors (i.e. sources) and m_i components per source

$$p(s_c^n | \varphi_c) = \prod_{i=1}^{L_c} \sum_{q_i=1}^{m_i} \pi_{i,q_i} N(s_{c,i}^n; \mu_{i,q_i}, \beta_{i,q_i}) \tag{6}$$

Equation (6) essentially describes the local features of cluster c, μ_{i,q_i} is the position of feature q_i, β_{i,q_i} is its size, and π_{i,q_i} is its prominence. The mixture proportions π_{i,q_i} are the prior probabilities of choosing component q_i of the i-th source of the c-th ICA model. q_i^n is a variable indicating which component of the i-th source is chosen for generating $s_{c,i}^n$. μ_{i,q_i} and β_{i,q_i} are the mean and covariance of Gaussian q_i in source i. The parameters of i-th source are $\varphi_{c,i} = \{\pi_{c,i}, \mu_{c,i}, \beta_{c,i}\}$ where bold face indicates the vector of m_i parameters. The complete parameter set of the source model is $\varphi_c = \{\varphi_{c,1}, \varphi_{c,2}, \cdots, \varphi_{c,L_c}\}$ [1].

2.2 Variational Bayesian Learning

The above defined ICA mixture model is trained using variational Bayesian method. The prior distributions over the hidden variables and model parameters are given based on the defined mixture model and some additional assumptions. The details are referred to [1]. Bayesian inference in such a model is computationally intensive and

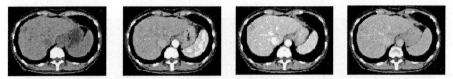

Fig. 1. Four-phase abdominal CT images. They are, from left to right, the pre-contrast image, image of early phase, portal phase, and late phase, respectively. These images are displayed within the range from -110 to 190 H.U.

intractable. To overcome the problem, the variational method [5, 6] is used to make assumptions about the posterior distributions and give tractability to the Bayesian model. The variational Bayesian method constructs a lower bound on the marginal likelihood, and attempts to optimize this bound using an iterative scheme that has intriguing similarities to the standard expectation-maximization algorithm. The parameters of model are learnt by alternating between estimating the posterior distribution over hidden variables for a particular setting of the parameters and then re-estimating the best-fit parameters given that distribution over the hidden variables.

3 ICA Analysis Result

We use the variational Bayesian mixture of ICA algorithm on a set of multi-phase CT images of human abdomen. The data was provided by the National Cancer Center Hospital East, which was collected at four phases before and after contrast material injected. Figure 1 shows the four phases CT images. They are the pre-contrast, early, portal and late images, respectively. The later three phase images were firstly registered to the pre-contrast image by template matching of the center of spine [7]. Then the four 512x512 pixel images were compressed to 170x170 pixel images.

The structure of model can be decided by calculating a term called negative free-energy (NFE) in the vbmoICA. The higher the NFE is, the better the structure that representing the data. Experimentally, we set the number of clusters equals to four, and each cluster is generated from a set of three latent independent components. The four images were vectorised, and 7000 samples were randomly drawn from the data. Then the sampled data were used to train the model. The trained models were then used to unmix the complete dataset into the corresponding independent features.

Figure 2 shows the derived independent components, which present a very meaningful result. The second class of independent components that consists of the components numbered 4-6 appear to be responsible for generating the liver, spleen and stomach areas with the muscle and fat tissue at the outside contour. The third class of ICs (7-9) seem to mainly highlight the ribs and spine, and the forth IC class (10-12) appear to emphasis the lower part of lung. One of the most attractive points is that, in the fifth component, the ribs and lung are completely removed, which makes the segmentation of liver or the spleen area much easier than the original CT images. Another interesting point is that there is a tumor at the left-up end of the liver, and it becomes more visible comparing to the original images.

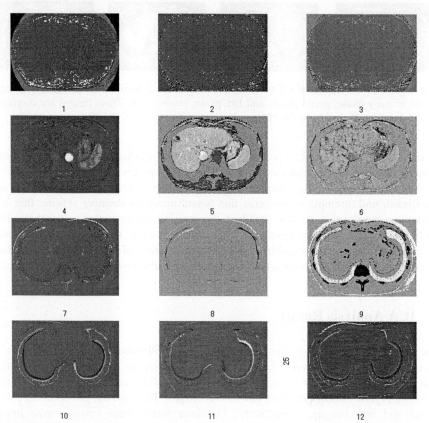

Fig. 2. ICA analysis result of four-phase abdominal CT images using vbmoICA. The data distribution in the vectorised CT images data is assumed to be consists of 4 clusters, and the each cluster is generated from a set of 3 latent independent components. The 4-6 ICs appear to highlight the internal organs, while the 7-9 seems to highlight the ribs and spine, and the 10-12 ICs seems to emphasis the lung. These images are displayed at their whole intensity ranges, respectively.

4   Applications

The anatomically and clinically meaningful result as shown in Fig.2 implies the prospects in various potential applications. Here we discuss its applications in segmentation and tumor detection.

4.1   Liver Area Segmentation

Segmentation of the organs, i.e., extracting boundary elements belonging to the same structure, from medical images is more difficult compared to other imaging fields due

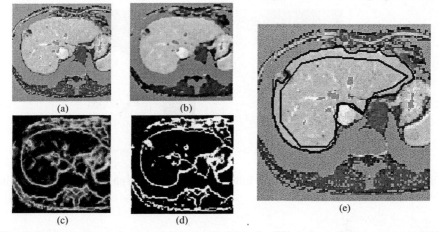

(a)   (b)

(c)   (d)

(e)

Fig. 3. Preprocessing and segmentation result. (a) is the fifth independent component, (b) is the image after smoothing, (c) is the feature image of phase congruency, (d) is the one after sigmoid filter. Figure 3(e) shows the segmentation result. The inner line shows the initial contour and the outer line shows the final reshaped contour of liver area.

to the large variability in shapes and complexity of anatomic structures. For example, the liver area is difficult to segment because surrounding tissues, such as stomach and muscle, have similar CT values and sometimes contact with each other, which may cause the boundaries of structures to be indistinct and disconnected. Although deformable models appear promising result because of their ability to match images of anatomic structures by exploiting constraints derived from the image data, it is still difficult to achieve a satisfying result. Consequently, preprocessing to simplify the complicity will be very helpful and expected.

The GVFSnake method proposed by Xu and Prince [8] is used in the segmentation test on the fifth feature. The difference of GVFSnake from the conventional Snake is that in GVFSnake the gradient vector field (GVF) is first calculated and used for increasing the capture range of the attracting image. The preprocessing includes the following three steps: 1) Smoothing by median filter (Fig.3(b)); 2) Detecting edge using phase congruency filter (Phase congruency is an illumination and contrast invariant measure of feature [9]. It is used here for emphasizing the edge reliably, see Fig.3(c)); 3) Suppressing unnecessary lines by sigmoid filter (Fig.3(d)).

After the processing, it is normal that the image does not only indicate the wanted border, but several others as well (see Fig.3(d)). There should be an initial contour that is quite close to the object to segment; otherwise it might get stuck on an irrelevant border. The initial contour may be obtained using some pixel-wised methods, for example [7]. Here we give it manually. Fig.3(e) shows the segmentation result. The inner line is the initial contour, where the outer line is the final contour. It shows that a good segmentation is easily achieved on the fifth component, which is often difficult on the original images. This is due to the fact that on the fifth feature, some of the tissues surrounding the liver have been removed and the contrast of CT intensities in liver area increased comparatively.

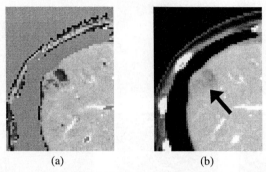

(a)   (b)

Fig. 4. Close-ups of the tumor in (a) the fifth IC, and (b) the portal phase image. The arrow in (b) indicates its location.

4.2   Contrast Variation Around Tumor

Another potential application of ICA analysis result is tumor detection. According to the doctor, there is a tumor at the left-up end of the liver. Fig.4(b) depicts its location. Fig.4 shows the close-ups of tumor on the fifth IC and portal phase image, respectively. It appears that the tumor has been emphasized in the fifth independent component comparing with the four original images, which means that the tumor becomes more detectable on IC than on the original images. For comparing the detectability of tumor quantitatively, we use the evaluation method [10], in which the detectability is quantified using the signal-to-noise ratio defined as below,

$$SNR = (P_{max} - \mu) / \sigma \qquad (7)$$

where, μ and σ denote the mean and standard deviation of the intensities of pixels surrounding the tumor within 10 mm Euclidean distance. P_{max} denotes the maximum intensity value within the tumor area. Table 1 shows the result. The fifth IC has a higher SNR value than the original images, which means the tumor is easier to be found using the independent component.

Table 1. Tumor detectability comparison

	Original CT images				5th IC
	Pre-contrast	Early	Portal	Late	
SNR	3.46	3.20	7.02	4.46	13.16

5   Conclusion

We performed the independent component analysis on several sets of data, and each achieved similar meaningful result. The reason why ICA mixture model can achieve such a meaningful results is not much clear. The explanation could be given is by Choudrey et. al. in [1] that the clusters in the model are learned to be represented by their own local coordinate systems that are constructed under the independent assumption. We once tried the standard ICA model on the CT images but failed to find any interesting phenomena. The reason is thought two: first, standard ICA has not the clustering ability; second, multi-phase CT images actually are highly similar with each other (except for the effect from the contrast material that whitens some particular organs or tissues in a sequence decided by flood circulation), i.e., in the ICA model $x = As$, x are quite similar. This equally means A is nearly singular because each channel of the observed variables is generated under similar mixing process. In such case, the latent features are difficult to be found. On the contrary, the clustering ability of ICA mixture model decreases the difficulty because the independent features are found within each decomposed cluster.

The anatomically and clinically meaningful results make us believe the promising prospect of ICA mixture model as preprocessing to increase the performance of organ segmentation and tumor detection. Currently, we are working on expanding its application on three-dimensional abdominal CT images.

References

[1]   R.A. Choudrey and S.J. Roberts, "Variational mixture of Bayesian independent component analyzers," *Neural Computation*, vol. 15(1), Jan. 2003.

[2]   T.W. Lee, M.S. Lewicki, "Upsupervised image classification, segmentation, and enhancement using ICA mixture models," *IEEE Trans. on Image Processing*, vol. 11, No. 3, March 2002.

[3]   T.W. Lee, M.S. Lewicki, and T.J. Sejnowski, "ICA mixture models for unsupervised classification and automatic context switching," *Proceeding of International workshop on Independent Component Analysis*, 1999, pp.209-214.

[4]   T.W. Lee, M. Girolami, and T.J. Sejnowski, "Independent component analysis using an extended infomax algorithm for mixed sub-Gaussian and super-Gaussian sources," *Neural Computation*, vol. 11, no. 2, pp.409-4333, 1999.

[5]   T. Jaakkola and M. Jordan, "Bayesian parameter estimation via variational methods," *Statistics and Computing*, vol. 10, pp. 25-37, 2000.

[6]   H. Attias, "Learning parameters and structure of latent variable models by variational Bayes," in *Electronic Proceedings of the Fifteenth Annual Conference on Uncertainty in Artificial Intelligence (UAI1999)*, http://www2.sis.pitt.edu/‾dsl/UAI/ uai.html.

[7]   T. Hitosugi, A. Shimizu, M. Tamura, and H. Kobatake, "Development of a liver extraction method using a level set method and its performance evaluation," *Journal of Computer Aided Diagnosis of Medical Images*, vol. 7, No. 4-2, Jun. 2003 (in Japanese).

[8]   C. Xu and J. L. Prince, "Snakes, shapes, and gradient vector flow," *IEEE Trans. on Image Processing*, 7(3), pp. 359-369, Mar. 1998.

[9]   Peter Kovesi, "Image Features From Phase Congruency". *Videre: A Journal of Computer Vision Research*. MIT Press. Volume 1, Number 3, 1999.

[10] Y. Okada, A. Shimizu, H. Kobatake, J. Hasegawa, and J. Toriwaki, "Evaluation of SN ratio of lung tumors in maximum intensity projection images and mean intensity projection images," *Medical Imaging Technology*. Vol. 21, No. 2, pp. 139-146, Mar. 2003 (in Japanese).

Volumetric Deformation Model for Motion Compensation in Radiotherapy

Kajetan Berlinger[1], Michael Roth[1], Jens Fisseler[3], Otto Sauer[2],
Achim Schweikard[3], and Lucia Vences[2]

[1] Technische Universität München, Image Understanding and Knowledge-Based
Systems, Boltzmannstr. 3 D-85748 Garching bei München
berlinge@in.tum.de,
http://www9.in.tum.de/research/med
[2] Universitätsklinikum Würzburg, Radiology Department,
Josef-Schneider-Str. 11 D-97080 Würzburg
[3] Universität Lübeck, Institute for Robotics and Cognitive Systems,
Ratzeburger Allee 160 D-23538 Lübeck

Abstract. A new system is described that can track tumors moving due
to respiratory motion, enabling specific and more effective irradiation of
the tumor. This spares healthy tissue, and allows for higher doses to
treat the tumor. To reach this goal a 3D motion picture of the lung of
the specific patient has to be computed before treatment, because of
the need to infer the respiratory state. This is done in a 4D registration
step, matching 2D radiographs with the computed synthetic 3D scans.
Morphing methods to calculate the deformation of the lung are described
and evaluated.

1 Introduction

To apply radiosurgical methods to tumors in the chest and abdomen, it is necessary to take into account respiratory motion, which can move the tumor by more
than 1 cm. Without compensation, it is unavoidable to enlarge the target volume
by a safety margin. As a consequence, healthy tissue is also affected. Therefore
lower doses must be used to treat the tumor. In [1] we described a method using
implanted fiducials to track the tumor. At the moment we are trying to achieve
our goal without these fiducials, in order to avoid the encumbering operation for
the patient and the medical staff. To solve this problem we need to compute a
correlation between respiratory state and tumor position.

2 Method

Prior to treatment two CT scans are taken. One scan during inhalation, one
during exhalation. From this data we then compute a series of intermediate synthetic CT scans. These are obtained by applying different interpolation methods,
as described in section 3, to the CT scans taken at maximum inhalation and exhalation. This yields a sequence of 3D scans, showing the respiration process as
a three-dimensional motion picture.

C. Barillot, D.R. Haynor, and P. Hellier (Eds.): MICCAI 2004, LNCS 3217, pp. 925–932, 2004.

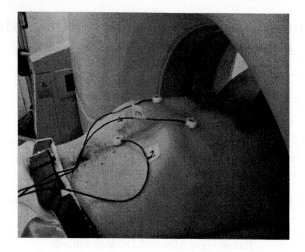

Fig. 1. The emitters, attached to the patient.

For each point in this time series, we compute a set of digitally reconstructed radiographs (DRR). A single DRR is computed by projecting a CT scan from a preselected angle using the known geometry of the imaging system. Thus a DRR can be regarded as a synthetic x-ray image, obtained by projecting through an existing CT volume. For each of the CT scans (synthetic or real), we compute a number of DRRs, each one for a preselected angle.

Before treatment, x-ray images are taken and compared to the set of DRRs we have created. (These x-ray images will be called live images). In these live images the tumor cannot be seen, but in the CT scans the target region is determined. After registration of the live image with the DRRs we know the best matching DRR in the series and therefore also the tumor position and the respiratory state, because of the stored association from a single DRR to its CT scan. Thus we acquire correlation from respiratory state to tumor position.

Instead of using pre-computed DRRs we are currently integrating a new method for online optimization using fast DRR calculation based on standard graphics hardware [2]. At the moment, registration time for a new live image is about 10 seconds for each stack.

This yields only intermittent information about the target location. At the time the comparison of all DRRs with the current live shot is completed, the target may already have moved. To solve this problem we use a sensor to report information on the current state of respiration in *real time*. This sensor is an infrared tracking system, with emitters attached to significant positions on the patient's chest and abdomen (figure 1). Kubo and Hill [7] compared various external sensors, like breath temperature sensor, strain gauge or spirometer, in matters of their applicability for respiratory gating. We use the infrared tracking method within our application, because of its high accuracy and speed as well as its stability under radiation exposure.

The information of the sensor is correlated to the target location computed by the comparison between the live shot and the DRRs. Therefore, the live shot has a time stamp, and we can determine which reading of the real time sensor corresponded to this point in time. Repeating this time stamp synchronization, a complete correlation model can be obtained, which correlates target motion to the readings of the real time sensor (internal to the external motion), without internal fiducials.

The correlation allows the computation of the position of the target volume only. However the therapeutical beam has to reach the target volume, which is in moving, early enough. Both synchronization (gating) and active tracking have latencies due to physical limitations of the particular technique. Therefore predictive tracking uses the periodicity of the particular anatomical signal (respiration or pulsation), in order to compensate for this latency [1].

In figure 2 the setup of the system described above is shown.

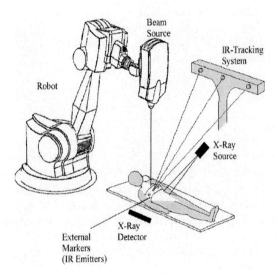

Fig. 2. The setup of our system, with an example of a linear accelerator, an infrared tracking camera and an x-ray device

3   Deformation of the Lung

Brock et al. [9] used finite element analysis to create a four-dimensional model of the liver. We considered two methods for the deformation of the lung, one based on tetrahedrization and the other on thin-plate splines. Both methods need as input:

1. Two initial CT scans, taken during inhalation respectively exhalation (figure 3)
2. The number of desired interpolation steps (number of image stacks of the resulting 3D motion picture)
3. An arbitrary amount of pairs of corresponding control points

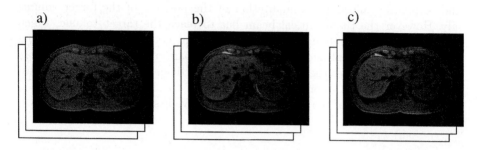

Fig. 3. a) MR scan taken at maximal inhalation. b) Intermediate scan (50% inhalation), only needed for evaluation of the method. c) MR scan taken at maximal exhalation. a and c are needed as input of our method.

3.1   Deformation by Barycentric Coordinates

First the two volumes are tessellated into tetrahedrons by Delaunay tetrahedrization. The control points and the 8 vertices of the bounding box of the volume are used as vertices for this tetrahedrization. During deformation, the vertices are linearly interpolated over time. In each interpolation step, the barycentric coordinates are calculated in relation to the enclosing tetrahedron, for all the points of the actual stack. Using these weights the positions of the corresponding pixels of the two source images are computed. The value of the new pixel is linearly interpolated between these pixels.

3.2   Deformation by Thin-Plate Splines

The second approach is based on thin-plate splines, which were introduced by Duchon in 1976 [3], but in the context of analysis of plane mappings they were first considered by Bookstein [4]. A thin-plate spline interpolates a surface that is constrained not to move at given control points. This surface represents a thin metal plate, which will be deformed into the most economic shape, in reference to its bending energy. The following quantity represents the bending energy of the thin-plate function in 3D space.

$$\int\int\int_{R^3}[(\frac{\partial^2 f}{\partial x^2})^2 + (\frac{\partial^2 f}{\partial y^2})^2 + (\frac{\partial^2 f}{\partial z^2})^2 + 2(\frac{\partial^2 f}{\partial x\partial y})^2 + 2(\frac{\partial^2 f}{\partial x\partial z})^2 + 2(\frac{\partial^2 f}{\partial y\partial z})^2]dxdydz$$

The thin-plate spline function is:

$$f(x, y, z) = a_1 + a_x x + a_y y + a_z z + \sum_{i=1}^{K} w_i U(|Z_i - (x, y, z)|)$$

The function consists of an affine part and a sum of functions $U(r)$, whereas in 3D space $U_{TPS}(r) = |r|$ is used.

In our approach we linearly interpolate the corresponding control point lines and in each interpolation step determine the coefficients of the thin-plate spline function. The number of interpolation steps depends on the number of desired target scans. This method deforms the inhalation scan into the exhalation scan step by step, yielding the 3D motion picture, needed to infer the respiratory state.

3.3   Results

To evaluate the warping algorithms, MR scans of the liver and lung were used. Tests with CT scans are in process. They are obligatory for the whole application of tracking tumors, because of the DRR based registration process.

Both of the methods were tested with 91 control point pairs selected manually by an expert and the two image stacks, one inhalation, one exhalation, (3) as input. 9 intermediate scans, for later registration, were calculated. Calculation times were 64 minutes for the thin-plate spline based method and 69 minutes for the tetrahedrization based method, respectively. Both computations were performed on a 2 GHz standard personal computer.

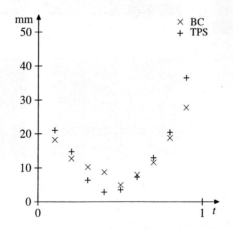

Fig. 4. The surfaces of the liver of all the synthetic intermediate scans were compared to the real intermediate scan. The best results are in the middle of the whole respiration, where the real intermediate scan is located. "TPS" stands for the thin-plate spline based method and "BC" for the tetrahedrization based method.

To evaluate the results we compared them with an intermediate scan, located right between the two initial scans (3). For evaluation, first the liver in the two input scans and in the intermediate scan was segmented. Then the calculations were performed on these images and the same control point pairs as before. After that the reconstructed surfaces of the synthetic intermediate scans were compared to the surface of the real intermediate scan, in order to get the average deviation of the surfaces in mm. The surfaces were reconstructed using the Marching Cubes Algorithm [11]. For each of the surface triangles' vertices of the real intermediate state, the distance to the nearest point on the nearest triangle of the computed intermediate state was calculated. The average deviation is taken to be the mean value of these distances.

As expected, the intermediate data set matches the artificial 4D model best at the middle of the time period of the respiratory cycle (cf. figure 4). The tetrahedrization based method lead to an average deviation of 4.94 mm and the thin-plate spline based method to an average deviation of 3.82 mm.

Additionally we generated some difference images to visualize the results. Figure 5 shows an example with the original image data, and in figure 6 with the segmented data.

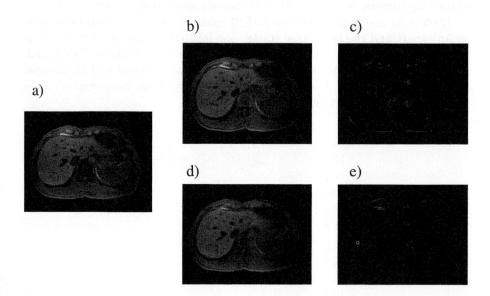

Fig. 5. a) Reference slice of the intermediate scan. b) Corresponding slice of the synthetic scan, same respiratory state, calculated with the thin-plate spline method. c) Difference between a and b. d) Corresponding slice of the synthetic scan, same respiratory state, calculated with the tetrahedrization based method. e) Difference between a and d.

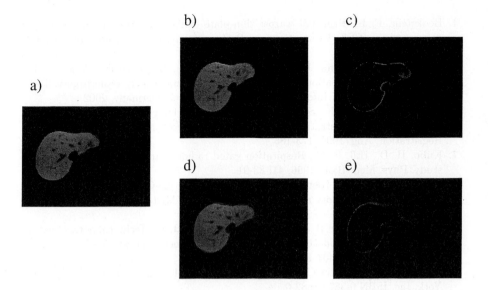

Fig. 6. a) Segmented liver of 5a b) Segmented liver of 5b c) Difference between a and b. d) Segmented liver of 5d e) Difference between a and d.

4   Conclusion and Future Work

We have shown that the computation of the deformation of internal organs due to respiration is feasible. Starting with two data sets, one at the inhal one at the exhal position, the prediction of the target position could be significantly improved using our approach. Our next steps are: Accomplishing a cohort study with a set of intermediate respiratory status CT scans. This will help us to refine our deformation models in order to reduce the residual deviations of artificial data compared to the true trajectories of organ movements.

A procedure is developed, which helps finding control points automatically or at least semi-automatically.

The next clinical goal is to create procedures for obtaining 4D CT images similar to Pan et al. in [8]. For inferring the respiratory state we also will consider the possibility of using portal images instead of radiographs.

References

1. Schweikard, A., Glosser, G., Bodduluri, M., Murphy, M., Adler, J. R., Robotic Motion Compensation for Respiratory Movement during Radiosurgery. Computer-Aided Surgery, Sept. 2000
2. Roth, M., Dötter, M., Burgkart, R., Schweikard, A., Fast intensity-based fluoroscopy-to-CT registration using pattern search optimization, 18th Int. Congress Computer Assisted Radiology and Surgery (CARS 2004), 2004
3. Duchon, J., Interpolation des fonctions de deux variables suivant le principe de la flexion des plaques minces. RAIRO Analyse Numérique, 1976

4. Bookstein, F. L., Principal warps: thin-plate splines and the decomposition of deformations. IEEE Transactions on Pattern Analysis an Machine Intelligence, 1989, 11:567-85
5. Schweikard, A., Shiomi, H., Dötter, M., Roth, M., Berlinger, K., Adler, J. R., Fiducial-less compensation of breathing motion in lung cancer radiosurgery. Technical Report A-02-23, Informatik, Universität Lübeck, Germany, 2002
6. Fornefett, M., Rohr, K., Stiehl, H. S., Radial Basis Functions with Compact Support for Elastic Registration of Medical Images. Workshop on Biomedical Image Registration, Aug. 1999, 173-185
7. Kubo, H. D., Hill, B. C., Respiration gated radiotherapy treatment: a technical study. Phys. Med. Biol., 1996, 41: 83-91
8. Pan, T., Lee, T.-Y., Rietzel, E., Chen, G. T. Y., 4D-CT imaging of a volume influenced by respiratory motion on multi-slice CT. Med. Phys., Feb 2004, Vol. 31 No. 2 333-340
9. Brock, K. K., Hollister, S. J., Dawson, L. A., Balter, J. M., Technical note: Creating a four-dimensional model of the liver using finite element analysis. Med. Phys., July 2002, Vol. 29 No. 7 1403-1405
10. Salomon, D., Computer Graphics and Geometric Modeling. Springer-Verlag New York, Inc. ISBN 0-387-98682-0
11. Lorensen, W. E., Cline, H. E., Marching cubes: A high resolution 3D surface construction algorithm. International Conference on Computer Graphics and Interactive Techniques, 1987, 163-169

Fast Automated Segmentation and Reproducible Volumetry of Pulmonary Metastases in CT-Scans for Therapy Monitoring

Jan-Martin Kuhnigk[1], Volker Dicken[1], Lars Bornemann[1], Dag Wormanns[2], Stefan Krass[1], and Heinz-Otto Peitgen[1]

[1] MeVis, 28359 Bremen, Germany, kuhnigk@mevis.de
[2] Institute for Clinical Radiology, University of Muenster, Germany

Abstract. The assessment of metastatic growth under chemotherapy belongs to the daily radiological routine and is currently performed by manual measurements of largest nodule diameters. As in lung cancer screening where 3d volumetry methods have already been developed by other groups, computer assistance would be beneficial to improve speed and reliability of growth assessment. We propose a new morphology and model based approach for the fast and reproducible volumetry of pulmonary nodules that was explicitly developed to be applicable to lung metastases which are frequently large, not necessarily spherical, and often complexly attached to vasculature and chest wall. A database of over 700 nodules from more than 50 patient CT scans from various scanners was used to test the algorithm during development. An in vivo reproducibility study was conducted concerning the volumetric analysis of 105 metastases from 8 patients that were subjected to a low dose CT scan twice within several minutes. Low median volume deviations in inter-observer (0.1%) and inter-scan (4.7%) tests and a negligible average computation time of 0.3 seconds were measured. The experiments revealed that clinically significant volume change can be detected reliably by the method.

1 Introduction

Since the entire cardiac output flows through the lungs, the risk of hematogenous metastases is very high. Apart from primary lung cancer, the most common tumors involving the lung parenchyma are breast cancer, gastrointestinal tumors, kidney cancer, melanoma, sarcomas, lymphomas and leukemias, and germ cell tumors. Because of the systemic character of the disease, chemotherapy is the standard treatment for lung metastases. To assess the effect of chemotherapy, a follow-up examination is performed typically 3-6 months after the start of the treatment. Tumor growth is the standard decision parameter on whether the current therapy is successful and to be continued, or not, in which case the therapy has to be modified. A similar question arises in the context of lung cancer screening, where nodule growth is used as an indicator for malignancy.

Being a 3-dimensional process, volume growth assessment is a challenging task in 2d CT slices. Current standard criteria (RECIST[1]) require the radiologist to locate the

---

[1] Response Evaluation Criteria in Solid Tumors, see http://ctep.cancer.gov/guidelines/recist.html for further information.

C. Barillot, D.R. Haynor, and P. Hellier (Eds.): MICCAI 2004, LNCS 3217, pp. 933–941, 2004.

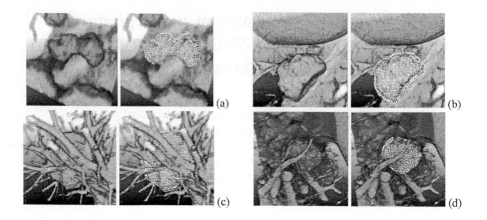

Fig. 1. 3d visualization of segmentation results for large metastases with irregular shape (a, b), extensive contact to the chest wall (a, d), a lobar fissure (b) and complex vasculature (c, d).

five largest tumors in the lung and find the axial slice where the tumor appears largest, in order to manually measure the greatest nodule diameter. Even if measuring errors are neglected, the 2d criteria are reliable only for spherical nodules and do generally fail for irregularly shaped nodules. Additionally, manually finding the correct slice and measuring 2d diameters for each of possibly many nodules not only leads to reproducibility issues but is also time-consuming. In order to assess nodule growth quickly and reliably, computer assistance for reproducible 3d volumetry is desirable.

The need for convenient and reliable growth estimation in the context of lung cancer screening has resulted in the development and evaluation of algorithms for volume assessment of small lesions. Examples of well evaluated algorithms specifically designed for the 3d segmentation of small pulmonary nodules can be found in [1] and [2]. For small nodules that consist mostly of partial volume in CT scans, the step from segmentation to volumetry is especially challenging. Ko et al. [3] compared different volume measurement methods in a phantom study and found that methods with an explicit model for partial volumes (*partial-volume methods, PVM*) perform significantly superior to fixed-threshold methods.

In contrast to the asymptomatic screening population the segmentation approaches mentioned above were primarily designed for, the population of patients undergoing chemotherapy typically suffers from advanced inoperable cancer. Metastatic tumors occur at all stages, so that algorithms have to deal with the full range of appearances, from small spherical nodules ($\varnothing < 10$ mm) consisting mostly of partial volume voxels, to large nodules ($\varnothing > 40$ mm) of irregular morphology. Due to their size, the latter are more likely to be complexly connected to vasculature and chest wall, structures which are in most cases indistinguishable from the nodule with respect to density values in CT scans. Additionally, performance issues arise, since the volume of interest to be analyzed for a 40 mm nodule is about $4^3 = 64$ times larger than for a 10 mm nodule.

Our approach does not include the *computer aided detection (CAD)* of nodules, but can be combined easily with existing CAD methods, examples of which can be found in [4] and [5]. Furthermore, the decision was made not to incorporate information from global lung structure analyses. Whilst robust methods in that area exist ([6], [7]) which could provide helpful information about the nodule location (such as proximity to the chest wall or a lobar fissure), any analysis performed by our method is restricted to the volume of interest. This allows for a simple integration into the workflow of existing clinical workstations.

In the following, the new segmentation procedure is explained in detail. Morphological methods are combined with model based considerations to achieve a robust separation of the nodule from attached structures. To assess the volume of the segmented lesion we developed a method similar to the procedure described by Ko et al. in [3].

2   Methods

2.1   Preliminaries

The algorithm works on a cubic input volume (*VOI, Volume of Interest*). The set V denotes the set of all voxels within the input volume. Density values range from -1024 Hounsfield Units (HU) to 3071 HU. The algorithm works under the assumption that V contains the complete nodule. The *seed point* s is required to be located in the nodule.

The elementary image processing methods included in the segmentation procedure, i. e., thresholding, region growing, connected component analysis, convex hull, Euclidean distance transform, are described and discussed in [8].

2.2   Preprocessing

An **initial segmentation** is performed using a region growing algorithm with a fixed lower threshold of -450 HU starting from the seed point s. The result is an initial set of voxels N_0, the first estimate of the nodule region (Figure 2b).

Subsequently, a *connected component analysis* (also called *region identification*) is performed on the complement of N_0. The largest connected non-segmented area P is extracted. It corresponds to the largest connected area of lung parenchyma in the VOI surrounding the nodule of interest (Figure 2c). For the segmentation, P is used in two ways: First, for nodules with no chest wall attachment, P is basically the complement of N_0, except for dark areas (such as necrosis or noise) within the nodule. We define a superset $N_1 := V - P$ of N_0, which is essentially N_0 with its gaps closed. Second, for nodules with chest wall attachment, P is crucial to the subsequent separation procedure.

2.3   Separation from the Chest Wall

As the example in Figure 2 shows, not only adjacent vasculature but also parts of the chest wall can be included in the initial segmentation result N_0. CT images generally do not show any visible density contrast between the nodule and the attached chest wall (2a). Even expert radiologists are usually unable to determine whether a nodule is still separated from the chest wall by the pleura, or if the chest wall was infiltrated. Thus, we decided to focus on reproducibly segmenting the part of the nodule surrounded by lung parenchyma. In order to achieve this goal, the algorithm makes use of the anatomical fact that the lungs are mostly[2] convex, while the surrounding parenchyma, defined by

---

[2] Noteworthy exceptions to this rule are the diaphragm and cardiac region.

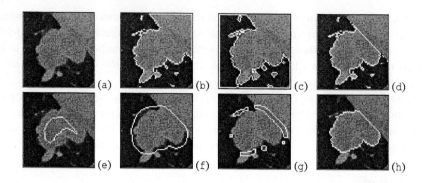

Fig. 2. The essential steps of the segmentation procedure visualized on a single slice. In each of the images (b) to (h), the area enclosed by highlighted boundaries corresponds to a specific set of voxels:

  (a) The situation: A pulmonary nodule with contact to both chest wall and vasculature.
  (b) N_0 : Result of the initial 3d region growing.
  (c) P : Complement of N_0 (in this case).
  (d) N_2 : Intersection of N_0 with the convex hull of P.
  (e) N_- : Result after the 3d erosion procedure.
  (f) N_+ : Result of the 3d dilation (using the secondary distance map D).
  (g) I_ε : Dilated intersection of the boundaries of N_+ (Fig. f) with the initial mask N_0
          (Fig.b).
  (h) $N_\star$: Refined segmentation result, obtained by combination of f and g.

P, shows at least one major concavity: the nodule itself. To remove concavities from an object, a *convex hull* operation can be used. It provides the minimal extension of a set S to a convex set that contains all points of S. The mask convex hull of P is used to mask out the chest wall part from N_1 and provide an improved estimate of the nodule region $N_2 := N_1 \cap \mathrm{convexHull}\,(P)$. The result can be seen in Figure 2d.

2.4 Separation from Attached Vasculature

Since the pleura separation is only capable of masking out structures that are not part of the lungs, adjacent vessels are still included in N_2. Since the algorithm aims specifically at the volumetry of large pulmonary metastases, extensive connections to vasculature are to be expected (as in Figures 1c and 1d).

    The density information in CT images does not suffice to allow a density-based separation procedure. However, nodules and vessels differ significantly in morphology. By making use of the fact that the nodule's connection to the vasculature is usually thinner than the nodule itself, a separation of the structures is performed by *morphological opening* (erosion followed by dilation). Two distance transformations were used to implement the erosion and dilation. A similar procedure was used to label aneurysm voxels in [9]. A *primary 3d Euclidean distance transform E* is performed to compute the minimum distance from each voxel in N_1 to the background. World coordinates are used in order to account for voxel anisotropy:

$$E(v) := \min \{\| \mathrm{world}(v) - \mathrm{world}(v') \|_2 : v' \notin N_1\}.$$

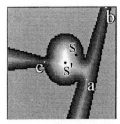

Schematic view of a nodule with vascular connection showing the primary distances in E represented by gray values, the initial seed point s, the corrected seed point s' as well as the three points a, b, c, indicating the minimum vessel radius on any path from s' to the VOI boundaries. The greatest distance value of all three points, in this case $E(a)$, provides the lower boundary for the erosion strength, since its application would remove the connections to any of the attached vessels.

Fig. 3. Vascular connectivity model.

The erosion is implemented by applying a threshold to the distance map. The crucial part of the operation is to find an optimal erosion threshold in order to cut off unwanted adjacent structures without clipping significant nodule boundary features. The determination of the threshold will be discussed in detail in the following.

Starting from the given seed point s, a local maximum search is performed on the distance map yielding a new seed point s' (Figure 3). For the determination of the optimal erosion threshold t_*, a model was established (see also Figure 3) which makes the following two assumptions with respect to vascular attachment: *(1) Each lung vessel is ultimately originating in the hilum region.* Hence, each vessel connected to the nodule is also connected to the VOI boundaries. *(2) Each vessel's diameter is monotonic decreasing with the increasing distance to the hilum.* Thus, if a vessel ends at the nodule, its diameter is smallest at its entry point into the nodule (point **c** in Figure 3). If a vessel only touches a nodule, the smallest diameters along the two possible paths from the touching point to the VOI boundaries are located directly at the boundaries (point **b** in Figure 3) and in close proximity to the nodule (point **a** in Figure 3). Given assumption (2), the latter is bigger than the former. Hence, by using the maximum of all minimal path diameters as a lower bound for the erosion strength parameter, we ensure that vessels are disconnected by the erosion in close proximity to their connection with the nodule. We will refer to this erosion threshold by t_*, since it is optimal with respect to the proposed model. The proposed procedure implies the limitation that a nodule cannot be separated from a broadly attached vessel that has a larger radius than the nodule itself. However, these cases appear to be extremely rare[3]. To actually compute t_*, a variable threshold region growing was performed on E which determines the highest threshold sufficient to reach the VOI boundaries from s'. To be less susceptible to noise and discretization artifacts, the actual erosion threshold t_- is chosen slightly greater than t_*.

To perform the second step of the opening, the dilation, a *secondary distance map* D is generated, mapping each voxel to its distance to the eroded nodule mask N_-:

$$D(v) := \min \{\| \text{ world}(v) - \text{world}(v') \|_2 : v' \in N_-\}.$$

2.5 Boundary Refinement

The dilation threshold t_+ is selected slightly larger than t_-, i.e., $t_+ := t_- + \varepsilon$ (Figure 2f) to include small irregularities in the nodule boundaries that were previously eradicated

---

[3] None was encountered during the described experiment, and our database of 700 pulmonary metastases included only a single case.

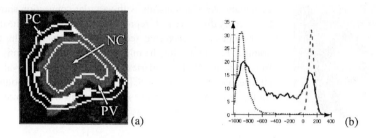

Fig. 4. (a) The white contour lines depict (from the inside to the outside) the nodule core (NC), partial volume (PV) and the parenchyma (PC) regions. The PV region is defined by the set of all voxels within 2 mm to the segmented nodule boundaries in either direction. The thick white areas (I_ε) are to be excluded from the PV region, since they were determined to be vascular attachments during the boundary refinement step (Figure 2g). (b) Histograms for the parenchyma region (dotted line), the nodule core region (dashed) and the partial volume area (solid).

by the erosion procedure. Previously removed vessel and chest wall parts are added in $N_+ := \{v \in V : D(v) < t_+\}$ as well. We therefore compute the intersection of the initial segmentation with the boundaries of the dilated mask, $I := N_0 \cap \partial N_+$. Dilating I by ε results in I_ε (see Figure 2g), which is used to removed unwanted structures. Our final segmentation result $N_\star$ (Figure 2h) is then defined as

$$N_\star := N_+ \setminus I_\varepsilon$$

2.6   Volumetry

The segmentation procedure described above performs its boundary refinement by using the initial fixed threshold segmentation results. As shown by Ko et al. in [3], fixed threshold methods are not suitable to reproducibly assess nodule volumes, especially for smaller nodules. In contrast to the experiments performed in [3], we have to deal with vasculature and chest wall regions within the volume of interest. Thus, a variation of the PVMA method described there was developed: Based on the segmentation result $N_\star$, three different areas, the nodule core (NC), a parenchyma area (PC) and a partial volume region (PV) are automatically identified (Figure 4). Average attenuation values are extracted from NC and PC to allow a weighted contribution of the voxels within PV to the nodule volume. In case the region NC is too small to extract a reliable average, we assume a fixed mean nodule density typical for solid nodules (i. e., 50 HU) instead.

3   Experiments and Results

During the development process, the segmentation method was repeatedly applied to a database containing over 700 lung nodules from various patients and CT scanners to ensure its robustness against the variety of nodule appearances in CT data. These nodules were not used in the reproducibility tests described in the following. Reproducibility of

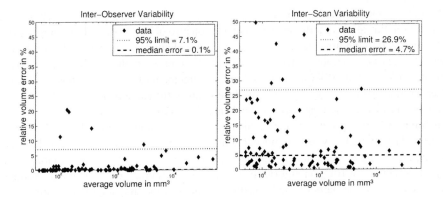

Fig. 5. Bland and Altman plots of absolute inter-observer and inter-scan variability.

volumetric results over different scans is essential with respect to tumor follow up. A study was performed using 16 CT scans (low-dose, 0.8 mm reconstruction increment, standard lung reconstruction kernel) from 8 patients with lung metastases acquired with a Siemens VolumeZoom CT scanner. After the first scan, the patient was asked to leave the scanner and the second low-dose scan was obtained independently from the first. The cases were processed by an expert radiologist and a radiological technician both unaware of the internals of the segmentation method. 105 lesions were identified by the radiologist with a minimum diameter of about 4.6 mm (the equivalent to 0.05 ml of volume for a spherical nodule). To ensure that seed points and surrounding volumes were selected without bias, the identified locations were used only for a rough indication of the nodule positions. In addition to the principal study comparing the measured volumes in the first and second scan, inter-observer repeatability tests were performed for the 8 primary scans.

For 96 of the total of 105 nodules (91.4%) the segmentation was classified as successful by the radiologist, the remaining 9 were excluded from the evaluation. The Bland and Altman statistic [10] was used to determine inter-observer variability as well as the agreement of volume measurement at both CT scans, called inter-scan variability in the following. The mean volume of the measurements was used to estimate the unknown true nodule volume. Median error and 95% limits of agreement (meaning that an increase of the measured volume by more than the computed limit has a 95% likelihood of being real growth rather than measurement inaccuracy) were computed and included in Figure 5. The volume differences are plotted as a percentage of the mean of the two measurements in Figure 5. Computation time measurements on a 3.2 GHz PC revealed a mean of 0.3 and a maximum of 4.1 seconds.

4   Discussion and Future Work

We have developed a new method for the volume assessment of lung tumors. One of the main features of the segmentation is the automated determination of an optimal erosion strength for the morphological opening procedure. In combination with the chest wall separation, this allows for the robust segmentation also of larger, irregularly shaped nodules attached to the lung surface and complex vasculature. An in vivo study conducted on 105 metastases demonstrated a small inter-observer variability (95% limit of agreement: 7.1%, median: 0.1%). The 95% limit of agreement of 26.9% (median: 4.7%) for measurements on two independent low-dose scans of the same patient shows that clinically significant volume increase can be detected reliably by the proposed method. The computation time on a PC was negligible (mean: 0.3 sec., maximum: 4.1 sec.). The evaluation of reproducibility on two independent low-dose patient CT scans is a challenging setting. Ongoing evaluation activities include phantom studies to assess variability under different reconstruction algorithms and absolute accuracy of the method. Nodules attached to concave parts of the lung surface (such as the diaphragm) appeared to be responsible for most of the larger measurement discrepancies, the improvement of their segmentation is subject of future methodological work.

By targeting the fast reproducible volumetric assessment of large pulmonary metastases, the presented method extends the applicability of 3d computer assisted lung nodule volumetry to chemotherapy monitoring. By the knowledge of the authors, no applications or algorithms designed for that purpose have previously been published.

The algorithm has been integrated into an application prototype using the research and development platform MeVisLab[11]. The prototype has been installed at six German and two North American clinics for further evaluation.

Acknowledgments. The research leading to this publication has been supported by the German Federal Ministry of Education and Research under grant number 01EZ0010. It was conducted as part of the cooperation project VICORA – Virtual Institute for Computer Assisted Radiology. Special thanks go to Dr. H. Bourquain and T. Schleef for their participation in the study.

References

1. Kostis WJ; Reeves AP; Yankelevitz DF; Henschke CI: *Three-dimensional segmentation and growth-rate estimation of small pulmonary nodules in helical CT images.* In: IEEE Trans. on Med. Imaging, **22(10)** (2003) 1259 – 1274
2. Wormanns D; Kohl G; Klotz E; et al: *Volumetric measurements of pulmonary nodules at multi-row detector CT: in vivo reproducibility.* In: Eur. Radiol. **14(1)** (2004) 86–92.
3. Ko JP; Rusinek H; Jacobs EL; et al: *Small Pulmonary Nodules: Volume Measurement at Chest CT – Phantom Study.* In: Radiology, **228(3)** (2003) 864–870
4. Armato SG III; Giger ML; Moran CJ; et al: *Computerized detection of pulmonary nodules on CT scans.* In: Radiographics, **19(5)** (1999) 1303–1311
5. Brown MS; McNitt-Gray MF; Goldin JG; et al: *Patient-specific models for lung nodule detection and surveillance in CT images.* In: IEEE Trans. on Med. Imaging, **20** (2001) 1242–1250
6. Reinhardt JM; Guo J; Zhang L; et al: *Integrated System for Objective Assessment of Global and Regional Lung Structure.* In: Proc. of MICCAI 2001, LNCS **2208** (2001) 1384–1385
7. Kuhnigk JM; Hahn HK; Hindennach M; et al: *Lung Lobe Segmentation by Anatomy-Guided 3D Watershed Transform.* In: Proc. of SPIE Medical Imaging 2003, **5032** (2003) 1482-1490

8. Sonka M; Hlavac V; Boyle R: *Image Processing, Analysis and Machine Vision*; 2nd Ed; International Thomson Publishing, (1998)

9. Bruijns J: *Fully-Automatic Lebelling of Aneurysm Voxels for Volume Estimation*. In: Proc. of Bildverarbeitung fuer die Medizin, (2003) 51–55

10. Bland JM, Altman DG: *Statistical methods for assessing agreement between two methods of clinical measurement*. In: Lancet 1 **(8476)** (1986) 307–310

11. Hahn HK, Link F, Peitgen HO: *Concepts for a Rapid Prototyping Platform in Medical Image Analysis and Visualization*. In: Proc. SimVis, SCS (2003) 283–298

Bone Motion Analysis from Dynamic MRI: Acquisition and Tracking

Benjamin Gilles[1], Rosalind Perrin[2], Nadia Magnenat-Thalmann[1], and Jean-Paul Vallée[2]

[1] MIRALab, University of Geneva, CH-1211 Geneva, Switzerland,
{gilles, thalmann}@miralab.unige.ch
[2] Geneva University Hospital, Radiology department, CH-1205 Geneva, Switzerland,

Abstract. For diagnosis, preoperative planning and postoperative guides, an accurate estimate of joints kinematics is required. We bring together MRI developments and new image processing methods in order to automatically extract active bone kinematics from multi-slice real-time dynamic MRI. We introduce a tracking algorithm based on 2D/3D registration and a procedure to validate the technique by using both dynamic and sequential MRI. We present how we optimize jointly the tracking method and the acquisition protocol to overcome the trade-off in acquisition time and tracking accuracy. As a case study, we apply this methodology on the human hip joint.

1 Introduction

Periacetabular osteotomy is an accepted surgical procedure to reorient the acetabulum in patients with hip symptoms of mechanical overload, impingement or femoral head instability. For both the diagnosis and the surgical planning, an accurate estimate of hip joint bone motion is required. Orthopedists can use animated 3D models, prior to joints surgeries, to evaluate their task and generally to reduce the overall time of the surgical operation. The long-term objective of our ongoing project is to model, analyze and visualize human joint motion in-vivo and non-invasively.

In order to deduce kinematical properties of the musculoskeletal system, techniques have been developed to measure internal motion of organs. The use of bone screws or implantable markers [1] provides a gold standard of bone motion measurement, although it is a very invasive approach. Optical motion capture consisting in recording markers trajectories attached to the skin leads to inaccuracy in the estimation of the position of internal organs because of fat/skin sliding artifacts [2]. Nowadays, medical imaging technology has reached a level where it is possible to capture internal motion with different modalities (CT, MRI, US). Several authors have reported kinematic studies of joints with sequential MRI acquisition techniques to evaluate the joint under passive motion, meaning the joint is stationary during acquisition. Brossmann et al. [3] reported the importance of acquiring joint motion actively, due to the existence of statistically significant variations between acquiring actively or passively. However,

C. Barillot, D.R. Haynor, and P. Hellier (Eds.): MICCAI 2004, LNCS 3217, pp. 942–949, 2004.

the problem of acquiring volumetric image data in real-time with MRI during active motion remains to be solved due to inherent trade-off in the MR imaging technique between Signal-to-Noise Ratio (SNR), spatial resolution and temporal resolution. Quick et al [4] published results on the use of the trueFISP (or b-FFE, FIESTA) imaging sequence for real-time imaging of active motion of the hand, ankle, knee and elbow (matrix 135 X 256, 6 frames/s) on a single slice. Bone motion tracking in 2D dynamic images, which are incomplete from a spatial point of view, is equivalent to a 2D/3D rigid registration between dynamic images and the static MRI volume used to reconstruct 3D models. Various registration methods have been proposed in the literature [5]. 2D/3D multimodal rigid registration has been investigated for intra-operative navigation using mainly X-rays and CT data. Tomazevic et al. [6] presented a technique based on bone surface matching; Zöllei et al. [7], a method based on mutual information optimization.

This paper presents the selection of the best dynamic imaging protocol available to our group and the adaptation of the technique to the joint motion extraction problem. We introduce a new technique to track bone motion automatically from real-time dynamic MRI based on the combination of temporal information of dynamic MRI and spatial information of static MRI by 2D/3D registration. Bone motion tracking in sequential MRI is used as a gold standard bone position measurement. Subsequently, we present how we optimized both the tracking method and the acquisition protocol to overcome the trade-off in acquisition time and tracking accuracy.

2   Real-Time Dynamic Images Acquisition

2.1   In Vitro Study

The acquisition was performed with a 1.5T Intera MRI system (Philips Medical Systems, Best NL). In a first step, the b-FFE (balanced Fast Field Echo, Philips Medical Systems, Best NL) imaging sequence (aka. trueFISP) was quantitatively compared to four other sequences, including Turbo Spin Echo (TSE), RF-spoiled FFE (T1-FFE) and a Field Echo, Echo Planar Imaging (FE-EPI) sequence. In order to quantify sequence performance, a phantom consisting of tubes of Gd-DTPA (Schering AG, Germany) at varying concentrations was used. Using this phantom, measurements of SNR could be made for a range of physiological T2/T1 values. The b-FFE sequence was found to outperform all other ultra-fast MR sequences available on the scanner in terms of SNR divided by the acquisition time, SNRt. The SNR and CNR (between muscle and fat) was optimal at a flip angle of 90deg for b-FFE sequence. Partial Fourier acquisition in the read-out direction was possible without significant reduction in image quality. This enabled the scan time to be reduced by 30%.

2.2   In Vivo Study

The imaging protocol was developed and optimized with reference to the limitations of the tracking algorithm. First, the trade off in image quality with

FOV and matrix was investigated qualitatively on healthy volunteers in order to achieve the optimum resolution, contrast and frame acquisition time. As scan duration was proportional to the phase encode matrix, the phase encode matrix was maintained <100 at the shortest repetition time possible (TR 3.5ms). It was found that reducing the FOV and hence the phase encode matrix, maintaining an in-plane resolution of 2mm, was not an effective way to reduce frame acquisition time, due to the need to use fold-over suppression to avoid aliasing in the phase encode direction. A parallel imaging technique, SENSE (Philips Medical Systems, Best NL), was found to reduce the scan time by a factor of 2 without significant reduction in image quality. A reference scan is acquired prior to the SENSE MR sequence to measure the sensitivity profile of the phased-array coil. The same reference scan is used for all the images of the dynamic series.

A positioning device was developed that facilitated reproducible abductive motion in both sequential and dynamic modes. A study was run with six healthy volunteers to optimize and evaluate the robustness of the registration-MRI protocol combination without the introduction of motion artifacts. Ethics approval was obtained from the local ethics committee for the study protocol. In a first session a complete static image data set of the pelvis and femur was acquired with a 2D multi-slice spin echo acquisition (TR/TE 578/18ms). In the second scan session the joint was stepped successively in abduction, and at a range of positions two scans were run. A 3D sequential acquisition at high spatial resolution (fast gradient echo sequence with radial reconstruction: FFE, TR/TE 6.4/3.1ms, Flip angle 15deg, FOV/matrix 500mm/410x512) was run to localize the hip position (gold standard) and secondly the optimized 2D dynamic protocol was run (seven imaging planes, gradient echo sequence with balanced gradients: bFFE, TR/TE 3.5/1.1ms, Flip angle 80deg, pixel size 2 x 2mm, slice thickness 10mm, partial Fourier reduction factor of 0.65 in read direction). The slice positions of the dynamic slices were required to be adjusted to intersect appropriate bony landmarks on each volunteer. These planes were set initially and maintained throughout the sequential motion protocol.

3   Bone Motion Tracking

3.1   Mathematical Definitions

Prior to tracking, the femur and the pelvis are automatically segmented and reconstructed from the static image data (three volumes rigidly registered in the static coordinate system W_s) using a deformable model-based method presented in [8] (see Fig. 1). We use a 3D simulation method based on bone-to-bone collision detection (see [9] for more details) to determine a fixed hip joint center of rotation C. Standard orthogonal coordinate systems of the femur (S_f) and the pelvis (S_p) are centered on C and oriented using anatomical landmarks [10] (see Fig.1). Let $M_f = M_{(S_f \to W_s)}$ (resp. $M_p = M_{(S_p \to W_s)}$) be the corresponding homogeneous transformation matrices.

The bone tracking problem is equivalent to rigidly registering at each instant t the 3D static volume where bony regions have been segmented and the 2D

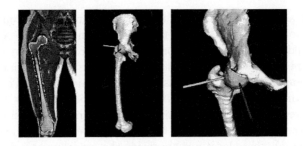

Fig. 1. Results of the automatic femur segmentation on a sample slice, reconstructed 3D models and standard coordinate system of the pelvis.

dynamic planes. A registration problem can often be stated as a functional energy minimization. The energy, calculated with a similarity metric [11], measures how good the matching is. Let θ_t^f (resp. θ_t^P) be the six registration parameters for translations and rotations of the femur (resp. the pelvis). Dynamic plane relative positions are defined from the acquisition parameters as a set of N (number of planes) coordinate systems P_i ($i \in [0.., N]$) in the dynamic acquisition system W_d corresponding to the homogeneous matrices $O_i = M_{(P_i \rightarrow W_d)}$. We define a transformation $\phi^f : \Re^2 X \aleph \rightarrow \Re^3$ (resp. $\phi^P : \Re^2 X \aleph \rightarrow \Re^3$) that maps a point of the plane z=0 in P_i to a point in Ws for the femur (resp. the pelvis) such as (method A):

$$\phi_{\theta_t^f}^f(x, y, i) = M_f.Q_t^f.O_i.[x, y, 0, 1]^T \text{ and } \phi_{\theta_t^P}^P(x, y, i) = M_p.Q_t^P.O_i.[x, y, 0, 1]^T$$

$$(1)$$

$Q_t^f = M_{(W_d \rightarrow S_f)}$ (resp. $Q_t^P = M_{(W_d \rightarrow S_p)}$) is defined by θ_t^f (resp. θ_t^P) using unit quaternions formulation for rotations [12]. It represents the position of the femur (pelvis) in W_d. ϕ can be expressed in different ways. For instance, we can use the relative position between the femur and the pelvis such as $Q_t^{rel} = Q_t^P(Q_t^f)^{-1}$ (method B). In this case, θ_t^{rel} (defining Q_t^{rel}) are the registration parameters. The conversion of Q_t^{rel} into standard hip joint angles gives normalized flexion, adduction and internal rotation angles which are medically relevant angles. Another way to represent ϕ is to use the variation of the relative transformations between the femur and the pelvis from one frame to the next one: $Q_t^{diff} = (Q_{t-1}^{rel})^{-1} Q_t^{rel}$ (method C).

The similarity metric aims at measuring the degree of alignment between the reference dataset (static MRI volume) and the transformed dataset (dynamic MRI images). In case of MR images, no similarity metric has proven to be superior especially when using different acquisition protocols with different tissues/intensity transfer functions. Roche et al. showed the importance of choosing an appropriate metric [13]. We have implemented three standard similarity metrics [11]: normalized cross-correlation (NCC), absolute differences (AD) and mutual information (MI). In addition, we use a metric we call "model matching"

(MM) that measures, independent of the static volume, the alignment of the re-constructed model and the edges of the dynamic images. Also, NCC, AD and MM are applied to the gradient vector images and are denoted by GNCC, GAD and GMM. Grey-scale values in the static volume are trilinearly interpolation at floating positions defined by the transformed dynamic images. The similarity is performed in the bone neighborhood where the motion is purely rigid. In other words, soft tissues that deform significantly are ignored. Considering a bone model reconstructed from the static MRI volume, we define a mask (subset of the static volume) where locations are inside the model or at a distance, deter-mined empirically, of 5mm from its surface. The mask is automatically generated using the ICP (Iterative Closest Point) algorithm.

3.2   Registration Procedure

The hip bone tracking problem to be resolved is to find, at each instant t and for each bone, the solution parameters θ_t^* that minimize the similarity measurement between the static volume and the transformed dynamic images. We can use ei-ther method A, B or C to define the rigid transformation. Given an optimization method Ψ and a solution search space Θ, we have:

$$\theta_t^* = argmin_{(\theta_t \in \Theta | \Psi)} \Delta(\phi_{\theta_t}(D_{r,t}), S_r) \qquad (2)$$

A coarse initialization is done manually. We use the amoeba optimizer, which is an implementation of the Nelder-Mead method [14] derived from simplex algorithm, as it is parameterizable (the number of iterations and the scale used when a parameter is modified can be set) and relatively robust in presence of local solutions. The three transformation parameters for rotations are the angle of the unit quaternion q defining Q_t and two orthogonal components used to modify the vectorial part of q.

Tracking bones in a real-time sequences, yields to the question of the ini-tialization: how to provide an accurate initialization for a particular frame t, knowing bones position in the preceding ones? The pelvis remains nearly immo-bile during movement implying that the user initialization for the first frame is suitable for the others. As a first step, we use method A to track the pelvis as it is independent to the position of the femur. To initialize the femur, we make the assumption that the movement is uniform. We tested two different initializations that led to comparable results: the spherical quaternion interpolation (so-called Slerp [12]) for Q_t^{rel} using frames $t-1$ and $t-2$ with an interpolation parame-ter equals to 2, and the use of the variation of relative transformation such as $Q_t^{diff} = Q_{t-1}^{diff}$. The tracking is done using method C as it is more convenient for the optimization. More precisely, if the motion of the femur with regards to the pelvis is planar, which is roughly correct, only one optimization parameter (quaternion angle Ω) defining Q_t^{diff} is modified. Obviously, for frames 0 and 1, where we cannot use method C formulation as it depends on $t-2$ frame, we use method B.

4   Results

4.1   Tracking in Sequential MRI

3D sequential acquisition gives a gold standard of bone positioning as it provides high spatial resolution. Because of acquisition time constraints, the sequential acquisition protocol (fast) is different to the initial static acquisition protocol. Bones tracking is done in two steps. First, bones positions are initialized for the first frame $t = 0$ assuming that there is no translation of the hip joint center (HJC) and using GMM metric which is computationally fast. At $t = 0$, the subject is in a neutral position (near zero position) and we have a good confidence that the HJC (estimated with method [9]) is correct as zero position is the reference for this calculation. It is corroborated by visual inspection of the alignment between bones contours in sequential MRI and 3D models. Second, the sequential volume at $t = 0$ is used as the reference (static) volume to track bones in the other frames, with AD metric. AD metric is accurate in this case because contrasts are the same. Translation parameters of the relative position between the pelvis and the femur represent the translation of the estimated HJC. Over 46 different positions (36 abductions, 5 flexions and 5 internal/external rotations) and 6 different subjects, the average translation is 0.53mm (standard deviation = 0.4mm, maximum = 2.4mm). It shows that the error in estimating the HJC (cumulated with possible translation of the real HJC) is minor.

4.2   Optimization and Validation of the Method

To measure the goodness of the tracking in dynamic MRI and hence to validate it, we compared, for a fixed subject position, pelvis/femur relative positions tracked in dynamic MRI with the ones tracked in sequential acquisition. The difference provides, similarly to [13], errors in rotation and translation. By minimizing these errors, we optimized tracking parameters. We determined empirically the parameters of the amoeba optimization procedure: scale of 1mm for translations, scales of 0.05mm and 0.05rad for rotations (defined with quaternions) and 200 iterations. We compared the seven different similarity metrics that we have implemented, keeping the same initial conditions (seven imaging planes, same initialization and same optimization parameters). For the mutual information metric, we estimated probability densities by using the joint histogram with 1000 random samples and 32 intensity bins in the range of 0-255. We found that normalized cross-correlation based on gradient vector images performs the best tracking in terms of accuracy: mean error in translation = 1.8mm (standard deviation = 1mm), mean error in rotation = 1.3deg (standard deviation = 0.7deg). Also it was found to be the most robust metric (the variation of the similarity around the solution was the sharpest).

In order to speed up the dynamic acquisition time, it is important to select the smallest number of planes and the smallest resolution that still preserve a acceptable accuracy (3deg of error in rotation). We measured the accuracy of the tracking (with the same tracking parameters) for all combinations of three planes from the initial configuration of seven imaging planes. For the tested abductive motion, optimal planes pass near the HJC and are approximately orthogonal as shown in Fig. 2. The mean error in translation is 2.4mm (standard deviation = 1mm) and the mean error in rotation is 2.1deg (standard deviation = 1.1deg). With this configuration, we simulated different resolutions by gaussian filtering and subsampling dynamic grey-scale images. A resolution of 4x4mm was found to be the limit: mean error in translation = 3.3mm (standard deviation = 1.7mm), mean error in rotation = 3.3deg (standard deviation = 1.5deg).

4.3   Application on Real-Time Dynamic MRI

We applied our method on real-time dynamic sequences (with motion artifacts) and obtained visually satisfactory results. The dynamic protocol was a fast gradient echo sequence with balanced gradients (bFFE, TR/TE 3.5/1.1ms, Flip angle 80deg, pixel size 4.7 x 2.6mm, partial Fourier reduction factor of 0.65 in read direction, SENSE acceleration factor of 2, frame rate = 6.7 frames/s). This protocol provides sufficient morphological data for bone tracking to be carried out. For the optimization we used the parameters: GNCC metric, 200 iterations, 1 mm for the translation scale, 0.05 mm and 0.05 rad for rotation scales. In case of a free abductive motion, with no positioning device, it was difficult to constrain the femur to remain in the coronal plane. Hence we used four planes by adding another coronal plane parallel to the previous one (Fig. 2).

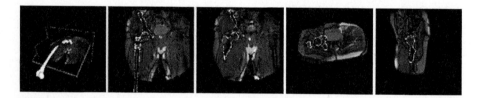

Fig. 2. 3D representation of the bones and the 4 dynamic acquisition planes, and corresponding MR images with tracked bones (in white)

5   Conclusion and Future Work

We present an automatic and optimized method to track bone motion from multi-slice dynamic MRI which was not previously available. This offers an accurate and non-invasive technique for the active kinematical analysis of human joints. We plan to improve the technique in terms of computational speed by using the multi-resolution approach in the optimization procedure and test the method on various movements like flexion/extension or internal/external rotation. Also, the study of the relative motion between skin markers and bones, with regards to joint angles, is under investigation. A possible application is the reduction of skin/fat sliding artifacts in optical motion capture.

Acknowledgments. This work is supported by CO-ME (Computer Aided and Image Guided Medical Interventions, www.co-me.ch) project funded by Swiss National Research Foundation. We would like to thank Dr. H. Sadri from the orthopedic surgery department of the Southern Hospital of Fribourg for his collaboration and the Geneva University Hospital for partial support.

References

1. Lafortune, M., Cavanagh, P., Sommer, H., Kalenak, A.: Threedimensional kinematics of the human knee during walking. Journal of Biomechanics **25** (1992) 347–357
2. Magnenat-Thalmann, N., Yahia-Cherif, L., Gilles, B., Molet, T.: Hip joint reconstruction and motion visualization using mri and optical motion capture. Proceeding of the Austrian, German and Swiss society for biomedical technology congress (EMB) (2003)
3. Brossmann, J., Muhle, C., Schroder, C., Metchert, U., Bull, C., Spielmann, R., Heller, M.: Patellar tracking patterns during active and passive knee extension: evaluation with motion-triggered cine mr imaging. Radiology **187** (1993) 205–212
4. Quick, H., Ladd, M., Hoevel, M., Bosk, S., Debatin, J., Laub, G., Schroeder, T.: Real-time mri of joint movement with truefisp. Journal of Magnetic Resonance Imaging **15** (2002) 710–715
5. Brown, L.: A survey of image registration techniques. ACM Computing Surveys **24** (1992) 325–376
6. Tomazevic, D., Likar, B., Slivnik, T., Pernus, F.: 3-d/2-d registration of ct and mr to x-ray images. IEEE Transactions on Medical Imaging **22** (2003) 1407–1416
7. Zöllei, L., Grimson, E., Norbash, A., Wells, W.: 2d-3d rigid registration of x-ray fluoroscopy and ct images using mutual information and sparsely sampled histogram estimators. IEEE CVPR (2001)
8. Yahia-Cherif, L., Gilles, B., Moccozet, L., Magnenat-Thalmann, N.: Individualized bone modeling from mri: Application to the human hip. Proceedings of Computer Assisted Radiology and Surgery (CARS) (2003)
9. Kang, M., Sadri, H., Moccozet, L., Magnenat-Thalmann, N.: Hip joint modeling for the control of the joint center and the range of motions. Proceedings of the IFAC symposium on modelling and control in biomedical systems (2003) 23–27
10. Wu, G., Siegler, S., Allard, P., Kirtley, C., Leardini, A., Rosenbaum, D., Whittle, M., D'Lima, D., Cristofolini, L., Witte, H., Schmid, O., Stokes, I.: Isb recommendation on definitions of joint coordinate system of various joints for the reporting of human joint motion-part i: ankle,hip, and spine. Journal of biomechanics **35** (2002) 543–548
11. Holden, M., Hill, D., Denton, E., Jarosz, J., Cox, T., Rohlfing, T., Goodey, J., Hawkes, D.: Voxel similarity measures for 3-d serial mr brain image registration. IEEE Transactions on Medical Imaging **19** (2000) 94–102
12. Shoemake, K.: Animating rotation with quaternion curves. Computer Graphics, Proceedings of SIGGRAPH 85 **19** (1985) 245–254
13. Roche, A., Malandain, G., Ayache, N.: Unifying maximum likelihood approaches in medical image registration. International Journal of Imaging Systems and Technology: Special Issue on 3D Imaging **11** (2000) 71–80
14. Nelder, J., Mead, R.: A simplex method for function minimization. Computer Journal **7** (1965) 308–313

Cartilage Thickness Measurement in the Sub-millimeter Range

Geert J. Streekstra[1], Pieter Brascamp[1], Christiaan van der Leij[2],
René ter Wee[1], Simon D. Strackee[3], Mario Maas[2], and Henk W. Venema[1]

[1] Dept. Medical Physics,
g.j.streekstra@amc.uva.nl
[2] Dept. Radiology,
[3] Dept. Plastic and Reconstructive Surgery,
Academic Medical Center, Meibergdreef 9, 1105 AZ, Amsterdam, The Netherlands

Abstract. We present a method to measure cartilage thickness from
CT images in the sub millimeter range. Current methods based on zero
crossings of second derivatives across the cartilage layers are known to
be biased in the sub millimeter range due to the finite width of the point
spread function (PSF) of the imaging system.

We developed a method for accurate thickness measurements of such
small layers by taking into account the effect of the PSF. To this end
the orientation of the cartilage layers is estimated using gradient vector
information in the cartilage region. Subsequently, a model of the attenuation profile across the cartilage layer is convolved with a measured PSF
to obtain an intensity profile that is fitted to the image data.

Results of thickness estimates from simulated image data reveal that our
method is unbiased in contrast to the method based on second derivative
zero crossings. We illustrate the usefulness of our method by comparing
measurement on CT arthrography images with results obtained from
high resolution anatomical sections that served as a reference.

We conclude that incorporation of the PSF in the measurement method
allows for accurate cartilage thickness estimates even in the sub millimeter range.

1 Introduction

In orthopaedics and musculoskeletal radiology detection of cartilage thickness is
of importance in both clinical practice and in research on biomechanics of joint
structures [1,2,3]. In clinical practise cartilage thickness estimates can be used to
stage joint disease in a primary diagnosis and in evaluation of pharmacological
or surgical procedures. Moreover, cartilage thickness is an essential parameter in
biomechanical models that describe the kinematic behavior of joint structures
[4].

A lot of effort has been put into detection of cartilage in the knee joint [1,
2,5,6,7,8,9]. In the knee cartilage thickness ranges typically from 2 to 5 mm.
Usually, the order of magnitude of the voxels size in the MR images used for

C. Barillot, D.R. Haynor, and P. Hellier (Eds.): MICCAI 2004, LNCS 3217, pp. 950–958, 2004.

cartilage measurement is 0.3x0.3x2.0 mm. In particular the slice thickness of 2 mm cause overestimation of cartilage thickness when the image plane cuts obliquely through the cartilage layer [2,6]. The relative inaccuracy caused by a slice thickness of several millimeters will increase with decreasing cartilage thickness.

Comparison of MR based methods for cartilage thickness measurements with estimates from anatomical sections show that roughly 10-50 % of the measurements have an inaccuracy of more than 0.5 mm [1,5]. These inaccuracies may be acceptable for measurements in the knee but are unacceptable when cartilage thickness is in the sub millimeter range like in most part of the wrist and in the ankle [10].

Since in the sub millimeter regime the size of the Point Spread Function (PSF) of the imaging system is also in the order of magnitude of the cartilage thickness the PSF should be taken into account when measuring cartilage thickness. In literature on image based thickness measurement in both CT and MRI it is generally acknowledged that the finite width of the PSF limits accuracy of measurement in thin sheet structures [11,12,13,14]. These methods utilize second derivative zero crossings for thickness measurement. The observed bias in the thickness estimates start to become significant in the sub millimeter regime even in high resolution CT protocols where the FWHM of the PSF is approximately 0.7 mm.

In this paper we propose a measurement procedure that strongly reduces PSF induced bias by incorporating the PSF directly into the thickness estimation method. The performance of the method is evaluated by thickness measurements in simulated images and images of cadaver wrists. In the cadaver wrists cartilage thickness estimates from CT arthrography images are compared to estimates in high resolution anatomical sections as obtained with an imaging cryomicrotome [15].

2   Cartilage Thickness Measurement Procedure

2.1   Cartilage Thickness Estimation

In a joint the cartilage layers are usually situated on the outer part of both bones to facilitate motion between two individual bones. As a result two parallel cartilage layers are close to each other. We can model the profile of X-ray attenuation coefficients by a series of step functions along a line perpendicular to the cartilage layers as depicted in Fig.1.

The profile reflects the different attenuation coefficients for trabecular bone, cortical bone, cartilage and the contrast medium that fills the gap between the two cartilage layers in CT arthrography images [16,17]. In a 2D image the cartilage layers appear as relatively dark line structures surrounded by the the cortical bone layers and the contrast agent that appear as bright lines (see Fig.2.).

In the image formation process the attenuation coefficient profile is blurred because of the limited resolution of the CT scanner. This means from a mathematical point of view that an intensity profile in the image across the cartilage

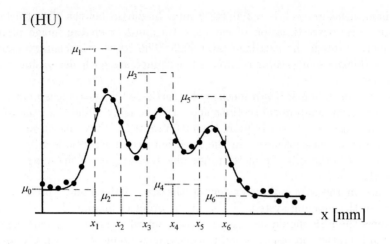

Fig. 1. Attenuation coefficient profile along a line perpendicular to the cartilage sheets (Dashed lines) and the convolution of the attenuation coefficient profile with the Point Spread Function (PSF) of the CT scanner (solid curve). The dots represent the noise corrupted discrete image points across the cartilage layers.

layers (Fig.1., solid curve.) is a 3D convolution of the attenuation coefficient profile (Fig.1., dashed lines.) with the PSF. Since in our case all relevant structures are approximately parallel with dimensions much larger than the size of the PSF the 3D convolution may be approximated by a 1D convolution along the attenuation coefficient profile. In the case that the PSF is isotropic and can be described by a 3D Gaussian [11] we find for the intensity profile across the cartilage layers:

$$I(x) = \int_{-\infty}^{x_1} \mu_0 g(x - \xi, \sigma) d\xi + \sum_{i=1}^{5} \int_{x_i}^{x_{i+1}} \mu_i g(x - \xi, \sigma) d\xi + \int_{x_6}^{\infty} \mu_6 g(x - \xi, \sigma) d\xi$$

$$(1)$$

In this equation μ_i, $(i = 0..6)$ represent the attenuation coefficients of the different materials across the profile and $g(x, \sigma)$ is a one dimensional Gaussian with scale σ:

$$g(x, \sigma) = \frac{1}{\sqrt{2\pi}\sigma} \exp(-\frac{1}{2}\frac{x^2}{\sigma^2})$$

$$(2)$$

Equation (1) shows that the intensity $I(x)$ at a certain x−position is influenced by the complete attenuation profile.

In the estimation of cartilage thickness the theoretical intensity profile as given in equation (1) is matched to a measured gray value profile in an image.

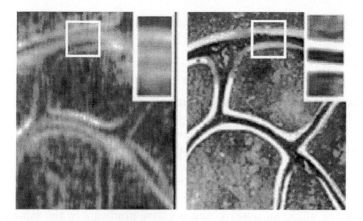

Fig. 2. Left: a slice of a 3D CT arthrography image showing the cartilage as dark lines between the bright cortical bone rims and contrast agent. Right: the corresponding anatomical section. The square regions are the positions of thickness estimates between radius and lunatum. The rectangular regions at the upper right corner of each image are magnifications of the ROI used for the thickness estimates.

For the matching a non-linear fit procedure is used to estimate the attenuation coefficients μ_i as well as the positions x_i of the interfaces between different materials. The thicknesses d_1 and d_2 of the two adjacent cartilage layers are calculated from the positions of the estimated interface positions between cartilage-cortical bone and cartilage-contrast medium.

2.2   Detection of Cartilage Sheet Orientation in 2D Image Slices

In order to determine the thickness of the cartilage sheets from intensity profiles we first select a small region of interest (ROI) in a 2D image of the cartilage (Fig.2.) that contains the 3D vector normal to the cartilage sheet.

In order to obtain intensity profiles perpendicular to the cartilage the normal vector of the cartilage sheets in the 2D image is determined. This can be done by utilizing intensity gradients in the ROI. The transitions for one material to another are all in the same direction orthogonal to the direction of the cartilage sheets. Therefore by determining the average gradient, one can find the direction of the intensity profile from which the cartilage thickness is extracted.

The gradient components of the image in two orthogonal directions, x and y, are calculated using Gaussian derivatives

$$I_x = \frac{\partial g_2(x, y, \sigma)}{\partial x} \otimes I(x, y) \quad , \quad I_y = \frac{\partial g_2(x, y, \sigma)}{\partial y} \otimes I(x, y) \tag{3}$$

where $\otimes$ is the 2D convolution operator and $g_2(x, y, \sigma)$ is the two-dimensional Gaussian

$$g_2(x, y, \sigma) = \frac{1}{2\pi\sigma^2} \exp(-\frac{x^2 + y^2}{2\sigma^2}) \tag{4}$$

with σ the scale of the Gaussian derivative kernel. By convolving the intensity with this Gaussian, the image is blurred for noise elimination while preserving derivative properties [18]. For every pixel in the ROI, the angle of the intensity gradient vector with the $x-$axis is calculated using

$$\theta = \arctan(\frac{I_y}{I_x}) \tag{5}$$

To prevent the angles of positive and negative gradients in the same direction to cancel each other out, the intensity derivatives in both x and y directions are multiplied by -1 for all pixels with a negative derivative in the y direction. Now a weighted average Θ of all angles with weight based on the magnitude of the gradients is made:

$$\Theta = \frac{\sum_{i=1}^{n} \sum_{j=1}^{m} [\sqrt{I_x(i,j)^2 + I_y(i,j)^2} \theta(i,j)]}{\sum_{i=1}^{n} \sum_{j=1}^{m} \sqrt{I_x(i,j)^2 + I_y(i,j)^2}} \tag{6}$$

where n and m are the width and height of the ROI, respectively. This is done because the largest gradients in the image are those on the edges of structures. Other (smaller) gradients are the result of noise. The influence of this noise is suppressed by taking a weighted average.

The local cartilage thickness is estimated by averaging the results of the fits of n lines in the the ROI with dimensions nxm. To estimate the error produced in this method, the bootstrap method [19] is used.

3   Experiments

3.1   Simulations

To gain insight into the potentials of the method we estimated the thickness of simulated 1D cartilage profiles. We compared our method with the commonly used method based on detection of second derivative zero crossings across the simulated cartilage layers [11,12,13,14].

The simulated profiles were constructed by convolving an attenuation profile of step functions with a Gaussian PSF (Eqs. (1) and (2)). The scale parameter σ of the PSF was chosen to be 0.25 mm which is a value obtained in the highest resolution mode of current CT scanners. The voxel size was set to 0.2 mm. We added random Gaussian noise to the simulated data with a SNR of 40.

Initially all distances between steps in the attenuation profile (i.e. distances between x_i and x_{i+1}, see Fig. 1.) were set to 1 mm. Subsequently, the thickness of one of the cartilage layers ($d = x_3 - x_2$) was varied between 0.5 and 1.5 mm. The signal to noise ration was set to 40.

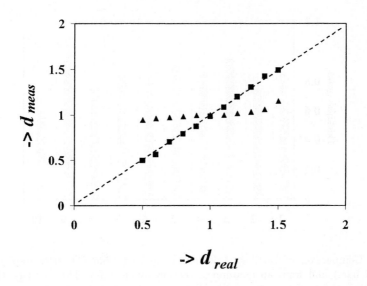

Fig. 3. Simulation based relationship between the real thickness of a cartilage layer (d_{real}) and the estimated thickness (d_{meas}). The triangles show the results of thickness estimated based on second derivative zero crossings across the cartilage layers. The squares show the results as obtained with our method that takes the PSF into account.

The results show that the method based on second derivative zero crossings show considerable bias in the estimated thickness (Fig. 3.). In comparison, thickness estimates with the present method shows virtually no bias. Only random variations appear to be present due to the small amount of noise added to the simulated intensity values.

3.2 Comparison of Thickness Estimation in CT and Anatomical Sections

To get an impression of the usefulness of our method in practise we compared thickness measurement from CT arthrography images with thickness estimates in high resolution anatomical sections as obtained with an imaging cryomicrotome [15] that served as a reference. The cryomicrotome images can be considered as an accurate reference since the width of the PSF of the cryomicrotome is approximately 20 times smaller than that of the CT-scanner (Mx8000, Philips) in the high resolution mode. The measured σ of the isotropic Gaussian PSF of the CT-scanner is 0.255 mm. The voxel size was set to 0.2x0.2x0.2 mm^3.

The cartilage thickness was estimated from layers situated between the radius and the ulna (See indicated square regions in Fig. 2.). The thickness was measured at 10 different positions along the cartilage where the two layers are parallel.

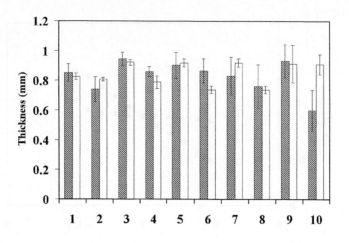

Fig. 4. Comparison of cartilage thickness estimated from CT arthography images (dashed bars) and from an anatomical section (open bars). The cartilage thickness was estimated from layers situated between the radius and the ulna (square regions in Fig. 2.)

As can be deduced from Fig. 4. the thickness estimated from the CT arthrography images correspond closely to those estimated from the cryomicrotome images in all cases except one.

4   Discussion

Measurement of thickness in sheet structures based on second derivative zero crossings is an accurate method if the size of the point spread function (PSF) of the imaging system is small compared to sheet thickness. In sheet structures below 1 mm, like cartilage sheets in the wrist joint or the ankle, the width of the PSF is in the same order of magnitude as the cartilage thickness. In that case second derivative methods show considerable bias as shown in Fig. 3.

We presented a method that yields a bias free thickness estimator of parallel cartilage layers with a attenuation profile as shown in Fig. 1. The agreement of thickness estimates from CT images with estimates from anatomical sections is most promising. Residual differences may be due to poor SNR of the CT images as well as slight differences in the the exact locations in CT and cryomicrotome images. For a definitive validation of the method special attention should be paid to these aspects.

References

1. Eckstein F., Sittek H., Gavazzeni A., Schulte E., Milz S., Kiefer B., Reiser M., Putz R. Magnetic resonance chondro-crassometry (MR CCM): A method for accurate determination of articular cartilage thickness. Magnetic Resonance in Medicine 35 (1), 89-96, 1996.
2. Losch A., Eckstein F., Haubner M., Englmeier K.H. A non-invasive technique for 3-dimensional assessment of articular cartilage thickness based on MRI Part 1: Development of a computational method. Magnetic Resonance Imaging 15 (7), 795-804, 1997.
3. Graichen H., Jakob J., von Eisenhart-Rothe R., Englmeier K.H., Reiser M., Eckstein F. Validation of cartilage volume and thickness measurements in the human shoulder with quantitative magnetic resonance imaging. Osteoarthritis and Cartilage 11(7), 475-482, 2003.
4. Blankevoort L., Kuiper J.H., Huiskes R., Grootenboer H.J. Articular Contact in a 3-Dimensional Model of the Knee. Journal of Biomechanics24 (11), 1019-1031, 1991.
5. Eckstein F., Gavazzeni A., Sittek H., Haubner M., Losch A., Milz S., Englmeier K.H., Schulte E., Putz R., Reiser M. Determination of knee joint cartilage thickness using three-dimensional magnetic resonance chondro-crassometry (3D MR-CCM). Magnetic Resonance in Medicine 36 (2), 256-265, 1996.
6. Haubner M., Eckstein F., Schnier M., Losch A., Sittek H., Becker C., Kolem H., Reiser M., Englmeier K.H. A non-invasive technique for 3-dimensional assessment of articular cartilage thickness based on MRI Part 2: Validation using CT arthrography. Magnetic Resonance Imaging 15 (7), 805-813, 1997.
7. Stammberger T., Eckstein F., Englmeier K.H., Reiser M. Determination of 3D cartilage thickness data from MR imaging: Computational method and reproducibility in the living. Magnetic Resonance in Medicine 41(3), 529-536, 1999.
8. Stammberger T., Eckstein F., Michaelis M., Englmeier K.H., Reiser M. Interobserver reproducibility of quantitative cartilage measurements: Comparison of B-spline snakes and manual segmentation. Magnetic Resonance Imaging 17 (7), 1033-1042, 1999.
9. Glaser C., Faber S., Eckstein F., Fischer H., Springer V., Heudorfer L., Stammberger T., Englmeier K.H., Reiser M. Optimization and validation of a rapid high-resolution T1-w 3D FLASH water excitation MRI sequence for the quantitative assessment of articular cartilage volume and thickness. Magnetic Resonance Imaging 19 (2), 177-185, 2001.
10. Shepherd D.E.T., Seedhom B.B. Thickness of human articular cartilage in joints of the lower limb. Annals of the Rheumatic Diseases 58 (1), 27-34, 1999.
11. Prevrhal S., Engelke K., Kalender W.A. Accuracy Limits for the Determination of Cortical Width and Density: The Influence of Object Size and CT Imaging Parameters. Physics in Medicine and Biology 44 (3), 751-764, 1999.
12. Prevrhal S., Fox J.C., Shepherd J.A., Genant H.K. Accuracy Of CT-Based Thickness Measurement of thin Structures: Modeling of Limited Spatial Resolution in all three Dimensions. Medical Physics 30 (1), 1-8, 2003.
13. Sato, Y., Nakanishi, K., Tanaka, H., Nishii, T., Sugano, N., Nakamura, H., Ochi, T., Tamura, S. Limits to the accuracy of 3D thickness measurement in magnetic resonance images. Lecture Notes in Computer Science 2208, 803-810, 2001.

14. Sato Y., Tanaka H., Nishii T., Nakanishi K., Sugano N., Kubota T., Nakamura H., Yoshikawa H., Ochi T., Tamura S. Limits on the accuracy of 3-D thickness measurement in magnetic resonance images - Effects of voxel anisotropy. IEEE Transactions on Medical Imaging 22 (9), 1076-1088, 2003.

15. Kelly J.J., Ewen J.R., Bernard S.L., Glenny R.W., Barlow C.H. Regional blood flow measurements from fluorescent microsphere images using an Imaging Cryo-Microtome. Review of Scientific Instruments 71 (1), 228-234, 2000.

16. Boven F., Bellemanns M.A., Geurts J., Potvliege R. A comparative study of the patellofemoral joint on axial roentgenogram axial arthrogram and computed tomography following arthrography. Skeletal Radiology 8, 179-181, 1982.

17. Ihara H. Double contrast CT arthrography of the cartilage of the patellofemoral joint. Clinical Orthopeadics 198, 50-55, 1985.

18. Ter Haar Romeny B.M. Front-End Vision and Multi-Scale Image Analysis. Kluwer Academic Publisher, Dordrecht 2003, p 102.

19. Press W.H., Teukolsky S.A., Vetterling W.T., Flannery, B.P. Numerical Recipes in C. Cambridge University Press, New York 1992, p. 691.

A Method to Monitor Local Changes in MR Signal Intensity in Articular Cartilage: A Potential Marker for Cartilage Degeneration in Osteoarthritis

Josephine H. Naish[1], Graham Vincent[2], Mike Bowes[2], Manish Kothari[3],
David White[3], John C. Waterton[4], and Chris J. Taylor[1]

[1] Imaging Science and Biomedical Engineering, University of Manchester, Manchester, UK
[2] imorphics Ltd., Incubator Building, Grafton Street, Manchester, UK
[3] Synarc Inc., 575 Market Street, San Francisco, USA
[4] AstraZeneca, Alderley Park, Macclesfield, Cheshire, UK

Abstract. Osteoarthritis (OA) involves changes in the composition and ultimately the loss of cartilage from articulating joints. MRI has the ability to non-invasively probe the compositional integrity of cartilage, thereby potentially identifying diseased cartilage before loss occurs. In this study we have developed a technique to compare local changes in signal intensity over time in fat suppressed 3D gradient echo MR images of articular cartilage in patients with OA. We have used an Active Appearance Model (AAM) based image registration to correspond locations within the cartilage in the same individual at different times. We have applied the technique to data taken over periods of 1 and 3 years in two groups of patients with established OA of the knee. In both these studies, no significant change in total cartilage volume could be detected but we were able to observe some significant changes in signal intensity. We conclude that in a study of cartilage structure the technique can provide additional information without the overhead of extra scans.

1 Introduction

Osteoarthritis (OA) is one of the principle causes of disability in elderly people. While a number of interventions that may slow the progression of the disease are becoming available, research has been hampered by a lack of accurate methods for assessing changes in articular cartilage in order to monitor disease progression and response to treatment. Of the available techniques, MRI would appear to be the optimal modality as it enables the (usually) non-invasive direct visualization of hyaline cartilage.

Techniques for accurately quantifying the volume of articular cartilage using fat suppressed 3D gradient echo magnetic resonance imaging have been developed and validated [1]. However, recent studies have cast doubt on the effectiveness of total cartilage volume as a measure of cartilage degeneration in OA [2] and suggest that future work should concentrate on assessing focal changes e.g. by mapping cartilage thickness. MRI also has the unique ability to non-invasively probe the compositional integrity of cartilage, thereby potentially identifying diseased cartilage before loss occurs. Measurements of cartilage quality may thus provide methods to monitor early disease progression and treatment response. These measurements include surrogates for hydration such as signal

C. Barillot, D.R. Haynor, and P. Hellier (Eds.): MICCAI 2004, LNCS 3217, pp. 959–966, 2004.

intensity, T_2 [3] and proton density [4], surrogates for protoglycan such as dGEMRIC [5] (which is an invasive technique) and sodium [6] (which requires a sodium coil), and surrogates for collagen such as magnetisation transfer [7]. Of these the simplest and hence most clinically useful techniques are those that monitor cartilage hydration. Several studies have shown that T_2 relaxation, measured using a multi-echo sequence, correlates with collagen matrix organisation and water content [3,8,9] but longitudinal studies have yet to be published. Calculation of absolute proton density requires multiple image acquisitions resulting in very long imaging times or compromising on image resolution. The technique also suffers from increased noise since it involves the calculation of secondary data sets from several primary acquisitions.

The raw signal intensity in a single fat suppressed gradient echo image is proportional to the proton density (and so related to hydration) but also affected by both T_1 and T_2^* relaxation, both of which may change with cartilage degeneration. Signal intensity does not therefore provide a direct measure of hydration but may still provide a marker for change in cartilage composition. The advantage of a signal intensity measurement is that, unlike other measurements of cartilage quality, it can be obtained from the structural scans so that with no additional scan time both the regional thickness and the cartilage composition may be assessed.

In this study we have developed an Active Appearance Model (AAM) based technique to compare local changes in signal intensity over time. We have applied the technique to data collected over 1 and 3 years in two groups of patients with established OA of the knee in order to investigate the usefulness of signal intensity as a marker for disease progression in OA.

2   Methods

2.1   Imaging

We have used data from two separate longitudinal studies of cartilage volume in patients with OA. In the first, eleven patients with established OA of the knee were imaged at baseline, 2 months, 1 year and 3 years using a 3D spoiled gradient-echo sequence with fat suppression. The imaging was performed using a 1.0T clinical scanner and the image sequence parameters were TR=50ms, TE=11ms, 40° flip angle, sagittal slices, slice thickness 1.56mm, in-plane resolution 0.55mm [2]. An example MR image from this data set is presented in Fig. 1. Volume measurements, made using a manual segmentation of the images at each time point, yielded no significant change over the three years in any of the cartilage compartments. See [2] for full details of the volume analysis.

The second study consisted of 50 patients, imaged at baseline, 3 months, 6 months and 1 year with some repeated measurements at the 3 and 6 month time points. Imaging was performed using a 1.5T clinical scanner and the sequence parameters were were TR=58ms, TE=6ms, 40° flip angle, sagittal slices, slice thickness 2mm, in-plane resolution 0.63mm. Volume measurements were made using a semi-automatic segmentation method based on the livewire algorithm. Again, no significant changes in volume could be detected over the timescale of the study.

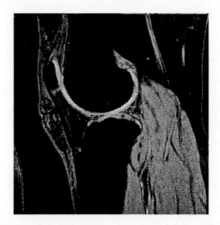

Fig. 1. Example 3D fat suppressed gradient echo magnetic resonance image. Slice shown is in the region of the lateral condyle. Note the hyper-intense signal in the regions of hyaline cartilage.

2.2   Image Registration

An image registration method was developed in order to compare the signal intensity at corresponding locations within the cartilage of the same individual at different times. An overall rigid registration (i.e. a global translation plus rotation) was not possible because the relative positions of the components of the knee joint can change as the knee flexes. However, a separate rigid registration for each cartilage compartment (femoral, patellar, tibial) provided a good approximation. This is only an approximation since cartilage may swell or be lost over time. Segmentations of each cartilage compartment for the data from both studies had been performed previously, either using a fully manual or semi-automated technique, as part of the cartilage volume calculations. Segmentations of the cartilage in the baseline images were used to construct a triangulated surface for each cartilage compartment. An example surface is presented in Fig. 2 for the femoral cartilage. For details of the surface building see [10]. Using this surface and the image signal intensities, a single example AAM [11] was built for each cartilage compartment for each individual. The models were then used to search the later time point images of each individual resulting in a translation and rotation for each compartment.

The registration was performed using Endpoint, a commercially available image analysis package written in a collaboration between the University of Manchester and imorphics.

2.3   Analysis

The image intensity was sampled at a set of corresponding points in each of the registered images using linear interpolation. In initial experiments these points were chosen as the grid of voxel locations in the baseline image ('rigid sampling') corresponding to the area inside the segmentation but in more recent experiments we have developed a method to sample at equidistant points along normals to the medial surface of the triangulation

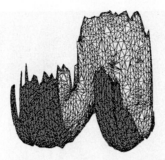

Fig. 2. Example triangulated surface built for the femoral cartilage compartment

('thickness sampling'). The final step was to correct for an overall scaling factor caused by changes in scanner settings. This was achieved by performing a robust fit (least median orthogonal distance) of a pair of sets of corresponding signal intensities. Once the scaling factor was determined in this way, differences in signal intensity over time could be investigated.

A qualitative local analysis was possible by comparing corresponding slices through the normalised 3D signal intensity at different times. We have also produced 2D maps of the signal intensity differences summed along normals to the medial surface which allow an overall spatial comparison of a cartilage segment over time.

For a more quantitative analysis, a global measure of signal intensity change was calculated by taking the average normalised difference for each cartilage compartment. The normalisation method we have used, based on a robust fit to corresponding pairs of intensity values, does not completely balance the mean signal intensity differences. The remaining global change in intensity tells us something about changes in the outliers of the distribution. These will include voxels subject to varying degrees of partial volume averaging but will also include those voxels for which a real change in signal intensity has occurred. Differences in signal intensity due to, for example, partial volume changes or differences in position in the coil will vary randomly over time whereas real differences in cartilage composition will change in some consistent way. Therefore, average net changes over time have been calculated by performing a linear regression of the average normalised signal intensity against time for each of the separate cartilage compartments for each individual. This results in values of percentage net change in total signal intensity per year.

3   Results

3.1   Signal Intensity Maps

Example results for a single slice through the cartilage are presented in Fig. 3a. These images demonstrate the effectiveness of the registration process and allow local comparisons of signal intensity and so cartilage quality to be made. Some focal changes can be seen in the tibial plateau in this example.

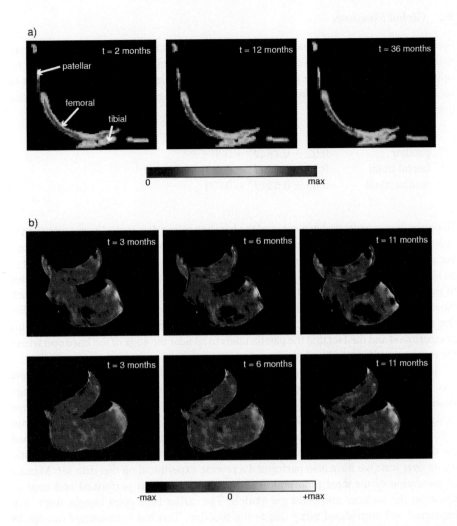

Fig. 3. a) Slice through registered and normalised cartilage compartments for three time points. b) 2D maps of signal intensity differences (i.e. signal intensity at time t minus baseline signal intensity) calculated by integrating along normals to the medial surface for the femoral cartilage compartment.

Two example 2D signal intensity difference maps are presented in Fig. 3b for the femoral cartilage compartment. The first example shows clear evidence of disease progression in the form of increasing regions of negative signal intensity change in both femoral condyles. In the second example an overall progression is more difficult to identify but some similar structures can be seen in the maps suggesting that regions of cartilage are changing in composition in some consistent manner over time.

3.2 Global Measures

For the 11 patients over 3 years two data sets could not be used because of problems with the images at one of the time points. For the 9 complete sets the following results were obtained using the rigid sampling method to sample corresponding pairs of values of signal intensity. Results are expressed as average percentage change per year (mean±standard error):

femoral	$-0.41 \pm 0.19 \, (P = 0.07)$
patellar	$-0.92 \pm 0.78 \, (P = 0.3)$
lateral tibial	$-0.22 \pm 0.10 \, (P = 0.06)$
medial tibial	$-0.65 \pm 0.34 \, (P = 0.09)$

To obtain these results we have not used the baseline image data in the linear regression to avoid introducing any bias. The probabilities quoted are for a two-tailed Student's t-test. For all four compartments we observe a mean decrease in overall signal intensity but in no single compartment does this reach statistical significance at a 5% level, perhaps due to the small number of individuals in this study. Note that the standard error is much larger in the case of the patellar cartilage than the other compartments; this is probably due to a combination of the increased error in registration because of the shape of this compartment and the fact that the patella tends to sit near the edge of the knee coil where the receive sensitivity is less homogeneous.

In the larger data set of 50 patients over one year we have 42 complete usable data sets. We have analysed these using the thickness sampling method to sample image intensities. The results for the femoral compartment show an annual percentage change in signal intensity of $-1.02 \pm 0.29 \, (P < 0.01)$ and in this case the result is significant statistically. This result is larger in magnitude but consistent with the results obtained for the small data set of 9 patients over three years. In order to check for systematic errors over time we have also performed a reverse experiment on this data set. Manual segmentation of the final time point (12 months) image was performed and used to construct the surfaces and build the models. The earlier time point images were then registered and normalised using this as the baseline. This has been carried out for 28 subjects. Linear regression produces an annual percentage change in signal intensity of -1.15 ± 0.39 which is consistent with the results from the forward experiment and so rules out a systematic error.

4 Discussion

By using an AAM based image registration we are able to correspond locations within the cartilage of the same individual in MR images taken at different times. Combined with normalisation, this allows a direct monitoring of the signal intensity of a region of cartilage over time. Manual (or semi-automatic) segmentation has to be performed at a single time point only, so that user input is minimised and errors resulting from inconsistent segmentation are eliminated. Focal changes in the structure of the cartilage can be directly visualised as focal changes in signal intensity.

By integrating the signal intensity change across normals to the medial surface of the cartilage compartments, information on the depth variation of signal intensity change is lost but the spatial distribution across the articulating surface may be more easily visualised. It is possible to identify regions of cartilage which change progressively and consistently over time suggesting that the method allows local changes in the composition of cartilage to be observed. One limitation of the technique presented is that in using a robust fit to the voxel signal intensities as the normalisation method we are assuming that the majority of the voxels within the cartilage do not change. If this assumption breaks down, i.e. if there is extensive and rapid disease progression, the method will tend to underestimate the overall change. This may be the cause of the regions of apparently increased signal intensity in the first example in Fig. 3b. This may be avoided in future studies by placing a signal intensity phantom in the field of view of the image and using this as a standard to calculate the scaling factor.

In order to carry out a more quantitative statistical analysis of the spatial variation of signal intensity change it will be necessary to correspond areas of cartilage across a population. A method to achieve this by modelling the underlying bone using statistical shape models has been presented in the context of cartilage thickness measurement [10] and we intend to apply this method to signal intensity measurement in a future study.

A statistical analysis of signal intensity change for this study has been carried out by calculating the global change for a cartilage compartment. We find a significant decrease in signal intensity over one year in 42 patients with established osteoarthritis. This change may be due to a reduction in hydration and hence proton density, changes in the structure (eg. collagen content) of the cartilage, an actual loss of cartilage or a combination of these factors. In future studies, compositional changes and cartilage loss may be separated by combining measurement of signal intensity with a measurement of local cartilage thickness, both of which may be obtained from a single MR scan.

5   Conclusions

Local signal intensity appears to offer important additional information in a study of cartilage quantity. The signal intensity in a gradient echo image is proportional to proton density (and hence cartilage hydration) but is also affected by T_1 and T_2^*, both of which may change with cartilage degeneration in osteoarthritis. It is therefore a non-specific marker for changes in cartilage composition but nevertheless should prove useful particularly when combined with studies of regional cartilage thickness.

Acknowledgements. We would like to thank the University of Bristol and GSK for the data used in this study. The work was supported by AstraZeneca, Synarc and imorphics.

References

1. Peterfy CG, van Dijke CF, Janzen DL, Gluer CC, Namba R, Majumdar S, Lang P, and Genant HK. Quantification of articular cartilage in the knee with pulsed saturation transfer subtraction and fat-suppressed mr imaging: optimization and validation. *Radiology*, 192(2):485–91, 1994.

2. Gandy SJ, Dieppe PA, Keen MC, Maciewicz RA, Watt I, and Waterton JC. No loss of cartilage volume over three years in patients with knee osteoarthritis as assessed by magnetic resonance imaging. *Osteoarthritis Cartilage*, 10(12):929–37, 2002.

3. Lüsse S, Claassen H, Gehrke T, Hassenpflug J, Schunke M, Heller M, and Gluer CC. Evaluation of water content by spatially resolved transverse relaxation times of human articular cartilage. *Magn Reson Imaging*, 18(4):423–30, 2000.

4. Selby K, Peterfy CG, Cohen ZA, Ateshian GA, Mow VC, Roos M, Wong S, Newitt DC, van Dijke CJ, Wendland M, and Genant HK. In vivo MR quantification of articular cartliage water content: a potential early indicator of arthritis. *Proc Intl Soc Magn Reson Med*, 3:204, 1995.

5. Gillis A, Gray M, and Burstein D. Relaxivity and diffusion of gadolinium agents in cartilage. *Magn Reson Med*, 48(6):1068–71, 2002.

6. Shapiro EM, Borthakur A, Gougoutas A, and Reddy R. 23Na MRI accurately measures fixed charge density in articular cartilage. *Magn Reson Med*, 47(2):284–91, 2002.

7. Kim DK, Ceckler TL, Hascall VC, Calabro A, and Balaban RS. Analysis of water-macromolecule proton magnetization transfer in articular cartilage. *Magn Reson Med*, 29(2):211–5, 1993.

8. Smith HE, Mosher TJ, Dardzinski BJ, Collins BG, Collins CM, Yang QX, Schmithorst VJ, and Smith MB. Spatial variation in cartilage T2 of the knee. *J Magn Reson Imaging*, 14(1):50–5, 2001.

9. Liess C, Lusse S, Karger N, Heller M, and Gluer CC. Detection of changes in cartilage water content using MRI T2-mapping in vivo. *Osteoarthritis Cartilage*, 10(12):907–13, 2002.

10. Williams TG, Taylor CJ, Gao ZX, and Waterton JC. Corresponding articular cartilage thickness measurements in the knee joint by modelling the underlying bone. *Lect Notes Comput Sc*, 2732:126–135, 2003.

11. Cootes TF, Edwards GJ, and Taylor CJ. Active Appearance Models. *IEEE Transactions on Pattern Analysis and Machine Intelligence*, 23(6):681–685, 2001.

Tracing Based Segmentation for the Labeling of Individual Rib Structures in Chest CT Volume Data

Hong Shen[1], Lichen Liang[2], Min Shao[3] , and Shuping Qing[1]

[1] Siemens Corporate Research, Inc., 755 College Road East, Princeton, NJ 08540, USA,
{shenh, sqing}@scr.siemens.com
[2] Electrical and Computer Engineering Department, University of Minnesota, Minneapolis,
MN 55455, USA, lianglc@ece.umn.edu
[3] Department of Electrical and Computer Engineering, University of Delaware, Newark, DE
19716, USA, 55298@udel.edu

Abstract. We propose a fast and robust segmentation algorithm for the extraction and labeling of individual rib structures in chest CT volume data. A diagnostic system based on this algorithm can display 3D rib centerlines, contours and surfaces. A click on a rib point in any slice image will have the system identify instantly the individual rib it belongs to. The algorithm is based on a recursive tracing approach. The geometrical properties of the rib structure are explored to set up valid assumptions and model. At each step, statistical analysis is combined with dynamic programming to estimate the outer surface contour from the detected edges. The algorithm works reliably on CT volume data of variant doses and resolutions. This algorithm can be extended to other modalities. The detected centerlines can also be used for reliable and fast registration of in or cross-modality volume data of chest scans.

1 Introduction

The advances in medical imaging equipment have brought efficiency and high capability to the screening, diagnosis and surgery of various kinds of diseases. The 3d imaging modalities, such as multi-slice CT scanners, produce large amount of digital data that is difficult and tedious to be interpreted merely by physicians. Computer Aided Diagnosis (CAD) systems will therefore play a critical role, especially in the visualization, segmentation, detection, registration, and reporting of medical pathologies.[1][2] Due to the large volume of the data involved and the on-time requirement of medical applications, feature based algorithms will be one of the most frequently applied methods to accomplish these tasks effectively and efficiently.

The extraction of the rib structure has significant meanings to achieve several of the above functionalities to be provided by a CAD system. There are 12 pairs of rib structures in the human body, with 8-10 pairs visible in a chest CT volume data. They are connected at one end with the spine, and the upper ribs are also connected to the sternum. As an anatomy, the visualization and labeling of rib structures are of great interest to radiologist, since they need to report any pathology pertaining to bones in a

C. Barillot, D.R. Haynor, and P. Hellier (Eds.): MICCAI 2004, LNCS 3217, pp. 967–974, 2004.
© Springer-Verlag Berlin Heidelberg 2004

chest CT scan. A mouse click on a rib in the volume data should have the system instantly identify the rib. This function is highly desirable by a chest radiologist.

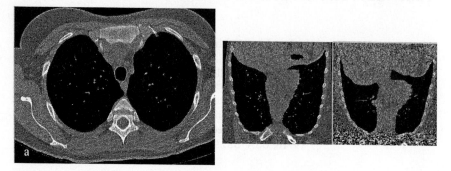

Fig. 1. (a) An axial slice image from a high dose chest CT volume data. The ellipsoid-like bright areas are the intersections of some of the individual ribs with this axial plane. Bottom left (b) and (c) Sagittal images of two volume data from high and low dose scans. Note the difference in noise level.

In the system viewpoint, the rib structures have high value in the reference and registration of other anatomies and pathologies.[3] The ribs have valuable properties common to bone tissues--rigid and stable in shape, and map to prominent intensities in CT data. Further, the rib structures enclose the complete chest area and part of lower abdomen, and are relatively less affected by lung surgery. Most importantly, they are highly ordered and symmetrical, and we observed that each pair of ribs roughly forms a plane—slanted plane that makes a significant angle with the axial plane. Because of these, the rib feature group can be used for reliable registration and reference. Certainly, to make full use of the structural advantage of the ribs, they should be extracted and labeled *individually*.

To our knowledge, there is little work in the 3D extraction of individual rib structures for the purpose of labeling or using them as features. In 3D volume data, efforts were spent on eliminating the ribs and other connected bone structures from the volume data by region-based approaches. [4]-[6] In the result, the ribs, spines and sternums were connected as one region. Moreover, the methods were semi-automatic—requires initial user input. In 2D x-ray images, works existed on extraction of ribs, by fitting curves [7][8] or using pixel-based statistical classification method [9].

Our algorithm uses a tracing based approach. It is designed to extract *individual* rib centerlines and boundaries reliably in 3D volume data. At first thought on this segmentation problem, one would easily think of a region grow approach based on intensity values. First, the separation of spines and sternum from the grown region of bones is itself a challenging problem. Second, due to the hollowness of ribs, region-based method followed by skeletonization [8][9] will have difficulties in obtaining reliable centerlines that are important for registration. Finally, it is hard to obtain good result using an intensity based approach. Although the vast majority of bone voxels have higher intensities (>1200) than surrounding tissues (700-1100), the lowest bone intensity and highest tissue intensity levels are quite close. With noise and partial volume effect, this narrow buffer zone is frequently crossed, and therefore no clear-cut intensity threshold exists between bone and other tissues.

The general principle of tracing has been widely explored, mostly in 2d, some in 3d situations.[11] The difficulty in the rib tracing includes the following. First, it is a 3d problem, with intrinsic issues to be handled. Second, the noise in low dose CT data can be high, leading to obscure and broken rib boundaries. The different noise levels can be seen from the pictures in Fig. 1(b) and (c). Third, the rib shapes vary greatly, making it hard to model. Fourth, the adjacent other bone structures may digress the tracing paths.

2 Methods

2.1 Model, Assumptions, and Basic Methods

An individual rib can be modeled as a tube-like structure, which is elongated, curved and internally hollow, as shown in Fig. 2(a). The cross-sections of a rib vary both in shape and size.

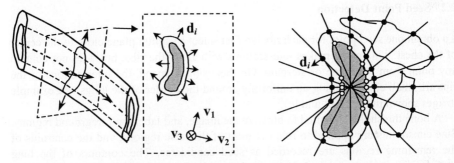

Fig. 2 (a) The geometric model of the rib structure. We assume the normals of the outer surface are perpendicular to the centerline direction (noted as v_3) everywhere. At each tracing step, contour is extracted in the cross-section plane with normal v_3. (b) At each step, all candidate edges are detected in each searching direction. The inner (white) edges are removed.

In our model, we assume that the outer surface is smooth everywhere, and more importantly, the surface normals d_i, $i=1\ldots n$ are roughly perpendicular to the centerline direction. This leads to our basic method of computing the tracing direction given the surface normals of detected edge points. Suppose the unit gradient vectors of n edge points on a local cross-section represent the local surface normals, and we compute a covariance matrix of all unit vectors d_i,

$$C = \sum_{i=1}^{n} (d_i - \overline{d})^t (d_i - \overline{d}), \tag{1}$$

where $\overline{\mathbf{d}}$ is average of all edge gradients. We compute the eigenvalues $\lambda_1 \geq \lambda_2 \geq \lambda_3$, with corresponding eigenvectors $\mathbf{v}_1$, $\mathbf{v}_2$, and $\mathbf{v}_3$. Since $\mathbf{v}_3$ is the new basis direction where the gradient vectors vary the least, it is perpendicular to the 2D subspace of the unit vectors. Therefore we take this vector as the centerline direction estimated from the gradient of local edges. The recursive tracing can then be described as

$$\mathbf{p}^{(i+1)} = \mathbf{p}^{(i)} + \alpha \mathbf{v}_3 \tag{2}$$

in which the current centerline point $\mathbf{p}^{(i+1)}$ is determined from the previous centerline point $\mathbf{p}^{(i)}$, and α is the step size.

At each step, we define a cross-section plane whose normal is the previous centerline direction. As shown in Fig. 2(a), the intersection points of this plane and the rib outer surface form a rib contour, which are extracted using 3d edge detection. . However, we do not perform edge detection on each pixel on the plane. Rather, as shown in Fig. 2(b), we extend 20 equal spaced search directions from the initial point $\mathbf{p}^{(i)}$ to look for strong edges. In many cases, more than one edge points are detected along each search direction.

2.2 Seed Point Detection

To obtain one seed point for each rib, we first select a sagittal plane close to the center of the chest. This plane makes intersections with all of the ribs, but does not contain any point from the spine or sternum. On this sagittal image, the intersections of the ribs are small ellipses lining up uniformly around the border of the lungs, see example images shown in Fig. 1(b) and (c).

A bone threshold is applied to binarize the image, and label the foreground regions. Size constraints are applied to rule out most of the false regions, and the centroids of the remaining regions are recorded as seed candidates. The contours of the lung boundaries are also extracted. Valid seed candidates are required to be close enough to the outer lung boundary, and uniformly distributed along the boundary.

Sometimes, due to partial volume effect and noises, the cross-section of a rib may split into more than one region. Hence, we merge the seed points that are very close to each other.

Using the above rules, all seed points are detected reliably from data of various noise levels. Depending on the range of the CT scan, we obtain 8-10 pairs of seed points. Starting at each seed point, we trace in both directions, and merge the two partial tracing results.

2.3 Extraction of Rib Contour in Cross-Section Plane

Instead of using a regular 3D edge operator to detect edges, we adapted the edge detector from the work of M. Brejl et al. [12] It is based on the fitting of the volume data in a small 3D voxel neighborhood by a polynomial. The resulting gradient computation yields accurate results, and has good performance at high noise levels. The algorithm can be implemented as a mask convolution with the mask size corresponding to the size of the voxel neighborhood within which the polynomial is fitted. We chose the mask size as 5×5×5, which proves to be the best compromise between accuracy and speed. The masks can be described as a function of position (x,y,z):

$$M_x(x,y,z) = (a + bx^2 - cy^2 - cz^2)x$$
$$M_y(x,y,z) = (a - cx^2 + by^2 - cz^2)y \qquad (3)$$
$$M_z(x,y,z) = (a - cx^2 - cy^2 + bz^2)z$$

where a=0.00214212, b=0.0016668, c=0.000952378, $x,y,z \in \{-2,-1,0,1,2\}$.

The above 3D masks are placed only around the points on the 20 search directions on the 2D cross-section plane whose normal is the previous tracing direction (Fig. 2). Edges are detected by convolution and non-maxima suppression along each search direction. Rib edge candidates are those edges that have high enough gradient magnitudes and with their gradient directions pointing out of the outer surface. Also, there must be enough high intensity bone voxels within their immediate neighborhood.

On each of the 20 search directions, there will be multiple edge candidates, only one of which is true. Some of the false edges are unfiltered inner edges and noise edges, but often they belong to nearby non-rib bone structures. A false edge can have a larger gradient magnitude than that of the true edge along a search direction.

To obtain the best contour, we use dynamic programming [13] to jointly estimate the best rib edge on each direction, taking into account both the shape and size of the rib contour.

From our model, the rib outer surface is smooth, and hence should result in compact and smooth contours in the cross-section plane. The energy function therefore contains terms measuring the length and total curvature of the contour. It is defined as

$$E = \sum_i (E_d(i) + \alpha E_c(i)), \qquad (4)$$

where $E_d(i)$ is the distance between the two selected candidates on the ith and $i+1^{th}$ search direction, $E_c(i)$ is the correlation between two tangential vectors of these two points, and α is a weight factor.

With the defined energy function, we regard each search direction as a stage, and each edge candidate on that search direction as a state. The true rib edges are determined by minimizing the total energy. The path associated with the minimum energy is selected as the optimal path. The states, or edge candidates on the path are recorded the final rib edge points.

The centroid of the final edges in this cross-section is then computed as the rib centerline point. The next tracing direction is also updated.

2.4 Trace Validation, Correction, and Termination

The rib structure signals, although prominent in CT data, can easily be deteriorated by noise, surrounding structures, and partial volume effect. Our assumptions and model do not hold for all points, when the rib shape is irregular. Due to these complications, the tracing validation at each step and the stopping criterions require careful design. They should be just lenient enough for a good trace to continue but terminate a trace when appropriate.

We record the tracing directions of the previous 10 steps, and require that the current direction be close enough to the average of these directions. We also require that the cross-section contour extracted at each step is associated with a high energy. A more basic rule requires that there should be valid edges in most of the search directions. In the paths from the initial center point to the rib edges there should be mostly high intensity voxels.

Failure to meet the above criterions usually indicates that the trace has entered the posterior or anterior terminals. However, a single event of failure will not terminate the trace. In such a case, we retrospectively make adjustments of the initial center location and the tracing direction estimated from the last step. The initial center location is allowed to move in the close neighborhood, and the initial tracing direction can be adjusted by adding small deviations. For each of these adjustments, we carry the tracing procedure once more to see it the stopping criterions are met.

If the retrospective test fails, then algorithm will decide that the trace should be terminated.

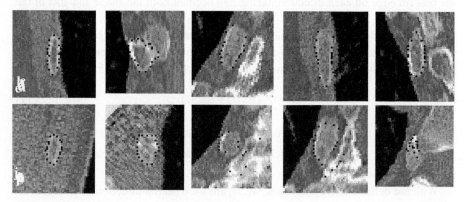

Fig. 3. Example cross-section contours. The black dots mark the contour edges determined by dynamic programming. (a)-(g): success cases (h-j): failure cases with energy values higher than threshold.

3   Results

We test the algorithm on around 40 multi-slice chest CT data sets. In our experiments, the data sets are super-sampled into isotropic data. The size of the slice image is 512×512, and each isotropic volume data set contains about 400~500 slices. The resolution is in the range of 0.5~0.8mm in each direction. Among these data sets, around half of them are from low-dose screening CT scans, and the rest is from high-dose diagnostic scans.

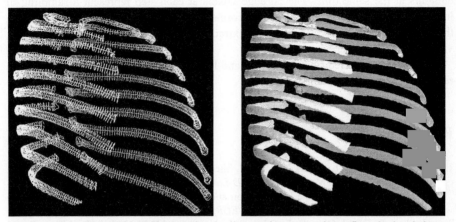

Fig. 4. An example result. (a) Extracted centerlines and contours that reflect the local shape. (b) Shaded surface display of the outer surface constructed from contours.

Shown in Fig. 3 are some example cross-section contours extracted during tracing. From pictures (a)-(g), we can see that the algorithm reliably extracts the contour edges despite noise and surrounding high intensity bone structures. Pictures (h)-(i) show cases where the energy function yields a high value, indicating a bad case. Some failure cases indicate that tracing has reached the spine terminals, and should be terminated; some are tolerated by the use of retrospective strategy. Generally, the edge detectors and dynamic programming techniques work well on convex and compact cross-section contours, but may have problem when the contours is very concave and even degenerate into a line-like structure.

The algorithm reliably extracts the centerlines, contours and outer surface of the rib structures, despite the various noise levels. Shown in Fig. 4 (a) and (b) is an example result. The surface in (b) is constructed with standard triangulation algorithms. The contours of the ribs reflect the local rib shapes, and the complete set of contours is an accurate description of the rib outer surface.

On a 2.8 GHz Dual Processor Pentium IV PC, the extraction of the complete set of rib structures takes about 10 seconds.

4 Conclusions

We have developed a fast and robust algorithm for extraction of individual rib structures from CT volume data. The algorithm uses mainly edges, but intensity information is also taken into account. Statistical analysis and dynamic programming techniques are combined to achieve good result despite high noise level and the disturbance of surrounding structures. Retrospective strategy with historical information is applied to help jumping through unfavorable cases.

The tracing algorithm has the advantage of extracting both the centerlines and contours at the same time. The 20 edge voxels at each step represent a sampling of local shape, forming the contour of the cross-section. All cross-section contours along the rib form the rib outer surface. These extracted features can be used for registration, visualization and other purposes.

Finally, the extracted ribs are ordered and labeled according to their relative spatial relationships and length ratios.

References

1. J. Qian, L. Fan, C. L. Novak, G. Wei, H. Shen, B. Odry G. Kohl D. P. Naidich, J. P. Ko, A. N. Rubinowitz, G. McGuinnes, "*ICAD-Lung*: An Interactive Computer Aided Diagnosis System for Lung Nodule Identification and Characterization" *the Matrix Presentation at the European Congress of Radiology (ECR2002)*, Vienna, March, 2002.
2. H. Shen, L. Fan, J. Qian, B. L. Odry, C. L. Novak, and D.P. Naidich, Real-Time Correspondence Between Lung Nodules in Follow-Up Multi-Slice High Resolution CT Studies, *the 2002 Conference of Radiological Society of North America*, November, 2002.
3. H. Shen, and M. Shao, A Thoracic Cage Coordinate System for Recording Pathologies in Lung CT Volume Data, *Proceedings of Nuclear Medicine Symposium and Medical Imaging Conference*, Portland, OR, 2003.
4. D. Kim, H. Kim, and H. Kang, Object-tracking segmentation method: vertebra and rib segmentation in CT images, *Proceedings of SPIE*, vol.4684, pt.1-3, p.1662-71, 2002.
5. F. Vogelsang, F. Weiler, J. Dahmen, M. Kilbinger, B. Wein, and R. Gunther, Detection and compensation of rib structures in chest radiographs for diagnose assistance, *Proceedings of SPIE*, vol.3338, p.774-785, 1998.
6. G. Bohm, C.J.Knoll, M.L. Alcaniz-Raya, and S.E.Albalat, Three-dimensional segmentation of bone structures in CT images, *Proceedings of Medical Imaging on Image Processing*, pp 277-286, 1999.
7. De. Souza P, Automatic rib detection in chest radiographs, *Computer Vision Graphics and Image Processing*, vol.23, no.2, p.129-61, Aug. 1983.
8. F.Volgelsang, F. Weiler, J. Dahmen, M.Kilbinger, B.Wein, and R.W.Gunther, Detection and compensation of rib structures in chest radiographs for diagnostic assistance, *Proceedings of the SPIE*, vol.3338, pt.1-2, p.774-85, 1998.
9. M. Loog, B. van Ginneken, M.A. Viergever, Segmenting the Posterior Ribs in Chest Radiographs by Iterated Contextual Pixel Classification, *Proceedings of SPIE*, San Diego, CA, US, 2003.
10. P.Dimitrov, J.N.Damon, and K.Siddiqi, Flux invariants for shape, *CVPR 2003: Computer Vision and Pattern Recognition Conference*, vol.1, Madison, WI, USA, 18-20 June 2003.
11. A. Can, H. Shen, J.N.Turner, H.L. Tanenbaum, and B. Roysam, "Rapid Automated Tracing and Feature Extraction from Retinal Fundus Images Using Direct Exploratory Algorithms", *IEEE Transactions on Information Technology in Biomedicine*, vol. 3, No.2, pp. 125-138, June 1999.
12. M. Brejl and M. Sonka, Directional 3D edge detection in anisotropic data: detector design and performance assessment, *Computer Vision and Image Understanding*, vol.77, no.2, p.84-110, Feb. 2000.
13. E.V.Denardo, *Models and Applications*, Dover Publications, May, 2003.

Automated 3D Segmentation of the Lung Airway Tree Using Gain-Based Region Growing Approach

Harbir Singh[1], Michael Crawford,[2], John Curtin[2], and Reyer Zwiggelaar[1]

[1] School of Computing Sciences, University of East Anglia, Norwich NR4 7TJ, England.
{Harbir.Singh, R.Zwiggelaar}@uea.ac.uk
[2] Norfolk and Norwich University Hospital, Norwich NR4 7UY, England.
{Michael Crawford, John.Curtin}@nnuh.nhs.uk

Abstract. In diagnosing lung diseases, it is highly desirable to be able to segment the lung into physiological structures, such as the intra-thoracic airway tree and the pulmonary structure. Providing an in-vivo and non-invasive tool for 3D reconstruction of anatomical tree structures such as the bronchial tree from 2D and 3D data acquisitions is a challenging issue for computer vision in medical imaging. Due to the complexity of the tracheobronchial tree, the segmentation task is non trivial. This paper describes a 3D adaptive region growing algorithm incorporating gain calculation for segmenting the primary airway tree using a stack of 2D CT slices. The algorithm uses an entropy-based measure known as information gain as a heuristic for selecting the voxels that are most likely to represent the airway regions.

1 Introduction

In diagnosing lung diseases, it is essential to be able to segment the lung into physiological structures, such as the intra-thoracic airway tree and the pulmonary structure. Once the airway tree is extracted, quantitative analysis can be performed to evaluate the tree structure and function. The tree structure is important in examining physiologic and pathological conditions such as stenosis and tumors. Given the complex branching of the airway tree, it is challenging to segment the tree manually. Such a manual annotation process is not free of problems. Image quality is compromised due to CT image acquisition process leading to intensity inhomogeneity. Partial volume effects make it difficult to identify small airways and minor detail clearly at the lower end of the tree. If the airway direction is parallel to the image plane, the density values in the airway lumen change, making the tracking of the airway regions difficult based on their intensity profile [1].

A number of automated approaches exist, covering segmentation and skeletonisation algorithms to extract all major airway branches and large parts of minor distal branches. Some of the approaches are based on mathematical morphology [2], central axis analysis [3], region growing [4], and knowledge-based techniques [5]. There is a trend towards hybrid approaches using a combination of techniques to give better results in terms of speed and detail of the extraction process [6]. A combination of morphological filtering, connection cost-based marking and a conditional watershed approach has been provided

C. Barillot, D.R. Haynor, and P. Hellier (Eds.): MICCAI 2004, LNCS 3217, pp. 975–982, 2004.

in [7] with use of fractal analysis and reconstruction. Other techniques are based on front propagation [8] to extract the major airway branches and parts of minor distal branches.

While 3D region growing is efficient, it suffers from partial volume effects, noise and global thresholding. The optimal threshold differs for large versus small airways, resulting in lack of finer details of the airways leading to incomplete structures and rough edges [6]. Similarly for method based on central axis analysis, selection of initial parameters, stopping criteria and forming of paths outside the airways warrants attention. For techniques based on morphology, the use and variation in morphological operators causes variation in the results obtained.

We have investigated the use of gain heuristic in 3D region growing for extracting the airway tree from a stack of volumetric CT data. The method has been evaluated against manually segmented tree obtained from the same data used for the automatic 3D method. The remainder of the paper is organized as follows. Section 2 explains the data and methods. Section 3 discusses the results and findings. Section 4 concludes with a few remarks and future directions.

2   Materials and Methods

2.1   Data

For each patient the data comprised of 125 transversal DICOM CT scans of 512×512 dimension obtained from Norfolk and Norwich University Hospital. The CT images are calibrated such that pure air voxel is represented by a value of about -1000 Hounsfield Units (HU), water is at 0 HU, soft tissue such as in the mediastinum is in the range of -100 HU to 200 HU and bone is represented by a value of +1000 HU [6]. These files were reduced to $256 \times 256 \times 125$ stack of images using lung window level settings. Fig. 1 shows image slices at the top, middle and lower sections of the lung cavity. In these images dark grey levels correspond to low density zones and light grey levels correspond to high density zones respectively. Bronchi appear as dark zones with bronchial lumen surrounded by medium-high thin grey level zones called bronchial walls.

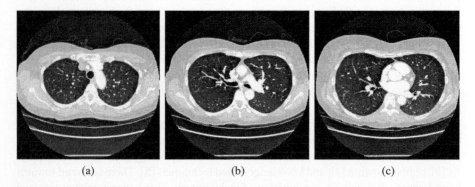

(a)   (b)   (c)

Fig. 1. Reconstructed transversal slices, where (a) CT slice showing the trachea, (b) branched airways at mid-section, and (c) airways in the lower-section.

2.2   Bronchus Structure

The bronchus has a pipe structure with air inside. Beginning from the end of the trachea, it extends into the lungs branching repeatedly like a tree. The splitting mainly occurs in bifurcations where the parent branch splits into two child branches with decreased diameters and lengths. The bronchi are classified into lobar bronchi which supply the five lobes, the segmental bronchi and the sub-segmental bronchi [8]. The contrast of the bronchus image is low and the bronchi is surrounded by a thin wall with inner area filled with air. This wall gets thinner as the branching increases and diameter of the bronchi decreases. The bronchus appears as a circular ring when it cuts orthogonal through a slice. CT values are lower inside the bronchus than those on the surrounding bronchus walls. This enables extraction of the bronchus area by following those areas in which the CT value is low and surrounded by walls of relatively higher CT values [4]. However, as the bronchi walls of the sub-segmental bronchi become very thin, the partial volume effect and image artifacts can break up the wall structure causing problems in the segmentation of the bronchi.

An example of manual segmentation of the airway tree can be found in Fig. 2.

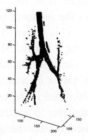

Fig. 2. Manual airway tree segmentation example.

2.3   3D Gain-Based Segmentation

The 3D segmentation method is based on regions growing using N_{26} voxel connectivity and incorporates information gain heuristic at the voxel processing stage. The details of the methods are given below.

At each candidate voxel, the gain at the voxels in the N_{26} neighborhood is calculated. The voxels with information gain higher than the threshold gain, are chosen for inclusion in the region growing process. These voxels with the highest information gain below the threshold gain, represent the greatest entropy reduction at the candidate voxel and reflect the least randomness or impurity at the candidate voxel [9].

Let set S consist of ns data points in the neighborhood of candidate voxel V. The intensity value of each voxel is $I(x_r, y_r, z_r)$. Considering N_{26} neighborhood, our sample S, will consist of 27 points. A voxel can be included in the region growing process or it can be excluded. Hence there are two classes which the sample points will be classified into. If I of each voxel is less than the threshold T, then that voxel is assigned a class of inclusion and if I of a voxel is more than the threshold T, then that voxel is assigned a class of exclusion. Given that our class label C has two values, (C=*include* or C=*exclude*), let s be the number of points belonging to class C_i in our sample.

The expected information for the whole sample S, is obtained as

$$EI(s_1, s_2, ...s_m) = -\sum_{i=1}^{m} p_i log_2(p_i) \tag{1}$$

where p_i is the probability of occurrence of voxel s_i with class C_i in the arbitrary sample and is given by s_i/ns.

The expected information E, at a given sample point s_i is given as

$$E(s_i) = p(s_i) * EI(s_i) \tag{2}$$

where $p(s_i)$ is the probability of sample point s_i in the sample.

Total gain is defined as

$$G = EI(s_1, s_2...s_m) - E(s_i) \tag{3}$$

The voxel with a gain higher than the threshold gain, is included in the region growing process. Fig. 3 shows the intensity profile of the airway region varies due to intensity homogeneity artifacts. This variation affects the 3D region growing algorithm based on a fixed threshold. Using a normal 3D segmentation approach leads to a large amount of variation in the area that gets included in the region growing process leading to an inaccurate segmentation. Often an adaptive thresholding approach is used where the threshold is dynamically adjusted in the region growing process as followed in [6, 10]. We introduced a gain parameter to control the 3D region growing process. In our approach no pre-processing such as smoothing or extraction of lung area was used. The results depend on the resolution and the quality of the underlying dataset.

2.4   Algorithm Outline

The steps of the algorithm are outlined below.
1. Initialize the algorithm providing a seed point $S(x_r, y_r, z_r)$, threshold value T, and a gain value G.
2. Perform 3D region growing using N_{26} connectivity with the seed $S(x_r, y_r, z_r)$, having intensity $I(x_r, y_r, z_r)$
3. For all voxels in the N_{26} neighborhood of seed point S, with intensity below threshold T, include in the region growing process.
4. For all voxels in the N_{26} neighborhood of seed point S, with intensity above threshold T, and intensity below an upper limit of the threshold T multiplied by a factor K, calculate gain G. (K=1.1$\times T$)
5. If the calculated gain G at the voxel is greater than the threshold gain G provided, include this voxel in the region growing process else ignore the voxel.
6. Goto step 3 until all voxels have been processed.
7. The output is a 3D binary subvolume of segmented airway tree.

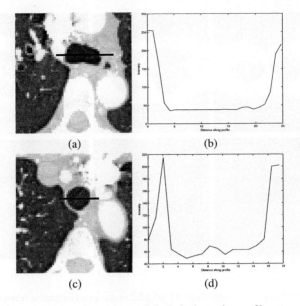

Fig. 3. (a,c) CT slice showing a bronchus and (b,d) the intensity profile across the bronchus.

3 Results

In this section we present and discuss the results obtained using the modified heuristic gain based 3D region growing algorithm.

Fig. 4 shows the processing results using 2D slices representing the top, middle and lower section of the bronchial tree. The 3D algorithm successfully identifies the bronchus area. Fig. 4a shows part of the trachea, Fig. 4b shows the trachea before splitting and Fig. 4c shows the airways when the trachea has split.

Fig. 5 shows the 3D visualization of the airway tree from the top, side and front angle segmented (threshold level equal to 53 and gain factor equal to 50%). The algorithm has been successful in identifying the branching and the structure of the airway tree on the given dataset to a high degree of accuracy.

We undertook a more detailed analysis, based on a single dataset, of sensitivity and specificity by plotting the values at different gain settings for different levels of thresholds, which can be found in Fig. 6. The automated results are compared to the manually segmented tree. It should be noted that the current evaluation methodology has a bias towards the initial levels in the airway tree as these contain relatively more pixels than the final levels of the tree. A level dependant evaluation is part of our future research directions. We see that in Fig. 6a sensitivity for T=47 is very low and in Fig. 6b specificity for T=47 very high (specificity=1) implying that the threshold setting was too low for the automated method to pick out the airway region. For these low threshold values the results are an under-segmentation of the tree. For higher levels of thresholds, the sensitivity is higher, with sensitivity=1 for T=60,63, while at the same level of thresholds, the specificity decreases as evident in Fig. 6b where the specificity curves shift downwards. This indicates an over-segmentation at these high threshold values.

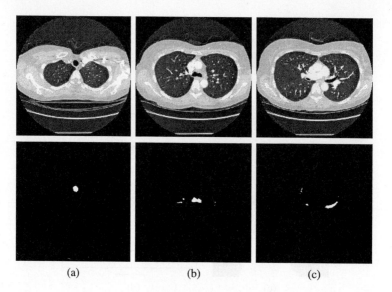

(a) (b) (c)

Fig. 4. 2D processing results showing original images and extracted bronchus area.

Using $(min((1 - sensitivity)^2 + (1 - specificity)^2))$, which takes both the sensitivity and specificity into account, the overall optimal segmentation parameters, for this dataset, are T=57 and G=70%.The segmentation is robust with respect to both parameters as all results for the ranges T=53-60 and G=10%-80% give acceptable results.

With respect to an increase in gain settings, Fig. 6a show almost constant sensitivity curves, with a slight decrease in sensitivity when the gain increases. However, Fig. 6b shows that the specificity gradually increases when the gain is increased. This implies that the use of gain heuristic has a larger influence on the specificity than on sensitivity.

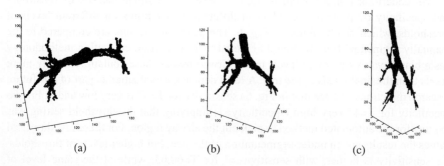

(a) (b) (c)

Fig. 5. Visualization of airway trees at T=53,G=50%, displaying (a) top view, (b) side view, and (c) front view.

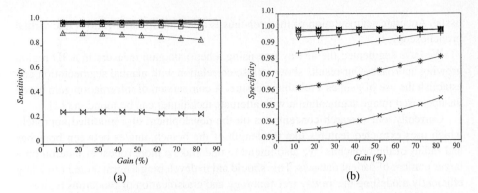

Fig. 6. Sensitivity and specificity graphs based on the following threshold values; ⋈: 47, △: 50, □: 53, ∇: 55, +: 57, *: 60 and ×: 63)

3.1 Limitations

However, as seen in Fig. 7, the algorithm is not fail proof as it encounters the problem of leakage which affects all segmentations of the airway tree based on the region growing approach. Even though the heuristic gain was used in this case, it was not able to prevent leakage of the grow process into the lung parenchyma. The heuristic gain at best introduces an additional control facility in the extraction process and combined with other parameters such as explosion of volume and other features of the regions of interest [11], can help in achieving better segmentation results.

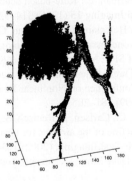

Fig. 7. Leakage, at T=63, G=10%, of the region grow process into the lung parenchyma.

4 Conclusion

The segmented bronchus area gives a measure of the volume of air in the lungs and can be subtracted from total lung volume to gauge a better estimate of volume of lung tissue. Accurate segmentation of the bronchus is also vital for applications like virtual bronchoscopy.

We have segmented the airway tree using a heuristic gain measure in a 3D region growing approach. Our results show a close correlation with manual segmentation and establish the use of gain as a reliable measure. A comparison of information gain based unsupervised image segmentation with alternate techniques can be found in [12].

Currently, our research concentrates on the development of a modified approach, which uses extracted features like the length of the branch, angles between branches and radius of the bronchus. We also intend to undertake a more robust evaluation on a larger number of patient datasets. This should aid in developing a normal lung model by efficiently modelling the airway tree topology and classification of cancerous regions.

References

1. Sonka, M., Fitzpatrick, J., eds.: Pulmonary Imaging and Analysis, Handbook Of Medical Imaging:Medical Image Processing and Analysis. Volume 2. SPIE - The International Society for Optical Engineering, Bellingham, Washington (2000)
2. Aykac, D., Hoffman, E., McLennan, G., Reinhardt, J.: Segmentation and analysis of the human airway tree from three-dimensional X-ray CT images. IEEE Transactions on Medical Imaging 22 (2003) 940–950
3. Swift, R., Kiraly, A., Sherbondy, A., Austin, A., Hoffman, E., McLennan, G., Higgins, W.: Automatic axes-generation for virtual bronchoscopic assessment of major airway obstructions. Computerized Medical Imaging and Graphics 26 (2002) 103–118
4. Mori, K., Hasegwawa, J., Toriwaki, J., Anno, H., Katada, K.: Automated extraction and visualisation of bronchus from 3D CT images of lung. In: CVRMed. Volume 905 of Lecture Notes in Computer Science. (1995) 542–548
5. Sonka, M., Park, W., Hoffman, E.: Rule-based detection of intrathoracic airway trees. IEEE Transactions on Medical Imaging 15 (1996) 314–326
6. Kiraly, A., Higgins, W., Hoffman, E., McLennan, G., Reinhardt, J.: 3D human airway segmentation for virtual bronchoscopy. In: Physiology and Function from Multidimensional Images. Volume 4683 of SPIE Medical Imaging. (2002) 16–29
7. Fetita, C., Preteux, F.: Three-dimensional reconstruction of human bronchial tree in HRCT. In: Proceedings SPIE Conference on Nonlinear Image Processing X. Volume 3646 of SPIE Electronic Imaging. (1999) 281–295
8. Schlatholter, T., Lorenz, C., Carlsen, I., Renisch, S., Deschamps, T.: Simultaneous segmentation and tree reconstruction of the airways for virtual bronchoscopy. In: Image Processing. Volume 4684 of SPIE Medical Imaging. (2002) 103–113
9. Han, J., Kamber, M.: Data Mining Concepts and Techniques. Morgan Kaufmann, San Francisco CA (2001)
10. Tschirren, J., Palagyi, K., Reinhardt, J., Hoffman, E., Sonka, M.: Segmentation, skeletonization and branchpoint matching - a fully automated quantitative evaluation of human intrathoracic airway trees. In: Medical Image Computing and Computer-Assisted Intervention,Part II. Volume 2489 of Lecture Notes in Computer Science. (2002) 12–19
11. Revol-Muller, C., Peyrin, F., Carrillon, Y., Odet, C.: Automated 3D region growing algorithm based on assessment function. Pattern Recognition Letters 23 (2002) 137
12. Singh, H., Zwiggelaar, R.: Unsupervised image segmentation using information gain. The Irish Machine Vision and Image Processing Conference (submitted) (2004)

Real-Time Dosimetry for Prostate Brachytherapy Using TRUS and Fluoroscopy

Danny French[1], James Morris[2], Mira Keyes[2], and S.E. Salcudean[1]

[1] Department of Electrical and Computer Engineering, University of British Columbia, 2356 Main Mall, Vancouver BC V6T 1Z4, Canada
[2] Vancouver Center, British Columbia Cancer Agency, 600 West 10th, Vancouver, BC V5Z 4EB, Canada

Abstract. A new approach for computing real-time dosimetry (RTD) for prostate brachytherapy is presented. Transrectal ultrasound (TRUS) and fluoroscopic images are fused to compute dosimetry. The frontal plane coordinates of the seeds are found in the fluoroscopic images and the remaining coordinate is computed from the TRUS. Our approach is verified on a phantom and tested on clinical data. A method for tracking intraoperative seed motion using TRUS is also presented.

1 Introduction

Prostate brachytherapy is frequently used to treat low-risk prostate cancer. Using transrectal ultrasound (TRUS) to guide needles between 80 and 150 small radioactive seeds are permanently implanted in the prostate.

Because of inaccuracies in needle placement and intraoperative prostate shifting and swelling, there is a need to provide accurate real-time dosimetric feedback. This feedback will allow radiation oncologists to intraoperatively modify the planned seed locations (i.e. interactive planning) ensuring the prostate receives sufficient radiation to destroy the cancerous cells [1] [2].

The need for real-time dosimetry (RTD) has resulted in several commercial systems. VariSeed (Varian Medical Systems, Palo Alto, CA), Prostate Implant Planning Engine for Radiotherapy (PIPER) system (RTek, Pittsford, NY), Interplant System (Burrdette Medical System, Champaign, IL), Strata System (Rosses Medical Systems, Columbia, MD), and SPOT (Nucletron Corporation, Veenandaal, Netherlands) all use ultrasound to locate needles or blood trails and assume seed spacing to compute dosimetry. Individual seed are not located because seeds cannot be reliably located in ultrasound images [7]. Therefore, another modality must be combined with TRUS to accurately compute dosimetry.

Because fluoroscopes are commonly used, in addition to TRUS, for prostate brachytherapy, several methods of fusing TRUS and fluoroscopic images to compute dosimetry have been reported. TRUS is used to identify the prostate contour and fluoroscopic images taken from three or more perspectives are used to locate individual seeds to compute dosimetry. In [3] TRUS and three fluoroscopic images are fused using four needle tips. In [5] the fluoroscopic images are registered to the TRUS image using five to seven noncoplanar reference points. Yet,

C. Barillot, D.R. Haynor, and P. Hellier (Eds.): MICCAI 2004, LNCS 3217, pp. 983–991, 2004.
© Springer-Verlag Berlin Heidelberg 2004

interactive planning is limited because the fluoroscope must be rotated to three different angles to update dosimetry, which is both time-consuming and inconsistent with the current procedure. A RTD system using intraoperative magnetic resonance (IMR) imaging is presented in [4]. This method cannot consistently locate individual seeds and is expensive.

This paper presents a new approach for RTD in prostate brachytherapy. Our system is fast enough to allow interactive planning and integrates into the current procedure with minimal change and without additional imaging equipment. TRUS is used to locate each needle tip and a single fluoroscopic image is used to locate individual seeds. The fluoroscopic image frame and TRUS image frame are registered, using a single fluoroscopic image of the TRUS probe. Knowing the location of each seed, dosimetry can be computed and displayed after each fluoroscopic image providing the radiation oncologist with the ability to confidently make modifications to the preoperative plan. A method of compensating for intraoperative seed motion is also presented.

2   TRUS and Fluoroscopic Based RTD – Methods

A flow chart of our approach is shown in Fig. 1. The coordinate systems used are described in Fig. 2a. Initially, as is current procedure at the Vancouver Cancer Center, the radiation oncologist positions the TRUS probe based on manual registration of preoperative TRUS images with intraoperative TRUS images. Once this is achieved, a single fluoroscopic image of the TRUS probe is used to register the fluoroscopic and TRUS images. The radiation oncologist continues with the current procedure by inserting each needle and locating its tip in the TRUS image (see Fig. 2b). From the tip location and the entry point of the needle, a needle path is computed by interpolating from the needle base to the tip. After each row of needles, a fluoroscopic image is taken to determine the (x,z)-coordinates of the seeds (see Fig. 2c). Using these coordinates and the needle path, the y-coordinates of the seeds are computed. Knowing the coordinates of each seed allows dosimetry to be displayed to the radiation oncologist after each row of needles, so the preoperative plan can be intraoperatively modified to reflect inaccuracies in seed placement and intraoperative seed motion.

Registration of TRUS and Fluoroscopic Images. The TRUS and fluoroscopic images are registered using a single fluoroscopic image of the TRUS probe. The edges of the probe are found in the fluoroscopic image using an intensity-based edge detector and a least squares fit. Knowing the corners of the probe in the fluoroscopic image, the physical dimensions of the probe and the source to image plane distance of the C-arm, a simple coordinate transform from the fluoroscopic image to the TRUS image can be found using similar triangles.

Fig. 3a shows the error in determining the height of the TRUS as a function of fluoroscopic image resolution. The accuracy of the height of an object above the image plane of the fluoroscope is primarily limited by the resolution of the

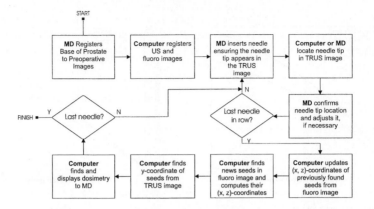

Fig. 1. A flow chart of our approach for computing RTD

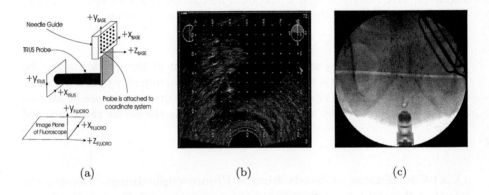

(a)   (b)   (c)

Fig. 2. (a) The coordinate systems used in our approach, (b) A TRUS image with needle artifact at C3, (c) A fluoroscopic image of implanted seeds

fluoroscope. While fluoroscopic image warping does contribute to error, it can be calibrated out [8]. In the data presented, image warping is ignored as it is not a determining factor in proving the feasibility of our approach. For simplicity, we assume that the C-arm and TRUS frames are parallel. The angular offsets between frames are small and contribute minimal errors. If necessary, they can be computed from the angles of edges that are known to be parallel.

The most significant error is in determining the height of the TRUS above the fluoroscopic image. Experimentally, the height of the TRUS was found using our registration algorithm for 15 different heights, with a mean absolute error of 2.16 mm and a maximum absolute error of 5.72 mm.

Locating the Needle Tip in TRUS Images. The needle tip artifact is a white flash in the TRUS image (see Fig. 2b). Currently, this is manually located in the TRUS image, but work is underway to automate this step. By doing

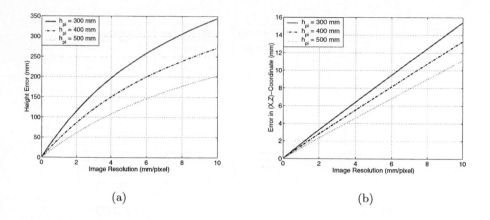

Fig. 3. (a) TRUS height error as a function of fluoroscopic image resolution, (b) Error in the (x,z)-coordinates of the seeds as a function of image resolution

a localized search of sequential frames the location of the needle tip can be approximated by finding a sudden clustered change in intensity between frames. However, identifying the exact location of the needle tip from the needle artifact is difficult [3]. This is why a manual step for locating the needle tip is included in Fig 1.

(X,Z)-Coordinates of Seeds from a Fluoroscopic Image. Because the height of the probe can be approximated reasonably well, fluoroscopic images can be back-projected to the TRUS frame to determine the (x,z)-coordinates of the seeds. Fig. 3b shows the error in the (x,z)-coordinates as a function of image resolution with an accuracy of less than 0.75 mm. The seeds are currently selected manually, but automation of this step using morphological operators has been demonstrated in [6], [5] and [3].

Because the seeds move, the intraoperative (x,z)-coordinates of the seeds must be updated with each fluoroscopic image. By searching in the regions near the coordinates of the previously found seeds, the seed coordinates can be updated. This step is done prior to searching for new seeds to simplify the search.

Y-Coordinate of Seeds from TRUS Images. It is obvious from Fig. 3a that the height of the seeds cannot be found from a single fluoroscopic image because of limited fluoroscopic image resolution (approximately 0.5 mm/pixel). In fact, even with a substantially higher resolution height errors are significant. However, the needle tip can be located in TRUS with much higher accuracy. So, knowing the entry point of the needle from the preoperative plan, a needle path is interpolated and the y-coordinates of the seeds calculated.

Computation of Dosimetry. Knowing the coordinates of each seed the dosimetry can be calculated. In this paper, each seed is modelled as a line source. The dosimetry results are displayed in the base frame which can easily be superimposed on TRUS images. This method of displaying dosimetry does not require the time-consuming step of segmenting the prostate, but allows the radiation oncologist to identify underdosed regions to do interactive planning.

3   TRUS and Fluoroscopic Based RTD – Experiments

3.1   Phantom

The phantom shown in Fig. 4a was constructed to validate the registration algorithm and to estimate the accuracy with which our system can locate seeds. The phantom is contained in a Plexiglas box (approximately 100 mm in each dimension). In one wall of the box there is one 32.5 mm diameter hole to insert a TRUS probe and four 1.5 mm diameter holes to insert needles. Mounted on the inside of the same wall is a metal needle guide to prevent needle deflection. On the inside of the opposite wall there is a Plexiglas shelf with four groves to hold seeds that are aligned with the holes in the needle guide. A latex condom filled with ultrasound gel extends from the 32.5 mm diameter hole to the opposite wall to simulate the rectum. Twelve seeds are secured in the groves of the Plexiglas shelf and the remaining space in the phantom is filled with gelatin (13 percent gelatin and 3 percent cellulose by mass).

A TRUS probe was inserted in the condom to a pre-determined depth between the metal needle guide and the Plexiglas shelf (the angle was measured to be approximately zero). A single fluoroscopic image was acquired (see Fig. 4b). The first needle was inserted until the needle tip appeared in the TRUS image (see Fig. 4c). The distance from the wall of the phantom to the hub of the needle was recorded. Using this distance and the fluoroscopic image of the TRUS probe, the TRUS image and fluoroscopic image spaces were registered. Three more needles were inserted until each needle tip appeared in the TRUS image.

The seed coordinates found by our system closely match the known seed locations. The mean error in the x,y,z directions is 0.47 mm, 0.52 and 0.78 mm, respectively, and the maximum error is 1.13 mm, 0.63 mm and 1.38 mm. These results support our approach for registering the TRUS and fluoroscopic image and our method for computing the coordinates of the seeds.

3.2   Clinical Data

Our approach was tested on clinical data collected during a prostate brachytherapy procedure. The ultrasound video was captured at 30 frames per second and fluoroscopic images were taken as described in Fig. 1. Both the seeds in the fluoroscopic images and the needle tips in the TRUS images were manually selected, but the feasibility of our approach is still proven. The results of our system are compared to the seed locations and dosimetry found from a computed tomography (CT) scan done 3-4 hours after the procedure.

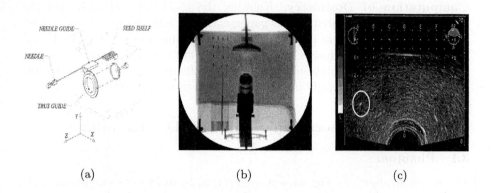

Fig. 4. (a) Diagram of the phantom, (b) Fluoroscopic image of the phantom, (c) TRUS image of the phantom (a needle artifact is enclosed by a circle)

Dosimetry was calculated for 3 mm^3 voxels for seed locations determined from the CT scan and our approach. Using CT as the gold standard, the error in dosimetry for each voxel was computed. The mean error was 14.4 percent with a standard deivation of 3.8 percent. The percent volume is plotted as a function of percent error in dosimetry in Fig. 6a.

Possible sources of error include lack of calibration and dewarping, errors in manually selecting seeds and needle tips, and errors in locating seeds in the CT images. However, a significant amount of error results from not compensating for intraoperative seed motion in the y-direction, which results from patient motion, probe motion and intraoperative prostate swelling and shifting.

4   Tracking Intraoperative Seed Motion

To compensate for motion in the y-direction, the motion of the prostate boundary or several seeds or blood trails is tracked in TRUS. Although seeds and blood trails cannot be consistently located or distinguished in TRUS, several image artifacts or the boundary of the prostate can be marked and cropped from a previous TRUS frame. The masks are correlated with a larger region having the same centroid in the new frame. The location of the maximum correlation coefficient is the new location of the mask. A weighted average based on the distance between the masks and the seeds is used to determine the vertical motion of each seed.

This seed tracking algorithm was also tested on clinical data. During the procedure the height of the probe was adjusted, the frames immediately before and after the adjustment are shown as Figs. 5a and 5b. The location of three seeds or blood trails was found in both the old and new frames, by finding the centroid of the artifact using a thresholding technique. Two seeds or blood trails and the posterior boundary of the prostate were selected as masks (see

Table 1. The results of tracking seed motion in clinical data

Seed	Motion in Image (mm)	Detected Seed Motion (mm)
1	−0.924	−0.947
2	−0.924	−0.912
3	−0.922	−0.995

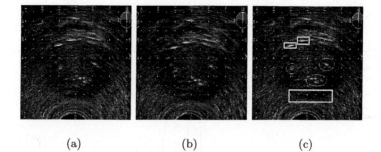

(a)   (b)   (c)

Fig. 5. (a) The old frame, (b) The new frame (note seed motion between frames), (c) The masks (enclosed in rectangles) and seeds (circled) used to verify the algorithm in clinical table

Fig. 5c). The motion detected by our algorithm was compared to the motion of the centroid of each seed or blood trail artifact. The results in Table 1 show that seed motion can be intraoperatively tracked in TRUS images of the prostate.

The dosimetry was also calculated for the same data presented in Section 3.2, with compensation for intraoperative seed motion. The mean error in dose was 11.2 percent with a standard deviation of 4.5 percent. The percent volume is plotted as a function of percent error in dosimetry in Fig. 6b.

In seed distributions that are compensated for motion in the y-direction the top rows of seeds more closely match the seed distribution found from the CT data. In our current system, masks are manually selected by the user, but work is ongoing to automate this process and determine the best choice of masks. It has been noted that TRUS frames recorded during a needle insertion cannot reliably identify seed motion because the needle forces temporarily cause motion beyond the actual resting point of the prostate.

5   Conclusion and Future Work

A new approach for computing RTD for prostate brachytherapy has been presented. The systems accounts for inaccuracies in needle placement and intraoperative seed motion. Dosimetry can be determined after each fluoroscopic image providing real-time dosimetric feedback and allowing interactive planning.

As this is a work in progress, improvements in automation and accuracy are possible. The best approach to selecting masks to track intraoperative seed motion needs to be determined. The accuracy with which the needle tip can be found in a TRUS image must be validated. Our approach could be better validated by comparing our results to the seed locations found from three fluoroscopic images, rather than seed locations determined from a CT scan.

The approach has been validated on a phantom and tested on clinical data with promising results.

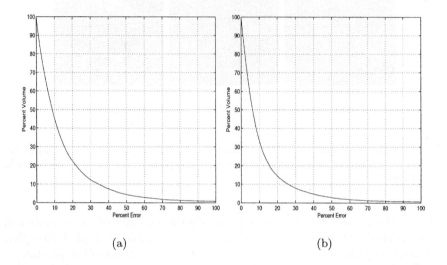

(a)   (b)

Fig. 6. The percent volume as a function of percent error in dosimetry without (a) and with (b) motion compensation for the y-coordinates of the seeds

References

[1] Subir Nag, Jay P. Ciezki, Robert Cormack, et al. Intraoperative planning and evalutation permanent prostate brachytherapy: Report of the American Brachytherapy Society. *Int. J. Radiation Oncology Biol Phys*, 51:1422-1430, 2001.
[2] L. Potter. Permanent prostate brachytherapy in men with clinically localised prostate cancer. *Clinical Oncology*, 15:301-315, 2003.
[3] L. Gong, P.S. Cho, B.H. Han, K.E. Wallner, et al. Ultrasonography and fluoroscopic fusion for prostate brachytherapy dosimetry *Int. J. Radiation Oncology Biol Phys*, 54:1322-1330, 2002.
[4] R.A. Cormack, H. Kooy, C.M. Tempany, A.V. D'Amico. A clinical method for real-time dosimetric guidance of transperineal ^{125}i prostate implants using interventional magnetic resonance imaging. *Int. J. Radiation Oncology Biol Phys*, 46:207-214, 2000.

[5] D.A. Todor, M. Zaider, G.N. Cohen, et al. Intraoperative dyanmic dosimetry for prostate implants. *Physics in Medicine and Biology*, 48:1153-1171, 2003.

[6] D. Tubic, A. Zaccarin, J. Pouliot, and L. Beaulieu. Automated seed detection and three-dimensional reconstruction I: Seed locatization from fluoroscopic images or radiographs. *Physics in Medicine and Biology*, 28:2265-2271, 2001.

[7] B.H. Han, K. Wallner, G. Merrick, et al. Prostate brachytherapy seed identification on post-implant TRUS images *Medical Physics*, 30:898-900, 2003.

[8] G. Gil and Y. Yoon. C-arm image distortion calibration method for computer-aided surgery. *International Journal of Human-friendly Welfare Robotic Systems*, 4:20-26, 2003.

Fiducial-Less Respiration Tracking in Radiosurgery

Achim Schweikard[1], Hiroya Shiomi[2], Jens Fisseler[1], Manfred Dötter[3], Kajetan Berlinger[3], Hans-Björn Gehl[4], and John Adler[5]

[1] Informatik, Universität Lübeck, 23538 Lübeck, Germany
[2] Div. of Multidisciplinary Radiotherapy, Osaka University Graduate School of Medicine, Japan
[3] Informatik, Technische Universität München, 85748 München, Germany
[4] Radiology, Universität Lübeck, 23538 Lübeck, Germany
[5] Neurosurgery, Stanford University Medical Center, Stanford, CA. 94304, USA

Abstract. Respiratory motion is difficult to compensate for with conventional radiotherapy systems. An accurate tracking method for following the motion of the tumor is of considerable clinical relevance. We investigate methods to compensate for respiratory motion using robotic radiosurgery. Infrared emitters are used to record the motion of the patient's skin surface. The position of internal gold fiducials is computed repeatedly during treatment, via x-ray image processing. We correlate the motion between external and internal markers. From this correlation model we infer the placement of the internal target. 15 patients with lung tumors have recently been treated with a fully integrated system implementing this new method. In this work we extend our method to tracking without implanted fiducials. We propose to use deformation algorithms on CT data sets combined with registration of digitally reconstructed radiographs to obtain intermittent information on the target location. This information is then combined with our basic correlation method to achieve real-time tracking. The term 7D registration is coined to describe the underlying method for performing this task.

1 Introduction

Radiosurgery uses a moving beam of photon radiation to destroy tumors. High precision radiosurgery has been limited to brain tumors, since stereotactic fixation is difficult to apply to tumors in the chest or abdomen. To apply radiosurgical methods to tumors in the chest and abdomen, it is necessary to take into account respiratory motion. Respiratory motion can move the tumor by more than 1 cm. Without compensation for respiratory motion, it is necessary to enlarge the target volume with a "safety margin". For small targets, an appropriate safety margin produces a very large increase in treated volume.

C. Barillot, D.R. Haynor, and P. Hellier (Eds.): MICCAI 2004, LNCS 3217, pp. 992–999, 2004.
© Springer-Verlag Berlin Heidelberg 2004

2   Related Work

Intra-treatment displacements of a target due to respiration have been reported
to exceed 3 cm in the abdomen, and 1 cm for the prostate [4], [8]. Conventional radiation therapy with medical linear accelerators (LINAC-systems) uses a gantry
with two axes of rotation movable under computer control [11]. This mechanical
construction was designed to deliver radiation from several different angles during a single treatment. It was not designed to track respiratory motion. Respiratory gating is a technique for addressing this problem with conventional LINAC
radiation therapy. Gating techniques do not directly compensate for breathing
motion. I.e., the therapeutic beam is not moved during activation. Instead the
beam is switched off whenever the target is outside a predefined window.

Tada and Minakuchi et. al. [9] report using an external laser range sensor
in connection with a LINAC-based system for respiratory gating. This device
is used to switch the beam off whenever the sensor reports that the respiratory
cycle is close to maximal inhalation or maximal exhalation.

In an earlier paper [7], we investigated a method for tracking a tumor during
treatment with a robotic arm. Stereo x-ray imaging is combined with infrared
tracking. x-ray imaging is used as an internal sensor, while infrared tracking
provides simultaneous information on the motion of the patient surface. While
x-ray imaging gives accurate information on the internal target location, it is
not possible to obtain real-time motion information from x-ray imaging alone.
In contrast, the motion of the patient surface can be tracked with commercially
available high speed infrared position sensors. The main idea of our approach is
to use a series of images from both sensors (infrared and x-ray) where signal acquisition is synchronized. From such a series of sensor readings and corresponding time-stamps, we can determine a motion pattern. This pattern correlates
external motion to internal motion.

Below we describe an integrated system using the new correlation method
from [7] (internal versus external fiducials), and outline a concept for extending
this work to tracking without implanted fiducials. A major obstacle for reaching
the goal of tracking without implanted fiducial markers is that image registration
must now be based solely on anatomic landmarks. The standard techniques
available are currently not suitable for real-time tracking. We thus present a
method for splitting the task of registration into a pre-operative computation
phase and an intra-operative phase. As a result, our method does not require
elastic registration.

3   System

Our system has the following components (Fig. 1). A robot arm (modified Cyberknife system) moves the therapeutic beam generator (medical linear accelerator). The component added to the standard Cyberknife system is an infrared
tracking system (BIG Inc., Boulder CO, USA). Infrared emitters are attached to
the chest and the abdominal surface of the patient. The infrared tracking system

records the motion of these emitters. A stereo x-ray camera system (two x-ray cameras with nearly orthogonal visual axes) records the position of internal gold markers, injected through an 18 gauge biopsy needle into the vicinity of the target area under CT monitoring.

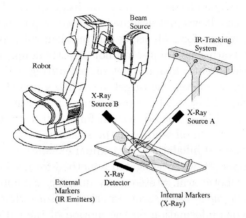

Fig. 1. System overview. A robotic arm moves the beam source to actively compensate for respiratory motion. Infrared surface tracking is correlated to internal x-ray imaging.

The correlation method for computing the position of the internal target has been described in more detail in [7] and is briefly summarized here. Prior to treatment, small gold markers are placed in the vicinity of the target organ. Stereo x-ray imaging is used during treatment to determine the precise spatial location of these gold markers once every 10 seconds.

External markers (placed on the patient's skin) can be tracked automatically with optical methods at very high speed. Updated positions can be transmitted to the control computer more than 20 times per second. However, external markers alone cannot adequately reflect internal displacements caused by breathing motion. Large external motion may occur together with very small internal motion, and vice versa. Similarly, the target may move much slower than the skin surface. Since neither internal nor external markers alone are sufficient for accurate tracking, x-ray imaging is synchronized with optical tracking of external markers. The external markers are small infrared emitters attached to the patient's skin. The first step during treatment is to compute the exact relationship between internal and external motion, using a series of x-ray snapshots showing external and internal markers simultaneously. Each snapshot has a time-stamp which is used to compute the correlation model.

4   Tracking Without Fiducials

The method described above requires x-ray opaque fiducials to be placed in the vicinity of the target. We extend our method in such a way that impanting fiducials is no longer needed. This extension works as follows:

Prior to treatment two CT scans are taken. One scan shows inhalation, one shows exhalation. From this data a series of intermediate CT scans is computed. This yields a series of 3D scans, showing the respiration process as a three-dimensional motion picture. For each point in this time series, we compute a set of digitally reconstructed radiographs (DRR), (see e.g. [6]). A single DRR is computed by projecting a CT scan from a preselected angle using the known geometry of the x-ray imaging system. Assume we have 12 time steps in our CT 3D motion picture. For each of the 12 time steps, we compute a number of DRRs for a preselected angle.

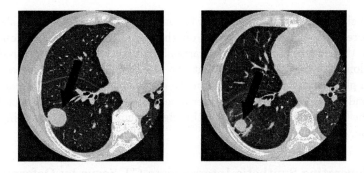

Fig. 2. Treatment of an adeno carcinoma with fiducial based respiration tracking. (Osaka university hospital. Treatment with 39 Gy / 3 Fractions).

During treatment, stereo x-ray images are taken with the stereo x-ray cameras. These images will be called live images. When a new live shot is taken, it is compared to each of the previously computed DRRs. This comparison selects the best matching DRR in the series. Assume this best matching DRR has index number n. Each DRR was computed from one CT scan. Then we can identify the CT scan from which this specific DRR (index number n) was generated. This allows for identifing a time step in the 3D CT series, i. e. a respiration state within the respiratory cycle. Furthermore the given DRR (index number n) represents a specific angle, under which the present CT scan is seen. This allows for determining the angle under which the patient was seen in the given live shot. Furthermore, computerized comparisons between the live shot and DRRs permit translational shifts to be determined. Overall, if the target is marked in each CT scan, we can identify the exact target location (position, orientation, respiration state) at the time the live shot was taken.

Notice that this gives only intermittent information on the target location. At the time the comparison of all DRRs with the current live shot is completed, the target may already have moved. However, our method is nonetheless capable of determining the real-time target position. As in the above fiducial-based correlation method, a real-time sensor is used to report information on the current state of respiration in real time. This information is correlated to the target location computed by the comparison between the live shot and DRRs.

5   Experiments and Clinical Trials

Clinical trials of the method in section 3 have been carried out at several institutions, including Cleveland Clinic Foundation and Osaka University Hospital. 15 patients have since been treated at Osaka University Hospital with the fiducial-based method described in section 3.

5.1   Clinical Trials

Figure 3 shows representative results for one clinical case. The figure shows the total correlation error. Thus, based on the correlation model (section 3), we compute the current position of the target based on the external infrared sensor signal alone. At this same time point, we also acquire a pair of x-ray images. We then plot the distance in mm from the placement inferred by the correlation model and the actual placement determined from the implanted fiducial markers in the image. The top curve in this figure shows the corresponding target excursion.

5.2   Generating Synthetic Intermediate CT Scans by Deformation

In vitro trials have been carried out to determine practicality of the fiducial-less method described above. In a first experiment, deformation methods for computing intermediate tomographic scans were tested. The goal of the experiment was to assess the practicality of the deformation sub-steps in terms of computing time and accuracy. A variety of methods for elastic registration and deformation (intensity or landmark-based) have been described in the literature (see e.g. [5] for a survey). Given two sets of tomographic data (CT or MR), one in inhale one in exhale position, plus a third "test set" of tomographic data (intermediate point in the respiratory cycle), we wish to verify that the test set indeed matches one of the synthetic 3D data sets computed by deformation. To this end liver liver data sets for several volunteers were acquired. For each of these volunteers, one inhale, one exhale, and up to three intermediate scans were aquired. The images were taken by a T1 sequence in a Siemens Symphony MRT scanner with 1.5 Tesla and gradients of 30 mTesla/m. In each case complete 3D image data sets (40 slices 0.65 mm of pixel distance within each layer, 2.5 mm thickness per layer and 2 mm slice distance) were taken. Aquisition time per complete data set is in the range of 15–25 seconds.

Three algorithms for deformation with various types of user interaction were implemented: Thirion's demons algorithm [10], thin plate spline warping based

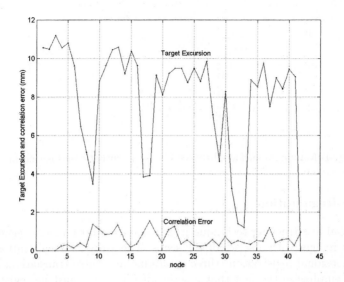

Fig. 3. Total target excursion (top curve), and correlation error (bottom curve) in mm for a clinical case. x-axis: treatment beam direction number (x-ray live shot number), y-axis: error in mm.

on control points placed at landmarks ([1]) and linear interpolation based on control points at landmarks ([2]). The liver volumes were segmented semi-automatically with a modified intelligent scissors algorithm to reconstruct the surface of the liver. This allows for measuring distances between deformed surfaces. Furthermore, given the segmentation, we compute the center of gravity of the segmented liver volume in each case. The total paths travelled by the center of gravity ranged from 21.8 mm to 46.7 mm for data stemming from distinct volunteers. From each algorithm we obtain a deformation field allowing to compute a continuous deformation between inhalation and exhalation. We consider the maximum surface distance between the intermediate data set obtained by actual imaging and the data set obtained synthetically by deformation.

Figure 4 shows the maximum surface distance between the synthetic data and the intermediate data set as a function of time, where the time parameter varies between 0 and 1, corresponding to exhalation and inhalation respectively. The figure shows a clear minimum for both thin-plate spline deformation and linear interpolation, with minima of 2.2 mm and 2.6 mm of maximum surface distance. The demon's algorithm gave similar results for maximum surface distances. Computing times were in the range of 50–70 minutes for all three algorithms. 80 control points (manually selected) were used for the control point oriented algorithms in each case.

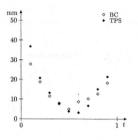

Fig. 4. Maximum surface distance between synthetic and actual image.

5.3   7D Registration

The fiducial-less tracking technique in section 4 requires a rigid registration of two x-ray images with a series of CT scans. The x-ray–CT registration alone is a six-dimensional registration (three rotational and three translational parameters). To emphasize the fact that a series of CT scans must be registered to a live x-ray image pair with respiration as an additional parameter, we will call this type of registration 7D registration. The experiments consisted of a series of 6D registrations between x-ray and CT images. We register two images of sizes $768/2 \times 576/2$ pixels against a CT image of 512×512 with 50 slices. (Thus original image size is 768×576 but only every second pixel was used in both directions for the registration). The original resolution is 3.4 pixels per millimeter, thus 1.7 pixels per millimeter in the images used for registration. Here CT resolution is 1.5 pixel per mm. This low resolution was used, since a large field of view was needed to allow for including a calibration plate. The volume registered was down-sampled to 128 by 128 by 128 voxels and describes a cube of size $128 \times 128 \times 128$ mm. The computing times for registration were 5 to 10 seconds with an average number of 150 to 300 function calls to a Hooke-Jeeves patterns search minimizer [3]. Hardware-accelerated volume rendering via 2D textures is used. Similarity measurement with the correlation coefficient gave best results over a variety of other similarity measures such as MI, NMI (see [5]). In order to lower the influence of regions outside the volumes to be registered, the following procedure was used: the rendered volume was threshold-segmented, and enlarged by 5 pixels via dilatation. Only the intersection of this 2D region with the "bulls-eye" stemming from the x-ray images was used for the registration. Computing times refer to a Pentium 3 processor with 1400 Mhz, running under Linux with 512 MB main storage and a 3D-card NVidia GeForce2.

6   Discussion and Conclusions

Clinical testing of the method in section 3 demonstrates an overall correlation error of below 2 mm throughout an entire 70 minutes treatment, while the total target motion was over 10 mm. This suggests that our method meets the definition of radiosurgcial accuracy and is capable of reducing safety margins by a very substantial amount.

A registration time of 5–10 seconds for a single simulated registration was determined in our experiments. To find the tomographic image best matching the given live shots, this registration must be repeated for a series of up to 8 synthetic or actual image 3D sets showing intermediate respiration states. Hence a total image processing time of under 100 seconds per live image pair is realistic in the given application. Notice that this would in practice allow for real-time tracking if combined with the correlation technique in section 3. Here 100 seconds is strictly intra-operative time. The reason why this is still fast enough to track is that the tracking relies solely on the external signal, which can be read in real-time.

References

1. F. L. Bookstein: Principal Warps: Thin-Plate Splines and the Decomposition of Deformations. *IEEE Transactions on Pattern Analysis and Machine Intelligence*, 11(6):565–587, 1989.
2. M. Fornefett, K. Rohr, H. S. Stiehl: Radial Basis Functions with Compact Support for Elastic Registration of Medical Images. In *Proc. Internat. Workshop Biomedical Image Registration (WBIR'99)*, pages 173–185, Aug. 1999.
3. R. A. Hooke, T. A. Jeeves: Direct Search Solution for Numerical and Statistical Problems. *Journal of the ACM*, 8(2):230–239, 1961.
4. S. M. Morrill, M. Langer, R. G. Lane: Real-Time Couch compensation for intra-treatment Organ Motion: Theoretical Advantages. *Medical Physics*, 23, 1083, 1996.
5. T. Rohlfing, C. R. Maurer, W. G. O'Dell, J. Zhong: Modeling liver motion and deformation during the respiratory cycle using intensity-based free-form registration of gated MR images. *Medical Imaging 2001*. In *Proc. of SPIE Vol. 4319*, pages 337–348, 2001.
6. D. B. Russakoff, T. Rohlfing et. al.: Fast calculation of digitally reconstructed radiographs using light fields. *Medical Imaging 2003*. In *Proc. of SPIE Vol. 5032*, 2003.
7. A. Schweikard, G. Glosser, M. Bodduluri, M. Murphy, J. R. Adler: Robotic Motion Compensation for Respiratory Movement during Radiosurgery. *Computer-Aided Surgery*, 5(4):263–277, 2000.
8. M. R. Sontag, Z. W. Lai et. al.: Characterization of Respiratory Motion for Pedriatic Conformal 3D Therapy. *Medical Physics*, 23, 1082, 1996.
9. T. Tada, K. Minakuchi et. al.: Lung Cancer: Intermittent Irradiation Synchronized with Respiratory Motion – Results of a Pilot Study. *Radiology*, 207(3): 779–783, 1998.
10. J.-P. Thirion: Non-Rigid Matching Using Demons. In *Proceedings of the 1996 Conference on Computer Vision and Pattern Recognition*, pages 245–251. IEEE Computer Society, 1996.
11. S. Webb: The Physics of Three-dimensional Radiation Therapy. *Institute of Physics Publishing*, Bristol and Philadelphia, 1993.

A Dynamic Model of Average Lung Deformation Using Capacity-Based Reparameterization and Shape Averaging of Lung MR Images

Tessa A. Sundaram, Brian B. Avants, and James C. Gee

University of Pennsylvania
Philadelphia PA 19104, USA tessa@mail.med.upenn.edu

Abstract. We present methods for extracting an average representation of respiratory dynamics from free-breathing lung MR images. Due to individual variations in respiration and the difficulties of real-time pulmonary imaging, time of image acquisition bears little physiologic meaning. Thus, we reparameterize each individual's expiratory image sequence with respect to normalized lung capacity (area, as a substitute for volume), where 1 represents maximal capacity and 0 minimal capacity, as measured by semi-automated image segmentation. This process, combined with intra-subject pairwise non-rigid registration, is used to interpolate intermediate images in the normalized capacity interval $[0, 1]$. Images from separate individuals with the same normalized capacity are taken to be at corresponding points during expiration. We then construct an average representation of pulmonary dynamics from capacity-matched image sequences. This methodology is illustrated using two coronal 2-D datasets from healthy individuals.

1 Introduction

The lung is a highly elastic organ composed of fibers connecting the large airways, intricate vasculature and pulmonary interstitium. A healthy lung is normally highly compliant, deforming easily during respiration, [1]. Pathological processes that affect the lung typically alter the normal mechanical properties of lung tissue, and manifest as observable changes in lung morphology and function. The ability to quantify differences in pulmonary deformation would be useful in early detection of disease, evaluation of treatment efficacy and improved assessment of disease staging and prognosis. Magnetic resonance (MR) imaging and other structural imaging modalities can be used to capture *in vivo* deformation of the lung between sequential images by harnessing the power of non-rigid registration algorithms, [2,3].

In prior studies, we have employed a variational registration algorithm with a linear elastic prior to quantify lung motion captured in serial image sequences, by registering sequential pairs of images I and J and examining the resulting displacement fields, [4]. We impose the linear elastic behavior of the image via a finite element mesh constructed over the domain of I. We have also applied this

C. Barillot, D.R. Haynor, and P. Hellier (Eds.): MICCAI 2004, LNCS 3217, pp. 1000–1007, 2004.
© Springer-Verlag Berlin Heidelberg 2004

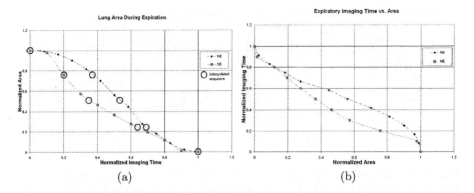

Fig. 1. (a) Evolution of pulmonary cross-sectional areas over imaging time in two healthy individuals. The decrement in area between each image pair is non-uniform throughout expiration. The large circles indicate the lung areas within the images interpolated via reparameterization. (b) At a fixed point in time, the extent of respiratory deformation will vary between individuals; this motivates our efforts toward establishing temporal correspondence.

technique to quantify the differences in pulmonary deformation between normal mice and transgenic mice with sickle cell disease, [5]. In related work, the original registration algorithm has been modified to yield the diffeomorphic fluid deformation framework which is assumed in this paper, [6]. The diffeomorphic component requires that the solution to the registration be continuous, differentiable and invertible. When combined with the fluid framework and approached from the Eulerian perspective, the total deformation between fixed image I and moving image J is considered to be a composition of incremental transformations, each of which is diffeomorphic.

One of the challenges in comparing the respiratory dynamics of two individuals is in achieving temporal correspondence between physiologically similar points of the respiratory cycle. Dynamic modeling as well as inter-subject matching are ongoing areas of research in cardiac imaging as well. Solutions have been proposed that include extending the B-spline framework used to perform pairwise registrations to simultaneous spatio-temporal image matching, as well as applying translation and scaling in the temporal domain as a precursor to nonrigid registration in the spatial domain, [7,8].

The images used in these experiments are acquired at a constant time interval while the volunteers breathe slowly and deeply, consciously controlling their respiration. Hence, even though the images are evenly spaced in time, the deformation of the lung is non-uniformly sampled during image acquisition (figure 1a). Consequently, the motion that occurs between one pair of images is not equivalent to the motion within the subsequent image pair. In order to be able to make accurate comparisons between individuals, it is necessary to correlate points during their respiratory cycles. Furthermore, we expect that at any fixed time during respiration, cross-sectional areas will differ between healthy subjects due to natural individual variations in respiratory deformation (figure 1b).

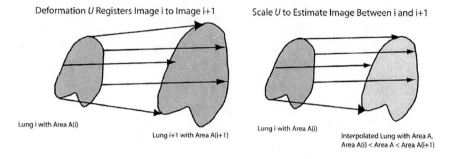

Fig. 2. Capacity-based reparameterization of the expiratory image sequences is performed as shown above. The desired intermediate image is acquired via linear search along the pre-computed deformation field between the two adjacent images.

In this work, we apply a novel capacity-based reparameterization to resample dynamic sequences of 2-D free-breathing lung MR images with the goal of achieving correspondence between individuals' respiratory cycles. Normalizing the lung capacity with respect to its maximum value at end-inspiration yields a "physiologic" time axis whose value is 1 at end-inspiration and zero at end-expiration. These two time points are selected manually by an expert user. The image sequence is then registered in time to find deformation fields (generally small) between an individual's lung state at time t_i and time t_{i+1}, with areas A_i and A_{i+1}, respectively. An interpolation method using these deformation fields and segmentations of both lungs is applied to estimate images which represent the lungs at desired area, A, where $A_i \leq A \leq A_{i+1}$. A dynamic average lung representation of the expiratory segment of breathing is then constructed by assuming inter-subject correspondence of images with identical relative areas, $\{A_0, \cdots, A_i, \cdots, A_1\}$, and computing the shape (or deformation) and intensity average between each area-coincident set of images.

2   Methods

We apply our method to two sequences of free-breathing coronal images collected from individuals with no known pulmonary disease (FIESTA, GE Signa, TR=3.22ms, TE=1.45ms, slice thickness=15mm, FOV=35cm, matrix=256x256). Volunteers were instructed to breathe as slowly and deeply as possible while images were continuously acquired every 1.4 seconds. In each dataset, approximately twenty-two images were acquired over one full breath (expiration followed by inspiration). Lung deformation was not smoothly sampled, since each individual was free to breathe at a comfortable pace. End-inspiration and end-expiration were determined by finding the maximal and minimal cross-sectional areas, respectively, of both lungs during the respiratory cycle. In these preliminary experiments, we focus on the expiratory phase of respiration alone.

In order to estimate the cross-sectional area of the lungs in each image, we stack the images into a volume and segment the lungs and vasculature using

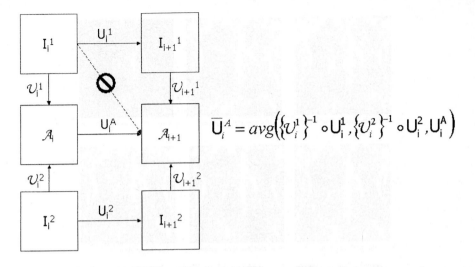

Fig. 3. Construction of dynamic atlases of lung deformation from sequences of images would proceed as shown above. Please refer to the text for further details.

ITK-SNAP, an open-source implementation of semi-automated level set segmentation, [9]. The segmentations are manually refined, smoothed with a median filter of radius 1, and post-processed using morphological closing (dilation followed by erosion) with a 6x6x6 structuring element. The resulting segmentations include the pulmonary parenchyma and most of the branches of the pulmonary vascular tree; however, some of the largest blood vessels remain as holes within the segmentation.

We first perform pairwise registration between consecutive images in each sequence of N images using the fluid registration discussed previously. The resulting set of deformation fields, $\{\mathbf{U}_1, \cdots, \mathbf{U}_{N-1}\}$ reveals the change in capacity between each image pair through the jacobian of the field, $\mathcal{J} = \int |\mathbf{D}\mathbf{U}_i| d\mathbf{x}$, with Ω the domain of the lung segmentation. By construction, $A_{i+1} = \int_\Omega |\mathbf{D}\mathbf{U}_i| d\mathbf{x}$. The non-uniform sampling of the imaging sequences (caused, in part, by each individual's voluntary modulation of respiration and illustrated in figure 1a) is also measured.

In order to appropriately compare the two sequences, we normalize the trend of capacities (i.e, cross-sectional areas) observed during expiration such that capacity has value 1 at end-inspiration and 0 at end-expiration. Within each sequence, intermediate images are reconstructed by solving the following minimization between consecutive images,

$$E(\gamma) = \frac{1}{2}\left(\int_\Omega |\mathbf{D}(\gamma \mathbf{U}_i)| d\mathbf{x} - A\right)^2, \qquad (1)$$

with $A_i \leq A \leq A_{i+1}$ and γ a scalar in $[0, 1]$. Linear scaling is used here because the deformation between images i and $i + 1$ is small, justifying a local linear approximation. We use normalized capacity values $A = \{0.25, 0.5, 0.75\}$

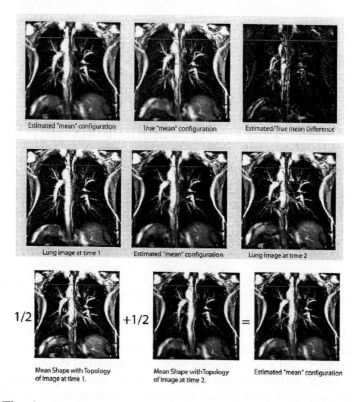

Fig. 4. The shape and intensity averaging evaluation process is illustrated above. Images taken at $t_1 = 1$ and $t_2 = 2$ from a single-subject image sequence are shape and intensity averaged. A third image, taken at time t, with $t_1 < t < t_2$ and with approximately equal deformation energy to each of its neighbors, is used as an estimate of ground truth to evaluate the quality of the mean image. The symmetric averaging method in [10] is used to estimate the mean shapes (shown in the bottom row on the left side of the equation), which are then intensity averaged to yield the image on the right side of the equation. The intensity difference between this average image and the image at time t was less than the difference with the images at t_1 and t_2. Similar results have been found with a set of slices from brain images.

to generate new sequences of five images each that represent the configuration of the pulmonary anatomy at particular values of the cross-sectional area. Note that each of the values between 1 and 0 represents a physiologic time during the expiratory phase, at which the lungs of all individuals have achieved the same reduction in capacity with respect to end-inspiration. Hence, we are now able to directly compare and match the images at these physiologic time points.

Using these capacity-coincident images, we are able to build a dynamic average lung model. First, the shape average of each set of capacity-coincident images is computed. This inter-subject average is determined by performing a simultaneous, symmetric registration of the two images, and traversing the gradient of the similarity at a constant step length, [10]. This produces a new sequence of five images representing the average respiratory deformation of the two individuals. The intensities of these symmetrically registered images are then averaged to give a least squares best representation of the database of anatomy at each of the five normalized capacity points $\{\mathcal{A}_i\}$.

The methodology for representing the average lung deformation relies on the composition of deformation fields, as shown in figure 3. The goal is to represent all deformation patterns with respect to the set of average configurations, $\{\mathcal{A}_i\}$, constructed from deformation- and intensity-averaging of the datasets for each capacity A_i. We only perform intra-subject registrations in time and inter-subject registrations at a given fixed normalized capacity. No registrations create a diagonal connection such as the one in figure 3. To illustrate, we denote the existing intra-subject transformation between a subject at end-inspiration, I_0^1, and its subsequent anatomy with capacity A_1, as $\mathbf{U}_0^1$. The same transformation from capacities A_0 to A_1 in a second subject, I_0^2, is $\mathbf{U}_0^2$. Then, the average end-inspiratory anatomy estimated from these two subjects would be $\mathcal{A}_0$, where transformations $\mathcal{U}_0^1$ and $\mathcal{U}_0^2$ map each subject, respectively, to $\mathcal{A}_0$. Each $\mathbf{U}_0^k$ is represented in the domain of $\mathcal{A}_0$ by composing $\mathcal{U}_0^{k-1}$ onto $\mathbf{U}_0^k$. In this domain, these fields (if small enough) may be averaged.

3   Results

The pairwise registrations between each sequence computed at the beginning of this paper quantify the non-uniform sampling of respiratory deformation that motivates this work. However, in each sequence, there is an image which is equidistant from its adjacent neighbors, where the distance is defined by deformation, [10]. We choose to reconstruct these images as validation of the shape averaging method (figure 4).

Figure 5 illustrates the results of the capacity reparameterization of both sequences. The newly interpolated images at equally spaced area fractions between end-inspiration and end-expiration are shown. Recall that these images do not represent physiologic conditions in each volunteer at the same point of elapsed time after end-inspiration, since each individual breathes at his or her own pace. Instead, the interpolated images represent a physiologic correspondence between the two individuals. The amount of time and respiratory deformation required to arrive at this anatomic configuration in each individual is different; however, they are proportionately at the same point in their respective breathing cycles. Achieving this correspondence enables us to make further quantitative comparisons between the two individuals with respect to deformation patterns and regional pulmonary strains. Furthermore, we can now construct the average lung deformation sequence using these correlated sequences. Despite the large intensity variations in the data associated with vascular and fluid-containing structures entering the imaging plane, we are still able to compute reasonable averages between the images, and produce a smooth representation of average lung deformation during expiration.

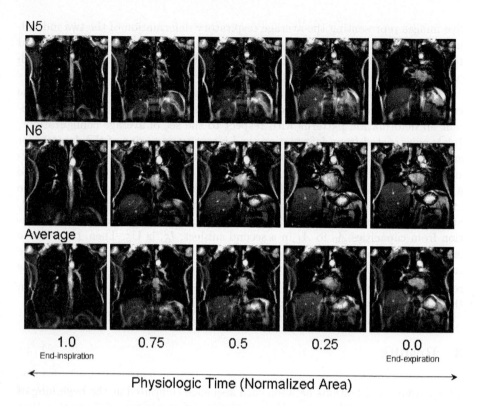

Fig. 5. Interpolated images are produced at specific physiologic times via area reparameterization in each individual, and the average lung deformation sequence can be computed via shape averaging of the area-coincident images.

4   Discussion and Future Work

We presented a method for reparameterizing images taken in time according to some physiologic function, in this case, lung capacity. In these experiments, we use cross-sectional area; in the three-dimensional case, we would naturally use lung volume. Given this reparameterization, we are able to bring images into correspondence with respect to this known physiologic reference. We can now confidently create an average model which will serve as the basis for further studies of normal and abnormal variations in lung deformation. Furthermore, we can use these techniques to perform inter-subject comparisons of deformation patterns and regional strains within the lung, by composing the incremental deformation fields required to arrive at the coincident anatomic configurations, and then making quantitative assessments of these total deformations. This technique is equally applicable if the data is acquired using breath-holding instead of free-breathing. The flexibility of the method is especially useful in volumetric MR studies, where the time necessary to image the whole chest exceeds the normal duration of a single breath (4-5 seconds).

We chose to focus on the expiratory phase of breathing in this paper to better illustrate the concepts presented. However, our approach can be extended to include the entire respiratory cycle, as well as to include more than two individuals in the mean deformation model. Furthermore, the quantitative information produced by our approach stimulates a number of interesting questions about respiratory deformation. In the future, we would like to explore the symmetry of the inspiratory and expiratory phases of respiration, and the disruption of any inherent symmetry as a result of disease. Additionally, we intend to investigate other physiological bases for reparameterization (e.g. deformation), extend this analysis to more than two individuals, and further explore the creation of 3-D dynamic atlases of the lung.

Acknowledgments. Hiroto Hatabu, M.D. Ph.D., Shigeru Kiryu, Ph.D., Masaya Takahashi, Ph.D. and colleagues for the data acquisition.

References

1. Kamm, R.D.: Airway Wall Mechanics. Ann. Rev. Biomed. Engr. **1** (1999) 47–72
2. Hatabu, H., Ohno, Y., Uematsu, H., Oshio, K., Gefter, W.B., Gee, J.C.: Lung biomechanics via non-rigid registration of serial MR images. Radiology **221 (P)** (2001) 630
3. Sundaram, T., Gee, J., Nishino, M., Kiryu, S., Mori, Y., Kuroki, M., Takahashi, M., Hatabu, H.: 3-D Lung Motion Estimation Via Non-Rigid Registration Using Volumetric MR and CT. In: Proc. ISMRM 12th Mtg. (2004) 2609
4. Gee, J.C., Sundaram, T., Hasegawa, I., Uematsu, H., Hatabu, H.: Characterization of Regional Pulmonary Mechanics from Serial MRI Data. Acad. Rad. **10** (2003) 1147–1152
5. Sundaram, T.A., Gee, J.C.: Biomechanical analysis of the lung: a feature-based approach using customized finite element meshes. In: Proc. ISMRM 11th Mtg. (2003) 410
6. Avants, B., Gee, J.C.: Non-rigid registration with general similarity, diffeomorphic and transient quadratic priors. (Submitted)
7. Ledesma-Carbayo, M.J., Kybic, J., Suhling, M., Hunziker, P., Desco, M., Santos, A., Unser, M.: Cardiac ultrasound motion detection by elastic registration exploiting temporal coherence. In: Proc. 1st IEEE ISBI. Volume 2. (2002) 585–588
8. Perperidis, D., Rao, A., Mohiaddin, R., Rueckert, D.: Non-rigid spatio-temporal alignment of 4D cardiac MR images. In Gee, J.C., Maintz, J.B.A., Vannier, M.W., eds.: Proc. 2nd Intl. WBIR. LNCS 2717 (2003) 191–200
9. Ho, S., Cody, H., Gerig, G.: SNAP: A Software Package for User-Guided Geodesic Snake Segmentation. Technical report, University of North Carolina (2003) http://www.cs.unc.edu/~gerig/publications/MICCAI03-Ho-snap.pdf.
10. Avants, B., Gee, J.C.: Shape averaging with diffeomorphic flows for atlas creation. In: International Symposium on Biomedical Imaging. (2004) in press

Prostate Shape Modeling Based on Principal Geodesic Analysis Bootstrapping

Erik Dam[1], P. Thomas Fletcher[2], Stephen M. Pizer[2],
Gregg Tracton[3], and Julian Rosenman[3]

[1] Image Analysis group, IT University of Copenhagen, and
Center for Clinical and Basic Research, erikdam@itu.dk
[2] Medical Image Display and Analysis Group, Uni. of North Carolina, Chapel Hill
[3] Dep. of Radiation Oncology, University of North Carolina, Chapel Hill

Abstract. The use of statistical shape models in medical image analysis is growing due to the ability to incorporate prior organ shape knowledge for tasks such as segmentation, registration, and classification.

Shape models are trained from collections of segmented organs. Though manual interaction during training can ensure correspondence, it also introduces bias and ruins reproducibility — automation is desirable.

We present a novel shape model construction method via a medial shape representation. The automatic method is based on an iterative bootstrap method that alternates between shape representation optimization and analysis of shape mean and variations.

The method is used to create a model from 46 segmented prostates with quantitatively and intuitively good results.

1 Introduction

Methods based on analysis of shape variation are widespread in medical imaging. These methods allow incorporation of statistical prior shape knowledge in tasks where image information alone is not enough to solve the task automatically. The classical example is the use of deformable models in segmentation.

Most statistical shape models consist of a mean shape with deformations that are constructed through statistical analysis of shapes from a training collection. Each shape is described partially by the chosen shape representation, and analysis of the parameters for the representation gives the mean and variations.

The best known is the *Active Shape Model* (ASM) [1] where the shapes are represented by a *point distribution model* (PDM) with given point-wise correspondence. The mean model is simply the mean of each point after Procrustes alignment. *Principal component analysis* (PCA) provides the variations.

This work pursues the medial shape representation *m-rep* [3]. The m-rep represents shape by means of the sheet of sampled medial atoms. This parameter space is not Euclidean but consists of a combination of position, scaling, and orientation parameters. Standard PCA is therefore not applicable. However, the analogue that applies to shape representations that form Lie groups is the *Principal Geodesic Analysis* (PGA) [4,5].

C. Barillot, D.R. Haynor, and P. Hellier (Eds.): MICCAI 2004, LNCS 3217, pp. 1008–1016, 2004.
© Springer-Verlag Berlin Heidelberg 2004

A key step in constructing shape models is the representation of the training shapes. This must define correspondence across the population. For a PDM the simplest method is manual selection of the boundary points by a medical expert. In 2D, and especially 3D, this is a time-consuming and non-reproducible. However, this is automated by Davies [6] by first generating boundary points from a spherical harmonics representation and then optimizing the boundary points and their correspondence in a *Minimum Description Length* (MDL) approach.

This work presents an essentially automatic shape modeling method. The essense is an automatic bootstrap process that iteratively fits the shape model to training shapes and then derives the PGA mean and modes of deformation. Through the bootstrap iterations, the PGA mean and variations are optimized to allow automatic fitting of all shapes in the training collection. The main difference compared to [6] is that the MDL approach starts the optimization process from representations with good training shape fit and poor correspondence. The MDL process then protects the shape fits while optimizing the correspondence. The PGA bootstrap starts from a generative model with explicit correspondence but with poor fit to the individual training shapes. The bootstrap process then keeps the correspondence while optimizing the fit to the training shapes.

Another method generates an m-rep mean model from training shapes through a spherical harmonics representation that is transformed to Voronoi skeletons [7]. Our approach provides modes of variation as well and is cleaner since the m-rep is the only representation in play. A similar bootstrapping approach that uses an atlas/registration methodology instead is presented in [8].

We evaluate the presented PGA bootstrap for construction of a prostate shape model. The training collection consists of 46 cases where the prostates were segmented in the course of prostate cancer external-beam radiation treatment. Especially in CT scans with slice thickness 2mm or larger, the boundaries of the prostate have low contrast — therefore, prior knowledge in a statistical shape model is essential to making automatic segmentation possible.

The contributions of this work are threefold: *a*) The PGA bootstrap method that allows essentially automatic generation of a shape model with mean and main modes of variation, *b*) Introduction of the necessary geometric regularization term for the m-rep, and *c*) The resulting prostate model that will be central in segmentation and analysis of prostates in radiation treatment planning.

2   The UNC Pelvis Collection

The slice-based segmentation programs, *MASK* [9] and *anastruct_editor*, from the PLan-UNC suite of radiotherapy treatment tools developed at UNC-CH Radiation Oncology, were used to manually produce binary segmentations. Prostatic fat is included in the prostate's shape, as is seen in clinical practise, both because of the difficulty of finding the border between these and the prostate and the chance that these will contain significant counts of cancer cells. Seminal vesicles are excluded from the prostate.

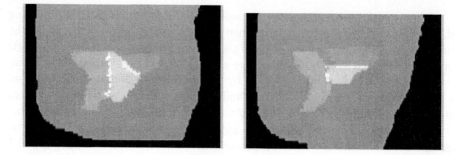

Fig. 1. Sagittal slices of the manual segmentations of rectum, prostate (brightest), and bladder (darkest) from two cases in the UNC pelvis collection. Notice the large variation in the shape of the segmented prostates. The volume varies from $12cm^3$ to $144cm^3$.

The ungated CT scans are acquired from non-immobilized supine patients at UNC Healthcare (Chapel Hill, NC, USA) and Western Wake Radiology (Cary, NC, USA) on Siemens Somotom 4+ scanners without contrast agents.

Retrospective patient images are selected from the archives based on technical criteria, such as adequate image quality and anatomical coverage (the entire bladder down through the prostate apex), as well as shape and anatomical considerations such as very large bladders, prosthetic hips, or surgical procedures proximal to the prostate, yielding "normal cancerous" prostates.

The collection has 46 sets with manual segmentations for prostate, bladder, and rectum (see figure 1). All cases are diagnosed with prostate cancer so the resulting shape model will not necessarily model prostates in general. For instance, an increase of the size of the prostate is common for prostate cancer patients. Since the shape model is to be used for analysis of patients diagnosed with prostate cancer, this bias towards cancerous prostates is desirable.

3   Medial Shape Representation: M-rep

We use a medial shape representation, m-rep, and here briefly review the geometry and the framework for image segmentation [10,11] and introduce a novel regularization term essential for the bootstrap framework.

The m-rep is based on the medial axis of Blum [12]. In this framework, a 3D geometric object is represented as a set of connected continuous medial sheets, which are formed by the centers of all spheres that are interior to the object and tangent to the object's boundary at two or more points. Here we focus on 3D objects that can be represented by a single medial sheet.

We sample the medial sheet $\mathcal{M}$ over a spatially regular lattice of *medial atoms* defined as a 4-tuple $\mathbf{m} = \{\mathbf{x}, r, \mathbf{F}, \theta\}$, consisting of: $\mathbf{x} \in \mathbb{R}^3$ and $r \in \mathbb{R}^+$, the center and radius of the sphere, $\mathbf{F} \in \mathbf{SO}(3)$ an orthonormal local frame parameterized by $(\mathbf{b}, \mathbf{b}^\perp, \mathbf{n})$, where $\mathbf{n}$ is the normal to the medial manifold, $\mathbf{b}$ is the direction in the tangent plane of the fastest narrowing of the implied boundary sections, and $\theta \in [0, \pi)$ the object angle determining the angulation of the two implied opposing boundary points to the local frame. Given an m-rep figure, we fit a smooth boundary surface to the model. We use a subdivision surface method [13] that interpolates the boundary positions and normals implied by each atom.

3.1 Segmentation Using m-reps

Following the deformable models paradigm, an m-rep model $\mathbf{M}$ is deformed into an image I by optimizing an objective function:
$$F(\mathbf{M}, I) = L(\mathbf{M}, I) + \alpha\, G(\mathbf{M}) + R(\mathbf{M})$$
The function L, the *image match*, measures how well the model matches the image information, while G, the *geometric typicality*, gives a prior on the possible variation of the geometry of the model weighted by $\alpha \geq 0$. The last term R, the *geometric regularization*, is a novel addition to the m-rep framework.

This objective function is optimized in a multiscale fashion. That is, it is optimized over a sequence of transformations that are successively finer in scale. Here we will only be concerned with the figural level and the medial atom level. At the figural level the transformation we use is a similarity transformation plus an elongation of the entire figure. At the atom level each medial atom is independently transformed by a similarity plus a rotation of the object angle.

M-rep models are fit to binary segmentation images of the prostates. These binary images are blurred slightly to smooth the objective function, which is optimized with a conjugate gradient method. The image match term of the objective function, L, is computed as a correlation with a Gaussian derivative kernel in the normal direction to the object boundary:
$$L(\mathbf{M}, I) = \int_{\mathcal{B}(\mathbf{M})} \int_{-\epsilon}^{\epsilon} \partial_t G(t)\, I\, (\mathbf{s} + (t/r)\mathbf{n})\, dt\, ds$$
where $\mathbf{s}$ is a parameterization of the boundary $\mathcal{B}(\mathbf{M})$, $\partial_t G$ is the Gaussian derivative kernel, r is the radius function, and $\mathbf{n}$ is the boundary normal.

The geometric typicality term, G, is defined as the change in the boundary from the previous level of scale (where $\mathbf{s}_0$ is the boundary position at that level):
$$G(\mathbf{M}) = - \int_{\mathcal{B}(\mathbf{M})} \frac{||\mathbf{s} - \mathbf{s}_0||^2}{r^2} ds$$
The geometric regularization term, R, essentially corresponds to the curvature and neighbor distance terms in the active contour model and is added during the bootstrap iterations that are introduced in section 5 at the atom scale level in order to keep the model nice. For a medial atom $\mathbf{m}$ with neighbor atoms $\mathbf{m_i}$:

$$R(\mathbf{m}) = \sum_{i=1}^{8} \gamma_{dist}\, rd[d(\mathbf{m}, \mathbf{m_i}), \overline{d(\cdot, \cdot)}]^2 \; + \; \gamma_{implode} \frac{diam^2}{(N+1)^2 d(\mathbf{m}, \mathbf{m_i})^2} +$$
$$\gamma_{grid}\, angle(\mathbf{m} - \mathbf{m_i}, \mathbf{m} - \mathbf{m_{-i}})^2 + \gamma_{swirl}\, angle(\mathbf{b}, \mathbf{b_{ideal}})^2 \quad (1)$$

Here $d(\cdot, \cdot)$ is the distance between atom centers (weighted by $1/\sqrt{2}$ for diagonal neighbors), $\overline{d(\cdot, \cdot)}$ is the mean distance for the model, and rd is the relative difference. Furthermore, $diam$ is the model diameter, N is the number of atoms, $\mathbf{m_{-i}}$ is the neighbor opposing $\mathbf{m_i}$ on the other side of $\mathbf{m}$, and $\mathbf{b_{ideal}}$ is the $\mathbf{b}$ vector as in an ideally oriented atom at that position in the lattice.

4   Principal Geodesic Analysis

Principal geodesic analysis (PGA) [5] is a generalization of principal component analysis (PCA) to curved manifolds. We briefly review the results here.

As shown in [5], the set of all medial atoms forms a Lie group $M = \mathbb{R}^3 \times \mathbb{R}^+ \times SO(3) \times SO(2)$, which we call the *medial group*. Likewise, the set of all m-rep models containing n medial atoms forms a Lie group M^n, i.e., the direct product of n copies of M. This allows the defintion of the exponential and logarithmic maps, $\exp(\cdot)$ and $\log(\cdot)$, that defines the geodesics of the medial group.

4.1   M-rep Means and PGA

The Riemannian distance between m-rep models $\mathbf{M}_1, \mathbf{M}_2 \in M^n$ is given by $d(\mathbf{M}_1, \mathbf{M}_2) = \|\log(\mathbf{M}_1^{-1}\mathbf{M}_2)\|$. Thus, the intrinsic mean of a set of m-rep models $\mathbf{M}_1, \dots, \mathbf{M}_N$ is the minimizer of the sum-of-squared geodesic distances:

$$\mu = \arg\min_{\mathbf{M} \in M^n} \sum_{i=1}^{n} \|\log(\mathbf{M}_i^{-1}\mathbf{M})\|^2$$

Principal components of Gaussian data in $\mathbb{R}^n$ are defined as the projection onto the linear subspace through the mean spanned by the eigenvectors of the covariance matrix. If we consider a general manifold, the counterpart of a line is a geodesic curve.

As shown in [4], the covariance structure of a Gaussian distribution on M^n may be approximated by a covariance matrix Σ in the Lie algebra $\mathfrak{m}^n$. The eigenvectors of this covariance matrix correspond via the exponential map to geodesics on M^n, called *principal geodesics*.

Algorithms for computing the m-rep mean and the principal geodesic analysis on a population of m-rep figures are given in [4].

Analogous to linear PCA models, we may choose a subset of the principal directions $\mathbf{u}^{(k)} \in \mathfrak{m}^n$ with corresponding variations λ_k that is sufficient to describe the variability of the m-rep shape space. New m-rep models may be generated within this subspace of typical objects. Given a set of coefficients $\{\alpha_1, \dots, \alpha_l\}$, we generate a new m-rep model by $\mathbf{M} = \mu \exp\left(\sum_{k=1}^{l} \alpha_k \mathbf{u}^{(k)}\right)$, where α_k is chosen to be within $[-3\sqrt{\lambda_k}, 3\sqrt{\lambda_k}]$.

5   Shape Model Bootstrapping

The segmentation program *Pablo* provides a user interface that allows construction of m-rep models and optimization of the parameters for fitting to a specific training case [10]. For this work, a batch version of Pablo was developed.

The shape model bootstrapping method is now strikingly simple. From a fiducial starting model, the batch fitting process is used to give rough representations of each shape. The PGA then generates the mean model and corresponding principal geodesics from the 46 fitted prostate models. This mean model is then used to fit the shapes using batch Pablo where the principal geodesics are now used during the figural stage. This bootstrapping procedure is iterated.

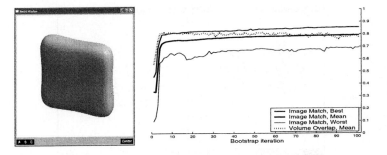

Fig. 2. The Generic model and the resulting bootstrap image match evolution. Image match is as defined in section 3.1 and DICE volume overlap is used (the volume of the intersection between model and manual segmentation divided by their mean volumes).

The idea is that the new mean of the fitted models is a better prototype than the initial model and as the bootstrap iterations progress the generated mean model converges to a good prototype.

5.1 Bootstrapping from the Generic Model

The *Generic* is the default 4x4 m-rep that Pablo generates as a starting model for building handcrafted models. The choice of the specific 4x4 grid of medial atom reflects a choice of sampling resolution combined with the intention of starting the bootstrap from a neutral, non-committed model. Figure 2 shows the starting model and the progression during bootstrap iterations.

5.2 Convergence

In this work, we address the question of convergence pragmatically. The image match and volume overlap values above appear to be converging. Formal proof of the necessary requirements (in terms of starting model and parameter choices) for convergence of the PGA mean and modes is left for future work.

Visual inspection of the mean models after up to 200 bootstrap iterations indicates that the mean is actually converging. Without formal convergence criteria, we use the heuristic approach of running the bootstrap until the image match values cease to improve significantly.

The geometrical regularization introduced in equation 1 is essential to achieving convergence. Without regularization the boundary converges but the medial grid becomes arbitrarily distorted and thereby ruins correspondence — see figure 3. The *grid* and *dist* terms keeps the sheet regular and evenly spaced, *implode* prevents the atoms from collapsing, and *swirl* keeps the boundary points in proximity to the related atoms. The constrained evolution that is achieved through the geometrical regularization ensures nice correspondence properties through a regular coordinate system on the boundary as well as inside and outside the resulting shape model.

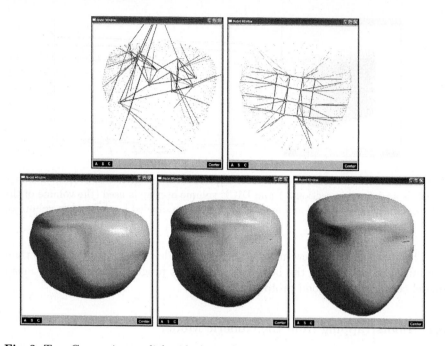

Fig. 3. Top: Comparing medial grid after 100 iterations without and with geometrical regularization ($\alpha = 0.25$, $\gamma_{dist} = 0.02$, $\gamma_{implode} = 0.0002$, $\gamma_{grid} = 0.002$, $\gamma_{swirl} = 0.03$). Bottom: Resulting Prostate Mean Model with ± 1 standard deviation of the first principal geodesic mode of variation — a Laurel/Hardy effect. All seen in anterior-posterior view.

5.3   Resulting Prostate Shape Model

The resulting Prostate mean shape model is compared to the result of running the bootstrap without geometrical penalty in figure 3. Without geometrical restrictions, the small deformations in each bootstrap iteration build up and distort the model arbitrarily.

The 10 modes of variation include 98% of the variation in the training collection. This ensures little need for atom optimization in the segmentation process which speeds up the segmentation method considerably. The automatic fitting achieves image match in the range 0.73–0.87 with mean 0.82 and a mean DICE volume overlap of 0.80. We consider this satisfying given the large variation in shape and the non-smooth boundary profiles in the binary segmentations in the training collection (see figure 1).

The shape model is here evaluated on binary images. In the full m-rep segmentation framework, the shape model is combined with profile models for the local boundary (as done in [14] that uses an experimental version of the PGA bootstrap method) instead of just using the Gaussian derivative profile.

Apart from being directly applicable for segmentation, the shape model and the condensed PGA parameterization is applicable for shape classification.

6   Conclusion

We present a novel shape model construction method using a medial shape representation. The method is essentially automatic based on an iterative bootstrap method that alternates between shape representation optimization and principal geodesic analysis of shape mean and variations. The method constructs an m-rep shape model consisting of a mean and corresponding main modes of variation. The non-automatic step is the choice of initial model — we have chosen a generic 4x4 atom grid that is a suitable compromise between compactness and accuracy.

The method is evaluated on a training collection of 46 manually segmented prostates. The resulting model is quantitatively and qualitatively satisfying.

Future work is centered on evaluating our method against the MDL approach that generate an ASM [6]. Central points to evaluate are compactness, correspondence, and legality (how likely are illegal models). Furthermore, modelling of kidneys, hearts and other anatomical structures is to come. Also, ongoing work explores representing medical atoms as a Riemannian symmetric space rather than a Lie group. We have extended the theory of PGA to this space, and future work will involve building the prostate shape model under this new framework.

Acknowledgement. We sincerely thank Per Halverson at Western Wake Radiology (Cary, NC, USA) for supplying pelvis scans for the collection.

References

1. Cootes, T., Taylor, C., Cooper, D., Graham, J.: Active shape models: Their training and application. CVIU (1995) 38–59
2. Cremers, D., Kohlberger, T., Schnörr, C.: Nonlinear shape statistics in mumford-shah based segmentation. In: 7th European Conference on Computer Vision. Volume 2351 of Springer LNCS. (2002)
3. Pizer, S., Fritsch, D., Yushkevich, P., Johnson, V., Chaney, E.: Segmentation, registration, and measurement of shape variation via image object shape. IEEE Transactions on Medical Imaging **18** (1996)
4. Fletcher, P.T., Joshi, S., Lu, C., Pizer, S.M.: Gaussian distributions on Lie groups and their application to statistical shape analysis. To appear *Information Processing in Medical Imaging* (2003)
5. Fletcher, P.T., Lu, C., Joshi, S.: Statistics of shape via principal geodesic analysis on Lie groups. To appear *Computer Vision and Pattern Recognition* (2003)
6. Davies, R., Twining, C., Cootes, T., Waterton, J., Taylor, C.: A minimum description length approach to statistical shape modeling. IEEE Transactions on Medical Imaging **21** (2002)
7. Styner, M., Gerig, G.: Medial models incorporating object variability for 3d shape analysis. In: Proc. of Information Processing in Medical Imaging. (2001)
8. Guimond, A., Meunier, J., Thirion, J.P.: Average brain models: A convergence study. Technical Report 3731, INRIA (1999)
9. Tracton, G., Chaney, E., Rosenman, J., Pizer, S.: Mask: combining 2d and 3d segmentation methods to enhance functionality. In: Proceedings of Mathematical Methods in Medical Imaging III. Volume SPIE Vol 2299. (1994)

10. Pizer, Chen, Fletcher, Fridman, Fritsch, Gash, Glotzer, Jiroutek, Joshi, Muller, Thall, Tracton, Yushkevich, Chaney: Deformable m-reps for 3d medical image segmentation. IJCV (2003)
11. Joshi, S., Pizer, S., Fletcher, P.T., Yushkevich, P., Thall, A., Marron, J.S.: Multiscale deformable model segmentation and statistical shape analysis using medial descriptions. Transactions on Medical Imaging **21** (2002)
12. Blum, H., Nagel, R.: Shape description using weighted symmetric axis features. Pattern Recognition **10** (1978) 167–180
13. Thall, A.: Fast C^2 interpolating subdivision surfaces using iterative inversion of stationary subdivision rules. Technical report, UNC (2002) http://midag.cs.unc.edu/pubs/papers/Thall_TR02-001.pdf.
14. Rao, M.: Analysis of a locally varying intensity template for segmentation of kidneys in ct images. Master's thesis, UNC, Chapel Hill (2003)

Estimation of Organ Motion from 4D CT for 4D Radiation Therapy Planning of Lung Cancer

Michael R. Kaus[1], Thomas Netsch[1], Sven Kabus[1,2], Vladimir Pekar[1], Todd McNutt[3], and Bernd Fischer[2]

[1] Philips Research Laboratories, Röntgenstr. 24–26, 22335 Hamburg, Germany
michael.kaus@philips.com
[2] Institute of Mathematics, University of Lübeck, Wallstraße 40, 23560 Lübeck, Germany
[3] Philips Medical Systems, 6400 Enterprise Lane, Madison, WI 53719, USA

Abstract. The goal of this paper is to automatically estimate the motion of the tumor and the internal organs from 4D CT and to extract the organ surfaces. Motion induced by breathing and heart beating is an important uncertainty in conformal external beam radiotherapy (RT) of lung tumors. 4D RT aims at compensating the geometry changes during irradiation by incorporating the motion into the treatment plan using 4D CT imagery. We establish two different methods to propagate organ models through the image time series, one based on deformable surface meshes, and the other based on volumetric B-spline registration. The methods are quantitatively evaluated on 8 3D CT images of the full breathing cycle of a patient with manually segmented lungs and heart. Both methods achieve good overall results, with mean errors of 1.02–1.33 mm and 0.78–2.05 mm for deformable surfaces and B-splines respectively. The deformable mesh is fast (40 seconds vs. 50 minutes), but accommodation of the heart and the tumor is currently not possible. B-spline registration estimates the motion of all structures in the image and their interior, but is susceptible to motion artifacts in CT.

Keywords: Radiation therapy, lung cancer, 4D CT, deformable registration, deformable surface models, B-splines

1   Introduction

External beam radiation therapy (RT) is one of the main cancer therapies for lung cancer, the leading cause of all cancer-related deaths with more than 150000 deaths in the USA each year [1]. Breathing and heart motion during irradiation causes significant variations in organ and target geometry in the order of several centimeters. This increases the dose to healthy tissue and reduces the dose to the target area, impairing the balance between complications and cure. 4D RT aims at compensating the deformation uncertainty by incorporating the motion characteristics into the dose calculation or gating the treatment device in phase with the motion pattern [2]. These techniques require a patient-specific motion model. With the advent of multi-slice CT, 4D image acquisition of dynamic processes such as breathing is now becoming possible.

Fully automated algorithms are desirable to estimate organ motion, but need to be sufficiently fast and with minimal user interaction [3]. A large variety of automated

C. Barillot, D.R. Haynor, and P. Hellier (Eds.): MICCAI 2004, LNCS 3217, pp. 1017–1024, 2004.

methods exists, including volumetric intensity-based registration techniques [4] and surface-based techniques [5]. Registration based on B-splines [6] has shown potential for medical applications such as breast MRI [7], brain [8] and cardiac [9]. Deformable surface models are computationally efficient, and their versatility has been demonstrated on a number of clinical applications including cardiac MRI time series [10,11] or brain mapping [12].

The goal of this paper is to establish and compare a volumetric and a surface based method for the estimation of internal organ motion as a first step towards 4D radiotherapy. The first method is a fast volumetric intensity-based B-spline registration method which has previously been applied to PET-CT registration and has not yet been quantitatively validated on clinical data [13]. The second approach is a deformable surface model algorithm which has previously been applied to bone segmentation in CT and left ventricle segmentation in MRI [14,11]. In the remainder of the text we will outline the two algorithms and their adaptation to 4D lung CT over the breathing cycle of one patient, and compare their results to manual segmentation of the lungs and the heart.

2   Methods

We apply two methods to automatically estimate organ motion in 4D images. The principle is to propagate 3D triangular surface meshes derived from a template image to the remaining images by re-calculation of the mesh vertex coordinates while leaving the mesh topology unchanged. The first approach is the volumetric grey-value based B-spline registration method described in [13], where the vertex coordinates are re-computed according to the 3D deformation field estimated for each voxel. The second method is the deformable surface mesh already proposed in [11], where the new vertex coordinates are calculated by minimization of the sum of an internal shape energy and an external feature energy.

2.1   Volumetric Grey-Value Based B-Spline Registration

For the transformation of a voxel position $\mathbf{x}_v = (x_1, x_2, x_3)^\mathsf{T}$ a grid G of $g_1 \times g_2 \times g_3$ control points with uniform spacing in each direction is defined. The displacement of a single control point is encoded by β_{ijk} and β is the collection of all these vectors. Following Rueckert et al. [6] the B-spline deformation $\mathbf{u}$ at position $\mathbf{x}_v$ can be described by a tensor product

$$\mathbf{u}(\mathbf{x}_v; \beta) = \sum_{i=1}^{g_1} \sum_{j=1}^{g_2} \sum_{k=1}^{g_3} \beta_{ijk} b_{i,3}(x_1) b_{j,3}(x_2) b_{k,3}(x_3) \tag{1}$$

where $b_{\cdot,3}$ refers to a cubic B-spline. The transformation itself is defined as the subtraction of a deformation $\mathbf{u}(\mathbf{x}_v; \beta)$ from its original position $\mathbf{x}_v$. The grid—and an extra layer of control points to avoid the use of boundary conditions—is placed on the image in such a way that the outmost grid controls coincide with the corners of the image.

For a given displacement field β, the quality of the match between the reference image R and the image to be registered T is determined by the sum f of squared differences (SSD) over the total number of voxels N:

$$f(\beta) = \frac{1}{2} \sum_{v=1}^{N} [F_v(\beta)]^2 = \frac{1}{2} \|\mathbf{F}(\beta)\|_2^2, \tag{2}$$

where $F_v(\beta) := T(\mathbf{x}_v - \mathbf{u}(\mathbf{x}_v)) - R(\mathbf{x}_v)$ and $\mathbf{F}(\beta) = (F_1(\beta), \ldots, F_N(\beta))^\mathsf{T}$. The optimization of the cost function f needs special attention since the large number of parameters involved may result in high computational cost. We therefore choose an iterative Levenberg-Marquardt method, one of the most efficient non-linear optimization schemes, generating a sequence (β^m) with starting value $\beta^0 \equiv 0$ and update rule $\beta^{m+1} := \beta^m + \alpha_m \mathbf{s}^m$. The parameter $\alpha_m \in [0, 1]$ denotes the step-size and $\mathbf{s}^m$ the search direction respectively. The search direction s^m is computed by solving the linear system

$$\left[J_F(\beta^m)^\mathsf{T} J_F(\beta^m) + \lambda_m I \right] \mathbf{s}^m = -J_F(\beta^m)^\mathsf{T} \mathbf{F}(\beta^m), \tag{3}$$

where $J_F(\beta^m)$ denotes the Jacobian of $\mathbf{F}(\beta^m)$ with entries $\partial F_v(\beta^m)/\partial \beta_i^m$. The diagonal matrix $\lambda_m I$ must be added to obtain a regular linear system since $J_F(\beta^m)$ is usually rank deficient: voxels in areas with constant or almost constant grey values yield zero partial derivatives [15]. The so-called trust region radius λ_m can be considered as an adaption of the step-length during the iteration.

In each iteration step the matrix and the right hand side of (3) is built. The partial derivatives $\partial F_v(\beta^m)/\partial \beta_i^m$ are approximated by finite differences. In practice, many of the partial derivatives have a small numerical value and can be set to zero without degrading the convergence rate, but leading to a much more favorable complexity. For a given λ_m the linear system is solved by a conjugate gradient scheme yielding the decent direction $\mathbf{s}^m$. Then the algorithm checks if the parameter update β^{m+1} for $\alpha_m = 1$ leads to a reduction in the cost function. If this is not the case α_m will be reduced stepwise until $f(\beta^m + \alpha_m \mathbf{s}^m) < 0.995 f(\beta^m)$ holds.

To determine λ_{m+1} for the next iteration step the predicted reduction of the cost function is compared to the actual decrease in f. This technique avoids additional time-consuming solving of the linear system during the trust region radius adaption. The control of λ_m is described in [13] in detail. For all registrations we start with $\lambda_0 = 16$. The iteration is stopped if the relative reduction of the cost function is less than 2%.

2.2   Deformable Surface Models

After initial positioning in a 3D image (see below), a triangular surface mesh is adapted to an image by iteratively carrying out surface detection in the image for each triangle, and reconfiguration of the vertex coordinates by minimizing $E = E_{\text{ext}} + \alpha E_{\text{int}}$. The parameter α weighs the relative influence of an external energy E_{ext}, which drives the mesh towards detected surface points, and an internal energy E_{int}, which maintains the vertex configuration of an initial mesh.

Surface detection is carried out for each triangle center $\mathbf{x}_i$. We seek the point $\tilde{\mathbf{x}}_i$ along the triangle normal $\mathbf{n}_i$ which maximizes the cost function consisting of a feature function F and the distance $j\delta$ to the triangle center according to

$$\tilde{\mathbf{x}}_i = \mathbf{x}_i + \delta \, \mathbf{n}_i \, \underset{j=-l, \ldots, l}{\arg\max} \left\{ F(\mathbf{x}_i + j\delta \, \mathbf{n}_i) - D j^2 \delta^2 \right\}, \tag{4}$$

where $2l + 1$ is the number of points investigated, δ specifies the distance between two points on the profile, and D controls the tradeoff between feature strength and distance.

The object specificity of F is crucial to the robustness and accuracy of deformable model adaptation. The image gradient is not a robust lung feature for 4D CT data due to noise, motion artifacts, and many false features inside the lungs. Instead, we search for the point where the grey-value transitions across a particular threshold according to

$$F(\mathbf{x}) = \begin{cases} 0 & \text{if } I_{j-1}(\mathbf{x}) < I_{\min} \text{ and } I_j(\mathbf{x}) < I_{\min}, \\ -1 & \text{if } I_{j-1}(\mathbf{x}) > I_T \text{ and } I_j(\mathbf{x}) < I_T, \\ 1 & \text{if } I_{j-1}(\mathbf{x}) < I_T \text{ and } I_j(\mathbf{x}) > I_T. \end{cases} \tag{5}$$

$I_{j-1}(\mathbf{x})$ and $I_j(\mathbf{x})$ are two successive grey values on the search profile from inside to outside of the organ, $I_{\min}$ is the minimum grey value of the lung parenchyma, and I_T is the transition grey value.

To compute the new vertex coordinates given the detected feature points, we minimize the weighted sum of the external and internal energies. E_{ext} drives the mesh towards the detected surface points:

$$E_{\text{ext}}(\mathbf{x}) = \sum_{i=1}^{T} w_i \|\tilde{\mathbf{x}}_i - \mathbf{x}_i\|_2^2, \quad w_i = \max\left\{0, F(\tilde{\mathbf{x}}_i) - Dj^2\delta^2\right\}, \tag{6}$$

T being the number of triangles. The weights w_i give the most promising surface points $\tilde{\mathbf{x}}_i$ the largest influence during mesh reconfiguration. The internal energy maintains the distribution of the mesh vertex coordinates $\mathbf{v}_j$ w.r.t. the edges of a given initial mesh $\tilde{\mathbf{v}}_{jk} = \tilde{\mathbf{v}}_j - \tilde{\mathbf{v}}_k$

$$E_{int} = \sum_{j=1}^{V} \sum_{k \in N(j)} \|\mathbf{v}_j - \mathbf{v}_k - s\mathbf{R}\tilde{\mathbf{v}}_{jk}\|_2^2, \tag{7}$$

where $N(j)$ is the set of neighbors of vertex j, and V is the number of vertex coordinates [14]. The rotation $\mathbf{R}$ and the scaling s between original and deforming mesh are estimated in each iteration using a fast closed-form point-based registration method based on singular value decomposition. Since the energies in (6) and (7) are quadratic, energy minimization results in the efficient solution of a sparse linear system using the conjugate gradient method.

3   Experiments

3.1   Image Data and Quantitative Validation Metric

We assessed the performance of the two algorithms based on a 4D CT study (512 × 512 × 165 voxels, 0.88 × 0.88 × 3.0 mm, Philips MX8000 IDT 16-line, retrospectively breathing gated helical cone-beam reconstruction) consisting of 8 3D volumes from end inspiration (CT 0) to end expiration (CT 4) to late inspiration (CT 7). Clinical experts carried out 2D slice-based contouring of the lungs and the heart with a commercial

Table 1. Mesh propagation from 7 CT volumes of different phases (1: early expiration, 7: late inspiration) to end inspiration phase image. Shown are surface distances between the triangulated manual segmentations and the deformed mesh surface before (Initialization) and after volumetric B-spline registration and deformable surface model adaptation respectively. The deformable surface method would require separate modeling of the heart and is not yet available.

CT No.	1	2	3	4	5	6	7
Right Lung (Mean Distance [mm] / 99%-Quantile Distance [mm])							
Initialization	1.0 / 6.0	2.0 / 11.8	2.9 / 18.9	3.8 / 29.1	3.4 / 23.3	2.1 / 11.4	1.3 / 9.3
B-spline	0.8 / 4.1	1.0 / 5.1	1.2 / 7.0	1.3 / 6.6	1.1 / 5.4	1.5 / 13.1	1.0 / 6.3
Deformable Models	1.2 / 6.4	1.3 / 6.8	1.3 / 7.8	1.3 / 8.2	1.3 / 8.5	1.3 / 8.1	1.2 / 6.5
Left Lung							
Initialization	0.4 / 1.8	1.4 / 5.5	1.9 / 6.3	1.5 / 6.1	1.8 / 6.3	1.8 / 5.7	1.1 / 4.2
B-spline	0.9 / 4.5	1.3 / 8.2	1.5 / 11.6	1.7 / 8.5	1.7 / 9.6	2.1 / 20.5	1.0 / 5.1
Deformable Models	1.0 / 4.7	1.1 / 6.1	1.1 / 4.5	1.0 / 4.4	1.1 / 5.1	1.0 / 4.3	1.0 / 4.3
Heart							
Initialization	5.4 / 25.9	2.7 / 10.1	3.2 / 8.4	3.6 / 12.3	3.4 / 13.4	3.3 / 10.9	3.5 / 10.7
B-spline	5.2 / 25.7	2.5 / 12.0	3.0 / 12.4	3.1 / 12.3	3.2 / 16.4	2.8 / 9.2	3.7 / 12.0

software package. The contours were subsequently transformed to binary masks and their surfaces triangulated. We quantified the difference between the deformed surface meshes and the expert segmentations by calculating the mean and 99%-quantile distance in mm between the vertices of the deformed mesh and the expert contours.

3.2 Experimental Setup

The CT volume of the end inspiration was used as the template. Patient-specific surface meshes were generated from the expert segmentations for validation. The meshes were deformed using the two methods to match the remaining CT volumes from early expiration to end expiration and compared to the triangulated manually segmented masks.

The B-spline registration was embedded into a multi-scale approach employing both an image pyramid and a parameter pyramid of three levels. The coarsest image resolution level used images of size $75 \times 57 \times 63$ voxels and a grid with $7 \times 7 \times 3$ control points, while the finest level used $256 \times 256 \times 165$ voxels and a $19 \times 19 \times 15$ mesh resulting in 17328 optimization parameters. The computation time was on the order of 50 minutes on average for the registration of two volumes (Intel Pentium IV, 2.66 GHz).

The deformable model was applied on the original image resolution with fixed parameters $l=40$, $\delta=1$ mm, $D=0.3$, $I_{min}=100$, $I_T=600$, and a coarse-to-fine parameter pyramid of $\alpha=1, 0.3, 0.2$, with 10 iterations on each level. The computation time for the entire adaptation of a high resolution mesh with 5000 vertices (i.e. 15004 parameters) to a volume was on the order of 40 seconds on average (Intel Pentium IV, 2.66 GHz).

3.3   Results

The deformation between end inspiration (CT 0) and the remaining phases was most prominent in the region of the diaphragm and the heart ventricles (Fig. 1 (a,b)). The geometric differences increased to a maximum at end expiration (CT 4) and decreased again towards late inspiration (CT 7) (Table 1, difference between manual segmentations (Initial)).

Both methods captured the overall deformation of the lungs between breathing phases well, with 1.06 ± 0.04 mm (1.26 ± 0.07 mm) mean difference for the left (right) lung with deformable surface models, 1.43 ± 0.41 mm (1.13 ± 0.25 mm) mean difference for the left (right) lung with B-spline registration, and 3.35 ± 0.90 mm mean difference for the heart with B-spline registration (the surface model approach would require separate modeling of the heart, which has not yet been done). A part of the error can be attributed to inaccuracies in the expert segmentations (inter- and intraobserver variations are typically in the order of 0.1 - 0.8 mm [16]). Small deformations < 1 mm mean surface distance are beyond the accuracy of both algorithms and cannot be recovered due to noise and the methods' smoothness and shape constraints.

The B-spline method produces partial errors at the diaphragm of the left lung and the heart (Fig. 1 (c,d)). These errors are due to image motion artifacts which cannot be distinguished well from the true lung surface with the SSD similarity measure. The motion artifacts are most severe in the area of the heart because the CT acquisition is breathing-gated, which is not well suited to compensate heart motion. The deformable surface model is more robust w.r.t. artifacts (consistent capturing of deformation for all phases), since the algorithm searches for a certain grey value transition and is thus not affected by motion artifacts. If the image artifacts are less severe (right lung), the B-spline registration outperforms the deformable models because volumetric registration takes more image information into account.

4   Discussion and Conclusions

Two alternative methods, a deformable surface method and a B-spline registration algorithm, were established and successfully applied to propagate organs in 4D CT of the chest with good overall mean accuracy of 1.02–1.33 mm and 0.78–2.05 for deformable surfaces and B-splines respectively.

The main advantage of volumetric registration is that the deformation for all organs, including the tumor, can be estimated with a single approach, while organ specific parameter settings and surface models must be designed for every new object addressed with the deformable models. However, the modeling effort pays off by a significant reduction of CPU time (40 seconds vs. 50 minutes) crucial for clinical applicability.

Improvement of the B-spline registration quality may be achieved by considering other similarity measures to better deal with missing image correspondences and image artifacts. Motion artifacts in 4D CT images may be reduced in the future by increased scanner speed and better gating and reconstruction schemes. We also plan to further explore the possibilities of deformable surface models by extension to other organs. An interesting question is the applicability to tumors where shape modeling is difficult.

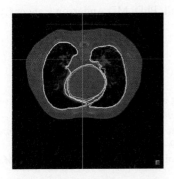

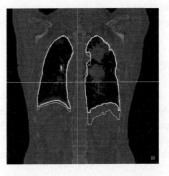

(a) Expert mesh (EE and EI), EE image   (b) Expert mesh (EE and EI), EE image

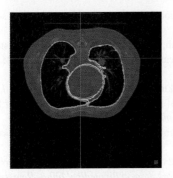

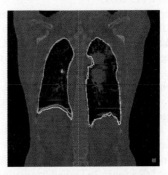

(c) Expert mesh, B-spline warped mesh at EI   (d) Expert mesh, B-spline warped mesh at EI

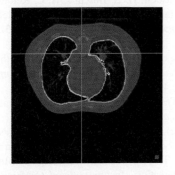

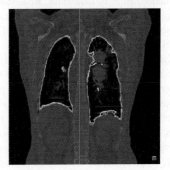

(e) Expert mesh, deformable model at EI   (f) Expert mesh, deformable model at EI

Fig. 1. Expert contours and contours generated by cutting the warped 3D surface meshes with the visible image planes. Significant deformation between end inspiration (EI) and end expiration (EE), (a,b) can be recovered with both the volumetric registration method (c,d) and the deformable surface method (e,f). The heart was only addressed with B-spline registration.

Finally, we need to evaluate more patients for a better understanding of organ and tumor motion and required clinical accuracy.

Acknowledgements. We thank George Starkshall, PhD, MD Anderson Cancer Center, for the preparation of the CT data of the lung.

References

1. L. A. G. Ries, M. P. Eisner, and C. L. Kosary et al. (eds). SEER cancer statistics review, 1975–2000. *NCI. Bethesda, Maryland, USA [http://www.cancer.gov/statistics]*.
2. S. S. Vedam, P. J. Keall, V. R. Kini, and R. Mohan. Determining parameters for respiration-gated radiotherapy. *Medical Physics*, 28(10):2139–2146, 2001.
3. L. E. Court and L. Dong. Automatic registration of the prostate for CT-guided RT. *Medical Physics*, 30(10):2750–2757, 2001.
4. J. V. Hajnal, D. L. Hill, and D. J. Hawkes, editors. *Medical Image Registration*. CRC Press, Boca Raton, FL, 2001.
5. T. McInerney and D. Terzopoulos. Deformable models in medical image analysis: A survey. *Medical Image Analysis*, 1(2):91–108, 1996.
6. D. Rueckert, L. I. Sonoda, D. L. Hill, M. O. Leach, and D. J. Hawkes. Nonrigid registration using free-form deformations: Application to breast MRI. *IEEE Transactions on Medical Imaging*, 18(8):712–721, 1999.
7. E. R. Denton, L. I. Sonoda, D. Rueckert, S. Rankin, C. Hayes, M. O. Leachand, D. L Hill, and D. J. Hawkes. Comparison and evaluation of rigid and non-rigid registration of breast MR images. *Journal of Computer Assisted Technology*, 23:800–805, 1999.
8. J. Kybic and M. Unser. Fast parametric elastic image registration. *IEEE Transactions on Image Processing*, 12(11):1427–1442, 2003.
9. D. Perperidis, A. Rao, R. Mohiaddin, and D. Rueckert. Non-rigid spatio-temporal alignment of 4D cardiac MR images. In *Second International Workshop on Biomedical Image Registration*, Philadelphia, PA, 2003.
10. S. C. Mitchell, B. P. F. Lelieveldt, R. J. van der Geest, H. G. Bosch, J. H. C. Reiber, and M. Sonka. Multistage hybrid active appearance model matching: Segmentation of left and right ventricles in cardiac MR images. *IEEE Transactions on Medical Imaging*, 20(5):415–423, 2001.
11. M. R. Kaus, J. von Berg, W. Niessen, and V. Pekar. Automated segmentation of the left ventricle in cardiac MRI. In *International Conference on Medical Image Computing And Computer Assisted Intervention (MICCAI)*, pages 432–439, 2003.
12. P. Thompson and A. W. Toga. A Surface-Based Technique for Warping Three-Dimensional Images of the Brain. *IEEE Transactions on Medical Imaging*, 15(4):402–417, 1996.
13. S. Kabus, T. Netsch, B. Fischer, and J. Modersitzki. B-spline registration of 3D images with Levenberg-Marquardt optimization. In *Image Processing*, SPIE Proceedings, 2004. In press.
14. J. Weese, M. R. Kaus, C. Lorenz, S. Lobregt, R. Truyen, and V. Pekar. Shape constrained deformable models for 3D medical image segmentation. In *International Conference on Information Processing in Medical Imaging*, pages 380–387, Davis, CA, USA, 2001.
15. P. Thévenaz and M. Unser. Spline pyramids for inter-modal image registration using mutual information. In *Image Processing*, volume 3169 of *SPIE Proceedings*, pages 236–247, 1997.
16. D. C. Collier, S. S. C. Burnett, M. Amin, S. Bilton, C. Brooks, A. Ryan, D. Roniger, D. Tran, and G. Starkschall. Assessment of consistency in contouring of normal-tissue anatomic structures. *Journal of Applied Clinical Medical Physics*, 4(1):17–24, 2003.

Three-Dimensional Shape-Motion Analysis of the Left Anterior Descending Coronary Artery in EBCT Images

Ioannis A. Kakadiaris*, Amol Pednekar, and Alberto Santamaría-Pang

Visual Computing Lab, Dept. of Computer Science, Univ. of Houston, Houston, TX

Abstract. In this paper, we present a physics-based deformable model framework for the quantification of shape and motion parameters of the Left Anterior Descending (LAD) coronary artery in the heart's local frame of reference. We define the long-axis of the heart as the local frame of reference. The shape of the LAD is modeled as a parametric curved axis with Frenet-Serret frame. The motion of the LAD (due to heart motion) is modeled as a composite of primitive shape-motion components: 1) longitudinal elongation, 2) radial displacement, and 3) twist with respect to the heart's local frame of reference. The three-dimensional shape-motion components are parameterized along the LAD's length. Results from simulated data and three asymptomatic subjects' Electron Beam Computed Tomography (EBCT) data are in agreement with the expected physiological trends.

1 Introduction

The significant increase in spatio-temporal resolution of computed tomography (CT) and magnetic resonance (MR) imaging has made it possible to acquire high-resolution volumetric cardiac image data over the cardiac cycle, thus enabling computer-assisted physiological analysis of the heart for diagnosis, prognosis, treatment planning, and monitoring [1]. The quantitative analysis of the volume, shape, deformation, and motion of the heart can help differentiate between normal and pathological hearts. The motion and deformation of the heart can be analyzed either by tracking the myocardium or by tracking anatomical, implanted, or induced landmarks. The complexity of the left ventricle (LV) nonrigid motion and the lack of reference landmarks within the myocardium make it difficult to extract the true motion trajectories of tissues. The LAD attached to the myocardium can be used as a natural landmark for tracking anterior-septal myocardial motion.

Previous approaches towards tracking of coronary arteries can broadly be classified as: 1) landmark-based [2,3,4], 2) template-based [5], and 3) geometric

---

* This material is based upon work supported in part by the National Science Foundation under Grants IIS-9985482 and IIS-0335578. Any opinions, findings, and conclusions or recommendations expressed in this material are those of the authors and do not necessarily reflect the views of the National Science Foundation.

C. Barillot, D.R. Haynor, and P. Hellier (Eds.): MICCAI 2004, LNCS 3217, pp. 1025–1033, 2004.

constraint-based methods [6,7,8]. Early coronary artery motion studies followed a landmark-based approach. Later, entire vessel analysis was performed using individual two-dimensional projections. Recent methods track the three-dimensional reconstruction of the arteries [6]. However, these methods do not accommodate radial displacement and axial torsion, as these parameters cannot be derived in a vessel's local frame of reference. This paper presents an extension of our previous work [9] in a physics-based deformable model framework for a clinically relevant parametric shape-motion analysis of the LAD. This new approach takes into consideration a common frame of reference for each subject by defining a local coordinate system for the heart [10]. Our main contribution is that our framework allows for three basic motion components that naturally describe the deformation of the LV that is imparted onto the LAD. This clinically relevant and anatomically normalized geometric reference frame allows comparison between various subjects.

2   Shape-Motion Modeling of the LAD

The shape-motion estimation of a non-rigid object poses challenges in terms of establishing point-to-point correspondences in space and over time. Furthermore, the shape modeling for anatomic structure poses the challenge of capturing the clinically relevant shape features along with the features' spatial variance [11], while motion modeling requires combining the clinical significance with the topological interdependence and spatial variance of the motion features. Thus, anatomy related shape-motion modeling requires: 1) an anatomy-relevant local frame of reference; 2) parameterization along the direction of the salient feature's spatial variation; and 3) decomposition of overall motion to capture interdependence of anatomical elements. To that effect, a physics-based deformable model of the LAD is used, where global deformation parameters represent the salient features of the shape changes and motion imparted by the myocardium onto the LAD. Then, shape-motion estimation for the LAD is performed using frame-by-frame tracking of the LAD over time. In this section, we provide a brief description of the deformable model framework [12,13], and its adaptation for shape-motion analysis of the LAD.

2.1   Model-Centered Frame of Reference

The definition of an object's own local coordinate system, effectively capturing its shape and motion specific features, is essential for the analysis of the shape, motion, and deformation of the object. Thus, determining the heart's local coordinate system is important for establishing the topological relationship between the heart and the coronary arteries. The local heart coordinate system enables the characterization of the coronary artery motion in terms of components relative to the medial axis of the heart.

Geometrically our LAD model consists of a 3D surface in space with intrinsic material coordinates, $\mathbf{u} = (u, v)$. The positions of the points on the model relative to an inertial frame of reference Φ in space are given by a vector-valued, time-varying function of $\mathbf{u}$: $\mathbf{x}(\mathbf{u}, t) = (x_1(\mathbf{u}, t), x_2(\mathbf{u}, t), x_3(\mathbf{u}, t))^\top$, where $\top$ denotes transposition. A non-inertial, model-centered reference frame ϕ is set up and the position function is expressed as: $\mathbf{x} = \mathbf{c} + \mathbf{R}\mathbf{p}$, where $\mathbf{c}(t)$ is the origin of ϕ at the center of the model and the rotation matrix $\mathbf{R}(t)$ gives the orientation of ϕ relative to Φ. Thus, $\mathbf{p}(\mathbf{u}, t)$ gives the positions of points on the model relative to the model frame.

We define the heart's coordinate system with its origin at the center of the base of the heart. The longitudinal axis of the heart's coordinate system is defined as the line between the midpoint of the split between ascending and descending pulmonary trunk and the LV apex (Figs. 1(a,b)). Thus, orientation and position of the long axis (with respect to the measured trans-axial images) are defined by two rotation angles and the origin's 3D coordinates, which are used to re-orient the trans-axial data to the local coordinates of the heart.

2.2 Parametric Shape Model

To incorporate global and local deformations, $\mathbf{p}$ is expressed as the sum of a global reference shape $\mathbf{s}(\mathbf{u})$ and a local displacement function $\mathbf{d}(\mathbf{u}, t)$: $\mathbf{p} = \mathbf{s} + \mathbf{d}$. The geometric model of the LAD is a tube-shaped parametric deformable model with a curved axis $\mathbf{e}(u)$ and Frenet-Serret (FS) frame oriented cross sectional planes $\mathbf{a}(u)$, defined as follows:

$$\mathbf{s}(u, v) = \begin{bmatrix} e_1(u) + a_1(u, v) \\ e_2(u) + a_2(u, v) \\ e_3(u) + a_3(u, v) \end{bmatrix}, \tag{1}$$

where $-\frac{\pi}{2} \leq u \leq \frac{\pi}{2}$, $-\pi \leq v \leq \pi$. The parametric curved axis is expressed as a 9th-degree polynomial to model the medial axis of the LAD. The degree of the polynomial was selected in order to capture the global shape of the tortuous medial axis of the LAD. The FS frame is used to capture the LAD along the medial axis since it provides a local frame of reference uniquely determined by a point on a curve and the curve's behavior around this point. A FS frame is independent of the curve's coordinate system, and the parameterization depends only on its local shape. The orthogonal system of axes that constitutes the FS frame is obtained from the axis derivatives:

$$\mathbf{T}(u) = \frac{\dot{\mathbf{e}}(u)}{|\dot{\mathbf{e}}(u)|}, \quad \mathbf{B}(u) = \frac{\dot{\mathbf{e}}(u) \times \ddot{\mathbf{e}}(u)}{|\dot{\mathbf{e}}(u) \times \ddot{\mathbf{e}}(u)|}, \quad \mathbf{N}(u) = \mathbf{B}(u) \times \mathbf{T}(u). \tag{2}$$

Thus, the cross sectional planes can be represented in a matrix form as follows:

$$\begin{bmatrix} a_1(u, v) \\ a_2(u, v) \\ a_3(u, v) \end{bmatrix} = r(u) \begin{bmatrix} N_1(u) & B_1(u) \\ N_2(u) & B_2(u) \\ N_3(u) & B_3(u) \end{bmatrix} \begin{bmatrix} cos(v) \\ sin(v) \end{bmatrix}, \tag{3}$$

where $r(u)$ is a radius of the circular cross section. Figure 1(c) illustrates the FS frames of an axis $\mathbf{e}(u)$ for various values of the parameter u.

2.3   Parametric Shape-Motion Estimation

The degrees of freedom of the model are incorporated into the vector $\mathbf{q} = (\mathbf{q}_c^\top, \mathbf{q}_\theta^\top, \mathbf{q}_s^\top, \mathbf{q}_d^\top)^\top$, which consists of the parameters necessary to define the translation $\mathbf{q}_c$, rotation $\mathbf{q}_\theta$, global deformation $\mathbf{q}_s$, and local deformation $\mathbf{q}_d$ of the model [13,14]. The aim here is to extract only the global shape change and motion imparted by myocardium onto the LAD. To that end, the degrees of freedom of the model are restricted to global deformation only. The motion of the LAD (due to the heart motion) is modeled as a composite sequence of primitive shape-motion components: 1) longitudinal elongation ($\mathbf{T_{LE}}$) along the length of the LAD; 2) radial displacement ($\mathbf{T_{RD}}$) with respect to the long axis of the heart; and 3) twist ($\mathbf{T_T}$) around the long axis of the heart. The axis of the LAD is initialized as the shape and position of the LAD over time, given by:

$$\mathbf{m}(u, v, t) = \mathbf{T_T}(u, t) \cdot (\mathbf{T_{RD}}(u, t) \cdot (\mathbf{T_{LE}}(u, t) \cdot (\mathbf{s}(u, v))))^\top, \qquad (4)$$

where $\mathbf{m}(u, v, t) = (m_1(u, v, t), m_2(u, v, t), m_3(u, v, t))^\top$ and $\mathbf{m}(u, v, 0) = \mathbf{s}(u, v)$. The longitudinal elongation (or shrinking) along the length of the artery can be parameterized as follows:

$$\mathbf{T_{LE}}(u, t) = [1, 1, c^l(u, t)]^\top, \qquad (5)$$

where $c^l(u, t)$ is a time-varying longitudinal elongation parameter function. The radial displacement with respect to the long axis of the heart can be parameterized as follows: $\mathbf{T_{RD}}(u, t) = [c_1^r(u, t), c_2^r(u, t), 1]^\top$, where $c_1^r(u, t)$ and $c_2^r(u, t)$ are the time-varying radial displacement parameter functions. Finally, the twist around the long axis of the heart can be parameterized as follows:

$$\mathbf{T_T}(u, t) = \begin{bmatrix} cos(c^t(u, t)) & -sin(c^t(u, t)) & 0 \\ sin(c^t(u, t)) & cos(c^t(u, t)) & 0 \\ 0 & 0 & 1 \end{bmatrix}, \qquad (6)$$

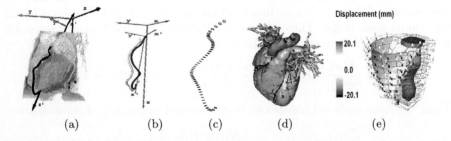

(a)   (b)   (c)   (d)   (e)

Fig. 1. (a) Local coordinate system of the heart. (b) Segmented LAD at end-systole (ES) and end-diastole (ED) and heart-centered coordinate system. (c) Shape model of the LAD with FS frames. (d) A geometric model of the heart from Visible Productions^{TM}. (e) A geometric model and motion data of a human subject's ventricles extracted using MRI-SPAMM data [15,16] (Courtesy: Prof. Dimitri Metaxas).

where $c^t(u, t)$ is the time-varying twisting parameter function along the LAD's length. Thus, the vector of motion parameters is defined as: $\mathbf{q}_m = (c^l, c_1^r, c_2^r, c^t)^\top$. Furthermore, the Jacobian matrix is computed as $\mathbf{J} = \frac{\partial \mathbf{m}}{\partial \mathbf{q_m}}$, in order to formulate the dynamics of the deformable model through the application of Lagrangian mechanics. The resulting Lagrangian equations for the LAD shape-motion estimation task are of the form $\dot{\mathbf{q}}_m + \mathbf{K}\mathbf{q}_m = \mathbf{f}_q$ where $\mathbf{K}$ is the stiffness matrix of the simulated elastic material [14], and the vector $\mathbf{f}_q$ represents the external forces that the LAD data apply to the model. Fitting is accomplished by integrating the Lagrangian equations through time using the physics-based modeling framework [12,13]. Once the equilibrium is reached, the values of $\mathbf{q}_m$ are the shape-motion parameters of the LAD.

2.4   Algorithm

The LAD tracking is comprised of the following three main steps:

Step 1 - Determine the local coordinate system of the heart: The long-axis of the heart is localized manually by selecting the center of the base and the apex of the heart. The splitting of the pulmonary trunk occurs two or three slices above the base of the heart (where the left main coronary artery starts) and serves as a landmark to locate the center of the base of the conical heart. The apex of the conical heart is localized about 6-8 slices below the first appearance of the liver in the EBCT data.

Step 2 - Fitting the data at the end-systole (ES): The parametric medial axis $\mathbf{e}(u)$ is computed from the center points corresponding to the LAD's 3D contours (currently, determined manually in each phase). Then, the deformable-model is initialized as: $\mathbf{m}(u, v, 0) = \mathbf{s}(u, v)$ to fit the LAD at ES [14].

Step 3 - Fitting of a deformable model from phase to phase: Global deformations are used to deform the fitted model at the ES from phase to phase, producing a vector of motion parameters $\mathbf{q}_m$ at every phase. Global deformations are computed from the corresponding LAD's 3D contours of each phase.

2.5   Experimental Data

We have performed a number of experiments to: 1) assess the validity of our LAD shape-motion estimation model, and 2) compare the range of shape-motion parameters computed by our method with the torsional measurements reported for LV through physiological experiments.

To simulate the LAD deformation over the cardiac cycle, we considered a prototype consisting of the following two components: 1) a geometric model of the heart from Visible Productions[TM]; these geometric models have been extracted using the Visible Human Data and include both the heart surface and the coronary artery tree (Fig. 1(d)); 2) the patient-specific ventricles motion data provided by Prof. Metaxas (Rutgers University); these motion data were obtained using the techniques detailed in [15,16] (Fig. 1(e)). The geometric model was animated using the patient-specific motion data from the LV and right ventricle (RV). To study the LAD motion on real data, three volunteer subjects'

EBCT images were acquired on a GE Imatron EBCT scanner. The acquisition parameters were: resolution 0.41x0.41x1.50 mm; 5 phases from ES to end-diastole (ED); 82 slices per phase, with presence of contrast agent.

3   Results and Discussion

Due to space limitation we present the estimated shape-motion parameters ($\mathbf{T_T}$, $\mathbf{T_{LE}}$, and $\mathbf{T_{RD}}$) of the LAD for the simulated data and for Subject-3. Figures 2(a,b) shows the twist angles for simulated data and Subject-3 around the long-axis of the heart. Positive twist angle represents counter-clockwise circumferential motion when looking from apex towards base from ES to ED. The twist angles for simulated data at the ED vary from $-3.26°$ in the basal third to $-0.34°$ in the apical third, taking a minimum value of $-22.67°$ in the apical third. While for Subject-3, twist angles at the ED phase range from $0.94°$ in the basal third to $3.56°$ in the apical third, with a minimum value of $-13.97°$ at the basal third. In both cases, the magnitude of torsional deformation increases from the base towards the apex. For Subject-3, an untwisting effect at the apex can be observed. It is important to mention that for Subject-3 the LAD's apical segment covers a longer portion of the apex compared to that of the simulated data, resulting in positive twist values for Subject-3 when the apex moves from ES to ED. These values and torsion patterns are consistent with those computed using biplane cineradiography of tantalum helices implanted within the LV midwall [17]. Figures 2(c-h) depict the estimated shape-motion parameters for Subject-3 with their corresponding rate of change. Positive-negative values for $\mathbf{T_{LE}}$, and $\mathbf{T_{RD}}$ represent longitudinal elongation-contraction and radial displacement away-towards the long-axis of the heart. The mean and standard deviation values per segment from ES to ED for $\mathbf{T_T}$, $\mathbf{T_{LE}}$, and $\mathbf{T_{RD}}$ are: $(-3.87° \pm 6.76°)$, (3.56 mm $\pm$2.71 mm), and (0.63 mm $\pm$1.43 mm) respectively.

Table 1 shows the mean, standard deviation, maximum, and minimum values for the shape-motion parameters in the basal, mid-ventricular, and apical segments for Subject-3. The $\mathbf{T_{RD}}$ values suggest that the overall LAD moves away from the long-axis of the heart. $\mathbf{T_{RD}}$ shows higher values in the basal segment, decreasing in the apical segment, moving towards the long-axis of the heart at the extreme apical segment. The increasing values of $\mathbf{T_{LE}}$ from base to apex indicate that the LAD's elongation takes place primarily from the mid-ventricular to the apical segment. These shape-motion parameters along with the rate of change from ES to ED, show physiological trends expected for asymptomatic hearts [10].

Our model provides a clinically relevant and anatomically normalized geometric reference frame, which allows comparison between various subjects. This suggests the possibility of classifying parameters associated with normal and pathological hearts. This model would serve as a detailed morphological model describing the interaction between coronary fluid flow and the vessel wall for the computational fluid dynamics simulations that will elucidate the biomechanical implications of the coronary arterial motion in vascular disease. The preoperative

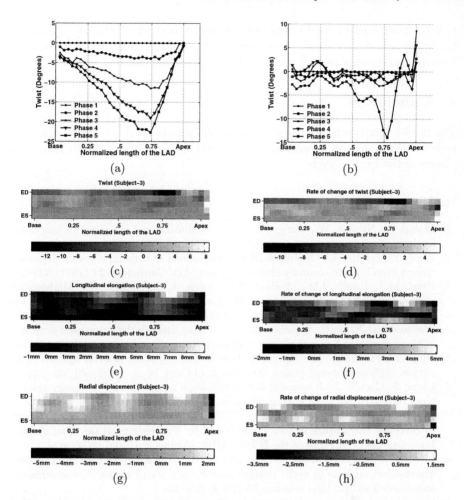

Fig. 2. Twist parameters from ES to ED for: (a) simulated data, and (b) Subject-3. Estimated parameters (Subject-3) for: (c) twist, (d) rate of change of twist, (e) longitudinal elongation, (f) rate of change of the longitudinal elongation, (g) radial displacement, and (h) rate of change of the radial displacement.

Table 1. Statistics corresponding to Subject-3's shape-motion parameters (ED) at three sections of the LAD: basal, mid-ventricular, and apical.

	Basal				Mid				Apical			
	mean	*std*	*max*	*min*	*mean*	*std*	*max*	*min*	*mean*	*std*	*max*	*min*
T_T	−2.33	0.94	−0.94	−3.70	−4.12	1.61	−2.08	−6.27	−4.42	6.26	3.56	−13.97
T_{RD}	1.40	0.54	2.29	0.50	0.44	0.90	1.83	−0.65	0.10	2.06	2.09	−5.50
T_{LE}	1.41	0.69	2.65	0.45	4.53	2.14	7.07	1.09	4.64	3.27	9.07	−0.74

patient-specific shape-motion parameters can be used for robotic surgery on the beating heart. Also, it can be used to compute geometric features like curvature, torsion, and discrete flexion points in the LAD's local frame of reference.

4   Conclusion

The model-based technique proposed provides a framework to extract clinically relevant shape-motion parameters of the LAD along its entire length for all the phases of the cardiac cycle.

References

1. Frangi, A., Niessen, W., Viergever, M.: Three-dimensional modeling for functional analysis of cardiac images: a review. IEEE TMI **20** (2001) 2–25
2. Kong, Y., Morris, J.J., McIntosh, H.D.: Assessment of regional myocardial performance from biplane coronary cineangiograms. Am. Cardiology **27** (1971) 529–537
3. Potel, M.J., Rubin, J.M., MacKay, S.A., Aisen, A.M., Al-Sadir, J.: Methods for evaluating cardiac wall motion in three-dimensions using bifurcation points of the coronary arterial tree. Investigative Radiology **18** (1983) 47–57
4. Stevenson, D.J., Smith, I., Robinson, G.: Working towards the automated detection of blood vessels in X-ray angiograms. Pattern Recognition Letters **2** (1987) 107–112
5. Ding, Z., Friedman, M.: Quantification of 3-D coronary arterial motion using clinical biplane cineangiograms. The Int. J. of Card. Imag. **16** (2000) 331–346
6. Chen, S., Carroll, J.: Kinematic and deformation analysis of 4-D coronary arterial trees reconstructed from cine angiograms. IEEE TMI **22** (2003) 710–721
7. Olszewski, M., Long, R., Mitchell, S., Wahle, A., Sonka, M.: A quantitative study of coronary vasculature in four dimensions. In: Proceedings of the 22nd Annual International Conference of the IEEE EMBS. Volume 4. (2000) 2621–2624
8. Liao, R., Chen, S.J., Messenger, J., Groves, B., Burchenal, J., Carroll, J.: Four-dimensional analysis of cyclic changes in coronary artery shape. Catheterization and Cardiovascular Interventions **55** (2002) 344–354
9. Kakadiaris, I., Pednekar, A., Zouridakis, G., Grigoriadis, K.: Estimating the motion of the LAD: A simulation-based study. In: MICCAI'01. Volume LNCS 2208., Utrecht,The Netherlands (2001) 1328–1331
10. Kwok, L., Miller, D.: Torsional deformation of the left ventricle. The Journal of the Heart Valve Disease **4** (1995) S214–222
11. Frangi, A., Niessen, W., Nederkoorn, P., Bakker, J., Mali, W., Viergever, M.: Quantitative analysis of vascular morphology from 3D MR angiograms: in vitro and in vivo results. Magnetic Resonance in Medicine **45** (2001) 311–322
12. Terzopoulos, D., Metaxas, D.: Dynamic 3D models with local and global deformations: Deformable superquadrics. IEEE Transactions on Pattern Analysis and Machine Intelligence **13** (1991) 703–714
13. Metaxas, D., Terzopoulos, D.: Shape and nonrigid motion estimation through physics-based synthesis. IEEE T-PAMI **15** (1993) 580–591
14. Metaxas, D., Kakadiaris, I.: Elastically adaptive deformable models. IEEE Transactions on Pattern Analysis and Machine Intelligence **24** (2002) 1310–1321
15. Park, J., Metaxas, D., Young, A., Axel, L.: Deformable models with parameter functions for cardiac motion analysis from tagged MRI data. IEEE Trans. Medical Imaging **15** (1996) 278–289

16. Haber, E., Metaxas, D., Axel, L.: Motion analysis of the right ventricle from MRI images. In: MICCAI'98. Number 1496, Cambridge, MA (1998) 177–188
17. Hansen, D., Daughters, G., Alderman, E., Ingels, N., Miller, D.: Torsional deformation of the left ventricular midwall in human hearts with intramyocardial markers: regional heterogeneity and sensitivity to the inotropic effects of abrupt rate changes. Circulation Research **62** (1988) 941–952

Automatic Detection and Removal of Fiducial Markers Embedded in Fluoroscopy Images for Online Calibration

Laurence Smith, Mike Pleasance, Rosalyn Seeton, Neculai Archip, and
Robert Rohling

University of British Columbia, Canada.
Software: http://www.ece.ubc.ca/~neculaia/Matlab_code_fluoroscopy.htm

1 Introduction

Computer assisted fluoroscopic navigation has received strong interest as a new tool for various medical interventions (e.g. spinal, orthopaedic and brachytherapy procedures). One of the challenges for the intraoperative use of c-arm imaging is on-line calibration [1,2]. Usually the method selected to perform this task involves placing a grid of fiducial markers in the x-ray path. The real geometry of the grid is known, so if the geometry of the grid in the image can be found then the real location of the other features in the image can be determined. Detection of the markers is the most important step in the calibration process [2]. This paper describes a new technique for automatic detection of markers. The purpose is to detect the highest number of markers as possible from a standard grid. As a convenience, removal of the detected markers is also proposed.

2 Methodology

Finding fiducial markers with an automatic algorithm is difficult because of the presence of tools and dark bones that obscure the markers, variability of the marker appearance and the arbitrary orientation of the grid. To allow the algorithm to work on a variety of c-arm scanners, the only assumptions are the approximate size and shape of the markers (small crosses between 5 and 20 pixels wide) and that they are regularly spaced. Given these assumptions, the following steps are performed. First, the outer portion of the image is masked using a circular Hough transform. This involves a search for two symmetric maximum to accommodate the slightly elliptical shape of the field-of-view from most c-arm scanners. Next, the image is convolved with a marker-shaped kernel and subtracted from the original image to emphasize the markers. Groups of pixels that exhibit full or partial marker shapes are flagged. The candidates are then pruned by rejecting flagged locations that do not fall at regular locations. The remaining candidates are assigned to bands by using a process similar to raster scanning. At this stage, the highly visible markers have been identified, and their regularly spaced locations can be used to recover weaker markers. So a virtual grid is constructed by fitting curves to the markers in each band and the virtual

C. Barillot, D.R. Haynor, and P. Hellier (Eds.): MICCAI 2004, LNCS 3217, pp. 1034–1035, 2004.
© Springer-Verlag Berlin Heidelberg 2004

grid intersections are used to recover the weaker markers. The complete list of markers is then used for on-line calibration. As an optional step, the markers are removed by replacing marker pixels with values obtained by spline-interpolation of nearby pixels. An example of marker detection and removal is given in Fig. 1.

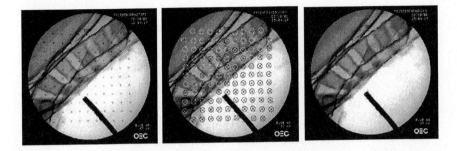

Fig. 1. The majority of the markers are located despite the presence of bones, tools and other obstructing features. The original image, circles around the detected markers, and the image after marker removal are shown.

3   Results and Conclusion

The algorithm was tested on 97 clinical images (768 × 576 pixels). The images are from both brachytherapy and orthopaedic surgeries. Various c-arm scanners were used including a Siemens Siremobil ISO C (Siemens Medical Solutions, Erlagen, Germany), GE/OEC Compact 7700 (General Electric, Milwaukee, WI) and Toshiba STX 650A (Toshiba America Medical Solutions, Tustin, CA). Of the 12066 possible fiducial markers, 11718 were successfully found, for a success rate of 96.28%. The success rate for each image is defined as the number of correctly located markers to the number of correctly located, extra and missing markers, so that 100% is only achieved if there are no extra or missing markers. Of the 97 images, only 16 had less than 95%. The best case identified 100% and the worst case identified 76%. This detection rate is comparable to manual marker identification and comparable to the number deemed sufficient for other grids [2]. Compared to manual identification, tests show the markers were located to within 1.30±0.89 pixels, which corresponds to 0.47±0.32 mm. Overall, the algorithm is suitable for clinical applications.

References

1. P. Tate, V. Lachine, L. Fu, H. Croitoru, M. Sati, *Performance and Robustness of Automatic Fluoroscopic Image Calibration in a New Computer Assisted Surgery System*, MICCAI 2001, LNCS 2208, pp. 1130-1136, 2001.
2. H. Livyatan, Z. Yaniv, L. Joskowicz, *Robust automatic C-arm calibration for fluoroscopy-based navigation: a practical approach*, MICCAI 2002, LNCS 2488, pp. 60-68, 2002.

Increasing Accuracy of Atrophy Measures from Serial MR Scans Using Parameter Analysis of the Boundary Shift Integral

Richard G. Boyes, Jonathan M. Schott, Chris Frost, and Nicholas C. Fox

Dementia Research Group, Institute of Neurology, University College London,
8-11 Queen Square, London WC1N 3BG, UK

Abstract. A statistical method is proposed to determine ideal window parameters for the boundary shift integral (BSI), based on comparing the BBSI to segmented volume differences for a range of windowing parameters. Upon application, new parameters were obtained to measure brain atrophy in 35 subjects (23 AD, 12 controls), and group separation measured. Group separation increased and the numbers required to power a treatment trial decreased.

1 Introduction

The boundary shift integral (BSI) is a measure of cerebral atrophy from serial MRI. It requires two parameters which specify the location and width of a sampling window. The BSI increases the precision of estimating atrophy (compared to segmented volume differences (SVDs)) but may slightly underestimate atrophy. We assumed we could choose parameters that would approximate the BSIs to the SVDs without reducing precision for a set of Alzheimer's disease (AD) and control subjects.

2 Methods

Twenty-three patients with AD and twelve age-matched controls had two volumetric T1-weighted MR scans acquired approximately one year apart. The repeat scan was rigidly registered brain-to-brain to the baseline.

The BSI [1] measures brain atrophy between a co-registered scan pair. It is calculated by subtracting normalised intensities between the borders of the co-registered brains to give a volume. I_c (window centre) and I_w (window width) are user defined normalised intensity parameters; they define an intensity window such that any intensity above or below the bounds of the window is set to the upper or lower bound, respectively.

In order to determine improved values of I_c and I_w, t-tests were used to assess the difference between volumes of the SVDs and BSIs (which should approximate each other) for all co-registered scans. Pitman's test was used to assess the difference in variance (BSI variance should be lower). The variability of these

C. Barillot, D.R. Haynor, and P. Hellier (Eds.): MICCAI 2004, LNCS 3217, pp. 1036–1037, 2004.

test statistics over the range of I_c and I_w allowed us to estimate evidence for differences in means or variances, and hence chose an improved I_c and I_w.

Changes in volume were calculated using the BSI and expressed as an annual % loss using the chosen parameters, group separation measured and power calculations [2] carried out for the original ($I_c = 0.5$, $I_w = 0.5$) and new parameters.

3   Results and Discussion

We chose an (I_c, I_w) of (0.6,0.2) because an I_c of 0.6 gave a close approximation to the SVDs (left figure) but also decreased BSI variability (right figure). An I_w of 0.2 was used as a trade off between the gain of the BSI and robustness.

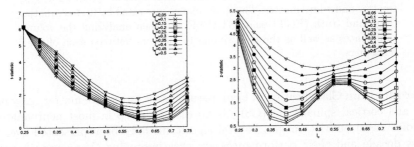

Using these parameters and comparing them to (I_c, I_w) = (0.5, 0.5) the mean atrophy rate increased from 1.98 ± 0.83 to 2.27 ± 0.83 for AD subjects, while controls increased to a lesser extent, from 0.48 ± 0.46 to 0.50 ± 0.46. Some evidence ($p = 0.06$) (using an unpaired t-test with unequal variances) was found that group separation had increased.

Applying methods for estimating numbers required to power a drug trial [2] for both old and new BSIs, for a drug anticipated to reduce excess atrophy by 20% over one year with 10% dropout, 22% fewer subjects would be required to achieve 90% statistical power for the new parameters.

By altering the parameters of the BSI, we have demonstrated that it is possible to increase the accuracy of whole brain atrophy measurements. The alteration in atrophy rates derived using this method in patients with AD and controls has clinical relevance: the numbers of patients required in trials of putative disease-modifying treatments are reduced, in this case by over 20%.

References

1. Freeborough, P.A., Fox, N.C.: The boundary shift integral: an accurate and robust measure of cerebral volume changes from registered repeat MRI. IEEE TOMI **16** (1997) 623–629
2. Fox, N.C., Cousens, S., Scahill, R.: Using serial registered brain magnetic resonance imaging to measure disease progression in Alzheimers Disease: Power calculations and estimates of sample size to detect treatment effects. Arch. Neurol. **57** (2000) 339–344

Evaluating Automatic Brain Tissue Classifiers

Sylvain Bouix, Lida Ungar, Chandlee C. Dickey, Robert W. McCarley, and
Martha E. Shenton

Surgical Planning Laboratory, Harvard Medical School, Boston, MA, USA.
Department of Psychiatry, Boston VA Healthcare System, Boston, MA, USA.

Abstract. We present a quantitative evaluation of MR brain images
segmentation. Five classifiers were tested. The task was to classify an MR
image into four different classes: background, cortical spinal fluid, gray
matter and white matter. The performance was rated by first estimating
a ground truth (EGT) using STAPLE and then analyzing the volume
differences as well as the Dice similarity measure between each of the 5
classifiers.

Introduction: Classification of brain tissue classes into white matter, gray matter and cortical spinal fluid (CSF) is an essential step in most neuroanatomy studies based on MR images. Several algorithms have been presented over the past decade and their performances are ever improving. Moreover, in recent years, novel evaluation procedures have been developed and it is now possible to rate accurately different methodologies even when a ground truth is not available. In an effort to improve our own segmentation pipeline, we have performed an evaluation of five different brain tissue classifiers. **Methods:** Our data set consisted of 24 pairs of MR volumes acquired on a GE 1.5T scanner. The first volume is a 0.9375x0.9375x1.5mm SPGR coronal scan, the second volume is a 0.9375x0.9375x3mm T2 weighted axial scan. All the classifiers use both volumes for the segmentation. The first algorithm (**1**) is an implementation of the seminal Expectation Maximization (EM) framework of Wells et al. [5]. The second algorithm (**2**) is the output of (**1**) manually edited by an expert to remove non brain tissues. The third algorithm (**3**) is also an EM segmenter, but one that uses spatial information provided by a probabilistic atlas as well as a hierarchical model for the tissue classes [1]. The fourth (**4**) is an implementation of the improved Watershed segmentation by [4]. In the fifth method (**5**) the bias field was corrected with [5] before running [4]. An approximate ground truth classification was estimated using STAPLE [3], and was later used to evaluate volumetric differences between each of the 5 classifiers and the estimated ground truth. The Dice similarity measure between the ground truth and the individual segmentations was also calculated [2].

Table 1. Performance scores of the different classifiers

	Gray Matter					CSF					White Matter				
	(1)	(2)	(3)	(4)	(5)	(1)	(2)	(3)	(4)	(5)	(1)	(2)	(3)	(4)	(5)
AVG($|X|-|EGT|$)	166	68	**-17**	141	119	-61	-116	**-5**	16	14	140	**6**	-16	-161	-138
STD($|X|-|EGT|$)	42	28	33	27	30	25	24	22	14	10	30	19	29	25	29
Dice	0.86	**0.93**	0.83	0.85	0.87	0.54	0.57	0.67	0.90	**0.91**	0.90	**1.00**	0.91	0.83	0.87

C. Barillot, D.R. Haynor, and P. Hellier (Eds.): MICCAI 2004, LNCS 3217, pp. 1038–1039, 2004.
© Springer-Verlag Berlin Heidelberg 2004

Results and Discussion: The results are shown in table 1. Figure 1 presents a box-and-whisker plot of the volume differences. The volumetric analysis ranks method (**3**) as the best method, but method (**5**) has the highest Dice scores. Our experts think method (**3**) is better but this judgment was not quantified. While it is difficult to know which is the best classifier, some conclusions can still be inferred: (i) thankfully, manual brain stripping always improves the results, (ii) bias field correction also always improves the segmentation, (iii) volumetric measurement and overlap measurements such as the Dice measure do not always agree, (iv) if one method is significantly different but better than all others, its score is likely to be low when compared to an *estimated* ground truth. In future work, we propose to investigate other measures, such as the sensitivity and specificity provided by STAPLE. We also plan to compare the different results to small regions of the brain previously manually segmented by experts.

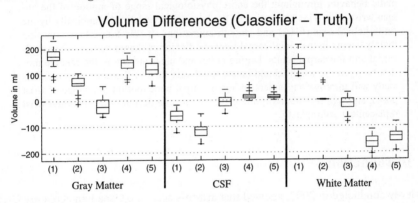

Fig. 1. Box-and-Whisker plot of the volume difference between each classifier and EGT

Acknowledgments. We acknowledge the support of NIH (K02 MH01110, R01 MH50747 to MES, R01 MH40799 to RWM), the Dept of Vet. Affairs Merit Awards (MES, RWM), Career Devel. Award (CCD).

References

1. K. M Pohl, W. M. Wells, A. Guimond, K. Kasai, M. E. Shenton, R. Kikinis, W. E. L. Grimson, S. K. Warfield. Incoperating non-rigid registration into expectation maximization algorithm to segment mr images. In *MICCAI*, pages 564–572, 2002.
2. L.R.Dice. Measure of the amount of ecological association between species. *Ecology*, 26:297–302, 1945.
3. S. K. Warfield, K. H. Zou, W. M. Wells. Validation of image segmentation and expert quality with an expectation-maximazation algorithm. In *MICCAI*, 2002.
4. V. Grau, A.J.U. Mewes,M. Alcaniz, R. Kikinis, S.K. Warfield. Improved watershed transform for medical image segmentation using prior information. *IEEE Trans Med Imag. In Press.*, 2003.
5. W.M. Wells III, W.E.L Grimson, R. Kikinis, F.A Jolesz. Adaptive segmentation of MRI data. *IEEE Transactions on Medical Imaging*, 15:429–442, 1996.

Wrist Kinematics from Computed Tomography Data

Maarten Beek, Carolyn F. Small, Steve Csongvay, Rick W. Sellens, R.E. Ellis, and
David R. Pichora

Human Mobility Research Centre
Kingston General Hospital
Kingston, ON, K7L 2V7
Canada
beek@me.queensu.ca

Abstract. Three-dimensional (3-d) surface models of human carpal bones obtained from Computed Tomography (CT) were used to investigate their kinematic behavior throughout the entire physiological range of motion of the human wrist joint. The 3-d motion of the bones was visualized graphically by the finite helical axis (FHA) and smooth animations. It was found that extension mainly occurs in the radial-carpal joint and flexion is shared between the radial-carpal and midcarpal joints. During radial and ulnar deviation, the relative motion between the scaphoid and lunate was larger than in flexion-extension. This study will improve our understanding of carpal bone motion in a range of wrist poses, and will provide morphological data for the design of a functional wrist replacement arthroplasty.

1 Introduction

A survey conducted in 2003, showed that arthritis costs the Canadian economy CAN$ 4.4 billion each year. The wrist joint is often involved and treatment options are limited. They include carpectomy, limited fusion or complete fusion. Wrist replacement is seldom performed due to the high failure rates of the presently available prostheses. An increased knowledge of the kinematics of the joint will assist in the design process of more successful arthroplasties.

2 Materials and Methods

Four fresh frozen human upper limbs were scanned in 11 different poses throughout their entire range of motion. Surface models of the carpal bones were created from the obtained CT images. Due to the small size and proximity of carpal bones, manual segmentation of the CT images was necessary. The Iterative Closest Point algorithm was applied to register the models of different poses to each other. The kinematics of each bone was described by a FHA [1]. Smooth animations of wrist motion were created to verify the kinematics visually[1]. The surface models were compared with point clouds generated by a laser scanner. The intra- and inter-operator variability was determined by comparing the surface areas and volumes of the models.

---

[1] http://me.queensu.ca/hmrc/research/KAJ_movie.html

C. Barillot, D.R. Haynor, and P. Hellier (Eds.): MICCAI 2004, LNCS 3217, pp. 1040–1041, 2004.

3 Results

The mean error between surface models and point clouds was less than 0.1 mm (n=9). The surface areas and volumes of the models were in agreement with other studies [2]. The kinematic analyses showed that extension mainly occurred in the radiocarpal joint and that flexion was shared between the radiocarpal and midcarpal joints. Compared with flexion-extension, the relative motion between the scaphoid and lunate was larger in radial-ulnar deviation, when the scaphoid moved out of the plane of motion. In pronation-supination motion, the inter-carpal motion was minimal.

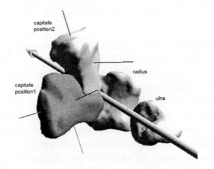

Fig. 1. The *finite helical axis* (*arrow*) describing the 3-d motion of the *capitate bone* when the wrist moves from neutral (*position1*) to 65° flexion (*position2*). The *principal axes*, shown in the models of the bone in both poses as *lines*, were used to determine its motion. The distal parts of the radius and the ulna are shown for reference

4 Discussion

Surface models obtained from CT images, were successfully applied to determine the kinematics of human wrists. Data from healthy and arthritic living subjects leading to more physiologically realistic results will be gathered once protocols and software tools are developed and validated. The created surface models can be applied in additional studies, like Finite Element analyses. Parts of the software can be used for pre-surgery planning, inter-operative guidance, and post-surgery evaluation.

References

1. Spoor CW, Veldpaus FE: Rigid body motion calculated from spatial co-ordinates of markers. Journal of Biomechanics 13(4), 391-393, 1980
2. Belsole RJ, Hilbelink DR, Llewellyn JA, Stenzler S, Greene TL, Dale M: Mathematical analysis of computed carpal models. Journal of Orthopaedic Research 6, 116-122, 1988

3D Analysis of Radiofrequency-Ablated Tumors in Liver: A Computer-Aided Diagnosis Tool for Early Detection of Local Recurrences

Ivan Bricault[1,2], Ron Kikinis[1], Eric vanSonnenberg[1],
Kemal Tuncali[1], and Stuart G. Silverman[1]

[1] Surgical Planning Lab / Department of Radiology, Brigham and Women's Hospital, 75
Francis Street, Boston, MA 02115, USA
[2] TIMC-IMAG laboratory, University Hospital, Grenoble, France
Ivan.Bricault@imag.fr

Abstract. Radiofrequency ablation is being used increasingly in the treatment of liver tumors, and the detection of local recurrences on follow-up imaging is an important and occasionally challenging task. When the tumor is not associated with nodular enhancement, recurrence detection only relies on a precise identification of shape changes in the post-ablation area. In order to better characterize subtle shape changes, we present a computer-aided diagnosis tool based on a semi-automatic segmentation of CT data with a watershed algorithm. The 3D moment of inertia of the segmented area is computed and provides a quantitative criterion for the study of post-ablation changes over time. Preliminary results on two clinical cases demonstrate that our tool can effectively improve the radiologist's ability to detect early tumor recurrence.

Radiofrequency (RF) ablation is a minimally invasive alternative to surgical resection of liver tumors. It delivers high-frequency alternating current in situ, inducing tumor thermal necrosis. In the follow-up of RF ablation, the most widely used imaging modality is contrast-enhanced computed tomography (CT). Successfully ablated tumors appear as low-attenuation areas with no enhancement; hence non-enhancing recurrences may be recognizable only by detecting subtle changes in the post-RF ablated area shape [1]. This detection on follow-up CT 2D slices constitutes a challenging task for the radiologist. Since it can have important consequences for patients, it motivated the development of our computer-aided diagnosis tool.

A method for the evaluation of RF ablations has been previously presented [2]. Whereas this study used an ellipsoid model for segmentation and was focused on the immediate post-ablation comparison between MRI and histological data, we address here the different clinical problem of long-term follow-up CT interpretation. Moreover, since we want to detect shape changes, our segmentation method is not restricted to a particular geometric model.

Our software is based on the National Library of Medicine's Insight toolkit (www.itk.org). A curvature flow filter is used for edge-preserving CT smoothing. A watershed algorithm, controlled by a user interactively defined segmentation level, is able to segment the post-RF ablated area. The resulting 3D object is post-processed by mathematical morphology erosion and dilatation filters. Because a normal post-ablation area usually shrinks and becomes smoother over time, the moment of inertia

C. Barillot, D.R. Haynor, and P. Hellier (Eds.): MICCAI 2004, LNCS 3217, pp. 1042–1043, 2004.
© Springer-Verlag Berlin Heidelberg 2004

has been chosen to characterize its shape in addition to 3D volume. The total procedure is fast (at most a few minutes) and requires minimal user interaction.

We retrospectively analyzed the case of a 47 year-old female presenting multiple liver metastases from a gastro-intestinal stromal tumor (patient **#1**). Follow-up axial CT scans were acquired at months M=1, 5, 6, 9, 12 and 15 after the RF ablation of one active metastasis. Whereas the radiologist detected an increase in size of the post-ablated area only at M=12, our computer tool demonstrated visually and quantitatively (Fig. 1) a definitive suggestion of recurrence at M=9. Tumor recurrence was confirmed by a PET scan at that time. In the case of patient #2, no recurrence was observed. The evolution chart in Fig. 1 confirms the success of this ablation. In both patients, Fig. 1 chart additionally shows that 3D moment of inertia can provide a more sensitive criterion than 3D volume, since inertia presents larger scale variations more dependent on peripheral shape deformations.

In conclusion, these preliminary results demonstrate the clinical effectiveness of 3D analysis for early recurrence detection. It is currently being further validated by studying the evolution patterns of post-RF areas in a larger series of patients.

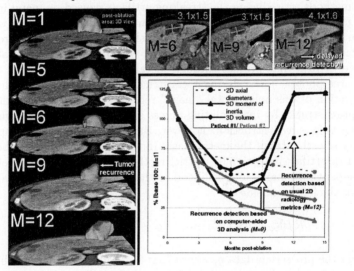

Fig. 1. Ablated area, **patient #1**: evolution of 3D segmented shape (*left*) and axial diameters (*top right*) over time (*M*=months after radiofrequency treatment).
Bottom right: Comparison of recurrence detection criteria, patients #1 and #2.

References

1. Choi, H., Loyer, E.M., DuBrow, R.A., Kaur, H., David, C.L., Huang, S., Curley, S., Charnsangavej, C.: Radio-frequency ablation of liver tumors: assessment of therapeutic response and complications. Radiographics 21 (2001) S41-S54
2. Lazebnik, R.S., Breen, M.S., Lewin, J.S., Wilson, D.L.: Automatic Model-Based Evaluation of Magnetic Resonance-Guided Radio Frequency Ablation Lesions with Histological Correlation. J. Magn. Reson. Imaging. 19 (2004) 245-354

This project was supported in part by a study grant from the French Radiological Society.

Fast Streaking Artifact Reduction in CT Using Constrained Optimization in Metal Masks

Jonas August and Takeo Kanade

Robotics Institute, Carnegie Mellon University, Pittsburgh, PA

Abstract. Here we accelerate computations that reduce CT metal artifacts by observing that metal projects to only a fraction of the X-ray detectors in each projection, and thus computations should focus on these metal "mask" regions. We propose that the penalized maximum likelihood optimization method for artifact reduction needs to be solved only within the metal mask, using the remaining non-mask regions as a constraint; we show that our approach leads to a 10x speedup.

Modern methods for reducing the streaking artifacts caused by metal in CT images (Fig. 1, top left) are based on solving an optimization problem where the unknown is the *entire* image [3]. Unfortunately, such solutions require computations far greater than the cause: the metal, which is typically a small area in the image. X-rays that project through metal are highly attenuated and thus have greater photon noise; during reconstruction the streaks form due to the backprojection of this noisy metal "mask" region. Projection completion methods suppress streaks by interpolating across such noisy metal portions of each projection before reconstruction; however, such ad-hoc techniques suffer from sensitivity to estimates of the metal mask. In this paper, we combine both ideas to accelerate artifact reduction by restricting the optimization to the metal mask.

In the penalized maximum likelihood method [2], one seeks that image f that minimizes the left hand side of

$$||g - \mathcal{R}f||_{\mathcal{W}}^2 + ||\nabla f||^2 \quad = \quad ||g - h||_{\mathcal{W}}^2 + \frac{1}{4\pi}||\mathcal{I}^{-3/2}h||^2, \qquad (1)$$

given only the projection data g, where $\mathcal{R}$ is the Radon transform (which takes line integrals) and $|| \cdot ||_{\mathcal{W}}$ is a weighted norm with a diagonal weight matrix $\mathcal{W}$ which is smaller in the metal regions of each projection. The first term ensures closeness to the data primarily in lower-attenuation regions, while the second enforces smoothness by penalizing gradients in f. Equivalently [1], one can instead minimize the right hand side of (1) with respect to $h = \mathcal{R}f$, where $\mathcal{I}^{-1}$ is the ramp filter used in filtered backprojection ($\mathcal{R}^{-1} \propto \mathcal{R}^T\mathcal{I}^{-1}$, where $\mathcal{R}^T$ is the backprojection operator). The advantage of optimizing over h is that the projections (one per angle) can be optimized separately without loss, since the ramp acts only along each projection. The final image is then $f = \mathcal{R}^{-1}h$.

Given a mask region $\mathcal{M}$, we accelerate the optimization over h by adding the equality constraint that $h = g$ outside of $\mathcal{M}$, where the data is less noisy. This gives rise to a much smaller set of equations for h within the noisy region $\mathcal{M}$ only, solved using a direct sparse solver in Matlab. The solution to the *un*constrained optimization problem for all projections for the image in Fig. 1 took 439 seconds

C. Barillot, D.R. Haynor, and P. Hellier (Eds.): MICCAI 2004, LNCS 3217, pp. 1044–1045, 2004.

on a 2.4 GHz Xeon, but only 42 seconds using the mask method, but the two solutions produce comparable images. These ideas also apply to regularized 3d cone-beam reconstruction, where we expect even greater speedup.

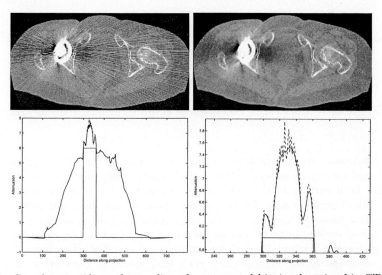

Fig. 1. Streaking artifacts that radiate from a metal hip implant in this CT image (top left) can be removed (top right) by solving optimization problem (1) along each projection (bottom left, with zoom of peak in bottom right). The dashed rough contour depicts the noisy CT projection data g corresponding to a single orientation from the sinogram (not shown); the solid smoother contour is the solution h to the optimization problem. These curves differ mostly near the peak where the noise is greatest. This noise is responsible for the streak artifacts produced by filtered backprojection. Here we propose a method to accelerate artifact reduction by solving the optimization problem only within the metal portion or "mask" along each projection where the data is most noisy; the mask is indicated with the rectangular impulse, and represents a fraction of the entire projection, since metal objects in CT tend to be small relative to the body. Thus the computation scales with the size of the metal, unlike other optimization approaches that solve for the entire image [4]. Note we do not require a precise mask, since it only limits the domain of smoothing. Here the mask is simply the data thresholded at an attenuation of 6; the constraint prevents mask-border effects.

References

1. J. August. Decoupling the equations of regularized tomography. In *International Symposium on Biomedical Imaging*, pages 653–656, 2002.
2. J. A. Fessler and S. D. Booth. Conjugate-gradient proconditioning methods for shift-variant pet image reconstruction. *IEEE Trans. on Image Proc.*, 8(5):688–699, 1999.
3. B. D. Man, J. Nuyts, P. Dupont, G. Marchal, and P. Suetens. Reduction of metal streak artifacts in x-ray computed tomography using a transmission maximum a posteriori algorithm. *IEEE Trans. on Nuclear Science*, 47(3):977–981, 2000.
4. G. Wang, T. Frei, and M. W. Vannier. Fast iterative algorithm for metal artifact reduction in x-ray ct. *Acad. Radiol.*, 7:607–614, 2000.

Towards an Anatomically Meaningful Parameterization of the Cortical Surface

Cédric Clouchoux[1], Olivier Coulon[1], Arnaud Cachia[2], Denis Rivière[2],
Jean-François Mangin[2], and Jean Régis[3]

[1] Laboratoire LSIS, UMR 6168, CNRS, Marseille, France,
[2] Equipe UNAF, SHFJ, CEA/DSV, Orsay, France,
[3] Service de Neurochirurgie Fonctionnelle et Stéréotaxique, Marseille, France

Abstract. We present here a method that aims at defining a surface-based coordinate system on the cortical surface. Such a system is needed for both cortical localization and intersubject matching in the framework of neuroimaging. We therefore propose an automatic parameterization based on the spherical topology of the grey/white matter interface of each hemisphere and on the use of organised and reproductible anatomical markers. From those markers used as initial constraints, the coordinate system is propagated via a PDE solved on the cortical surface. Preliminary work and results are presented here as well as further directions of research.

Introduction. In the context of inter-subject brain data matching and localization, the most common methods deal with 3-dimensional images and consider the problem as an inter-subject registration one, known as *spatial normalization*. Nevertheless there is great interest in analyzing data projected on the cortical surface [1]. In this context, matching cortical surfaces implies facing several problems, the main one being the lack of an implicit coordinate system, such as the voxel grid in 3 dimensions. Therefore the problem can be approached in terms of localization more than registration. Few methods aim at building a surface referential by parameterizing the cortical surface in a reproductible way [1,2]. In this framework, we propose here a method to automatically provide an anatomically meaningful parameterization, based on the definition of invariant and organised anatomical features, and which does not require any warping of the surface (e.g. to a sphere [1,2]).

Method. The outline of our method is to build a complete parameterization, in a longitude/latitude manner, starting from a few anatomical markers and propagating a coordinate systems from those original constraints over the whole cortical surface of each hemisphere. From MR anatomical images, a triangulation of the cortical surface is extracted and all the major sulci are automatically labelled [3]. A subset of parts of these sulci is projected on the surface, which are anatomically reproducible and geometrically organised as subparts of meridians or parallels on the cortical surface of each hemisphere [4], topologically equivalent to a sphere. Those projections are attributed a constant longitude (meridians)

C. Barillot, D.R. Haynor, and P. Hellier (Eds.): MICCAI 2004, LNCS 3217, pp. 1046–1047, 2004.

or latitude (parallels). Those markers are then used as sources of a surfacic heat-equation diffusion process [5] that drives the propagation of both longitude and latitude over the whole hemisphere surface (figure 1), resulting in a global coordinate system that complies with the initial constraints.

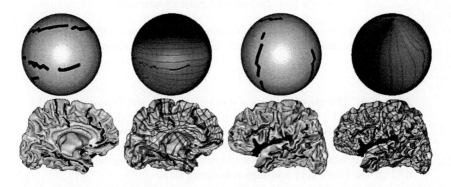

Fig. 1. Results on (top) synthetic spherical data (constraints and resulting isoparameter lines for longitude and latitude); (bottom) real brain data (constraints and isoparameter lines).

Further work. From this preliminary work, several line of research arise : the definition of the set of anatomical markers, the possible coupling between the two diffusion systems (longitude and latitude), and validation in a neuroimaging experimental context. Future applications are surfacic analysis of functional brain data, surface morphometry, or localization for the integration of modalities such as EEG and MEG.

References

1. Fischl, B., Sereno, M.I., Tootell, R., Dale, A.M. : Cortical surface-based analysis, II: Inflation, flattening, and a surface-based coordinate system. NeuroImage **9** (1999) 195–207
2. Toro, R., Burnod, Y. : Geometric atlas: modeling the cortex as an organized surface. NeuroImage **20(3)** (2003) 1468–1484
3. Rivière, D., Mangin, J.F., Papadopoulos-Orfanos, D., Martinez, J.M., Frouin, V., Régis, J. : Automatic recognition of cortical sulci of the Human Brain using a congregation of neural networks. Medical Image Analysis **6(2)** (2002) 77–92
4. Régis, J., Mangin, J.F., Ochiai, T., Frouin, V., Riviére, D., Cachia, A., Do, L., Samson, Y. : The Sulcal roots generic model: a hypothesis to overcome the variability of the human cortex folding patterns. Submitted (2004)
5. Brechbuhler, C., Gerig, G., Kobler, O. : Parameterization of closed surfaces for 3D shape description. Computer Vision and Image Understanding **61** (1995) 154–170

Nodule Detection in Postero Anterior Chest Radiographs

Paola Campadelli and Elena Casiraghi

Universitá degli Studi di Milano, Dipartimento di Scienze dell'Informazione
http://www.dsi.unimi.it, {Campadelli,Casiraghi}@dsi.unimi.it

Abstract. The use of image processing techniques and Computer Aided Diagnosis (CAD) systems has proved to be effective for the improvement of radiologists' diagnosis, especially in the case of lung nodules detection. In this paper we describe a method for processing Postero Anterior chest radiographs which extracts a set of nodule candidate regions characterized by low cardinality and high sensitivity ratio.

1 Introduction

Chest radiography is by far the common type of procedure for the initial detection and diagnosis of lung cancer. This motivates the great deal of research aimed to the creation of CAD systems aimed to lung nodules detection in chest radiographs [1]; however the problem is still open due to the significant loss of true positives. The multiscale method described in this paper has been tested on a standard database acquired by the Japanese Society of Radiological Technology [5] and extracts a set of candidate regions with an high sensitivity ratio.

2 Method

We work on images down-sampled to 256×256 pixels and use the lung area obtained in [1] but extended in order to include the parts behind the heart, near the spinal column and behind the diaphragm. To enhance the conspicuity of nodules of different size and brightness we use a multiscale approach. We start creating 11 *Difference Images* by subtracting from the original one the result of its convolution with a gaussian filter with standard deviation $s (s \in [2, 12])$. The result of subtracting to a nodule sub-image its smoothed version is an image with a positive peak in the central part of the nodule, and negative values in the neighborhood. The histogram of each *Difference Image* always shows a peak on the set of the positive values; we then create 11 binary images by selecting for each *Difference Image* all the pixels with a value bigger than the one corresponding to this peak; they are the pixels corresponding to the details identified at the scale s. The sum of all the binary images is a *Sum Image*, where the nodules appear as circular regions of different sizes, characterized by the highest values and surrounded by a much darker ring. To detect these regions we repeat

C. Barillot, D.R. Haynor, and P. Hellier (Eds.): MICCAI 2004, LNCS 3217, pp. 1048–1049, 2004.

the procedure described below for each possible radius value $R (R \in [2, 12])$. Having fixed the radius R, we calculate for each pixel $P = P(x, y)$ a coefficient $P_R = MEAN(Circle_R(P)) - MEAN(Ring_R(P))$, where $Circle_R(P)$ is the region composed by the pixels in the circle of radius R and centered in P, $Ring_R(P)$ is the region composed by the pixels in the 2-pixel-thick ring around the circle $Circle_R(P)$, $MEAN(X)$ is the mean of the gray values of the pixels in a region X. The thickness of the ring is fixed for every radius since what allows to identify a circular region is a darker ring surrounding it, no matter which is the thickness of the ring itself. To select the pixels which are potential nodule centers, we automatically find a threshold on the set of coefficients P_R with the algorithm described in [2]. For each connected region in the obtained *Binary Image*, we calculate its circularity, the biggest diagonal D of the minimum ellipse containing the region itself, and discard it either if the circularity is lower than 0.5 or D is bigger than $2R$. Repeating the procedure for all the 11 radius values we obtain a set of 11 *Binary Images* which are combined to extract a final set of candidates. All the regions appearing in only one of the *Binary Images* are taken as candidates. If some regions in different *Binary Images* overlap we choose as representative the one with the most circular shape.

The result is a set of about 24000 regions on all the 247 images of the database and only 7 true positives lost out of 153. We compared these results with those of other two extraction schemes tested on the same database. The first method, [4], extracts a set with 33000 candidates loosing 20 true positives; furthermore the authors apply a classification method that selects 5028 candidates, loosing other 15 true positives, for a total of 35 false negatives. We implemented the second method, [3] obtaining poor results in terms of true positive lost.

To prune the set of extracted candidates we calculated a set of 21 most representative features, based on the shape, the position, the gray level distribution in the original image, and the values of the coefficients P_R calculated during the candidates extraction. Applying to these features simple rules describing the relationships observed between pairs of features, we can reach a total number of candidates equal to 11500 loosing no true positive (sensitivity ratio= 0.95).

This high ratio demonstrates the efficiency of the method; further works will focus on the trimming of the false positive set to obtain a clinically useful system.

References

1. B. van Ginneken, A.: Computer-Aided Diagnosis in Chest Radiographs. P.h.D. dissertation, Utrecht Univ., Utrecht, The Nederlands. (2001)
2. Kapur,Sahoo,Woong, A.: A new method for gray level picture thresholding using the entropy of the histogram. Comp.Vis. Grap.and Im.Proc. **29** (1985) 273–285
3. Keserci,Bilgin and Yoshida, Hiroyuki, A.:Computerized detection of pulmonary nodules in chest radiographs based on morphological features and wavelet snake model. Med. Image Analisys. **6** (2002) 431–447
4. A.Schilham, B.Van Ginneken, M.Loog, A.:Multi-scale nodule detection in chest radiographs. Proc. MICCAI. (2003)
5. Web address: http://www.macnet.or.jp/jsrt2/cdrom_nodules.html

Texture-Based Classification of Hepatic Primary Tumors in Multiphase CT*

Dorota Duda[1,2], Marek Krętowski[2], and Johanne Bézy-Wendling[1]

[1] LTSI-INSERM, Université de Rennes 1, France
[2] Faculty of Computer Science, Białystok Technical University, Poland

Abstract. A new approach to the hepatic primary tumor recognition from dynamic CT images is proposed. In the first step of the proposed method, texture features are extracted from manually traced ROI-s to objectively characterize lesions. The second step consists in applying decision tree classifier. For the first time, the parameters obtained in subsequent acquisition moments are analyzed simultaneously.

Introduction. Computed Tomography (CT) is now widely applied for diagnosis of hepatic tumors. Typical visual inspection of scans enables radiologists to localize pathological regions and to recognize, to a certain extent, the type of lesion. Nevertheless, the definitive diagnosis usually requires invasive procedures like needle biopsy. More accurate computer-aided image analysis allows obtaining reliable predictions and avoiding these undesirable interventions [2].

In the paper texture-based classification of hepatic lesions from CT images is investigated. So far, the proposed diagnostic systems, which combine texture analysis with classification methods (e.g. [3,4]) were applied to non-enhanced CT scans of the liver. In our previous contribution [5] it was shown that considering the acquisition moments could improve classification accuracy in case of hepatic metastasis. In this paper, for the first time, the texture characteristics obtained in subsequent acquisition moments are analyzed simultaneously.

Method. In clinical practice, when dynamic CT of the liver is performed, three scan series are usually acquired: non-enhanced images and after contrast product injection, in arterial and portal phases. Radiologists commonly exploit an evolution of the tissue region appearance in different acquisition moments as a discriminating factor in the tumor diagnosis. An analogous idea is adopted in the proposed approach. Not only the texture characteristics of the considered region are analyzed, but also their changes in the three acquisition moments.

The first step in applying any classification tool is preparation of a learning set, which is used to generate the classifier. In our approach, the learning set is composed of texture feature vectors, each describing the same region of interest (ROI) in the three corresponding images. The regions are visually detected and manually drawn. As the classifier, Dipolar Decision Tree [1] is applied. When the classifier is created it can be used in prediction of suspected ROI-s.

* This work was supported by the grant W/WI/1/02 from Białystok Technical University

Results. The proposed approach was applied to recognizing the normal liver and its two main primary malignant lesions: hepato-carcinoma and cholangio-carcinoma. The database of 495 images from 22 patients was gathered in Eugene Marquis Center in Rennes, France. Acquisitions were performed with a GE HiSpeed CT device and the standardized acquisition protocol was applied: helical scanning, slice thickness 7 mm, 100 ml of contrast material injected at 4 m/s. For each phase and each tissue class 150 non-overlapped ROIs (diameters from 30 to 70 pixels) were traced. In our experiments the following texture features were extracted: (*i*) 4 first order parameters, (*ii*) entropy of image after filtering it with 24 zero-sum 5x5 Laws' filters, (*iii*) 8 Run-Length Matrix features and (*iv*) 11 Co-occurrence Matrix parameters. For the two last methods, features computed in 4 standard directions ($0°$, $45°$, $90°$, $135°$) and for 5 distances (from 1 to 5) were averaged. The 5-times repeated 10-fold cross-validation procedure was applied to estimate the classification accuracy (Table 1).

It could be observed that regardless of texture analysis method, the classification quality is significantly increased, when feature vectors are composed of parameters from subsequent acquisition moments.

Table 1. Classification accuracy obtained for different groups of texture features

Method	No contrast (N)	Arterial (A)	Portal (P)	N + A + P
First order	90.16 ± 1.31	85.82 ± 1.48	90.40 ± 1.69	98.76 ± 0.73
Laws' filters	94.16 ± 0.87	95.56 ± 1.23	94.53 ± 1.37	97.33 ± 1.50
Run length	95.53 ± 1.02	93.89 ± 1.28	95.45 ± 1.59	99.73 ± 0.42
Co-occurrence	96.36 ± 0.88	94.29 ± 1.79	94.87 ± 0.83	99.67 ± 0.37

Conclusion. In the paper, texture characteristics derived from images corresponding to three typical acquisition moments in dynamic CT of the liver are analyzed simultaneously. The experimental validation shows that the proposed approach improves the capability of hepatic primary tumor recognition.

References

1. Bobrowski, L., Krętowski, M.: Induction of multivariate decision trees by using dipolar criteria. Lecture Notes in Computer Science, **1910** (2000) 331–336
2. Bruno, A., Collorec, R., Bézy-Wendling, J., Reuzé, P., Rolland, Y.: Texture analysis in medical imaging. In: Roux, C., Coatrieux, J.L. (eds.): Contemporary Perspectives in Three-dimensional Biomedical Imaging. IOS Press (1997) 133–164
3. Chen, E.L., Chung, P.C., Chen, C.L., Tsai, H.M., Chang, C.I.: An automatic diagnostic system for CT liver image classification. IEEE T-BE, **45(6)** (1998) 783–794
4. Gletsos, M., Mougiakakou, S.G., Matsopoulos, G.K., Nikita, K.S., Nikita, A.S., Kelekis, D.: Classification of hepatic lesions from CT images using texture features and neural networks. Proc. of 23rd Int Conf of the IEEE EMBS (2001) 2748–2751
5. Krętowski, M., Bézy-Wendling, J., Duda, D.: Classification of hepatic metastasis in enhanced CT images by dipolar decision tree. Proc. of GRETSI (2003) 327–330

Construction of a 3D Volumetric Probabilistic Model of the Mouse Kidney from MRI

Hirohito Okuda[1,2,3], Pavel Shkarin[3], Kevin Behar[4], James S. Duncan[2,3], and Xenophon Papademetris[2,3]

[1]Production Engineering and Research Lab., Hitachi Ltd., Kanagawa, Japan,
[2] Department of Biomed. Engineering,
[3]Diag. Radiology and [4]Phsychiatry
Yale University New Haven, CT 06520-8042

Abstract. We present the results of constructing a probabilistic volumetric model of 3D MR kidney images. The ultimate goal of this work is the mouse kidney segmentation based on a probabilistic volumetric model. The kidneys were aligned into the base shape using an extended robust point matching algorithm. The registration step consists of the global linear transformation and the local B-spline based free form deformation. Shape modeling is performed with globally aligned shape and template volumetric image is generated with locally aligned images. We are currently working on developing a segmentation algorithm using our model.

1 Introduction

The ultimate goal of this work is to automate the segmentation of kidneys, and to quantify kidney volume in transgenic mouse models [1] of polycystic kidney disease. Toward this goal, here we present the result of constructing a probabilistic volumetric model which is the first key component of our strategy for the segmentation process. A general drawback of the model constructing methods proposed so far [2,5] is the correspondence problem where the definition of one-to-one mapping across data are needed. To solve this problem, we apply the extended robust point matching algorithm (RPM)[3] which can automatically compute the correspondences. Here we present a result of probabilistic volumetric model of both kidneys constructed using RPM .

2 Method and Results

Figure 1(a) shows an example of training image data. Ten postmortem eight-week old C57BL6 wild type mice were scanned. All imaging was performed on a Bruker 4.0T/40 cm bore animal system using a T2-weighted 3D Multi-spin multi-echo sequence (MSME), with a TE=15ms,FOV=4x2.5x1.8cm and an imaging matrix of 256x128x64.

An expert user performed the original surface extraction of both kidneys from the images with a software platform originally designed for segmenting the left ventricle

C. Barillot, D.R. Haynor, and P. Hellier (Eds.): MICCAI 2004, LNCS 3217, pp. 1052–1054, 2004.

of the heart. Segmented surfaces are aligned into the common base shape with RPM, first by a global linear transformation and next, by a local B-spline based free form deformation[4]. An example of this registration process is shown in Figure 1. The target kidney in Figure 1(b) is aligned into the base shape with a global linear transformation. The shape difference which remains after the linear transformation (Figure 1(c)) shows the shape variation to be modeled that is invariant to affine transformation. The final result of the registration after the local free form deformation (Figure 1(d)) indicates the RPM registration is enough accurate to construct an intensity model on the base shape. This yields an explicit volumetric deformable model as opposed to a model of simple surface shape.

The free form deformation is parameterized by concatenating the displacement vectors on grid points, and is used as an implicit representation of the kidney shape. The shape modeling is done by performing principal component analysis (PCA). The mean shape and first three modes of PCA are shown in Figure 2 (a) and (c). The modes of model are sorted in decreasing magnitude of their corresponding eigenvalues. The result shows the large variability included in the kidney model. Also, the template volumetric image is generated by transforming training data set into the base shape and averaging the transformed training data (Figure 2 (b)). This volumetric template image with statistical shape model could be used as the probabilistic volumetric model in the segmentation process.

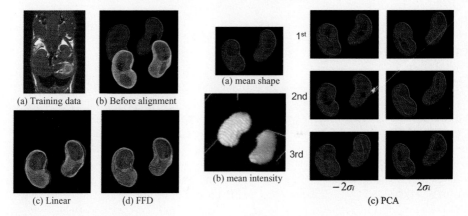

Fig. 1. Model construction step. (red) target, (yellow) base

Fig. 2. Result of Model construction

3   Conclusion

We demonstrate the feasibility of applying the RPM registration technique for the construction of probabilistic volumetric model of mouse kidney. We are currently working on developing a segmentation algorithm using the model proposed here.

Acknowledgments. We would like to thank Production Engineering Research Lab., Hitachi Ltd. for giving the opportunity of this research.

References

1. G.Wu *et al*, Somatic inactivation of PKD2 results in polycystic kidney disease. *Cell*, 93:177- 188, 1998
2. T.F. Cootes, C. Beeston, G. Edwards, and C. Taylor : Unified framework for atlas matching using active appearance models. IPMI, (1999).
3. Xenophon. Papademetris, Andrea P. Jackowski. Robert T. Schultz, Lawrence H. Staib, James S.Duncan : Computing 3D Non-rigid Brain Registration Using Extended Robust Point Matching for Composite Multisubject fMRI Analysis. MICCAI2003, 788-795.
4. Daniel Rueckert, Alejandro F. Frangi, Julia A. Schnabel : Automatic Construction of 3-D Statistical Deformation Models of the Brain Using Nonrigid Registration, *IEEE Transactions On Medical Imaging*,vol.22,No.8.Aug. 2003.
5. S. S. Gleason, H. Sari-Sarraf, M. A. Abidi, O. Karakashian, and F. Morandi. A new deformable model for analysis of X-ray CT images in preclinical studies of mice for polycystic kidney desease. IEEE Transactions on Medical Imaging, 21(10):1302-1309, October 2002.

Fluid Deformation of Serial Structural MRI for Low-Grade Glioma Growth Analysis

Bernard Cena[1], Nick Fox[1], and Jeremy Rees[2]

[1] Dementia Research Group, Institute of Neurology, University College London,
8-11 Queen Square, London WC1N 3BG, UK
{bcena,nfox}@dementia.ion.ucl.ac.uk
[2] Department of Molecular Neuroscience, Institute of Neurology, National Hospital
for Neurology and Neurosurgery, London, UK

Abstract. We apply fluid model non-rigid registration of serial structural T1 weighted MR images to obtain deformation-based measurements of low-grade glioma growth. Preliminary experimental results from ten patients show that measurements of tumour regions, together with visual inspection, provide insight into glioma growth characteristics.

1 Introduction and Method

Gliomas are the most common primary brain tumours. The management of low-grade gliomas (LGG) is difficult because they grow slowly, infiltrate diffusely and patient survival time is highly variable. Most cases of LGG progress to high-grade glioma (HGG) by a process of malignant transformation, which is an unpredictable event in the individual patient [1]. This study aims to measure LGG growth using serial T1-weighted MR imaging. Our imaging protocol includes structural T1 and fast spin echo T2, fFLAIR, sequences. Ten patients were chosen from a glioma imaging project of whom five were clinically and radiologically stable (defined as non-transforming), the others progressed clinically or developed a new area of gadolinium enhancement (transforming). All patients have had biopsies to confirm the diagnosis and have been imaged at 6 monthly intervals with a minimum of 4 studies.

For each study, the tumour region was roughly segmented by simple semi-automated thresholding on a fFLAIR image to provide a region of interest (ROI) and then co-registered with the corresponding T1 image. The fFLAIR image provides good contrast for anatomy affected by the tumour, but suffers from poor axial resolution (6 mm slices). For each patient, all T1 studies were resampled to cubic voxels ($2\,\mathrm{mm}^3$) and rigidly registered (with rescaling) to baseline T1. For each consecutive pair of studies, the later study was non-rigidly registered to the earlier using a fluid model deformation [2]. Tumour growth was assessed by integration of the Jacobian determinant of the deformation field at all voxels over the union of tumour regions at all time points for each patient. Malignant transformation was assessed by connected component analysis of the top 5% of Jacobians inside the composite ROI.

C. Barillot, D.R. Haynor, and P. Hellier (Eds.): MICCAI 2004, LNCS 3217, pp. 1055–1056, 2004.
© Springer-Verlag Berlin Heidelberg 2004

2   Results and Discussion

Table 1 shows growth rates in mm^3 for each subject adjusted for time (6 month interval). These growth rates correspond to the total contribution of connected components of the top 5% (empirical choice) of Jacobian values. Transforming patients (T) show steady or accelerating expansion of the tumour. The data for the non-transforming (NT) group suggests static or steady growth.

Table 1. Growth rates of highest growth clusters for transforming (T) and non-transforming (NT) subjects in mm^3 adjusted for time interval. † Patient T1 had chemotherapy between time points 5 and 6.

interval	T1	T2	T3	T4	T5	NT1	NT2	NT3	NT4	NT5
1 → 2	1.14	3.42	1.30	1.48	1.22	0.51	3.21	1.00	1.79	0.64
2 → 3	1.40	3.49	4.33	1.30	2.74	0.51	1.38	2.36	3.40	1.13
3 → 4	1.06	3.34	4.45	2.59	5.58	0.36	1.68	2.87	1.78	0.98
4 → 5	2.91	5.06		3.43		0.80	2.51	3.25	1.13	0.98
5 → 6	† 0.16	7.80		9.17		0.36				

We chose a very high degree of freedom (DOF) non-rigid registration algorithm based on a fluid model [2] to avoid making assumptions about the unknown glioma growth characteristics. The fluid model enables measurement of both displacing and, to some degree, infiltrating tumour growth, but suffers from slow convergence in areas of large displacement. We monitored the convergence of all registrations by visual analysis of transformed images.

The pattern of glioma growth is unique for every patient. Analysis of the highest growth areas has potential for predicting foci of malignant transformation. We plan to introduce a medium DOF registration between the rigid and fluid stages in order to normalise large scale deformations and achieve faster and better convergence of the fluid stage. Correlation of these preliminary results with perfusion and diffusion studies, and more sophisticated analysis of the deformation fields, is expected to provide further information about the process of LGG to HGG transformation.

Currently, the regional measurements combined with visual analysis of the deformations provide valuable clinical insight into glioma growth progression.

Acknowledgment. The authors thank Mr. Chris Benton for the MRI data.

References

1. Rees, J.: Advances in magnetic resonance imageing of brain tumours. Current Opinion in Neurology **16** (2003) 643–650
2. Freeborough, P.A., Fox, N.C.: Modeling brain deformation in Alzheimer Disease by fluid registration of serial 3D MR images. J. Comput. Assist. Tomogr. **22** (1998) 838–843

Cardiac Motion Extraction Using 3D Surface Matching in Multislice Computed Tomography

Antoine Simon[1], Mireille Garreau[1], Dominique Boulmier[2], Jean-Louis Coatrieux[1], and Herve Le Breton[1,2]

[1] LTSI, INSERM U642, Université de Rennes 1, Campus de Beaulieu, 35042 Rennes, France
antoine.simon@univ-rennes1.fr
[2] Centre Cardio-Pneumologique, CHU Pontchaillou, 35033 Rennes, France

Abstract. A new generation of Multislice Computed Tomography (MSCT) scanners, which allows a complete heart coverage and offers new perspectives for cardiac kinetic evaluation, is becoming widely available. A new method has been developed for the left ventricle motion analysis from dynamic MSCT images. It is based on a 3D surface matching process applied to left cavity volumes. It provides 3D velocity fields which can express contraction or expansion movements. First results obtained on real data show that MSCT imaging could be of great clinical interest for cardiac applications.

1 Introduction

The recent significant advances of spiral computed tomography, with the introduction of ultra-fast rotating gantries (-0.5s/tr-) along with multi-rows detectors, allow a huge progress toward the imaging of moving organs providing higher spatial and temporal resolutions. Non-rigid motion extraction methods are classified into three types: geometric or parametric deformable models, optical flow estimation and feature matching methods. Some of them have been applied in cardiac imaging [1,2,3], but nothing has been done for MSCT.

We propose a first method to extract elastic motion from cardiac human MSCT images. This approach is based on local 3D surface feature matching, under global constraints. First results obtained on real data show the great potential of this new imaging system for cardiac motion evaluation in non invasive imaging.

2 Method and Results

The proposed approach is based on surface primitive matching. It estimates local motion with global constraints providing 3D displacement vectors between two surfaces (corresponding to times t and $t + 1$) previously extracted by a 3D region growing [4]. This process requires to define: (1) the entities and their descriptive parameters; (2) the energy function for local feature matching; (3) the global matching process. The entities chosen have to regularly describe the whole surface, to be easily accessible and to enable the computation of descriptive parameters. Taking this into account, mesh nodes have been considered as entities. The mean curvature computed on the local geometry of the nodes

C. Barillot, D.R. Haynor, and P. Hellier (Eds.): MICCAI 2004, LNCS 3217, pp. 1057–1059, 2004.

has highlighted a spatial and temporal coherence and so has been retained as the main descriptive parameter. The energy function defined to match two nodes is composed of two terms: a data term (based on descriptive parameters and euclidian distance), a regularization term (based on the coordinates of a node, of its neighbours, and of their respective corresponding nodes) which allows to preserve spatio-temporal coherence. A simulated annealing is used to locally minimize the weighted summation of that two energy terms resulting in a global optimization of the correspondences.

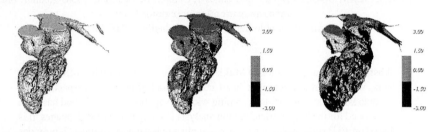

Fig. 1. Surface visualization (left anterior view)   **Fig. 2.** Extracted motion (diastole)   **Fig. 3.** Extracted motion (systole)

This method has been tested with one temporal database acquired by a Siemens SOMATOM PLUS 4 - VZ with ten volumes representing a whole cardiac cycle. The motion extraction process has been applied to two consecutive endocardial surfaces (previously smoothed (cf. Fig.1)) resulting in a set of displacement vectors defined at each surface node. From this 3D velocity field, some descriptive parameters related to cardiac kinetics can be extracted. As illustration, Fig.2 and 3 show the motion amplitude and direction corresponding to the beginning of main cardiac phases (contraction/null or very small/expansion movements are respectively represented with white/grey/black colour). These first results show coherence between motion extracted and physiological information, and highlight the issue of contractile function evaluation.

3   Conclusion

A first solution has been proposed for the 3D motion extraction of the left ventricle in cardiac MSCT images. Our approach is applied on extracted volumes and provides first 3D velocity fields for the left cavity surface. These displacement vectors can represent accurate informations related to contraction and expansion movements. These first results confirm the great potential of MSCT imaging for cardiac applications.

Acknowledgement. This work is supported by Brittany region and the French Medical Research and Health National Institute (INSERM). The authors express their thanks to Siemens, Medical Division, France.

References

1. Frangi *et al.*, 2001, Three-Dimensionnal Modeling for Functionnal Analysis of Cardiac Images: A Review, *IEEE Trans. on Medical Imaging*, 20(1):2-25.
2. Kambhamettu C. *et al.*, 2000, 3D non-rigid motion analysis under small deformations, *Image and Vision Computing*, 21(3):229-245
3. Eusemann *et al.*, 2003, Parametric Visualization Methods for the Quantitative Assesment of Myocardial Motion, *Acad. Radiol.*, 10:66-76
4. Guillaume *et al.*, 2003, Segmentation de cavités cardiaques en imagerie scanner multi-barettes, *12ème Forum des Jeunes Chercheurs en Génie Biologique et Médical*, Nantes, France.

Automatic Assessment of Cardiac Perfusion MRI

Hildur Ólafsdóttir[1], Mikkel B. Stegmann[1,2], and Henrik B.W. Larsson[2,3]

[1] Informatics and Mathematical Modelling, Technical University of Denmark
[2] Danish Research Centre for Magnetic Resonance, H:S Hvidovre Hospital, Denmark
[3] Dept. of Diagnostic Imaging, St. Olavs Hospital, Trondheim University, Norway

Abstract. In this paper, a method based on Active Appearance Models (AAM) is applied for automatic registration of myocardial perfusion MRI. A semi-quantitative perfusion assessment of the registered image sequences is presented. This includes the formation of perfusion maps for three parameters; maximum up-slope, peak and time-to-peak.

1 Introduction

Myocardial perfusion MRI has proven to be a powerful method to assess coronary artery diseases. The ultimate goal of the analysis is to obtain a full quantification of the perfusion in ml/(g·min), see e.g. [3]. A step towards this goal is a semi-quantitative perfusion assessment obtained by generating perfusion maps from a registered sequence of images, see e.g. [4]. This paper presents an automatic registration of multi-slice perfusion sequences and a preliminary clinical validation in terms of perfusion maps.

2 Methods and Results

The data material comprises 500 myocardial perfusion, multi-slice, short-axis, magnetic resonance images (MRI) obtained from ten freely breathing patients with acute myocardial infarction. Each image is composed of four spatial slices. The registration method is based on Active Appearance Models (AAMs) [1]. AAMs establish a compact parameterisation of object variability, as learned from a representative training set. Objects are defined by marking up each training example with points of correspondence, i.e. landmarks. Here, landmark positions are optimised by an MDL approach [2]. Subsequently, AAMs can be registered rapidly to unseen images. Modifications to the standard AAM framework include slice-coupled modelling, sequence priors and clustering of texture vectors. For further details, refer to [5].

Given the per-pixel point correspondences of each slice of the myocardium, a semi-quantitative perfusion assessment is carried out. Signal-intensity (SI) curves (plot of intensity vs. time frame) for each pixel position are generated and from those, three perfusion parameters are derived, the *maximum upslope*, *peak* and *time-to-peak*.

Registration of the perfusion data was carried out in a leave-one-out cross validation. Quantitative comparison to ground-truth (manual) registration showed

C. Barillot, D.R. Haynor, and P. Hellier (Eds.): MICCAI 2004, LNCS 3217, pp. 1060–1061, 2004.
© Springer-Verlag Berlin Heidelberg 2004

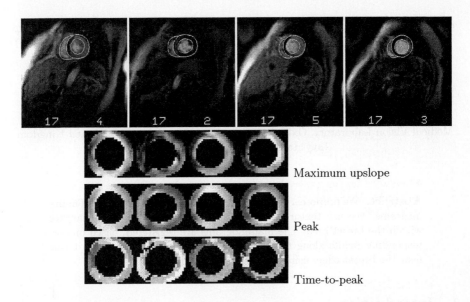

Maximum upslope

Peak

Time-to-peak

Fig. 1. Above: Registration of multi-slice time frame 17 from patient 8 (Slice 1–4 left to right). Below: Perfusion maps for patient 8 generated from the automatic registration.

a mean registration accuracy of 1.25 ± 0.36 pixels in terms of point to curve distance. Qualitative registration results and perfusion maps for patient 8 are given in Figure 1. The figure reveals a severe perfusion deficit at the anteroseptal and inferoseptal wall judged from the original multi-slice frame. This is confirmed by the perfusion maps for all slices for the maximum upslope parameter and slices 1, 3 and 4 for the remaining two parameters. Same regions were identified by the perfusion maps for the ground-truth registration.

Based on the preliminary clinical validation, it is concluded that the automatic registration method holds great promise for the automation of quantitative perfusion examinations.

References

1. T. F. Cootes, G. J. Edwards, and C. J. Taylor. Active appearance models. *IEEE Trans. on Pattern Analysis and Machine Intelligence*, 23(6):681–685, 2001.
2. R. H. Davies, C. J. Twining, T. F. Cootes, J. C. Waterton, and C. J. Taylor. A minimum description length approach to statistical shape modeling. *Medical Imaging, IEEE Transactions on*, 21(5):525–537, 2002.
3. H. B. W. Larsson, T. Fritz-Hansen, E. Rostrup, L. Søndergaard, P. Ring, and O. Henriksen. Myocardial perfusion modeling using MRI. *Magnetic Resonance in Medicine*, 35:716–726, 1996.
4. E. Nagel, N. Al-Saadiand, and E. Fleck. Cardiovascular magnetic resonance: Myocardial perfusion. *Herz*, 25(4):409–416, 2000.
5. M. B. Stegmann, H. Ólafsdóttir, and H. B. W. Larsson. Unsupervised motion-compensation of multi-slice cardiac perfusion MRI. *Invited contribution for the FIMH special issue in Medical Image Analysis*, 2004 (accepted for publication).

Texture Based Mammogram Registration Using Geodesic Interpolating Splines

Styliani Petroudi and Michael Brady

Medical Vision Laboratory, Oxford University, Oxford, OX2 7DD, United Kingdom
{styliani, jmb}@robots.ox.ac.uk

Abstract. We propose a new approach for nonrigid registration of mammograms. We use texture models for the mammographic appearance within the breast area. The mammograms are registered, based on corresponding points along the boundaries of the region of adipose tissue near the breast edge, using geodesic interpolating splines.

1 Introduction

Registration of mammograms is required for analysis of bilateral, temporal, and different view mammograms, and for multi-subject studies. Mammogram registration has proven a difficult problem, not least because of the enormous diversity in the appearance of mammograms. Various classes of image transformations for registration have been investigated, including flow and thin plate splines. Recent progress in the estimation of flows of diffeomorphisms have resulted in the development of geodesic interpolating splines (GIS) [1]. These provide an unambiguous one-to-one correspondence between all points in any pair of images. Registration results can be used to detect changes in the breast tissue that are characteristic of cancer. Most algorithms compare registered image intensities or a representation derived from image intensities, which requires some form of normalization. However, we have shown that it is possible to compute a representation of textures within a mammogram; these are known to be significant in the evaluation of disease.

2 Method and Results

In this paper we propose an approach to matching mammograms which combines texture classes as image descriptors and GIS. Texture classes are used to establish control points for the geodesic warps and to evaluate the outcomes for temporal matching. The preliminary results are very encouraging. Textons are defined as clustered filter responses, where the set of filters used, mirrors a non-parametric representation of Markov Random Fields. First we construct a texton dictionary by processing a large number of segmented mammograms and then aggregating and clustering filter responses using k-means analysis. Given the texton dictionary, each image pixel in the breast region is assigned a label by the texton which lies closest to it in the filter space. A texture based classifier

C. Barillot, D.R. Haynor, and P. Hellier (Eds.): MICCAI 2004, LNCS 3217, pp. 1062–1063, 2004.

segments the image in different tissue types of varying parenchymal density as in Figure 1(d) and (e). One of these classes corresponds to the fatty breast edge which can be consistently observed in all the mammograms. The boundary of the transition from the fatty breast edge to dense tissue, along with the nipple, the axilla and the rib, and other points on the breast boundary provide the control points. After mapping the points in both views onto each other the warped image is obtained by interpolating between the control points using geodesic interpolating splines. The GIS uses, instead of one large step, a succession of small diffeomorphic steps to warp the image [2]. A pair of registered mammograms is shown in Figure 1(a),(b) and (c). To compare the registered mammograms, the warped image is also segmented into the different tissue types, using the presented texture model followed by a texture-based classifier. A region is labelled suspicious if it corresponds to tissue that has evolved to be very dense. We are still developing a more robust system for evaluating the tissue changes. The complete algorithm has so far been applied to 10 pairs of temporal mammograms with excellent results.

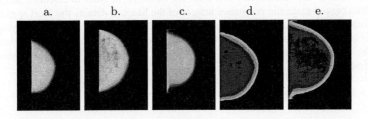

Fig. 1. (a)The mammogram that needs registration. (b)The base mammogram. (c)The geodesically registered mammogram. (d-e)The texture based representation of (a-b) respectively.

3   Conclusions

We have presented an algorithm for nonrigid mammogram registration which investigates the combination of texture models with GIS. The use of texture models provides a reliable framework for establishing correspondences and detecting comparative changes in mammograms. The method overcomes the difficulty arising form the degree of involution in the breast tissue.

References

1. V. Camion and L. Younes. Geodesic interpolating splines. In *Proceedings of EMM-CVPR'01*, volume 2134, pages 513–527, 2001.
2. C. J. Twining and S. Marsland. Constructing diffeomorphic representations of nonrigid registrations of medical images. In *IPMI 2003*, 2003.

Gabor Filter-Based Automated Strain Computation from Tagged MR Images

Tushar Manglik[1], Alexandru Cernicanu[2], Vinay Pai[1], Daniel Kim[1], Ting Chen[1], Pradnya Dugal[1], Bharathi Batchu[1], and Leon Axel[1]

[1] Department of Radiology, New York University, NY, USA
[2] Department of Electrical Engineering, University of Pennsylvania, PA, USA

Abstract. Myocardial tagging is a non-invasive MR imaging technique; it generates a periodic tag pattern in the magnetization that deforms with the tissue during the cardiac cycle. It can be used to assess regional myocardial function, including tissue displacement and strain. Most image analysis methods require labor-intensive tag detection and tracking. We have developed an accurate and automated method for tag detection in order to calculate strain from tagged magnetic resonance images of the heart. It detects the local spatial frequency and phase of the tags using a bank of Gabor filters with varying frequency and phase. This variation in tag frequency is then used to calculate the local myocardial strain. The method is validated using computer simulations.

1 Introduction

Conventional tag analysis techniques, such as finite element and B-spline models, require tag tracking [1-2] that often rely on active contours. The purpose of this study was to develop an automated Gabor filter-based tag analysis method. Previously, Gabor filters have been used for quantifying displacement and to enhance or suppress either the tags or the non-tagged regions of the image [3-5].

2 Methods

In image domain, a set of 2D Gabor filters is used for convolution with tagged image. A two dimensional Gabor filter (Fig. 1) h(x,y) is mathematically defined as

$$h(x,y) = g(x',y').s(x,y) .\tag{1}$$
$$g(x',y') = 1/(2\pi\,\sigma_{x'}\sigma_{y'})exp\,(-\,((x'/\,\sigma_{x'}\,)^2 + (y'/\,\sigma_{y'}\,)^2)/2)\,.\tag{2}$$
$$s(x,y)\ \ = sin(2\pi d/\lambda + \Phi),\ d = x\ cos(\xi) + y\ sin(\xi)\tag{3}$$
$$x' = x\ cos(\theta) + y\ sin(\theta), y' = x\ sin(\theta) + y\ cos(\theta)\tag{4}$$

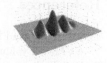

Fig. 1. *2D Gabor filter*

where $\sigma_{x'}$, $\sigma_{y'}$ are the standard deviations of the 2D Gaussian envelope along the x and the y directions, θ is the orientation of the Gaussian envelope, ξ is the orientation of the sinusoid and Φ

C. Barillot, D.R. Haynor, and P. Hellier (Eds.): MICCAI 2004, LNCS 3217, pp. 1064–1066, 2004.

is the phase offset of the sinusoid. The spatial wavelength and phase of the Gabor filter are determined by the wavelength, λ, and phase, $(2\pi d/\lambda + \Phi)$, of the sinusoidal function. The response of each individual filter centered at a given image pixel measures how well the wavelength and phase of the filter match with the spatial tag spacing and phase of the tags in the vicinity of this pixel. For strain calculations, we used a numerically generated annular 2D phantom with superimposed sinusoidal tags as an approximation of a tagged short axis image slice of the human heart (Fig. 2(a)), and applied a radially symmetric deformation with known longitudinal strain, E_{YY}, (Fig. 2(c)) to generate a sequence of nine images that simulates ventricular contraction (Fig. 2(b)). The Gaussian envelope was made eccentric so that it was elongated in a direction θ. The orientation, θ, of the Gaussian envelope and the orientation, ξ, of the sinusoid were set normal to the direction of the tags. The longitudinal strain in y-direction in each of these images was computed at every pixel as

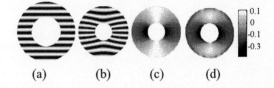

(a)   (b)   (c)   (d)

$$E_{YY} = (\ \Delta L / L). \qquad (5)$$

where L is the original tag spacing and ΔL is change in tag spacing (as detected by Gabor filter)

Fig. 2. (a) 2D numerical phantom (b) the phantom after a series of radial contractions (c) known longitudinal strain E_{YY} applied to simulate these ventricular contractions (d) strain calculated from Gabor filter-observed tag spacing

3 Results and Discussion

We calculated the percentage error and the standard deviation in Gabor filter-observed tag spacing (Fig. 3) for the phantom deformation sequence. This error was observed to be less than 5%. In this study we have demonstrated that Gabor filter-based detection of tag spacing and phase allows us to locally analyze the tag pattern in simulated tagged MRI. The study indicates that this technique may be useful for fast and automated strain calculations. Future work will apply this technique to analyze *in-vivo* cardiac images.

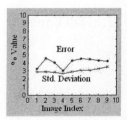

Fig. 3. *Error and std. deviations* in the Gabor filter-observed tag spacing values

References

[1] Young, A., Axel, L.: Three-dimensional motion and deformation of the heart wall: Estimation with spatial modulation of magnetization - A model based approach. Radiology, 185 (1992) 241-247

[2] Chen, Y., Amini., A.: A MAP Framework for tag line detection in SPAMM data using Markov random fields on the B-spline solid. IEEE Tran. Md. Img. 21(9) (2002 Sep) 1110-22

[3] Qian Z., Montillo, A., Metaxas, D., Axel, L.: Segmenting cardiac MRI tagging lines using Gabor filter banks. Proc. of 25th Anl. Intl. Conf. of the IEEE EMBS (2003 Sep), 630-633

[4] Montillo, A., Axel, L., Metaxas, D.: Extracting tissue deformation using Gabor filter banks. Proc. of SPIE, Vol. 5369 (2004) pp.1 -9

[5] Manglik, T., Axel, L., Pai, V. M., Kim, D., Dugal, P., Montillo, A., Zhen, Q.: Use of bandpass Gabor filters for enhancing blood-myocardium contrast and filling-in tags in tagged MR images. Proc. Intl. Soc. Mag. Reson. Med. 11 (2004) 1793

Non-invasive Derivation of 3D Systolic Nonlinear Wall Stress in a Biventricular Model from Tagged MRI

Aichi Chien[1], J. Paul Finn[2], and Carlo D. Montemagno[1]

[1] Dept. of Biomedical Engineering, University of California Los Angeles, CA 90095, USA
aichi@seas.ucla.edu
[2] Dept. of Radiological Sciences, University of California, Los Angeles, CA 90095, USA

Abstract. We present a nonlinear finite element method to calculate the local myocardial wall stress in a reconstructed biventricular MRI model. Nonlinear formulations are utilized in order to describe the ventricular large deformation. Using incremental force computation, a dynamic model showing the change of myocardium wall stress during systolic contraction was established. The preliminary results show that in the normal human heart the local stress increases by a factor of 10^4 from the end of diastole to the end of systole. Furthermore, during the systolic process the left ventricle develops three times more inner wall stress than the right ventricle, and the peak inner wall stress areas in both ventricles are located at the apex.

1 Introduction

To gain insight into the mechanisms of heart failure, it is necessary to elucidate the dynamic forces generated by the ventricles. Abnormal heart wall stress (WS) is known to be an important factor leading to cardiac dysfunction. Evidence for this is that regional ventricular remodeling is closely related to ventricular stress [1]. The goal of this paper is to present a nonlinear finite element (FE) model based on tagged MRI to calculate the 3D WS and provide information necessary to better understand the mechanisms of cardiac dysfunction. We believe this is the first attempt to solve human biventricular WS using a nonlinear large deformation formulation in a gross model. The benefit of this method is that it avoids the breakdown of linear theory which usually happens when the strain is larger than 10% — the type of deformation typical in cardiac contraction [2].

2 Method and Results

A 3D biventricular gross model representing normal heart geometry was constructed based on published MRI data [2]. Then, using the FE program COSMOS, we divided the gross model into 29,136 tetrahedral mesh elements. The formulations included nonlinear myocardium material properties with large deformation equations [3]. Furthermore, we defined five time intervals in a 450 msec contraction process and as-

C. Barillot, D.R. Haynor, and P. Hellier (Eds.): MICCAI 2004, LNCS 3217, pp. 1067–1068, 2004.
© Springer-Verlag Berlin Heidelberg 2004

signed incremental force on these intervals. The force representing blood resistance and the torsion/contraction force were both considered in our simulation. The total number of equations was 1,359,105 and the overall calculation time was 24,998 sec.

The ventricular local stress changes in systole show that the stress increases as the ventricles contract (Fig.1). The WS, on average, increases by a factor of 10^4 during the contraction. A nonuniform stress distribution is observed which suggests pumping efficiency may drop if the muscle in this high stress area develops defects. The calculation also indicates that the left ventricle (LV) has three times higher inner WS compared to the right ventricle (RV) and that the maximum local stress of 1.6356×10^5 Pa occurs in the apex of the LV. This high stress area is more likely to change the myocardium elasticity and may explain that infarction expansion tends to occur more frequently among patients with infractions involving the apex of the ventricles [4]. Comparing the calculated inner and outer ventricular WS, the results show that inner ventricular WS increases more during the contraction. It may suggest that myocardium contractive force is mainly produced by the inner region of the ventricular wall.

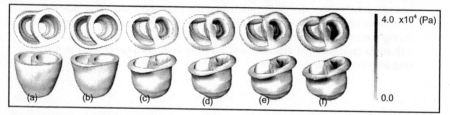

Fig. 1. 3D stress distribution on ventricles from the end of diastole (a) to the end of systole (f).

3 Conclusion

The model presented here uses 3D MRI to reconstruct the ventricular geometry, coupled with nonlinear FE methods. Preliminary results show the stress distribution in the normal heart contraction, providing unique insight into cardiac function in an entirely non-invasive way. However, a more accurate stress calculation will require correct data for the material properties of the myocardium *in-vivo*. Further material formulation and clinical model validation are currently in progress.

References

1. Grossman, W., Jones, D. & McLaurin, L.P. Wall stress and patterns of hypertrophy in the human left ventricle. J Clin Invest 56, 56-64 (1975).
2. Haber, I., Metaxas, D.N. & Axel, L. Three-dimensional motion reconstruction and analysis of the right ventricle using tagged MRI. Med Image Anal 4, 335-55 (2000).
3. Hunter, P.J., McCulloch, A.D. & ter Keurs, H.E. Modelling the mechanical properties of cardiac muscle. Prog Biophys Mol Biol 69, 289-331 (1998).
4. Pfeffer, M.A. Left ventricular remodeling after acute myocardial infarction. Annu Rev Med 46, 455-66 (1995).

MRI Compatible Modular Designed Robot
for Interventional Navigation
– Prototype Development and Evaluation –

Hiroaki Naganou[1], Hiroshi Iseki[2], and Ken Masamune[1]

[1]Tokyo Denki University, Ishizaka, Hatoyama-cho, Hiki, Saitama
[2]Tokyo Women's Medical University, Kawada-cho8-1, Shinjyuku-ku ,Tokyo

Abstract. Interventional MRI therapy has started in these years, and many researchers are focusing on surgical robots operated under the MRI environment to achieve most effective image guided surgery. In this paper, the prototype development of MRI compatible modular-designed navigation robot is proposed as the basic components of the future MRI-guided robot surgery. System features and the evaluation testing are described

1 Introduction

The surgical procedures that perform drilling such as a biopsy or inject drugs, requires accurate positioning, and in case of interventional MRI therapy, engineering technologies are considered useful to give surgeon precise orientation information to reach to the target tumor more precisely [1]. In this research, we proposed and developed the prototype of simple two D.O.F. robot for needle guidance surgery, that characteristics are followings: intended to use inside the MRI gantry, modular design for apply many kinds of surgical procedure, well-consideration of sterilization, considering usability with 2DOF active arm and 14 DOF passive arm which materials are MRI-compatible. We describe the design strategy, and the evaluation testing of the image distortion caused by the robot.

2 Description of the Robot Design

To support navigation surgery, we decided to give only two DOF, that are indispensable for drilling. The robot performs only positioning of an angle, and compensate surgeon's hand tremor. The developed robot is shown in a Fig.1. The robot is composed of a linear actuator and a rotary actuator. It has two arms and small free joints on the arms' tip for guiding a needle. A surgeon locates the arm 1 at the insertion point, then the insertion angle is fixed by arm 2 which is moved by the actuators. Finally, the surgeon punctures the needle by himself. A cleanliness of the mechatronics part can be maintained by sterilization cover sheet. Instead of using a ferromagnetic metal, we adopted the non-ferro magnetic metal, the reinforced plastic, and the synthetic resin. The ultrasonic motor (Shinsei Kogyo, Japan) was adopted as an actuator.

C. Barillot, D.R. Haynor, and P. Hellier (Eds.): MICCAI 2004, LNCS 3217, pp. 1069–1070, 2004.

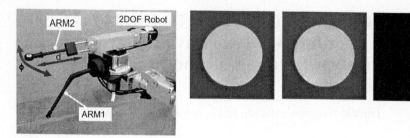

Fig. 1. MRI compatible modular designed robot for interventional navigation

Fig. 2. From left to right: MR-image when nstalling robot, Control image, Subtraction image

3   Experiments, Results, and Discussion

Mechanical accuracy evaluation : Backlash, positioning accuracy and repeatability are measured subject to JIS standard method. The backlash was 0.37[mm], the positioning accuracy 0.14 [mm], and the repeatability ±0.085[mm]. Evaluation about a rotation mechanism has not been carried out.

Image distortion study : To evaluate the influence of the navigation robot installed into MR gantry, we evaluated the image distortion with the cylindrical phantom filled with MR-enhance solution, which is used for the initial set-up calibration of the MRI system. We calculated the subtraction image to evaluate noise caused by the manipulator. The subtraction image was calculated from the image with a robot, and the image without installation (Fig. 2.).

Discussion: Considering the MR image resolution of 1mm, the results of mechanical accuracy was enough as the surgical robot for needle guidance surgery. We calculated the Signal-to-Noise ratio (It defines as the ratio of average of pixel intensity of ROI and standard deviation of the noise area) of an images, in order to evaluate the noise caused by the navigation robot. S/N ration of MR-image when installing robot is 108.65. S/N ration of Control image is 153.21. From here onwards, we can evaluate the quality of image which is debased by installed robot.

4   Conclusion

In this study, 2-DOF MRI compatible modular designed navigation robot is proposed and the fundamental evaluations are performed. This robot will be useful for the MRI image guided therapy performed inside the MRI gantry in the future.

References

1.   K Masamune, et al.: Development of an MRI compatible Needle Insertion Manipulator for Stereotactic Neurosurgery, J Image Guided Surgery, Vol.1, pp.242-248, 1995

A Model for Some Subcortical DTI Planar and Linear Anisotropy

Song Zhang and David Laidlaw

Brown University, Providence, RI 02912, USA

1 Introduction

Linear anisotropy, planar anisotropy and isotropy [1] are used as metrics for different kinds of diffusion in diffusion imaging. While linear anisotropy is reported to correlate to coherent neural fiber structures, the cause for planar anisotropy remains ambiguous. We hypothesize that overlapping linear structures and partial-volume averaging generate the planar anisotropy. We identify a subcortical region containing both linear and planar anisotropy in a human volumetric diffusion tensor image (DTI), propose a model of the anatomy and of the imaging process, and calculate simulated diffusion images of the anatomical model that qualitatively agree with the human DTI. Regions of planar anisotropy are common immediately beneath the cortex. Choosing one such region as representative, we model the anatomy with isotropic regions and linearly anisotropic structures. From the possibly overlapping model structures we simulate the diffusion imaging process, generating a series of diffusion weighted images (DWIs) of the anatomical structures. We then fit the DTI from these simulated DWIs and visualize it. The visualization agrees qualitatively with the visualization of a subcortical human DTI.

2 Method

We first identified an immediately subcortical region in the most superior part of the brain just adjacent to the interhemispheric fissure. Figure 1 shows a visualization of the white-matter structures in the region. The red streamtubes run along the direction of fastest diffusion in regions of linear anisotropy; the green surfaces show regions of planar anisotropy [2]. Our anatomical model comprises isotropic structures and linear structures. We represent isotropic regions like gray matter and fluid with isotropic diffusion tensors, and model linear structures with a cubic B-spline curve and a constant circular cross section. We then simulate DWIs from this anatomical model. In the simulation, we use isotropic tensors to represent isotropic structures; we use linear diffusion tensors whose major eigenvectors align with the tangent of the curve to represent linear structures. We generate DWIs from the anatomical model based on the relationship between the echo intensity and diffusion tensor given in [3].

To simulate the partial-volume effect, we supersample our anatomical model and then average the echo intensity over all the subsamples within one voxel.

C. Barillot, D.R. Haynor, and P. Hellier (Eds.): MICCAI 2004, LNCS 3217, pp. 1071–1073, 2004.

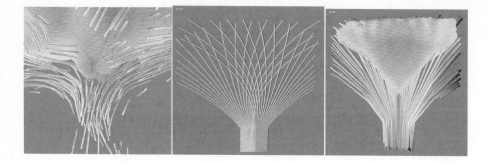

Fig. 1. In a subcortical region, complicated anisotropy patterns result in discontinuous fiber pathways. The dimensions of this feature are about 8 × 9 × 3 mm. Image resolution is 1.70 mm isotropic

Fig. 2. We specify a qualitative model (shown here in 2D) with crossing fiber structures to represent the anatomy in Figure 1.

Fig. 3. A visualization of the DTI/DWIs generated from the anatomical model in Figure 2. Note that the planar anisotropy in the middle forms a pattern similar to Figure 1.

We constructed the phantom model shown in Figure 2 to be analogous to the region shown in Figure 1. We use the same visualization method that helped us identify the subcortical region of anisotropy to visually analyze our synthetic images.

3   Results and Discussion

Figure 1 shows a small subcortical region in which fibers emerge from the bottom, then splay out and cross each other, creating the planar anisotropy in the middle of the figure. Figure 2 shows our anatomical model. After synthesizing 25 DWIs (12 directions with b values of 500 and 1000 and a non-weighted diffusion image) from the model and fitting the DWIs to create a DTI, we visualize the DTI as in Figure 3. Note that the partial-volume effect in the region of crossing fibers creates planar anisotropy similar to that in Figure 1. The various crossing patterns and fiber densities result in various planar anisotropies, reflected by the different shades of green in the results. We also found that the streamtubes in the crossing area lie between the two crossing fibers. The result supports our hypothesis that overlapping structures and partial-volume averaging generate the planar anisotropy and also bias the direction of fastest diffusion in some regions of linear anisotropy away from the underlying fiber direction. Compensating for these distortions may be important in synthesizing accurate quantitative DTI analyses.

Acknowledgments. Support from NSF CCR-0086065, the Human Brain Project (NIBIB and NIMH), NIMH, Alzheimer's Assoc, and the Ittleson Fund at Brown.

References

[1] Westin et al. ISMRM97
[2] Zhang et al. IEEE TVCG. 9:454-462(2003)
[3] Basser et al. J. Magn. Reson. B 103:247-254(1994)

A 3D Model of the Human Lung

Tatjana Zrimec[1,2], Sata Busayarat[2], and Peter Wilson[3]

[1] Centre for Health Informatics
[2] School of Computer Science and Engineering
University of New South Wales
Sydney 2052, Australia
{tatjana,satab}@cse.unsw.edu.au
[3] Pittwater Radiology
Sydney, Australia

Abstract. This paper presents a method for modelling human lungs using knowledge of lung anatomy and High Resolution CT images. The model consists of a symbolic anatomical structure map and an annotated 3D atlas. The model is implemented using Frame structures. Frames provide a good platform for the comprehensive description of anatomical features and for enabling communication between the image data and the symbolic knowledge. A few important landmarks have been determined and used to divide the lung into clinically meaningful regions, which enable accurate mapping of the model to patient data.

1 Introduction

A 3D model of the human lung is used in an image understanding system for interpreting HRCT images. The model consists of a qualitative component - a semantic model of lung anatomy and a quantitative component - a 3D atlas. From a set of segmented axial 2D images, a 3D model of the lung is constructed for easy visualization and manipulation (See Fig 1). Relationships among objects in the 3D model are represented using a spatial coordinate system. Our approach differs from the approach proposed in [1] in that we are developing a complete lung model that includes also anatomical information.

2 Modelling and Representation

An anatomical model should have the ability to encode the shape of anatomical features and to include normal cases and variations [2]. To assist image processing, a model should include knowledge at both the image level and the anatomical level. Consequently, the knowledge includes descriptions of anatomical components and the relations between them. At the image level, the knowledge includes information about the expected appearance of an anatomical feature in an image. We use a Frame

C. Barillot, D.R. Haynor, and P. Hellier (Eds.): MICCAI 2004, LNCS 3217, pp. 1074–1075, 2004.

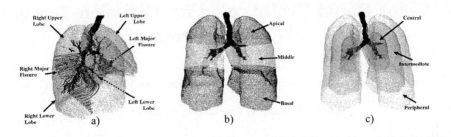

Fig. 1. (a) Lung lobes; Regions: (b) Apex, Medial, Basal; (c) Central, Intermediate, Peripheral.

representation to implement the model, since Frames allow easy representation of the hierarchical structures that are found in the human anatomy [2]. The model includes appearances of the modelled structures from different views. The following Frame types represent the domain knowledge:

Anatomy frame – stores anatomical information about the properties and organization of the lungs and surrounding anatomical structures (for example, spine, lungs, mediastinum).

Structure frame – stores information of the lung structure and lung division: Left lung, Right lung; lung lobes, see Fig. 1. a, and subdivisions down to a particular Bronchopulmonary Segment.

Spatial frame – stores 3D spatial organization and spatial relations of the lung features (apex, hilum, base, borders and surfaces (see Fig. 1. b, c).

View frame - Volume and *2D* - contains a description of a set of axial images as produced by HRCT, and a set of images as produced by X-ray.

Pathology frame - contains knowledge of diseases patters, their expected location and distribution in the lungs.

Currently, we have developed a model of the lung with a 3D lung atlas using a set HRCT volume data from eight cases with 300 to 400 images per study. The lungs were segmented automatically using "Active contour" snakes and morphological operator. Segmented fissures enable division of the lung model into lobes (See Fig. 1. a). A few important landmarks in HRCT images: trachea, sternum, vertebrae, spinal canal, Carina and hilum were segmented automatically and used for lung division into clinically meaningful regions: Apex, Medial, and Base (see Fig. 1. b), Central, Intermediate and Peripheral (see Fig. 1. c). The model facilitates image interpretation and evaluation of the methods for automatic feature segmentation.

References

1. Li, B., Christensen, E.G., Hoffman, E.A., et.al.: Establishing a Normative Atlas of the Human Lung: Intersubject Warping and Registration of Volumetric CT Images, *Acad Radiol,* **10** (2003) 255–265
2. Zrimec, T., Sammut, C. "A Medical Image Understanding System", *Engineering applications of Artificial Intelligence* **10** (1) (1997) 31-39

Color Rapid Prototyping for Diffusion-Tensor MRI Visualization

Daniel Acevedo, Song Zhang, David H. Laidlaw, and Christopher W. Bull

Brown University, Providence, RI 02912, USA

We describe work toward creating color rapid prototyping (RP) plaster models as visualization tools to support scientific research in diffusion-tensor (DT) MRI analysis. We currently give surgeons and neurologists virtual-reality (VR) applications to visualize different aspects of their brain data, but having physical representations of those virtual models allows them to review the data with a very robust, natural, and fast haptic interface: their own hands. Our initial results are encouraging, and end users are excited about the possibilities of this technique. For example, using these models in conjunction with digital models on the computer screen or VR environment provides a static frame of reference that helps keep users oriented during their analysis tasks.

RP has been used in visualization largely for building molecular models to test assembly possibilities [1]. Nadeau et al. [4] created models of the human brain surface with the same RP techniques we use. Our approach, however, enables us to build inner brain structures.

1   Method

We examine the geometric models generated from a DTI dataset using tractography [5,2,6]. In our models, red streamtubes represent the diffusion in regions of linear anisotropy, where water diffuses primarily in one direction [6]. The streamtube direction represents the principal direction of diffusion along the tube. Studies show a correlation between the structures of neural fibers in white matter and the tracts derived from the principal direction of diffusion in linear

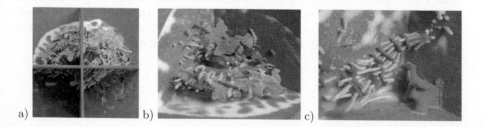

Fig. 1. (a,b) A plaster model showing areas of linear and planar water self-diffusion obtained from DT-MR images. (c) Detail of support structures (dark gray surfaces around tubes) for the streamtubes; these surfaces are created using the second and third eigenvectors of the tensors that produce the tubes.

C. Barillot, D.R. Haynor, and P. Hellier (Eds.): MICCAI 2004, LNCS 3217, pp. 1076–1078, 2004.
© Springer-Verlag Berlin Heidelberg 2004

anisotropy regions [3]. Green streamsurfaces are generated in regions of planar anisotropy, where water diffuses primarily in a small plane at any given point. These planar structures could result from crossing fibers or laminar structures [6]. In addition to tubes and surfaces, we show anatomical features for context: blue surfaces show ventricles, and the images on the three orthogonal planes show slices of T2-weighted images collected with DTI.

To create our color models we use Z-Corp's Z406 printer. The digital model, in VRML format, is subdivided into horizontal layers by the printer software. These layers are then manufactured by putting down a thin layer of plaster powder and dropping colored binder at the boundaries of the model at that level. Once all the layers are built, the powder outside the boundaries of the model is vacuumed out and loose powder is removed using a fine blower. Finally, the piece is bathed in hot wax to strengthen it and enhance its colors.

The structures in the DT-MRI models require very careful treatment. Because the long thin streamtubes often fail to support themselves during powder removal, we inserted some supporting surfaces that interconnect neighboring streamtubes without occluding interesting features. These supports are created from the second and third eigenvectors of the diffusion tensor that creates the streamtubes, so they are perpendicular by definition (see Figure 1(c)). We arrived at this methodology after several tests, including building thicker tubes and increasing their number so they supported one another. Using information already present in the DT-MRI data, we have been able to create models with better structural stability.

2   Results and Conclusions

These early stages of development have highlighted some important issues. For example, our visualizations involve organic, free-form shapes, whereas current RP technology is designed for models with more regular shapes, such as mechanical parts and molecular models. Also, the printing and cleaning process can take as much as 12 hours for complicated brain models measuring up to $8'' \times 8'' \times 10''$. However, our initial experiments suggest that this technology has the great advantage of exploiting users' familiarity with physical models: they recognize the utility of holding them in their hands when studying them. Providing scientists with these models enhances the use and analysis of their digital counterparts. To quote one of the doctors who experimented with these models: *"These physical models complement displays in digital format by providing a hard-copy frame of reference that can be touched and manipulated with optimum hand-eye coordination and immediate results."* We believe this type of physical model can be very useful in preoperative planning when used as a quick reference for structure identification.

Acknowledgments. DT-MRI data provided by Dr. Susumu Mori (Johns Hopkins U.) Support from NSF (CCR-0086065, CCR-0093238) and Human Brain Project (NIDA, NIMH).

References

1. M.J. Bailey et al. Curr. Op. Str. Bio., 8(2), 1998.
2. P.J. Basser et al. MR in Medicine, 44:625-632, 2000.
3. E.W. Hsu et al. Am. J. Physiol, 274, 1998.
4. D.R. Nadeau et al. IEEE Visualization 2000.
5. R. Xue et al. MR in Medicine, 42:1123-1127, 1999.
6. S. Zhang et al. IEEE TVCG, 9(4), 2003.

Process of Interpretation of Two-Dimensional Densitometry Images for the Prediction of Bone Mechanical Strength

Laurent Pothuaud

INSERM, University Victor Segalen, Bordeaux, France
Pothuaud@aol.com

1 Introduction

The *in vivo* evaluation of Trabecular Bone Structure (TBS) is a major challenge in bone study. The modern definition of osteoporosis involves low Bone Mineral Density (BMD) and TBS alterations. BMD is well measured in clinical practice by DEXA (Double Energy X-ray Absorptiometry). On the other hand, TBS cannot be measured in routine at the present time. The aim of the present process is to exploit the increased quality of DEXA bone images in order to characterize the gray level properties of such bone projection images and to evaluate a parameter TBS by considerations of projection effects. Moreover, a mathematical model is proposed that allows to evaluate a combined parameter BDS (Bone Density Structure).

2 *In Vitro* Validation

In a preliminary *in vitro* study, it has been showed the potential of the new parameter BDS for the prediction of the ultimate constraint of bone (Cu).

3 Preliminary Results in Normal Postmenopausal Women

The aim of this preliminary clinical study was to evaluate the changes in TBS and BDS parameters in two BMD matched groups with significant age difference. Two groups of 12 subjects each (G_Y and G_O) were constituted with mean age of 54.9+/-7.7 years (G_Y) and 70.1+/-6.6 years (G_O), while neck-BMD was matched for the two groups: 0.647+/-0.072 (G_Y) and 0.646+/-0.071 (G_O). Significant differences were obtained between the two groups for both TBS and BDS parameters, with: TBS=0.631+/-0.079 (G_Y) versus TBS=0.798+/-0.055 (G_O), $p<0.0001$ (t-test); BDS=0.222+/-0.022 (G_Y) versus BDS=0.190+/-0.036 (G_O), $p=0.015$ (t-test). These differences, in accordance with the exponential model, showed that with BMD constant an increase of TBS was associated with a decrease of BDS (aimed to predict the mechanical strength of bone). This result was in agreement with the fact that the older

C. Barillot, D.R. Haynor, and P. Hellier (Eds.): MICCAI 2004, LNCS 3217, pp. 1079–1080, 2004.
© Springer-Verlag Berlin Heidelberg 2004

group (G_O) would be less strong than the younger one (G_Y), although their bone mineral densities (BMD) were identical.

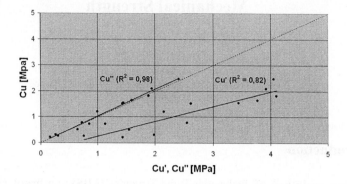

Fig. 1. The parameter BMD makes it possible to explain a relatively great part of the ultimate constraint (Cu). The linear model - Cu'=a_0+a_1*BMD – allows to explain approximately 82% of the variations of Cu – experimental results obtained from a set of 13 trabecular bone samples. This relationship is however limited by the fact that various samples with very close densities can have different mechanical properties, just as control and osteoporotic subjects can have very close values of BMD. The exponential model - Cu"=BDS=b_0+b_1*exp(b_2*BMD)*TBS – makes it possible to increase the accuracy of the prediction of Cu explaining up to 98% of its variations.

4 Discussion

In this preliminary study, it has been firstly demonstrated the technical feasibility to evaluate a new parameter TBS directly from DEXA bone images. Furthermore, it has been showed the potential interest of the new proposed method of interpretation (BDS) to evaluate, more accurately than BMD alone, the quality of bone. This is a very new and original approach that does not necessitate supplementary exam for patient in benefiting from a well-standardized and well-reproducible imaging technique. This approach can be exploited in retrospective study as well. At present, only BMD is used to quantify the quality of bone. The prevention strategy then consists to compare the BMD value of a subject to two "age-matched" and "young normals" standards, giving a comparative indication on the remained amount of bone and on the kinetics of bone loss respectively. Nevertheless, it is well recognized that BMD alone is not sufficient to accurately predict the risk of fracture in individual subject. Further investigations, aimed to establish normative references of TBS and BDS in larger normal women population are in progress. Such normative references would permit to define more reliable risk factor to increase the prevention strategy of osteoporotic fractures.

Transient MR Elastography: Modeling Traumatic Brain Injury

Paul McCracken, Armando Manduca, Joel P. Felmlee, and Richard L. Ehman

MRI Research Lab, Mayo Clinic and Foundation, Rochester, MN 55905, USA
mccracken.paul@mayo.edu

Abstract. Current theory holds that the mechanisms by which head trauma causes hemorrhage, cerebral contusions and diffuse axonal injury result from angular acceleration and its resulting shear motion. We have developed a method for phase contrast MR imaging of small amplitude transient shear displacements as they traverse through the brain *in vivo*. This technique was successfully implemented and preliminary results suggest that it has promise as a tool for studying the underlying biomechanics of brain trauma and for detailed analysis of injury mechanism models.

1 Introduction

More than 1.5 million people sustain a traumatic brain injury each year in the United States, at a treatment cost of over $4 billion [1]. Since 1943, it has been theorized that angular acceleration, rotational forces, and the resulting propagating shear waves are the predominant mechanism causing diffuse axonal injury [2]. However, there are no existing methods to non-destructively test this theory on an *in vivo* human brain. The existing research has ranged from destructive experimental animal and cadaver models, to advanced mathematical models and finite-element simulations [3]. There still exists little data about how the human brain actually reacts during impact.

Magnetic Resonance Elastography is a technique that non-invasively measures displacements from propagating shear waves [5]. This technique typically uses applied harmonic motion and has been used to study breast, prostate and skeletal muscle *in vivo*. More recently, the idea of using a mechanical transient impulse as the excitation for MR elastography was introduced [6]. Using transient elastography, the goals of this work were to measure *in vivo* brain displacements resulting from a small amplitude impact, determine the displacement pattern or path of the particles during and immediately after impact, and calculate the resulting shear strains within the brain.

2 Methods and Results

All experiments were run on a 1.5 T GE Signa MRI scanner (GE Medical Systems, Milwaukee, WI). We applied a low amplitude rotational mechanical shear transient of 5 msec duration to the heads of volunteers by means of an electromechanical driver coupled to a bite bar. This generated shear transients in the brain with a maximum

C. Barillot, D.R. Haynor, and P. Hellier (Eds.): MICCAI 2004, LNCS 3217, pp. 1081–1082, 2004.

displacement of approximately 40 microns. We performed phase contrast imaging using a gradient echo sequence with additional motion encoding gradients to detect and measure the shear wave propagation. The experiment measured displacements every 4 msec for a 60 msec time period at MR pixel resolution (~1 mm). Measurements of 1-2 micron displacements are readily achievable, and the technique can in principle measure all three components of displacement in 3D space over time. From the measured displacements, the strain tensor can be calculated, and from it the principal strains and the maximum shear strain and maximum shear angle at each point in space and time can be derived. The maximum shear strain is a quantity of interest in the literature that is hypothesized to indicate possible regions of injury.

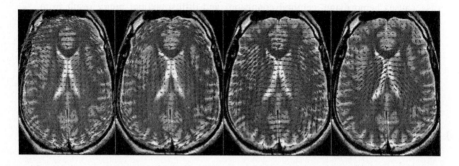

Fig. 1. Measured 2D displacement field at 4 points in time after initial counter-clockwise rotation (left) and clockwise restoring rotation (second image) mapped onto an anatomical image. The largest arrows represent approximately 40 micron displacements.

Future work includes (1) the validation of transient MR measurements of displacement in phantoms in which the displacement can be simultaneously measured with other techniques such as laser vibrometry, (2) the use of such transient data to refine and test existing finite element and biomechanical models of the brain, and (3) the exploration of what quantities are most predictive of actual location and severity of brain injury. The results suggest that it may be possible to use transient wave imaging to directly study the biomechanics of head trauma using *in vivo* models.

References

1. Sosin, D.M., et al.: Incidence of mild and moderate brain injury in the United States, 1991. Brain Injury (1996) 10:47-54.
2. Holbourn, A.H.S.: Mechanics of head injuries. The Lancet (1943). ii: p. 438-441.
3. Muthupillai, R., Lomas, D.J., Rossman, P.J., Greenleaf, J.F., Manduca, A., Ehman, R.L.: Magnetic Resonance Elastography by Direct Visualization of Propagating Acoustic Strain Waves. Science 269 (1995) 1854–1857.
4. Ruan, J.S., et al.: Dynamic response of the human head to impact by three-dimensional finite element analysis. Journal of Biomechanical Engineering, 1994, 116:44-50.
5. McCracken, P.J., et al.: Mechanical Transient-Based MR Elastography. Proc. ISMRM2002.

Study on Evaluation Indexes of Surgical Manipulations with a Stereoscopic Endoscope

Yasushi Yamauchi [1] and Kazuhiko Shinohara [2]

[1] Surgical Assist Technology Group, National Institute of Advanced Industrial Science and Technology (AIST), AIST Tsukuba Central 6, 1-1-1 Higashi, Tsukuba 305-8566, Japan
y.yamauchi@aist.go.jp, http://staff.aist.go.jp/y.yamauchi/
[2] School of Bionics, Tokyo University of Technology,
1404 Katakura, Hachioji, Tokyo 192-0982, Japan
fwpa6707@mb.infoweb.ne.jp

Abstract. We compared stereoscopic displays (3D) with monocular displays (2D) by experimenting on the manipulation of forceps with a laparoscope. The task consisted of repetitive movements of the tip of the forceps under both conditions to targets. Time for manipulation with a 3D display was significantly shorter than for a 2D display. Little significant difference was observed for the psychological indexes.

1 Introduction

For medical stereoscopic imaging, the usefulness of the presentation of depth information and the issues of fatigue have been discussed. The report on an endoscopic trainer [1] revealed a remarkable improvement in the accuracy of forceps manipulation by a stereoscopic endoscope than a monocular endoscope. Clinical findings on cholecystectomy [2], however, revealed no difference in performance between them.

This study attempted to measure and to evaluate surgical manipulations performed by using a stereoscopic endoscope. Evaluation indexes consisted of a physical index (task execution time) and psychological indexes on depth perception.

2 Methods

We used a stereoscopic laparoscope (SK-1057-3D-A, Shinko Optical, Japan) and a forceps (5-mm EndoGrasp, AutoSuture). Stereoscopic (3D) images were presented in a 120-Hz time-sharing display system and a polarized glasses. The system was also capable of providing 2D images by presenting the left (or right) images to both eyes.

24 subjects were asked to move a conductive rubber chip fixed on the end of the forceps. Ten numbered holes were randomly drilled on the surface of a curved pegboard (Fig. 1) placed inside a laparoscope trainer (Limbs & Things). A target number was randomly displayed on a PC screen and the subject was required to insert the chip

C. Barillot, D.R. Haynor, and P. Hellier (Eds.): MICCAI 2004, LNCS 3217, pp. 1083–1084, 2004.
© Springer-Verlag Berlin Heidelberg 2004

into the hole of the corresponding number. This procedure was repeated for five minutes in both 2D/3D displays. The subject was not told which was being presented ('blind test').

For measurement of the psychological indexes, a questionnaire was conducted after the experiment, including a question of fatigue and the order of 2D/3D displays.

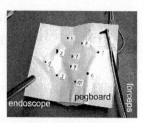

Fig. 1. Pegboard

3   Results and Discussion

As a performance index (Table 1), the ratio of the average time required in the first trial to the time in the second trial to manipulate the forceps was used. In Group B, the time for manipulation with a 3D display was shorter than for a 2D display. In contrast, Group A showed no statistically significant difference between two trials. This is probably because the subjects in Group A improved their manipulation performance by observing a 3D display to such an extent as to compensate for the learning effect.

Table 2 shows the results of the questionnaire investigation. Only in "Fatigue," significance was found, but the difference was small. 9 of the 24 subjects were not able to correctly discern a 3D image from a 2D image.

Table 1. Results on performance index

Group (trial order)	# of subjects	Avg. time per procedure (ratio)	
A (3D before 2D)	11	$2D/3D = 0.88 \pm 0.19$	$p > 0.10$
B (2D before 3D)	13	$3D/2D = 0.69 \pm 0.17$	$p < 0.01$

Table 2. Questions and results on psychological indexes

Questions (4:very strong 1:none)	3D	2D	
Did you have a sense of depth?	3.0	2.5	$p > 0.05$
Did you have a feeling similar to motion sickness?	1.2	1.1	$p > 0.05$
Did you have eye fatigue?	1.7	1.5	$p < 0.05$
Which of the two trials involved 3D image presentation?	15	5	(# of 24)

References

1. Taffinder, N., et al.: The effect of a second-generation 3D endoscope on the laparoscopic precision of novices and experienced surgeons. Surg Endosc 13 (1999) 1087-1092
2. Hanna, G.B., et al.: Randomised study of influence of two-dimensional versus three-dimensional imaging on performance of laparoscopic cholecystectomy. Lancet 351 (1998) 248-251

A Modular Scalable Approach to Occlusion-Robust Low-Latency Optical Tracking

Andreas Köpfle[1], Markus Schill[2], Markus Schwarz[3],
Peter Pott[3], Achim Wagner[4], Reinhard Männer[1], Essameddin Badreddin[4],
Hans-Peter Weiser[5], and Hanns-Peter Scharf[3]

[1] Institute of Computer Science V, University of Mannheim, Germany
[2] VRmagic GmbH, Mannheim, Germany
[3] Department of Orthopedic Surgery, University Clinic of Mannheim, Germany
[4] Automation Laboratory, University of Mannheim, Germany
[5] Institute for CAE, University of Applied Sciences, Mannheim, Germany

Abstract. An advanced optical tracking system for computer assisted surgery (CAS) is presented. The system supports an arbitrary number of cameras that may be placed at suitable positions e.g. fixed cameras at the ceiling of the operating theater or movable cameras on the operating lamps. The modular scalable system architecture reduces occlusion problems and allows adaptation to tracking scenarios of different complexity. The camera modules each integrate hardware-based image processing to allow for low latency of 10ms required in demanding applications like robot control. As a first application tracking of a handheld robotic manipulator has been implemented.

1 Introduction

The usage of navigation systems in image guided surgery aims at supporting the surgeon, enhancing his or her capabilities, without negative influences to the work flow during operation. This goal is only partly fullfilled by current optical tracking systems. They are extremely susceptible to occlusion problems because the tracking process involves no redundancy. As the systems are placed next to the operation area they are blocking a position normally used by the surgeon's assistants, necessitating modified operation procedures. Low update frequencies and high system latencies impede the employment in demanding fields like online robotics control. Recent studies also show negative effects of operating time and aging on tracking accuracy. We are developing MOSCOT — an advanced optical tracking system that will reduce the afore mentioned deficiencies.

2 Materials and Methods

MOSCOT uses a new modular scalable approach to the tracking system architecture. Independent camera modules, with the capability to do fast online image processing, can be freely positioned around the tracking space. Number and type

C. Barillot, D.R. Haynor, and P. Hellier (Eds.): MICCAI 2004, LNCS 3217, pp. 1085–1086, 2004.
© Springer-Verlag Berlin Heidelberg 2004

of the cameras are chosen according to the complexity of the problem. The camera modules each track the positions of markers attached to the observed objects. Each module is composed of a camera with an attached proprietary image processing hardware. This dedicated hardware uses an FPGA chip to extract the marker positions on the tracked object in real-time, including all steps of filtering, segmentation and classification. It transmits the detected marker positions to a central reconstruction module, thus reducing data bandwidth and necessary processing resources. This module collects the data and reconstructs the 3D pose of the tracked objects. By providing redundancy in the camera information the system can tolerate partial camera occlusions.

3   Results

After integration of the major hardware & software modules the prototype system was calibrated by Zhang's standard calibration procedures. The first prototype camera modules do not support IR-reflective markers but use passive color markers instead. System setups with 2 and 3 cameras at different locations were used to demonstrate the scalability of the system. Using 3 cameras the system proved robust against occlusion of one arbitrary camera. The latency between image read-out from the camera sensor to the availability of the reconstructed 3D position was measured as 10ms. The RMS error within an tracked volume of approx. $(0.5m)^3$ was 1.0-1.5mm. To show the performance of the MOSCOT tracking system in a real world scenario we used it successfully to track positions of the newly developed handheld robotic manipulator ITD [1].

4   Discussion

The results obtained from our first prototype setup show that a modular scalable approach to optical tracking is appropriate to circumvent some of the deficiencies of standard tracking systems. The easy extension of the system by more cameras together with free configuration of cameras provided flexible adaptation to different tracking tasks. The low system latency allowed the use for robotics control. During these first tests the accuracy of tracked marker positions was impaired by the use of color markers which are more difficult to extract from the image background under environmental lighting changes, and the use of off-the shelf video cameras of low image quality combined with low image resolution.

In the next steps we will improve the tracking accuracy by the use of enhanced image processing hardware and high-resolution CMOS cameras along with IR-reflective markers. We also plan to implement a dynamic online recalibration process of the MOSCOT system as recent studies show influences of power-on time and aging on the accuracy of optical tracking systems.

References

1. Pott, PP et al.: ITD - A Handheld Manipulator for Medical Applications: Concept and Design. Proc of 3rd Annual Meeting of CAOS, Marbella, Spain, 2003

Distance Measurement for Sensorless 3D US

Peter Hassenpflug, Richard Prager, Graham Treece, and Andrew Gee

Department of Engineering, University of Cambridge, Trumpington Street,
Cambridge, UK, CB2 1PZ, ph305@cam.ac.uk

Abstract. Previously it was thought that speckle-based distance measurement techniques worked best over very small distances. We show that this is not necessarily the case. This result has significance for the design of accurate sensorless freehand 3D ultrasound systems that are convenient to use in a clinical setting.

1   Introduction

Freehand 3D ultrasound, in which B-scan slices and probe trajectory are simultaneously recorded, provides a valuable clinical tool for volume measurement and the analysis of complex geometry. However, the need for a position sensor with a fixed transmitter or cameras external to the ultrasound probe is inconvenient in a clinical environment. The goal is thus to use less intrusive techniques for probe tracking without compromising the spatial accuracy of the overall system.

In this paper, we are concerned with estimating the probe motion perpendicular to the plane of the 2D B-scan (in the elevational direction). Speckle decorrelation [1] and speckle regression [2] can both be used to measure the distance between neighbouring B-scan slices in this direction provided that the spacing of the slices is less than the width of the ultrasound beam. In our previous work we regarded this as the only restriction on the usefulness of these algorithms. In this paper we show that this is not the whole story and there is also a lower limit to the useful working range of the speckle-based algorithms.

2   Distance Measurement

Speckle-based distance measurement is based on the fact that there is a roughly Gaussian relationship between the correlation (or regression gradient) of the echo envelope intensities of a pair of patches of speckle, and their distance apart. The precise shape of this relationship depends on the beam profile, but it is usually of the form shown in the top left graph in figure 1. For very small distances, the shallow gradient of the curve means that small errors in either the curve shape, or the measured correlation coefficient, result in large percentage errors in the predicted distance.

A speckle phantom was scanned with a 5–10 MHz linear array probe. The radio frequency data was recorded at 66.67 MHz for sixty parallel slices 0.02 mm apart. Models were built of the elevational decorrelation rate for 136 patches of about 2500 intensity samples spread across the slice. Distance measurements

C. Barillot, D.R. Haynor, and P. Hellier (Eds.): MICCAI 2004, LNCS 3217, pp. 1087–1088, 2004.
© Springer-Verlag Berlin Heidelberg 2004

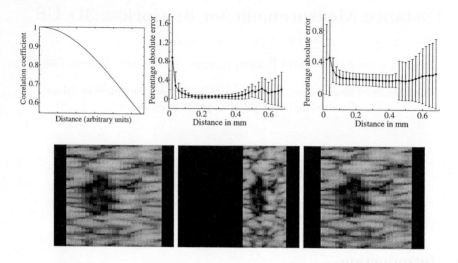

Fig. 1. Top left: a typical speckle decorrelation curve. Top mid & right: percentage errors for training and test data *vs.* size of distance measured. Bottom left: correct reslice of 2 mm diameter void. Bottom mid & right: reslices based on decorrelation measurements over 0.04 mm and 0.16 mm respectively.

were made over various ranges from 0.02 mm up to 0.68 mm using one patch with beam width ≈ 1 mm. The mean and standard deviation of the absolute errors are shown in the top middle graph for the data that was used to build the model, and in the top right graph for different data of a similar phantom.

The bottom left figure shows an accurate reslice through a 2 mm diameter anechoic void in the phantom. The horizontal spacing of the slices is 0.16 mm. The bottom right figure shows the same reslice with positions calculated using decorrelation between all the patches on the slices. The spacing is similar to the correct answer. The bottom middle reslice uses positions derived from the sum of four decorrelation calculations between slices 0.04 mm apart, by using three extra slices between each of those shown. Here, the horizontal spacing is poor.

3   Conclusions

The accuracy of speckle-based distance measurement techniques degrades for distances less than about 10% of the beam width.

References

1. J-F. Chen, J. B. Fowlkes, P. L. Carson, and J. M. Rubin. Determination of scan-plane motion using speckle decorrelation: theoretical considerations and initial test. *International Journal of Imaging Systems Technology*, 8:38–44, 1997.
2. R. W. Prager, A. H. Gee, G. M. Treece, C. J. C. Cash, and L. H. Berman. Sensorless freehand 3D ultrasound using regression of the echo intensity. *Ultrasound in Medicine and Biology*, 29(3):437–446, March 2003.

An Analysis Tool for Quantification of Diffusion Tensor MRI Data

Hae-Jeong Park[1,2,3], Martha E. Shenton[3], and Carl-Fredrik Westin[2]

[1]Division of Nuclear Medicine, Dept. of Diagnostic Radiology, Yonsei University, College
of Medicine, Shinchon-dong, Seodaemun-gu, Seoul 120-749, Korea
parkhj@yumc.yonsei.ac.kr
[2]Laboratory of Mathematics in Imaging, Dept. of Radiology, Brigham and Women's Hospital,
Harvard Medical School, 75 Francis Str. Boston, MA 02115, USA
westin@bwh.harvard.edu
[3]Clinical Neuroscience Division, Laboratory of Neuroscience, Boston VA Health Care System-Brockton Division, Dept. of Psychiatry, Harvard Medical School, Boston, MA 02115,
USA
martha_shenton@hms.harvard.edu

Abstract. A software tool for analyzing Diffusion Tensor MRI (DT-MRI) data
is presented. The tool includes methods for segmentation of white matter for
automatic definition of seed points for fiber tractography, and methods for 2D
slice visualization using different types of tensor glyphs and color-coding
schemes.

1 Introduction

DT-MRI is rapidly gaining clinical importance but tools for exploring and analyzing
data from DT-MRI are still not widely available. In this paper, we introduce a diffusion tensor analysis tool developed with the aim of meeting current demands in both
research and clinical applications.

2 Methods

This software tool, DoDTI, is implemented in Matlab (Mathworks Inc., USA), which
is available for a wide range of platforms. The basic features of this tool are:

1) 2D slice visualization of DT-MRI data with several types of tensor glyphs and
coloring schemes displayed on a background of fractional anisotropy, T2-weighted
MRI data, or the apparent diffusion coefficient (ADC).

2) Automated or semi-automated methods for whole brain tractography where seedpoints and stopping criteria may be assigned, either from automated segmentation
using SPM2, or in a user-configurable manner. The tractography algorithm is based on
a 4th order Runge-kutta integration solver with a choice of several regularization
schemes to better handle crossing fiber bundles.

C. Barillot, D.R. Haynor, and P. Hellier (Eds.): MICCAI 2004, LNCS 3217, pp. 1089–1090, 2004.

3) 3D visualization of fiber bundles using streamlines or streamtubes with optional, orthogonal, gray-level reference images superimposed. In addition, parcellations of gray matter can be used for classifying fiber bundles with specific colors.

4) Selection of fiber bundles based on user-defined criteria, such as a combination of the length of a fiber, maximal angle difference, and minimum distance between end points of a fiber. Manually or semi-automatically drawn regions of interest (ROIs) can be used for the selection of fibers of interest intersecting those ROIs. Visualization of fiber bundles with renderings of ROIs is available for better understanding of the fiber connection between ROIs.

5) Information about the properties of fiber bundles of interest, such as the mean fractional anisotropy along the fiber, can be calculated, which is useful for further evaluation of white matter abnormality.

6) Integration of functional MRI activation maps derived using SPM2 can be used as ROIs to enable the exploration of brain function or functional abnormality in relation with anatomical connectivity.

3   Conclusion

The software tool DoDTI has been developed to provide analysis and quantification of DT-MRI data and includes methods for visualization and automated methods for fiber tractography. More information and directions on how to download this tool can be found at the following URL: http://neuroimage.yonsei.ac.kr/dodti.

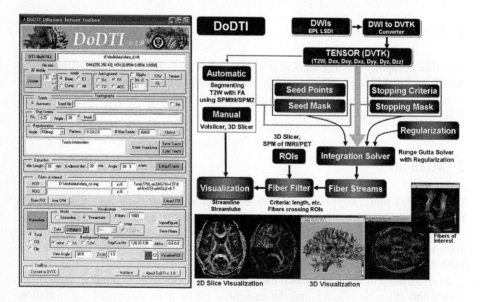

Fig. 1. Analysis flow of DoDTI

A Cross-Platform Software Framework for Medical Image Processing

Koen Van Leemput and Janne Hämäläinen

HUS Helsinki Medical Imaging Center
University of Helsinki
P.O.B. 340, FIN-00029 HUS, Finland
{ koen.vanleemput, janne.hamalainen }@hus.fi

Abstract. In this paper we present a cross-platform software framework for medical image analysis that we make freely available to the medical imaging community [1]. It allows individual software modules to be loaded on demand, providing ad hoc extensibility and maximal software reusability across multiple application areas. We implemented a number of such software modules, and describe their application in research projects and clinical applications at our hospital.

1 Introduction

With the ever-increasing quantity and quality of data produced by medical imaging devices, post-processing of acquired images is increasingly finding its way into clinical practice and medical research. While modern radiological workstations offer tools for manipulating and visualizing images in three dimensions, specific clinical applications and research projects in our hospital require tailor-made image analysis software that implements more advanced techniques. Since a considerable amount of functionality is shared by many of these applications, we implemented a highly modular software framework for medical image processing that allows common software modules to be re-used in different projects. The framework provides both an end-user application for medical researchers and clinicians, as well as a rapid development environment for emerging algorithms.

2 Materials and Methods

The software is centered around the National Library of Medicine Insight Segmentation and Registration Toolkit (ITK). To make ITK operational in our hospital environment, we developed a number of accompanying tools:

- An ITK image class that describes the position of the image grid with respect to the patient using a fully affine transformation. This allows, among other things, to correctly process and visualize oblique MR scans or CT images acquired with the gantry tilted.

---

[1] Interested readers should contact the first author.

C. Barillot, D.R. Haynor, and P. Hellier (Eds.): MICCAI 2004, LNCS 3217, pp. 1091–1092, 2004.

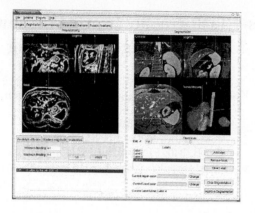

Fig. 1. Specific image analysis tasks can be accomplished by loading a combination of plug-ins that provide the required functionality. This figure shows the plug-in for interactive watershed segmentation.

- An advanced image viewer that can be connected directly to ITK, implemented using the Visualization Toolkit (VTK). It provides arbitrarily oriented multi-planar reconstructions, linked cursors, tracking of curved anatomical structures, as well as 3-D surface and volume rendering.
- ITK classes that use the DICOM Toolkit (DCMTK) to read and write images in the DICOM file format, and to query, retrieve, and send images from and to the hospital PACS system and radiological workstations.

We use the Fast Light Toolkit (FLTK) for the graphical user interface, and provide a mechanism to load so-called plug-ins at run time. Each such a plug-in implements specific image processing routines provided by ITK, along with associated user interface and visualization components. The software runs on Windows, Linux and Sun Solaris platforms.

3   Results and Conclusion

To date, we have implemented plug-ins for DICOM connectivity, multi-modal registration, deformable registration, interactive watershed segmentation, registration based on internal and external markers, fMRI analysis, and visualization of MEG and EEG source localizations along with structural and functional image data.

The software is currently being used at our hospital in research projects involving morphometry of brain MRI, as well as in treatment planning for boron neutron capture therapy (BNCT). Application and clinical validation in epilepsy surgery planning is scheduled for the forthcoming months. Due to the modular software architecture, future applications will be able to rely on previously implemented plug-ins for common image manipulation tasks, considerably reducing development efforts.

Detection of Micro- to Nano-Sized Particles in Soft Tissue

Helmut Troster[3], Stefan Milz[2], Michael F. Trendelenburg[3], F. Jorder[1],
Hanns-Peter Scharf[1], and Markus Schwarz[1]

[1] Lab. of Biomechanics and Exptl. Orthopaedics, Dep. of Orthopaedic Surgery, Faculty of
Clinical Medicine Mannheim, University Heidelberg, Theodor-Kutzer-Ufer 1-3, D-68167
Mannheim, markus.schwarz@ortho.ma.uni-heidelberg.de
[2] University of Munich, Anatomical Institute, Pettenkofer Strasse 11, D-80336 München
[3] German Cancer Research Center (DKFZ), Biomedical Structure Analysis, Dep. A120, Im
Neuenheimer Feld 280, D-69120 Heidelberg

Abstract. The demand is growing to study particulate debris in the human organism. This task is time-consuming. Therefore it is important to find an efficient way of particle identification and analysis. Carriers of hip replacement implants are exposed to particulate wear debris close to and even far away from the implantation sites. This could ease the study of particle transport in the human organism because detectable amounts of particulate matter are likely to arrive in distant organs with regard to the implant. A feasible approach for particle analysis down to the level of electron microscopy is presented here.

Loosening of hip replacement implants, but even normal use causes abrasion setting free particles from the interacting surfaces (Fig. 1 a; [1]). Wear debris is accumulating near by and in inguinal lymph nodes (ILN). Moreover, implant wear debris in liver, spleen and paraaortal lymph nodes was found [2] suggesting systemic distribution. To study their transport and consequences of particle distribution, these structures were focused on in different organs. Since this is like seeking after a pin in a haystack, a protocol for their efficient localisation and analysis had to be elaborated.

It was found that light microscopy (LM) for the visualisation of most of the wear debris (Fig. 1 b), excluding polyethylene particles, had to be completed by transmission electron microscopy (TEM; EM 912 Omega from LEO Elektronenmikroskopie GmbH, Oberkochen, Germany) for two reasons: i) particles in the range of 10-100 nanometer (nm) can form aggregates which would mimic single particles in the LM (e.g.: aggregation of approx. 1 µm in Fig. 1 c), as well as small single particles (e.g.: 66 nm particle in c) cannot be resolved by LM; ii) elemental analyses can better be performed on the EM level. Therefore, targets as identified by LM have to be further processed for TEM by embedding and cementing the LM section of interest to the surface of an EM specimen and sectioning it for EM use. TEM and additional elemental analyses are feasible now because EM types like the EM 912 Omega are energy-filtering TEMs (EFTEMs) with this extra-option of elemental analysis. This is necessary for the proof of tracer elements within particles being suspicious of originating from the implant. Since normal EM grids are symmetric, defining the particles' positions was the objective. The so-called finder grid (Fig. 1 d) allows to relocate a structure to be analysed later on. Finally, elemental analysis based on energy-filtering TEM (EFTEM) can be performed with the same LEO EM 912 Omega.

C. Barillot, D.R. Haynor, and P. Hellier (Eds.): MICCAI 2004, LNCS 3217, pp. 1093–1094, 2004.
© Springer-Verlag Berlin Heidelberg 2004

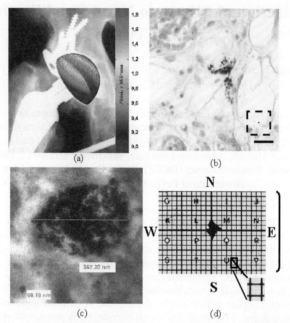

Fig. 1. Search for and characterisation of prosthesis wear particles in soft tissues. (a) Wear particles' origin: projection of an implant's acetabulum (ac) onto an x-ray image from a total hip prosthesis. Abrasion varies from high (ac, proximal) to low intensity (ac, distal; values, right, in mm), is found on both the head and the ac, and where the implant was cemented into the bone. (b) Target structures: LM specimen (ILN) from the body of an implant carrier showing an aggregation of dark particulate debris (centre). Regarding dimensions, the dashed square (right bottom) corresponds to one grid mesh area (emphasized in d) and the black dot in its centre covers the image area in c; bar: 55 μm. (c) Hard particulate matter: EM section of an ILN from a hip implant carrier (sector width: 1.4 μm). The particle aggregation (centre) would be resolved as one particle by LM; the single particle in the left bottom would be invisible. (d) Recovery of structures for TEM: LM image of a finder EM grid (Maxtaform, Plano, Wetzlar, Germany); the right parenthesis symbol spans 1 mm (grid diameter: 3 mm). Letters define interesting positions (symbolized by compass points N, W, S, E); extension piece (right bottom) emphasizes one mesh (width: 60 μm).

References

1. Schwarz M.L.R., Jörder F., Pustornakova K., Menges S., Milz S., Knaak W., Ritter A., Kaiser E., Moriggl B., Selinger T., Claus A., Scharf H.-P.: Determination of femoral head penetration and main wear direction of autopsy retrieved well-functioning total hip replacements using a 3d-coordinate measuring machine. 50th Annual Meeting of the Orthopaedic Research society. March 7-10, 2004, San Francisco, USA, Poster presentation.
2. Urban, R.M., Jacobs, J.J., Tomlinson, M.J., Gavrilovic, J., Black, J., Peoc'h, M.: Dissemination of wear particles to the liver, spleen, and abdominal lymph nodes of patients with hip or knee replacement. J. Bone Joint Surg. Am. 82 (2000) 457-476

We thank Prof. V. Mersch-Sundermann (Univ. Giessen, Germany) and Prof. W. Probst (Essingen, Germany) for support and helpful discussions.

Hardware-Assisted 2D/3D Intensity-Based Registration for Assessing Patellar Tracking

T.S.Y. Tang[1], N.J. MacIntyre[2], H.S. Gill[3], R.A. Fellows[2], N.A. Hill[2], D.R. Wilson[4], and R.E. Ellis[12]

[1] School of Computing, Queen's University, Kingston, Canada
{ttang, ellis}@cs.queensu.ca
[2] Department of Mechanical Engineering, Queen's University, Kingston, Canada
[3] Nuffield Orthopaedic Center, University of Oxford, Oxford, UK
[4] Department of Orthopaedics, University of British Columbia, Vancouver, Canada

1 Introduction

The problem in 2D/3D intensity-based registration of computed tomography (CT) images is to find a pose such that a digitally reconstructed radiograph (DRR) of the 3D image matches a given 2D image. Generating DRRs, a computationally intensive process, can be accelerated by precomputation [1], or by using custom hardware that accelerates volume rendering. Recent algorithmic advances for 3D texture mapping using off-the-shelf video cards have further improved volume rendering. We propose to generate DRRs generated in real time, without any precomputation, for 2D/3D registration.

This work is a continuation of the point-based fluoroscopic technique for assessing patellar tracking [4], in which a cadaver patellofemoral joint was tracked by a single-plane fluoroscope using a point-based registration method [3] with accuracy determined by comparison to Roentgen Stereophotogrammetric Analysis (RSA). We have developed a hardware-assisted intensity-based registration method and applied it to the same set of data.

2 Materials and Methods

Details of the experimental set-up can be found in [4]. The original CT scan of the knee was roughly divided into three volumes corresponding to each of the femur, patella and tibia, so that only one of the bone would show up in a DRR. To generate a DRR, the CT slices were first transferred to the texture memory of the video card; then, a particular pose could be rendered by setting the camera geometry according to the information from fluoroscope calibration. An NVidia GeForce FX 5800 video card on a 2.4 GHz PC was used. For registration purposes, soft-tissue was not rendered, although this can be done easily by adjusting the transfer function according the Hounsfield units of the CT voxels.

A *single* fluoroscopic image was used in the intensity-based registration. Each of the femur, patella, and tibia was registered separately. For the similarity measure, which estimated how similar the original fluoroscopic image was to the DRR, we used the weighted gradient correlation (a modified version of gradient

C. Barillot, D.R. Haynor, and P. Hellier (Eds.): MICCAI 2004, LNCS 3217, pp. 1095–1096, 2004.

correlation [2]). A rough region of interest was specified in the fluoroscopic image, and when a DRR was generated, pixels in the DRR that were outside the ROI had a negative weight added. To find a registration pose that maximized the similarity measure we used the downhill simplex algorithm in a multiscale manner: given an initial guess, it was perturbed m times and registration was done at a low resolution (128^2), the n best answers were used as initial guesses at a medium resolution (512^2), and its result was used for registering in full resolution (980^2). We used $m = 5$ and $n = 2$.

3   Results and Discussion

With a $512^2 \times 160$ CT, a DRR of size 128^2, 512^2, and 980^2 took about 0.01, 0.11, and 0.38 seconds, respectively, to generate. A registration with a single volume took 3 to 5 minutes to complete. Results were compared with the ground truth obtained from RSA. The table shows the mean absolute errors and standard deviations for the variables describing patellar orientation and translation.

Patella Motion	Point-Based		Intensity-Based	
	Error	SD	Error	SD
Orientation (degrees)				
Flexion	1.71	0.64	1.81	0.63
Internal Rotation	1.75	0.64	1.80	0.80
Lateral Tilt	0.84	0.55	0.79	0.57
Translation (mm)				
Lateral	0.99	0.81	1.29	0.77
Proximal	0.51	0.35	0.97	0.64
Anterior	2.09	1.35	2.49	1.65

Hardware generation of DRRs did not need precomputation and was about 25 times faster than software computation, yet preserved the image quality. It worked well with intensity-based registration, and it made the implementation straightforward. Also, in less than 5% of all instances, an incorrect registration was found with a similarity value greater than that of the correct registration. This situation could perhaps be resolved by using another similarity measure [2].

Errors in our intensity-based registration were comparable to those reported in literature. The main advantage of our method is that only a single fluoroscopic image is used, while most others use at least two. It allows the assessment of patellar tracking to be done using commonly available graphics hardware.

References

1. D. A. LaRose et al. Transgraph: interactive intensity based 2D/3D registration of X-ray and CT data. In *SPIE Image Processing*, 2000.
2. G. P. Penney et al. A comparision of similarity measures for use in 2-D–3-D medical image registration. *IEEE Transactions on Medical Imaging*, 17(4):586–595, 1998.
3. T. S. Y. Tang et al. Fiducial registration from a single X-Ray image: a new technique for fluoroscopic guidance and radiotherapy. In *MICCAI 2000*, pages 502–511.
4. T. S. Y. Tang and N. J. MacIntyre et al. Accuracy of a fluoroscopy technique for assessing patellar tracking. In *MICCAI 2003*, pages I:319–326.

Multiple Coils for Reduction of Flow Artefacts in MR Images

David Atkinson[1], David J. Larkman[2], Philipp G. Batchelor[1], Derek L.G. Hill[1], and Joseph V. Hajnal[2]

[1] Imaging Sciences, Guy's Hospital, King's College London, SE1 9RT, UK,
David.Atkinson@kcl.ac.uk,
[2] Robert Steiner MRI Unit, Imaging Sciences Department, Clinical Sciences Centre, Hammersmith Hospital, Imperial College London, W12 0NN, UK.

Abstract. Flowing blood can cause streak or blob artefacts in MR images and these may degrade subsequent image analysis. Multiple MRI receiver coils enable the reconstruction of images using data from different combinations of coils. The artefact intensities differ in these images due to the differing coil sensitivities. The artefact cause is parameterised and an optimisation routine is used to find self-consistent image reconstructions which have reduced artefacts.

1 Introduction

Blood flow and other physiological processes can result in the ghosting and blurring of MR images. In addition to the blurring, these artefacts can introduce additional features that are not present in the object. This can be problematic, for example, difference images from registered serial brain volumes can be corrupted by flow artefacts from the carotid and middle cerebral arteries.

Multiple coils have previously been used to detect and reject motion-corrupted phase encode lines [1]. The remaining data was then reconstructed using a generalised SMASH [2] approach. Odd and even echos in EPI images have been used for flow artefact reduction [3]. Here we apply a new, more general, technique to the problem of artefacts from flowing blood.

2 Method

In the absence of any artefacts, the image s^γ obtained from coil γ with spatial sensitivity c^γ is given by

$$s^\gamma = c^\gamma \cdot r \tag{1}$$

where r is the underlying object. This can be expressed in k-space as a convolution which in turn can be written as the matrix multiplication $\mathbf{S} = \mathbf{CR}$. Here $\mathbf{S}$ and $\mathbf{C}$ can contain data relating to either one or all coils. In the presence of flow artefacts, the k-space representation of the object and the acquired k-space change to $\bar{\mathbf{R}}$ and $\bar{\mathbf{S}}$ respectively. If the artefact can be parameterised as a change

C. Barillot, D.R. Haynor, and P. Hellier (Eds.): MICCAI 2004, LNCS 3217, pp. 1097–1098, 2004.

to the coils, rather than the object, we can write $\bar{\mathbf{S}} = \mathbf{C}\bar{\mathbf{R}} = \bar{\mathbf{C}}\mathbf{R}$. In the case of flowing blood, we assume that the coil profile at the position of the artery can be multiplied by one complex term for each discrete time step during the scan. Solving for $\mathbf{R}$ with one or all coils [2] enables us to minimise the cost function

$$F = \sum_{\gamma,n} |r^\gamma - r^G|^2, \tag{2}$$

where the reconstructed object has been Fourier transformed to the image domain and the sum is over all coils and all image-domain pixels.

3   Results and Conclusions

Figure 1 shows an axial slice from a volunteer acquired on a Philips 1.5T Eclipse using a 4-element body array coil (128×128, TR/TE of 250/10 ms, breath-hold, no cardiac gating, 128 discrete time points). Ghosts can be seen in the spinal body and intestine region as well as outside the body. We use the MATLAB [The MathWorks] least squares nonlinear optimisation routine with 256 unknowns (128 complex multiplicative factors). After processing with our algorithm, the ghosts are reduced and image quality is comparable to a similar slice acquired with saturation bands (which would not be effective for multi-slice acquisitions).

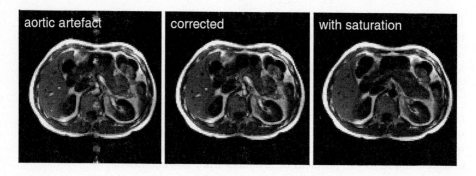

Fig. 1. Slice corrupted by flow in aorta (left), corrected (middle) and a similar slice acquired using saturation slabs in a different breath-hold (right).

References

1. M. Bydder et al. *Magn. Reson. Med.*, 47:677–686, 2002.
2. M. Bydder et al. *Magn. Reson. Med.*, 47:160–170, 2002.
3. Y. Mashida et al. *Proc. ISMRM* 9(2001), p. 1810.

Freely Available Software for 3D RF Ultrasound

Graham Treece*, Richard Prager, and Andrew Gee

Dept. Engineering, Univ. Cambridge, Cambridge, UK, CB2 1PZ, gmt11@cam.ac.uk

Abstract. We present a 3D radio frequency (RF) ultrasound (US) system capable of acquiring real-time RF data at a sustained rate of 30-60 frames per second with 60 dB real dynamic range and typical phase error of only $\pm 2.3°$ at 6 MHz. The software is freely available to other researchers, and opens up the possibility of extending elastography, deconvolution, spectral processing and other RF analysis into 3D.

1 Introduction

The availability of radio frequency (RF) ultrasound (US) data enables the study of elastography [4], flow detection, deconvolution [2], spectral processing [3] and other important topics. Many of these require real-time acquisition, and all are considerably enhanced by the availability of 3D data. However, access to such data is currently limited: RF analysis is often based on single frames acquired at only 8-bits sampling resolution, with several minutes delay to download the data to an external PC [3]. A 3D RF system using 16-bit acquisition at 20MHz has been reported [2], but not in real-time. Similarly a real-time system using 12-bit acquisition at 30 MHz has been reported [4], but not in 3D. Commercial RF systems are generally neither real-time nor 3D.

We present a real-time 3D RF system, using 14-bit (60 dB useful dynamic range) acquisition, synced to the US machine clock at 66.6 MHz, which is capable of recording 30-60 frames of RF data per second (fps). The software[1] [1] requires a Gage CompuScope 14100 PCI analogue to digital converter. Each frame is downloaded from on-board Gage memory to a 3 GHz Pentium 4 PC in real-time, hence storage is only limited by PC RAM. The system will work with any ultrasound machine from which analogue focused RF data and some simple timing signals are available: we use a Dynamic Imaging Diasus US machine.

2 Validation

3D point precision of the non-RF system has been demonstrated as 0.6 mm [1]. A high sampling resolution is crucial to preserving signal-to-noise at depth, since the RF data is acquired before log-compression: Fig. 1(a) demonstrates a similar noise floor for B-scans derived from acquired RF data to those from the US machine. Repeatability of the RF phase from vector to vector is also critical for analysing 3D RF data. This was assessed at 2 cm depth by scanning a planar

---

* Graham Treece is supported by an EPSRC/RAEng Postdoctoral Fellowship
[1] Stradx, freely available from http://mi.eng.cam.ac.uk/~rwp/stradx/

C. Barillot, D.R. Haynor, and P. Hellier (Eds.): MICCAI 2004, LNCS 3217, pp. 1099–1100, 2004.

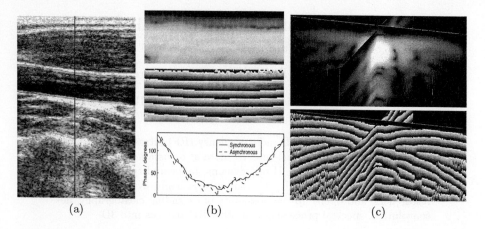

(a)   (b)   (c)

Fig. 1. (a) B-scan from US machine (left) and derived from RF data (right). (b) B-scan and phase image of a plane, magnified x20 axially, with corresponding intra-vector phase variation. (c) 3D RF amplitude and phase of the tip of a 0.15 mm wire, showing the elevational (left to right) and lateral (front to back) point spread function.

target with a 5-10 MHz probe, as in Fig. 1(b). The inter-vector phase had 2.3° standard deviation at the centre frequency, compared to 8.0° for asynchronous 100 MHz sampled data. Intra-vector variation was similar, as shown in graphical form in Fig. 1(b). High accuracy 3D RF data is demonstrated in Fig. 1(c).

Speed of acquisition is an equally important factor. Data is transfered from the Gage card to the PC at 75 Mb/s, hence for 66.6 MHz sampling, every third frame can be stored. This typically gives full-frame rates of 30-60 fps, dependent on probe frequency, assuming a single transmit focus. This rate can be increased upwards of 1000 fps if not all of the RF vectors are acquired. RF-derived B-scans can be displayed in real-time, though at a reduced frame rate of typically 15 fps.

3   Conclusions

We have presented a real-time 3D RF US system which is fast and accurate enough to form a solid basis for the study of RF US processing in 3D, yet available at only the cost of an acquisition card and a suitable US machine.

References

1. Treece, G.M., Gee, A.H., Prager, R.W., Cash, C.J.C., Berman, L.H.: High definition freehand 3D ultrasound. Ultrasound Med Biol **29** (2003) 529–546
2. Taxt, T.: Three-dimensional blind deconvolution of ultrasound images. IEEE T Ultrason Ferr **48** (2001) 867–871
3. Watson, R.J., McLean, C.C., Moore, M.P., Spencer, T., Salter, D.M., Anderson, T., Fox, K.A.A., McDicken, W.N.: Classification of arterial plaque by spectral analysis of in vitro RF intravascular ultrasound data. Ultrasound Med Biol **26** (2000) 73–80
4. Pesavento, A., Lorenz, A., Siebers, S., Emmert, H.: New real-time strain imaging concepts using diagnostic ultrasound. Phys Med Biol **45** (2000) 1423–1435

A Study of Dosimetric Evaluation and Feasibility of Image Guided Intravascular Brachytherapy in Peripheral Arteries

Julien Bellec[1], Jean-Pierre Manens[1], Cemil Göksu[2], Cécile Moisan[3], and Pascal Haigron[2]

[1] CRLCC Eugène Marquis, CS 44229 35042 Rennes, France
[2] LTSI, INSERM U642, Université de Rennes 1, 35042 Rennes, France
[3] Service de Chirurgie Vasculaire, CHRU, Rennes, France

Abstract. This work involves the conception of the experimental dosimetric testing setup of an image based procedure for intravascular brachytherapy by ^{192}Ir seed in peripheral arteries. After making sure of the suitability of the basis dosimetry data used for dose calculation, the treatment sequence as a whole has been tested in a customized tissue-equivalent phantom. The method is based on the use of CT preoperative images and 2D intra-operative radiographs. Experimental dosimetric results agree with the planning and demonstrate the feasibility of the procedure.

1 Introduction

Intravascular Brachytherapy (IVB) constitutes a new therapeutic solution to avoid iterative redilations practiced after minimally invasive treatment of peripheral arterial stenoses. Following percutaneous transluminal angioplasty procedure, IVB aims at preventing intimal hyperplasia / restenosis. Its application to peripheral arteries by means of a high dose rate (HDR) [192]Ir seed remains at a preliminary stage. Peripheral arteries present some specific features compared to coronary arteries as for their shape, geometrical characteristics (length, diameter, curvature) and the presence of surrounding anatomical structures. Based on AAPM TG 43/60 formalism [1, 2] and a dedicated phantom model this work focuses on the dosimetric evaluation of the treatment sequence relating to the dose prescription with respect to the arterial wall as well as the precise localization of the seed from preoperative CT and intra-operative fluoroscopic images.

2 Methods and Material

First, in order to validate dose calculation, the TG 43 dosimetry parameters from our own ^{192}Ir seed have been experimentally evaluated (i.e. air kerma strength, dose rate constant, radial dose function and anisotropy function). Since no gold standard exists

C. Barillot, D.R. Haynor, and P. Hellier (Eds.): MICCAI 2004, LNCS 3217, pp. 1101–1102, 2004.

for dosimetry in IVB, different types of detectors have been analysed : a Nuclear Farmer cylindrical ionization chamber ; a PTW-Frieburg 31006 pinpoint chamber ; a PTW-Frieburg 60003 diamond detector and GR-100M Fimel LiF (Mg, Ti) thermoluminescent dosimeters (TLD). A water phantom from PTW-Frieburg and a polystyrene phantom have been used. The dosimetric evaluation of the whole treatment sequence (planning and tracking) has been carried out on a dedicated polystyrene phantom. In it, a simplified tubular model (straight cylindrical paths) has been digged. In order to measure the dose actually applied around the source train, a batch of TLD type GR-100M has been inserted into the phantom. To minimize uncertainties due to extremely large dose gradient near the ^{192}Ir source, these measurements have been conducted at a distance larger than 1 cm. An intravascular navigation guidance method already presented in [3] has been implemented in order to locate the ^{192}Ir seed intra-operatively. The framework involves the simulation of 2D fluoroscopy images from both the CT data and the virtual C-arm pose. Anatomical feature-based 2D/3D registration between a single 2D fluoroscopic view, reproduced from the planned pose, and the preoperative volume, is performed by minimizing the distance between the projection of a selected set of centerlines and the 2D vascular skeleton by means of a chamfer distance map.

3   Results and Discussion

Regarding the dose calculation validation, the maximum standard deviation between the experimental dosimetric parameters and those used in the treatment planning system is within 5 % : the results are suitable with the recommandations [1]. In the same way, the measured dose around the source train during the simulated treatment are within 3 % of the computed dose.

Therefore, the results demonstrate that IVB treatment sequence is valid in simplified experimental conditions (straight and centered source path). However, further in-phantom investigations based on the artery model are necessary to complete the validation. An overall evaluation of the method should include both the curvature and the centering guide-catheter system.

References

1. Nath R, Anderson LL, Luxton G, Weaver KA, Williamson J Fand, Meigooni AS. Dosimetry of interstitial brachytherapy sources : Recommendations of the AAPM Radiation Therapy Committee Task Group No. 43. *Med. Phys.* 22: 209-234 ; 1995.
2. Nath R, Amols H, Coffey C, Jani S, Li Z, Schell MC, Soares C, Whiting J, Cole P, Crocker I, Schwartz R. Intravascular brachytherapy physics : Report of the AAPM Radiation Therapy Committee Task Group No. 60. *Med. Phys.* 26 (2): 119-152 ; 1999.
3. Göksu C, Haigron P, Zhang H, Soulas T, Le Certen G, Lucas A. 3D intraoperative localization for endovascular navigation guidance. In *Surgetica'2002, Computer-Aided Medical Interventions: tools and applications*, J Troccaz, Ph Merloz, eds., Sauramps Medical: 323-329 ; 2002.

3D Elastography Using Freehand Ultrasound

Joel Lindop, Graham Treece, Andrew Gee, and Richard Prager

Department of Engineering, University of Cambridge, Trumpington Street,
Cambridge, UK, CB2 1PZ, jel35,gmt11,ahg,rwp@eng.cam.ac.uk

Abstract. We present a novel technique for 3D elastography using free-hand ultrasound. The scan is straightforward to perform, requiring just a single sweep over the area of interest with an unmodified 2D probe. The 3D elastogram is constructed in real time and can be visualised immediately following the sweep. Results are presented for a jelly phantom containing a hard inclusion.

1 Introduction

The term "elastography" refers to the imaging of tissue stiffness. One way of performing elastography is by ultrasonic strain imaging, whereby a sequence of ultrasound images is used to quantify tissue deformation under applied pressure. The clinical motivation for this sort of imaging is well rehearsed: hard inclusions, such as certain types of tumour, are often far easier to detect in elastograms than in conventional B-mode images. Manufacturers of ultrasound equipment are beginning to offer 2D elastography on their top-end machines. 3D elastography has been reported using a mechanically swept 3D probe [1]. Here, we present an alternative approach to 3D elastography using an unmodified 2D probe and a freehand scanning protocol. To the best of our knowledge, this is the first time such a system has been reported in the literature.

2 Freehand 3D Elastography

There are several ways to apply the time-varying pressure required for ultrasonic strain imaging. For instance, the probe can be modified to incorporate a mechanical vibrator. Here, we adopt the simplest approach whereby the clinician applies the pressure manually. For 2D elastography, the clinician holds the probe over the area of interest and applies a varying contact pressure. Pesavento et al [2] describe how the resulting radio frequency (RF) image sequence can be analysed in real time to produce a set of 2D elastograms showing axial stiffness.

For our 3D system, we use a 5-10 MHz linear array probe connected to a Dynamic Imaging Diasus ultrasound machine. The RF echo signal is digitised at 67 MHz, 30 frames per second using a Gage CompuScope 14100 analogue to digital converter. Sequential frames are compared to produce 2D elastograms in real time using Pesavento's phase root seeking algorithm [2]. The position and orientation of the probe are tracked using a Northern Digital Polaris optical position sensor: the 2D elastograms can therefore be located in space and reconstructed in 3D using the Stradx freehand 3D ultrasound system. The 3D point precision of this system has been measured at around 0.6 mm [3].

C. Barillot, D.R. Haynor, and P. Hellier (Eds.): MICCAI 2004, LNCS 3217, pp. 1103–1104, 2004.
© Springer-Verlag Berlin Heidelberg 2004

The freehand scanning protocol for 3D elastography is surprisingly simple: it transpires that a single sweep is sufficient. Compared with the axial resolution, the elevational and lateral resolutions are poor. Given the high acquisition rate, speckle decorrelation between neighbouring frames is due almost entirely to axial strain and not elevational or lateral movement. Thus, meaningful 2D elastograms can be constructed between neighbouring frames, even though the motion is predominantly elevational and not axial. The operator need make no special effort to vary the contact pressure: the system is sufficiently sensitive to detect the involuntary variations implicit in a freehand scan. Figure 1 shows 3D elastography of a hard inclusion (an olive) embedded in a jelly phantom.

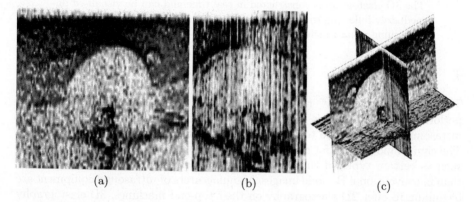

(a)	(b)	(c)

Fig. 1. 3D elastography of jelly/olive phantom. (a) is a 2D elastogram, (b) is a perpendicular reslice through the elastograms, (c) shows an elastogram and two such reslices.

3   Conclusions

We have presented a novel system for freehand 3D elastography. The scanning protocol is simple and the elastograms are constructed in real time using a standard PC and unmodified freehand 3D ultrasound equipment.

References

1. Lorenz, A., Pesavento, A., Pesavento, M., Ermert, H.: Three-dimensional strain imaging and related strain artifacts using an ultrasonic 3D abdominal probe. In: Proceedings of the 1999 IEEE Ultrasonics Symposium. Volume 2. (1999) 1657–1660
2. Pesavento, A., Perrey, C., Krueger, M., H., E.: A time efficient and accurate strain estimation concept for ultrasonic elastography using iterative phase zero estimation. IEEE T Ultrason Ferr **46** (1999) 1057–1067
3. Treece, G.M., Gee, A.H., Prager, R.W., Cash, C.J.C., Berman, L.: High definition freehand 3D ultrasound. Ultrasound Med Biol **29** (2003) 529–546

Author Index

Lecture Notes in Computer Science

For information about Vols. 1–3122

please contact your bookseller or Springer

Vol. 3179: F.J. Perales, B.A. Draper (Eds.), Articulated Motion and Deformable Objects. XI, 270 pages. 2004.

Vol. 3178: W. Jonker, M. Petkovic (Eds.), Secure Data Management. VIII, 219 pages. 2004.

Vol. 3177: Z.R. Yang, H. Yin, R. Everson (Eds.), Intelligent Data Engineering and Automated Learning – IDEAL 2004. XVIII, 852 pages. 2004.

Vol. 3176: O. Bousquet, U. von Luxburg, G. Rätsch (Eds.), Advanced Lectures on Machine Learning. IX, 241 pages. 2004. (Subseries LNAI).

Vol. 3175: C.E. Rasmussen, H.H. Bülthoff, B. Schölkopf, M.A. Giese (Eds.), Pattern Recognition. XVIII, 581 pages. 2004.

Vol. 3174: F. Yin, J. Wang, C. Guo (Eds.), Advances in Neural Networks - ISNN 2004. XXXV, 1021 pages. 2004.

Vol. 3173: F. Yin, J. Wang, C. Guo (Eds.), Advances in Neural Networks – ISNN 2004. XXXV, 1041 pages. 2004.

Vol. 3172: M. Dorigo, M. Birattari, C. Blum, L. M. Gambardella, F. Mondada, T. Stützle (Eds.), Ant Colony, Optimization and Swarm Intelligence. XII, 434 pages. 2004.

Vol. 3170: P. Gardner, N. Yoshida (Eds.), CONCUR 2004 - Concurrency Theory. XIII, 529 pages. 2004.

Vol. 3166: M. Rauterberg (Ed.), Entertainment Computing – ICEC 2004. XXIII, 617 pages. 2004.

Vol. 3163: S. Marinai, A. Dengel (Eds.), Document Analysis Systems VI. XI, 564 pages. 2004.

Vol. 3162: R. Downey, M. Fellows, F. Dehne (Eds.), Parameterized and Exact Computation. X, 293 pages. 2004.

Vol. 3160: S. Brewster, M. Dunlop (Eds.), Mobile Human-Computer Interaction – MobileHCI 2004. XVII, 541 pages. 2004.

Vol. 3159: U. Visser, Intelligent Information Integration for the Semantic Web. XIV, 150 pages. 2004. (Subseries LNAI).

Vol. 3158: I. Nikolaidis, M. Barbeau, E. Kranakis (Eds.), Ad-Hoc, Mobile, and Wireless Networks. IX, 344 pages. 2004.

Vol. 3157: C. Zhang, H. W. Guesgen, W.K. Yeap (Eds.), PRICAI 2004: Trends in Artificial Intelligence. XX, 1023 pages. 2004. (Subseries LNAI).

Vol. 3156: M. Joye, J.-J. Quisquater (Eds.), Cryptographic Hardware and Embedded Systems - CHES 2004. XIII, 455 pages. 2004.

Vol. 3155: P. Funk, P.A. González Calero (Eds.), Advances in Case-Based Reasoning. XIII, 822 pages. 2004. (Subseries LNAI).

Vol. 3154: R.L. Nord (Ed.), Software Product Lines. XIV, 334 pages. 2004.

Vol. 3153: J. Fiala, V. Koubek, J. Kratochvíl (Eds.), Mathematical Foundations of Computer Science 2004. XIV, 902 pages. 2004.

Vol. 3152: M. Franklin (Ed.), Advances in Cryptology – CRYPTO 2004. XI, 579 pages. 2004.

Vol. 3150: G.-Z. Yang, T. Jiang (Eds.), Medical Imaging and Augmented Reality. XII, 378 pages. 2004.

Vol. 3149: M. Danelutto, M. Vanneschi, D. Laforenza (Eds.), Euro-Par 2004 Parallel Processing. XXXIV, 1081 pages. 2004.

Vol. 3148: R. Giacobazzi (Ed.), Static Analysis. XI, 393 pages. 2004.

Vol. 3146: P. Érdi, A. Esposito, M. Marinaro, S. Scarpetta (Eds.), Computational Neuroscience: Cortical Dynamics. XI, 161 pages. 2004.

Vol. 3144: M. Papatriantafilou, P. Hunel (Eds.), Principles of Distributed Systems. XI, 246 pages. 2004.

Vol. 3143: W. Liu, Y. Shi, Q. Li (Eds.), Advances in Web-Based Learning – ICWL 2004. XIV, 459 pages. 2004.

Vol. 3142: J. Diaz, J. Karhumäki, A. Lepistö, D. Sannella (Eds.), Automata, Languages and Programming. XIX, 1253 pages. 2004.

Vol. 3140: N. Koch, P. Fraternali, M. Wirsing (Eds.), Web Engineering. XXI, 623 pages. 2004.

Vol. 3139: F. Iida, R. Pfeifer, L. Steels, Y. Kuniyoshi (Eds.), Embodied Artificial Intelligence. IX, 331 pages. 2004. (Subseries LNAI).

Vol. 3138: A. Fred, T. Caelli, R.P.W. Duin, A. Campilho, D.d. Ridder (Eds.), Structural, Syntactic, and Statistical Pattern Recognition. XXII, 1168 pages. 2004.

Vol. 3137: P. De Bra, W. Nejdl (Eds.), Adaptive Hypermedia and Adaptive Web-Based Systems. XIV, 442 pages. 2004.

Vol. 3136: F. Meziane, E. Métais (Eds.), Natural Language Processing and Information Systems. XII, 436 pages. 2004.

Vol. 3134: C. Zannier, H. Erdogmus, L. Lindstrom (Eds.), Extreme Programming and Agile Methods - XP/Agile Universe 2004. XIV, 233 pages. 2004.

Vol. 3133: A.D. Pimentel, S. Vassiliadis (Eds.), Computer Systems: Architectures, Modeling, and Simulation. XIII, 562 pages. 2004.

Vol. 3132: B. Demoen, V. Lifschitz (Eds.), Logic Programming. XII, 480 pages. 2004.

Vol. 3131: V. Torra, Y. Narukawa (Eds.), Modeling Decisions for Artificial Intelligence. XI, 327 pages. 2004. (Subseries LNAI).

Vol. 3130: A. Syropoulos, K. Berry, Y. Haralambous, B. Hughes, S. Peter, J. Plaice (Eds.), TeX, XML, and Digital Typography. VIII, 265 pages. 2004.

Vol. 3129: Q. Li, G. Wang, L. Feng (Eds.), Advances in Web-Age Information Management. XVII, 753 pages. 2004.

Vol. 3128: D. Asonov (Ed.), Querying Databases Privately. IX, 115 pages. 2004.

Vol. 3127: K.E. Wolff, H.D. Pfeiffer, H.S. Delugach (Eds.), Conceptual Structures at Work. XI, 403 pages. 2004. (Subseries LNAI).

Vol. 3126: P. Dini, P. Lorenz, J.N.d. Souza (Eds.), Service Assurance with Partial and Intermittent Resources. XI, 312 pages. 2004.

Vol. 3125: D. Kozen (Ed.), Mathematics of Program Construction. X, 401 pages. 2004.

Vol. 3124: J.N. de Souza, P. Dini, P. Lorenz (Eds.), Telecommunications and Networking - ICT 2004. XXVI, 1390 pages. 2004.

Vol. 3123: A. Belz, R. Evans, P. Piwek (Eds.), Natural Language Generation. X, 219 pages. 2004. (Subseries LNAI).